Medical and Health Information Directory

Volume 3:
Health Services

ISSN 0749-9973

TWENTY-NINTH EDITION

Medical and Health Information Directory

A Guide to Organizations, Agencies, Institutions, Programs, Publications, Services, and Other Resources Concerned with Clinical Medicine, Basic Biomedical Sciences, and the Technological and Socioeconomic Aspects of Health Care

Volume 3:

Health Services
Including Clinics, Treatment Centers, Care Programs, and Counseling/Diagnostic Services

Part 4
Chapters 34-35
Index

Donna Batten
Project Editor

GALE
CENGAGE Learning

Farmington Hills, Mich • San Francisco • New York • Waterville, Maine
Meriden, Conn • Mason, Ohio • Chicago

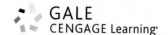

**Medical and Health Information Directory,
29th Edition, Volume 3**

Project Editor: Donna Batten

Editorial Support Services: Emmanuel
Barrido

Composition and Electronic Capture: Gary
Oudersluys

Manufacturing: Rita Wimberley

Gale
27500 Drake Rd.
Farmington Hills, MI, 48331-3535

ISBN-13: 978-1-56995-948-0 (set)
ISBN-13: 978-1-56995-949-7 (vol. 1 set)
ISBN-13: 978-1-56995-950-3 (vol. 1, part 1)
ISBN-13: 978-1-56995-951-0 (vol. 1, part 2)
ISBN-13: 978-1-56995-952-7 (vol. 1, part 3)
ISBN-13: 978-1-56995-953-4 (vol. 1, part 4)
ISBN-13: 978-1-56995-954-1 (vol. 2 set)
ISBN-13: 978-1-56995-955-8 (vol. 2, part 1)
ISBN-13: 978-1-56995-956-5 (vol. 2, part 2)
ISBN-13: 978-1-56995-957-2 (vol. 3 set)
ISBN-13: 978-1-56995-958-9 (vol. 3, part 1)
ISBN-13: 978-1-56995-959-6 (vol. 3, part 2)
ISBN-13: 978-1-56995-960-2 (vol. 3, part 3)
ISBN-13: 978-1-56995-961-9 (vol. 3, part 4)

ISSN 0749-9973

Printed in the United States of America
1 2 3 4 5   18 17 16 15 14

Contents

Volume 3 of the *Medical and Health Information Directory (MHID)*, a three-part softcover resource, is now in its twenty-ninth edition. *MHID* is a convenient one-stop source of information on clinics, treatment centers, care programs, and counseling/diagnostic services. It directs health care professionals and the public alike to a wide variety of health services in the United States, including:

- AIDS Programs
- Amyotrophic Lateral Sclerosis Clinics
- Audiology & Speech/Language Services
- Cancer Programs
- Community & Migrant Health Centers
- Cystic Fibrosis Centers
- Clinical Programs for the Developmentally Disabled
- Domestic Violence and Sexual Assault Programs
- Eating Disorders Clinics
- Family Planning Services
- Genetic Services Centers
- Headache Clinics
- Home Health Care Agencies
- Hospices
- In Vitro Fertilization Clinics
- Kidney Dialysis & Transplant Services
- Mental Health Services
- Multiple Sclerosis Centers & Clinics
- Organ & Tissue Banks
- Pain Management Programs
- Runaway & Homeless Youth Centers
- Sickle Cell Anemia Centers
- SIDS Information & Counseling Programs
- Sleep Disorders Centers & Laboratories
- Substance Abuse Services
- Suicide Prevention & Crisis Intervention Centers

Comprehensive Coverage

There are many published and unpublished directories of service agencies that provide specialized health care in the United States; however, these directories are usually limited in coverage to a single health issue or to a particular geographic area. In contrast, Volume 3 of *MHID* is broad in scope, presenting resources, a significantly larger compilation of programs that provide treatment and care for, or information on, a wide range of medical and health-related conditions and issues on a national level.

Content and Arrangement

Volume 3 consists of Descriptive Listings and an Alphabetical Name and Keyword Index.

- The Descriptive Listings are organized within 35 chapters, according to type of health service, as outlined on the "Contents" pages.

- The Alphabetical Name and Keyword Index speeds access to Volume 3 entries through a consolidated listing of all clinics, treatment centers, care programs, and counseling/diagnostic services included in the book.

For additional information on the content, arrangement, and indexing of Volume 3, consult the "User's Guide" following this introduction.

Method of Compilation

The twenty-ninth edition of Volume 3 represents a complete revision and updating of all material presented in the previous edition, incorporating thousands of changes to addresses, telephone numbers, personnel, and other key details.

Many sources were used to update this edition, including federal and state government documents and publications, and lists and directories supplied by numerous national organizations.

Companion Volumes Profile Organizations and Information Resources

The companion volumes in this set complement Volume 3's coverage of health services:

- **Volume 1** covers organizations, agencies, and institutions

- **Volume 2** covers publications, libraries, and other information resources

Together, these volumes provide complete coverage of the medical and health care information and delivery system.

Available in Electronic Formats

Licensing. The *Medical and Health Information Directory* is available for licensing. The complete database is provided in a fielded format and is deliverable on such media as disk or CD-ROM. For more information, contact Gale's Business Development Group at 1-800-877-GALE, or visit us on our web site at http://gale.cengage.com/bizdev.

Online. The Directory is also available online as part of the *Gale Directory Library*. For more information, call 1-800-877-GALE.

Comments Welcome

We encourage users to bring new or unlisted resources to our attention. Every effort will be made to include them in subsequent editions of *MHID*. Comments and suggestions for improving the directory are also welcome. Please contact:

Medical and Health Information Directory
Gale
27500 Drake Rd.
Farmington Hills, MI 48331-3535
Telephone: (248)699-GALE
Toll-Free: (800)877-4253
Fax: (248)699-8865

Volume 3 of the *Medical and Health Information Directory (MHID)* consists of a main body of Descriptive Listings grouped within separate chapters by type of health service, and an Alphabetical Name and Keyword Index, which provides a convenient alphabetical listing of all clinics, treatment centers, care programs, and counseling/diagnostic services included in Volume 3. Each section is described below.

Listings are numbered sequentially within 35 separate chapters, as outlined on the "Contents" pages. Details on the content, arrangement, indexing, and sources for each chapter are provided in the following descriptions.

AIDS Programs

- Scope: Clinical research programs sponsored by the National Institute of Allergy and Infectious Diseases (NIAID) at sites across the country to evaluate promising therapies, drugs, and vaccines for people infected with the human immunodeficiency virus (HIV), the cause of AIDS. The chapter comprises three sections: 1) AIDS Clinical Trials Units (ACTU), 2) Community Programs for Clinical Research on AIDS (CPCRA), and 3) AIDS Vaccine Evaluation Units. ACTUs, which conduct large, multi-center studies at U.S. universities and medical centers, evaluate therapies for all aspects of HIV disease in adults and children. CPCRA studies bring clinical trials to HIV-infected patients in such community settings as hospitals, health centers, private practices and clinics, and drug treatment facilities. They complement studies in the ACTUs by focusing on how to use available treatments most effectively and determining the long-term consequences of different treatments. AVEUs conduct clinical trials of experimental vaccines to prevent HIV infection.

- Entries Include: Institution and/or program name, address, telephone number, fax number, e-mail address, and web site.

- Arrangement: Geographical by states, then alphabetical by institution/program names within each state.

- Indexed by: Institution or program names.

- Source: The National Institute of Allergy and Infectious Diseases (National Institutes of Health, U.S. Department of Health and Human Services).

Amyotrophic Lateral Sclerosis Clinics

- Scope: Clinics certified by the ALS Association that specialize in the care and treatment of people suffering from Amyotrophic Lateral Sclerosis (ALS).

- Entries Include: Institution and/or program name, address, telephone number, fax number, e-mail address, web site, and contact name.

- Arrangement: Geographical by states, then alphabetical by institution/program names within each state.

- Indexed by: Institution or program names.

- Source: List provided by the ALS Association (1275 K St. NW, Ste. 1050, Washington, DC 20005; 202-407-8580; http://www.alsa.org).

Arthritis & Musculoskeletal Diseases Centers

- Scope: Multipurpose Arthritis and Musculoskeletal Diseases Centers that conduct research on the causes, treatment, and prevention of arthritis and musculoskeletal diseases. With grant support from the National Institute of Arthritis and Musculoskeletal and Skin Diseases (NIAMS), these centers develop and carry out programs in basic and/or clinical research, epidemiology and health services research, and research related to professional, patient, and public education.

- Entries Include: Institution name, address, and telephone number.

- Arrangement: Geographical by states, then alphabetical by institution names within states.

- Indexed by: Institution names.

- Source: The National Institute of Arthritis and Musculoskeletal and Skin Diseases (National Institutes of Health, U.S. Department of Health and Human Services).

Audiology and Speech/Language Services

- Scope: Services for the deaf and hearing-impaired comprising two sections: 1) Educational Programs, including residential and day schools that offer pre-school through secondary-level education for deaf children, and 2) Rehabilitation Programs that provide clinical services in audiology, speech-language pathology, or both.

- Entries Include: Organization or institution name, address, telephone number, fax number, e-mail address, and web site.

- Arrangement: Geographical by states and cities, then alphabetical by organization or institution names within cities.

- Indexed by: Organization or institution names.

- Source: Original research by the editorial staff.

Services for the Blind and Sight Impaired

- Scope: Institutions in two sections: 1) Educational Programs for blind and visually impaired children, pre-school through high school, and 2) Libraries for the Blind and Physically Handicapped. Libraries are part of a national network established by The Library of Congress to provide free recorded and Braille materials to persons who are unable to read or use standard printed materials because of visual or physical impairment.

- Entries Include: Institution name, address, telephone number, fax number, e-mail address, and web site.

- Arrangement: Educational Programs are geographical by states, then alphabetical by institution names within states. Libraries for the Blind and Physically Handicapped are geographical by states, then alphabetical by library names within states.

- Indexed by: Institution names.

- Source: National Library Service for the Blind and Physically Handicapped (a service of the Library of Congress) and original research by the editorial staff.

Brain and Spinal Cord Injury Programs

- Scope: Institutions that provide services for brain and spinal cord injured persons. Included, among others, are programs administered by the Spinal Cord Injury Service of the U.S. Department of Veterans Affairs and programs that receive funding as model spinal cord injury systems from the National Institute on Disability and Rehabilitation Research (NIDRR).

- Entries Include: Parent institution and/or program name, address, and telephone number, as well as a notation identifying programs supported by NIDRR.

- Arrangement: Geographical by states, then alphabetical by institution/program names within states.

- Indexed by: Parent institution and/or program names.

- Source: Original research by the editorial staff.

Burn Care Services

- Scope: Hospitals that offer specialized burn care services.

- Entries Include: Institution name, address, telephone number, fax number, e-mail address, and the number of designated burn care beds in each hospital.

- Arrangement: Geographical by states, then alphabetical by institution names within states.

- Indexed by: Institution names.

- Source: Original research by the editorial staff.

Cancer Programs

- Scope: Hospital cancer programs approved by the Commission on Cancer of the American College of Surgeons.

- Entries Include: Institution name, address, and telephone number.

- Arrangement: Geographical by states and cities, then alphabetical by institution names within cities.

- Indexed by: Institution names.

- Source: *Commission on Cancer Approved Cancer Programs* (published by the American College of Surgeons, 633 N. St. Clair St., Chicago, IL 60611, http://www.facs.org, 800-621-4111) and the National Cancer Institute, National Institutes of Health, U.S. Department of Health and Human Services.

Community & Migrant Health Centers

- Scope: Community and/or migrant health centers that receive funding through two federal grant programs administered by the Bureau of Primary Health Care (Health Resources and Services Administration, Public Health Service, U.S. Department of Health and Human Services). Community health centers provide basic primary medical services to persons located in rural and urban areas with financial, geographic, or cultural barriers to care. Migrant health centers provide a comprehensive range of primary health services to migrant and seasonal farm workers and their dependents.

- Entries Include: Organization name, address, telephone number, and the type of funding (community health center, migrant health center, or both) provided to each grantee organization.

- Arrangement: Geographical by states and cities, then alphabetical by organization names within cities.

- Indexed by: Organization names.

- Source: Original research by the editorial staff.

Cystic Fibrosis Centers

- Scope: Centers affiliated with the Cystic Fibrosis Foundation. These centers, located at institutions throughout the country, specialize in diagnosis and comprehensive care for children and young adults who suffer from the disease.

- Entries Include: Institution name, address, telephone number, and fax number.

- Arrangement: Geographical by states, then alphabetical by institution names within states.

- Indexed by: Institution names.

- Source: List provided by the Cystic Fibrosis Foundation (6931 Arlington Rd., 2nd Floor, Bethesda, MD 20814; 800-FIGHT-CF; http://www.cff.org).

Clinical Programs for the Developmentally Disabled

- Scope: Programs that provide comprehensive diagnosis/evaluation, counseling, treatment, and follow-up services to children and adults who have or are at risk of having a developmental disability, including intellectual disabilities, cerebral palsy, epilepsy, autism, or other conditions closely related to mental retardation.

- Entries Include: Institution and/or program name, address, and telephone number.

- Arrangement: Geographical by states, then alphabetical by institution/program names within states.

- Indexed by: Institution or program names.

- Source: Original research by the editorial staff.

Domestic Violence and Sexual Assault Programs

- Scope: Community resources nationwide for victims of domestic violence. Each of these programs offers some or all of the following services: shelters for battered women and their children, 24-hour crisis lines, information and referrals, support groups, counseling, and legal advocacy.

- Entries Include: Parent organization and/or program name, address, telephone number, fax number,

e-mail address and, for most, crisis phone number(s) (24-hour hotlines, unless noted otherwise).

- Arrangement: Geographical by states and cities, then alphabetical by organization/program names within cities.

- Indexed by: Parent organization and/or program names.

- Source: Original research by the editorial staff.

Down Syndrome Clinics

- Scope: Clinics that specialize in the care and treatment of people suffering from Down Syndrome.

- Entries Include: Institution and/or program name, address, telephone number, and contact name.

- Arrangement: Geographical by states, then alphabetical by organization names within states.

- Indexed by: Institution or program names.

- Source: List provided by the National Down Syndrome Congress (30 Mansell Ct., Ste. 108, Roswell, GA 30076; 800-232-NDSC; http://www.ndsccenter.org).

Eating Disorders Clinics

- Scope: Clinics that specialize in the care and treatment of people suffering from Eating Disorders.

- Entries Include: Institution and/or program name, address, telephone number, fax number, e-mail address, and web site.

- Arrangement: Geographical by states, then alphabetical by organization names within states.

- Indexed by: Institution or program names.

- Source: Original research by the editorial staff.

Family Planning Services

- Scope: Offices, affiliates, and chapters of the Planned Parenthood Federation of America.

- Entries Include: Organization name, address, telephone number, and fax number.

- Arrangement: Geographical by states, then alphabetical by organization name within states.

- Indexed by: Organization names.

- Source: Directory provided by the Planned Parenthood Federation of America (434 W. 33rd St., New York, NY 10001; (212)541-7800; http://www.plannedparenthood.org).

Genetic Services Centers

- Scope: Clinical genetic services centers that offer comprehensive diagnostic services, medical management, counseling, and follow-up care for a range of genetic conditions. (Specialized clinics and programs, such as those for cystic fibrosis, hemophilia, and sickle cell anemia, are covered in separate chapters of this publication.)

- Entries Include: Institution name, address, telephone number, fax number, e-mail address, and web site.
- Arrangement: Geographical by states then alphabetical by institution names within states.
- Indexed by: Institution names.
- Source: Original research by the editorial staff.

Headache Clinics

- Scope: Clinics that specialize in the treatment of migraine headaches.
- Entries Include: Institution name, address, telephone number, fax number, web site, and contact person.
- Arrangement: Geographical by states then alphabetical by institution names within states.
- Indexed by: Institution names.
- Source: List provided by the National Headache Foundation (820 N Orleans St., Ste. 411, Chicago, IL 60610; (312) 274-2650; http://www.headaches.org)

Hemophilia Centers

- Scope: Federally funded hemophilia treatment facilities.
- Entries Include: Parent institution and/or center name, address, telephone number, fax number, email address, and web site.
- Arrangement: Geographical by states, then alphabetical by institution/center names within states.
- Indexed by: Parent institution and/or center names.
- Source: Maternal and Child Health Bureau (Health Resources and Services Administration, U.S. Department of Health and Human Services).

Home Health Care Agencies

- Scope: Home health agencies accredited by The Joint Commission, formerly named the Joint Commission on Accreditation of Healthcare Organizations. These hospitals, public health departments, and various for-profit and nonprofit organizations provide skilled nursing, home health aids, and other therapeutic services in patients' own homes.
- Entries Include: Parent organization and/or agency name, address, telephone number, contact person, and current accreditation status.
- Arrangement: Geographical by states and cities, then alphabetical by organization/agency names within cities.

- Indexed by: Parent organization and/or agency names.
- Source: List provided by The Joint Commission (One Renaissance Blvd., Oakbrook Terrace, IL 60181; (630) 792-5000; http://www.jointcommission.org).

Hospices

- Scope: Hospices that are Medicare certified. These organizations, which may be independent units, sponsored by hospitals, or affiliated with home health care agencies, focus on managing the pain and discomfort of terminally ill persons and provide emotional support to family members as well. Services usually take place in the home, but are sometimes provided in hospital or nursing home units.
- Entries Include: Parent organization and/or hospice name, address, and telephone number.
- Arrangement: Geographical by states and cities, then alphabetical by organization names within cities.
- Indexed by: Parent organization and/or hospice names.
- Source: Original research by the editorial staff.

In Vitro Fertilization Clinics

- Scope: Clinics that specialize in in vitro fertilization procedures.
- Entries Include: Organization and/or facility name, address, telephone number, and contact person.
- Arrangement: Geographical by state, then alphabetical by organization and/or facility name within state.
- Indexed by: Organization and/or facility name.
- Source: Original research by the editorial staff.

Kidney Dialysis & Transplant Services

- Scope: Facilities approved by the Centers for Medicare and Medicaid Services, U.S. Department of Health and Human Services, to provide kidney dialysis and transplant services under the Medicare program.
- Entries Include: Parent organization and/or facility name, address, telephone number, and the number of dialysis treatment stations at each facility.
- Arrangement: Geographical by states and cities, then alphabetical by organization/facility names within cities.
- Indexed by: Parent organization and/or facility names.
- Source: *National Listing of Medicare Providers Furnishing Kidney Dialysis and Transplant Services*

(published by the Office of Clinical Standards and Quality, Centers for Medicare and Medicaid Services, U.S. Department of Health and Human Services).

Mental Health Services

- Scope: Governmental, public, or private organizations, agencies, and institutions that provide services to persons with mental disorders. The chapter comprises three sections: 1) Multiservice Mental Health Organizations, which provide two or more of the following care services: inpatient, residential, partial care (day/evening), outpatient, and residential supportive care; 2) Psychiatric Hospitals, which provide 24-hour inpatient care to mentally ill persons; and 3) Residential Treatment Centers for Emotionally Disturbed Children, which serve children and adolescents under age 18.

- Entries Include: Organization, agency, or institution name, address, telephone number, and toll-free and fax numbers.

- Arrangement: Geographical by states and cities, then alphabetical by organization/agency/institution names within each of the sections noted above.

- Indexed by: Organization, agency, or institution names.

- Source: Original research by the editorial staff.

Multiple Sclerosis Centers & Clinics

- Scope: MS Comprehensive Care Centers and MS Care Centers. The Comprehensive Care Centers, established throughout the country by neurologists specializing in the field of MS, provide a broad range of services to meet the medical, psychosocial, educational and rehabilitation needs of people with multiple sclerosis and their families. The Care Clinics are affiliated with local chapters of the National Multiple Sclerosis Society. Many are also part of the Consortium of MS Centers, which has established guidelines for the type and quality of programs needed.

- Entries Include: Organization or institution name, address, and telephone number.

- Arrangement: Geographical by states, then alphabetical by organization/institution names within states.

- Indexed by: Organization or institution names.

- Source: List provided by the National Multiple Sclerosis Society (733 3rd Ave., 3rd Floor, New York, NY 10017; 800-FIGHT-MS; http://www.nmss.org).

Muscular Dystrophy Clinics

- Scope: Clinics sponsored by the Muscular Dystrophy Association at hospitals nationwide to provide diagnostic examinations, as well as follow-up care, to patients afflicted with any of the 40 neuromuscular diseases covered by the association's programs.

- Entries Include: Institution name, address, telephone number, toll-free number, fax number, e-mail address, and web site.

- Arrangement: Geographical by states, then alphabetical by institution names within states.

- Indexed by: Institution names.

- Source: Original research by the editorial staff.

Organ and Tissue Banks

- Scope: Tissue and organ banks that obtain, evaluate, and distribute eye tissue for use in corneal transplantation, research, and education; and blood cord banks.

- Entries Include: Parent organization and/or eye bank name, address, telephone number, fax number, e-mail address, and web site.

- Arrangement: Geographical by states, then alphabetical by organization names within states.

- Indexed by: Parent organization and/or bank names.

- Source: Original research by the editorial staff.

Pain Management Programs

- Scope: Inpatient and/or outpatient centers and clinics concerned with improving the quality of life for persons suffering acute chronic pain (i.e., headaches, backaches, arthritis, etc.).

- Entries Include: Parent organization and/or program name, address, and telephone number.

- Arrangement: Geographical by states, then alphabetical by organization/program names within states.

- Indexed by: Parent organization and/or program names.

- Source: Original research by the editorial staff.

Runaway & Homeless Youth Centers

- Scope: Grantees that receive federal funding through the Runaway and Homeless Youth Program administered by the U.S. Administration on Children, Youth and Families. These community-based centers provide a range of services, including temporary shelter, counseling, legal aid, and referrals to medical care.

- Entries Include: Organization name, address, telephone number, fax number, e-mail address, and web site.
- Arrangement: Geographical by states, then alphabetical by organization names within states.
- Indexed by: Organization names.
- Source: Original research by the editorial staff.

Sickle Cell Anemia Centers

- Scope: Sickle cell programs, including comprehensive sickle cell centers funded by the National Heart, Lung, and Blood Institute, as well as programs located in Veterans Affairs Medical Centers.
- Entries Include: Institution name, address, telephone number, and fax number.
- Arrangement: Geographical by states, then alphabetical by institution names within states.
- Indexed by: Institution names.
- Source: Lists provided by the U.S. Department of Veterans Affairs and the National Heart, Lung, and Blood Institute (National Institutes of Health, U.S. Department of Health and Human Services).

SIDS Information & Counseling Programs

- Scope: State agencies and programs funded by the Maternal and Child Health Bureau (Public Health Service, U.S. Department of Health and Human Services) to disseminate public information and counsel families affected by SIDS (Sudden Infant Death Syndrome).
- Entries Include: Agency and/or program name, address, and telephone number.
- Arrangement: Geographical by states, then alphabetical by agency/program names within states.
- Indexed by: Agency and/or program names.
- Source: Original research by the editorial staff.

Sleep Disorders Centers & Laboratories

- Scope: Accredited members of the American Academy of Sleep Medicine, including centers which provide full diagnostic and treatment services for all types of sleep-related disorders, and laboratories which specialize only in sleep-related breathing disorders.
- Entries Include: Parent institution and/or center/laboratory name, address, telephone number, and fax number.
- Arrangement: Geographical by states, then alphabetical by institution or center/laboratory names within states.

- Indexed by: Parent institution and/or center/laboratory names.
- Source: Membership roster provided by the American Academy of Sleep Medicine (2501 N. Frontgate Rd., Darien, IL 60561; (630) 737-9790; http://www.aasmnet.org).

Sports Medicine Clinics

- Scope: Organizations and institutions that provide a variety of services aimed at the diagnosis, treatment, and prevention of injuries resulting from participation in professional or recreational sports.
- Entries Include: Organization or institution name, address, telephone number, e-mail address, and web site.
- Arrangement: Geographical by states and cities, then alphabetical by organization/institution names within cities.
- Indexed by: Organization or institution names.
- Source: Original research by the editorial staff.

Substance Abuse Services

- Scope: Federal, state, local, and privately-funded organizations, agencies, and organizations that provide alcoholism and/or drug abuse treatment services.
- Entries Include: Organization, agency, or institution name, address, telephone number, toll-free and fax numbers, e-mail address and web site.
- Arrangement: Geographical by states and cities, then alphabetical by organization/agency/institution names within cities.
- Indexed by: Organization, agency, or institution names.
- Source: Substance Abuse and Mental Health Services Administration, U.S. Department of Health and Human Services.

Suicide Prevention & Crisis Intervention Centers

- Scope: Organizations that provide suicide prevention and crisis intervention services.
- Entries Include: Parent organization and/or center name, address, business telephone number, and one or more crisis phone numbers. (Most crisis lines are available 24 hours a day, seven days a week, unless otherwise noted.)
- Arrangement: Geographical by states and cities, then alphabetical by organization/center names within cities.

- Indexed by: Parent organization and/or center names.

- Source: Original research by the editorial staff.

Veterans Services

- Scope: Veterans services comprising three sections: 1) Veterans Affairs Medical Centers; 2) Post-Traumatic Stress Disorder (PTSD) Programs that provide a variety of inpatient, outpatient, and residential treatment services to veterans suffering from PTSD or co-existing PTSD/substance abuse; and 3) Vietnam Vet Centers that provide a broad range of psychological and vocational counseling, as well as other assistance to Vietnam-era veterans and their families. (Other veterans services covered in separate Volume 3 chapters include sickle cell anemia programs, spinal cord injury programs, and substance abuse treatment programs.)

- Entries Include: Facility name, address, and telephone number.

- Arrangement: Geographical by states and cities, then alphabetical by facility names within each of the sections noted above.

- Indexed by: Facility names.

- Source: Lists provided by the U.S. Department of Veterans Affairs.

Alphabetical Name and Keyword Index

The Alphabetical Name and Keyword Index provides access to all clinics, treatment centers, care programs, and counseling/diagnostic services included in Volume 3. Index references are to book entry numbers rather than to page numbers.

Many of the entries in Volume 3 use a hierarchical organization name structure, with a parent organization and often intermediate sub-units preceding the specific unit name. The Alphabetical Name and Keyword Index offers access to all multiple-part organization names via the parent organization name. Some entries are also referenced under the specific unit name and some under a significant intermediate unit name. Multiple parts of names are separated in index citations by a bullet (•). If several entries have the same parent organization, as is the case with many of the health services listed in Volume 3, the related units appear as a group under the name of the parent organization.

Alphabetizing Rules

In both the descriptive listings chapters and the index, organization names are sorted on a word-by-word basis, so that "New York Easter Seal Society" comes before "Newark Beth Israel Medical Center." Initial articles ("A," "An," or "The") are ignored for sorting purposes. Conjunctions, articles, and most prepositions elsewhere in the names are also not considered in alphabetizing. In addition:

- Numbers are sorted as if spelled-out and interfiled alphabetically with other non-number words.

- Abbreviations such as "U.S.," "St.," "Mt.," "Ft.," and "Dr." are sorted as if spelled-out and interfiled with names in which the full version of those words are used.

- Personal names are sorted under the first name, or initial, within the descriptive listings chapters. In the index, they can be accessed under both the first and last names.

Act.	Acting	Dr.	Drive	MN	Minnesota
Adj.	Adjutant	E.	East	MO	Missouri
Admin.	Administrator	Educ.	Education	MS	Mississippi
AFB	Air Force Base	Exec.	Executive	MT	Montana
AK	Alaska	Expy.	Expressway	Mt.	Mount
AKA	Also Known As	Ext.	Extension	N.	North
AL	Alabama	First Pub	First Published	Natl.	National
Alt. Contact	Alternate Contact	FL	Florida	NC	North Carolina
Apt.	Apartment	Flr.	Floor	ND	North Dakota
AR	Arkansas	Fnded	Founded	NE	Nebraska, Northeast
Assoc.	Associate	Freq	Frequency	NH	New Hampshire
Asst.	Assistant	Frmly	Formerly	NJ	New Jersey
Ave.	Avenue	Ft.	Fort	No.	Number
AZ	Arizona	Fwy.	Freeway	NV	Nevada
Bldg.	Building	GA	Georgia	NW	Northwest
Blvd.	Boulevard	Gen.	General	NY	New York
Br.	Branch	Geo. Dist.	Geographical Distribution	Off.	Officer
CA	California			OH	Ohio
Cat. No.	Catalogue Number	GU	Guam	OK	Oklahoma
CEO	Chief Executive Officer	Hd.	Head	OR	Oregon
Chf.	Chief	HI	Hawaii	PA	Pennsylvania
Chm.	Chairman	Hwy.	Highway	Pgs	Pages
Cir.	Circle	IA	Iowa	Pkwy.	Parkway
Clghse.	Clearinghouse	ID	Idaho	Pl.	Place
c/o	Care of	IL	Illinois	Plz.	Plaza
CO	Colorado	IN	Indiana	PO Box	Post Office Box
Co.	Company	Inc.	Incorporated	PR	Puerto Rico
Coll.	Collection	Info.	Information	Pres.	President
Comdr.	Commander	KS	Kansas	Prog.	Program
Commun.	Communication	KY	Kentucky	Pub	Publication
Coord.	Coordinator	LA	Louisiana	RD	Rural Delivery
Corp.	Corporation	Lang	Language	Rd.	Road
Couns.	Counselor	Lib.	Library	Ref.	Reference
CT	Connecticut	Libn.	Librarian	Reg.	Regional
Ct.	Court	Ln.	Lane	Res.	Research
Ctr.	Center	MA	Massachusetts	RFD	Rural Free Delivery
DC	District of Columbia	MD	Maryland	RI	Rhode Island
DE	Delaware	ME	Maine	Rm.	Room
Dept.	Department	Med.	Medical	RR	Rural Route
Desc	Description	Mem	Members	Rte.	Route
Dir.	Director	Mgr.	Manager	S.	South
		MI	Michigan		

SC	South Carolina	Sta.	Station	U.S.	United States
Sci.	Science	Ste.	Suite, Sainte	U.S. Dist	U.S. Distributor
SD	South Dakota	Subscript	Subscription(s)	UT	Utah
SE	Southeast	Supv.	Supervisor	VA	Virginia
Sec.	Secretary	SW	Southwest	VI	Virgin Islands
Sect.	Section	Telecom	Telecommunications	VP	Vice President
Serv.	Service	Ter.	Terrace	VT	Vermont
Soc.	Social	TN	Tennessee	W.	West
Spec.	Specialist	Tpke.	Turnpike	WA	Washington
Sq.	Square	Trl.	Trail	WV	West Virginia
Sr.	Senior	TX	Texas	WY	Wyoming
St.	Saint, Street	Univ.	University		

This chapter lists organizations that provide suicide and crisis intervention services. Entries are arranged geographically by states and cities, then alphabetically by organization names within cities. See the "User's Guide" located at the front of this directory for additional information.

ALABAMA

Alexander City

50608 ■ Nan Coley Murphy Counseling Center
1508 Hwy. 22 W
Alexander City, AL 35010
Ph: (256)329-8463
URL: http://www.eastalabamamhc.org/locations.htm

Auburn

50609 ■ Crisis Center of East Alabama, Inc.
PO Box 1053
Auburn, AL 36831-1053
Ph: (334)821-8600
E-mail: crisiscenter@earthlink.net
URL: http://www.home.earthlink.net/~crisiscenter/

Birmingham

50610 ■ Crisis Center--Birmingham
3600 8th Ave. S, Ste. 501
Birmingham, AL 35222
Ph: (205)323-7782
Fax: (205)328-6225
URL: http://www.CrisisCenterBham.com

Brewton

50611 ■ Southwest Alabama Behavioral Health Care System--Brewton
1321 McMillian St., Ste. A
Brewton, AL 36426
Ph: (251)867-3242
Fax: (251)867-7151
URL: http://www.swamh.com

Decatur

50612 ■ Mental Health of North Central Alabama
4110 Hwy. 31 S
Decatur, AL 35603
Ph: (256)355-6091
Fax: (256)355-6092
E-mail: mentalhealth@mhcnca.org
URL: http://www.mhcnca.org

Evergreen

50613 ■ Southwest Alabama Behavioral Health Care System--Evergreen
220 Magnolia Ave.
Evergreen, AL 36401
Ph: (251)578-4545
Fax: (251)578-4583
URL: http://www.swamh.com

Gadsden

50614 ■ 13th Place, Inc.
405 S 12th St.
Gadsden, AL 35901

Ph: (256)547-9505
Fax: (256)547-8979
URL: http://www.facebook.com/group.php?gid=60456647586

Grove Hill

50615 ■ Southwest Alabama Behavioral Health Care System--Grove Hill
129 Clarke St.
Grove Hill, AL 36451
Ph: (251)275-4165
Fax: (251)275-4807
URL: http://www.swamh.com

Huntsville

50616 ■ Crisis Services of North Alabama, Inc.
PO Box 368
Huntsville, AL 35804
Ph: (256)716-1000
URL: http://www.csna.org/

50617 ■ HELPline--Huntsville
PO Box 368
Huntsville, AL 35804
Ph: (256)716-1000
URL: http://www.csna.org/HELPline.php

Mobile

50618 ■ Contact Mobile Helpline, Inc.
PO Box 66608
Mobile, AL 36660-1608
Ph: (334)431-5111
E-mail: helpline@acan.net
URL: http://www.helplinemobile.org

Monroeville

50619 ■ Southwest Alabama Behavioral Health Care System--Monroeville
530 Hornady Dr.
Monroeville, AL 36460
Ph: (251)575-4837
Fax: (251)575-4837
URL: http://www.swamh.com

50620 ■ Southwest Alabama Mental Health Center
328 W Claiborne St.
Monroeville, AL 36460
Ph: (251)575-4203
Fax: (251)575-9459
E-mail: swamh@frontiernet.net
URL: http://www.swamh.com

Muscle Shoals

50621 ■ C.R.U.T.C.H., Inc.
PO Box 2487
Muscle Shoals, AL 35662
URL: http://www.themereproject.org

Phoenix City

50622 ■ East Alabama Mental Health Center
2400 10th St.
Phoenix City, AL 36869
Ph: (334)298-2405
URL: http://www.themereproject.org

Tuscaloosa

50623 ■ Indian River Mental Health Center
PO Box 2190
Tuscaloosa, AL 35401
Ph: (205)345-1600
URL: http://www.themereproject.org

Valley

50624 ■ Alsobrook Counseling Center
6376 Fairfax Bypass
Valley, AL 36854
Ph: (334)756-4117
URL: http://www.themereproject.org

ALASKA

Akiak

50625 ■ Akiak Native Community Suicide Prevention
PO Box 52127
Akiak, AK 99552
Ph: (907)765-7911
Fax: (907)765-7512

Alakanuk

50626 ■ Alakanuk Suicide Prevention
PO Box 167
Alakanuk, AK 99554
Ph: (907)238-3313

Anchorage

50627 ■ North Star Behavioral Health System
2530 DeBarr Rd.
Anchorage, AK 99508
Ph: (907)258-7575
Free: 800-478-7575
E-mail: info@northstarbehavioral.com
URL: http://www.northstarbehavioral.com/

50628 ■ South Central Counseling Center
4020 Folker St.
Anchorage, AK 99508
Ph: (907)563-1000
Fax: (907)563-2045
URL: http://www.acmhs.com

Barrow

50629 ■ North Slope Borough Community Mental Health Center
PO Box 69
Barrow, AK 99723
Ph: (907)852-0260

Bethel

50630 ■ Yukon Kuskokwim Health Corp.--Behavioral Health
PO Box 528
Bethel, AK 99559
Ph: (907)543-6104
URL: http://www.ykhc.org/

Cordova

50631 ■ Sound Alternatives
602 Chase Ave.
Cordova, AK 99574
Ph: (907)424-8300

Dillingham

50632 ■ Bristol Bay Counseling Center
Box 130
Dillingham, AK 99576
Ph: (907)842-5301
Free: 800-478-5201
URL: http://www.bbahc.org/mental.html

Fairbanks

50633 ■ Fairbanks Crisis Line
PO Box 70908
Fairbanks, AK 99707
Ph: (907)451-8600
URL: http://www.cityoffairbanks.com

Hooper Bay

50634 ■ Sunshine Suicide Prevention
Hooper Bay Native Village
Hooper Bay, AK 99604
Ph: (907)758-4917
URL: http://www.themereproject.org

Juneau

50635 ■ Suicide Prevention--Juneau
3406 Glacier Hwy.
Juneau, AK 99801
Ph: (907)586-4357
Free: 877-266-4357
URL: http://www.juneausuicideprevention.org/

Kenai

50636 ■ Central Peninsula Counseling Services
506 Lake St.
Kenai, AK 99611
Ph: (907)283-7501
Fax: (907)283-9006

Kipnuk

50637 ■ Kipnuk Traditional Council Community Suicide Prevention Program
Kipnuk, AK 99614
Ph: (907)896-5555
URL: http://www.themereproject.org

Kotlik

50638 ■ Kotlik City Council Suicide Prevention Program
Kotlik, AK 99620
Ph: (907)899-4040
Fax: (907)899-4826
URL: http://www.themereproject.org

Minto

50639 ■ Minto Village Council Suicide Prevention Line
Minto, AK 99758
Ph: (907)798-7400
Fax: (907)798-7627
URL: http://www.themereproject.org

Nondalton

50640 ■ Nondalton Suicide Prevention
Nondalton, AK 99640
Ph: (907)294-2300
URL: http://www.themereproject.org

Toksook

50641 ■ Suicide Prevention Services--Toksook
PO Box 37008
Toksook, AK 99637
Ph: (907)427-7016
URL: http://www.themereproject.org

Wasilla

50642 ■ Mat-Su Health Services
1363 W Spruce Ave.
Wasilla, AK 99654-5327
Ph: (907)376-2411
Free: 800-478-2410
E-mail: info@matsuhealth.org
URL: http://www.bhs-mat-su.com/
Formerly: Life Quest.

ARIZONA

Gila Bend

50643 ■ Suicide Prevention Center--Gila Bend
220 N Martin Ave.
Gila Bend, AZ 85337
Ph: (520)683-2346
URL: http://www.themereproject.org

Holbrook

50644 ■ Community Counseling Centers, Inc.--Holbrook
105 N 5th Ave.
Holbrook, AZ 86025-2817
Ph: (928)524-6126
URL: http://www.themereproject.org

Mesa

50645 ■ Teens Talk To Teens
570 W Brown Rd.
Mesa, AZ 85201
Ph: (480)461-8888

Phoenix

50646 ■ Arizona Teen Crisis Solutions
Phoenix, AZ
Free: 800-818-6228
URL: http://arizonateenhelp.com/

50647 ■ Southwest Behavioral Health Service
3450 N 3rd St.
Phoenix, AZ 85014
Ph: (602)265-8338
E-mail: info@sbhservices.org
URL: http://www.sbhservices.org/

50648 ■ Teen Lifeline
PO Box 10745
Phoenix, AZ 85064
Ph: (602)248-8337
Free: 800-248-8336
Fax: (602)266-1958
E-mail: nikki@teenlife.org
URL: http://www.teenlifeline.org

50649 ■ TriWest Healthcare Alliance
15451 N 28th Ave.
Phoenix, AZ 85053
Ph: (602)564-2339
URL: http://www.triwest.com/

Saint Johns

50650 ■ Little Colorado Behavioral Health Centers, Saint Johns
470 W Cleveland St.
Saint Johns, AZ 85936
Ph: (928)337-4301
Fax: (928)337-2269
URL: http://www.lcbhc.org/

Show Low

50651 ■ Community Counseling Centers, Inc.--Show Low
2500 Show Low Lake Rd.
Show Low, AZ 85901
Ph: (928)537-2951
Fax: (928)537-8520
URL: http://www.themereproject.org

Springerville

50652 ■ Little Colorado Behavioral Health Centers, Springerville
50 N Hopi St.
Springerville, AZ 85938
Ph: (928)333-2683
URL: http://www.themereproject.org

Tempe

50653 ■ EMPACT Suicide Prevention Center
1232 E Broadway Rd., Ste. 120
Tempe, AZ 85282
Ph: (480)784-1514
E-mail: info@empact-spc.com
URL: http://www.empact-spc.com

Tucson

50654 ■ Excel Program
1930 E 6th St.
Tucson, AZ 85719
Ph: (520)622-6000

50655 ■ Help on Call Crisis Line
101 N Stone Ave.
Tucson, AZ 85701
Ph: (520)594-5600

50656 ■ SAMHC Behavioral Health Services
2502 N Dodge Blvd., Ste. 190
Tucson, AZ 85716
Ph: (520)622-6000
Free: 800-796-6762
URL: http://www.samhc.com

Winslow

50657 ■ Community Counseling Centers, Inc.--Winslow
1015 E 3rd St.
Winslow, AZ 86047
Ph: (928)289-4658
URL: http://www.themereproject.org

Yuma

50658 ■ Excel Group
3250 E 4th St.
Yuma, AZ 85365
Ph: (520)782-7273
Free: 800-880-8901
URL: http://www.excelgroup.org

ARKANSAS

Clarksville

50659 ■ Counseling Associates, Inc.--Clarksville
1021 E Poplar St.
Clarksville, AR 72830
Ph: (479)754-8610
Fax: (479)754-8788
URL: http://www.caiinc.org/

Conway

50660 ■ Counseling Associates Inc.--Conway
350 Salem Rd., Ste. 1
Conway, AR 72034
Ph: (501)336-8300
Fax: (501)329-5508
URL: http://www.caiinc.org/

Copper City

50661 ■ Copper River Native Association--Behavioral Health Services
Copper City, AR 99573
Ph: (907)822-5241
Fax: (907)822-8801
URL: http://www.crnative.org/bhs.html

Hot Springs

50662 ■ Community Counseling Services--Hot Springs
700 South Ave.
Hot Springs, AR 71902
Ph: (501)624-7111
URL: http://www.communitycounselingservices.org/

Morrilton

50663 ■ Counseling Associates Inc.--Morrilton
8 Hospital Dr.
Morrilton, AR 72110
Ph: (501)354-1561
Fax: (501)364-1564
URL: http://www.caiinc.org/

Russellville

50664 ■ Counseling Associates Inc.--Russellville
110 Skyline Dr.
Russellville, AR 72801
Ph: (479)968-1298
Fax: (479)968-6053
URL: http://www.caiinc.org/

Springdale

50665 ■ Northwest Arkansas Crisis Intervention Center
614 E Emma Ave.
Springdale, AR 72764
Ph: (479)756-1995
Fax: (479)756-2338
E-mail: rhill@jtlshop.jonesnet.org
URL: http://www.nwacrisiscenter.org

CALIFORNIA

Anaheim

50666 ■ Hotline Help Center
PO Box 110
Anaheim, CA 92815
Ph: (714)441-2099

Burlingame

50667 ■ Youth and Family Assistance Crisis Intervention and Suicide Prevention Center
1860 El Camino Real, Ste. 400
Burlingame, CA 94010
Ph: (650)692-6662
Fax: (650)652-9745

Capitola

50668 ■ Suicide Prevention Services of Santa Cruz County
1395 41st Ave., Ste. B
Capitola, CA 95010
Ph: (831)462-6831

Culver City

50669 ■ Didi Hirsch Community Mental Health Center Suicide Prevention Center
4760 S Sepulveda Blvd.
Culver City, CA 90230
Ph: (310)390-6612
Fax: (310)398-5690
E-mail: info@didihirsch.org
URL: http://www.didihirsch.org

Davis

50670 ■ Suicide Prevention of Yolo County
PO Box 622
Davis, CA 95617
Ph: (530)756-7542
Fax: (530)756-2931
URL: http://www.suicidepreventionyolocounty.org/

El Cajon

50671 ■ Crisis House
1034 N Magnolia
El Cajon, CA 92020
Ph: (619)444-9926
URL: http://www.crisishouse.org/

El Centro

50672 ■ Sure Help Line Center
395 Broadway St., Ste. 2
El Centro, CA 92243
Ph: (760)352-7873
URL: http://www.themereproject.org

Garden Grove

50673 ■ New Hope Telephone Counseling Center
12141 Lewis St.
Garden Grove, CA 92640
Ph: (714)639-4673
URL: http://www.newhopeonline.org

Lafayette

50674 ■ Contact Care Center
PO Box 901
Lafayette, CA 94549
Ph: (925)284-2207
URL: http://www.themereproject.org

Lakeport

50675 ■ Lake County Mental Health Emergency Service
922 Bevins Ct.
Lakeport, CA 95453
Ph: (707)263-2258

Los Alamitos

50676 ■ Hotline of Southern California
PO Box 32
Los Alamitos, CA 90720
Ph: (562)596-5548

Los Angeles

50677 ■ Psychological Trauma Center
8730 Alden Dr., Rm. C-106A
Los Angeles, CA 90048
Ph: (310)855-3506
URL: http://www.ptcweb.org/

50678 ■ Teen Line
PO Box 48750
Los Angeles, CA 90048
Ph: (310)423-3401
URL: http://www.teenlineonline.org

Mariposa

50679 ■ Mariposa Counseling Center
5037 Stroming Rd.
Mariposa, CA 95338
Ph: (209)966-2000
Free: 800-549-6741
Fax: (209)966-8415

Modesto

50680 ■ CrossRoads Psychological Health Center
Memorial Hospital Association
1700 Coffee Rd.
Modesto, CA 95355
Ph: (209)572-7238

Napa

50681 ■ Suicide Prevention/Crisis Line of Volunteer Center of Napa County
1820 Jefferson St.
Napa, CA 94559
Ph: (707)422-2555

Newark

50682 ■ Second Chance, Inc.
6330 Thornton Ave.
Newark, CA 94560
Ph: (510)792-4357
URL: http://www.secondchanceinc.com

Oakland

50683 ■ Crisis Support Services of Alameda County
PO Box 3120
Oakland, CA 94609
Ph: (510)420-2460
URL: http://www.crisissupport.org

Pacific Grove

50684 ■ Suicide Prevention and Crisis Center
PO Box 52078
Pacific Grove, CA 93950
Ph: (831)375-6966
URL: http://www.themereproject.org

Pasadena

50685 ■ Kaiser Permanente Behavioral Healthcare Helpline
CCC, 3rd Fl.
393 E Walnut St.
Pasadena, CA 91188
Ph: (626)405-3682
URL: http://www.kp.org

Port Hueneme

50686 ■ Anacupa Hospital Stanislaus County Behavioral Health and Recovery Center
307 E Clara
Port Hueneme, CA 93041
Ph: (805)488-4900

Redding

50687 ■ Help, Inc.
PO Box 992498
Redding, CA 96099-2498
Ph: (530)225-5255
Free: 800-891-5252
E-mail: help@helpshasta.org
URL: http://www.helpshasta.org/

Sacramento

50688 ■ Suicide Prevention--Crisis Services, Sacramento
8912 Volunteer Ln., Ste. 100
Sacramento, CA 95826
Ph: (916)368-3118

Salinas

50689 ■ Suicide Prevention and Crisis
371 Main St.
Salinas, CA 93901
Ph: (408)649-8008

San Bernardino

50690 ■ Family Service Agency of San Bernardino
1669 North E St.
San Bernardino, CA 92405
Ph: (909)886-6737
Fax: (909)881-3871

San Carlos

50691 ■ Youth and Family Enrichment Services Crisis Center
610 Elm St., Ste. 212
San Carlos, CA 94070
Ph: (650)591-9623
URL: http://www.yfes.org

San Diego

50692 ■ United Behavioral Health--Access and Crisis Line
3111 Camino del Rio N
San Diego, CA 92108
Ph: (619)641-6800

San Francisco

50693 ■ Center for Elderly Suicide Prevention and Grief Related Services
3626 Geary Blvd.
San Francisco, CA 94118
Ph: (415)750-5348
URL: http://www.growthhouse.org/cesp.html

50694 ■ San Francisco Suicide Prevention
PO Box 191350
San Francisco, CA 94119-1350
Ph: (415)984-1900
E-mail: info@sfsuicide.org
URL: http://www.sfsuicide.org

San Jose

50695 ■ Santa Clara County Suicide and Crisis Service
2220 Moorpark Ave.
San Jose, CA 95128
Ph: (408)885-6250

San Luis Obispo

50696 ■ Hotline of San Luis Obispo
PO Box 5456
San Luis Obispo, CA 93403
Ph: (805)544-6065
URL: http://www.slohotline.org

San Rafael

50697 ■ Family Service Agency of Marin
555 Northgate Dr.
San Rafael, CA 94903
Ph: (415)491-5700
Fax: (415)491-5750
E-mail: fsa@fsamarin.org
URL: http://www.themereproject.org

50698 ■ Suicide Prevention and Community Counseling Service of Marin
PO Box 4369
San Rafael, CA 94913-4369
Ph: (415)499-1195
URL: http://www.fsamarin.org

Santa Cruz

50699 ■ Crisis Intervention Service
Santa Cruz Mental Health Service
1060 Emeline Ave.
Santa Cruz, CA 95060

Ph: (831)454-4170

50700 ■ Family Service Agency of the Central Coast
104 Walnut Ave., Ste. 208
Santa Cruz, CA 95060
Ph: (831)459-9373
URL: http://www.fsa-cc.org/

50701 ■ Family Service Association of Santa Cruz
Suicide Prevention Service
PO Box 1222
Santa Cruz, CA 95061
Ph: (831)459-9373
Free: 877-663-5433
URL: http://www.fsa-cc.org/programs/suicide_prev. html

50702 ■ Suicide Prevention Service of the Central Coast
PO Box 1222
Santa Cruz, CA 95061-1222
Ph: (831)458-5300
URL: http://www.fsa-cc.org/programs/suicide_prev. html

Stockton

50703 ■ San Joaquin County Behavioral Health Services
1212 N California St.
Stockton, CA 95202-1594
Ph: (209)468-8700
Formerly: San Joaquin County Mental Health Services.

Ventura

50704 ■ The Behavioral Health Crisis Team
200 N Hillmont Ave.
Ventura, CA 93003
Ph: (805)652-6565
Formerly: Mobile Crisis Team.

Victorville

50705 ■ First Call for Help--Victorville
Victor Valley Community Service Council
15476 6th St.
Victorville, CA 92392
Ph: (760)245-8592

Walnut Creek

50706 ■ Contra Costa Crisis Center
PO Box 3364
Walnut Creek, CA 94598
Ph: (925)939-1916
Fax: (925)939-1933
E-mail: admin@crisis-center.org
URL: http://www.crisis-center.org

West Hollywood

50707 ■ Trevor Project
8704 Santa Monica Blvd., Ste. 200
West Hollywood, CA 90069
Ph: (310)271-8845
Fax: (310)271-8846
URL: http://www.thetrevorproject.org

Yuba City

50708 ■ Sutter-Yuba Mental Health Crisis Clinic
1965 Live Oak Blvd.
Yuba City, CA 95991
Ph: (530)822-7200
Fax: (530)822-7508
URL: http://sutter.networkofcare.org/mh/home/index. cfm

COLORADO

Arvada

50709 ■ Jefferson Center for Mental Health
5265 Vance St.
Arvada, CO 80002
Ph: (303)425-0300
URL: http://www.jeffersonmentalhealth.org

Aurora

50710 ■ Comitis Crisis Center
9840 E 17th Ave.
Aurora, CO 80010
Ph: (303)343-9890
URL: http://www.comitis.org/

Boulder

50711 ■ Broomfield Mental Health Center
Emergency Psychiatric Service
12 Garden Centre Suite
Boulder, CO 80301
Ph: (303)447-1665

50712 ■ Mental Health Center of Boulder, Inc.
Emergency Psychiatric Services
1100 Balsam Ave.
Boulder, CO 80304
Ph: (303)447-1665
URL: http://www.mhcbc.org

50713 ■ Mental Health Center of Broomfield County
12 Garden Centre, Ste. 210
Boulder, CO 80020
Ph: (303)447-1665

Colorado Springs

50714 ■ Suicide Prevention Partnership
704 N Tejon St.
Colorado Springs, CO 80903
Ph: (719)573-7447
E-mail: prevent@codenet.com
URL: http://sppppr.org

Denver

50715 ■ American Red Cross - Mile High Chapter
444 Sherman St.
Denver, CO 80203
Ph: (303)722-7474
Fax: (303)722-7588
E-mail: questions@denver-redcross.org
URL: http://www.redcross.org/co/denver/about-us/ leadership/mile-high-leadership
Gino Greco, Chief Executive Officer

50716 ■ Suicide and Crisis Control--Denver
2459 S Ash
Denver, CO 80222
Ph: (303)756-8485

Fort Collins

50717 ■ Suicide Resource Center of Larimer County
619 S College Ave. No. 12
Fort Collins, CO 80524
Ph: (970)482-2209
URL: http://www.suicideresourcecenter.org/

Grand Junction

50718 ■ Colorado West Mental Health Center
740 Gunnison Ave.
Grand Junction, CO 81501
Ph: (970)241-6022
Fax: (970)255-1266
URL: http://www.cwrmhc.org

Greeley

50719 ■ **Suicide Education and Support Services of Weld County**
1260 H St.
Greeley, CO 80631
Ph: (970)313-1089
E-mail: Kristen.jernigan@northrange.org
URL: http://www.endsuicide.org

Pueblo

50720 ■ **Pueblo Suicide Prevention Center, Inc.**
1925 E Orman, Ste. G-25
Pueblo, CO 81004
Ph: (719)564-6642
Fax: (719)564-7975

Steamboat Springs

50721 ■ **Colorado West Regional Mental Health**
407 S Lincoln Ave.
Steamboat Springs, CO 80477
Ph: (970)879-2141
Fax: (970)879-7912
URL: http://www.cwrmhc.org/sboat.htm

50722 ■ **Steamboat Mental Health Center**
2025 Shield Dr.
Steamboat Springs, CO 80477
Ph: (970)879-1090

Westminster

50723 ■ **Light for Life Foundation of America**
PO Box 644
Westminster, CO 80030
Ph: (303)429-3530
URL: http://www.yellowribbon.org/

CONNECTICUT

Bristol

50724 ■ **Wheeler Clinic Helpline**
632 King St.
Bristol, CT 06010
Ph: (860)747-3434
URL: http://www.wheelerclinic.org

Derby

50725 ■ **Griffin Hospital Psychiatric Crisis Team**
130 Division St.
Derby, CT 06418
Ph: (203)735-7421
Fax: (203)732-1551
URL: http://www.griffinhealth.org

Enfield

50726 ■ **North Central Counseling Services**
153 Hazard Ave.
Enfield, CT 06082
Ph: (860)253-5020
Fax: (860)253-5030
URL: http://www.chrhealth.org/

Greenwich

50727 ■ **Hotline/Family Centers**
20 Bridge St.
Greenwich, CT 06830
Ph: (203)661-4378

Hartford

50728 ■ **The Samaritans of The Capital Region**
PO Box 12004
Hartford, CT 06112
Ph: (860)232-9559
Fax: (860)673-1614
URL: http://ctsamaritans.org/

Meriden

50729 ■ **Midstate Behavioral Health System Crisis Stablization Program**
883 Paddock Ave.
Meriden, CT 06450
Ph: (203)630-5305
Fax: (203)630-5335

Middletown

50730 ■ **Middlesex Hospital Crisis Assessment and Triage Service**
28 Crescent St.
Middletown, CT 06457
Ph: (860)344-6765
Fax: (860)358-8858
URL: http://www.midhosp.org/go/85A7B9D9-97C0-80AF-9DE0119CCA323A7E/

50731 ■ **River Valley Services Mobile Crisis Team**
Silver St.
Middletown, CT 06457
Ph: (860)344-2100

Milford

50732 ■ **Bridges--A Community Support System**
949 Bridgeport Ave.
Milford, CT 06460
Ph: (203)878-6365
URL: http://www.bridgesmilford.org/

New Haven

50733 ■ **Clifford W. Beers Guidance Clinic CAMPES**
93 Edwards St.
New Haven, CT 06511
Ph: (203)772-1270
Fax: (203)772-0051
URL: http://www.cliffordbeers.org/

50734 ■ **Connecticut Mental Health Center Acute Care Services**
34 Park St.
New Haven, CT 06519
Ph: (203)974-7713
Fax: (203)974-7234
URL: http://www.ct.gov/dmhas/site/default.asp

Plainville

50735 ■ **Wheeler Clinic Emergency Services**
91 Northwest Dr.
Plainville, CT 06062
Ph: (888)793-3500
E-mail: jmingel@wheelerclinic.org
URL: http://www.wheelerclinic.org

Rocky Hill

50736 ■ **United Way of Connecticut /INFOLINE**
1344 Silas Deane Hwy.
Rocky Hill, CT 06067
Ph: (860)571-7557
URL: http://www.infoline.org/

Trumbull

50737 ■ **Trumbull Counseling Center**
4632 Madison Ave.
Trumbull, CT 06611
Ph: (203)452-5082
URL: http://www.trumbullct.com/counselingcenter-info.htm

Waterbury

50738 ■ **Waterbury Hospital Psychiatric Center**
64 Robbins St.
Waterbury, CT 06708

Ph: (203)573-6500
Fax: (203)573-7007
URL: http://www.waterburyhospital.org

West Mystic

50739 ■ **Contact of Southeast Connecticut**
PO Box 249
West Mystic, CT 06388
Ph: (860)572-8143

DELAWARE

Dover

50740 ■ **Delaware Health and Social Services Division of Substance Abuse and Mental Health Crisis Intervention Service**
805 River Rd.
Dover, DE 19901
Ph: (302)739-4275
URL: http://dhss.delaware.gov/dhss/dsamh/crisis_intervention.html

Georgetown

50741 ■ **Delaware Health and Social Services--Georgetown Division of Substance Abuse and Mental Health Crisis Intervention Service**
546 S Bedford St.
Georgetown, DE 19947
Ph: (302)856-5490
URL: http://dhss.delaware.gov/dhss/dsamh/crisis_intervention.html

Milford

50742 ■ **Kent/Sussex Mobile Crisis Unit**
PO Box 912
Milford, DE 19963
Ph: (302)422-1395
Fax: (302)422-1320

New Castle

50743 ■ **Delaware Health and Social Services--New Castle Division of Substance Abuse and Mental Health Crisis Intervention Service**
14 Central Ave.
New Castle, DE 19720
Ph: (302)577-2484
Free: 800-652-2929
URL: http://dhss.delaware.gov/dhss/dsamh/crisis_intervention.html

Wilmington

50744 ■ **CONTACT Delaware, Inc.**
PO Box 9525
Wilmington, DE 19809
Ph: (302)761-9800
Fax: (302)761-4280
E-mail: sadeghee@contactdelaware.org
URL: http://www.contactlifeline.org

50745 ■ **Mobile Crisis Intervention Service New Castle CMHC**
801 West St., 2nd Fl.
Wilmington, DE 19801
Ph: (302)577-2484
Fax: (302)577-6498

50746 ■ **Tressler Brandywine Program Center of Delaware**
240 N James St., Ste. 200
Wilmington, DE 19804
Ph: (302)995-2002
Fax: (302)995-2121

DISTRICT OF COLUMBIA

Washington

50747 ■ Comprehensive Psychiatric Emergency Program
Commission on Mental Health Services
Crisis Helpline
1905 E St. SE
Washington, DC 20003
Ph: (202)673-9307

50748 ■ Suicide Prevention Action Network (SPAN USA)
1010 Vermont Ave. NW, Ste. 408
Washington, DC 20005
Ph: (202)449-3600
Free: 800-273-8255
Fax: (202)449-3601
E-mail: info@spanusa.org
URL: http://www.capwiz.com/spanusa/home/
Michael Ballard, Director
Description: Works to increase awareness of the toll of suicide in the nation. Advances public policies that help prevent suicide. Develops political will to ensure that government effectively addresses the problem of suicide.

FLORIDA

Bartow

50749 ■ Peace River Center Crisis Line
PO Box 1559
Bartow, FL 33831
Ph: (863)519-0575
Free: 800-627-5906
URL: http://www.peace-river.com/locations.html

Bonifay

50750 ■ Life Management Center of Northwest Florida Inc.--Bonifay
801 S Weeks St.
Bonifay, FL 32425
Ph: (850)638-6185
URL: http://www.lifemanagementcenter.org

Bradenton

50751 ■ Family Resources, Inc.--Bradenton
361 6th Ave. W
Bradenton, FL 34205
Ph: (941)741-3575
Fax: (941)741-3578
URL: http://www.family-resources.org/

50752 ■ Manatee Glens Corp. HELPline
2020 26th Ave. E
Bradenton, FL 34208
Ph: (941)741-3805
URL: http://www.manateeglens.com

Cocoa

50753 ■ 2-1-1 Brevard
PO Box 417
Cocoa, FL 32923
Ph: (321)631-9290
Fax: (321)631-9291
E-mail: ldonoghue@211brevard.org
URL: http://www.211brevard.org
Libby Donoghue, Executive Director

Daytona Beach

50754 ■ ACT Corporation
1220 Willis Ave.
Daytona Beach, FL 32114-2897
Ph: (386)947-3200
Free: 800-539-4228
Fax: (386)947-4238
URL: http://www.actcorp.org/

DeFuniak Springs

50755 ■ COPE Center Beachside Counseling
3686 US Hwy. 331 S
DeFuniak Springs, FL 32435
Ph: (850)892-8035
URL: http://www.copecenter.org/
Formerly: Cope Center.

Fort Lauderdale

50756 ■ First Call for Help/Broward County
16 SE 13th St.
Fort Lauderdale, FL 33301
Ph: (954)524-8371
Fax: (954)524-0852
URL: http://www.211-broward.org/

Fort Myers

50757 ■ Lee Mental Health Center
Crisis Stabilization Unit
10140 Deer Run Farms Rd.
Fort Myers, FL 33966
Ph: (239)275-3222
URL: http://www.rccbhc.org/vistors.html

50758 ■ Ruth Cooper Center
2789 Ortiz Ave SE
Fort Myers, FL 33905
Ph: (941)275-3222
URL: http://www.rccbhc.org/vistors.html

Fort Pierce

50759 ■ New Horizons of the Treasure Coast, Inc.
4500 W Midway Rd.
Fort Pierce, FL 34951
Ph: (561)468-5600
E-mail: nhtcadm@aol.com
URL: http://www.nhtcinc.org

Fort Walton Beach

50760 ■ Crisis Line/Bridgeway Center, Inc.
137 Hospital Dr.
Fort Walton Beach, FL 32548
Ph: (850)833-9204
Fax: (850)833-7439
E-mail: shobbs@bridgeway.org
URL: http://www.bridgewaycenter.org

Gainesville

50761 ■ Alachua County Crisis Center
218 SE 24th St.
Gainesville, FL 32641
Ph: (352)264-6789
Fax: (352)264-6777
URL: http://www.alachuacounty.us/government/depts/css/crisis/

50762 ■ Meridian Behavioral Healthcare
4300 SW 13th St.
Gainesville, FL 32608
Ph: (352)374-5600
URL: http://www.mbhci.org

50763 ■ Suicide and Crisis Intervention Service
730 NE Waldo Rd.
Gainesville, FL 32641
Ph: (352)372-3659
URL: http://www.themereproject.org

Hialeah

50764 ■ Northwest Dade Community Mental Health Center
Children/Adolescent Crisis Service
4175 W 20th Ave.
Hialeah, FL 33012
Ph: (305)558-0151

Jacksonville

50765 ■ First Call For Help/United Way
PO Box 41428
Jacksonville, FL 32203-1428
Fax: (904)390-3278
URL: http://www.nefl211.org

50766 ■ Florida Suicide Prevention Coalition
PO Box 16841
Jacksonville, FL 32246
Ph: (907)742-6403
E-mail: rczipperer@aol.com
URL: http://www.floridasuicideprevention.org/region_4.htm

Key West

50767 ■ Helpline, Inc.
PO Box 2186
Key West, FL 33045-2186
Ph: (305)292-8445
Fax: (305)292-8447
URL: http://www.keyshelpline.org/

Lantana

50768 ■ Center for Information and Crisis Services
Crisis Line
PO Box 3588
Lantana, FL 33465
Ph: (561)547-8637
Fax: (561)547-8639
URL: http://www.211palmbeach.org/

Largo

50769 ■ 2-1-1 Tampa Bay Cares
Largo, FL
Ph: (727)210-4233
URL: http://www.211tampabay.org

50770 ■ Tampa Cares 211
PO Box 5164
Largo, FL 33779
Ph: (727)562-1543
URL: http://www.211tampabay.org/
Formerly: Pinellas Cares, Inc. 211.

Lecanto

50771 ■ Marion-Citrus Mental Health Center--Lecanto Campus
3238 S Lecanto Hwy.
Lecanto, FL 34461
Ph: (325)726-7155
URL: http://www.marion-citrusmhc.org/

Maitland

50772 ■ Central Florida Helpline
PO Box 941524
Maitland, FL 32794-1524
Ph: (407)333-9028
URL: http://www.centralfloridahelpline.org

Marianna

50773 ■ Life Management Center of Northwest Florida Inc.--Marianna
4094 Lafayette St.
Marianna, FL 32446
Ph: (850)482-7441
URL: http://www.lifemanagementcenter.org/

Miami

50774 ■ Institute for Child & Family Health
Sunset Clinic
9380 Sunset Dr., Ste. B120
Miami, FL 33173
Ph: (305)274-3172
URL: http://www.icfhinc.org/
Formerly: Children's Psychiatric Center.

50775 ■ Switchboard of Miami, Inc.
444 Brickell Ave., Ste. 450
Miami, FL 33131
Ph: (305)358-1640
Fax: (305)377-2269
E-mail: info@switchboardmiami.org
URL: http://www.switchboardmiami.org

Middleburg

**50776 ■ Clay County Behavioral Health
Center**
3292 County Rd. 220
Middleburg, FL 32068
Ph: (904)284-2887
URL: http://www.ccbhc.org/

Naples

**50777 ■ Hotline and Referral/Project Help,
Inc.**
PO Box 7804
Naples, FL 34101
Ph: (239)649-1404
E-mail: michelle@projecthelpnaples.org
URL: http://www.projecthelpnaples.org/

Pensacola

**50778 ■ Baptist Hospital
Adolescent Stress Treatment Program**
1000 W Moreno St.
Pensacola, FL 32501
Ph: (850)434-4866
Fax: (850)469-7514
URL: http://www.ebaptisthealthcare.org/Homepage/

50779 ■ First Call for Help--Pensacola
1301 W Government
Pensacola, FL 32502
Ph: (850)595-5905
URL: http://www.fcfh.info/

**50780 ■ Lakeview Center, Inc.
Pensacola Help Line**
1221 W Lakeview St.
Pensacola, FL 32501
Ph: (850)432-1222
URL: http://www.ebaptisthealthcare.org/Lakeview-Center/

Pinellas Park

**50781 ■ Family Resources, Inc.--Pinellas
Park**
5180 62nd Ave. N
Pinellas Park, FL 33781
Ph: (727)521-5200
Fax: (727)521-2510
URL: http://www.family-resources.org/

**50782 ■ Personal Enrichment through Mental
Health Services, Inc.**
11254 58th St. N
Pinellas Park, FL 33782
Ph: (727)545-6477
Fax: (727)545-6467
URL: http://www.pemhs.org

Port Richey

50783 ■ First Call for Help--Port Richey
10934 US Hwy. 19
Port Richey, FL 34668
Ph: (727)863-3255
URL: http://www.themereproject.org

Rockledge

50784 ■ Circles of Care
1770 Cedar St.
Rockledge, FL 32955
Ph: (321)634-6264
URL: http://www.circlesofcare.org

50785 ■ Helpline Brevard 211
PO Box 561108
Rockledge, FL 32956
Ph: (321)632-6688
URL: http://www.211brevard.org/

Saint Petersburg

50786 ■ Helpline/Family Resources, Inc.
PO Box 13087
Saint Petersburg, FL 33733
Ph: (813)893-1141
URL: http://www.family-resources.org/

**50787 ■ Pinellas Emergency Mental Health
Services**
11254 58th St., N
Saint Petersburg, FL 33701
Ph: (727)541-4628
URL: http://www.themereproject.org

Tallahassee

50788 ■ 2-1-1 Big Bend
PO Box 10950
Tallahassee, FL 32302
Ph: (850)617-6348
Fax: (850)561-3443
URL: http://www.211bigbend.net
Randy Nicklaus, President

Tampa

50789 ■ Crisis Center of Tampa Bay
1 Crisis Center Plz.
Tampa, FL 33613
Ph: (813)964-1964
Fax: (813)964-1564
URL: http://www.crisiscenter.com/

50790 ■ Hillsborough County Crisis Center
2214 E Henry Ave.
Tampa, FL 33610
Ph: (813)238-8411
URL: http://www.crisiscenter.com/

50791 ■ Mental Health Care
5707 N 22nd St.
Tampa, FL 33610
Ph: (813)272-2244
URL: http://www.mhcinc.org

**50792 ■ Tampa Help Line/Christian Helpline
Network**
PO Box 9565
Tampa, FL 33674-9565
Ph: (813)251-4040

Vero Beach

**50793 ■ Mental Health Association
Indian Res./Saint Lucie Crisis Line**
2101 14th Ave.
Vero Beach, FL 32960
Ph: (561)569-9788
Fax: (561)569-2088

GEORGIA

Atlanta

50794 ■ Emergency Mental Health Services
141 Pryor St. SW, Ste. 4035
Atlanta, GA 30303
Ph: (404)730-1600

Augusta

50795 ■ Integrated Health Resources
961 Broad St.
Augusta, GA 30901
Ph: (706)722-1708
Fax: (706)722-6963
E-mail: bhlwebl@ihrcorp.com
URL: http://www.integratedhealthresources.com/

**50796 ■ Serenity Behavioral Health Systems
Crisis Line**
3421 Mike Padgett Hwy.
Augusta, GA 30906
Ph: (877)554-4897
URL: http://www.cmhc.us/
Formerly: Community Mental Health Center.

Austell

**50797 ■ Cobb and Douglas Counties
Community Services Board--Austell**
6133 Love St.
Austell, GA 30168
Ph: (770)819-9229
URL: http://www.cadissoftware.com/

Blairsville

50798 ■ Union County Mental Health Clinic
41 Hospital St., Ste. 134
Blairsville, GA 30512
Ph: (706)745-5911
E-mail: Stephen.Sorrells@avitapartners.org
URL: http://www.gamtns.org/about/locations.php

Cleveland

50799 ■ White County Mental Health Center
1241 Helen Hwy., Ste. 180
Cleveland, GA 30528
Ph: (706)865-7886

Columbus

50800 ■ CONTACT Chattahoochee Valley
PO Box 12002
Columbus, GA 31907
Ph: (706)327-0199
E-mail: helpline@contact211.org
URL: http://www.contact211.org

Conley

**50801 ■ Clayton Center--Behavioral Health
Services**
1800 Slate Rd.
Conley, GA 30288
Ph: (404)366-1529
Fax: (404)366-9698
URL: http://www.claytoncenter.org/contact_us.htm

Decatur

**50802 ■ Winn Way Mental Health
Center--Central Access**
445 Winn Way
Decatur, GA 30030
Ph: (404)892-4646
URL: http://www.dekcsb.org/

Demorest

**50803 ■ Habersham County Mental Health
Center**
Scoggins Dr.
Demorest, GA 30535
Ph: (706)778-4474
URL: http://www.themereproject.org

Gainesville

50804 ■ CONTACT Helpline Hall County
PO Box 1616
Gainesville, GA 30503
Ph: (770)536-7145
URL: http://www.hallcounty.org/living/links.asp

Homer

50805 ■ Banks County Mental Health
667 Thompson St.
Homer, GA 30547
Ph: (706)677-5261
URL: http://www.co.banks.ga.us/

Jonesboro

50806 ■ Clayton Center--Community Support Services
217 Stockbridge Rd.
Jonesboro, GA 30236
Ph: (770)471-4617
Fax: (770)471-7817
URL: http://www.claytoncenter.org/contact_us.htm

50807 ■ Clayton Mental Health Center
112 Broad St.
Jonesboro, GA 30236
Ph: (770)478-2280
Fax: (770)478-8722
URL: http://www.claytoncenter.org

Marietta

50808 ■ Cobb and Douglass Counties Community Service Board--Crisis Line--Marietta
Intake Information and Referral
361 N Marietta Pkwy, Ste. 200
Marietta, GA 30060
Ph: (770)422-0202
URL: http://www.cobbcsb.com/

Riverdale

50809 ■ Clayton Center--Flint River Center
6315 Garden Walk Blvd.
Riverdale, GA 30274
Ph: (770)991-7420
Fax: (770)991-7429
URL: http://www.claytoncenter.org/contact_us.htm

Statesboro

50810 ■ Pineland Mental Health
PO Box 745
Statesboro, GA 30459
Ph: (912)764-6906
Free: 800-746-3526
E-mail: info@pinelandcsb.org
URL: http://www.pinelandcsb.org/

Toccoa

50811 ■ Georgia Mountains Community Services
Stephens County Mental Health Clinic
1020 E Tugalo St.
Toccoa, GA 30577
Ph: (706)282-4542

Warner Robins

50812 ■ Helpline Georgia
2762 Watson Blvd.
Warner Robins, GA 31093
Ph: (478)953-5675
Fax: (478)953-5674
URL: http://www.hodac.org/index.php/about-hodac/contact-hodac.html

HAWAII

Hilo

50813 ■ American Red Cross--Hilo
55 Ululani St.
Hilo, HI 96720
Ph: (808)326-7528
Fax: (808)969-3673
URL: http://www.redcross.org

Honolulu

50814 ■ Helping Hands Hawaii Bilingual Access Line
680 Iwilei Rd., Ste. 430
Honolulu, HI 96817
Ph: (808)526-9724
URL: http://www.helpinghandshawaii.org/

50815 ■ Suicide and Crisis Center--Honolulu
Honolulu, HI 96813

Lihue

50816 ■ American Red Cross--Lihue
4365 Hardy St., Ste. A
Lihue, HI 96766
Ph: (808)245-4919
URL: http://www.redcross.org

Wailuku

50817 ■ American Red Cross--Wailuku
1063 Lower Main St., Apt. 207
Wailuku, HI 96793
Ph: (808)244-0051
URL: http://www.redcross.org

IDAHO

Boise

50818 ■ Idaho Suicide Prevention Hotline Service
1810 W State St., Ste. 122
Boise, ID 83702
Ph: (208)385-3532

50819 ■ Region IV Mental Health Center
Boise Emergency Line
1720 Westgate Dr.
Boise, ID 83704
Ph: (208)334-0894
Fax: (208)334-0788

Bonners Ferry

50820 ■ Boundary County Youth Crisis and Domestic Violence Hotline
PO Box 633
Bonners Ferry, ID 83805
Ph: (208)267-3355
Fax: (208)267-3355
URL: http://www2.state.id.us/crimevictim/olddirectoryinfo/pr/Boundary/index.html

Coeur D'Alene

50821 ■ Region I Mental Health Emergency Service
W. George Moody Health Center
2195 Ironwood Ct.
Coeur D'Alene, ID 83814
Ph: (208)769-1406
Fax: (208)769-1430

Idaho Falls

50822 ■ Region VII Mental Health Center
150 Shoup St., Ste. 19
Idaho Falls, ID 83402
Ph: (208)528-5700

Kellogg

50823 ■ Region I Mental Health - Kellogg/Wallace
35 Wildcat Way, Ste. B
Kellogg, ID 83837
Ph: (208)784-1351

Lewiston

50824 ■ YWCA Crisis Service--Lewiston
300 Main St.
Lewiston, ID 83501
Ph: (208)746-9655
Fax: (208)746-1510
E-mail: ywcacscharleyfleet@lewiston.com
URL: http://www.ywcaidaho.org/EmergServices.htm

Mountain Home

50825 ■ Regional Mental Health Services
24-Hour Crisis Line
Mountain Home, ID

Twin Falls

50826 ■ Region V Mental Health Center
Twin Falls Emergency Service
823 Harrison
Twin Falls, ID 83301
Ph: (208)736-2177
Fax: (208)736-2113

ILLINOIS

Anna

50827 ■ Union County Counseling Service
204 South St.
Anna, IL 62906
Ph: (618)833-8551

Aurora

50828 ■ Association for Indian Development
Crisis Line of the Fox Valley
309 W New Indian Trl. Ct.
Aurora, IL 60506
Ph: (630)966-4000
URL: http://the-association.org

Bartonville

50829 ■ Mental Health Association of Illinois Valley--Bartonville
5032 W Burns Ave.
Bartonville, IL 61607
Ph: (309)692-1766
URL: http://www.mhai.org

Batavia

50830 ■ Suicide Prevention Services, Inc.--Batavia
Crisis Line of the Fox Valley
528 S Batavia Ave.
Batavia, IL 60510
Ph: (630)482-9696
E-mail: spsinfo@spsfv.org
URL: http://www.spsfv.org

Bloomington

50831 ■ McLean County Center for Human Services
Emergency Crisis Intervention Team
108 W Market St.
Bloomington, IL 61701
Ph: (309)827-5351

50832 ■ Providing Access to Help
201 E Grove
Bloomington, IL 61701
Ph: (309)828-1022
URL: http://pathcrisis.org/

Cairo

50833 ■ Cairo Crisis Line
Mental Health Center
1001 Washington Ave.
Cairo, IL 62914
Ph: (618)734-2665

Carbondale

50834 ■ Southern Illinois Regional Social Services
604 E College, Ste. 101
Carbondale, IL 62901
Ph: (618)457-6703
URL: http://www.sirss.org/

Chicago

50835 ■ Community Counseling Centers of Chicago
4740 N Clark St.
Chicago, IL 60640
Ph: (773)769-0205
URL: http://www.c4chicago.org

50836 ■ **University of Illinois at Chicago Counseling Center**
In-Touch Hotline
1200 W Harrison St.
MC 333
Chicago, IL 60607
Ph: (312)996-3490
Fax: (312)996-7645
URL: http://www.uic.edu/depts/counselctr/counseling/intouch.htm

Clinton

50837 ■ **DeWitt County Human Resource Center**
PO Box 616
Clinton, IL 61727
Ph: (217)935-9496

DeKalb

50838 ■ **Ben Gordon Center**
12 Health Services Dr.
DeKalb, IL 60115
Ph: (815)756-4875
Free: 866--BGC0111
URL: http://www.bengordoncenter.org/

Decatur

50839 ■ **Heritage Behavioral Health Center Inc.**
151 N Main St.
Decatur, IL 62523
Ph: (217)362-6262
URL: http://www.heritagenet.org/

East Moline

50840 ■ **Robert Young Center for Community Health**
465 Ave. of the Cities
East Moline, IL 61244
Ph: (309)779-2999
URL: http://www.trinityqc.com/body.cfm?id=92

East Saint Louis

50841 ■ **Call for Help**
Suicide and Crisis Intervention
9400 Lebanon Rd.
East Saint Louis, IL 62203
Ph: (618)397-0975
URL: http://www.callforhelpinc.org/

Elgin

50842 ■ **Community Crisis Center**
PO Box 1390
Elgin, IL 60121
Ph: (847)697-2381
Fax: (847)742-4182
URL: http://www.crisiscenter.org/

50843 ■ **Ecker Center for Mental Health**
1845 Grandstand Pl.
Elgin, IL 60123
Ph: (847)695-0484
Fax: (847)695-1265
URL: http://www.eckercenter.org

Elk Grove

50844 ■ **Talkline Help Lines Inc.**
PO Box 1321
Elk Grove, IL 60009
Ph: (708)981-1271

Evanston

50845 ■ **Evanston Hospital Crisis Intervention**
2650 Ridge Ave.
Evanston, IL 60201
Ph: (847)570-2500
URL: http://www.enh.org/

Freeport

50846 ■ **Contact Stephenson County**
PO Box 83
Freeport, IL 61032
Ph: (815)233-4402

Galesburg

50847 ■ **Bridgeway, Inc.--Galesburg**
2323 Windish Dr.
Galesburg, IL 61401
Ph: (309)344-2323
Free: 800-344-2331
Fax: (309)344-4281
URL: http://www.bway.org

Granite

50848 ■ **Community Counseling Services/Chestnut Health Systems**
50 Northgate Industrial Dr.
Granite, IL 62040
Ph: (618)656-8721
URL: http://www.chestnut.org/

Hillsboro

50849 ■ **Montgomery County Health Department**
Division of Mental Health Helpline
Rte. 185
Hillsboro, IL 62049
Ph: (217)532-2001
Fax: (217)532-2089
URL: http://www.montgomeryco.com/health/

Hoffman Estates

50850 ■ **Institute for Stress Management and Psychotherapy**
2500 W Higgins Rd., Ste. 1080
Hoffman Estates, IL 60195
Ph: (708)519-0890

Joliet

50851 ■ **Crisis Line of Will County**
PO Box 2354
Joliet, IL 60434
Ph: (815)744-5280
Fax: (815)744-7782

50852 ■ **Will County Mental Health Center**
Intervention Program
1550 Plainfield Rd.
Joliet, IL 60431
Ph: (630)759-4555
URL: http://www.willcountyhealth.org

Kewanee

50853 ■ **Bridgeway--Kewanee**
137 E College
Kewanee, IL 61443
Ph: (309)852-4331
Free: 800-728-0985
URL: http://www.bway.org/content/view/57/49/

Libertyville

50854 ■ **Connection Telephone**
Crisis Intervention and Referral
PO Box 906
Libertyville, IL 60048
Ph: (847)362-3381
URL: http://www.communityresources.net/telephonecrisis.html

Lincoln

50855 ■ **Logan-Mason Mental Health Center**
Lincoln Crisis Clinic
304 8th St.
Lincoln, IL 62656

Ph: (217)732-2161
Fax: (217)732-9847

Lombard

50856 ■ **Du Page County Health Department**
Mental Health Division
Access and Crisis Center
440 S Finley Rd.
Lombard, IL 60148
Ph: (630)627-1700
URL: http://www.dupagehealth.org/services/access_crisis.html

Macomb

50857 ■ **Bridgeway--Macomb**
900 S Deer Rd.
Macomb, IL 61455
Ph: (309)837-4876
Free: 800-475-4226
URL: http://www.bway.org/content/view/57/49/

Mattoon

50858 ■ **Coles County Mental Health Center**
1300 Charleston Ave.
Mattoon, IL 61938
Ph: (217)234-6405
Fax: (217)234-6786
E-mail: lweiss@ccmhc.org

Moline

50859 ■ **Robert Young Center**
4600 3rd St.
Moline, IL 61265
Ph: (309)779-2031
URL: http://www.trinityqc.com/body.cfm?id=92

Mount Vernon

50860 ■ **Comprehensive Services, Inc.**
Mount Vernon Crisis Line
Rte. 37 N
Mount Vernon, IL 62864
Ph: (618)242-1510
Fax: (618)242-6392
URL: http://jccsinc.info/Services.asp

Normal

50861 ■ **Illinois State University--Student Counseling Services**
Campus Box 2420
Normal, IL 61790
Ph: (309)438-3655
E-mail: counseling@illinoisstate.edu
URL: http://www.counseling.ilstu.edu/about/

North Pekin

50862 ■ **Bridgeway--North Pekin**
2077 Edgewater Dr.
North Pekin, IL 61554
Ph: (309)382-2006
URL: http://www.bway.org/content/view/57/49/

Orland Park

50863 ■ **Meyer Medical Group**
Mental Health Services
10000 W 151st St.
Orland Park, IL 60462
Ph: (708)349-6200

Paris

50864 ■ **Human Resources Center**
PO Box 1118
Paris, IL 61944
Ph: (217)465-4118
URL: http://www.hrcec.org

Paxton

50865 ■ Community Resource and Counseling Center
1510 W Ottawa St.
Paxton, IL 60957
Ph: (217)359-4141
URL: http://www.themereproject.org

Pekin

50866 ■ Tazwood Mental Health Center--Pekin
3248 Vandever Ave.
Pekin, IL 61554
Ph: (309)347-5522
Free: 877-579-5112
URL: http://www.tazwoodmentalhealth.org/

Peoria

50867 ■ Mental Health Association of Illinois Valley--Peoria
5407 N University
Peoria, IL 61614
Ph: (309)692-1766
Fax: (309)692-2966
E-mail: mhaiv@mhaiv.org
URL: http://www.mhaiv.org

50868 ■ Suicide Prevention - Crisis Intervention Service
1015 W McBean St.
Peoria, IL 61605
Ph: (309)673-7373
URL: http://www.themereproject.org

50869 ■ Tazwood Mental Health Center--Peoria
100 N Main E, Lower Level
Peoria, IL 61614
Ph: (309)694-6462
URL: http://www.tazwoodmentalhealth.org/locations.html

50870 ■ Teens Need Teens Hotline
5407 N University St.
Peoria, IL 61614
Ph: (309)637-8336
URL: http://www.mhaiv.org/

Princeton

50871 ■ Options EAP
1000 E Backbone Rd.
Princeton, IL 61356
Ph: (815)879-0327

Quincy

50872 ■ Transitions of Western Illinois Suicide Prevention and Crisis Service
4409 Maine
Quincy, IL 62305
Ph: (217)223-0413
Fax: (217)223-0461
URL: http://www.twi.org

Rockford

50873 ■ Contact of Rockford
PO Box 1976
Rockford, IL 61110
Ph: (815)636-5001
Fax: (815)636-5009

Springfield

50874 ■ Memorial Behavioral Health Group
710 N 8th St.
Springfield, IL 62702
Ph: (217)525-1064
URL: http://memorialmedical.com/AboutUs/

50875 ■ Mental Health Centers of Central Illinois
1 Center Dr.
Springfield, IL 62701
Ph: (217)525-1064
URL: http://www.themereproject.org

50876 ■ Mental Health Centers of Illinois Crisis Hotline
200 W Lake Shore Dr.
Springfield, IL 62703
Ph: (217)525-1064
URL: http://www.mhcci.org/

Sullivan

50877 ■ Moultree County Counseling Center Sullivan Crisis Line
2 W Adams
Sullivan, IL 61951
Ph: (217)728-4358
Fax: (217)728-2270

Taylorville

50878 ■ Christian County Mental Health Center Taylorville Helpline
730 N Pawnee
Taylorville, IL 62568
Ph: (217)824-4905
Fax: (217)824-3070
URL: http://www.ccmha.net/program_crisis.html

Watseka

50879 ■ Iroquois Mental Health Center
908 E Cherry St.
Watseka, IL 60970
Ph: (815)432-5241
URL: http://www.themereproject.org

Winfield

50880 ■ Central Dupage Hospital--Crisis Stabilization Program
25 N Winfield Rd.
Winfield, IL 60190
Ph: (630)933-4000
URL: http://www.cdh.org/medical-services/services-A-Z/behavioral-health/crisis-stabiliz ation.aspx

Wood River

50881 ■ Behavioral Health Alternative, Inc. of Madison County
337 E Ferguson
Wood River, IL 62095
Ph: (618)251-4073
URL: http://www.bha-inc.org/

Woodstock

50882 ■ McHenry County Crisis Program
PO Box 1990
Woodstock, IL 60098
Free: 800-892-8900
URL: http://www.mchenry-crisis.org/

INDIANA

Anderson

50883 ■ Contact/Help
PO Box 303
Anderson, IN 46015
Ph: (765)649-4939
URL: http://www.centralindiana.com/netdirect/contact.htm

Avon

50884 ■ Cummins Mental Health Center Inc.
Central Switchboard
6655 E US Hwy. 36
Avon, IN 46123

Ph: (317)272-3330
URL: http://www.cumminsmhc.com

Batesville

50885 ■ Community Mental Health Center, Inc.
215 E George St.
Batesville, IN 47006
Ph: (812)537-1302
URL: http://www.themereproject.org

Evansville

50886 ■ Southwestern Indiana Mental Health Center, Inc.
415 Mulberry St.
Evansville, IN 47713-1298
Ph: (812)423-7791
URL: http://www.southwestern.org

Fort Wayne

50887 ■ Switchboard, Inc.
227 E Washington Blvd., Ste. 101
Fort Wayne, IN 46802
Ph: (260)424-3551

Gary

50888 ■ Crisis Center-Rap Line
101 N Montgomery
Gary, IN 46403
Ph: (219)938-7070
Fax: (219)938-7502
URL: http://www.crisiscenterysb.org/staff.htm

Greencastle

50889 ■ Cummins Mental Health Center, Inc.
308 Medic Way
Greencastle, IN 46135
Ph: (765)420-0938
URL: http://www.vectren.com

Greenwood

50890 ■ Valle Vista Hospital Access Center
898 E Main St.
Greenwood, IN 46143
Ph: (317)887-1348
URL: http://www.psysolutions.com/facilities/valle-vista/

Indianapolis

50891 ■ Community Hospital North--Psychiatric Pavilion
7165 Clearvista Way
Indianapolis, IN 46256
Ph: (317)621-5100
URL: http://www.ecommunity.com/behavioralcare/index.aspx?pg=203

50892 ■ Indianapolis Community Hospital, Inc.
Access Services
7150 Clearvista Dr.
Indianapolis, IN 46256
Ph: (317)841-5100
URL: http://www.ecommunity.com/

50893 ■ Mental Health Association of Marion County
Crisis and Suicide Intervention Service
301 E 38th St.
Indianapolis, IN 46205
Ph: (317)251-0005
URL: http://www.mhaindy.net/

Lafayette

50894 ■ Lafayette Crisis Center
1244 N 15th St.
Lafayette, IN 47904-2114
Ph: (765)742-0247
Fax: (765)742-0247
URL: http://www.lafayettecrisiscenter.org/

Lawrenceburg

50895 ■ **Community Mental Health Center Lawrenceburg Crisis Line**
285 Bielby Rd.
Lawrenceburg, IN 47025
Ph: (812)537-1302
Fax: (812)537-0194
URL: http://www.cmhcinc.org

Lebanon

50896 ■ **Mental Health America of Boone County**
c/o Ms. Jane Taylor
1122 N Lebanon St., No. A
Lebanon, IN 46052-1759
Ph: (765)482-3020
Fax: (765)482-9001
E-mail: janetaylor@ilines.net
URL: http://www.mhai.net
Formerly: (2007) Mental Health Association in Boone County.

Merrillville

50897 ■ **Contact-Cares Inc. of Northwest Indiana**
PO Box 10247
Merrillville, IN 46411
Ph: (219)769-0611
Fax: (219)769-3286

Monticello

50898 ■ **Twin Lakes Contact-Help**
PO Box 67
Monticello, IN 47960
Ph: (219)583-4357

Terre Haute

50899 ■ **Vigo County Lifeline, Inc.**
PO Box 1017
Terre Haute, IN 47808
Ph: (812)238-2620
URL: http://www.wvlifeline.org/

IOWA

Ames

50900 ■ **Runaway-Youth and Shelter Services**
703 Burnett Ave.
Ames, IA 50010
Ph: (515)233-2330
Free: 800-600-2330
E-mail: gbelitsos@yss.ames.ia.us
URL: http://www.yss.ames.ia.us

Cedar Rapids

50901 ■ **Foundation II Crisis Center**
1540 2nd Ave. SE
Cedar Rapids, IA 52403
Ph: (319)362-1170
Fax: (319)398-7006
E-mail: f2crisis@aol.com
URL: http://www.F2online.org

Des Moines

50902 ■ **American Red Cross--Des Moines Community Telephone Service Crisis Line**
2116 Grand Ave.
Des Moines, IA 50312
Ph: (515)244-6700
Fax: (515)244-8012
URL: http://www.desmoines-redcross.org/

50903 ■ **First Call For Help--Des Moines**
1111 9th St., No. 300
Des Moines, IA 50314
Ph: (515)246-6555
URL: http://65.166.193.134/IFTWSQL4/iowa/public.aspx

Dubuque

50904 ■ **Phone-a-Friend Crisis Line**
3505 Stoneman Rd., Ste. 5
Dubuque, IA 52002
Ph: (319)557-8331

Iowa City

50905 ■ **Johnson County Crisis Center**
1121 Gilbert Ct.
Iowa City, IA 52240
Ph: (319)351-2726
Fax: (319)351-4671
URL: http://www.jccrisiscenter.org/
Formerly: Iowa City Crisis Center.

Keokuk

50906 ■ **Bridgeway--Keokuk**
208 Bank St.
Keokuk, IA 52632
Ph: (319)524-3873
URL: http://www.bway.org/content/view/57/49/

Mason City

50907 ■ **North Iowa Crisis Center**
1631 4th St. SW
Mason City, IA 50401
Ph: (641)494-1758

Sioux City

50908 ■ **AID--Assistance Information Direction Center**
715 Douglas St.
Sioux City, IA 51101
Ph: (712)252-1861

Waterloo

50909 ■ **Family Service League Crisis Services**
3830 W 9th St.
Waterloo, IA 50702
Ph: (319)233-8484

KANSAS

Andover

50910 ■ **South Central Mental Health Counseling Center--Andover**
217 W Ira Ct.
Andover, KS 67002
Ph: (316)733-5047
URL: http://www.scmhcc.org/

Anthony

50911 ■ **Horizons Mental Health Center**
125 N Jennings Ave.
Anthony, KS 67003
Ph: (620)665-2299

Augusta

50912 ■ **South Central Mental Health Counseling Center--Augusta**
2821 S Brookside
Augusta, KS 67010
Ph: (316)425-0073
URL: http://www.scmhcc.org/

Dodge City

50913 ■ **Area Mental Health Center--Dodge City**
2101 W Hwy. 50
Dodge City, KS 67801
Ph: (620)227-8566
Fax: (620)225-5824
URL: http://www.areamhc.org/

El Dorado

50914 ■ **South Central Mental Health Counseling Center--El Dorado**
2365 W Central
El Dorado, KS 67042
Ph: (316)321-6036
Fax: (316)321-6336
URL: http://www.scmhcc.org/

Emporia

50915 ■ **Mental Health Center of East Central Kansas**
Emporia Emergency Services
1000 Lincoln St.
Emporia, KS 66801
Ph: (316)342-0548
Fax: (316)342-1021
URL: http://www.mhceck.org

Garden City

50916 ■ **Area Mental Health Center--Garden City**
1111 E Spruce
Garden City, KS 67846
Ph: (620)276-7689
Fax: (620)276-6117
URL: http://www.areamhc.org/

Greensburg

50917 ■ **Iroquois Center for Human Development**
Crisis Line
610 E Grant Ave.
Greensburg, KS 67054
Ph: (620)723-2272
URL: http://www.irqcenter.com

Humboldt

50918 ■ **Southeast Kansas Mental Health Services**
Emergency Line
1106 S 9th St.
Humboldt, KS 66748
Ph: (316)473-2241
Fax: (316)473-3334

Kansas City

50919 ■ **Mental Health America of the Heartland - Kansas City, Kansas**
739 Minnesota Ave.
Kansas City, KS 66101
Ph: (913)281-2221
Free: 866-927-6327
Fax: (913)281-3977
E-mail: info@mhah.org
URL: http://www.mhah.org
Susan Crain Lewis, President

50920 ■ **Wyandot Mental Health Center**
757 Armstrong Ave.
Kansas City, KS 66101
Ph: (913)831-9500
URL: http://www.wyandotcenter.org/

Lawrence

50921 ■ **Headquarters Counseling Center**
1419 Massachusetts
Lawrence, KS 66044
Ph: (785)841-2345
E-mail: hqcc@lawrence.ks.us
URL: http://www.hqcc.lawrence.ks.us

Manhattan

50922 ■ **Crisis Center, Inc.**
PO Box 1526
Manhattan, KS 66502
Ph: (913)539-2785
URL: http://www.thecrisiscenterinc.org/contact.htm

Salina

**50923 ■ HOTLINE--Salina
Crisis, Information, and Referral Program**
227 N Santa Fe, Ste. 203
Salina, KS 67401
Ph: (785)827-4803
Fax: (785)827-6654
E-mail: hotline@salhelp.org

Scott City

**50924 ■ Area Mental Health Center--Scott
City**
210 W 4th
Scott City, KS 67871
Ph: (620)872-5338
Fax: (620)872-2879
URL: http://www.areamhc.org

Ulysses

50925 ■ Ulysses Area Mental Health Center
102 W Flower
Ulysses, KS 76880
Ph: (620)356-3198
Fax: (620)356-3101
URL: http://www.areamhc.org

Wichita

**50926 ■ COMCARE of Sedgewick County
Wichita Crisis Intervention Services**
934 N Water
Wichita, KS 67203
Ph: (316)660-7525
URL: http://www.sedgwickcounty.org/comcare/crisis.
 asp

50927 ■ Comcare of Sedgwick County
635 N Main
Wichita, KS 67203
Ph: (316)660-7600
URL: http://www.sedgwickcounty.org/comcare

KENTUCKY

Ashland

**50928 ■ Pathways, Inc. of Ashland
Crisis Service**
201 22nd St.
Ashland, KY 41105
Ph: (606)324-1141
URL: http://www.pathways-ky.org/

Bowling Green

**50929 ■ Life Skills Helpline--E Main Street,
Bowling Green**
707 E Main St.
Bowling Green, KY 42101
Ph: (502)843-4357
Fax: (502)843-4685
URL: http://www.lifeskills.com/cs.html

**50930 ■ Life Skills Helpline--Suwannee Trail,
Bowling Green**
380 Suwannee Trail St.
Bowling Green, KY 42103
Ph: (270)901-5000
URL: http://www.lifeskills.com/cs.html

Corbin

**50931 ■ Cumberland River Comprehensive
Mental Health Board
Corbin Emergency Services**
PO Box 568
Corbin, KY 40701
Ph: (606)528-7010
Fax: (606)528-5401

Elizabethtown

50932 ■ Elizabethtown Crisis Line
1311 N Dixie
Elizabethtown, KY 42701
Ph: (270)765-2605
URL: http://www.communicare.org/

Hazard

50933 ■ Kentucky River Community Care
PO Box 794
Hazard, KY 41339
Ph: (606)666-9006
URL: http://www.krccnet.com/welcomepage.html

Hopkinsville

**50934 ■ Pennyroyal Regional Mental Health
Center
Hopkinsville Crisis Line**
735 North Dr.
Hopkinsville, KY 42240
Ph: (502)886-5163
Fax: (502)885-5871
URL: http://www.pennyroyalcenter.org/

Lexington

50935 ■ Bluegrass Regional Mental Health
201 Mechanic St.
Lexington, KY 40507-1096
Ph: (859)253-1686
URL: http://www.bluegrass.org

Louisville

**50936 ■ Seven Counties Services Inc.
Crisis and Information Center**
101 W Muhammad Ali Blvd.
Louisville, KY 40202-1429
Ph: (502)589-8630
Fax: (502)589-8756
URL: http://www.sevencounties.org

Middlesboro

**50937 ■ Comprehensive Care Center,
Cumberland River**
203 W Chester Ave.
Middlesboro, KY 40965
Ph: (606)248-4949

Owensboro

**50938 ■ River Valley Behavioral Health
Crisis and Information Line**
1001 Frederica St.
Owensboro, KY 42301
Ph: (270)689-6500
E-mail: help@rvbh.com
URL: http://www.rvbh.com

Pineville

**50939 ■ Cumberland River Comprehensive
Care Center**
215 E Tennessee Ave.
Pineville, KY 40977
Ph: (606)337-6137

Prestonsburg

**50940 ■ Mountain Comprehensive Care
Center
Prestonburg Helpline**
18 S Front Ave.
Prestonsburg, KY 41653
Ph: (606)886-8572
Fax: (606)886-8577
URL: http://www.mtcomp.org

LOUISIANA

Alexandria

50941 ■ First Call For Help--Alexandria
c/o United Way of Central Louisiana
Alexandria, LA 71309

Ph: (318)443-7203

Baton Rouge

**50942 ■ Baton Rouge Crisis Intervention
Center, Inc.**
4837 Revere Ave.
Baton Rouge, LA 70808
Ph: (225)924-1431
Fax: (225)924-6964
URL: http://www.brcic.org

DeRidder

**50943 ■ Beauregard De Ridder Community
Help Line**
PO Box 815
DeRidder, LA 70634
Ph: (318)462-1452

Lafayette

**50944 ■ Charter Cypress Behavioral Health
System**
302 Dulles Dr.
Lafayette, LA 70506
Ph: (318)233-9024

50945 ■ The Jacob Crouch Foundation
2851 Johnston St., PMB 282
Lafayette, LA 70503
Ph: (337)234-1828
E-mail: info@injacobsmemory.org
URL: http://www.injacobsmemory.org/

**50946 ■ Southwest Louisiana Education and
Reference Center**
PO Box 52763
Lafayette, LA 70505
Ph: (318)232-4357

Lake Charles

50947 ■ 310 info
1023 Common St.
Lake Charles, LA 70601
Ph: (337)310-INFO
Free: 866-310-4636
URL: http://cg.servicept.com/lakecharles/

Metairie

**50948 ■ Jewish Family Services
Copeline Crisis Line**
3330 W Esplanade Ave. S, Ste. 600
Metairie, LA 70002
Ph: (504)831-8475

Monroe

50949 ■ Mainline
PO Box 1322
Monroe, LA 71210
Ph: (318)343-3585
Fax: (318)343-0396

**50950 ■ Young Women's Christian
Association of Northeast Louisiana**
1515 Jackson St.
Monroe, LA 71202
Ph: (318)323-1505
Fax: (318)323-1361

New Orleans

**50951 ■ River Oaks Hospital
Admission and Referral Service**
1525 River Oaks Rd. W
New Orleans, LA 70123-2199
Ph: (504)734-1740
Fax: (504)733-7020
URL: http://www.riveroakshospital.com

50952 ■ Volunteer and Information Agency
4747 Earhart Blvd., Ste. 111
New Orleans, LA 70125
Ph: (504)895-5575
Fax: (504)895-5560

Opelousas

50953 ■ Suicide Prevention Hotline
526 E Prudhomme Ln.
Opelousas, LA 70570
Ph: (318)942-4673

MAINE

Augusta

**50954 ■ Kennebec Behavioral
Health--Augusta**
66 Stone St.
Augusta, ME 04330
Free: 888-322-2136
URL: http://www.kbhmaine.org/locations.html

Bangor

50955 ■ Youth Crisis Stabilization Program
PO Box 425
Bangor, ME 04402
Ph: (207)947-0366
URL: http://www.umaine.edu/peered/resources.htm

Biddeford

50956 ■ Crisis Response Services
409 Alfred Rd.
Park 111
Biddeford, ME 04005
Ph: (207)284-1087
URL: http://www.suicidology.org

Farmington

50957 ■ Evergreen Behavioral Services
RR4, Box 5122A
Farmington, ME 04984
Ph: (207)778-0035
Free: 800-394-1900
Fax: (207)778-6879
URL: http://www.fchn.org

Lewiston

**50958 ■ Tri County Mental Health Service
Crisis Intervention Unit**
1155 Lisbon St.
Lewiston, ME 42401
Ph: (207)783-9141
URL: http://tcmhs.org/pages/androscoggin.php

Machias

**50959 ■ Washington County Psychotherapy
Associates**
PO Box 29
Machias, ME 04654
Ph: (207)255-4990
Fax: (207)255-8748
URL: http://www.wcpa.net

Portland

50960 ■ Ingraham
PO Box 1868
Portland, ME 04104
Ph: (207)874-1055
Fax: (207)774-5901
URL: http://www.yimaine.org/

Rumford

50961 ■ Greater Rumford AMI
150 Congress St.
Rumford, ME 04276
Ph: (207)364-3549
Fax: (207)364-2143
E-mail: admin@oxford.org

Saco

**50962 ■ Sweetser Children's Services
Crisis Intervention and Stabilization**
50 Moody St.
Saco, ME 04072
Ph: (207)284-5981
Free: 800-434-3000
E-mail: info@sweetser.org
URL: http://www.sweetser.org/

Skowhegan

50963 ■ Crisis Stabilization Unit
PO Box 588
Skowhegan, ME 04976
Ph: (207)474-2564

**50964 ■ Kennebec Behavioral
Health--Skowhegan**
30 High St.
Skowhegan, ME 04976
Ph: (207)474-8368
Free: 888-322-2136
URL: http://www.kbhmaine.org/locations.html
Formerly: Kennebec Valley Mental Health.

Waterville

**50965 ■ Kennebec Behavioral
Health--Waterville**
67 Eustis Pkwy.
Waterville, ME 04901
Ph: (207)873-2136
Free: 888-322-2136
URL: http://www.kbhmaine.org/?q=node/27
Formerly: Kennebec Valley Mental Health.

Winthrop

**50966 ■ Kennebec Behavioral
Health--Winthrop**
736 Old Lewiston Rd.
Winthrop, ME 04364
Free: 888-322-2136
URL: http://www.kbhmaine.org/locations.html

MARYLAND

Baltimore

50967 ■ Baltimore Crisis Response, Inc.
2041 E Fayette St.
Baltimore, MD 21231
Ph: (410)433-5255

50968 ■ First Step
8303 Liberty Rd.
Baltimore, MD 21244
Ph: (410)521-4141
URL: http://www.firststepmd.com

**50969 ■ Sinai Hospital
Baltimore Crisis Line**
Belvedere & Greenspring Ave.
Baltimore, MD 21215
Ph: (410)601-5457

Cambridge

50970 ■ For All Seasons, Inc.--Cambridge
208 Cedar St.
Cambridge, MD 21613
Ph: (410)822-1018
Fax: (410)820-5884
URL: http://forallseasonsinc.org/

Chestertown

50971 ■ For All Seasons, Inc.--Chestertown
516 Washington Ave., Ste. 4
Chestertown, MD 21620
Ph: (410)822-1018
Fax: (410)820-5884
URL: http://forallseasonsinc.org/

Columbia

**50972 ■ Grassroots Crisis Intervention
Center, Inc.**
6700 Freetown Rd.
Columbia, MD 21044
Ph: (410)531-6006
Fax: (410)531-3487
E-mail: info@grassrootscrisis.org
URL: http://www.grassrootscrisis.org

Denton

50973 ■ For All Seasons, Inc.--Denton
322 Market St.
Denton, MD 21629
Ph: (410)822-1018
Fax: (410)820-5884
URL: http://forallseasonsinc.org/

Easton

50974 ■ For All Seasons, Inc.--Easton
6 W Dover St.
Easton, MD 21601
Ph: (410)822-1018
Fax: (410)820-5884
URL: http://forallseasonsinc.org/

Frederick

**50975 ■ Mental Health Association of
Frederick County Hotline**
263 W Patrick St.
Frederick, MD 21701
Ph: (301)663-0011
Fax: (301)695-4747
URL: http://www.fcmha.org/

Hyattsville

50976 ■ Community Crisis Services, Inc.
PO Box 149
Hyattsville, MD 20781
Ph: (301)864-7095
Fax: (301)864-7146
URL: http://www.communitycrisis.org/

**50977 ■ Prince George's County Hotline and
Suicide Prevention Center**
PO Box 149
Hyattsville, MD 20781
Ph: (301)864-7095
Fax: (301)864-7146
URL: http://www.communitycrisis.org/

Lanham

50978 ■ Suicide Prevention Center--Lanham
5012 Rhode Island Ave.
Lanham, MD 20706
Ph: (301)731-0004

Rockville

**50979 ■ Montgomery County Hotline
Mental Health Association**
1000 Twinbrook Pkwy.
Rockville, MD 20851
Ph: (301)424-0656
E-mail: info@mhamc.org
URL: http://www.mhamc.org

Salisbury

50980 ■ Life Crisis Center
PO Box 387
Salisbury, MD 21803
Ph: (410)749-0771
E-mail: eharris@lifecrisiscenter.org
URL: http://www.lifecrisiscenter.org

Waldorf

50981 ■ Center for Abused Persons
2670 Crane Hwy, Ste. 303
Waldorf, MD 20601

Ph: (301)645-8994
Fax: (301)645-8342
URL: http://www.centerforabusedpersons.com/

White Plains
50982 ■ Center for Abused Persons
4305 Charles Crossing Dr.
White Plains, MD 20695
Ph: (301)645-8994
URL: http://www.centerforabusedpersons.com/

MASSACHUSETTS
Attleboro
50983 ■ New Hope/Attleboro
140 Park St.
Attleboro, MA 02703
Ph: (508)226-4015
Fax: (508)226-6917
URL: http://www.new-hope.org

Boston
50984 ■ American Foundation for Suicide Prevention
56 Broad St.
Boston, MA 02109
Ph: (617)439-0940
URL: http://www.afsp.org/

50985 ■ Samaritans of Boston
141 Tremont St., 7th Fl.
Boston, MA 02111
Ph: (617)536-2460
E-mail: samaritans@mindspring.com
URL: http://www.samaritansofboston.org

Brockton
50986 ■ Brockton Helpline
47 W Elm St.
Brockton, MA 02301
Ph: (508)584-4357
Free: 866-621-4747
URL: http://www.bamsi.org/services/helpline.html

Fall River
50987 ■ Samaritans of Fall River/New Bedford
386 Stanley St.
Fall River, MA 02720
Ph: (508)673-3777
Free: 866-508-4357
E-mail: samsfrnb@aol.com
URL: http://www.samaritans-fallriver.org/

Falmouth
50988 ■ Samaritans on Cape Cod and the Islands, Inc.
PO Box 65
Falmouth, MA 02541
Ph: (508)548-7999
Fax: (508)548-7999
URL: http://www.capesamaritans.org

Framingham
50989 ■ Samaritans, Suburban West
276 Union Ave.
Framingham, MA 01702
Ph: (508)872-1780
Fax: (508)875-4910
E-mail: rhurtig@samaritanshope.org
URL: http://www.samaritansofboston.org/pr_050503.html

Haverhill
50990 ■ North Essex Mental Health Center Crisis Service and Central Intake
60 Merrimack St.
Haverhill, MA 01830

Ph: (978)462-4644
URL: http://www.hes-inc.org/

Holyoke
50991 ■ City Clinic
230 & 235 Maple St.
Holyoke, MA 01040
Ph: (413)532-0389
URL: http://www.bhninc.org/mount-tom-city-clinic.html

50992 ■ Mount Tom Mental Health Center
40 Bobala Rd.
Holyoke, MA 01040
Ph: (413)536-5473
URL: http://www.bhninc.org/

Methuen
50993 ■ Samaritans of Merrimack Valley
169 East St.
Methuen, MA 01844
Ph: (978)688-0030
Fax: (978)688-6009
E-mail: gamiller@samaritans-mass.org

Northampton
**50994 ■ Service Net
Emergency Service of Northampton**
129 King St.
Northampton, MA 01060
Ph: (413)586-5555
Fax: (413)585-1352
URL: http://www.servicenetinc.org/

Norwood
50995 ■ Riverside Community Care
190 Lenox St.
Norwood, MA 02062
Ph: (781)769-8670
Fax: (781)769-6717
URL: http://www.riversidecc.com

Pittsfield
50996 ■ First Call For Help/Berkshire United Wayfield
200 South St.
Pittsfield, MA 01201
Ph: (413)442-6948
Free: 877-211-6277
URL: http://www.mass211.org/

Southbridge
50997 ■ Y.O.U., Inc. Family Services
52 Charlton St.
Southbridge, MA 01550
Ph: (508)765-9101
URL: http://www.youinc.org

Springfield
50998 ■ Psychiatric Crisis Services
503 State St.
Springfield, MA 01109
Ph: (413)746-3758
Fax: (413)733-7841

Stoneham
50999 ■ Boston Medical Center Psychiatric Services
5 Woodland Rd.
Stoneham, MA 02180
Ph: (781)979-7025
URL: http://www.bmc.org/psychiatry.htm

Taunton
51000 ■ New Hope--Taunton
39 Taunton Green S, Ste. 203
Taunton, MA 02780
Ph: (508)824-5205
URL: http://www.new-hope.org/contact.html

Webster
51001 ■ New Hope--Webster
6 River Ct.
Webster, MA 01570
Ph: (508)949-0452
URL: http://www.new-hope.org/contact.html

Westfield
51002 ■ Westfield Crisis Team
77 Mill St.
Westfield, MA 01085
Ph: (413)568-6386
URL: http://www.masspreventssuicide.org/resources/ch16.html

Worcester
51003 ■ MJ Leadenham Center
91 Prescott St.
Worcester, MA 01605
Ph: (508)753-3146
URL: http://www.new-hope.org/contact.html

**51004 ■ Y.O.U., Inc.
Crisis Center**
81 Plantation St.
Worcester, MA 01604
Ph: (508)849-5600
URL: http://www.youinc.org

MICHIGAN
Ann Arbor
51005 ■ Dawn Farm
544 N Division St.
Ann Arbor, MI 48103
Ph: (734)669-8265
URL: http://www.dawnfarm.org/index.html

51006 ■ Ozone House Youth and Family Services
1705 Washtenaw Ave.
Ann Arbor, MI 48104
Ph: (734)662-2265
Fax: (734)662-9724
URL: http://ozonehouse.org

51007 ■ University of Michigan Health Systems
1500 E Medical Center Dr.
Ann Arbor, MI 48109-0120
Ph: (734)936-4960
URL: http://www.med.umich.edu/

Benton Harbor
51008 ■ Link Crisis Intervention Center
2480 M-139
Benton Harbor, MI 49022
Ph: (269)927-1422
E-mail: info@cfsswmi.org
URL: http://www.linkforteens.org

Bloomfield Hills
51009 ■ Common Ground Sanctuary
1410 S Telegraph
Bloomfield Hills, MI 48302
Ph: (248)456-8150
Fax: (248)456-8147
E-mail: contactus@commongroundsanctuary.org
URL: http://www.commongroundhelps.org/

Cadillac
51010 ■ North Central Community Mental Health
527 Cobbs
Cadillac, MI 49601
Ph: (616)775-3463

Chesterfield Township

51011 ■ Macomb County Community Mental Health Access Center
Survivors of Suicide
43740 N Groesbeck Hwy.
Chesterfield Township, MI 48036
Ph: (586)948-0222
URL: http://www.mhweb.org/macomb/maccmh.htm

Coldwater

51012 ■ Pines Behavioral Health Services
200 Orleans Blvd.
Coldwater, MI 49036
Ph: (517)278-2129
Fax: (517)279-8172
E-mail: mail@pinesbhs.org
URL: http://www.pinesbhs.org/

Detroit

51013 ■ Neighborhood Service Organization
220 Bagley, Ste. 626
Detroit, MI 48226
Ph: (313)961-1060
Fax: (313)963-3108
E-mail: jeasley@nso-mi.org
URL: http://www.nso-mi.org

East Lansing

51014 ■ Gateway Community Services
910 Abbott Rd., Ste. 100
East Lansing, MI 48823
Ph: (517)351-4000
Fax: (517)351-4094
E-mail: info@gatewayservices.org
URL: http://www.gatewayservices.org

51015 ■ The Listening Ear, Inc.
313 W Grand River Ave.
East Lansing, MI 48823
Ph: (517)337-1728
E-mail: theear@msu.edu
URL: http://www.thelisteningear.net

Flint

51016 ■ Genesee County Community Mental Health Services
Mental Health Crisis Clinic
918 Patrick St.
Flint, MI 48503
Ph: (810)232-5850
Fax: (810)233-5925
URL: http://www.gencmh.org

Fort Gratiot

51017 ■ Blue Water Mental Health Clinic
1501 Krafft Rd.
Fort Gratiot, MI 48059
Ph: (810)985-5125
URL: http://www.bluewaterclinic.com/

Holland

51018 ■ Ottawa County Community Mental Health Services
Crisis Intervention Services
Help-Line
12265 James St.
Holland, MI 49424
Ph: (616)392-1873
E-mail: info@county.ottawa.mi.us
URL: http://www.co.ottawa.mi.us/healthcomm/cmh/cmhhome.htm

Houghton

51019 ■ Dial Help
Copper Country Mental Health Services
609 Shelden Ave.
Houghton, MI 49931

Ph: (906)482-4357
URL: http://www.cccmh.org/home.html

Jackson

51020 ■ Lifeways--Jackson
1198 N West Ave.
Jackson, MI 49202
Ph: (517)789-1200
Free: 800-284-8288
URL: http://www.lifewaysmco.com/
Formerly: Behavioral Health Connections.

Kalamazoo

51021 ■ Gryphon Place
1104 S Westnedge
Kalamazoo, MI 49008
Ph: (269)381-1510
Fax: (269)381-0935
E-mail: gryphon@telecity.org
URL: http://www.gryphon.org

Lapeer

51022 ■ Lapeer County Community Mental Health Center
1570 Suncrest Dr.
Lapeer, MI 48446
Ph: (810)667-0500
URL: http://www.county.lapeer.org/CMH/

Mount Pleasant

51023 ■ Community Mental Health for Central Michigan
301 S Crapo
Mount Pleasant, MI 48858
Ph: (989)772-5938
Fax: (989)773-1968
URL: http://www.cmhcm.org/

51024 ■ Listening Ear Crisis Center, Inc.--Mount Pleasant
PO Box 65
Mount Pleasant, MI 48858
Ph: (517)772-2918
URL: http://www.listeningear.com

Muskegon

51025 ■ Community Mental Health of West Michigan
141 E Apple
Muskegon, MI 49442
Ph: (231)720-3200

Pontiac

51026 ■ Common Ground Crisis Services
7 S Perry
Pontiac, MI 48342
Ph: (248)456-1991
URL: http://www.commongroundhelps.org/

Port Huron

51027 ■ Saint Clair County Community Mental Health Services
1011 Military
Port Huron, MI 48060
Ph: (810)985-8900
Fax: (810)987-2336
E-mail: scccmh@cccmh.org
URL: http://www.scccmh.org/hi_res_crisis.htm

Saginaw

51028 ■ Saginaw City Mental Health Center
Crisis Intervention Services
500 Hancock
Saginaw, MI 48602
Ph: (989)797-3400
URL: http://www.sccmha.org/

Three Rivers

51029 ■ Saint Joseph County Community Mental Health
210 S Main St.
Three Rivers, MI 49093
Ph: (616)273-5000
URL: http://www.stjoecmh.org/

Traverse City

51030 ■ Third Level Crisis Center
1022 E Front St.
Traverse City, MI 49685
Ph: (231)922-4802
E-mail: info@thirdlevel.org
URL: http://www.thirdlevel.org

Troy

51031 ■ Cranbrook Counseling and Crisis Services
2555 Crooks Rd., Ste. 110
Troy, MI 48084
Ph: (248)981-0498
Free: 800-509-8460
Fax: (248)857-8465
E-mail: cranbrookcounseling@compuserve.com

Ypsilanti

51032 ■ SOS Crisis Center
101 S Huron
Ypsilanti, MI 48197
Ph: (734)485-8730
Fax: (734)485-8739
E-mail: info@soscs.org
URL: http://www.soscs.org/

51033 ■ Washtenaw County Community Mental Health Center
555 Towner, Box 915
Ypsilanti, MI 48198
Ph: (734)544-3000
URL: http://www.ewashtenaw.org/government/departments/community_mental_health

Zeeland

51034 ■ Suicide Prevention Service--Zeeland
21 S Elm St.
Zeeland, MI 49464
Ph: (616)396-4357

MINNESOTA

Alexandria

51035 ■ Listening Ear Crisis Center--Alexandria
700 Cedar St., Ste. 204
Alexandria, MN 56308
Ph: (320)763-6638
Fax: (320)763-6639

Apple Valley

51036 ■ Dakota County Crisis Response Unit
14955 Galaxie Ave.
Apple Valley, MN 55124
Ph: (952)891-7400
Free: 800-247-1056
E-mail: Emily.Schug@co.dakota.mn.us
URL: http://www.co.dakota.mn.us/Departments/SocialServices/Services/default.htm

Austin

51037 ■ Crime Victims Resource Center
101 14th St. NW
Austin, MN 55912
Ph: (507)437-6680
URL: http://mayohealthsystem.org
Program(s): Crisis Nursery; Children's Visitation Center; Crime Victims Resource Center; Domestic Violence Intervention Program; Crisis Intervention; Advocacy; Education Programs; Support Groups. **Re-**

marks: Makes arrangements for emergency shelter and transportation. Services are free.

Brainerd

51038 ■ Crisis Line and Referral Service
PO Box 192
Brainerd, MN 56401
Ph: (218)828-4515
URL: http://crisislineandreferralservice.org/

Grand Rapids

51039 ■ First Call For Help--Itasca County
1211 SE 2nd Ave.
Grand Rapids, MN 55744
Ph: (218)326-8565
URL: http://www.firstcall211.net/

51040 ■ Northland Recovery Center
1215 SE 7th Ave.
Grand Rapids, MN 55744
Ph: (218)327-1026
Free: 800-626-0377
URL: http://www.northlandrecovery.com/

Minneapolis

51041 ■ Hennepin County Medical Center Crisis Intervention Center
701 Park Ave. S
Minneapolis, MN 55415
Ph: (612)873-3161
URL: http://www.hcmc.org/depts/psych/cic.htm

51042 ■ Love Lines Crisis Center
2535 Central Ave.
Minneapolis, MN 55418
Ph: (612)379-1199
Fax: (612)782-8880
E-mail: counselor@lovelines.org
URL: http://www.lovelines.org

Owatonna

51043 ■ CONTACT, Serving Steele and Waseca Counties
PO Box 524
Owatonna, MN 55060
Ph: (507)451-1897
Fax: (507)451-1897
E-mail: info@contacthelp.org
URL: http://www.contacthelp.org/

Richfield

51044 ■ Crisis Connection
PO Box 23090
Richfield, MN 55423
Ph: (612)852-2201
Fax: (612)379-6391
E-mail: jenn@crisis.org
URL: http://www.crisis.org

Saint Paul

51045 ■ Ramsey County Adult Mental Health Services
Crisis Center
1919 University
Saint Paul, MN 55101
Ph: (651)266-7890
URL: http://www.co.ramsey.mn.us/hs/mhc/adultmentalhealth.htm

51046 ■ Regions Hospital
CRISIS Program
640 Jackson St.
Saint Paul, MN 35101
Ph: (615)221-2055
URL: http://www.regionshospital.com/Regions/Menu/0,1640,4197,00.html

MISSISSIPPI

Columbus

51047 ■ CONTACT Helpline--Columbus
PO Box 1304
Columbus, MS 39703
Ph: (601)327-2968
URL: http://unitedwaylowndescounty.org/community-resources.html

51048 ■ Mississippi State Community Counseling Services
1001 Main St.
Columbus, MS 39701
Ph: (662)328-0200

Jackson

51049 ■ CONTACT Crisis Line
PO Box 5192
Jackson, MS 39296-5192
Ph: (601)713-4099
Fax: (601)713-4098
URL: http://www.contactthecrisisline.org/

51050 ■ Suicide Anonymous
E South St.
Jackson, MS 39201
Ph: (601)713-4357

Starkville

51051 ■ Community Counseling Services--Starkville
Contact Helpline
302 N Jackson St.
Starkville, MS 39759
Ph: (662)323-4357
URL: http://www.ccsms.org/

MISSOURI

Arnold

51052 ■ Provident Jefferson County
3675 W Outer Rd., Ste. 203
Arnold, MO 63010
Ph: (314)371-6500
Fax: (314)647-1762
URL: http://providentstl.org/

Cape Girardeau

51053 ■ Community Counseling Center
402 S Silver Springs Rd.
Cape Girardeau, MO 63703
Ph: (573)334-1100
URL: http://www.cccntr.com/

Fredericktown

51054 ■ Community Counseling Center of Madison County
311 Garrett St.
Fredericktown, MO 63645
Ph: (573)783-4104
Fax: (573)783-4572
URL: http://www.cccntr.com/
Formerly: Community Counseling Center at Fredericktown.

Joplin

51055 ■ Ozark Center
3006 McClelland Blvd.
Joplin, MO 64804
Ph: (417)781-4031
URL: http://www.freemanhealth.com/ozarkcenter

Kansas City

51056 ■ Western Missouri Mental Health Center
Kansas City Suicide Prevention Line
600 E 22nd St.
Kansas City, MO 64108

Ph: (816)512-4000

Marble Hill

51057 ■ Community Counseling Center of Bollinger County
208 Broadway
Marble Hill, MO 63764
Ph: (573)238-1027
Fax: (573)238-1171
URL: http://www.cccntr.com/

Maryland Heights

51058 ■ Behavioral Health Response--Maryland Heights
PO Box 1125
Maryland Heights, MO 63043
Ph: (314)469-4908
Fax: (314)469-2795
E-mail: barrys@bhrstl.org
URL: http://www.bhrstl.org

Perryville

51059 ■ Community Counseling Center of Perry County
406 N Spring St., Ste. 2
Perryville, MO 63775
Ph: (573)547-8305
Fax: (573)547-8306
URL: http://www.cccntr.com/

Saint Joseph

51060 ■ Family Guidance Center for Behavioral Health Care
510 Francis St.
Saint Joseph, MO 64501
Ph: (816)364-1501
URL: http://www.familyguidance.org/

Saint Louis

51061 ■ Behavioral Health Response--Saint Louis
12647 Olive Blvd., Ste. 200
Saint Louis, MO 63141
Ph: (314)638-6218
URL: http://www.bhrstl.org/crisishotline.htm

51062 ■ Kids Under Twenty One
2718 S Brentwood
Saint Louis, MO 63144
Ph: (314)963-7571
Fax: (314)963-7574
URL: http://www.kuto.org

51063 ■ Provident Central City
2650 Olive St.
Saint Louis, MO 63103
Ph: (314)371-6500
Fax: (314)647-1762
URL: http://providentstl.org/
Formerly: Life Crisis Services, Inc.

51064 ■ Provident South City
6555 Chippewa, Ste. 150
Saint Louis, MO 63109
Ph: (314)371-6500
Fax: (314)647-1762
URL: http://providentstl.org/

51065 ■ Provident West County
12755 Olive St., Ste. 115
Saint Louis, MO 63141
Ph: (314)371-6500
Fax: (314)647-1762
URL: http://providentstl.org/

Sainte Genevieve

51066 ■ Community Counseling Center of Sainte Genevieve County
820 Park Dr.
Sainte Genevieve, MO 63670

Ph: (573)883-7407
Fax: (573)883-7537
URL: http://www.cccntr.com/

Springfield

51067 ■ Burrell Center, Inc.
Crisis Assist Team
930 S Robberson
Springfield, MO 65807
Ph: (417)269-0410
URL: http://www.burrellcenter.com/services/crisissta-bilization.aspx

MONTANA

Billings

51068 ■ Department of Family Services
Billings Helpline
2508 3rd Ave. N
Billings, MT 59101
Ph: (406)657-3120

51069 ■ Mental Health Center
Helpline
1245 N 29th St.
Billings, MT 59101
Ph: (406)252-5658
URL: http://www.mhcbillings.org/

Bozeman

51070 ■ Bozeman Help Center
421 E Peach St.
Bozeman, MT 59715
Ph: (406)586-3333
Fax: (406)587-2034
E-mail: info@bozemanhelpcenter.org
URL: http://www.bozemanhelpcenter.org/
Formerly: Network Against Sexual and Domestic Violence.

Great Falls

51071 ■ Crisis Line
PO Box 6644
Great Falls, MT 59405
Ph: (406)771-8648
URL: http://www.voicesofhope.info/

Helena

51072 ■ Mental Health Services--Helena
1101 Missola
Helena, MT 59601
Ph: (406)443-4922

Kalispell

51073 ■ First Call For Help, Inc.--Kalispell
Help Net
PO Box 8181
Kalispell, MT 59904
Ph: (406)752-7266

NEBRASKA

Boys Town

51074 ■ Father Flanagan's Boy's Home
Boys Town National Hotline
13940 Gutowski Rd.
Boys Town, NE 68010
Ph: (402)498-1900
Free: 800-989-0000
Fax: (402)498-1875
URL: http://www.boystown.org

Lincoln

51075 ■ Personal Crisis Service
PO Box 80083
Lincoln, NE 68501
Ph: (402)475-5171

North Platte

51076 ■ Heartland Counseling and Consulting Clinic
110 N Bailey Ave.
North Platte, NE 69101
Ph: (308)534-6029
Fax: (308)534-6961
URL: http://www.r2hs.com/

NEVADA

Las Vegas

51077 ■ Suicide Prevention Center of Clark County, Inc.
3342 S Sandhill Rd.
Box 9-528
Las Vegas, NV 89121

Reno

51078 ■ Crisis Call Center
PO Box 8016
Reno, NV 89507
Ph: (775)784-8085
Fax: (775)784-8083
E-mail: admin@crisiscallcenter.org
URL: http://www.crisiscallcenter.org

NEW HAMPSHIRE

Berlin

51079 ■ Androscoggin Valley Mental Health Clinic
Berlin Emergency Service
Riverside Courtyard
3 12th St.
Berlin, NH 03570
Ph: (603)752-7404
Fax: (603)752-5194
URL: http://www.nnhmhds.org

Concord

51080 ■ Community Services Council of New Hampshire
PO Box 2338
Concord, NH 03302
Ph: (603)225-9000
Fax: (603)225-4033
URL: http://www.cscnh.org/

51081 ■ Riverbend Community Mental Health Services
278 Pleasant St.
Concord, NH 03302
Ph: (603)228-1551
URL: http://www.riverbendcmhc.org

Derry

51082 ■ Center for Life Management
43 Birch St.
Derry, NH 03038
Ph: (603)434-1577
URL: http://www.cimbehav.org/

Dover

51083 ■ Strafford Guidance Center, Inc.
Emergency Crisis Team
130 Central Ave.
Dover, NH 03820
Ph: (603)742-0630
Fax: (603)749-6304

Keene

51084 ■ Samaritans
103 Roxbury St., Ste. 304
Keene, NH 03431
Ph: (603)357-5510

Free: 877-583-8336
Fax: (603)357-5506
E-mail: rill@samaritansnh.org
URL: http://www.samaritansnh.org
Formerly: (2004) Samaritans of the Monadnock Region.

Laconia

51085 ■ Genesis - The Counseling Group
111 Church St.
Laconia, NH 03246
Ph: (603)524-1100

Lebanon

51086 ■ Headrest, Inc.
14 Church St.
Lebanon, NH 03766
Ph: (603)448-4872
Fax: (603)448-1829
URL: http://www.headrest.org

Manchester

51087 ■ Mental Health Center of Greater Manchester
401 Cypress St.
Manchester, NH 03103
Ph: (603)668-4111
Fax: (603)669-1131
E-mail: info@mhcgm.org
URL: http://www.mhcgm.org
Remarks: Residential program serving ages 18 and up; clinic serving all ages.

Portsmouth

51088 ■ Seacoast Mental Health Services
1145 Sagamore Ave.
Portsmouth, NH 03801
Ph: (603)431-6703
URL: http://www.smhc-nh.org/

Salem

51089 ■ CLM Behavioral Health Systems
44 Stiles Rd.
Salem, NH 03079
Ph: (603)432-2253
URL: http://www.clmbehav.org

NEW JERSEY

Annandale

51090 ■ Hunterdon Helpline
14 Mine St.
Annandale, NJ 08802
Ph: (908)735-4357
E-mail: info@helplinehc.org
URL: http://www.helplinehc.org

Atlantic City

51091 ■ Atlantic City Medical Center
Psychiatric Intervention Program
1925 Pacific Ave.
Atlantic City, NJ 08401
Ph: (609)344-1118
URL: http://www.state.nj.us/humanservices/dmhs/services/centers/

Bridgeton

51092 ■ Cumberland County Guidance Center
Crisis Hotline
423 Manheim Ave.
Bridgeton, NJ 08302
Ph: (609)455-8088
URL: http://www.state.nj.us/humanservices/dmhs/services/centers/

51093 ■ Jersey Hospital--Cumerland County Guidance Center
333 Irving Ave.
Bridgeton, NJ 08302
Ph: (856)455-5555
URL: http://www.state.nj.us/humanservices/dmhs/
services/centers/

Cape May Court House

51094 ■ Cape Regional Medical Center
2 Stone Harbor Blvd.
Cape May Court House, NJ 08210
Ph: (609)465-5999
URL: http://www.state.nj.us/humanservices/dmhs/
services/centers/

Carney's Point

51095 ■ Primary Screening Center of Salem County
Healthcare Commons, Inc. at Memorial Hospital of Salem County
500 S Pennsville-Auburn Rd.
Carney's Point, NJ 08079
Ph: (856)299-3001
URL: http://www.state.nj.us/humanservices/dmhs/
services/centers/

Cherry Hill

51096 ■ Contact Community Services
PO Box 8563
Cherry Hill, NJ 08002
Ph: (856)795-5073
Fax: (856)795-2103
URL: http://www.contacthelplines.org/

Denville

51097 ■ Primary Screening Center for Morris County
Saint Clare's Hospital
25 Pocono Rd.
Denville, NJ 07834
Ph: (973)625-0280
URL: http://www.state.nj.us/humanservices/dmhs/
services/centers/

East Orange

51098 ■ East Orange General Hospital--Primary Screening Center
Essex County
300 Central Ave.
East Orange, NJ 07019
Ph: (973)266-4478
URL: http://www.state.nj.us/humanservices/dmhs/
services/centers/

Elizabeth

51099 ■ Primary Screening Center of Union County
Trinitas Hospital
655 E Jersey St.
Elizabeth, NJ 07201
Ph: (908)994-7131
URL: http://www.state.nj.us/humanservices/dmhs/
services/centers/

Ewing

51100 ■ Contact of Mercer County, NJ Inc.
1985 Pennington Rd.
Ewing, NJ 08618
Ph: (609)883-2880
E-mail: contactofmercercounty@verizon.net
URL: http://www.contactofmercer.org

Fair Lawn

51101 ■ Fair Lawn Mental Health Center
17-07 Romaine St.
Fair Lawn, NJ 07410
Ph: (201)797-2660
URL: http://www.careplusnj.org/

Flemington

51102 ■ Primary Screening Center for Hunterdon County
Hunterdon Medical Center
2100 Wescott Dr.
Flemington, NJ 08822
Ph: (908)788-6400
URL: http://www.state.nj.us/humanservices/dmhs/
services/centers/

Hoboken

51103 ■ Hoboken University Medical Center Community Mental Health Center
314 Clinton St.
Hoboken, NJ 07030
Ph: (201)792-8200
Fax: (201)792-8655
URL: http://www.hobokenumc.com/main/contents.
php?Id=14
Formerly: Saint Mary's Community Mental Health Center.

Jersey City

51104 ■ Primary Screening Center for Hudson County
Christ Hospital
176 Palisade Ave.
Jersey City, NJ 07304
Ph: (201)795-8374
URL: http://www.state.nj.us/humanservices/dmhs/
services/centers/

51105 ■ Primary Screening Center for Hudson County
Jersey City Medical Center
355 Grand St.
Jersey City, NJ 07340
Free: 866-367-6023
URL: http://www.state.nj.us/humanservices/dmhs/
services/centers/

Lakewood

51106 ■ Primary Screening Center for Ocean County
Kimball Medical Center
600 River Ave.
Lakewood, NJ 08701
Ph: (732)886-4474
URL: http://www.state.nj.us/humanservices/dmhs/
services/centers/

Long Branch

51107 ■ Primary Screening Center for Monmouth County
Monmouth Medical Center
300 2nd Ave.
Long Branch, NJ 07740
Ph: (732)923-6999
URL: http://www.state.nj.us/humanservices/dmhs/
services/centers/

Lyndhurst

51108 ■ Comprehensive Behavioral Healthcare, Inc.
516 Valley Brook Ave.
Lyndhurst, NJ 07071
Ph: (201)935-3322
Fax: (201)935-9196
URL: http://www.cbhcare.com/

Margate

51109 ■ Contact Cape Atlantic
9500 Ventnor, Bldg. 2
Margate, NJ 08402
Ph: (609)823-1850
Fax: (609)823-1938
URL: http://contactcapeatlantic.org/index.html

Montclair

51110 ■ Mental Health Resource Center
60 S Fullerton Ave., Ste. 210
Montclair, NJ 07042
Ph: (973)744-6522
URL: http://www.careplusnj.org/

Moorestown

51111 ■ Contact Burlington County
PO Box 333
Moorestown, NJ 08057
Ph: (856)234-5484
URL: http://www.contactburlco.org

Morristown

51112 ■ Morristown Memorial Hospital Psychiatric Emergency Service
Crisis Hotline
100 Madison Ave.
Morristown, NJ 07960
Ph: (973)540-0100
URL: http://www.state.nj.us/lps/dcj/victimwitness/
mental.htm

Mount Holly

51113 ■ Virtua Memorial Hospital Screening and Crisis Intervention Program
175 Madison Ave.
Mount Holly, NJ 08060
Ph: (609)261-8000
Fax: (609)261-3416
URL: http://www.virtua.org/locations/hospitals-and-
locations/virtua-memorial.aspx
Formerly: Memorial Hospital of Burlington County.

Newark

51114 ■ Emergency Psychiatric Services
100 Bergen St.
Newark, NJ 07103
Ph: (973)982-6134
URL: http://www.state.nj.us/humanservices/dmhs/
services/centers/

51115 ■ Newark Beth Israel Medical Center--Primary Screening Center
Essex County
201 Lyons Ave.
Newark, NJ 07112
Ph: (973)926-7444
URL: http://www.state.nj.us/humanservices/dmhs/
services/centers/

Newton

51116 ■ Primary Screening Center of Sussex County
Newton Memorial Hospital
175 High St.
Newton, NJ 07860
Ph: (973)383-0973
URL: http://www.state.nj.us/humanservices/dmhs/
services/centers/

North Bergen

51117 ■ Primary Screening Center for Hudson County
Palisades Medical Center
7600 River Rd.
North Bergen, NJ 07047
Ph: (201)854-6300
URL: http://www.state.nj.us/humanservices/dmhs/
services/centers/

Paramus

51118 ■ Mid-Bergen Center, Paramus
610 Valley Health Plz.
Paramus, NJ 07652
Ph: (201)265-8200
URL: http://www.careplusnj.org/

Paterson

51119 ■ Primary Screening Center of Passaic County
Saint Joseph's Hospital & Medical Center
646 Broadway
Paterson, NJ 07514
Ph: (973)684-7792
URL: http://www.state.nj.us/humanservices/dmhs/services/centers/

Pequannock

51120 ■ Contact Hotline
PO Box 219
Pequannock, NJ 07440
Ph: (973)831-1879
Fax: (973)831-8728

Phillipsburg

51121 ■ Primary Screening Center of Warren County
Family Guidance Center of Warren County
370 Memorial Pkwy.
Phillipsburg, NJ 08865
Ph: (908)454-5141
URL: http://www.state.nj.us/humanservices/dmhs/services/centers/

Red Bank

51122 ■ Riverview Medical Center
Helpline - Crisis Unit
1 Riverview Plz.
Red Bank, NJ 07701
Ph: (732)530-2438
Fax: (732)530-2540
URL: http://www.riverviewmedicalcenter.com/index.cfm/Services/BehavioralHealth/crisis.c fm

Somerville

51123 ■ Primary Screening Center of Somerset County
Somerset County PESS
110 Rehill Ave.
Somerville, NJ 08876
Ph: (908)526-4100
URL: http://www.state.nj.us/humanservices/dmhs/services/centers/

Trenton

51124 ■ Primary Screening Center for Mercy County
Capital Health System at Fuld
750 Brunswick Ave.
Trenton, NJ 08638
Ph: (609)396-4357
URL: http://www.state.nj.us/humanservices/dmhs/services/centers/

Westfield

51125 ■ CONTACT We Care, Inc.
PO Box 2376
Westfield, NJ 07091
Ph: (908)301-1899
URL: http://www.contactwecare.org

Woodbury

51126 ■ Primary Screening Center for Gloucester County
Newpoint Behavioral Health Care, Underwood Memorial Hospital
509 N Broad St.
Woodbury, NJ 08096
Ph: (856)845-9100
URL: http://www.state.nj.us/humanservices/dmhs/services/centers/

NEW MEXICO

Albuquerque

51127 ■ University of New Mexico
Agora Crisis Center
1716 Las Lomas NE
Albuquerque, NM 87131
Ph: (505)277-7855
E-mail: agora@unm.edu
URL: http://www.unm.edu/~agora/contact.htm

Deming

51128 ■ Border Area Mental Health Services Inc.
901 W Hickory St.
Deming, NM 88030
Ph: (505)538-3488
URL: http://www.bamhs.org/

Espanola

51129 ■ Crisis Center of Northern New Mexico
577 El Llano Rd.
Espanola, NM 87532
Ph: (505)753-1656
Free: 800-206-1656
E-mail: ccnnm@crisis-centers.com
URL: http://www.crisis-centers.com

Portales

51130 ■ Mental Health Resources
300 E 1st St.
Portales, NM 88130
Ph: (505)359-1221

Santa Fe

51131 ■ Presbyterian Medical Services
Crisis Response of Santa Fe
1422 Paseo de Peralta
Santa Fe, NM 87501
Ph: (505)820-1440
URL: http://quasar.pmsnet.org/hub/index.php

NEW YORK

Albany

51132 ■ Capital District Psychiatric Center
75 New Scotland Ave.
Albany, NY 12208-3474
Ph: (518)447-9611
Fax: (518)434-0041
URL: http://www.omh.state.ny.us/omhweb/facilities/cdpc/facility.htm

51133 ■ Family and Children's Service of the Capital Region
The Samaritans of The Capital District
PO Box 5228
Albany, NY 12205
Ph: (518)459-0196
URL: http://www.orgsites.com/ny/samaritans-albany/
Formerly: The Dutchess County Department of Mental Hygiene.

Batavia

51134 ■ Regional Action Phone, Inc.
PO Box 281
Batavia, NY 14021
Ph: (585)343-1212
E-mail: rapinc1@verizon.net
URL: http://www.geneseeny.com/rap

Bellmore

51135 ■ Long Island Crisis Center
2740 Martin Ave.
Bellmore, NY 11710
Ph: (516)826-0244
URL: http://www.longislandcrisiscenter.org/

Buffalo

51136 ■ Crisis Services, Inc.
2969 Main St.
Buffalo, NY 14214
Ph: (716)834-2310
Fax: (716)834-9881
URL: http://www.crisisservices.org

East Syracuse

51137 ■ Contact Community Services
6520 Basile Rowe
East Syracuse, NY 13057
Ph: (315)251-1400
Fax: (315)251-2218
E-mail: contact@contactsyracuse.org
URL: http://www.contactsyracuse.org

Ellenville

51138 ■ Family of Ellenville
14 Church St.
Ellenville, NY 12428
Ph: (845)647-2443
Fax: (845)647-2460
E-mail: foeh@familyofwoodstockinc.org
URL: http://www.familyofwoodstockinc.org/

Elmsford

51139 ■ Mental Health Association of Westchester County
Sterling Center
2269 Saw Mill River Rd., Bldg. A
Elmsford, NY 10523
Ph: (914)345-5900
E-mail: help@mhawestchester.org
URL: http://www.mhawestchester.org/

Goshen

51140 ■ Mental Health Association in Orange County, Inc.
Help Line
20 John St.
Goshen, NY 10924
Ph: (845)294-7411
E-mail: mha@mhaorangeny.com
URL: http://www.mhaorangeny.com

Ithaca

51141 ■ Suicide Prevention and Crisis Service of Tompkins County
124 E Court St.
Ithaca, NY 14850
Ph: (607)272-1505
Fax: (607)272-1839
E-mail: info@suicidepreventionandcrisisservice.org
URL: http://suicidepreventionandcrisisservice.org/

Jamestown

51142 ■ Jones Memorial Health Center
Adult Mental Health Unit
Jamestown Crisis Line
207 Foote Ave.
Jamestown, NY 14701
Ph: (716)487-0140
Fax: (716)664-8607

New Paltz

51143 ■ Family of New Paltz
51 N Chestnut St.
New Paltz, NY 12561
Ph: (845)255-8801
Fax: (845)255-3498
E-mail: fnph@familyofwoodstockinc.org
URL: http://www.familyofwoodstockinc.org

51144 ■ State University College
Psychological Counseling Center
Deyo Hall G13c
1 Hawk Dr.
New Paltz, NY 12561
Ph: (845)257-4930
URL: http://www.newpaltz.edu/counseling/

New York

51145 ■ Covenant House-NineLine
460 W 41st St.
New York, NY 10036-6801
Ph: (212)613-0300

Free: 800-999-9999
E-mail: info@covenanthouseny.org
URL: http://www.covenanthouseny.org
Pauline Heslop, Director

51146 ■ The Samaritans of New York
PO Box 1259
New York, NY 10159
Ph: (212)673-3000
URL: http://www.samaritansnyc.org/

Niagara Falls

51147 ■ Niagara County Mental Health Hotline and Crisis Intervention
Trott Access Ctr.
1001 11th St.
Niagara Falls, NY 14301
Ph: (716)285-3518
URL: http://www.healthyniagara.com/

Plattsburgh

51148 ■ Crisis Center of Clinton, Essex, and Franklin Counties, Inc.
36 Brinkerhoff St.
Plattsburgh, NY 12901
Ph: (518)561-2330
Fax: (518)561-1813
E-mail: crisisline@aol.com
URL: http://www.nctrc.plattsburgh.edu/hrdirectory/agency.php?id=1865

Potsdam

51149 ■ REACHOUT of Saint Lawrence County, Inc.
PO Box 5051
Potsdam, NY 13676
Ph: (315)265-2422
Fax: (315)265-1752
URL: http://www.reachouthotline.org/

Poughkeepsie

51150 ■ The Dutchess County Department of Mental Hygiene Helpline
230 North Rd.
Poughkeepsie, NY 12601
Ph: (845)486-2896
E-mail: kmg@dcdmh.org
URL: http://www.co.dutchess.ny.us/CountyGov/Departments/Mentalhygiene/MHIndex.htm

Rochester

51151 ■ 2-1-1 Fingerlakes
1 Mt. Hope Ave.
Rochester, NY 14620
Ph: (716)423-9490
URL: http://www.211Fingerlakes.org
Formerly: Health Association of Rochester, Lifeline.

Stony Brook

51152 ■ Response of Suffolk County, Inc.
PO Box 300
Stony Brook, NY 11790
Ph: (631)751-7620
Fax: (631)751-7420
E-mail: info@responsehotline.org
URL: http://www.responsehotline.org

Utica

51153 ■ Saint Elizabeth Medical Center Crisis Evaluation Team
2209 Genesee St.
Utica, NY 13501
Ph: (315)798-8100
Fax: (315)734-3423
URL: http://www.stemc.org/healthcare_services/

Valhalla

51154 ■ Westchester Medical Center Behavioral Health Center Crisis Intervention Unit
Valhalla, NY 10595
Ph: (914)493-7075
Fax: (914)493-1553
URL: http://www.worldclassmedicine.com/home_specialty.cfm?id=60

Woodstock

51155 ■ Family of Woodstock
16 Rock City Rd.
Woodstock, NY 12498
Ph: (845)679-2485
Fax: (845)679-8490
E-mail: fowh@familyofwoodstockinc.org
URL: http://www.familyofwoodstockinc.org

NORTH CAROLINA

Ahoskie

51156 ■ Roanoke-Chowan Human Services Center
Rte. 2, Box 22-A
Ahoskie, NC 27910
Ph: (252)332-4137
Fax: (252)332-8457

Asheboro

51157 ■ Randolph Helpline
PO Box 4397
Asheboro, NC 27204
Ph: (336)625-5551
Free: 877-235-8177
URL: http://mharandolph.org/

Buies Creek

51158 ■ Lee-Harnett Emergency Crisis and Suicide Intervention Service
5841 US 421 S
Buies Creek, NC 27506
Ph: (910)893-2118

Burlington

51159 ■ Suicide and Crisis Service of Alamance County
319 N Graham-Hopedale Rd., Ste. a
Burlington, NC 27217
Ph: (336)513-4200
URL: http://www.acmhddsa.org

Chapel Hill

51160 ■ Crisis Central/OPC Area Program
412B Caldwell St.
Chapel Hill, NC 27516
Ph: (919)929-2528
URL: http://www.opcareaprogram.com/

Charlotte

51161 ■ Alexander Youth Nework--The Relatives, Inc.
PO Box 30186
Charlotte, NC 28203
Ph: (704)335-0203
Fax: (704)355-0207
URL: http://www.alexanderyouthnetwork.org

Clinton

51162 ■ Eastpointe Sampson County
207A W Main St.
Clinton, NC 28328
Free: 800-913-6109
URL: http://www.eastpointe.net/aboutus/crisiswalkin-centers.aspx

Clyde

51163 ■ Parents Against Teen Suicide/T.E.A.C.H.
81 Main St.
Clyde, NC 28721
Ph: (828)627-1001
Fax: (828)627-1005
URL: http://www.teachhotline.org

Durham

51164 ■ CONTACT Helpline--Durham
2706 N Roxboro Rd.
Durham, NC 27704
Ph: (919)220-2534

Goldsboro

51165 ■ Eastpointe Wayne County
1706 Wayne Memorial Dr.
Goldsboro, NC 27534
Free: 800-913-6109
URL: http://www.eastpointe.net/aboutus/crisiswalkin-centers.aspx

51166 ■ Wayne County Mental Health Center Hotline
301 N Herman St.
Goldsboro, NC 27530
Ph: (919)731-1133
Fax: (919)731-1333

Greensboro

51167 ■ Youth Focus, Inc.
Teen Crisis Line
301 E Washington St., Ste. 201
Greensboro, NC 27401
Ph: (336)333-6853
URL: http://www.youthfocus.org/

Greenville

51168 ■ REAL Crisis Intervention, Inc.
600 E 11th St.
Greenville, NC 27858
Ph: (252)946-0294
Fax: (252)758-0455
E-mail: realcrisis@embarqmail.com
URL: http://www.realcrisis.org

Hope Mills

51169 ■ CONTACT of Fayetteville, Inc.
3507 Hill St.
Hope Mills, NC 28348
Ph: (910)483-8970
E-mail: contactcrisishelp@gmail.com
URL: http://www.contactcrisishelp.com/

Lexington

51170 ■ Pastor's Pantry
208 E Center St.
Lexington, NC 27293
Ph: (336)249-8824
Fax: (336)249-8974
URL: http://www.taste-of-lexington.com/charities/pastors_pantry.php

Manteo

51171 ■ Outer Banks Hotline
PO Box 1490
Manteo, NC 27954
Ph: (252)473-5121
Fax: (252)473-9895
E-mail: info@obhotline.org
URL: http://www.obhotline.org/

Morehead

51172 ■ Helpline of Carteret County, Inc.
209 N 35th St.
Morehead, NC 28557
Ph: (252)240-0540

Raleigh

51173 ■ Hopeline
PO Box 20152
Raleigh, NC 27619
Ph: (919)231-7991
URL: http://www.hopeline-nc.org/

Roanoke

51174 ■ Halifax County Mental Health Roanoke Rapids Crisis Line
PO Box 1199
Roanoke, NC 27870
Ph: (252)537-2909
E-mail: glane@halifaxrmc.org

Roanoke Rapids

51175 ■ Riverstone Counseling and Personal Development
210 Smith Church Rd.
Roanoke Rapids, NC 27870
Ph: (252)537-6174

Salisbury

51176 ■ Salisbury Dial Help
165 Mahaley
Salisbury, NC 28144
Ph: (704)633-3616
Fax: (704)633-5902

Sanford

51177 ■ Lee County Mental Health Crisis Line
130 Carbonton Rd.
Sanford, NC 27330
Ph: (919)774-6521
Fax: (919)776-6179

Smithfield

51178 ■ Contact Johnston County
140 Market St.
Smithfield, NC 27577
Ph: (919)934-6979
Fax: (919)934-6979

Statesville

51179 ■ Counseling Center of Iredell
503 Brookdale Dr.
Statesville, NC 28677
Ph: (704)872-7638
Fax: (704)872-7639
E-mail: cci125@conninc.com
URL: http://www.unitedwayofiredell.org/partners.htm#CCI

Wilmington

51180 ■ Open House of Coastal Horizons Center, Inc.
Crisis Line
615 Shipyard Blvd.
Wilmington, NC 28412
Ph: (910)392-6936
URL: http://www.coastalhorizons.org

Wilson

51181 ■ Wilson Crisis Center
PO Box 8026
Wilson, NC 27893
Ph: (252)237-5156
URL: http://www.nc-van.org/directory/wilson/Wilson-CrisisCenter.html

Winston Salem

51182 ■ Contact Helpline of the Triad
851 W 5th St.
Winston Salem, NC 27101
Ph: (336)722-5153

NORTH DAKOTA

Bismarck

51183 ■ Mental Health America of North Dakota
PO Box 4106
Bismarck, ND 58502-4106
Ph: (701)255-3692
Free: 800-472-2911
Fax: (701)255-2411
E-mail: mharrv@juno.org
URL: http://www.mhand.org
Tom Regan, President (Acting)
Formerly: National Mental Health Association of North Dakota.

51184 ■ Mental Health Association in North Dakota (MHAND)
523 N 4th St.
Bismarck, ND 58502-4106
Ph: (701)255-3692
Fax: (701)255-2411
URL: http://www.mhand.org
Susan Helgeland, Executive Director
Formerly: North Dakota Mental Health Association.

51185 ■ West Central Human Service Center Crisis and Emergency Services
600 S 2nd St., Ste. 5
Bismarck, ND 58504
Ph: (701)255-3090
Fax: (701)328-8900

Devils Lake

51186 ■ Lake Region Human Service Center
200 Hwy. 2 SW
Devils Lake, ND 58301
Ph: (701)665-2200
E-mail: dhslrhsc@nd.gov
URL: http://www.nd.gov/dhs/locations/regionalhsc/lakeregion/index.html

Dickinson

51187 ■ Badlands Human Service Center
300 13th Ave. W, Ste. 1
Dickinson, ND 58601
Ph: (701)227-7500
Free: 888-227-7525
URL: http://www.nd.gov/dhs/locations/regionalhsc/badlands/index.html

Fargo

51188 ■ Hotline--Fargo
PO Box 447
Fargo, ND 58107
Ph: (701)293-6462
Fax: (701)237-0982

51189 ■ North Dakota Southeast Human Service Center
2624 9th Ave. SW
Fargo, ND 58103
Ph: (701)298-4500
URL: http://www.nd.gov/dhs/locations/regionalhsc/southeast/index.html

Grand Forks

51190 ■ Northeast Human Service Center
151 S 4th St., Ste. 401
Grand Forks, ND 58201
Ph: (701)795-3000
Free: 800-845-3731
Fax: (701)795-3050
E-mail: dhsnehsc@nd.gov
URL: http://www.nd.gov/dhs/locations/regionalhsc/northeast/index.html

Jamestown

51191 ■ South Central Human Service Center
520 3rd St. NW
Jamestown, ND 58402
Ph: (701)253-6300
Free: 800-260-1310
E-mail: dhsschsc@nd.gov
URL: http://www.nd.gov/dhs/locations/regionalhsc/southcentral/index.html

Minot

51192 ■ Trinity Mental Health Services Minot Suicide Prevention Service
407 3rd St. NE
Minot, ND 58701
Ph: (701)857-5000
Fax: (701)857-2187
URL: http://www.trinityhealth.org/
Formerly: Unimed Medical Center.

Valley City

51193 ■ Wellness in the Valley
570 Chautauqua Blvd.
Valley City, ND 58072
Ph: (701)845-6504
URL: http://www.wellnessinthevalley.com

Williston

51194 ■ Northwest Human Service Center
316 2nd Ave. W
Williston, ND 58802
Ph: (701)774-4600
Free: 800-231-7724
URL: http://www.nd.gov/dhs/locations/regionalhsc/northwest/index.html

OHIO

Akron

51195 ■ Portage Path Community Mental Health Center
10 Penfield Ave.
Akron, OH 44310
Ph: (330)434-1214
Fax: (330)434-2818
URL: http://www.portagepath.org

Athens

51196 ■ Tri-County Mental Health and Counseling Services
Careline
90 Hospital Dr.
Athens, OH 45701
Ph: (740)592-3091
URL: http://www.athensohio.com/community/index.php?page=216&item=1740

Bowling Green

51197 ■ The Link of Behavioral Connections
315 Thurstin Ave.
Bowling Green, OH 43402
Ph: (419)352-5387
Fax: (419)352-3430
URL: http://www.behavioralconnections.org/

Bucyrus

51198 ■ CONTACT Crawford County
PO Box 631
Bucyrus, OH 44820
Ph: (419)562-9099
URL: http://www.contactcrawfordcounty.org/

Caldwell

51199 ■ Six County, Inc.
Noble Counseling Center
44020 Marietta Rd.
Caldwell, OH 43724

Ph: (740)732-5233
Fax: (740)732-4777
E-mail: info@sixcounty.org
URL: http://www.sixcounty.org

Cambridge

51200 ■ Six County, Inc.
Noble Counseling Center
2500 John Glenn Hwy.
Cambridge, OH 43725
Ph: (740)439-4428
Fax: (740)439-3389
E-mail: info@sixcounty.org
URL: http://www.sixcounty.org

Canton

51201 ■ Crisis Intervention Center of Stark County, Inc.
2421 13th St. NW
Canton, OH 44708
Ph: (330)588-2204
URL: http://www.circstark.org/

Carrollton

51202 ■ Community Mental Healthcare, Inc.
Carrollton Office
331 W Main St.
Carrollton, OH 44615
Ph: (330)627-4313
Fax: (330)627-1141
E-mail: carrollton@cmhdover.org
URL: http://www.cmhdover.org/carrolltonoffice.html

Chillicothe

51203 ■ Scioto-Paint Valley Mental Health Center
Chillicothe Crisis Center
4449 State Rte. 159
Chillicothe, OH 45601
Ph: (740)775-1260
Fax: (740)773-8322
URL: http://www.spvmhc.org/poc/view_doc.php?type=doc&id=3195

Cincinnati

51204 ■ 281-CARE: Crisis Care Center
Talbert House
3891 Reading Rd.
Cincinnati, OH 45229
Ph: (513)281-2866
Fax: (513)281-9866

Cleveland

51205 ■ The Free Medical Clinic of Greater Cleveland
12201 Euclid Ave.
Cleveland, OH 44106
Ph: (216)721-4010
URL: http://www.thefreeclinic.org/

51206 ■ Mobile Crisis Team
1744 Payne Ave.
Cleveland, OH 44114
Ph: (216)623-6555
URL: http://mhs-inc.org/mobilecrisisteam.asp

Columbus

51207 ■ Ohio State University--Suicide Prevention Services
Younkin Success Ctr., 4th Fl.
1640 Neil Ave.
Columbus, OH 43210
Ph: (419)529-9941
URL: http://reach.osu.edu/help/

51208 ■ Suicide Prevention Services--Columbus
1301 N High St.
Columbus, OH 43201
Ph: (614)299-6600
Fax: (614)421-3111
E-mail: sps@ncmhs.org
URL: http://suicidepreventionservices.org/site/

Connellsville

51209 ■ Six County, Inc.
Morgan Counseling Center
915 S Riverside Dr.
Connellsville, OH 43756
Ph: (740)962-5204
E-mail: info@sixcounty.org
URL: http://www.sixcounty.org

Coshocton

51210 ■ Six County, Inc.
Coshocton Counseling Center
710 Main St.
Coshocton, OH 43812
Ph: (740)622-3404
Fax: (740)622-3412
E-mail: info@sixcounty.org
URL: http://www.sixcounty.org

Dayton

51211 ■ Samaritan Behavioral Health-- Crisis Care
Elizabeth Pl., NW Bldg., 1st Fl.
601 Edwin C. Moses Blvd.
Dayton, OH 45408
Ph: (937)224-4646
URL: http://www.sbhihelp.org/html/locations.htm

51212 ■ Samaritan Behavioral Health--Youth Resources
Elizabeth Pl., NW Bldg., 4th Fl.
601 Edwin C. Moses Blvd.
Dayton, OH 45408
Ph: (937)276-8333
URL: http://www.sbhihelp.org/html/locations.htm

51213 ■ Suicide Prevention Center--Dayton
PO Box 1393
Dayton, OH 45401
Ph: (937)226-0818
Fax: (937)837-2708
URL: http://www.suicidepreventioncenter.tk/

Delaware

51214 ■ HelpLine of Delaware and Morrow Counties, Inc.--Delaware
11 N Franklin St.
Delaware, OH 43015
Ph: (740)363-1835
Fax: (740)369-0358
E-mail: helpline@midohio.net
URL: http://www.helplinedelmor.org

Dover

51215 ■ Community Mental Healthcare, Inc.
Dover Office
201 Hospital Dr.
Dover, OH 44622
Ph: (330)343-6631
Fax: (330)343-8188
E-mail: cmh@cmhdover.org
URL: http://www.cmhdover.org/doveroffice.html

Eaton

51216 ■ Preble County Counseling Center Hotline
225 N Barron St.
Eaton, OH 45320
Ph: (937)456-6201
URL: http://mentalhealth.ohio.gov/

51217 ■ Samaritan Behavioral Health--Preble County
PO Box 267
Eaton, OH 45320
Ph: (937)456-1915
Free: 800-453-3386
URL: http://www.sbhihelp.org/html/locations.htm

Fairborn

51218 ■ The Community Network--Fairborn
600 Dayton-Yellow Springs Rd.
Fairborn, OH 45324
Ph: (937)879-3400
URL: http://www.tcn-bhs.org

Gallipolis

51219 ■ Woodland Centers, Inc.
3086 St. Rte. 160
Gallipolis, OH 45631
Ph: (740)446-5500
Fax: (740)441-4431
URL: http://www.woodlandcenters.org

Hopedale

51220 ■ Community Mental Health Services Inc.
400 Lahm Dr.
Hopedale, OH 43976
Ph: (740)695-0032

Kent

51221 ■ Townhall II Helpline
123 S Water St.
Kent, OH 44240
Ph: (330)678-4357
URL: http://www.townhall2.com/

Lancaster

51222 ■ Information and Crisis Service
PO Box 1054
Lancaster, OH 43130
Ph: (740)687-0500
Fax: (740)689-9827
URL: http://www.fairfieldcounty211.org/

Mansfield

51223 ■ Help Line/Adapt
741 Sholl Rd.
Mansfield, OH 44907
Ph: (419)756-1717
Fax: (419)756-5832
E-mail: info@cifscenter.org
URL: http://www.richlandthecenter.com/

Marion

51224 ■ Marion Area Counseling Center, Inc.
CONTACT Care Line
320 Executive Dr.
Marion, OH 43302
Ph: (740)387-5210
Fax: (740)383-3472
E-mail: info@maccsite.com
URL: http://www.maccsite.com/

Martins Ferry

51225 ■ Hillcrest of Ohio Valley Medical Center
9090 N 4th St.
Martins Ferry, OH 43935
Ph: (304)234-1666

Medina

51226 ■ Alternative Paths, Inc.
246 Northland Dr., Ste. 200A
Medina, OH 44256

Ph: (330)725-9195
Fax: (330)725-9187
E-mail: apgilroy@bright.net
URL: http://www.alternativepaths.org/

Mount Gilead

51227 ▪ HelpLine of Delaware and Morrow Counties, Inc.--Mount Gilead
950 Meadow Dr.
Mount Gilead, OH 43338
Ph: (419)946-1350
E-mail: outreach@helplinedelmor.org
URL: http://www.helplinedelmor.org/contactus.php

Napoleon

51228 ▪ First Call for Help, Inc.--Napoleon
600 Freedom Dr.
Napoleon, OH 43545
Ph: (419)599-1660
Fax: (419)592-8336
E-mail: firstcall@bright.net
URL: http://www.firstcallnwo.org

New Lexington

51229 ▪ Six County, Inc.
Perry Counseling Center
1375 Commerce Dr.
New Lexington, OH 43764
Ph: (740)342-5154
Fax: (740)342-6704
E-mail: info@sixcounty.org
URL: http://www.sixcounty.org

New Philadelphia

51230 ▪ Community Mental Healthcare, Inc.
New Philadelphia Office
567 Wabash Ave.
New Philadelphia, OH 44663
Ph: (330)343-3050
Fax: (330)343-3150
E-mail: newphila@cmhdover.org
URL: http://www.cmhdover.org/newphilaoffice.html

51231 ▪ Cornerstone Support Services
344 W High Ave.
New Philadelphia, OH 44663
Ph: (330)339-7850
Fax: (330)339-7844

Oxford

51232 ▪ Community Counseling and Crisis Center
110 S College Ave.
Oxford, OH 45056
Ph: (513)523-4149
Fax: (513)523-4145
URL: http://www.helpandhealing.org/

Toledo

51233 ▪ Rescue Mental Health Services
3350 Collingwood Blvd.
Toledo, OH 43610
Ph: (419)255-9585
Fax: (419)255-2801
URL: http://www.rescuemhs.com/

Warren

51234 ▪ CONTACT Community Connection
1569 Woodland NE, Ste. 10
Warren, OH 44483-5346
Ph: (330)395-5255
Fax: (330)395-9437

51235 ▪ Trumbull 2aa
320 High St. NE
Warren, OH 44481
Ph: (330)394-9090
E-mail: info@trumbull211.org
URL: http://www.trumbull211.org/

Xenia

51236 ▪ The Community Network--Xenia Greene County Crisis Services
452 W Market St.
Xenia, OH 45385
Ph: (937)376-8700
Fax: (937)376-8793
URL: http://www.tcn-bhs.org

Youngstown

51237 ▪ Help Hotline Crisis Center, Inc.
PO Box 46
Youngstown, OH 44501-0046
Ph: (330)747-5111
Fax: (330)747-4055
E-mail: hhcc@helphotline.org
URL: http://www.helphotline.org/

Zanesville

51238 ▪ Six County, Inc.
Crisis Hotline
2845 Bell St.
Zanesville, OH 43701
Ph: (740)454-9766
E-mail: info@sixcounty.org
URL: http://www.sixcounty.org

OKLAHOMA

Ada

51239 ▪ Southeastern Oklahoma 211 Helpline
PO Box 355
Ada, OK 74820
Ph: (580)427-4121
E-mail: harcher@wilnet1.com
URL: http://www.211seok.org/

Lawton

51240 ▪ United Way Helpline, Inc.
PO Box 66
Lawton, OK 73502
Ph: (580)355-0218
Fax: (580)355-0810
URL: http://www.uwlawton.org/

Oklahoma City

51241 ▪ Contact Telephone Helpline
PO Box 12832
Oklahoma City, OK 73157
Ph: (405)840-9396
Fax: (405)840-9552
URL: http://www.heartlineoklahoma.org

51242 ▪ Lighthouse Counseling Service Inc.
3837 NW 23rd St.
Oklahoma City, OK 73107
Ph: (405)942-8115
Fax: (405)942-1028
E-mail: lighthouse3837@spcglobal.net

51243 ▪ Oklahoma City Department of Mental Health
Teenline
PO Box 53277
Oklahoma City, OK 73152
Ph: (405)271-8336
Free: 800-522-8336
URL: http://www.odmhsas.org/hotlines.htm#ir1

Ponca City

51244 ▪ Helpline/Ponca City
PO Box 375
Ponca City, OK 74602
Ph: (580)765-5552

Tulsa

51245 ▪ Tulsa Helpline
PO Box 52847
Tulsa, OK 74152

Ph: (918)838-0195
E-mail: 211info@csctulsa.org
URL: http://www.211tulsa.org/

OREGON

Albany

51246 ▪ Linn County Crisis Services
445 3rd Ave. SW
Albany, OR 97321
Ph: (541)967-3866
Free: 800-304-7468
URL: http://www.co.linn.or.us/health/mental_health/mh_crisis.htm

Astoria

51247 ▪ Clatsop Behavioral Healthcare
2120 Exchange Street
Astoria, OR 97103
Ph: (503)325-5722
Fax: (503)325-8678
E-mail: health@co.clatsop.or.us
URL: http://www.clatsopbh.org/contact/
Remarks: Clinic serving all ages.

Baker City

51248 ▪ Mountain Valley Mental Health Programs, Inc.
Crisis Intervention
2200 4th St.
Baker City, OR 97814
Ph: (541)523-3646
E-mail: info@mvmhp.org
URL: http://www.mvmhp.org/

Bend

51249 ▪ Deschutes County Mental Health--Crisis Line
2577 NE Courtney Dr.
Bend, OR 97701
Ph: (541)322-7500
URL: http://www.co.deschutes.or.us/index.cfm?objectid=FFE263DF-874E-67E2-D350EB9AC8D999 A8

Corvallis

51250 ▪ Benton County Mental Health--Crisis Line
530 NW 27th St.
Corvallis, OR 97330
Ph: (541)766-6835
URL: http://www.co.benton.or.us/health/mentalhealth/adult.php

Dallas

51251 ▪ Sable House
PO Box 783
Dallas, OR 97338
Ph: (503)623-6703
Fax: (503)623-7971
URL: http://www.sablehouse.org

Eugene

51252 ▪ White Bird Clinic
341 E 12th St.
Eugene, OR 97401
Ph: (541)342-4357
URL: http://www.whitebirdclinic.org
Program(s): Community Health Center.

Grants Pass

51253 ▪ Helpline Referral Services
317 NW B St.
Grants Pass, OR 97526
Ph: (541)474-5446

51254 ■ Josephine County Mental Health
Grants Pass, OR
Ph: (541)474-5365
URL: http://www.co.josephine.or.us/SectionIndex.
asp?SectionID=116

Hillsboro

**51255 ■ Washington County Mental Health
Services**
155 N 1st Ave., Ste. 160
Hillsboro, OR 97124
Ph: (503)846-8881
URL: http://www.co.washington.or.us/HHS/Mental-
Health/

Hood River

51256 ■ Mid-Columbia Center for Living
1610 Woods Ct.
Hood River, OR 97031
Ph: (541)386-2620
E-mail: info@mccfl.org
URL: http://www.mccfl.org/

John Day

**51257 ■ Burns Paiute Reservation Health
Program
Suicide Prevention Service**
Grant County Community Health Department
528 E Main St.
John Day, OR 97845
Ph: (541)575-1466
Free: 541-575-3607

Lebanon

**51258 ■ Linn County Mental Health
Services--Crisis Services, Lebanon**
1600 S Main
Lebanon, OR 97355
Ph: (541)451-5932
Free: 888-451-2631
URL: http://www.co.linn.or.us/health/mental_health/
mh_crisis.htm

Medford

51259 ■ Centerpoint Crisis Line
801 O'Hare Pkwy., Ste. 101
Medford, OR 97504
Ph: (541)245-0789
Free: 866-287-0789
URL: http://www.centerpointonline.com/

51260 ■ Community Works Help Line
PO Box 819
Medford, OR 97501
Ph: (541)779-2393
Fax: (541)779-3317
URL: http://www.community-works.org

Milton-Freewater

51261 ■ Mental Health of Umatilla County
810 S Main St.
Milton-Freewater, OR 97862
Ph: (541)938-3988
URL: http://www.communityofcare.org/counties/uma-
tilla_mhp.htm

Ontario

51262 ■ Lifeways--Ontario
702 Sunset Dr.
Ontario, OR
Ph: (541)889-9167
Fax: (541)889-7873
URL: http://www.lifeways.org/

Portland

51263 ■ Oregon Partnership
6443 SW Beaverton-Hillsdale Hwy., Ste. 200
Portland, OR

Ph: (503)244-5211
URL: http://www.orpartnership.org/

Prinevile

**51264 ■ Lutheran Community Services
Northwest**
365 NE Court St.
Prineville, OR 97754
Ph: (541)447-7441
URL: http://www.lcsnw.org/offices/prineville.html

Saint Helens

**51265 ■ Columbia County Mental Health
Crisis Intervention**
58646 McNulty Way
Saint Helens, OR 97051
Ph: (503)397-5211
Free: 800-294-5211
URL: http://www.columbiacommunitymentalhealth.
com/

Salem

**51266 ■ Northwest Human Services--Crisis &
Information Hotline**
335 Belmont St. NE
Salem, OR 97301
Ph: (503)581-5535
Fax: (503)391-5291
URL: http://www.northwesthumanservices.org/

Sweet Home

**51267 ■ Linn County Mental Health
Services--Crisis Services, Sweet Home**
799 Long St.
Sweet Home, OR 97386
Ph: (541)367-3888
Free: 800-920-7571
URL: http://www.co.linn.or.us/health/mental_health/
mh_crisis.htm

The Dalles

51268 ■ Mid-Columbia Center for Living
419 E 7th St., Annex A
The Dalles, OR 97058
Ph: (541)296-5452
E-mail: info@mccfl.org
URL: http://www.mccfl.org/

Tillamook

51269 ■ Tillamook Family Counseling Center
906 Main Ave.
Tillamook, OR 97141
Ph: (503)842-8201
Free: 800-962-2851
Fax: (503)815-1870
E-mail: frankhw@tfcc.org
URL: http://www.tfcc.org/index.html

PENNSYLVANIA

Allentown

51270 ■ Crisis Intervention of Lehigh County
501 W Hamilton St.
Allentown, PA 18101
Ph: (610)820-3127

Altoona

**51271 ■ Altoona Hospital Center for Mental
Health Services**
620 Howard Ave.
Altoona, PA 16601
Ph: (814)946-2141
Fax: (814)949-3115
E-mail: info@altoonahospital.org
URL: http://www.altoonaregional.org/medicalser-
vices_behave.htm

51272 ■ CONTACT Altoona
Admin. Offices
2729 8th Ave.
Altoona, PA 16602
Ph: (814)946-9050
Fax: (814)946-4573
URL: http://www.contactaltoona.com
Paula J. Crew, Director
Description: Services offered: Crisis intervention or
hotline and referral. Office: (814)946-0531.

Bala Cynwyd

**51273 ■ Contact Careline for Greater
Philadelphia**
PO Box 2516
Bala Cynwyd, PA 19004-6516
Ph: (215)877-9099

Beaver

51274 ■ CONTACT Beaver Valley
PO Box 584
Beaver, PA 15009
Ph: (724)728-3650
Fax: (724)728-6830
E-mail: don.cbv@verizon.net
URL: http://contactbv.org/

Butler

**51275 ■ Center for Community Resources
Inc.**
111 Sunnyview Circle
Butler, PA 16001
Ph: (724)431-0242
Fax: (724)431-0099
URL: http://www.ccrinfo.org/

**51276 ■ Irene Stacy Community Mental
Health Center**
112 Hillvue Dr.
Butler, PA 16001
Ph: (724)287-0791
Fax: (724)287-2730
URL: http://www.irenestacy.com/

Camp Hill

**51277 ■ Holy Spirit Hospital
Crisis Intervention/Teenline**
503 N 21st St.
Camp Hill, PA 17011
Ph: (717)763-2219
Fax: (717)763-3040
URL: http://www.hsh.org/patients/services/our-
services.aspx

Cherry Tree

51278 ■ The Open Door--Cherry Tree
71 S Main St.
Cherry Tree, PA 15724
Ph: (724)465-2605
Fax: (724)425-2610
URL: http://www.theopendoor.org

Easton

**51279 ■ Northampton County Crisis
Intervention**
45 N 2nd St.
Easton, PA 18042
Ph: (610)252-9060
URL: http://www.northamptoncounty.org/northamp-
ton/cwp/view.asp?a=1528&Q=620679

Erie

51280 ■ Erie Hotline, Inc.
PO Box 6556
Erie, PA 16512
Ph: (814)453-2937
Fax: (814)454-0180

Gettysburg

51281 ■ Adams/Hanover Counseling Services, Inc.--Gettysburg
Crisis Intervention Program
44 S Franklin St.
Gettysburg, PA 17325
Ph: (717)334-9111
URL: http://ahcsinc.com/

Hanover

51282 ■ Adams/Hanover Counsel Service--Hanover
Crisis Intervention Program
625 W Elm Ave.
Hanover, PA 17331
Ph: (717)632-4900

Harrisburg

51283 ■ Contact Helpline--Harrisburg
PO Box 90035
Harrisburg, PA 17109-0035
Ph: (717)652-4987
Fax: (717)652-5017
E-mail: contact@paonline.com
URL: http://www.contacthelpline.org

51284 ■ Dauphin County Crisis Intervention
25 S Front St.
Harrisburg, PA 17101
Ph: (717)255-2705
Fax: (717)255-2960
E-mail: kstumpp@microserve.net
URL: http://www.dauphincounty.org/human-services/mental-health-retardation/crisis-inter vention/

Indiana

51285 ■ The Open Door--Indiana
334 Philadelphia St.
Indiana, PA 15701
Ph: (724)465-2605
Fax: (724)425-2610
URL: http://www.theopendoor.org

Lancaster

51286 ■ Contact Lancaster Helpline
447 E King St.
Lancaster, PA 17602
Ph: (717)291-2261
Fax: (717)291-6403
URL: http://www.contact-lancaster.org/

51287 ■ Lancaster County Helpline
Family Services
1120 Francis Ave.
Lancaster, PA 17601
Ph: (717)394-2631
Fax: (717)399-7357
URL: http://it.co.lancaster.pa.us/linc/ViewProgram.aspx?id=729&catid=833

Nanticoke

51288 ■ Northeast Counseling Services
130 W Washington St.
Nanticoke, PA 18634-3113
Ph: (717)735-7590
URL: http://www.northeastcounseling.org/

New Castle

51289 ■ CONTACT EARS HELPLINE
PO Box 7804
New Castle, PA 16107
Ph: (724)658-5529
URL: http://www.lawrencecountycares.org/ContactE-ARS.htm
Shirley J. Senko, Director
Description: Services offered: Counseling, crisis intervention or hotline, referral. Teen Talkline: (724)657-8255.

Norristown

51290 ■ Montgomery County Emergency Service Inc.
50 Beech Dr.
Norristown, PA 19403
Ph: (610)279-6100
Free: 800-452-4189
Fax: (610)279-0978
E-mail: mail@mces.org
URL: http://www.mces.org/

Philadelphia

51291 ■ Covenant House of Pennsylvania
31 E Armat St.
Philadelphia, PA 19144
Ph: (215)951-5411
URL: http://www.covenanthouse.org/programs/crisis-care

51292 ■ Philadelphia Suicide and Crisis Center
1101 Market, 7th Fl.
Philadelphia, PA 19107
Ph: (215)685-6440
Fax: (215)735-2508

Pittsburgh

51293 ■ Contact Pittsburgh, Inc.
PO Box 111294
Pittsburgh, PA 15238
Ph: (412)820-0100
E-mail: contact@contactpgh.org
URL: http://www.contactpgh.org

51294 ■ Helpline--Pittsburgh
c/o Carnagie Library of Pittsburgh
4400 Forbes Ave.
Pittsburgh, PA 15213
Ph: (412)578-2450
URL: http://www.unitedwaypittsburgh.org

Richboro

51295 ■ Contact Bucks County
PO Box 167
Richboro, PA 18954
Ph: (215)355-6611
Fax: (215)355-6824
URL: http://contactgreaterphiladelphia.org

Scranton

51296 ■ Telephone FIRST
Free Information and Referral System
Scranton Life Bldg.
538 Spruce St., Ste. 420
Scranton, PA 18503-1816
Ph: (570)961-1234
URL: http://www.vacnepa.org/

Tunkhannock

51297 ■ Counseling Services of Northeast Pennsylvania--Tunkhannock
99 Bridge St.
Tunkhannock, PA 18657
Ph: (570)836-3118
URL: http://www.bhswv.org/community_counseling.html

Upland

51298 ■ Delaware County Crisis Intervention--West Side
Crozer Medical Center
Upland, PA 19013
Ph: (610)565-6000
URL: http://www.crozer.org/

West Chester

51299 ■ Chester County Mental Health
Crisis Intervention Services
222 N Walnut St.
West Chester, PA 19380

Ph: (610)918-2100
URL: http://dsf.chesco.org/mhmr/cwp/view.asp?A=3&Q=607729

Wilkes Barre

51300 ■ Counseling Services of Northeast Pennsylvania--Wilkes Barre
110 S Pennsylvania Ave.
Wilkes Barre, PA 18701
Ph: (570)552-6000
URL: http://www.bhswv.org/community_counseling.html

51301 ■ Helpline--Wilkes Barre
1195 Hwy. 315
Wilkes Barre, PA 18702
Ph: (570)829-1341
Free: 888-829-1341

Williamsport

51302 ■ Williamsport YWCA Helpline
815 W 4th St.
Williamsport, PA 17701
Ph: (570)323-8555
Fax: (570)322-3029
URL: http://www.ywcawilliamsport.org/ywcawlmsprt/site/default.asp

York

51303 ■ CONTACT York
PO Box 1865
York, PA 17405
Ph: (717)854-9504
Fax: (717)843-5295

51304 ■ York Hospital
Crisis Intervention Services
1001 S George St.
York, PA 17405
Ph: (717)851-3156
Fax: (717)851-5324
URL: http://www.wellspan.org/body.cfm?id=416&oTopID=416

RHODE ISLAND

Coventry

51305 ■ NRI Community Services, Inc.
50 Wood St.
Coventry, RI 02816
Ph: (401)235-7121
URL: http://www.nricommunityservices.org/

Johnston

51306 ■ Gateway Healthcare--Adult Crisis Services
1443 Hartford Ave.
Johnston, RI 02919
Ph: (401)273-8100
URL: http://www.gatewayhealth.org/ad_crisis.asp

Middletown

51307 ■ Clinical Services for Youth
654 Green End Ave.
Middletown, RI 02842
Ph: (401)848-0758
URL: http://www.211ri.org/find/Details.aspx?OrgId=29717

Pawtucket

51308 ■ About Families CEDARR Center--Pawtucket
203 Concord St., Ste. 335
Pawtucket, RI 02860
Ph: (401)365-6855
E-mail: info@aboutfamilies.org
URL: http://www.aboutfamilies.org/

51309 ■ Gateway Healthcare--Adult Crisis Services
101-103 Bacon St.
Pawtucket, RI 02919
Ph: (401)722-3560
URL: http://www.gatewayhealth.org/ad_crisis.asp

51310 ■ Kid's Link Rhode Island
160 Beechwood Ave.
Pawtucket, RI 02860
Ph: (401)722-5573
URL: http://www.sprc.org/stateinformation/statep-ages/showstate.asp?stateID=39

Providence

51311 ■ Samaritans of Rhode Island
2 Magee St.
Providence, RI 02906
Ph: (401)272-4243
Fax: (401)272-4516
URL: http://www.samaritansri.org/

51312 ■ United Way 211 in Rhode Island
50 Valley St.
Providence, RI 02909
Ph: (401)444-0600
E-mail: 211info@uwri.org
URL: http://www.211ri.org/

Wakefield

51313 ■ Sympatico
57 Columbia St.
Wakefield, RI 02879
Ph: (401)783-0782
Fax: (401)783-1154

Woonsocket

51314 ■ About Families CEDARR Center--Woonsocket
1 Cumberland St., 4th Fl.
Woonsocket, RI 02895
Ph: (401)671-6533
E-mail: info@aboutfamilies.org
URL: http://www.aboutfamilies.org/

SOUTH CAROLINA

Aiken

51315 ■ Aiken--Barnwell Mental Health Center
1135 Gregg Hwy.
Aiken, SC 29801
Ph: (803)641-7700
URL: http://www.state.sc.us/dmh/ab/index.html

51316 ■ Aiken County Help Line, Inc.
1579 Edgefield Hwy.
Aiken, SC 29802
Ph: (803)641-4143
Free: 866-648-9900
Fax: (803)641-4169
URL: http://www.aikenhelpline211.org/main/

Allendale

51317 ■ Coastal Empire Community Mental Health Center--Allendale Crisis Intervention Center
438 Barnwell Rd.
Allendale, SC 29810
Ph: (803)584-4636
URL: http://www.cecmhc.org/services.htm

Anderson

51318 ■ Anderson-Oconee-Pickens Mental Health Center Teen Suicide Prevention
200 McGee Rd.
Anderson, SC 29625
Ph: (864)260-2220
URL: http://www.aopmentalhealth.org/

51319 ■ Crisis Ministries
PO Box 1925
Anderson, SC 29622
Ph: (864)226-0297
Fax: (864)224-4873

Beaufort

51320 ■ Coastal Empire Community Mental Health Center--Beaufort Crisis Intervention Center
1050 Ribaut Rd.
Beaufort, SC 29902
Ph: (843)524-3378
URL: http://www.cecmhc.org/services.htm

Charleston

51321 ■ Charleston Dorchester Mental Health Center Assessment/Mobile Crisis
2100 Charlie Hall Blvd.
Charleston, SC 29414
Ph: (843)414-2350
URL: http://www.cdcmhc.org/

Columbia

51322 ■ Columbia Area Mental Health Services Adult Crisis Services
10 Medical Park
1618 Sunset Dr.
Columbia, SC 29203
Ph: (803)898-4800
URL: http://www.state.sc.us/dmh/cmhc.htm

51323 ■ Helpline of the Midlands, Inc.
PO Box 6336
Columbia, SC 29260
Ph: (803)782-3771
Free: 866-892-9211

51324 ■ Impact
1800 Colonial Dr.
Columbia, SC 29202
Ph: (803)898-9835
Fax: (803)898-2194
URL: http://www.state.sc.us/dmh/cmhc.htm

51325 ■ United Way of the Midlands
1800 Main St.
Columbia, SC 29201
Ph: (803)733-7312
E-mail: info@uway.org
URL: http://www.uway.org
Mr. Mac Bennett, President

Conway

51326 ■ Coastal Carolina Hospital
152 Waccamaw Medical Park Dr.
Conway, SC 29526
Ph: (803)347-7156

Florence

51327 ■ Pee Dee Mental Health Center Adult Crisis Services
125 E Cheves St.
Florence, SC 29506
Ph: (843)317-4089
Fax: (843)317-4096
URL: http://www.state.sc.us/dmh/peedee/

51328 ■ Pee Dee Mental Health Center Child Crisis Services
125 E Cheves St.
Florence, SC 29506
Ph: (843)317-4073
Fax: (843)317-4080
URL: http://www.state.sc.us/dmh/peedee/

Gaffney

51329 ■ Helpline--Gaffney
PO Box 1231
Gaffney, SC 29342
Ph: (864)487-4357

Greenville

51330 ■ Greenville Mental Health Center Crisis Intervention
124 Mallard St.
Greenville, SC 29601
Ph: (864)241-1040
URL: http://www.greenvillementalhealth.org/

51331 ■ Mental Health America of Greenville County
429 N Main St., Ste. 2
Greenville, SC 29601
Ph: (864)467-3344
Fax: (864)467-3547
E-mail: mhagc@mhagc.org
URL: http://www.mhagc.org
Eric Wall, President

Greenwood

51332 ■ Beckman Center--Crisis Intervention
1547 Parkway, Ste. 100
Greenwood, SC 29646
Ph: (864)229-7120
Fax: (864)229-5526
URL: http://www.beckmancenter.com/

Hilton Head

51333 ■ Coastal Empire Community Mental Health Center--Hilton Head Crisis Intervention Center
151 Dillon Rd.
Hilton Head, SC 29925
Ph: (843)681-4865
URL: http://www.cecmhc.org/services.htm

51334 ■ HelpLine--Hilton Head
PO Box 22538
Hilton Head, SC 29925
Ph: (843)681-6420

Moncks Corner

51335 ■ Berkeley Community Mental Health Center
PO Box 1030
Moncks Corner, SC 29461
Ph: (843)761-8282
URL: http://www.bcmhc.org/

North Charleston

51336 ■ Trident United Way's 211 Hotline
PO Box 63305
North Charleston, SC 29419
Ph: (843)747-3007
Fax: (843)566-7193
E-mail: 211@tuw.org

Ridgeland

51337 ■ Coastal Empire Community Mental Health Center--Ridgeland Crisis Intervention Center
1510 Grays Hwy.
Ridgeland, SC 29936
Ph: (843)726-8030
URL: http://www.cecmhc.org/services.htm

Simpsonville

51338 ■ Piedmont Mental Health Clinic
20 Powderhorn Rd.
Simpsonville, SC 29681
Ph: (864)271-8888
URL: http://www.pcmhs.org/

Varnville

**51339 ■ Coastal Empire Community Mental
Health Center--Varnville
Crisis Intervention Center**
65 Forrest Dr.
Varnville, SC 29944
Ph: (803)943-2828
URL: http://www.cecmhc.org/services.htm

Walterboro

**51340 ■ Coastal Empire Community Mental
Health Center--Walterboro
Crisis Intervention Center**
507 Forest Cir.
Walterboro, SC 29488
Ph: (843)549-1551
URL: http://www.cecmhc.org/services.htm

SOUTH DAKOTA

Huron

**51341 ■ Community Counseling
Services--Care Program**
357 Kansas Ave. SE
Huron, SD 57350
Ph: (605)352-8596
URL: http://www.ccs-sd.org/pages/care.htm

Lake Andes

**51342 ■ Lewis & Clark Behavioral Health
Services, Inc.--Lake Andes
CARE Program & Crisis Intervention**
51 S 3rd
Lake Andes, SD 57356
Ph: (605)487-6082
URL: http://www.lcbhs.com/outpatient.shtml

Madison

**51343 ■ Community Counseling
Services--Care Program**
914 NE 3rd St.
Madison, SD 57042
Ph: (605)256-9656
URL: http://www.ccs-sd.org/pages/care.htm

Mitchell

**51344 ■ Dakota Counseling Institute
C.A.R.E. Services & Crisis Intervention**
910 W Havens
Mitchell, SD 57301
Ph: (605)996-9686
URL: http://www.dakotacounseling.com/services.html

Pierre

51345 ■ Capital Area Counseling Service
803 E Dakota Ave.
Pierre, SD 57501
Ph: (605)224-5811
URL: http://www.cacsnet.org

Rapid City

**51346 ■ Behavior Management Systems
Crisis Intervention and Suicide Stabilization**
350 Elk St.
Rapid City, SD 57701
Ph: (605)343-7262
E-mail: info@behaviormanagement.org
URL: http://www.behaviormanagement.org

Sioux Falls

51347 ■ Avera Behavioral Health Center
800 E 21st St.
Sioux Falls, SD 57117
Ph: (605)224-3100
URL: http://www.averamckennan.org/amck/abhc/
conditions/Adult-Senior/adult_riskofsuicide

**51348 ■ Volunteer Information
Center/HELPLINE**
1000 N West Ave., Ste. 310
Sioux Falls, SD 57104
Ph: (605)334-6646
Fax: (605)332-1333
E-mail: helpline@helplinecenter.org
URL: http://www.helplinecenter.org

Vermillion

**51349 ■ Lewis & Clark Behavioral Health
Services, Inc.--Vermillion
CARE Program & Crisis Intervention**
28 E Cherry St.
Vermillion, SD 57069
Ph: (605)624-9148
URL: http://www.lcbhs.com/outpatient.shtml

Yankton

**51350 ■ Lewis & Clark Behavioral Health
Services, Inc.--Yankton
CARE Program & Crisis Intervention**
1028 Walnut St.
Yankton, SD 57078
Ph: (605)665-4606
URL: http://www.lcbhs.com/outpatient.shtml

TENNESSEE

Athens

51351 ■ McMinn/Meigs/Monroe CONTACT
PO Box 69
Athens, TN 37371-0069
Ph: (423)745-1042
Fax: (423)745-4292

Chattanooga

51352 ■ Contact of Chattanooga
6221 Vance Rd.
Chattanooga, TN 37421-2979
Ph: (423)899-5719
Fax: (423)899-5814
URL: http://contactofchattanoogahelpline.org/

Clarksville

**51353 ■ Clarksville/Montgomery County
Crisis Intervention Center**
PO Box 212
Clarksville, TN 37041
Ph: (931)647-8099
URL: http://www.tennhelp.com/tennHelpView?th_
id=3453

Hendersonville

51354 ■ Jason Foundation Inc.
116 Maple Row Blvd., Ste. C
Hendersonville, TN 37075
Ph: (615)264-2323
Free: 888-881-2323
URL: http://www.jasonfoundation.com/

Johnson City

51355 ■ Contact Ministries
PO Box 1403
Johnson City, TN 37605
Ph: (423)926-0140
Fax: (423)926-0145
URL: http://www.contactministries.org

**51356 ■ Frontier Health
Crisis Helpline**
200 W Fairview Ave.
Johnson City, TN 37604
Ph: (423)467-3600
URL: http://www.frontierhealth.org/
Formerly: Woodbridge Hospital.

Kingsport

**51357 ■ CONTACT-CONCERN of Northeast
Tennessee, Inc.**
PO Box 3336
Kingsport, TN 37664
Ph: (423)247-7763
Fax: (423)247-7761
E-mail: contactconcern@chartertn.net
URL: http://www.contactconcern.org
D. Lynn Sorrell, Executive Director

Knoxville

51358 ■ Contact Telephone of Knoxville
PO Box 11234
Knoxville, TN 37939-1234
Ph: (423)523-9108
Fax: (423)521-7797

**51359 ■ Helen Ross McNabb Center
Adult Services**
1520 Cherokee Trl.
Knoxville, TN 37920
Ph: (865)637-9711
Free: 800-255-9711
Fax: (865)637-1278
URL: http://www.mcnabbcenter.org/

51360 ■ Mobile Crisis Unit
104 Suburban
Knoxville, TN 37919
Ph: (423)584-9911
URL: http://www.peninsulabehavioralhealth.org/
?id=1689&sid=15

51361 ■ Overlook Mobile Crisis Unit
3001 Lakebrook Blvd.
Knoxville, TN 37909
Ph: (423)588-2933

Memphis

51362 ■ The Crisis Center
PO Box 40068
Memphis, TN 38174
Ph: (901)276-1111
Fax: (901)726-9505

51363 ■ Lakeside Behavioral System
2911 Brunswick Rd.
Memphis, TN 38133
Ph: (901)377-4700
URL: http://www.lakesidebhs.com/

Nashville

**51364 ■ Centerstone Community Health
Centers, Inc.**
633 Thompson Ln.
Nashville, TN 37204-0406
Ph: (615)460-4372
Fax: (615)460-4434
URL: http://centerstone.org

51365 ■ Crisis Intervention Center
PO Box 40752
Nashville, TN 37204-0752
Ph: (615)298-3359
URL: http://www.fcsnashville.org

Oak Ridge

51366 ■ CONTACT Helpline, Inc.
PO Box 4641
Oak Ridge, TN 37831-4641
Ph: (865)482-5040
Fax: (865)482-5040
E-mail: contact@contact-helpline.org
URL: http://www.discoveret.org/orhelp/

Tullahoma

51367 ■ Tullahoma CONTACT Life Line
PO Box 1614
Tullahoma, TN 37388
Ph: (931)455-7150
Fax: (931)455-3440
E-mail: contactlifeline@mudtnn.net

TEXAS

Abilene

51368 ■ Betty Hardwick Center: A Community Mental Health Resource
2616 S Clack
Abilene, TX 79606
Ph: (325)690-5100
Fax: (325)690-5136
URL: http://www.bhcmhmr.org

51369 ■ Mental Health Association in Abilene (MHAA)
500 Chestnut, Ste. 1807
Abilene, TX 79602
Ph: (325)673-2300
Free: 800-273-TALK
Fax: (325)673-2671
E-mail: mhaa@bitstreet.com
URL: http://www.abilenementalhealth.org
Kirk W. Hancock, Executive Director

Amarillo

51370 ■ Texas Panhandle Mental Health Authority
1501 S Polk St.
Amarillo, TX 79116
Ph: (806)359-2025
URL: http://www.tpmhmr.org

Athens

51371 ■ East Texas Crisis Center--Athens
PO Box 847
Athens, TX 75751
Ph: (903)675-2137
URL: http://www.etcc.org

Austin

51372 ■ Austin-Travis Counties Mental Health Center
Hotline to Help
PO Box 3548
Austin, TX 78764-3548
Ph: (512)703-1300
Fax: (512)703-1394
URL: http://www.atcmhmr.com

Beaumont

51373 ■ Crisis Center of Southeast Texas
PO Box 5011
Beaumont, TX 77726
Ph: (409)832-6530
Fax: (409)832-4324
URL: http://www.rapesuicidebeaumont.org/web/default.aspx
Formerly: Rape and Suicide Crisis of Southeast Texas.

Clarendon

51374 ■ Suicide Prevention--Clarendon
111 S Kearny
Clarendon, TX 79226
Ph: (806)874-3504

Conroe

51375 ■ Montgomery County United Way
Tri County Mental Health Dept.
Conroe, TX 77301
Ph: (936)525-2700
URL: http://www.mcuw.org/index.cfm?fuseaction=needhelp.main

Dallas

51376 ■ CONTACT Counseling and Crisis Line
PO Box 800742
Dallas, TX 75380-0742
Ph: (972)233-0866
Fax: (972)233-2427
URL: http://www.contactdallas.org

51377 ■ Suicide and Crisis Center--Dallas
2808 Swiss Ave.
Dallas, TX 75204
Ph: (214)828-1000
Fax: (214)828-1627
URL: http://www.sccenter.org

Fort Worth

51378 ■ Mental Health/Mental Retardation of Tarrant County
3840 Hulen St., N Tower
Fort Worth, TX 76107
Ph: (817)569-4300
URL: http://www.mhmrtc.org/MHSD/

Graham

51379 ■ Helen Farabee Regional MHMR Center
1720 4th St.
Graham, TX 76450
Ph: (940)549-4896
URL: http://www.helenfarabee.org

Houston

51380 ■ Crisis Intervention of Houston, Inc.
PO Box 130866
Houston, TX 77219
Ph: (713)527-9864
Fax: (713)527-0435
URL: http://www.crisishotline.org

51381 ■ Cypress Creek Hospital
17750 Cali Dr.
Houston, TX 77090
Ph: (281)586-7600
Fax: (281)586-5925
URL: http://www.psysolutions.com/facilities/cypress-creek/

51382 ■ Intracare Hospital
7601 Fannin
Houston, TX 77054
Ph: (713)790-0949
Fax: (713)790-0456
URL: http://www.intracarehospital.com/

51383 ■ Mental Health/Mental Retardation Association of Harris County NeuroPsychiatric Center
1502 Taub Loop
Houston, TX 77030
Ph: (713)970-7020
URL: http://www.mhmraharris.org/

51384 ■ West Oaks Hospital
6500 Hornwood
Houston, TX 77074
Ph: (713)995-0909
Fax: (713)778-5253
URL: http://www.psysolutions.com/facilities/westoaks/

Laredo

51385 ■ Lifeline of Laredo, Inc.
1803 Juarez Ave.
Laredo, TX 78040
Ph: (956)722-0063

Lubbock

51386 ■ Contact Lubbock
PO Box 6477
Lubbock, TX 79493-6477
Ph: (806)765-7272
Free: 800-886-4351
Fax: (806)765-7209
URL: http://www.contactlubbock.org

51387 ■ Lubbock Regional MHMR Center
1602 10th St.
Lubbock, TX 79408
Ph: (806)766-0310
Fax: (806)766-0250
URL: http://www.lubbockmhmr.org

Midland

51388 ■ Permian Basin Community Centers
401 E Illinois
Midland, TX 79701
Ph: (915)570-3333
Fax: (915)570-3346
URL: http://www.pbmhmr.com

Plainview

51389 ■ Central Plains Center Crisis Hotline
Plainview, TX
Ph: (806)296-2726
URL: http://www.clplains.org

Richardson

51390 ■ Texas Council on Problem and Compulsive Gambling
PO Box 835895
Richardson, TX 75083
Ph: (972)889-2331
Fax: (972)889-2383
E-mail: tcpcg@ruff.com
URL: http://www.problemgambling.com/links.html#

Richmond

51391 ■ Fort Bend County Women's Center
PO Box 183
Richmond, TX 77406
Ph: (281)344-5750
Fax: (281)232-5041
E-mail: mail@fortbendwomenscenter.org
URL: http://fortbendwomenscenter.org
Vita Rogers, Executive Director

San Angelo

51392 ■ Concho Valley Crisis Hotline
244 N Magdalen
San Angelo, TX 76903
Ph: (325)655-8965
URL: http://www.mhmrcv.org

San Antonio

51393 ■ United Way of San Antonio Information and Referral Department
700 S Alamo
San Antonio, TX 78205
Ph: (210)352-7000
E-mail: helpline@unitedwaysatx.org
URL: http://www.unitedwaysatx.org

Tyler

51394 ■ East Texas Crisis Center--Tyler
PO Box 7060
Tyler, TX 75711
Ph: (903)509-2526
Fax: (903)509-2283
URL: http://www.etcc.org

Victoria

51395 ■ Gulf Bend Center
6502 Nursery Dr., Ste. 100
Victoria, TX 77904
Ph: (361)575-0611

Free: 800-421-8825
Fax: (361)578-0506
URL: http://www.gulfbend.org

51396 ■ Hope of South Texas
2701 N Azalea, Ste. 24
Victoria, TX 77902
Ph: (361)573-5868
Fax: (361)573-5913

Wichita Falls

51397 ■ Concern, Inc.
PO Box 1945
Wichita Falls, TX 76307
Ph: (817)723-8231

51398 ■ Helen Farabee Regional MHMR Center
1000 Brook
Wichita Falls, TX 76301
Ph: (940)397-3143
URL: http://www.helenfarabee.org

UTAH

Magna

51399 ■ England Counseling Services
3564 S 7200 West
Magna, UT 84044
Ph: (801)250-2909

Midvale

51400 ■ Valley Mental Health--Midvale
7434 S State St.
Midvale, UT 84047
Ph: (801)566-4423
URL: http://www.vmh.com

Murray

51401 ■ Valley Mental Health--Murray
5965 S 900 East
Murray, UT 84121
Ph: (801)273-6395
URL: http://www.vmh.com

Orem

51402 ■ Utah County Crisis Line
PO Box 1493
Orem, UT 84059
Ph: (801)226-4433
Fax: (801)226-2578
URL: http://www.unitedwayuc.org/crisisline/faq.htm

Park City

51403 ■ Valley Mental Health--Park City
1753 Sidewinder Dr.
Park City, UT 84060
Ph: (435)649-9079
URL: http://www.vmh.com

Provo

51404 ■ Wasatch Mental Health Crisis Line
750 N Freedom Blvd.
Provo, UT 84601
Ph: (801)373-4760
URL: http://www.wasatch.org

Salt Lake City

51405 ■ Suicide Prevention--Crisis Center, Salt Lake City
3944 S 400 East
Salt Lake City, UT 84107
Ph: (801)261-1442

51406 ■ Valley Mental Health Crisis Service--Salt Lake City
1020 S Main, Ste. 100
Salt Lake City, UT 84101
Ph: (801)539-7000
URL: http://www.vmh.com

Tooele

51407 ■ Valley Mental Health--Tooele
100 S 1000 West
Tooele, UT 84074
Ph: (435)843-3520
URL: http://www.vmh.com

VERMONT

Brattleboro

51408 ■ Healthcare and Rehabilitation Service of Southeast Vermont
HELPLINE
4 High St., Ste. 6
Brattleboro, VT 05301
Ph: (802)257-7989
Fax: (802)257-4715
E-mail: helpline@sover.net
URL: http://www.unitedwaywindham.org

Randolph

51409 ■ Clara Martin Center
Emergency Services
PO Box G
Randolph, VT 05060
Ph: (802)728-4466
Fax: (802)728-4197
E-mail: claramartin@connriver.net
URL: http://www.claramartin.org/

Saint Albans

51410 ■ Northwestern Counseling & Support Services, Inc.
8 Ferris St.
Saint Albans, VT 05478
Ph: (802)524-6554
Fax: (802)527-7801
E-mail: info@ncssinc.org
URL: http://www.ncssinc.org/

VIRGINIA

Alexandria

51411 ■ MHMRSA of Alexandria
720 N St. Asaph St.
Alexandria, VA 22314
Ph: (703)746-3400
URL: http://alexandriava.gov/mhmrsa/info/default.aspx?id=2472

Arlington

51412 ■ Northern Virginia Hotline
PO Box 7563
Arlington, VA 22207-0563
Ph: (703)527-6603
Fax: (703)516-6767
E-mail: info@crisislink.org
URL: http://www.crisislink.org

Belle Haven

51413 ■ Eastern Shore Community Services Board
Emergency Services
10106 Pine Ave.
Belle Haven, VA 23306
Ph: (757)442-7707

Blacksburg

51414 ■ New River Valley Community Services
ACCESS Services
700 University City Blvd.
Blacksburg, VA 24060

Ph: (540)961-8300
Fax: (540)961-8469
URL: http://www.nrvcs.org/

Bristol

51415 ■ Crisis Center--Bristol
PO Box 642
Bristol, VA 24203
Ph: (276)466-2218
Fax: (276)466-5481
E-mail: srsnake@crisiscenterinc.org
URL: http://www.crisiscenterinc.org

Charlottesville

51416 ■ Madison House
170 Rugby Rd.
Charlottesville, VA 22903
Ph: (434)977-7051
Fax: (434)977-7339
URL: http://scs.student.virginia.edu/~madison/

Chester

51417 ■ Chesterfield County Crisis Intervention
6801 Lucy Corr Ct.
Chester, VA 23831
Ph: (804)748-1227
URL: http://www.chesterfield.gov/content.aspx?id=3192

Danville

51418 ■ Contact Crisis Line of Danville/Pittsylvania County
PO Box 41
Danville, VA 24543
Ph: (804)793-4940
Fax: (804)792-4359

Dumfries

51419 ■ ACTS Helpline
PO Box 74
Dumfries, VA 22026
Ph: (703)368-4141
Fax: (703)368-6544
URL: http://www.actspwc.org/

Lynchburg

51420 ■ Crisis Line of Central Virginia
PO Box 3074
Lynchburg, VA 24503
Ph: (804)947-5921
Fax: (804)947-5501
URL: http://www.crisislineofcentralvirginia.org/

Martinsville

51421 ■ Contact Martinsville/Henry County
PO Box 1287
Martinsville, VA 24114
Ph: (276)638-8980
URL: http://www.contactmartinsville.org/

Norfolk

51422 ■ The Crisis Line of The Planning Counsel
130 W Plume St., Ste. 400
Norfolk, VA 23510
Ph: (757)622-1256
URL: http://www.theplanningcouncil.org/

Portsmouth

51423 ■ Suicide--Crisis Center, Inc.
PO Box 7428
Portsmouth, VA 23707
Ph: (757)393-0502

Richmond

51424 ■ West End Behavioral Healthcare System
12800 W Creek Pkwy.
Richmond, VA 23238
Ph: (804)819-4000
Fax: (804)819-4263

Winchester

51425 ■ Concern Hotline, Inc.
PO Box 2032
Winchester, VA 22601
Ph: (540)667-8208
Fax: (540)667-8239
URL: http://www.concernhotline.com

51426 ■ Crisis Care of Winchester Medical Center
1890 Amherst St.
Winchester, VA 22601
Ph: (540)536-8140
Fax: (540)536-8139
URL: http://www.valleyhealthlink.com/?id=315&sid=1

Woodbridge

51427 ■ Community Mental Health and Substance Abuse Services Board Prevention Division
15941 Cardinal Dr.
Woodbridge, VA 22191
Ph: (703)792-4900
URL: http://www.co.prince-william.va.us/default.aspx-?topic=010009000890000647

WASHINGTON

Bellingham

51428 ■ Whatcom County Mental Health Program
509 Girard St.
Bellingham, WA 98225
Ph: (360)676-6724
URL: http://www.co.whatcom.wa.us/health/human/mental_health/index.jsp

Bremerton

51429 ■ Crisis Clinic of Kitsap County
5455 Almira Dr. NE
Bremerton, WA 98311
Ph: (360)415-5816
Fax: (360)415-5891
URL: http://crisisclinicofthepeninsulas.org/

Cathlamet

51430 ■ Wahkiakum County Mental Health
42 Elochoman Valley Rd.
Cathlamet, WA 98612
Ph: (360)795-8630
Fax: (360)795-6224
URL: http://www.co.wahkiakum.wa.us/depts/health/MentalHealthServices.htm

Chehalis

51431 ■ Human Response Network
125 NW Chehalis Ave., PO Box 337
Chehalis, WA 98532
Ph: (360)748-6601
Free: 800-244-7414
Fax: (360)748-6630
E-mail: info@hrnlc.org
URL: http://www.hrnlc.org/

Clarkston

51432 ■ Rogers Counseling Center
900 7th St.
Clarkston, WA 99403
Ph: (509)758-3341

Free: 888-475-5665
Fax: (509)758-8009
URL: http://www.qualitybehavioralhealth.com/

51433 ■ YWCA Crisis Services--Clarkston
Clarkston, WA 99403
Ph: (208)743-1535
E-mail: ywcacs@lewiston.com
URL: http://www.ywcaidaho.org/Contact.htm

Colville

51434 ■ NorthEast Washington Alliance Counseling Services--Colville
165 E Hawthorne Ave.
Colville, WA 99114
Ph: (509)684-4597
Fax: (509)684-5286
URL: http://www.co.stevens.wa.us/counseling/index.htm
Formerly: Stevens County Counseling Services.

Davenport

51435 ■ Lincoln County Counseling Center
PO Box 278
Davenport, WA 99122
Ph: (509)725-3001
Fax: (509)725-1609
E-mail: jlippold@co.lincoln.wa.us

Dayton

51436 ■ Blue Mountain Counseling of Columbia County
221 E Washington St.
Dayton, WA 99328
Ph: (509)382-1164
Fax: (509)382-1164
URL: http://bmc.homestead.com/

Ellensburg

51437 ■ Crisis Line of Kittitas County
110 W 6th Ave.
Ellensburg, WA 98926
Ph: (509)925-2881
Fax: (509)925-2166
E-mail: crisisln@eburg.com

51438 ■ Ellensburg Crisis Line
507 Nanum
Ellensburg, WA 98926
Ph: (509)925-2166

Ephrata

51439 ■ North Central Washington Regional Support Network
119 Basin St. SW
Ephrata, WA 98823
Ph: (509)754-6577
Free: 800-251-5350
URL: http://www.dshs.wa.gov/mentalhealth/ncentral.shtml

Everett

51440 ■ Snohomish County Mental Health Services
Crisis Intervention and Referral
Care Crisis Response Services
Everett, WA 98201
Ph: (425)258-4357
URL: http://www.voaww.org

51441 ■ Volunteers of America
Care Crisis Line
PO Box 839
Everett, WA 98206-0839
Ph: (425)259-3191
Free: 800-747-8654
Fax: (425)259-3073
URL: http://www.voaww.org

Friday Harbor

51442 ■ North Islands Counseling and Psychotherapy
Crisis Service
PO Box 247
Friday Harbor, WA 98250
Ph: (360)378-2669
Fax: (360)378-5669

Grandview

51443 ■ Yakima Valley Farm Workers Clinic--Grandview
Child & Adolescent Crisis Intervention
1000 Wallace Way
Grandview, WA 98930
Ph: (509)882-3444
Free: 800-500-0934
URL: http://www.yvfwc.com/yakima_bhs.html

Hoquiam

51444 ■ Evergreen Counseling Center
205 8th St.
Hoquiam, WA 98550
Ph: (360)532-8629
Free: 800-548-0558
Fax: (360)538-0124
URL: http://karisable.com/ghc/mh.htm

Kennewick

51445 ■ Benton and Franklin Counties Crisis Response Unit
2635 W Deschutes Ave.
Kennewick, WA 99336
Ph: (509)783-0500

51446 ■ Greater Columbia Behavioral Health RSN
101 N Edison St.
Kennewick, WA 99336
Free: 800-795-9296
URL: http://www.gcbh.org/

Lakewood

51447 ■ Greater Lakes Mental Healthcare
9330 59th Ave. SW
Lakewood, WA 98499
Ph: (253)581-7020
URL: http://www.glmhc.org/

Long Beach

51448 ■ Willapa Counseling Center--Long Beach
PO Box 863
Long Beach, WA 98631
Ph: (360)642-3787
Fax: (360)642-2096
URL: http://willapabh.org/

Longview

51449 ■ Lower Columbia Mental Health
600 Broadway, Ste. 200
Longview, WA 98632
Ph: (360)425-5380
Fax: (360)423-2311
URL: http://www.ccgacares.com/index.php?q=node/4

Moses Lake

51450 ■ Grant Mental Health and Family Service
Crisis Line
840 E Plum
Moses Lake, WA 98837
Ph: (509)765-9239
Fax: (509)765-1582
URL: http://www.gmhealthcare.org/

Mount Vernon

51451 ■ Skagit Mental Health
208 Kincaid St.
Mount Vernon, WA 98273
Ph: (360)416-7520
Fax: (360)416-7095

Newport

51452 ■ Pend Oreille County Mental Health
PO Box 5055
Newport, WA 99156
Ph: (509)447-5651
Free: 800-404-5151
Fax: (509)447-2671
URL: http://www.pendoreilleco.org/county/cs.asp

Olympia

51453 ■ Crisis Clinic of Thurston and Mason Counties
PO Box 2463
Olympia, WA 98507
Ph: (360)586-2888
Fax: (360)586-2808
URL: http://www.crisis-clinic.org

51454 ■ Department of Social & Health Services--Mental Health Division
PO Box 45320
Olympia, WA 98504
Ph: (360)902-0790
Free: 888-713-6010
URL: http://www.biawa.org/eresources/emental-health.htm

Omak

51455 ■ Okanogan Behavioral Healthcare
1007 Koala Dr.
Omak, WA 98841
Ph: (509)826-6191
Fax: (509)826-8416
URL: http://www.okbhc.org/
Formerly: Okanogan County Counseling Service.

Othello

51456 ■ Community Counseling Services of Adams County--Othello
425 E Main, Ste. 600
Othello, WA 99344
Ph: (509)488-5611
URL: http://www.co.adams.wa.us/departments/counseling.asp

Port Angeles

51457 ■ Peninsula Community Mental Health Center
118 E 8th St.
Port Angeles, WA 98362
Ph: (360)457-0431
Fax: (360)457-0493
E-mail: info@pcmhc.org
URL: http://www.pcmhc.org/

Port Townsend

51458 ■ Jefferson Mental Health Services Community Counseling Service
884 W Park St.
Port Townsend, WA 98368
Ph: (360)385-0321
URL: http://www.jeffersonmhs.org/

Pullman

51459 ■ Palouse Regional Crisis Line
340 NE Maple, Ste. 1
Pullman, WA 99163
Ph: (509)332-1505

Raymond

51460 ■ Willapa Counseling Center--Raymond
North Pacific County Crisis
300 Ocean Ave.
Raymond, WA 98577
Ph: (360)942-2303
URL: http://willapabh.org/

Republic

51461 ■ Ferry County Community Services
42 Klondike Rd.
Republic, WA 99166
Ph: (509)775-3341
Fax: (509)775-3341
E-mail: timberli@televar.com

Richland

51462 ■ Lourdes Counseling Center
1175 Carondelet Dr.
Richland, WA 99352
Ph: (509)943-9104
Fax: (509)943-7206
URL: http://www.lourdeshealth.net/counseling.html

Ritzville

51463 ■ Community Counseling Services of Adams County--Ritzville
120 E 1st Ave.
Ritzville, WA 99169
Ph: (509)659-4357
URL: http://www.co.adams.wa.us/departments/counseling.asp

Seattle

51464 ■ Children's Crisis Outreach Response System (CCORS)
401 5th Ave., Ste. 400
Seattle, WA 98104
Ph: (206)263-9000
URL: http://www.kingcounty.gov/healthServices/MentalHealth/Services/Youth/CrisisOutreach.aspx

51465 ■ Crisis Clinic of King County
1515 Dexter Ave. N, Ste. 300
Seattle, WA 98109
Ph: (206)461-3210
Fax: (206)461-8368
E-mail: info@crisisclinic.org
URL: http://www.crisisclinic.org

51466 ■ Seattle Counseling Service for Sexual Minorities
1216 Pine St., Ste. 300
Seattle, WA 98101
Ph: (206)323-1768
Fax: (206)323-2184
E-mail: info@seattlecounseling.org
URL: http://www.seattlecounseling.org/Services.htm

51467 ■ Sound Mental Health
1600 E Olive St.
Seattle, WA 98122
Ph: (206)302-2200
Fax: (206)302-2210
URL: http://www.smh.org/
Formerly: Seattle Mental Health.

Sequim

51468 ■ Peninsula Community Mental Health Center
490 N 5th Ave.
Sequim, WA 98382
Ph: (360)681-0585
URL: http://www.pcmhc.org/

South Bend

51469 ■ Willapa Counseling Center--South Bend
North Pacific County Crisis
PO Box 65
South Bend, WA 98586
Ph: (360)942-2303
URL: http://willapabh.org/

Spokane

51470 ■ Spokane Mental Health
First Call for Help
107 S Division
Spokane, WA 99202
Ph: (509)838-4651
URL: http://www.smhca.org/

Stevenson

51471 ■ Skamania County Counseling Center
PO Box 790
Stevenson, WA 98648
Ph: (509)427-9488
URL: http://www.skamaniacounty.org/Juvenile/local-resources.htm

Tacoma

51472 ■ Crisis Clinic of Pierce County
Comprehensive Mental Health
1201 S Proctor St.
Tacoma, WA 98405
Ph: (253)404-3503
URL: http://www.compmh.org

Toppenish

51473 ■ Yakima Valley Farm Workers Clinic--Toppenish
Child & Adolescent Crisis Intervention
518 W 1st Ave., Bldg. 602-A
Toppenish, WA 98948
Ph: (509)865-5898
Free: 800-500-0934
URL: http://www.yvfwc.com/yakima_bhs.html

Vancouver

51474 ■ Lutheran Community Services Northwest
3600 Main St., Ste. 200
Vancouver, WA 98663
Ph: (360)694-5624
Fax: (360)694-8515
URL: http://www.lcsnw.org/services.html

Walla Walla

51475 ■ Walla Walla Crisis Response Team
1520 Kelly Pl.
Walla Walla, WA 99362
Ph: (509)524-2920
E-mail: croberts@co.walla-walla.wa.us
URL: http://www.co.walla-walla.wa.us/departments/hrs/CrisisUnit.shtml

51476 ■ Walla Walla Mental Health
Inland Counseling Center
209 S 2nd St.
Walla Walla, WA 99362
Ph: (509)525-0241

Wenatchee

51477 ■ Chelan-Douglas Behavioral Health Clinic
701 N Miller St.
Wenatchee, WA 98801
Ph: (509)662-7195
Free: 800-852-2923
Fax: (509)662-1269
URL: http://www.biawa.org/eresources/emental-health.htm

Yakima

51478 ■ Central Washington Comprehensive Mental Health (CWCMH)
402 S 4th Avenue
Yakima, WA 98907
Ph: (509)575-4084
URL: http://www.cwcmh.org
Rick Weaver, President

51479 ■ Children's Village
Child & Adolescent Crisis Intervention
3801 Kern Rd.
Yakima, WA 98902
Ph: (509)574-3220
Free: 800-500-0934
URL: http://www.yvfwc.com/yakima_bhs.html

51480 ■ Yakima Valley Farm Workers Clinic
Child & Adolescent Crisis Intervention
918 E Mead Ave.
Yakima, WA 98903
Ph: (509)453-1344
Free: 800-500-0934
Fax: (509)453-2209
URL: http://www.yvfwc.com/yakima_bhs.html

WEST VIRGINIA

Branchland

51481 ■ Prestera Center for Mental Health Services, Lincoln County
Crisis Helpline
25 Lincoln Plz.
Branchland, WV 25506
Ph: (304)824-5790
Fax: (304)824-2632
URL: http://www.prestera.org/

Charleston

51482 ■ Prestera Center for Mental Health Services, Kanawha County
Crisis Helpline
511 Morris St.
Charleston, WV 25301
Ph: (304)341-0511
Fax: (304)345-8163
URL: http://www.prestera.org/

Clarksburg

51483 ■ United Summit Center Crisis Line
No. 6 Hospital Plz.
Clarksburg, WV 26301
Free: 800-786-6480
URL: http://www.uscwv.org/

Clay

51484 ■ Prestera Center for Mental Health Services, Clay County
Crisis Helpline
163 Main St.
Clay, WV 25043
Ph: (304)587-4205
Fax: (304)587-2978
URL: http://www.prestera.org/

Danville

51485 ■ Prestera Center for Mental Health Services, Boone County
Crisis Helpline
376 Kenmore Dr.
Danville, WV 25053
Ph: (304)369-1930
Fax: (304)369-1978
URL: http://www.prestera.org/

Franklin

51486 ■ Potomac Highlands Mental Health Guild Crisis Unit--Franklin
100 Maple Ave.
Franklin, WV 26807

Ph: (304)358-2351
URL: http://thephg.org/

Huntington

51487 ■ Contact Huntington, Inc.
PO Box 2963
Huntington, WV 25728
Ph: (304)523-3447
Fax: (304)523-0558
E-mail: contacth@contacthuntington.com
URL: http://www.contacthuntington.com/

51488 ■ Prestera Center for Mental Health Services, Cabell County
Crisis Helpline
3375 US Rte. 60 E
Huntington, WV 25705
Ph: (304)525-7851
Fax: (304)525-1504
URL: http://www.prestera.org/

Lewisburg

51489 ■ Seneca Behavioral Health Center
100 Church St.
Lewisburg, WV 24901
Ph: (304)645-3319
Fax: (304)645-6532
URL: http://www.shsinc.org/

Morgantown

51490 ■ Valley HealthCare System
301 Scott Ave.
Morgantown, WV 26508
Ph: (304)296-1731
Free: 304-225-2288
URL: http://www.valleyhealthcare.org

Mullens

51491 ■ Southern Highlands Community Mental Health Center--Mullens
Mullens Clinic
102 Howard Ave.
Mullens, WV 25882
Ph: (304)294-5353
URL: http://www.shcmhc.com/

New Creek

51492 ■ Potomac Highlands Mental Health Guild Crisis Unit--New Creek
PO Box 128
New Creek, WV 26743
Ph: (304)788-2241
URL: http://thephg.org/

Petersburg

51493 ■ Potomac Highlands Mental Health Guild Crisis Unit--Petersburg
PO Box 1119
Petersburg, WV 26847
Ph: (304)257-1155
URL: http://thephg.org/

Point Pleasant

51494 ■ Prestera Center for Mental Health Services, Mason County
Crisis Helpline
715 Main St.
Point Pleasant, WV 25550
Ph: (304)675-2361
Fax: (304)675-8086
URL: http://www.prestera.org/

Princeton

51495 ■ Southern Highlands Community Mental Health Center--12th Street, Princeton
200 12th St. Ext.
Princeton, WV 24740
Ph: (304)425-9541
URL: http://www.shcmhc.com/

51496 ■ Southern Highlands Community Mental Health Center--Mercer Street, Princeton
Crisis Respite Unit
329 Mercer St.
Princeton, WV 24740
Ph: (304)487-1488
URL: http://www.shcmhc.com/

Wayne

51497 ■ Prestera Center for Mental Health Services, Wayne County
Crisis Helpline
145 Kenova Ave.
Wayne, WV 25570
Ph: (304)272-3466
Fax: (304)272-6418
URL: http://www.prestera.org/

Welch

51498 ■ Southern Highlands Community Mental Health Center--Welch
Welch Clinic
787 Virginia Ave.
Welch, WV 24801
Ph: (304)436-2106
URL: http://www.shcmhc.com/

Winfield

51499 ■ Prestera Center for Mental Health Services, Putnam County
Crisis Helpline
3389 Winfield Rd.
Winfield, WV 25213
Ph: (304)586-0670
Fax: (304)586-0671
URL: http://www.prestera.org/

WISCONSIN

Antigo

51500 ■ Langlade Health Care Center
Emergency Mental Health
1225 Langlade Rd.
Antigo, WI 54409
Ph: (715)845-4326
URL: http://www.norcen.org/

Appleton

51501 ■ Outagamie County Crisis Intervention Center
401 Elm St.
Appleton, WI 54911
Ph: (920)832-5270
Fax: (920)832-5488
URL: http://www.co.outagamie.wi.us/human_ services/mental_health/hhs-mh-home.html

Cedarburg

51502 ■ Cope Hotline Ozaukee County
PO Box 723
Cedarburg, WI 53012
Ph: (414)377-1477
URL: http://www.coperesources.net

Eau Claire

51503 ■ Omni Clinic
2005 Highland Ave.
Eau Claire, WI 54701
Ph: (715)832-5030
Fax: (715)832-2991
URL: http://www.omneclinic.com/

Elkhorn

51504 ■ Walworth County Department of Human Services
Box 1005, W4051
Elkhorn, WI 53121

Ph: (262)741-3200
URL: http://www.co.walworth.wi.us/

Fond du Lac

51505 ■ CIC/Fond du Lac County Health Center
459 E 1st St.
Fond du Lac, WI 54935
Ph: (920)929-3500
Fax: (920)929-3129
URL: http://www.fdlco.wi.gov/index.aspx?page=271

Green Bay

51506 ■ Family Services of Northeast Wisconsin, Inc.
Crisis Center
300 Crooks St.
Green Bay, WI 54305-2308
Ph: (920)436-6800
Fax: (920)432-5966
E-mail: intake@familyservicesnew.org
URL: http://www.familyservicesnew.org

Kenosha

51507 ■ Rogers Memorial Hospital--Kenosha
9916 75th St.
Kenosha, WI 53142
Ph: (262)942-4000
Fax: (262)942-7740
URL: http://www.rogershospital.org/

La Crosse

51508 ■ Gundersen--Lutheran Memorial Center
1900 South Ave.
La Crosse, WI 54601
Ph: (608)775-2287
Free: 800-362-9567
URL: http://www.gundluth.org/

Madison

51509 ■ Emergency Service Mental Health Center of Dane County
625 W Washington Ave.
Madison, WI 53703
Ph: (608)280-2580
Fax: (608)280-2703
URL: http://www.mhcdc.org/Services/ESUFrameset.html

Merrill

51510 ■ Lincoln Health Care Center
607 N Sales St.
Merrill, WI 54452
Ph: (715)536-9482
URL: http://www.norcen.org/

Milwaukee

51511 ■ Aurora Family Service
3200 W Highland Blvd.
Milwaukee, WI 53208
Ph: (414)342-4560
URL: http://www.aurorahealthcare.org/services/familysocial/index.asp

51512 ■ Helpline--Milwaukee
PO Box 510465
Milwaukee, WI 53203
Ph: (414)276-8487

51513 ■ Mental Health America of Wisconsin
600 W Virginia St., Ste. 502
Milwaukee, WI 53204-1551
Ph: (414)276-3122
Free: 866-948-6483
Fax: (414)276-3124
E-mail: info@mhawisconsin.org
URL: http://www.mhawisconsin.org
Judy McGregor, President
Formerly: (2007) Mental Health Association in Milwaukee County.

51514 ■ Transitional Living Services, Inc.
Crisis Resource Center
2057 S 14th St.
Milwaukee, WI 53214
Ph: (414)643-8778
Fax: (414)643-8708
URL: http://www.tlservices.org/Content/crisis_resource_center.asp

Onalaska

51515 ■ First Call for Help--Great Rivers 211
PO Box 426
Onalaska, WI 54650
Ph: (608)775-6339
Fax: (608)775-4766
URL: http://www.firstcallforhelp.org/

Rhinelander

51516 ■ Community Mental Health Services--Crisis Link
1831 N Stevens St.
Rhinelander, WI 54501
Ph: (715)365-7000

Sturgeon Bay

51517 ■ HELP of Door County, Inc.
Helpline
219 Green Bay Rd.
Sturgeon Bay, WI 54235
Ph: (920)743-8785
Fax: (920)743-9984
E-mail: help@helpofdoorcounty.org
URL: http://www.helpofdoorcounty.org

Tomahawk

51518 ■ Lincoln Health Care Center
310 W Wisconsin Ave.
Tomahawk, WI 54487
Ph: (715)453-5381
URL: http://www.norcen.org/

Waukesha

51519 ■ Mental Health Association in Waukesha County, Inc.
First Call for Help
S22 W22660 E Broadway, Ste. 5S
Waukesha, WI 53186

Ph: (262)547-0769
Fax: (262)547-1609
E-mail: mail@mhawauk.org
URL: http://www.mhawauk.org

Wausau

51520 ■ Marathon Health Care Center
North Central Health Care-Crisis Intervention
1100 Lake View Dr.
Wausau, WI 54403
Ph: (715)845-4326
URL: http://www.norcen.org/

Wauwatosa

51521 ■ Milwaukee Community Mental Health Complex
Psychiatric Crisis Service
9455 W Watertown Plank Rd.
Wauwatosa, WI 53226
Ph: (414)257-7665
URL: http://www.mcw.edu/psychiatry/clinicalsites.htm

Wisconsin Rapids

51522 ■ Suicide Prevention--Wisconsin Rapids
Crisis Intervention and Referral Service
2611 12th St. S
Wisconsin Rapids, WI 54494
Ph: (715)421-2345

WYOMING

Casper

51523 ■ Wyoming Behavioral Institute
2521 E 15th St.
Casper, WY 82609
Ph: (307)237-7444
Free: 800-457-9312
URL: http://www.wbihelp.com/

Cheyenne

51524 ■ Cheyenne Helpline
PO Box 404
Cheyenne, WY 82001
Ph: (307)634-4469
Denise E. Vigil, Executive Director

51525 ■ Needs, Inc.
900 Central Ave.
Cheyenne, WY 82007
Ph: (307)632-4132
Fax: (307)634-7147
URL: http://needsincorporate.qwestoffice.net/

Worland

51526 ■ Victims of Violence Center
101 N. 19th
Worland, WY 82401
Ph: (307)347-4992
Fax: (307)347-4992
E-mail: vovc@rtconnect.net

This chapter includes three sections: (1) Veterans Affairs Medical Centers, (2) Post-Traumatic Stress Disorder Programs, and (3) Vet Centers. Entries in each section are arranged geographically by states and cities, then alphabetically by organization names within cities. Consult the "User's Guide" located at the front of this directory for additional information.

VETERANS AFFAIRS MEDICAL CENTERS

ALABAMA

Birmingham

51527 ■ Veterans Affairs Medical Center Birmingham AL
700 S 19th St.
Birmingham, AL 35233
Ph: (205)933-8101
Free: 866-487-4243
Fax: (205)933-4484
URL: http://www.birmingham.va.gov

Montgomery

51528 ■ Central Alabama Veterans Health Care System
West Campus
215 Perry Hill Rd.
Montgomery, AL 36109-3798
Ph: (334)272-4670
Free: 800-214-8387
Fax: (334)260-4143
URL: http://www.centralalabama.va.gov/

Tuscaloosa

51529 ■ Veterans Affairs Medical Center Tuscaloosa AL
3701 Loop Rd. E
Tuscaloosa, AL 35404
Ph: (205)554-2000
Free: 888-269-3045
Fax: (205)554-2034
URL: http://www.tuscaloosa.va.gov/

Tuskegee

51530 ■ Central Alabama Veterans Health Care System
East Campus
2400 Hospital Rd.
Tuskegee, AL 36083-5001
Ph: (334)727-0550
Free: 800-214-8387
Fax: (334)724-2793
URL: http://www.centralalabama.va.gov

ALASKA

Anchorage

51531 ■ Alaska Veterans Affairs Healthcare System
1201 N Muldoon Rd.
Anchorage, AK 99504
Ph: (907)257-4700
Free: 888-353-7574
Fax: (907)257-6774
URL: http://www.visn20.med.va.gov/Alaska

ARIZONA

Phoenix

51532 ■ Phoenix Veterans Affairs Health Care System
650 E Indian School Rd.
Phoenix, AZ 85012
Ph: (602)277-5551
Free: 800-554-7174
URL: http://www.phoenix.va.gov
Beds: 299. **Formerly:** Department of Veterans Affairs Integrated Service Network VISN 18; Carl T. Hayden Veterans Affairs Medical Center.

Prescott

51533 ■ Northern Arizona Veterans Affairs Health Care System
500 N Hwy. 89
Prescott, AZ 86313
Ph: (928)445-4860
Free: 800-949-1005
Fax: (928)768-6076
URL: http://www.prescott.va.gov

ARKANSAS

Fayetteville

51534 ■ Veterans Health Care System of the Ozarks
1100 N College Ave.
Fayetteville, AR 72703
Ph: (479)443-4301
Free: 800-691-8387
URL: http://www.fayettevillear.va.gov/

Little Rock

51535 ■ Central Arkansas Veterans Healthcare System
John L. McClellan Memorial Veterans Hospital
4300 W 7th St.
Little Rock, AR 72205-5484
Ph: (501)257-1000
URL: http://www.littlerock.va.gov/

North Little Rock

51536 ■ Central Arkansas Veterans Healthcare System
Eugene J. Towbin Healthcare Center
2200 Fort Roots Dr.
North Little Rock, AR 72114-1706
Ph: (501)257-1000
URL: http://www.littlerock.va.gov/

CALIFORNIA

Livermore

51537 ■ Veterans Affairs Medical Center Palo Alto Health Care System
Livermore Division
4951 Arroyo Rd.
Livermore, CA 94550
Ph: (925)373-4700
URL: http://www.paloalto.va.gov/

Loma Linda

51538 ■ Veterans Affairs Loma Linda Healthcare System
11201 Benton St.
Loma Linda, CA 92357
Ph: (909)825-7084
Free: 800-741-8387
Fax: (909)422-3106
URL: http://www.lomalinda.va.gov

Los Angeles

51539 ■ Veterans Affairs Greater Los Angeles (GLA) Healthcare System
11301 Willshire Blvd.
Los Angeles, CA 90073
Ph: (310)478-3711
Free: 800-952-4852
Fax: (310)268-3494
URL: http://www.losangeles.va.gov
Charles M. Dorman, Director

Mather

51540 ■ Veterans Affairs Northern California Health Care System
Sacramento Medical Center
10535 Hospital Way
Mather, CA 95655
Ph: (916)843-7000
Free: 800-382-8387
Fax: (916)843-9001
URL: http://www.northerncalifornia.va.gov

Menlo Park

51541 ■ Veterans Affairs Medical Center Palo Alto Health Care System
Menlo Park Division
795 Willow Rd.
Menlo Park, CA 94025
Ph: (650)614-9997
URL: http://www.paloalto.va.gov/

Palo Alto

51542 ■ Palo Alto Health Care System
3801 Miranda Ave.
Palo Alto, CA 94304-1290
Ph: (650)493-5000
Free: 800-455-0057
Fax: (650)852-3228
URL: http://www.paloalto.va.gov

San Diego

51543 ■ Veterans Affairs San Diego Healthcare System
3350 La Jolla Village Dr.
San Diego, CA 92161

Ph: (858)552-8585
Free: 800-331-8387
Fax: (858)552-7452
URL: http://www.sandiego.va.gov/

San Francisco

51544 ■ Veterans Affairs Medical Center
San Francisco CA
4150 Clement St.
San Francisco, CA 94121-1598
Ph: (415)221-4810
Fax: (415)750-2185
URL: http://www.sanfrancisco.va.gov

COLORADO

Denver

51545 ■ Veterans Affairs Eastern Colorado
Health Care System
1055 Clermont St.
Denver, CO 80220
Ph: (303)399-8020
Free: 888-336-8262
Fax: (303)393-2861
URL: http://www2.va.gov/directory/guide/facility.
asp?ID=39&dnum=All
Formerly: Department of Veterans Affairs Integrated
Service Network VISN 19.

Grand Junction

51546 ■ Veterans Affairs Medical Center
Grand Junction CO
2121 North Ave.
Grand Junction, CO 81501
Ph: (970)242-0731
Free: 866-206-6415
Fax: (970)244-1303
URL: http://www.grandjunction.va.gov/

CONNECTICUT

Newington

51547 ■ Veterans Affairs Connecticut
Healthcare System
Newington Campus
555 Willard Ave.
Newington, CT 06111
Ph: (860)666-6951
Fax: (860)667-6764
URL: http://www2.va.gov/directory/guide/facility.
asp?ID=914&dnum=All

West Haven

51548 ■ Veterans Affairs Connecticut
Healthcare System
West Haven Campus
950 Campbell Ave.
West Haven, CT 06516
Ph: (203)932-5711
Fax: (203)937-3868
URL: http://www.connecticut.va.gov/

DELAWARE

Wilmington

51549 ■ Veterans Affairs Medical Center
Wilimington DE
1601 Kirkwood Hwy.
Wilmington, DE 19805
Ph: (302)994-2511
Free: 800-461-8262
Fax: (302)633-5591
URL: http://www.wilmington.va.gov/

DISTRICT OF COLUMBIA

Washington

51550 ■ Washington DC Veterans Affairs
Medical Center
50 Irving St. NW
Washington, DC 20422

Ph: (202)745-8000
Free: 877-328-2621
Fax: (202)745-8530
URL: http://www.washingtondc.va.gov/

FLORIDA

Bay Pines

51551 ■ Bay Pines Veterans Affairs Health
Care System
10000 Bay Pines Blvd.
Bay Pines, FL 33744
Ph: (727)398-6661
Free: 888-820-0230
Fax: (727)398-9442
URL: http://www.baypines.va.gov/

Gainesville

51552 ■ North Florida/South Georgia
Veterans Health System
Gainesville Division
Malcolm Randall VAMC
1601 SW Archer Rd.
Gainesville, FL 32608-1197
Ph: (352)376-1611
Free: 800-324-8387
Fax: (352)374-6113
URL: http://www.northflorida.va.gov/

Lake City

51553 ■ North Florida/South Georgia
Veterans Health System
Lake City Division
619 S Marion St.
Lake City, FL 32025-5808
Ph: (386)755-3016
Free: 800-308-8387
Fax: (386)758-3209
URL: http://www.northflorida.va.gov/

Miami

51554 ■ Veterans Affairs Medical Center
Miami FL
1201 NW 16th St.
Miami, FL 33125
Ph: (305)575-7000
Free: 888-276-1785
Fax: (305)575-3232
URL: http://www.miami.va.gov/

Orlando

51555 ■ Orlando Veterans Affairs Medical
Center
5201 Raymond St.
Orlando, FL 32803
Ph: (407)629-1599
Free: 800-922-7521
Fax: (407)599-1591
URL: http://www.orlando.va.gov/

Tampa

51556 ■ Tampa (James A. Haley) Veterans
Hospital
13000 Bruce B. Downs Blvd.
Tampa, FL 33612
Ph: (813)972-2000
Free: 888-811-0107
Fax: (813)972-7673
URL: http://www.tampa.va.gov/

West Palm Beach

51557 ■ Veterans Affairs Medical Center
West Palm Beach FL
7305 N Military Trl.
West Palm Beach, FL 33410-6400
Ph: (561)422-8262
Free: 800-972-8262
Fax: (561)422-8613
URL: http://www.westpalmbeach.va.gov/

GEORGIA

Augusta

51558 ■ Charlie Norwood Veterans Affairs
Medical Center
1 Freedom Way
Augusta, GA 30904
Ph: (706)733-0188
Free: 800-836-5561
Fax: (706)823-3934
URL: http://www2.va.gov/directory/guide/facility.
asp?ID=9&dnum=All

Decatur

51559 ■ Atlanta Veterans Affairs Medical
Center
1670 Clairmont Rd.
Decatur, GA 30033
Ph: (404)321-6111
Free: 800-944-9726
Fax: (404)728-7733
URL: http://www.atlanta.va.gov
Beds: 291. Formerly: Department of Veterans Affairs Integrated Service Network VISN 7.

Dublin

51560 ■ Carl Vinson Veterans Affairs Medical
Center
1826 Veteran's Blvd.
Dublin, GA 31021
Ph: (478)272-1210
Free: 800-595-5229
Fax: (478)272-2717
URL: http://www.dublin.va.gov/

HAWAII

Honolulu

51561 ■ Veterans Affairs Pacific Islands
Health Care System
459 Patterson Rd.
Honolulu, HI 96819
Ph: (803)433-0600
Free: 800-214-1406
Fax: (808)433-0390
URL: http://www.hawaii.va.gov/

IDAHO

Boise

51562 ■ Veterans Affairs Medical Center
Boise ID
500 Fort St.
Boise, ID 83702
Ph: (208)422-1000
Free: 866-437-5093
Fax: (208)422-1326
URL: http://www.boise.va.gov/

ILLINOIS

Danville

51563 ■ Veterans Affairs Illiana Health Care
System
1900 E Main St.
Danville, IL 61832
Ph: (217)554-3000
Free: 888-838-6446
Fax: (217)554-4552
URL: http://www.danville.va.gov/

Hines

51564 ■ Edward Hines Jr. Veterans Affairs
Hospital
5000 S 5th Ave.
Hines, IL 60141
Ph: (708)202-8387
Fax: (708)202-7998
URL: http://www.hines.va.gov/

Marion

51565 ■ Veterans Affairs Medical Center
Marion IL
2401 W Main St.
Marion, IL 62959
Ph: (618)997-5311
Free: 866-289-3300
URL: http://www.marion.va.gov

North Chicago

51566 ■ Veterans Affairs Medical Center
Captain James A. Lovell Federal Health Care Center
3001 Green Bay Rd.
North Chicago, IL 60064
Ph: (224)688-1900
Free: 800-393-0865
Fax: (224)610-3806
URL: http://wwww.lovell.fhcc.va.gov/

INDIANA

Fort Wayne

51567 ■ Veterans Affairs Northern Indiana Health Care System
Fort Wayne Campus
2121 Lake Ave.
Fort Wayne, IN 46805
Ph: (260)426-5431
Free: 888-838-6446
Fax: (260)460-1336
URL: http://www.northernindiana.va.gov/

Marion

51568 ■ Veterans Affairs Northern Indiana Health Care System
Marion Campus
1700 E 38th St.
Marion, IN 46953
Ph: (765)674-3321
Free: 888-838-6446
Fax: (765)677-3124
URL: http://www.northernindiana.va.gov/

IOWA

Des Moines

51569 ■ Des Moines Division
Veterans Affairs Central Iowa Health Care System
3600 30th St.
Des Moines, IA 50310-5774
Ph: (515)699-5999
Free: 800-294-8387
Fax: (515)699-5862
URL: http://www.centraliowa.va.gov

Iowa City

51570 ■ Veterans Affairs Medical Center
Iowa City IA
601 Hwy. 6 W
Iowa City, IA 52246-2208
Ph: (319)338-0581
Free: 866-687-7382
Fax: (319)339-7171
URL: http://www.iowacity.va.gov/

KANSAS

Leavenworth

51571 ■ Veterans Affairs Eastern Kansas Health Care System
Dwight D. Eisenhower Veterans Affairs Medical Center
4101 S 4th St.
Leavenworth, KS 66048-5055
Ph: (913)682-2000
Free: 800-952-8387
URL: http://www.leavenworth.va.gov

Topeka

51572 ■ Veterans Affairs Eastern Kansas Health Care System
Colmery-O'Neil Veterans Affairs Medical Center
2200 SW Gage Blvd.
Topeka, KS 66622
Ph: (785)350-3111
Free: 800-574-8387
Fax: (785)350-4336
URL: http://www.topeka.va.gov

Wichita

51573 ■ Robert J. Dole Medical and Regional Office Center
Veterans Affairs Medical Center
5500 E Kellogg
Wichita, KS 67218
Ph: (316)685-2221
Free: 888-878-6882
Fax: (316)651-3666
URL: http://www.wichita.va.gov

KENTUCKY

Lexington

51574 ■ Lexington Veterans Affairs Medical Center
Leestown Division
2250 Leestown Rd.
Lexington, KY 40511
Ph: (859)281-4900
Free: 888-824-3577
URL: http://www.lexington.va.gov

51575 ■ Veterans Affairs Medical Center
Lexington KY
1101 Veterans Dr.
Lexington, KY 40502
Ph: (859)281-4900
URL: http://www.lexington.va.gov

Louisville

51576 ■ Robley Rex Veterans Affairs Medical Center
800 Zorn Ave.
Louisville, KY 40206
Ph: (502)287-4000
Free: 800-376-8387
Fax: (502)287-6225
URL: http://www.louisville.va.gov/

LOUISIANA

New Orleans

51577 ■ Veterans Affairs Medical Center
New Orleans LA
1601 Perdido St.
New Orleans, LA 70112
Ph: (504)412-3700
Free: 800-935-8387
Fax: (504)565-4835
URL: http://www.neworleans.va.gov/

Pineville

51578 ■ Veterans Affairs Medical Center
Pineville LA
2495 Shreveport Hwy. 71 N
Pineville, LA 71360
Ph: (318)473-0010
Free: 800-375-8387
Fax: (318)483-5029
URL: http://www4.va.gov/502alexandria/

MARYLAND

Baltimore

51579 ■ Baltimore Veterans Affairs Medical Center
Veterans Affairs Maryland Health Care System
10 N Greene St.
Baltimore, MD 21201

Ph: (410)605-7000
Free: 800-463-6295
Fax: (410)605-7901
URL: http://www.maryland.va.gov/

51580 ■ Loch RavenVeterans Affairs Rehabilitation and Extended Care Center
3900 Loch Raven Blvd.
Baltimore, MD 21218
Ph: (410)605-7000
Free: 800-463-6295
Fax: (410)605-7900
URL: http://www.maryland.va.gov/

51581 ■ Veterans Affairs Medical Center
Veterans Affairs Maryland Health Care System
10 N Greene St.
Baltimore, MD 21201
Ph: (410)605-7000
Free: 800-463-6295
URL: http://www.maryland.va.gov/

MASSACHUSETTS

Bedford

51582 ■ Edith Nourse Rogers Memorial Veterans Hospital
200 Springs Rd.
Bedford, MA 01730
Ph: (781)687-2000
Free: 800--VETMED1
Fax: (781)687-2101
URL: http://www.bedford.va.gov/

Brockton

51583 ■ Veterans Affairs Boston Healthcare System
Brockton Division
940 Belmont St.
Brockton, MA 02301
Ph: (508)583-4500
Free: 800-865-3384
URL: http://www.boston.va.gov/

Jamaica Plain

51584 ■ Veterans Affairs Boston Healthcare System
Jamaica Plain Division
150 S Huntington Ave.
Jamaica Plain, MA 02130
Ph: (617)232-9500
Free: 800-865-3384
Fax: (617)278-4508
URL: http://www.boston.va.gov/

Leeds

51585 ■ Northampton Veterans Affair Medical Center
421 N Main St.
Leeds, MA 01053-9764
Ph: (413)584-4040
Free: 800-893-1522
Fax: (413)582-3121
URL: http://www.northampton.va.gov/

West Roxbury

51586 ■ Veterans Affairs Boston Healthcare System
West Roxbury Division
1400 VFW Pkwy.
West Roxbury, MA 02132
Ph: (617)323-7700
Free: 800-865-3384
URL: http://www.boston.va.gov/

MICHIGAN

Ann Arbor

51587 ■ Veterans Affairs Medical Center
Ann Arbor MI
2215 Fuller Rd.
Ann Arbor, MI 48105

Ph: (734)769-7100
Free: 800-361-8387
Fax: (734)845-3245
URL: http://www.annarbor.va.gov

Battle Creek

51588 ■ Veterans Affairs Medical Center
Battle Creek MI
5500 Armstrong Rd.
Battle Creek, MI 49037
Ph: (269)966-5600
Free: 888-214-1247
Fax: (269)966-5483
URL: http://www.battlecreek.va.gov

Iron Mountain

51589 ■ Oscar G. Johnson Veterans Affairs
Medical Center
325 E H St.
Iron Mountain, MI 49801
Ph: (906)774-3300
Free: 800-215-8262
Fax: (906)779-3188
URL: http://www.ironmountain.va.gov/

Saginaw

51590 ■ Aleda E. Lutz Veterans Affairs
Medical Center
1500 Weiss St.
Saginaw, MI 48602
Ph: (989)497-2500
Free: 800-406-5143
Fax: (989)321-4903
URL: http://www.saginaw.va.gov

MINNESOTA

Minneapolis

51591 ■ Veterans Affairs Medical Center
Minneapolis MN
1 Veterans Dr.
Minneapolis, MN 55417
Ph: (612)725-2000
Free: 866-414-5058
Fax: (612)725-2049
URL: http://www.minneapolis.va.gov/

Saint Cloud

51592 ■ Veterans Affairs Medical Center
Saint Cloud MN
4801 Veterans Dr.
Saint Cloud, MN 56303
Ph: (320)252-1670
Free: 800-247-1739
Fax: (320)255-6494
URL: http://www.stcloud.va.gov

MISSISSIPPI

Biloxi

51593 ■ Veterans Affairs Gulf Coast Veterans
Health Care System
400 Veterans Ave.
Biloxi, MS 39531
Ph: (228)523-5000
Free: 800-296-8872
Fax: (228)523-5719
URL: http://www.biloxi.va.gov/

Jackson

51594 ■ GV Sonny Montgomery Veterans
Affairs Medical Center
1500 E Woodrow Wilson Dr.
Jackson, MS 39216
Ph: (601)362-4471
Free: 800-949-1009
Fax: (601)364-1359
URL: http://www.jackson.va.gov

MISSOURI

Columbia

51595 ■ Harry S Truman Memorial
800 Hospital Dr.
Columbia, MO 65201-5297
Ph: (573)814-6000
Free: 800-349-8262
Fax: (573)814-6600
URL: http://www.columbiamo.va.gov/

Kansas City

51596 ■ Veterans Affairs Medical Center
Kansas City MO
4801 Linwood Blvd.
Kansas City, MO 64128
Ph: (816)861-4700
Free: 800-525-1483
URL: http://www.kansascity.va.gov

Poplar Bluff

51597 ■ John J. Pershing Veterans Affairs
Medical Center
1500 N Westwood Blvd.
Poplar Bluff, MO 63901
Ph: (573)686-4151
Free: 888-557-8262
Fax: (573)778-4559
URL: http://www.poplarbluff.va.gov/

Saint Louis

51598 ■ Veterans Affairs Medical Center
Jefferson Barracks Division
1 Jefferson Barracks Dr.
Saint Louis, MO 63125
Ph: (314)652-4100
Free: 800-228-5459
URL: http://www.stlouis.va.gov/

51599 ■ Veterans Affairs Medical Center
John Cochran Division
915 N Grand Ave.
Saint Louis, MO 63106
Ph: (314)652-4100
Free: 800-228-5459
Fax: (314)289-6557
URL: http://www.stlouis.va.gov/

MONTANA

Fort Harrison

51600 ■ Veterans Affairs Montana Healthcare
System
Fort Harrison MT
3687 Veterans Dr.
Fort Harrison, MT 59636
Ph: (406)442-6410
Free: 877-468-8387
Fax: (406)447-7916
URL: http://www.montana.va.gov/

NEBRASKA

Omaha

51601 ■ Omaha Division
Veterans Affairs Nebraska Western Iowa
Health Care System
4101 Woolworth Ave.
Omaha, NE 68105
Ph: (402)346-8800
Free: 800-451-5796
URL: http://www.nebraska.va.gov

NEVADA

North Las Vegas

51602 ■ Veterans Affairs Southern Nevada
Healthcare System
901 Rancho Ln.
North Las Vegas, NV 89106
Ph: (702)636-3000

Free: 888-633-7554
URL: http://www.lasvegas.va.gov/

NEW HAMPSHIRE

Manchester

51603 ■ Veterans Affairs Medical Center
Manchester NH
718 Smyth Rd.
Manchester, NH 03104
Ph: (603)624-4366
Free: 800-892-8384
Fax: (603)626-6579
URL: http://www.manchester.va.gov/

NEW JERSEY

East Orange

51604 ■ East Orange Campus of the
Veterans Affairs
New Jersey Healthcare System
385 Tremont Ave.
East Orange, NJ 07018
Ph: (973)676-1000
Fax: (973)676-4226
URL: http://www.newjersey.va.gov/

Lyons

51605 ■ Lyons Campus of the Veterans
Affairs
New Jersey Healthcare System
151 Knollcroft Rd.
Lyons, NJ 07939
Ph: (908)647-0180
Fax: (908)676-4226
URL: http://www.newjersey.va.gov/

NEW MEXICO

Albuquerque

51606 ■ New Mexico Veterans Affairs Health
Care System
1501 San Pedro Dr. SE
Albuquerque, NM 87108-5153
Ph: (505)265-1711
Free: 800-465-8262
Fax: (505)256-2855
URL: http://www.albuquerque.va.gov

NEW YORK

Albany

51607 ■ Veterans Affairs Medical Center
Samuel S. Stratton
113 Holland Ave.
Albany, NY 12208
Ph: (518)626-5000
Free: 800-223-4810
Fax: (518)626-5500
URL: http://www.albany.va.gov/

Batavia

51608 ■ Veterans Affairs Western New York
Healthcare System at Batavia
222 Richmond Ave.
Batavia, NY 14020
Ph: (585)297-1000
Free: 888-798-2302
URL: http://www.buffalo.va.gov/batavia.asp

Bath

51609 ■ Veterans Affairs Medical Center
Bath NY
76 Veterans Ave.
Bath, NY 14810
Ph: (607)664-4000
Free: 877-845-3247
Fax: (607)664-4511
URL: http://www.bath.va.gov/

Bronx

51610 ■ James J. Peters Veterans Affairs Medical Center
130 W Kingsbridge Rd.
Bronx, NY 10468
Ph: (718)584-9000
Free: 800-877-6976
Fax: (718)741-4269
URL: http://www.bronx.va.gov
Remarks: Spinal cord and brain injuries.

Brooklyn

51611 ■ Brooklyn Campus of the Veterans Affairs
New York Harbor Healthcare System
800 Poly Place
Brooklyn, NY 11209
Ph: (718)836-6600
Fax: (718)630-2840
URL: http://www.nyharbor.va.gov/

Buffalo

51612 ■ Veterans Affairs Western New York Healthcare System at Buffalo
3495 Bailey Ave.
Buffalo, NY 14215
Ph: (716)834-9200
Free: 800-532-8387
Fax: (716)862-8759
URL: http://www.buffalo.va.gov/

Canandaigua

51613 ■ Veterans Affairs Medical Center Canandaigua NY
400 Fort Hill Ave.
Canandaigua, NY 14424
Ph: (585)394-2000
Free: 800-204-9917
Fax: (585)393-8328
URL: http://www.canandaigua.va.gov/

Castle Point

51614 ■ Veterans Affairs Hudson Valley Healthcare System--Castle Point Campus
Rte. 9D
Castle Point, NY 12511
Ph: (845)831-2000
Free: 800-269-8749
Fax: (845)838-5193
URL: http://www.hudsonvalley.va.gov/

Montrose

51615 ■ Veterans Affairs Hudson Valley Healthcare System--Montrose Campus
2094 Albany Post Rd.
Montrose, NY 10548
Ph: (914)737-4400
Free: 800-269-8749
Fax: (914)788-4244
URL: http://www.hudsonvalley.va.gov/

New York

51616 ■ Veterans Affairs New York Harbor Healthcare System
Veterans Affairs Medical Center Manhattan
423 E 23rd St.
New York, NY 10010
Ph: (212)686-7500
Fax: (212)951-3487
URL: http://www.nyharbor.va.gov/

Northport

51617 ■ Veterans Affairs Medical Center Northport NY
79 Middleville Rd.
Northport, NY 11768
Ph: (631)261-4400
URL: http://www.northport.va.gov/

Syracuse

51618 ■ Veterans Affairs Medical Center Syracuse NY
800 Irving Ave.
Syracuse, NY 13210
Ph: (315)425-4400
Free: 800-792-4334
Fax: (315)425-4375
URL: http://www.syracuse.va.gov/

NORTH CAROLINA

Asheville

51619 ■ Veterans Affairs Medical Center Asheville NC
1100 Tunnel Rd.
Asheville, NC 28805
Ph: (828)298-7911
Free: 800-932-6408
Fax: (828)299-2502
URL: http://www.asheville.va.gov/

Durham

51620 ■ Veterans Affairs Medical Center Durham NC
508 Fulton St.
Durham, NC 27705
Ph: (919)286-0411
Free: 888-878-6890
Fax: (919)286-6805
URL: http://www.durham.va.gov/

Fayetteville

51621 ■ Veterans Affairs Medical Center Fayetteville NC
2300 Ramsey St.
Fayetteville, NC 28301
Ph: (910)488-2120
Free: 800-771-6106
Fax: (910)822-7093
URL: http://www.fayettevillenc.va.gov/

Salisbury

51622 ■ WG Hefner Veterans Affairs Medical Center
1601 Brenner Ave.
Salisbury, NC 28144
Ph: (704)638-9000
Free: 800-469-8262
URL: http://www.salisbury.va.gov

NORTH DAKOTA

Fargo

51623 ■ Veterans Affairs Medical Center Fargo ND
2101 N Elm St.
Fargo, ND 58102
Ph: (701)232-3241
Free: 800-410-9723
Fax: (701)239-3705
URL: http://www.fargo.va.gov/

OHIO

Brecksville

51624 ■ Louis Stokes Cleveland Veterans Affairs Medical Center--Brecksville Campus
10000 Brecksville Rd.
Brecksville, OH 44141
Ph: (440)526-3030
URL: http://www.cleveland.va.gov

Chillicothe

51625 ■ Veterans Affairs Medical Center Chillicothe OH
17273 State Rte. 104
Chillicothe, OH 45601
Ph: (740)773-1141

Free: 800-358-8262
Fax: (740)773-1141
URL: http://www.chillicothe.va.gov

Cincinnati

51626 ■ Veterans Affairs Medical Center Cincinnati OH
3200 Vine St.
Cincinnati, OH 45220
Ph: (513)861-3100
Free: 888-267-7873
Fax: (513)475-6500
URL: http://www.cincinnati.va.gov/

Cleveland

51627 ■ Louis Stokes Cleveland Veterans Affairs Medical Center--Wade Park Campus
10701 East Blvd.
Cleveland, OH 44106
Ph: (216)791-3800
Fax: (216)421-3217
URL: http://www.cleveland.va.gov

Columbus

51628 ■ Veterans Affairs Medical Center
Chalmers P. Wylie Veterans Affairs Ambulatory Care Center
420 N James Rd.
Columbus, OH 43219
Ph: (614)257-5200
Free: 888-615-9448
URL: http://www.columbus.va.gov/

Dayton

51629 ■ Veterans Affairs Medical Center Dayton OH
4100 W 3rd St.
Dayton, OH 45428
Ph: (937)268-6511
Free: 800-368-8262
URL: http://www.dayton.va.gov

OKLAHOMA

Muskogee

51630 ■ Jack C. Montgomery Veterans Affairs Medical Center
1011 Honor Heights Dr.
Muskogee, OK 74401
Ph: (918)577-3000
Free: 866-397-8387
URL: http://www.muskogee.va.gov/
License Status: Accredited. **Program(s):** Medical Services; Speech Pathology; Pathology and Lab Services; Nutrition and Food Service; Surgical Services.

Oklahoma City

51631 ■ Veterans Affairs Medical Center Oklahoma City OK
921 NE 13th St.
Oklahoma City, OK 73104
Ph: (405)456-1000
URL: http://www.oklahoma.va.gov/

OREGON

Portland

51632 ■ Veterans Affairs Medical Center Portland OR
3710 S W US Veterans Hospital Rd.
Portland, OR 97239
Ph: (503)220-8262
Free: 800-949-1004
Fax: (503)273-5319
URL: http://www.portland.va.gov/

White City

51633 ■ Veterans Affairs Southern Oregon Rehabilitation Center and Clinics
8495 Crater Lake Hwy.
White City, OR 97503
Ph: (541)830-3515
Free: 800-809-8725
Fax: (541)830-3500
URL: http://www.visn20.med.va.gov/southern-oregon/index.asp
License Status: Accredited.

PENNSYLVANIA

Altoona

51634 ■ James E. van Zandt Veterans Affairs Medical Center - Altoona
2907 Pleasant Valley Blvd.
Altoona, PA 16602-4377
Free: 877-626-2500
URL: http://www.altoona.va.gov/

Butler

51635 ■ Veterans Affairs Butler Health Care
325 New Castle Rd.
Butler, PA 16001
Ph: (724)287-4781
Free: 800-362-8262
Fax: (724)282-4408
URL: http://www.butler.va.gov/

Coatesville

51636 ■ Veterans Affairs Medical Center Coatesville PA
1400 Black Horse Hill Rd.
Coatesville, PA 19320
Ph: (610)384-7711
Free: 800-290-6172
URL: http://www.coatesville.va.gov

Erie

51637 ■ Veterans Affairs Medical Center Erie PA
135 E 38th St.
Erie, PA 16504
Ph: (814)868-8661
Free: 800-274-8387
Fax: (814)860-2120
URL: http://www.erie.va.gov/

Lebanon

51638 ■ Veterans Affairs Medical Center Lebanon PA
1700 S Lincoln Ave.
Lebanon, PA 17042
Ph: (717)272-6621
Free: 800-409-8771
URL: http://www.lebanon.va.gov/

Philadelphia

51639 ■ Veterans Affairs Medical Center Philadelphia PA
3900 Woodland Ave.
Philadelphia, PA 19104
Ph: (215)823-5800
Free: 800-949-1001
Fax: (215)823-6007
URL: http://www.philadelphia.va.gov

Pittsburgh

51640 ■ Veterans Affairs Health Care System--Pittsburgh PA
H. John Heinz III Progressive Care Center
1010 Delafield Rd.
Pittsburgh, PA 15260
Ph: (412)822-2222
Free: 866-482-7488
Fax: (412)784-3724
URL: http://www.pittsburgh.va.gov/

51641 ■ Veterans Affairs Pittsburgh Healthcare System
Highland Drive Division
7180 Highland Dr.
Pittsburgh, PA 15206
Ph: (412)688-6000
Free: 866-482-7488
Fax: (412)365-4213
URL: http://www.pittsburgh.va.gov/

51642 ■ Veterans Affairs Pittsburgh Healthcare System
University Drive Division
University Dr.
Pittsburgh, PA 15240
Ph: (412)688-6000
Free: 866-482-7488
URL: http://www.pittsburgh.va.gov/

Wilkes Barre

51643 ■ Veterans Affairs Medical Center Wilkes Barre PA
1111 E End Blvd.
Wilkes Barre, PA 18711
Ph: (570)824-3521
Free: 877-928-2621
Fax: (570)821-7278
URL: http://www.wilkes-barre.va.gov/

PUERTO RICO

San Juan

51644 ■ Veterans Affairs Medical Center Caribbean Healthcare System
10 Casia St.
San Juan, PR 00921
Ph: (787)641-7582
Free: 800-449-8729
Fax: (787)641-4557
URL: http://www.caribbean.va.gov/

RHODE ISLAND

Providence

51645 ■ Veterans Affairs Medical Center Providence RI
830 Chalkstone Ave.
Providence, RI 02908-4799
Ph: (401)273-7100
Free: 866-363-4486
URL: http://www.providence.va.gov/

SOUTH CAROLINA

Columbia

51646 ■ William Jennings Bryan Dorn Veterans Administration Hospital
6439 Garners Ferry Rd.
Columbia, SC 29209
Ph: (803)776-4000
Free: 800-293-8262
Fax: (803)695-6739
URL: http://www.va.gov/columbiasc/

SOUTH DAKOTA

Fort Meade

51647 ■ The Veterans Affairs Black Hills Health Care System
Fort Meade Campus
113 Comanche Rd.
Fort Meade, SD 57741
Ph: (605)347-2511
Free: 800-743-1070
URL: http://www.blackhills.va.gov/

Hot Springs

51648 ■ The Veterans Affairs Black Hills Health Care System
Hot Springs Campus
500 N 5th St.
Hot Springs, SD 57747

Ph: (605)745-2000
Free: 800-764-5370
Fax: (605)745-2091
URL: http://www.blackhills.va.gov

Sioux Falls

51649 ■ Royal C. Johnson Veterans Affairs Medical Center
2501 W 22nd St.
Sioux Falls, SD 57105
Ph: (605)336-3230
Free: 800-316-8387
URL: http://www.siouxfalls.va.gov/

TENNESSEE

Memphis

51650 ■ Veterans Affairs Medical Center Memphis TN
1030 Jefferson Ave.
Memphis, TN 38104
Ph: (901)523-8990
Free: 800-636-8262
Fax: (901)577-7251
URL: http://www.memphis.va.gov

Mountain Home

51651 ■ Mountain Home Veterans Affairs Medical Center
Corner of Lamont & Veterans Way
Mountain Home, TN 37684
Ph: (423)926-1171
Free: 877-573-3529
Fax: (423)979-3519
URL: http://www.mountainhome.va.gov/

Murfreesboro

51652 ■ Tennessee Valley Healthcare System Alvin C. York Veterans Affairs Medical Center
3400 Lebanon Pike
Murfreesboro, TN 37129
Ph: (615)867-6000
Free: 800-876-7093
Fax: (615)225-4901
URL: http://www.tennesseevalley.va.gov
Formerly: Veterans Affairs Tennessee Valley Healthcare System.

Nashville

51653 ■ Tennessee Valley Healthcare System Veterans Affairs Medical Center
Nashville Campus
1310 24th Ave. S
Nashville, TN 37212-2637
Ph: (615)327-4751
Free: 800-228-4973
Fax: (615)321-6350
URL: http://www.tennesseevalley.va.gov

TEXAS

Amarillo

51654 ■ Veterans Affairs Medical Center Amarillo TX
6010 Amarillo Blvd. W
Amarillo, TX 79106
Ph: (806)355-9703
Free: 800-687-8262
Fax: (806)354-7860
URL: http://www.amarillo.va.gov/

Big Spring

51655 ■ West Texas Veterans Affairs Health Care System
300 Veterans Blvd.
Big Spring, TX 79720
Ph: (432)263-7361

Free: 800-472-1365
Fax: (432)264-4834
URL: http://www.bigspring.va.gov
License Status: Accredited.

Bonham

51656 ■ Veterans Affairs North Texas Health Care System
Sam Rayburn Memorial Veterans Center
1201 E 9th St.
Bonham, TX 75418
Ph: (903)583-6692
Free: 800-924-8387
Fax: (903)583-6692
URL: http://www.northtexas.va.gov
Remarks: Spinal cord injuries.

Dallas

51657 ■ Veterans Affairs North Texas Health Care System
Dallas Veterans Affairs Medical Center
4500 S Lancaster Rd.
Dallas, TX 75216
Ph: (214)742-8387
Free: 800-849-3597
Fax: (214)857-1171
URL: http://www.northtexas.va.gov

El Paso

51658 ■ Veterans Affairs Health Care System--El Paso TX
5001 N Piedras St.
El Paso, TX 79930-4211
Ph: (915)564-6100
Free: 800-672-3782
Fax: (915)564-7920
URL: http://www.elpaso.va.gov/

Harlingen

51659 ■ Veterans Affairs Valley Coastal Bend Health Care System
2701 S 77 Sunshine Strip
Harlingen, TX 78550
Ph: (957)430-9325
Free: 800-752-0650
URL: http://www.va.gov

KerrvilleTemple

51660 ■ South Texas Veterans Affairs Health Care System
Kerrville Division
3600 Memorial Blvd.
KerrvilleTemple, TX 78028
Ph: (830)896-2020
Free: 866-487-1653
Fax: (254)743-2338
URL: http://www.southtexas.va.gov/KD.asp

San Antonio

51661 ■ South Texas Veterans Health Care System
Audie Murphy Veterans Affairs Hospital
7400 Merton Minter Blvd.
San Antonio, TX 78229
Ph: (210)617-5300
Free: 877-469-5300
URL: http://www.southtexas.va.gov/

Temple

51662 ■ Central Texas Veterans Affairs Health Care System
1901 Veterans Memorial Dr.
Temple, TX 76504
Ph: (254)778-4811
Free: 800-423-2111
URL: http://www.centraltexas.va.gov

Waco

51663 ■ Central Texas Veterans Health Care System
Waco Veterans Affairs Medical Center
4800 Memorial Dr.
Waco, TX 76711
Ph: (254)752-6581
Free: 800-423-2111
URL: http://www.centraltexas.va.gov/

UTAH

Salt Lake City

51664 ■ Veterans Affairs Salt Lake City Health Care System
George E. Whalen Department of Veterans Affairs Medical Center
500 Foothill Dr.
Salt Lake City, UT 84148
Ph: (801)582-1565
Free: 800-613-4012
URL: http://www.saltlakecity.va.gov

VERMONT

White River Junction

51665 ■ Veterans Affairs Medical Center White River Junction VT
215 N Main St.
White River Junction, VT 05009
Ph: (802)295-9363
Free: 866-687-8387
Fax: (802)296-6354
URL: http://www.whiteriver.va.gov/

VIRGINIA

Hampton

51666 ■ Veterans Affairs Medical Center Hampton VA
100 Emancipation Dr.
Hampton, VA 23667
Ph: (757)722-9961
Fax: (757)723-6620
URL: http://www.hampton.va.gov/

Salem

51667 ■ Veterans Affairs Medical Center Salem VA
1970 Roanoke Blvd.
Salem, VA 24153
Ph: (540)982-2463
Free: 888-982-2463
Fax: (540)983-1096
URL: http://www.salem.va.gov/

WASHINGTON

Seattle

51668 ■ Veterans Affairs Puget Sound Health Care System
1660 S Columbian Way
Seattle, WA 98108
Ph: (206)762-1010
Free: 800-329-8387
Fax: (206)764-2224
URL: http://www.pugetsound.va.gov/

Spokane

51669 ■ Veterans Affairs Medical Center Spokane WA
4815 N Assembly St.
Spokane, WA 99205
Ph: (509)434-7000
Free: 800-325-7940
Fax: (509)434-7119
URL: http://www.spokane.va.gov/

Tacoma

51670 ■ Veterans Affairs Puget Sound Healthcare System
American Lake Division
9600 Veterans Dr.
Tacoma, WA 98493
Ph: (253)582-8440
Free: 800-329-8387
URL: http://www.pugetsound.va.gov/

Walla Walla

51671 ■ Jonathan M. Wainwright Memorial Veterans Affairs Medical Center
77 Wainwright Dr.
Walla Walla, WA 99362
Ph: (509)525-5200
Free: 888-687-8863
Fax: (509)527-3452
URL: http://www.visn20.med.va.gov/walla-walla/
License Status: Accredited.

WEST VIRGINIA

Beckley

51672 ■ Veterans Affairs Medical Center Beckley WV
200 Veterans Ave.
Beckley, WV 25801
Ph: (304)255-2121
Free: 877-902-5142
Fax: (304)255-2431
URL: http://www.beckley.va.gov/

Huntington

51673 ■ Veterans Affairs Medical Center Huntington WV
1540 Spring Valley Dr.
Huntington, WV 25704
Ph: (304)429-6741
Free: 800-827-8244
Fax: (304)429-6713
URL: http://www.huntington.va.gov/

Martinsburg

51674 ■ Veterans Affairs Medical Center Martinsburg WV
510 Butler Ave.
Martinsburg, WV 25405
Ph: (304)263-0811
Free: 800-817-3807
Fax: (304)262-7433
URL: http://www.martinsburg.va.gov

WISCONSIN

Madison

51675 ■ William S. Middleton Memorial Veterans Affairs Medical Center
2500 Overlook Ter.
Madison, WI 53705-2286
Ph: (608)256-1901
Free: 888-478-8321
URL: http://www.madison.va.gov/

Milwaukee

51676 ■ Clement J Zablocki Veterans Affairs Medical Center
5000 W National Ave.
Milwaukee, WI 53295
Ph: (414)384-2000
Free: 888-469-6614
Fax: (414)382-5319
URL: http://www.milwaukee.va.gov/

Tomah

51677 ■ Veterans Affairs Medical Center Tomah WI
500 E Veterans St.
Tomah, WI 54660

Ph: (608)372-3971
Free: 800-872-8662
URL: http://www.tomah.va.gov/

WYOMING

Cheyenne

51678 ■ Veterans Affairs Medical Center
Regional Office Center
2360 E Pershing Blvd.
Cheyenne, WY 82001
Ph: (307)778-7550
Free: 888-483-9127
Fax: (307)778-7336
URL: http://www.cheyenne.va.gov/

Sheridan

51679 ■ Veterans Affairs Medical Center
Sheridan WY
1898 Fort Rd.
Sheridan, WY 82801
Ph: (307)672-3473
Free: 866-822-6714
Fax: (307)672-1900
URL: http://www.sheridan.va.gov/

POST-TRAUMATIC STRESS DISORDER PROGRAMS

ALABAMA

Birmingham

51680 ■ Veterans Affairs Medical Center--Birmingham AL
PTSD Clinical Team
700 S 19th St.
Birmingham, AL 35233
Ph: (205)933-8101
E-mail: jose.vazquez@va.gov
URL: http://www.birmingham.va.gov

Tuscaloosa

51681 ■ Tuscaloosa Veterans Affairs Medical Center
Residential Rehabilitation Program
Intensive/Inpatient
PTSD Clinical Team
3701 Loop Rd. E
Tuscaloosa, AL 35404
Ph: (205)554-2000
Free: 888-269-3045
E-mail: david.gay2@va.gov
URL: http://www.tuscaloosa.va.gov

Tuskegee

51682 ■ Central Alabama Veterans Affairs Health Care System
PTSD Clinical Team
East Campus
2400 Hospital Rd.
Tuskegee, AL 36083
Ph: (334)727-0550
Free: 800-214-8387
E-mail: Stephen.Sams@va.gov
URL: http://www.westcentralalabama.va.gov

ALASKA

Anchorage

51683 ■ Alaska Veterans Affairs Health Care System
PTSD Clinical Team Outpatient
1201 N Muldoon Rd.
Anchorage, AK 99504
Ph: (907)257-4700
Free: 888-353-7574
E-mail: laura.gambone@va.gov
URL: http://www.alaska.va.gov

ARIZONA

Phoenix

51684 ■ Carl T. Hayden Veterans Affairs Medical Center
PTSD Clinical Team
650 E Indian School Rd.
Phoenix, AZ 85012
Ph: (602)277-5551
E-mail: Karen.Kattar@va.gov
URL: http://www.phoenix.va.gov

51685 ■ Carl T. Hayden Veterans Affairs Medical Center
Substance Abuse PTSD Clinical Team
650 E Indian School Rd.
Phoenix, AZ 85012
Ph: (602)277-5551
E-mail: Karen.Kattar@va.gov
URL: http://www.phoenix.va.gov

Prescott

51686 ■ Northern Arizona Veterans Affairs Health Care System
PTSD Clinical Team
500 N Hwy. 89
Prescott, AZ 86313
Ph: (928)445-4860
E-mail: james.hall4@va.gov
URL: http://www.prescott.va.gov

Tucson

51687 ■ Veterans Affairs Southern Arizona Health Care System
PTSD Clinic
3601 S 6th Ave.
Tucson, AZ 85723
Ph: (520)792-1450
E-mail: david.bell-adaskin@va.gov
URL: http://www.tuscon.va.gov

ARKANSAS

North Little Rock

51688 ■ Central Arkansas Veterans Affairs Health Care System
PTSD Program
2200 Fort Roots Dr.
North Little Rock, AR 72114
Ph: (501)257-1000
E-mail: john.roca@va.gov
URL: http://www.littlerock.va.gov

CALIFORNIA

East Los Angeles

51689 ■ Greater Los Angeles Veterans Affairs Medical Center
PTSD Clinical Team
5426 E Olympic Blvd., Ste. 150
East Los Angeles, CA 90022
Ph: (323)725-7557
E-mail: Rachel.stone2@va.gov
URL: http://www.losangeles.va.gov

Livermore

51690 ■ Veterans Affairs Palo Alto Healthcare System--Livermore Division
PTSD Clinical Team
Bldg. 66, Rm. 418
4951 Arroyo Rd.
Livermore, CA 94550
Ph: (925)373-4700
URL: http://www.paloalto.va.gov

Loma Linda

51691 ■ Veterans Affairs Loma Linda Healthcare System
PTSD Clinical Team
11201 Benton St.
Loma Linda, CA 92357

Ph: (909)825-7084
E-mail: Cheryl.Hardcastle@va.gov
URL: http://www.lomalinda.va.gov

51692 ■ Veterans Affairs Loma Linda Healthcare System
Women's Stress Disorder Treatment Team
11201 Benton St.
Loma Linda, CA 92357
Ph: (909)583-6046
E-mail: Cheryl.Hardcastle@va.gov
URL: http://www.lomalinda.va.gov

Long Beach

51693 ■ Veterans Affairs Long Beach Healthcare System
PTSD Clinical Team
5901 E 7th St.
Long Beach, CA 90822
Ph: (562)826-5604
Free: 888-769-8387
E-mail: Richard.Hanson@va.gov
URL: http://www.longbeach.va.gov

Mather

51694 ■ Northern California Veterans Affairs Healthcare System
Mather Mental Health Outpatient Clinic
PTSD Clinical Team
10535 Hospital Way
Mather, CA 95655
Ph: (916)366-5434
E-mail: Jeanette.Giorgio@va.gov
URL: http://www.northerncalifornia.gov

Menlo Park

51695 ■ Veterans Affairs Palo Alto Healthcare System
PTSD Clinical Team
795 Willow Rd.
Menlo Park, CA 94025
Ph: (650)614-9997
E-mail: Ann.LeFevre@va.gov
URL: http://www.paloalto.va.gov

51696 ■ Veterans Affairs Palo Alto Healthcare System
PTSD Residential Rehabilitation Program
795 Willow Rd.
Menlo Park, CA 94025
Ph: (650)493-5000
E-mail: Marion.Gautschi@va.gov
URL: http://www.paloalto.va.gov

San Diego

51697 ■ Veterans Affairs San Diego Healthcare System
PTSD Clinical Team
8810 Rio San Diego Dr.
San Diego, CA 92108
Ph: (619)400-5000
E-mail: john.mcquaid@va.gov
URL: http://www.sandiego.va.gov

San Francisco

51698 ■ Veterans Affairs Medical Center--San Francisco
PTSD Clinical Team
4150 Clement St.
San Francisco, CA 94121
Ph: (415)221-4810
E-mail: Eduardo.Ramirez2@va.gov
URL: http://www.sanfrancisco.va.gov
Program(s): Post-Traumatic Stress Disorder Program.

51699 ■ Veterans Affairs Medical Center--San Francisco
Substance Abuse PTSD Team
4150 Clement St.
San Francisco, CA 94121

Ph: (415)221-4810
E-mail: Ben.Ramos@va.gov
URL: http://www.sanfrancisco.va.gov
Program(s): Post-Traumatic Stress Disorder Program.

COLORADO

Colorado Springs

51700 ■ Denver Veterans Affairs Medical
  Center
Colorado Springs Clinic
Women's Stress Disorder Treatment Team
Outpatient
25 N Spruce St.
Colorado Springs, CO 80905
Ph: (719)327-5660
Free: 800-278-3883
E-mail: nancy.galbraith@va.gov
URL: http://www.denver.va.gov

Denver

51701 ■ Eastern Colorado Veterans Affairs
  Healthcare System
PTSD Residential Rehabilitation Program
1055 Clermont St.
Denver, CO 80220
Ph: (303)399-8020
E-mail: renee.labor@va.gov
URL: http://www.denver.va.gov

Grand Junction

51702 ■ Veterans Affairs Medical
  Center--Grand Junction CO
PTSD Clinical Team
2121 North Ave.
Grand Junction, CO 81501
Ph: (970)263-2824
Free: 866-206-6415
E-mail: heather.martinez@va.gov
URL: http://www.grandjunction.va.gov

CONNECTICUT

Newington

51703 ■ Veterans Affairs Connecticut
  Healthcare System
PTSD Residential Rehabilitation Program
555 Willard Ave.
Newington, CT 06111
Ph: (860)666-6951
E-mail: Robin.Gilmartin@va.gov
URL: http://www.connecticut.va.gov

West Haven

51704 ■ Veterans Affairs Connecticut
  Healthcare System
PTSD Clinical Team
950 Campbell Ave.
West Haven, CT 06516
Ph: (203)932-5711
URL: http://www.connecticut.va.gov

51705 ■ Veterans Affairs Connecticut
  Healthcare System
Substance Abuse PTSD Team
950 Campbell Ave.
West Haven, CT 06516
Ph: (203)932-5711
URL: http://www.connecticut.va.gov

DISTRICT OF COLUMBIA

Washington

51706 ■ Veterans Affairs Medical
  Center--Washington DC
PTSD Clinical Team
50 Irving St. NW
Washington, DC 20422

Ph: (202)745-8000
E-mail: David.Cueva@va.gov
URL: http://www.washingtondc.va.gov

FLORIDA

Bay Pines

51707 ■ Veterans Affairs Medical Center--Bay
  Pines FL
PTSD Clinical Team
10000 Bay Pines Blvd.
Bay Pines, FL 33744
Ph: (727)398-6661
Free: 888-820-0230
E-mail: Anthony.Taylor@va.gov
URL: http://www.baypines.va.gov

51708 ■ Veterans Affairs Medical Center--Bay
  Pines FL
PTSD Domiciliary
10000 Bay Pines Blvd.
Bay Pines, FL 33744
Ph: (727)398-6661
Free: 888-820-0230
E-mail: Anthony.Taylor@va.gov
URL: http://www.baypines.va.gov

Gainesville

51709 ■ Malcolm Randall Veterans Affairs
  Medical Center
North Florida--South Georgia Healthcare
System
PTSD Clinical Team
1601 SW Archer Rd.
Gainesville, FL 32608
Ph: (352)376-1611
E-mail: Thomas.Hundersmarck2@va.gov
URL: http://www.northflorida.va.gov

Lake City

51710 ■ Veterans Affairs North Florida--South
  Georgia Healthcare System
PTSD Clinical Team
619 S Marion Ave.
Lake City, FL 32025
Ph: (386)755-3016
Free: 800-308-8387
E-mail: april.drewing@va.gov
URL: http://www.northflorida.va.gov

Miami

51711 ■ Miami Veterans Affairs Healthcare
  System
PTSD Clinical Team
1201 NW 16th St.
Miami, FL 33125
Ph: (305)575-7000
Free: 888-276-1785
E-mail: Nicole.Larkin@va.gov
URL: http://www.miami.va.gov

Port Saint Lucie

51712 ■ Veterans Affairs Medical Center--Port
  Saint Lucie
Saint Lucie County PTSD Clinical Team
126 SW Chambers Ct.
Port Saint Lucie, FL 34986
Ph: (772)878-7876
E-mail: Raymond.Pierson@va.gov
URL: http://www.va.gov

Tampa

51713 ■ James A. Haley Veterans Hospital
PTSD Clinical Team
13000 Bruce Downs Blvd.
Tampa, FL 33612
Ph: (813)631-7135
E-mail: Narine.Karakashian@va.gov
URL: http://www.tampa.va.gov

West Palm Beach

51714 ■ West Palm Beach Veterans Affairs
  Medical Center
Women's Stress Disorder Treatment Team
Outpatient
7305 N Military Trail
West Palm Beach, FL 33410
Ph: (561)422-8262
Free: 800-972-8262
URL: http://www.westpalmbeach.va.gov

GEORGIA

Atlanta

51715 ■ Atlanta Veterans Affairs Medical
  Center
PTSD Clinical Team
1670 Clairmont Rd.
Atlanta, GA 30033
Ph: (404)321-6111
E-mail: Larry.Folson@va.gov
URL: http://www.atlanta.va.gov

Augusta

51716 ■ Charles Norwood Veterans Affairs
  Medical Center
PTSD Clinical Team
1 Freedom Way
Augusta, GA 30904
Ph: (706)733-0188
E-mail: Lorraine.Braswell@va.gov
URL: http://www.augusta.va.gov

Dublin

51717 ■ Carl Vinson Veterans Affairs Medical
  Center
PTSD Clinical Team
1826 Veterans Blvd.
Dublin, GA 31021
Ph: (478)277-1210
E-mail: fay.fennel@va.gov
URL: http://www.dublin.va.gov

HAWAII

Honolulu

51718 ■ Veterans Affairs Pacific Islands
  Healthcare System
PTSD Clinical Team
459 Patterson Rd.
Honolulu, HI 96819
Ph: (808)433-0672
E-mail: Nadine.Shigezawa@va.gov
URL: http://www.hawaii.va.gov

51719 ■ Veterans Affairs Pacific Islands
  Healthcare System
PTSD Residential Rehabilitation Program
459 Patterson Rd.
Honolulu, HI 96819
Ph: (808)433-0062
E-mail: Kenneth.Hirsch2@va.gov
URL: http://www.hawaii.va.gov

IDAHO

Boise

51720 ■ Veterans Affairs Medical
  Center--Boise ID
PTSD Clinical Team
500 W Fort St.
Boise, ID 83702
Ph: (208)422-1110
E-mail: Margaret.Blandford@va.gov
URL: http://www.boise.va.gov

51721 ■ Veterans Affairs Medical
  Center--Boise ID
PTSD Evaluation and Brief Treatment Unit
500 W Fort St.
Boise, ID 83702

Ph: (208)422-1125
E-mail: Anne.Flickinger@va.gov
URL: http://www.boise.va.gov

ILLINOIS

Chicago

51722 ■ Jesse Brown Veterans Affairs Medical Center
PTSD Clinical Team
820 S Damen Ave.
Chicago, IL 60612
Ph: (312)569-8387
E-mail: Evelyn.Harris2@va.gov
URL: http://www.chicago.va.gov

Danville

51723 ■ Veterans Affairs Illiana Healthcare System
PTSD Clinical Team
1900 E Main St.
Danville, IL 61832
Ph: (217)554-4257
Free: 800-320-8387
E-mail: Jody.Marshall@va.gov
URL: http://www.danville.va.gov

Hines

51724 ■ Edward Hines Jr. Veterans Affairs Medical Center
PTSD Clinical Team
5000 S 5th Ave.
Hines, IL 60141
Ph: (708)202-8387
E-mail: Kelly.Maieritsch@va.gov
URL: http://www.hines.va.gov

Marion

51725 ■ Veterans Affairs Medical Center--Marion IL
PTSD Clinical Team
2401 W Main St.
Marion, IL 62959
Ph: (618)997-5311
E-mail: Steven.Hurst@va.gov
URL: http://www.marion.va.gov

North Chicago

51726 ■ Captain James A. Lovell Federal Health Care Center
PTSD Residential Rehabilitation Program
3001 N Greenbay Rd.
North Chicago, IL 60064
Ph: (847)688-1900
E-mail: Benita.Perez@va.gov
URL: http://www.lovell.fhcc.va.gov

51727 ■ Veterans Affairs Medical Center--North Chicago IL
PTSD Clinical Team
3001 N Greenbay Rd.
North Chicago, IL 60064
Ph: (224)610-5789
E-mail: Carla.Bachmann@va.gov
URL: http://www.ptsd.va.gov

INDIANA

Fort Wayne

51728 ■ Veterans Affairs Northern Indiana Healthcare System
PTSD Clinical Team
2121 Lake Ave.
Fort Wayne, IN 46805
Ph: (260)426-5431
Free: 800-498-8792
E-mail: Donald.Wilson3@va.gov
URL: http://www.northernindiana.va.gov

Indianapolis

51729 ■ Richard L. Roudebush Veterans Affairs Medical Center
PTSD Clinical Team
1481 W 10th St.
Indianapolis, IN 46202
Ph: (317)988-4329
Free: 888-342-7602
E-mail: David.Tarr@va.gov
URL: http://www.indianapolis.va.gov

Marion

51730 ■ Veterans Affairs Northern Indiana Healthcare System
PTSD Clinical Team
1700 E 38th St.
Marion, IN 46953
Ph: (765)674-3321
Free: 800-498-8792
E-mail: James.Lowery1@va.gov
URL: http://www.northernindiana.va.gov

IOWA

Des Moines

51731 ■ Veterans Affairs Central Iowa Healthcare System
PTSD Clinical Team
3600 30th St.
Des Moines, IA 50310
Ph: (515)699-5999
E-mail: John.Wallace4@va.gov
URL: http://www.centraliowa.va.gov

Iowa City

51732 ■ Veterans Affairs Health Care System--Iowa City
PTSD Clinical Team
601 Hwy. 6 West
Iowa City, IA 52246
Ph: (319)688-3405
E-mail: Mary.Schmeichel@va.gov
URL: http://www.iowacity.va.gov

Knoxville

51733 ■ Veterans Affairs Central Iowa Healthcare System
PTSD Domiciliary
1515 W Pleasant St.
Knoxville, IA 50138
URL: http://www.ptsd.va.gov

KANSAS

Topeka

51734 ■ Veterans Affairs Eastern Kansas Healthcare System
PTSD Clinical Team
2200 SW Gage Blvd.
Topeka, KS 66622
Ph: (785)350-3111
E-mail: timothy.rot@va.gov
URL: http://www.topeka.va.gov

51735 ■ Veterans Affairs Eastern Kansas Healthcare System
Specialized Inpatient PTSD Unit
2200 SW Gage Blvd.
Topeka, KS 66622
Ph: (785)350-3111
E-mail: terry.falck@va.gov
URL: http://www.topeka.va.gov

Wichita

51736 ■ Robert J. Dole Veterans Affairs Medical Center
PTSD Clinical Team
5500 E Kellogg
Wichita, KS 67218

Ph: (316)685-2221
Free: 888-685-2221
E-mail: Barbara.Harrison@va.gov
URL: http://www.wichita.va.gov

KENTUCKY

Lexington

51737 ■ Veterans Affairs Medical Center--Lexington KY
PTSD Clinical Team
1101 Veterans Dr.
Lexington, KY 40502
Ph: (859)281-3817
E-mail: Deborah.Tharpe@va.gov
URL: http://www.lexington.va.gov

51738 ■ Veterans Affairs Medical Center--Lexington KY
PTSD Residential Rehabilitation Program
1101 Veterans Dr.
Lexington, KY 40502
Ph: (859)281-3949
E-mail: Alma.Perkins@va.gov
URL: http://www.lexington.va.gov

Louisville

51739 ■ Robley Rex Veterans Affairs Medical Center
PTSD Clinical Team
DuPont Clinic
800 Zorn Ave.
Louisville, KY 40206
Ph: (502)287-4000
E-mail: Karen.Grantz@va.gov
URL: http://www.louisville.va.gov

LOUISIANA

Alexandria

51740 ■ Veterans Affairs Medical Center--Alexandria LA
PTSD Clinical Team
PO Box 69004
Alexandria, LA 71306
Ph: (318)473-0010
Free: 800-375-8387
E-mail: Leslie.Drew@va.gov
URL: http://www.alexandria.va.gov

New Orleans

51741 ■ Southeast Louisiana Veterans Healthcare System
New Orleans Veterans Affairs Outpatient Clinic
PTSD Clinical Team
1601 Perdido St.
New Orleans, LA 70112
Ph: (504)571-8326
Free: 800-935-8387
E-mail: carlette.porter@va.gov
URL: http://www.neworleans.va.gov

Shreveport

51742 ■ Overton Brooks Veterans Affairs Medical Center
PTSD Clinical Team
510 E Stoner Ave.
Shreveport, LA 71101
Ph: (318)990-5419
E-mail: david.montgomery@va.gov
URL: http://www.shreveport.va.gov

MAINE

Augusta

51743 ■ Togas Veterans Affairs Medical Center
PTSD Clinical Team
1 VA Center
Augusta, ME 04330

Ph: (207)623-8411
E-mail: Chantel.Mihm@va.gov
URL: http://www.togus.va.gov

51744 ■ Togus Veterans Affairs Medical Center
PTSD Day Hospital
1 VA Center
Augusta, ME 04330
Ph: (207)623-8411
E-mail: Joseph.Andrews4@va.gov
URL: http://www.togus.va.gov

MARYLAND

Baltimore

51745 ■ Veterans Affairs Maryland Healthcare System
PTSD Clinical Team
10 N Greene St.
Baltimore, MD 21201
Ph: (410)605-7422
E-mail: Aaron.Jacoby@va.gov
URL: http://www.maryland.va.gov

51746 ■ Veterans Affairs Maryland Healthcare System
PTSD Day Hospital
10 N Greene St.
Baltimore, MD 21201
Ph: (410)605-7418
E-mail: Andrew.Santanello@va.gov
URL: http://www.maryland.va.gov

Perryville

51747 ■ Veterans Affairs Maryland Healthcare System
PTSD Clinical Team
515 Broad St.
Perryville, MD 21903
E-mail: Christina.Watlington2@va.gov
URL: http://www.maryland.va.gov

MASSACHUSETTS

Boston

51748 ■ Veterans Affairs Boston Healthcare System
PTSD Clinical Team
150 S Huntington Ave.
Boston, MA 02130
Ph: (617)364-4122
E-mail: Karen.Ryabchenko@va.gov
URL: http://www.boston.va.gov

51749 ■ Veterans Affairs Boston Healthcare System
Women's Stress Disorder Treatment Team
150 S Huntington Ave.
Boston, MA 02130
Ph: (857)364-4012
E-mail: Eve.Davison@va.gov
URL: http://www.boston.va.gov

Brockton

51750 ■ Veterans Affairs Boston Healthcare System
PTSD Clinical Team
940 Belmont St.
Brockton, MA 02301
Ph: (508)826-1727
E-mail: Julie.Klunkgillis@va.gov
URL: http://www.boston.va.gov

Leeds

51751 ■ Northampton Veterans Affairs Medical Center
PTSD Clinical Team
421 N Main St.
Leeds, MA 01053

Ph: (413)584-4040
E-mail: Wayne.Lynch@va.gov
URL: http://www.northampton.va.gov

MICHIGAN

Ann Arbor

51752 ■ Veterans Affairs Ann Arbor Healthcare System
PTSD Clinical Team
2215 Fuller Rd.
Ann Arbor, MI 48105
Ph: (734)845-3044
E-mail: Edward.McPhee@va.gov
URL: http://www.annarbor.va.gov

Battle Creek

51753 ■ Veterans Affairs Medical Center--Battle Creek MI
PTSD Clinical Team
5500 Armstrong Rd.
Battle Creek, MI 49037
Ph: (269)966-5600
E-mail: Annie.Ingram@va.gov
URL: http://www.battlecreek.va.gov

51754 ■ Veterans Affairs Medical Center--Battle Creek MI
PTSD Residential Rehabilitation Program
5500 Armstrong Rd.
Battle Creek, MI 49037
Ph: (269)966-5600
E-mail: wendy.johnson@va.gov
URL: http://www.battlecreek.va.gov

Detroit

51755 ■ John D. Dingell Veterans Affairs Medical Center
PTSD Clinical Team
4646 John R
Detroit, MI 48201
Ph: (313)576-4962
E-mail: Christina.Hall@va.gov
URL: http://www.detroit.va.gov

Saginaw

51756 ■ Aleda E. Lutz Veterans Affairs Medical Center
PTSD Clinical Team
1500 Weiss St.
Saginaw, MI 48602
Ph: (989)497-2500
E-mail: lisa.garabelli-smith@va.gov
URL: http://www.saginaw.va.gov

MINNESOTA

Minneapolis

51757 ■ Veterans Affairs Medical Center--Minneapolis MN
PTSD Clinical Team
1 Veterans Dr.
Minneapolis, MN 55417
Ph: (612)725-2125
E-mail: Christopher.Erbes@va.gov
URL: http://www.minneapolis.va.gov

Saint Cloud

51758 ■ Saint Cloud Veterans Affairs Health Care System
Women's Stress Disorder Treatment Team Outpatient
4801 Veterans Dr.
Saint Cloud, MN 56303
Ph: (320)252-1670
E-mail: Jeremy.maurstad@va.gov
URL: http://www.stcloud.va.gov

MISSISSIPPI

Biloxi

51759 ■ Veterans Affairs Gulf Coast Veterans Healthcare System
PTSD Program
400 Veterans Ave.
Biloxi, MS 39531
Ph: (228)523-4215
Free: 800-296-8872
E-mail: amy.walters@va.gov
URL: http://www.biloxi.va.gov

Jackson

51760 ■ G.V. Sonny Montgomery Veterans Affairs Medical Center
PTSD Residential Rehabilitation Program
1500 E Woodrow Wilson Dr.
Jackson, MS 39216
Ph: (601)362-4471
E-mail: Randy.Burke@va.gov
URL: http://www.jackson.va.gov

51761 ■ G.V. Sonny Montgomery Veterans Affairs Medical Center
Substance Use PTSD Team
1500 E Woodrow Wilson Dr.
Jackson, MS 39216
Ph: (601)362-4471
E-mail: Randy.Burke@va.gov
URL: http://www.jackson.va.gov

MISSOURI

Columbia

51762 ■ Harry S. Truman Memorial Veterans Hospital
PTSD Clinical Team
800 Hospital Dr.
Columbia, MO 65201
Ph: (573)814-6000
E-mail: Grant.Oneal@va.gov
URL: http://www.columbiamo.va.gov

Kansas City

51763 ■ Veterans Affairs Medical Center--Kansas City MO
PTSD Clinical Team
4801 Linwood Blvd.
Kansas City, MO 64128
Ph: (816)861-4700
E-mail: Hemant.Thakus@va.gov
URL: http://www.kansascity.va.gov

Poplar Bluff

51764 ■ John J. Pershing Veterans Affairs Medical Center
PTSD Clinical Team
1500 N Westwood Blvd.
Poplar Bluff, MO 63901
Ph: (537)686-4151
E-mail: Kevin.Wagner@va.gov
URL: http://www.poplarbluff.va.gov

Saint Louis

51765 ■ Saint Louis Veterans Affairs Medical Center
Jefferson Barracks Division
PTSD Clinical Team
1 Jefferson Barracks Dr.
Saint Louis, MO 63125
Ph: (314)894-6639
Free: 800-228-5459
E-mail: Mary.Lages@va.gov
URL: http://www.stlouis.va.gov

NEBRASKA

Lincoln

51766 ■ Veterans Affairs Nebraska--Western Iowa Healthcare System
Community-Based Outpatient Clinic
PTSD Clinical Team
600 S 70th St.
Lincoln, NE 68510

Ph: (402)486-7923
E-mail: Stanley.Moore2@va.gov
URL: http://www.nebraska.va.gov

Omaha

51767 ■ Veterans Affairs Nebraska--Western Iowa Medical Center
PTSD Clinical Team
4101 Woolworth Ave.
Omaha, NE 68105
Ph: (402)346-8800
E-mail: Terry.North@va.gov
URL: http://www.nebraska.va.gov

NEVADA

Las Vegas

51768 ■ Veterans Affairs Southern Nevada Healthcare System
Healthcare for Homeless Veterans
PTSD Clinical Team
926 W Owens Ave.
Las Vegas, NV 89106
Ph: (702)636-4060
E-mail: Martha.Bacon@va.gov
URL: http://www.lasvegas.va.gov

Reno

51769 ■ Veterans Affairs Sierra Nevada Healthcare System
PTSD Clinical Team
1000 Locust St.
Reno, NV 89502
Ph: (775)786-7200
E-mail: George.Daforno@va.gov
URL: http://www.reno.va.gov

NEW JERSEY

East Orange

51770 ■ Veterans Affairs New Jersey Healthcare System
East Orange Campus
PTSD Unit
385 Tremont Ave.
East Orange, NJ 07018
Ph: (973)676-1000
E-mail: saila.donepudi@va.gov
URL: http://www.newjersey.va.gov

Lyons

51771 ■ Veterans Affairs New Jersey Healthcare System
PTSD Clinical Team
151 Knollcroft Rd.
Lyons, NJ 07939
Ph: (908)647-1080
Fax: (908)647-3452
E-mail: Bradler.Sussner@va.gov
URL: http://www.newjersey.va.gov

51772 ■ Veterans Affairs New Jersey Healthcare System
PTSD Residential Rehabilitation Program
151 Knollcroft Rd.
Lyons, NJ 07939
Ph: (908)647-0180
E-mail: Mia.Downing@va.gov
URL: http://www.newjersey.va.gov

51773 ■ Veterans Affairs New Jersey Healthcare System
Women's Trauma Recovery Program
151 Knollcroft Rd.
Lyons, NJ 07939
Ph: (908)647-0180
E-mail: Suzanne.Loftus@va.gov
URL: http://www.newjersey.va.gov

NEW MEXICO

Albuquerque

51774 ■ Veterans Affairs New Mexico Healthcare System
PTSD Clinical Team
1501 San Pedor Dr. SE
Albuquerque, NM 87108
Ph: (505)265-1711
E-mail: Tammy.Lamere@va.gov
URL: http://www.albuquerque.va.gov

51775 ■ Veterans Affairs New Mexico Healthcare System
Women's Stress Disorder Treatment Team
1501 San Pedro Dr. SE
Albuquerque, NM 87108
Ph: (505)265-1711
E-mail: maria.rodriguez@va.gov
URL: http://www.albuquerque.va.gov

NEW YORK

Batavia

51776 ■ Veterans Affairs Western New York Healthcare System
PTSD Day Hospital
222 Richmond Ave.
Batavia, NY 14020
Ph: (585)297-1000
E-mail: Harold.Rybak@va.gov
URL: http://www.buffalo.va.gov/

51777 ■ Veterans Affairs Western New York Healthcare System
PTSD Women's Trauma Recovery Program
222 Richmond Ave.
Batavia, NY 14020
Ph: (585)297-1000
E-mail: Terri.Julian@va.gov
URL: http://www.buffalo.va.gov

51778 ■ Veterans Affairs Western New York Healthcare System
Women's Trauma Recovery Program
222 Richmond Ave.
Batavia, NY 14020
Ph: (585)297-1216
E-mail: Joanne.Shreder-Robinson@va.gov
URL: http://www.buffalo.va.gov

Bronx

51779 ■ Veterans Affairs Medical Center--Bronx NY
PTSD Clinical Team
130 W Kingsbridge Rd.
Bronx, NY 10468
Ph: (718)584-9000
E-mail: lisa.kluepfel@va.gov
URL: http://www.bronx.va.gov

Brooklyn

51780 ■ Veterans Affairs New York Harbor Healthcare System
PTSD Clinical Team
800 Poly Pl.
Brooklyn, NY 11209
Ph: (718)630-3713
E-mail: marie.deteskey@va.gov
URL: http://www.nyharbor.va.gov

Canandaigua

51781 ■ Veterans Affairs Medical Center--Canandaigua NY
PTSD Clinical Team
400 Fort Hill Ave.
Canandaigua, NY 14424
Ph: (585)393-7225
Free: 800-204-9917
E-mail: Khamkay.Chitaphong@va.gov
URL: http://www.canandaigua.va.gov

Castle Point

51782 ■ Veterans Affairs Hudson Valley Healthcare System
Castle Point Campus
PTSD Program
100 Rte. 9D Castle Point Rd.
Castle Point, NY 12511
Ph: (914)737-4400
E-mail: debra.tolliver2@va.gov
URL: http://www.hudsonvalley.va.gov

Montrose

51783 ■ Veterans Affairs Hudson Valley Healthcare System
PTSD Domiciliary
2094 Albany Post Rd.
Montrose, NY 10548
Ph: (914)737-4400
E-mail: debra.tolliver@va.gov
URL: http://www.hudsonvalley.va.gov

New York

51784 ■ Veterans Affairs New York Harbor Healthcare System
PTSD Clinical Team
423 E 23rd St.
New York, NY 10010
Ph: (212)686-7500
E-mail: Evelyn.Quinones@va.gov
URL: http://www.nyharbor.va.gov

Northport

51785 ■ Northport Veterans Affairs Medical Center
PTSD Clinical Team Outpatient
79 Middleville Rd.
Northport, NY 11768
Ph: (631)261-4400
E-mail: Ganesan.Krishanmoorthy@va.gov
URL: http://www.northport.va.gov

51786 ■ Northport Veterans Affairs Medical Center
PTSD Clinical Team Residential Rehabilitation Program Intensive/Inpatient
79 Middleville Rd.
Northport, NY 11768
Ph: (631)261-4400
E-mail: ganesan.krishnamoorthy@va.gov
URL: http://www.northport.va.gov

Syracuse

51787 ■ Veterans Affairs Medical Center--Syracuse NY
PTSD Clinical Team
800 Irving Ave.
Syracuse, NY 13210
Ph: (315)425-3486
Free: 800-792-4334
E-mail: shawne.steiger@va.gov
URL: http://www.syracuse.va.gov

NORTH CAROLINA

Asheville

51788 ■ Veterans Affairs Medical Center--Asheville NC
PTSD Clinical Team
1100 Tunnel Rd.
Asheville, NC 28805
URL: http://www.ashville.va.gov

Durham

51789 ■ Veterans Affairs Medical Center--Durham NC
PTSD Clinical Team
1824 Hillandale Rd.
Durham, NC 27705

Ph: (919)383-6107
E-mail: Josephine.Allen@va.gov
URL: http://www.durham.va.gov

Fayetteville

51790 ■ Veterans Affairs Medical Center--Fayetteville NC
PTSD Clinical Team
2300 Ramsey St.
Fayetteville, NC 28301
Ph: (910)488-2120
Fax: (910)488-5589
E-mail: Tammy.Foster2@va.gov
URL: http://www.fayettevillenc.va.gov

Salisbury

51791 ■ W.G. Bill Hefner Veterans Affairs Medical Center
Specialized Inpatient PTSD Unit
1601 Brenner Ave.
Salisbury, NC 28144
Ph: (704)638-9000
E-mail: Jo.Cooley@va.gov
URL: http://www.salisbury.va.gov

51792 ■ W.G. Bill Hefner Veterans Affairs Medical Center
Women's Trauma Recovery Program
1601 Brenner Ave.
Salisbury, NC 28144
Ph: (704)638-9000
E-mail: Kristen.Humphrey@va.gov
URL: http://www.salisbury.va.gov

OHIO

Brecksville

51793 ■ Louis Stokes Veterans Affairs Medical Center
PTSD Clinical Team
10000 Brecksville Rd.
Brecksville, OH 44141
Ph: (440)526-3030
E-mail: John.Hrovat@va.gov
URL: http://www.ohio.va.gov

51794 ■ Veterans Affairs Medical Center
Women's Stress Disorder Treatment Team
10000 Brecksville Rd.
Brecksville, OH 44141
Ph: (440)526-3030
E-mail: tina.brown@va.gov
URL: http://www.ohio.va.gov

Chillicothe

51795 ■ Veterans Affairs Medical Center--Chillicothe OH
PTSD Clinical Team
17273 State Rte. 104
Chillicothe, OH 45601
Ph: (740)773-1141
Free: 800-358-8262
E-mail: Carrie.Robinson@va.gov
URL: http://www.chillicothe.va.gov

Cincinnati

51796 ■ Veterans Affairs Medical Center--Cincinnati OH
PTSD Clinical Team
1000 S Ft. Thomas Ave.
Cincinnati, OH 41075
Ph: (859)572-6208
E-mail: ryan.faulkner@va.gov
URL: http://www.cincinnati.va.gov

51797 ■ Veterans Affairs Medical Center--Cincinnati OH
PTSD Day Hospital
1000 S Ft. Thomas Ave.
Cincinnati, OH 41075

Ph: (859)572-6238
E-mail: Susan.Mcilvain@va.gov
URL: http://www.cincinnati.va.gov

Columbus

51798 ■ Chalmers P. Wylie Veterans Affairs Ambulatory Care Center
PTSD Clinical Team
420 N James Rd.
Columbus, OH 43219
Ph: (614)257-5420
E-mail: Chan.Bowman@va.gov
URL: http://www.columbus.va.gov

Dayton

51799 ■ Veterans Affairs Medical Center--Dayton OH
PTSD Clinical Team
4100 W 3rd St.
Dayton, OH 45428
Ph: (937)268-6511
E-mail: Kristin.Rodzinka@va.gov
URL: http://www.dayton.va.gov

51800 ■ Veterans Affairs Medical Center--Dayton OH
PTSD Day Hospital
4100 W 3rd St.
Dayton, OH 45428
Ph: (937)268-6511
E-mail: Deborah.Downey2@va.gov
URL: http://www.dayton.va.gov

OKLAHOMA

Muskogee

51801 ■ Jack C. Montgomery Veterans Hospital
PTSD Clinical Team
1011 Honor Heights Dr.
Muskogee, OK 74401
Ph: (918)577-3698
E-mail: Jane.Swan2@va.gov
URL: http://www.muskogee.va.gov

Oklahoma City

51802 ■ Veterans Affairs Medical Center--Oklahoma City OK
PTSD Clinical Team
921 NE 13th St.
Oklahoma City, OK 73104
Ph: (405)456-5367
E-mail: William.Parker@va.gov
URL: http://www.oklahoma.va.gov

OREGON

Portland

51803 ■ Veterans Affairs Medical Center--Portland OR
PTSD Clinical Team
3710 SW US Veterans Hospital Rd.
Portland, OR 97239
Ph: (503)220-8262
E-mail: tammy.lewis2@va.gov
URL: http://www.portland.va.gov

Roseburg

51804 ■ Veterans Affairs Roseburg Healthcare System
PTSD Clinical Team
913 NW Garden Valley Blvd.
Roseburg, OR 97470
Ph: (541)440-1000
E-mail: Stella.Faas@va.gov
URL: http://www.roseburg.va.gov

PENNSYLVANIA

Coatesville

51805 ■ Veterans Affairs Medical Center--Coatesville PA
PTSD Clinical Team
1400 Black Horse Hill Rd.
Coatesville, PA 19320
Ph: (610)384-7711
URL: http://www.coatesville.va.gov

51806 ■ Veterans Affairs Medical Center--Coatesville PA
PTSD Domiciliary
1400 Black Horse Hill Rd.
Coatesville, PA 19320
Ph: (610)384-7711
URL: http://www.coatesville.va.gov

Lebanon

51807 ■ Veterans Affairs Medical Center--Lebanon PA
PTSD Clinical Team
1700 S Lincoln Ave.
Lebanon, PA 17042
Ph: (717)272-6621
E-mail: jill.roling@va.gov
URL: http://www.lebanon.va.gov

Philadelphia

51808 ■ Veterans Affairs Medical Center--Philadelphia PA
PTSD Clinical Team
3900 Woodland Ave.
Philadelphia, PA 19104
Ph: (215)823-5800
E-mail: Andrew.Stone2@va.gov
URL: http://www.philadelphia.va.gov

Pittsburgh

51809 ■ Veterans Affairs Pittsburgh Healthcare System
PTSD Clinical Team
7180 Highland Dr.
Pittsburgh, PA 15206
Ph: (412)954-4322
E-mail: Daniel.ziff@va.gov
URL: http://www.pittsburgh.va.gov

PUERTO RICO

San Juan

51810 ■ Veterans Affairs Caribbean Healthcare System--San Juan Division
PTSD Clinical Team
10 Casia St.
San Juan, PR 00912
E-mail: Angie.Zayas-Ortiz@va.gov
URL: http://www.caribbean.va.gov

RHODE ISLAND

Providence

51811 ■ Veterans Affairs Medical Center--Providence RI
PTSD Clinical Team
830 Chalkstone Ave.
Providence, RI 02908-4799
Ph: (401)273-7100
E-mail: William.Unger@va.gov
URL: http://www.providence.va.gov

SOUTH CAROLINA

Charleston

51812 ■ Ralph H. Johnson Veterans Affairs Medical Center
PTSD Clinical Team
109 Bee St.
Charleston, SC 29401

Ph: (843)789-7721
E-mail: carol.denier@va.gov
URL: http://www.charleston.va.gov

Columbia

51813 ■ WJB Dorn Veterans Affairs Medical Center
PTSD Clinical Team
6439 Garners Ferry Rd.
Columbia, SC 29209
Ph: (803)776-4000
E-mail: Joanna.Plunkett@va.gov
URL: http://www.columbiasc.va.gov

SOUTH DAKOTA

Fort Meade

51814 ■ Veterans Affairs Black Hills Healthcare System
Fort Meade Campus
PTSD Residential Program
113 Comanche Rd.
Fort Meade, SD 57747
Ph: (605)720-7480
Free: 800-743-1070
E-mail: Stacy.Sondreal@va.gov
URL: http://www.blackhills.va.gov

Hot Springs

51815 ■ Veterans Affairs Black Hills Healthcare System
Hot Springs Campus
PTSD Domiciliary
500 N 5th St.
Hot Springs, SD 57747
Ph: (605)745-2000
E-mail: RoseMary.Slater@va.gov
URL: http://www.va.gov

Sioux Falls

51816 ■ Sioux Falls Veterans Affairs Health Care System
PTSD Domiciliary Program Intensive/Inpatient
2501 W 22nd St.
Sioux Falls, SD 57117
Ph: (605)336-3230
Free: 800-764-5370
E-mail: alyce.clasen@va.gov
URL: http://www.siouxfalls.va.gov

51817 ■ Sioux Falls Veterans Affairs Medical Center
PTSD Residential Rehabilitation Program Intensive/Inpatient
2501 W 22nd St.
Sioux Falls, SD 57117
Free: 800-764-5370
E-mail: alyce.clasen@va.gov
URL: http://www.siouxfalls.va.gov

TENNESSEE

Memphis

51818 ■ Veterans Affairs Medical Center--Memphis TN
PTSD Clinical Team
1030 Jefferson Ave.
Memphis, TN 38104
Ph: (901)523-8990
Free: 800-636-8262
E-mail: lisa.gilliam@va.gov
URL: http://www.memphis.va.gov

51819 ■ Veterans Affairs Medical Center--Memphis TN
PTSD Domiciliary
1030 Jefferson Ave.
Memphis, TN 38104

Ph: (901)523-8990
E-mail: ernie.samuel@va.gov
URL: http://www.memphis.va.gov

Mountain Home

51820 ■ James H. Quillen Veterans Affairs Medical Center
PTSD Clinical Team
Veterans Way & Lamont Sts.
Mountain Home, TN 37684
Ph: (423)926-1171
E-mail: steve.herrin@va.gov
URL: http://www.mountainhome.va.gov

Murfreesboro

51821 ■ Tennessee Valley Veterans Affairs Health Care System
PTSD Clinical Team Outpatient
Alvin C. York Campus
3400 Lebanon Pke.
Murfreesboro, TN 37129
Ph: (615)904-7227
Free: 800-876-7093
E-mail: nikki.mcclellan@va.gov
URL: http://www.tennesseevalley.va.gov

51822 ■ Tennessee Valley Veterans Affairs Health Care System
Women's Stress Disorder Treatment Team
Alvin C. York Campus
3400 Lebanon Pke.
Murfreesboro, TN 37129
Ph: (615)873-3010
Free: 800-876-7093
E-mail: Michele.Panucci@va.gov
URL: http://www.tennesseevalley.va.gov

Nashville

51823 ■ Tennessee Valley Veterans Affairs Healthcare System
Nashville Campus
PTSD Clinical Team
1310 24th Ave. S
Nashville, TN 37212
Ph: (615)327-4751
E-mail: Sonya.Jones2@va.gov
URL: http://www.tennesseevalley.va.gov

TEXAS

Austin

51824 ■ Central Texas Veterans Healthcare System
PTSD Clinical Team
Southcliff Bldg.
2115 S Interstate 35, Ste. 101
Austin, TX 78741
Ph: (512)433-2038
E-mail: shaun.perkins@va.gov
URL: http://www.va.gov

Dallas

51825 ■ Veterans Affairs North Texas Healthcare System
PTSD Clinical Team
4500 Lancaster Rd.
Dallas, TX 75216
Ph: (214)857-0722
E-mail: Thelma.Lowe@va.gov
URL: http://www.northtexas.va.gov

51826 ■ Veterans Affairs North Texas Healthcare System
Women's Stress Disorder Treatment Team
4500 S Lancaster Rd.
Dallas, TX 75216
Ph: (214)857-0722
E-mail: Alina.Suris@va.gov
URL: http://www.northtexas.va.gov

El Paso

51827 ■ El Paso Veterans Affairs Healthcare System
PTSD Clinical Team
5001 N Piedras St.
El Paso, TX 79930
Ph: (915)564-6100
E-mail: Kevin.Pannell@va.gov
URL: http://www.elpaso.va.gov

Houston

51828 ■ Michael E. Debakey Veterans Affairs Medical Center
PTSD Clinical Team
2002 Holcombe Blvd.
Houston, TX 77030
Ph: (713)791-1414
Free: 800-553-2278
E-mail: McGavin.JillK@va.gov
URL: http://www.houston.va.gov

San Antonio

51829 ■ South Texas Veterans Affairs Healthcare System
Frank M. Tejeda Outpatient Clinic
PTSD Clinical Team
5788 Eckerd Rd.
San Antonio, TX 78240
Ph: (210)699-2139
E-mail: Donald.Glover@va.gov
URL: http://www.southtexas.va.gov

Temple

51830 ■ Veterans Affairs Central Texas Healthcare System
PTSD Program
1901 Veterans Memorial Dr.
Temple, TX 76504
Ph: (254)778-4811
URL: http://www.centraltexas.va.gov

Waco

51831 ■ Central Texas Veterans Affairs Healthcare System
PTSD Clinical Team
4800 Memorial Dr.
Waco, TX 76711
Ph: (254)297-3890
Free: 800-423-2111
E-mail: Karen.Boyd-Wuertz@va.gov
URL: http://www.centraltexas.va.gov

51832 ■ Veterans Affairs Medical Center--Waco TX
PTSD Residential Rehabilitation Program
4800 Memorial Dr.
Waco, TX 76711
Ph: (254)292-3668
E-mail: Robert.Huggins@va.gov
URL: http://www.centraltexas.va.gov

UTAH

Salt Lake City

51833 ■ Veterans Affairs Salt Lake City Healthcare System
PTSD Clinical Team
500 Foothill Blvd.
Salt Lake City, UT 84148
Ph: (801)582-1565
E-mail: charlotte.erickson@va.gov
URL: http://www.saltlakecity.va.gov

VERMONT

White River Junction

51834 ■ White River Junction Veterans Affairs Medical Center
PTSD Clinical Team
215 N Main St.
White River Junction, VT 05009

Ph: (802)295-9363
Free: 866-687-8387
E-mail: Lisa.Harmon@va.gov
URL: http://www.whiteriver.va.gov

VIRGINIA

Hampton

51835 ■ Veterans Affairs Medical Center--Hampton VA
PTSD Clinical Team
100 Emancipation Dr.
Hampton, VA 23667
Ph: (757)722-9961
Fax: (757)723-6620
E-mail: tribia.kennedy@va.gov
URL: http://www.hampton.va.gov

51836 ■ Veterans Affairs Medical Center--Hampton VA
PTSD Domiciliary
100 Emancipation Dr.
Hampton, VA 23667
Ph: (757)722-9961
E-mail: Stephanie.eppinger@va.gov
URL: http://www.hampton.va.gov

Richmond

51837 ■ Hunter Holmes Maguire Veterans Affairs Medical Center
PTSD Clinical Team
1201 Broad Rock Blvd.
Richmond, VA 23249
Ph: (804)675-5000
E-mail: marilyn.royster@va.gov
URL: http://www.richmond.va.gov

Salem

51838 ■ Veterans Affairs Medical Center--Salem VA
PTSD Clinical Team
1970 Roanoke Blvd.
Salem, VA 24153
Ph: (540)982-2463
Free: 888-982-2463
E-mail: Dana.Holohan@va.gov
URL: http://www.salem.va.gov

51839 ■ Veterans Affairs Medical Center--Salem VA
Specialized Inpatient PTSD Unit
1970 Roanoke Blvd.
Salem, VA 24153
Ph: (540)982-2463
Free: 888-982-2463
Fax: (540)983-1096
E-mail: Robert.Guthrie@va.gov
URL: http://www.salem.va.gov

WASHINGTON

Lakewood

51840 ■ Veterans Affairs Puget Sound Health Care System
PTSD Domiciliary Intensive/Inpatient
9600 Veterans Dr.
Lakewood, WA 98493
Ph: (253)583-1670
Free: 800-329-8387
E-mail: dale.smith1@va.gov
URL: http://www.pugetsound.va.gov

51841 ■ Veterans Affairs Puget Sound Health Care System
Women's Stress Disorder Treatment Team Outpatient
9600 Veterans Dr.
Lakewood, WA 37129
Ph: (415)221-4810

Free: 800-329-8387
E-mail: Caitlin.hasser@va.gov
URL: http://www.pugetsound.va.gov

Seattle

51842 ■ Veterans Affairs Puget Sound Healthcare System
Evaluation and Brief Treatment PTSD Unit
1660 S Columbian Way
Seattle, WA 98108
Ph: (206)277-3007
E-mail: Aura.Jones@va.gov
URL: http://www.pugetsound.va.gov

51843 ■ Veterans Affairs Puget Sound Healthcare System
PTSD Clinical Team
1660 S Columbian Wy.
Seattle, WA 98108
Ph: (206)277-3007
E-mail: Aura.Jones@va.gov
URL: http://www.pugetsound.va.gov

Spokane

51844 ■ Veterans Affairs Medical Center--Spokane WA
PTSD Clinical Team
4815 N Assembly St.
Spokane, WA 99205
Ph: (509)434-7277
E-mail: John.Miller14@va.gov
URL: http://www.spokane.va.gov

WEST VIRGINIA

Clarksburg

51845 ■ Louis A. Johnson Veterans Affairs Medical Center
PTSD Residential Rehabilitation Program
1 Medical Center Dr.
Clarksburg, WV 26301
Ph: (304)623-3461
E-mail: Heather.Meit@va.gov
URL: http://www.clarksburg.va.gov

Huntington

51846 ■ Veterans Affairs Medical Center--Huntington WV
PTSD Clinical Team
1540 Spring Valley Dr.
Huntington, WV 25704
Ph: (304)429-6755
E-mail: Linda.Pennington2@va.gov
URL: http://www.huntington.va.gov

Martinsburg

51847 ■ Veterans Affairs Medical Center--Martinsburg WV
PTSD Clinical Team
510 Butler Ave.
Martinsburg, WV 25405
Ph: (304)263-0811
E-mail: Theodore.Hughes@va.gov
URL: http://www.martinsburg.va.gov

51848 ■ Veterans Affairs Medical Center--Martinsburg WV
PTSD Domiciliary
510 Butler Ave.
Martinsburg, WV 25405
Ph: (304)263-0811
Free: 800-817-3807
Fax: (304)262-7433
E-mail: Theodore.Hughes@va.gov
URL: http://www.martinsburg.va.gov

WISCONSIN

Madison

51849 ■ William S. Middleton Veterans Affairs Hospital
PTSD Clinical Team
2500 Overlook Terr.
Madison, WI 53705

Ph: (608)256-1901
E-mail: Nathan.Miller@va.gov
URL: http://www.madison.va.gov

Milwaukee

51850 ■ Clement J. Zablocki Veterans Affairs Medical Center
PTSD Clinical Team
5000 W National St.
Milwaukee, WI 53295
Ph: (414)384-2000
E-mail: Karen.Berte@va.gov
URL: http://www.milwaukee.va.gov

51851 ■ Clement J. Zablocki Veterans Affairs Medical Center
PTSD Domiciliary
5000 W National Ave.
Milwaukee, WI 53295
Ph: (414)384-2000
E-mail: Catherine.Deyoung@va.gov
URL: http://www.milwaukee.va.gov

Tomah

51852 ■ Veterans Affairs Medical Center--Tomah WI
PTSD Residential Rehabilitation Program
500 E Veterans St.
Tomah, WI 54660
Ph: (608)372-3971
E-mail: cathy.komiskey@va.gov
URL: http://www.tomah.va.gov

WYOMING

Cheyenne

51853 ■ Veterans Affairs Medical Center--Cheyenne WY
PTSD Clinical Team
2360 E Pershing Blvd.
Cheyenne, WY 82001
Ph: (307)778-7650
E-mail: Irena.Danczik@va.gov
URL: http://www.cheyenne.va.gov

VET CENTERS

ALABAMA

Birmingham

51854 ■ Vet Center
Birmingham AL
1201 2nd Ave. S
Birmingham, AL 35233
Ph: (205)212-3122
Fax: (205)212-3123
URL: http://www2.va.gov

Huntsville

51855 ■ Vet Center
Huntsville AL
Bldg. H
415 Church St., Ste. 101
Huntsville, AL 35801
Ph: (256)539-5775
Fax: (256)533-1973
URL: http://www2.va.gov

Mobile

51856 ■ Vet Center
Mobile AL
Bldg. 2, Ste. C
3221 Springhill Ave.
Mobile, AL 36607
Ph: (251)478-5906
Fax: (251)478-2237
URL: http://www2.va.gov

Montgomery

51857 ■ Vet Center
Montgomery AL
4405 Atlanta Hwy.
Montgomery, AL 36109
Ph: (334)273-7796
Fax: (334)277-8376
URL: http://www2.va.gov

ALASKA

Anchorage

51858 ■ Vet Center
Anchorage AK
4201 Tudor Centre Dr., Ste. 115
Anchorage, AK 99508
Ph: (907)563-6966
Fax: (907)561-7183

Fairbanks

51859 ■ Vet Center
Fairbanks AK
540 4th Ave., Ste. 100
Fairbanks, AK 99701
Ph: (907)456-4238
Fax: (907)456-0475

Soldotna

51860 ■ Vet Center
Kenai Vet Center Satellite
Red Diamond Center
Bldg. F, Ste. 4
43335 Kalifornsky Beach Rd.
Soldotna, AK 99669
Ph: (907)260-7640
Fax: (907)260-7642

Wasilla

51861 ■ Wasila Vet Center
Wasilla AK
851 E West Point Ave., Ste. 111
Wasilla, AK 99654
Ph: (907)376-4318
Fax: (907)373-1883

ARIZONA

Chinle

51862 ■ Vet Center
Chinle AZ
Navajo Rte. 7
Chinle, AZ 86503
Ph: (928)674-3682
Fax: (928)674-5640
URL: http://www2.va.gov

Hotevilla

51863 ■ Vet Center
Hopi Vet Center Outstation 2
1 Main St.
Hotevilla, AZ 86030
Ph: (928)734-5166
Fax: (928)738-5531
URL: http://www2.va.gov

Mesa

51864 ■ Phoenix East Valley Vet Center
1303 S. Longmore, Ste. 5
Mesa, AZ 85202
Ph: (480)610-6727
Fax: (480)464-3526
URL: http://www2.va.gov

Peoria

51865 ■ West Valley Vet Center
Peoria AZ
14050 N 83rd Ave., Ste. 170
Peoria, AZ 85381

Ph: (623)398-8854
Fax: (623)398-6478
URL: http://www2.va.gov

Phoenix

51866 ■ Vet Center
Phoenix AZ
77 E Weldon, Ste. 100
Phoenix, AZ 85012
Ph: (602)640-2981
Fax: (602)640-2967
URL: http://www2.va.gov

Prescott

51867 ■ Vet Center
Prescott AZ
3180 Stillwater Dr.
Prescott, AZ 86305
Ph: (928)778-3469
Fax: (928)776-6042
URL: http://www2.va.gov

Tucson

51868 ■ Vet Center
Tucson AZ
3055 N 1st Ave.
Tucson, AZ 85719
Ph: (520)882-0333
Fax: (520)670-5862
URL: http://www2.va.gov

Yuma

51869 ■ Yuma Vet Center
Yuma AZ
3939 S Ave SE, Ste. 122
Yuma, AZ 85365
Ph: (928)271-8700
Fax: (928)304-7446
URL: http://www2.va.gov

ARKANSAS

Fayetteville

51870 ■ Vet Center
Fayetteville AR
1416 N College Ave.
Fayetteville, AR 72703
Ph: (479)582-7152
Fax: (479)251-1823
URL: http://www2.va.gov

North Little Rock

51871 ■ Little Rock Vet Center
201 W Broadway, Ste. A
North Little Rock, AR 72114
Ph: (501)324-6395
Fax: (501)324-6928
URL: http://www2.va.gov
Formerly: North Little Rock Vet Center.

CALIFORNIA

Bakersfield

51872 ■ Bakersfield Vet Center
1110 Golden State Ave.
Bakersfield, CA 93301
Ph: (661)323-8387
Fax: (661)325-8387
URL: http://www2.va.gov

Bonita

51873 ■ Chula Vista Vet Center
180 Otay Lakes Rd., Ste. 108
Bonita, CA 91902
Ph: (858)618-6534
Free: 877-618-6534
Fax: (619)479-8539
URL: http://www2.va.gov

Capitola

51874 ■ Santa Cruz County Vet Center
1350 41st Ave., Ste. 201
Capitola, CA 95010
Ph: (831)464-4575
Fax: (831)464-6597
URL: http://www2.va.gov

Chico

51875 ■ Vet Center
Chico CA
280 Cohasset, Ste. 100
Chico, CA 95928
Ph: (530)899-8549
Fax: (530)899-0581
URL: http://www2.va.gov

Citrus Heights

51876 ■ Citrus Heights Vet Center
5650 Sunrise Blvd., Ste. 150
Citrus Heights, CA 95610
Ph: (916)535-0420
Fax: (916)535-0419
URL: http://www2.va.gov

Colton

51877 ■ Vet Center
Colton CA
1325 E Cooley Dr., Ste. 101
Colton, CA 92324
Ph: (909)801-5762
Fax: (909)801-5767
URL: http://www2.va.gov

Commerce

51878 ■ Vet Center
Commerce CA
5400 E Olympic Blvd., No. 140
Commerce, CA 90022
Ph: (323)728-9966
Fax: (323)887-1082
URL: http://www2.va.gov

Concord

51879 ■ Vet Center
Concord CA
1333 Willow Pass Rd., Ste. 106
Concord, CA 94520
Ph: (925)680-4526
Fax: (925)680-0410
URL: http://www2.va.gov

Corona

51880 ■ Vet Center
Corona CA
800 Magnolia Ave., Ste. 110
Corona, CA 92879
Ph: (951)734-0525
Fax: (951)734-0063
URL: http://www2.va.gov

Culver City

51881 ■ Vet Center
Culver City CA
5730 Uplander Way, Ste. 100
Culver City, CA 90230
Ph: (310)641-0326
Fax: (310)641-2653
URL: http://www2.va.gov

Eureka

51882 ■ Vet Center
Eureka CA
2830 G St., Ste. A
Eureka, CA 95501
Ph: (707)444-8271
Fax: (707)444-8391
URL: http://www2.va.gov

Fairfield

51883 ■ Vet Center
Fairfield CA
420 Executive Ct. N, Ste. A
Fairfield, CA 94534
Ph: (707)646-2988
Fax: (707)646-2960
URL: http://www2.va.gov

Fresno

51884 ■ Vet Center
Fresno CA
3636 N 1st St., Ste. 112
Fresno, CA 93726
Ph: (559)487-5660
Fax: (559)487-5399
URL: http://www2.va.gov

Garden Grove

51885 ■ Orange County Vet Center
12453 Lewis St., Ste. 101
Garden Grove, CA 92840
Ph: (714)776-0161
Fax: (714)748-4573
URL: http://www2.va.gov

Gardena

51886 ■ Los Angeles Vet Center
1045 W Redondo Beach Blvd., Ste. 150
Gardena, CA 90247
Ph: (310)767-1221
Fax: (310)767-1403
URL: http://www2.va.gov

Mission Viejo

51887 ■ Vet Center
Mission Viejo CA
26431 Crown Valley Pkwy., Ste. 100
Mission Viejo, CA 92691
Ph: (949)348-6700
Fax: (949)348-6719
URL: http://www2.va.gov

Modesto

51888 ■ Vet Center
Modesto CA
1219 N Carpenter Rd., Ste. 12
Modesto, CA 95351
Ph: (209)569-0713
Fax: (209)569-0718
URL: http://www2.va.gov

Oakland

51889 ■ Vet Center
Oakland CA
1504 Franklin St., Ste. 200
Oakland, CA 94612
Ph: (510)763-3904
Fax: (510)763-5631
URL: http://www2.va.gov

Palmdale

51890 ■ Vet Center
Palmdale CA
38925 Trade Center Dr., Ste. J
Palmdale, CA 93551
Ph: (661)267-1026
Fax: (661)267-2045
URL: http://www2.va.gov

Redwood City

51891 ■ Peninsula Vet Center
2946 Broadway St.
Redwood City, CA 94062
Ph: (650)299-0672
Fax: (650)299-0677
URL: http://www2.va.gov

Rohnert Park

51892 ■ Vet Center
Rohnert Park CA
6225 State Farm Dr., Ste. 101
Rohnert Park, CA 94928
Ph: (707)586-3295
Fax: (707)586-9055
URL: http://www2.va.gov

Sacramento

51893 ■ Vet Center
Sacramento CA
1111 Howe Ave., Ste. 390
Sacramento, CA 95825
Ph: (916)566-7430
Fax: (916)566-7433
URL: http://www2.va.gov

San Diego

51894 ■ Vet Center
San Diego
2790 Truxton Rd., Ste. 130
San Diego, CA 92106
Ph: (858)642-1500
Fax: (619)294-2535
URL: http://www2.va.gov

San Francisco

51895 ■ Vet Center
San Francisco CA
505 Polk St.
San Francisco, CA 94102
Ph: (415)441-5051
Fax: (415)441-5092
URL: http://www2.va.gov

San Jose

51896 ■ Vet Center
San Jose CA
278 N 2nd St.
San Jose, CA 95112
Ph: (408)993-0729
Fax: (408)993-0829
URL: http://www2.va.gov

San Marcos

51897 ■ Vet Center
San Marcos CA
1 Civic Center Dr., Ste. 140
San Marcos, CA 92069
Ph: (760)744-6914
Fax: (760)744-6919
URL: http://www2.va.gov

Sepulveda

51898 ■ Vet Center
Sepulveda CA
9737 Haskell Ave.
Sepulveda, CA 91343
Ph: (818)892-9227
Fax: (818)892-0557
URL: http://www2.va.gov

Temecula

51899 ■ Vet Center
Temecula CA
40935 County Center Dr., Ste. A
Temecula, CA 92591
Ph: (951)302-4849
Fax: (951)296-0598
URL: http://www2.va.gov

Ventura

51900 ■ Vet Center
Ventura CA
790 E Santa Clara St., Ste. 100
Ventura, CA 93001

Ph: (805)585-1860
Fax: (805)585-1864
URL: http://www2.va.gov

Victorville

51901 ■ Vet Center
Victorville CA
15095 Amargosa Rd., Ste. 107
Victorville, CA 92394
Ph: (760)261-5925
Fax: (760)241-7828
URL: http://www2.va.gov

COLORADO

Boulder

51902 ■ Vet Center
Boulder CO
2336 Canyon Blvd., St. 103
Boulder, CO 80302
Ph: (303)440-7306
Fax: (303)449-3907
URL: http://www2.va.gov

Colorado Springs

51903 ■ Vet Centers
Colorado Springs CO
602 S Nevada Ave.
Colorado Springs, CO 80903
Ph: (719)471-9992
Fax: (719)632-7571
URL: http://www2.va.gov
Program(s): Individual, group, marital/family, alcohol/ drug, and employment counseling services; job referral; community education programs.

Denver

51904 ■ Vet Center
Denver CA
789 Sherman St., Ste. 570
Denver, CO 80203
Ph: (303)393-2897
Fax: (303)860-7614
URL: http://www2.va.gov

Fort Collins

51905 ■ Fort Collins Vet Center
Bldg. C
702 W Drake
Fort Collins, CO 80526
Ph: (970)221-5176
Fax: (970)482-9428
URL: http://www2.va.gov

Grand Junction

51906 ■ Grand Junction Vet Center
2472 F Rd., Unit 16
Grand Junction, CO 81505
Ph: (970)245-4156
Fax: (970)245-7623
URL: http://www2.va.gov

Pueblo

51907 ■ Vet Center
Pueblo CO
1515 Fortino Blvd., Ste. 130
Pueblo, CO 81001
Ph: (719)583-4058
Fax: (719)583-4074
URL: http://www2.va.gov

CONNECTICUT

Danbury

51908 ■ Danbury Vet Center
457 N Main St.
Danbury, CT 06811
Ph: (203)790-4000
URL: http://www2.va.gov

Norwich

51909 ■ Vet Center
Norwich CT
2 Cliff St.
Norwich, CT 06360
Ph: (860)887-1755
Fax: (860)887-2444
URL: http://www2.va.gov

Rocky Hill

51910 ■ Hartford Vet Center
25 Elm St., Ste. A
Rocky Hill, CT 06067
Ph: (860)563-8800
Fax: (860)563-8805
URL: http://www2.va.gov

West Haven

51911 ■ Vet Center
West haven CT
141 Captain Thomas Blvd.
West Haven, CT 06516
Ph: (203)932-9899
Fax: (203)937-9419
URL: http://www2.va.gov

DELAWARE

Wilmington

51912 ■ Vet Center
Wilmington DE
2710 Centerville Rd., Ste. 103
Wilmington, DE 19808
Ph: (302)994-1660
Fax: (302)994-8361
URL: http://www2.va.gov

DISTRICT OF COLUMBIA

Washington

51913 ■ Washington DC Vet Center
Washington DC
1250 Taylor St. NW
Washington, DC 20011
Ph: (202)726-5212
Fax: (202)726-8968
URL: http://www2.va.gov

FLORIDA

Bay Pines

51914 ■ Vet Center
Bay Pines CA
Bldg. T203
10000 Bay Pines Blvd.
Bay Pines, FL 33744
Ph: (727)398-9343
Fax: (727)398-9444
URL: http://www2.va.gov

Clearwater

51915 ■ Vet Center
Clearwater FL
29259 US Hwy. 19 N
Clearwater, FL 33761
Ph: (727)549-3600
Fax: (727)549-6701
URL: http://www2.va.gov

Coral Springs

51916 ■ Pompano Beach Vet Center
2300 W Sample Rd.
Coral Springs, FL 33073
Ph: (954)357-5555
Fax: (954)357-5710
URL: http://www2.va.gov

Daytona Beach

51917 ■ Vet Center
Daytona Beach FL
1620 Mason Ave., Ste. C
Daytona Beach, FL 32117
Ph: (386)366-6600
Fax: (386)274-5700
URL: http://www2.va.gov

Fort Lauderdale

51918 ■ Vet Center
Fort Lauderdale FL
713 NE 3rd Ave.
Fort Lauderdale, FL 33304
Ph: (954)356-7926
Fax: (954)356-7609
URL: http://www2.va.gov

Fort Myers

51919 ■ Vet Center
Fort Myers FL
4110 Center Pte. Dr., Unit 204
Fort Myers, FL 33916
Ph: (239)479-4401
Fax: (239)277-5817
URL: http://www2.va.gov

Gainesville

51920 ■ Vet Center
Gainesville FL
105 NW 75th St., Ste. 2
Gainesville, FL 32607
Ph: (352)331-1408
Fax: (352)331-1962
URL: http://www2.va.gov

Greenacres

51921 ■ Palm Beach Vet Center
4996 10th Ave. N, Ste. 6
Greenacres, FL 33463
Ph: (561)422-1201
Fax: (561)439-5877
URL: http://www2.va.gov

Jacksonville

51922 ■ Vet Center
Jacksonville FL
300 E State St., Ste. J
Jacksonville, FL 32202
Ph: (904)232-3621
Fax: (904)232-3167
URL: http://www2.va.gov

Jupiter

51923 ■ Jupiter Vet Center
6650 W Indiantown Rd., Ste. 120
Jupiter, FL 33458
Ph: (561)422-1220
Fax: (561)746-1458
URL: http://www2.va.gov

Key Largo

51924 ■ Vet Center
Key Largo FL
105662 Overseas Hwy.
Key Largo, FL 33037
Ph: (305)451-0164
Fax: (305)451-4864
URL: http://www2.va.gov

Melbourne

51925 ■ Vet Center
Melbourne FL
2098 Sarno Rd.
Melbourne, FL 32935
Ph: (321)254-3410
Fax: (321)254-9138
URL: http://www2.va.gov

Miami

51926 ■ Vet Center
Miami FL
8280 NW 27th St., Ste. 511
Miami, FL 33122
Ph: (305)718-3712
Fax: (305)718-8712
URL: http://www2.va.gov

Orlando

51927 ■ Vet Center
Orlando FL
5575 S Semoran Blvd, Ste. 36
Orlando, FL 31406
Ph: (407)857-2800
Fax: (407)857-5005
URL: http://www2.va.gov

Pensacola

51928 ■ Vet Center
Pensacola FL
4504 Twin Oaks
Pensacola, FL 32506
Ph: (850)456-5886
Fax: (850)456-9403
URL: http://www2.va.gov

Saint Petersburg

51929 ■ Vet Center
Saint Petersburg FL
Gaslight Sq., Bldg. A
6798 Crosswinds
Saint Petersburg, FL 33710
Ph: (727)549-3633
Fax: (727)299-6700
URL: http://www2.va.gov

Sarasota

51930 ■ Vet Center
Sarasota FL
4801 Swift Rd., Ste. A
Sarasota, FL 34231
Ph: (941)927-8285
Fax: (941)927-8307
URL: http://www2.va.gov

Tallahassee

51931 ■ Vet Center
Tallahassee FL
548 Bradford Rd.
Tallahassee, FL 32303
Ph: (850)942-8810
Fax: (850)942-8814
URL: http://www2.va.gov

Tampa

51932 ■ Vet Center
Tampa FL
Fountain Oaks Business Plz.
4747 W Waters Ave., Ste. 600
Tampa, FL 33614
Ph: (813)228-2621
Fax: (813)228-2868
URL: http://www2.va.gov

GEORGIA

Atlanta

51933 ■ Vet Center
Atlanta GA
1440 Dutch Valley Pl., Ste. 1100
Box 55
Atlanta, GA 30324
Ph: (404)347-7264
Fax: (404)347-7274
URL: http://www2.va.gov

Lawrenceville

51934 ■ North Atlantic Vet Center
930 River Cte. Pl.
Lawrenceville, GA 30043
Ph: (404)728-4195
URL: http://www2.va.gov

Macon

51935 ■ Vet Center
Macon GA
750 Riverside Dr.
Macon, GA 31201
Ph: (478)477-3813
Fax: (478)746-7023
URL: http://www2.va.gov

Marietta

51936 ■ Vet Center
Marietta GA
40 Dodd St., Ste. 700
Marietta, GA 30060
Ph: (404)327-4954
Fax: (770)419-1314
URL: http://www2.va.gov

Savannah

51937 ■ Vet Center
Savannah GA
321 Commercial Dr.
Savannah, GA 31406
Ph: (912)961-5800
Fax: (478)274-5751
URL: http://www2.va.gov

GUAM

Hagatna

51938 ■ Guam Vet Center
222 Chalan Santo Papast
Reflection Center, Ste. 201
Hagatna, GU 96910
Ph: (671)472-7160
Fax: (671)472-7162
URL: http://www2.va.gov

HAWAII

Hilo

51939 ■ Vet Center
Hilo HI
70 Lanihuli St., Ste. 102
Hilo, HI 96720
Ph: (808)969-3833
Fax: (808)969-2025
URL: http://www2.va.gov

Honolulu

51940 ■ Vet Center
Honolulu HI
1680 Kapiolani Blvd., Ste. F-3
Honolulu, HI 96814
Ph: (808)973-8387
Fax: (808)973-5295
URL: http://www2.va.gov

Lihue

51941 ■ Kauai Vet Center
33367 Kuhio Hwy., Ste. 101
Lihue, HI 96766
Ph: (808)246-1163
Fax: (808)246-4625
URL: http://www2.va.gov

Wailuku

51942 ■ Maui Vet Center
35 Lunalilo St., Ste. 101
Wailuku, HI 96793

Ph: (808)242-8557
Fax: (808)242-8559
URL: http://www2.va.gov

IDAHO

Boise

51943 ■ Vet Center
Boise ID
2424 Bank Dr., Ste. 100
Boise, ID 83705
Ph: (208)342-3612
Fax: (208)342-0327
URL: http://www2.va.gov

Pocatello

51944 ■ Vet Center
Pocatello ID
1800 Garrett Way
Pocatello, ID 83201
Ph: (208)232-0316
Fax: (208)232-6258
URL: http://www2.va.gov

ILLINOIS

Aurora

51945 ■ DuPage County Vet Center
750 Shoreline Dr., Ste. 150
Aurora, IL 60504
Ph: (630)585-1853
Fax: (630)585-1956
URL: http://www2.va.gov

Chicago

51946 ■ Chicago Veterans Resource Center
7731 S Halsted St.
Chicago, IL 60620
Ph: (773)962-3740
Fax: (773)962-3750
URL: http://www2.va.gov

Chicago Heights

51947 ■ Vet Center
Chicago Heights IL
1600 Halsted St.
Chicago Heights, IL 60411
Ph: (708)754-0340
Fax: (708)754-9882
URL: http://www2.va.gov

East Saint Louis

51948 ■ East Saint Louis Vet Center
1265 N 89th St., Ste. 5
East Saint Louis, IL 62203
Ph: (618)397-6602
Fax: (618)397-6541
URL: http://www2.va.gov

Evanston

51949 ■ Vet Center
Evanston IL
565 Howard St.
Evanston, IL 60202
Ph: (847)332-1019
Fax: (847)332-1024
URL: http://www2.va.gov

Moline

51950 ■ Quad Cities Vet Center
1529 46th Ave., No. 6
Moline, IL 61265
Ph: (309)762-6954
Fax: (309)762-8298
URL: http://www2.va.gov

Oak Park

51951 ■ Vet Center
Oak Park IL
155 S Oak Park Ave.
Oak Park, IL 60302
Ph: (708)383-3225
Fax: (708)383-3247
URL: http://www2.va.gov

Orland Park

51952 ■ Vet Center
Orland Park IL
8651 W 159th St., Ste. 1
Orland Park, IL 60462
Ph: (708)444-0561
Fax: (708)444-0588
URL: http://www2.va.gov

Peoria

51953 ■ Vet Center
Peoria IL
8305 N Allen Rd., Ste. 1
Peoria, IL 61615
Ph: (309)689-9708
Fax: (309)689-9720
URL: http://www2.va.gov

Rockford

51954 ■ Vet Center Outstation
Rockford IL
7015 Rote Rd., Ste. 105
Rockford, IL 61107
Ph: (815)395-1276
Fax: (815)395-1280
URL: http://www2.va.gov

Springfield

51955 ■ Vet Center
Springfield IL
1227 S 9th St.
Springfield, IL 62703
Ph: (217)492-4955
Fax: (217)492-4963
URL: http://www2.va.gov

INDIANA

Evansville

51956 ■ Vet Center
Evansville IN
311 N Weinback Ave.
Evansville, IN 47711
Ph: (812)473-5993
Fax: (812)473-4028
URL: http://www2.va.gov

Fort Wayne

51957 ■ Vet Center
Fort Wayne IN
5800 Fairfield Ave., Ste. 265
Fort Wayne, IN 46807
Ph: (260)460-1456
Fax: (260)456-0829
URL: http://www2.va.gov

Indianapolis

51958 ■ Vet Center
Indianapolis IN
8330 Naab Rd., Ste. 103
Indianapolis, IN 46268
Ph: (317)988-1600
Fax: (317)988-1617
URL: http://www2.va.gov

Merrillville

51959 ■ Vet Center
Merrillville IN
6505 Broadway
Merrillville, IN 46410

Ph: (219)736-5633
Fax: (219)736-5937
URL: http://www2.va.gov

IOWA

Cedar Rapids

51960 ■ Vet Center Satellite
Cedar Rapids IA
1642 42nd St. NE
Cedar Rapids, IA 52402
Ph: (319)378-0016
Fax: (319)378-8145
URL: http://www2.va.gov

Des Moines

51961 ■ Vet Center
Des Moines IA
2600 Martin Luther King Jr. Pkwy.
Des Moines, IA 50310
Ph: (515)284-4929
Fax: (515)277-4949
URL: http://www2.va.gov

Sioux City

51962 ■ Vet Center
Sioux City IA
1551 Indian Hills Dr., Ste. 214
Sioux City, IA 51104
Ph: (712)255-3808
Fax: (712)255-3725
URL: http://www2.va.gov

KANSAS

Manhattan

51963 ■ Vet Center
Manhattan KS
205 S 4th St., Ste. B
Manhattan, KS 66502
Ph: (785)350-4920
Fax: (785)350-4939
URL: http://www2.va.gov

Wichita

51964 ■ Vet Center
Wichita KS
5500 E Kellogg
Wichita, KS 67218
Ph: (316)265-2221
Fax: (316)265-0190
URL: http://www2.va.gov

KENTUCKY

Lexington

51965 ■ Vet Center
Lexinington KY
301 E Vine St., Ste. C
Lexington, KY 40507
Ph: (859)253-0717
Fax: (859)281-4801
URL: http://www2.va.gov

Louisville

51966 ■ Vet Center
Louisville KY
1347 S 3rd St.
Louisville, KY 40208
Ph: (502)634-1916
Fax: (502)625-7082
URL: http://www2.va.gov

LOUISIANA

Alexandria

51967 ■ Rapides Parish Vet Center
5803 Coliseum Blvd., Ste. D
Alexandria, LA 70303

Ph: (318)466-4327
Fax: (318)427-8044
URL: http://www2.va.gov

Baton Rouge

51968 ■ Vet Center
Baton Rouge LA
5207 Essen Ln., Ste. 2
Baton Rouge, LA 70809
Ph: (225)761-3440
Fax: (225)757-0054
URL: http://www2.va.gov

Kenner

51969 ■ New Orleans Veterans Resource
  Center
2200 Veterans Memorial Blvd., Ste. 114
Kenner, LA 70062
Ph: (504)565-4977
Fax: (504)464-6710
URL: http://www2.va.gov

Shreveport

51970 ■ Vet Center
Shreveport LA
Bldg. 1
2800 Youree Dr., Ste. 105
Shreveport, LA 71104
Ph: (318)861-1776
Fax: (318)868-1788
URL: http://www2.va.gov

MAINE

Bangor

51971 ■ Vet Center
Bangor ME
In-Town Plaza
368 Harlow St.
Bangor, ME 04401
Ph: (207)947-3391
Fax: (207)941-8195
URL: http://www2.va.gov

Caribou

51972 ■ Vet Center
Caribou ME
York Street Complex
456 York St.
Caribou, ME 04736
Ph: (207)496-3900
Fax: (207)493-6773
URL: http://www2.va.gov

Lewiston

51973 ■ Vet Center
Lewiston ME
Parkway Complex
29 Westminster St.
Lewiston, ME 04240
Ph: (207)783-0068
Fax: (207)783-3505
URL: http://www2.va.gov

Portland

51974 ■ Vet Center
Portland ME
475 Stevens Ave.
Portland, ME 04103
Ph: (207)780-3584
Fax: (207)780-3545
URL: http://www2.va.gov

Springvale

51975 ■ Vet Center
Springvale ME
628 Main St.
Springvale, ME 04083

Ph: (207)490-1513
Fax: (207)490-1609
URL: http://www2.va.gov

MARYLAND

Aberdeen

51976 ■ Vet Center
Aberdeen Outstation
223 W Belair Ave.
Aberdeen, MD 21001
Ph: (410)272-6771
Fax: (410)297-9041
URL: http://www2.va.gov

Annapolis

51977 ■ Vet Center
Annapolis MD
100 Annapolis St., Ste. 102
Annapolis, MD 21401
Ph: (410)605-7826
Fax: (410)267-0129
URL: http://www2.va.gov

Baltimore

51978 ■ Vet Center
Baltimore MD
1777 Reisterstown Rd., Ste. 199
Baltimore, MD 21208
Ph: (410)764-9400
Fax: (410)764-7780
URL: http://www2.va.gov

Bethesda

51979 ■ Silver Spring Vet Center
10411 Motor City Dr., 5th Fl.
Bethesda, MD 20817
Ph: (240)395-1425
Fax: (240)395-1424
URL: http://www2.va.gov

Cambridge

51980 ■ Vet Center Outstation 1
Cambridge MD
830 Chesapeake Dr.
Cambridge, MD 21613
Ph: (410)228-6305
Fax: (410)901-4011
URL: http://www2.va.gov

Elkton

51981 ■ Vet Center
Elkton MD
103 Chesapeake Blvd.
Ste. A
Elkton, MD 21921
Ph: (410)392-4485
Fax: (410)392-6381
URL: http://www2.va.gov

Silver Spring

51982 ■ Vet Center
Silver Spring MD
1015 Spring St., Ste. 101
Silver Spring, MD 20910
Ph: (301)589-1073
Fax: (301)588-4882
URL: http://www2.va.gov

Towson

51983 ■ Vet Center Mid Atlantic
Towson MD
305 W Chesapeake Ave., Ste. 300
Towson, MD 21204
Ph: (410)828-6619
Fax: (410)962-5151
URL: http://www2.va.gov

MASSACHUSETTS

Boston

51984 ■ **Vet Center**
Boston MA
665 Beacon St., Ste. 100
Boston, MA 02215
Ph: (617)424-0665
Fax: (617)424-0254
URL: http://www2.va.gov

Brockton

51985 ■ **Vet Center**
Brockton MA
1041-L Pearl St.
Brockton, MA 02301
Ph: (508)580-2730
Fax: (508)586-8414
URL: http://www2.va.gov

Fairhaven

51986 ■ **Vet Center**
Fairhaven MA
73 Huttleton Ave., Unit 2
Fairhaven, MA 02719
Ph: (508)999-6920
Fax: (508)997-3348
URL: http://www2.va.gov

Hyannis

51987 ■ **Vet Center**
Hyannis MA
474 W Main St.
Hyannis, MA 02601
Ph: (508)778-0124
Fax: (508)775-3014
URL: http://www2.va.gov

Lowell

51988 ■ **Vet Center**
Lowell MA
Gateway Center
10 George St.
Lowell, MA 01852
Ph: (978)453-1151
Fax: (978)441-1271
URL: http://www2.va.gov

Springfield

51989 ■ **Vet Center**
Springfield MA
1985 Main St.
Springfield, MA 01103
Ph: (413)737-5167
Fax: (413)733-0537
URL: http://www2.va.gov

Worcester

51990 ■ **Vet Center**
Worcester MA
691 Grafton St.
Worcester, MA 01604
Ph: (508)753-7902
Fax: (508)753-4296
URL: http://www2.va.gov

MICHIGAN

Clinton Township

51991 ■ **Macomb County Vet Center**
42621 Garfield Rd., Ste. 105
Clinton Township, MI 48038
Ph: (586)412-0107
Fax: (586)412-0196
URL: http://www2.va.gov

Dearborn

51992 ■ **Vet Center**
Dearborn MI
2881 Monroe St., Ste. 100
Dearborn, MI 48124
Ph: (313)277-1428
Fax: (313)277-5471
URL: http://www2.va.gov

Detroit

51993 ■ **Vet Center**
Detroit MI
4161 Cass Ave.
Detroit, MI 48201
Ph: (313)831-6509
Fax: (313)831-6919
URL: http://www2.va.gov

Escanaba

51994 ■ **Vet Center**
Escanaba MI
3500 Ludington St., Ste. 110
Escanaba, MI 49829
Ph: (906)233-0244
Fax: (906)233-0217
URL: http://www2.va.gov

Grand Rapids

51995 ■ **Vet Center**
Grand Rapids MI
2050 Breton Rd. SE
Grand Rapids, MI 49546
Ph: (616)285-5795
Fax: (616)285-5898
URL: http://www2.va.gov

Pontiac

51996 ■ **Vet Center**
Pontiac MI
44200 Woodward Ave., Ste. 108
Pontiac, MI 48341
Ph: (248)874-1015
Fax: (248)874-0813
URL: http://www2.va.gov

Saginaw

51997 ■ **Vet Center**
Saginaw MI
4048 Bay Rd.
Saginaw, MI 48603
Ph: (989)321-4650
Fax: (989)791-7507
URL: http://www2.va.gov

Traverse City

51998 ■ **Traverse City Vet Center**
3766 N US 31 S
Traverse City, MI 49684
Ph: (231)935-0051
Fax: (231)935-0071
URL: http://www2.va.gov

MINNESOTA

Brooklyn Park

51999 ■ **Vet Center**
Brooklyn Park MN
7001 78th Ave. N, Ste. 300
Brooklyn Park, MN 55445
Ph: (763)503-2220
Fax: (763)503-6179
URL: http://www2.va.gov

Duluth

52000 ■ **Vet Center**
Duluth MN
405 E Superior St.
Duluth, MN 55802
Ph: (218)722-8654
Fax: (218)723-8212
URL: http://www2.va.gov

New Brighton

52001 ■ **Saint Paul Vet Center**
550 County Rd. D, Ste. 10
New Brighton, MN 55112
Ph: (651)644-4022
Fax: (651)917-2555
URL: http://www2.va.gov

MISSISSIPPI

Biloxi

52002 ■ **Vet Center**
Biloxi MS
288 Veterans Ave.
Biloxi, MS 39531
Ph: (228)388-9938
Fax: (228)388-9253
URL: http://www2.va.gov

Jackson

52003 ■ **Vet Center**
Jackson MS
1755 Lelia Dr., Ste. 104
Jackson, MS 39216
Ph: (601)965-5727
Fax: (601)965-4023
URL: http://www2.va.gov

MISSOURI

Columbia

52004 ■ **Columbia Vet Center**
4040 Rangeline Rd., Ste. 105
Columbia, MO 65202
Ph: (573)814-6206
Fax: (573)814-2608
URL: http://www2.va.gov

Kansas City

52005 ■ **Kansas City Vet Center**
4800 Main St., Ste. 107
Kansas City, MO 64111
Ph: (816)753-1866
Fax: (816)753-2328
URL: http://www2.va.gov

Saint Louis

52006 ■ **Central Vet Center**
2122 Kratky Rd.
Saint Louis, MO 63114
Ph: (314)426-5460
Fax: (314)426-4725
URL: http://www2.va.gov

52007 ■ **Vet Center**
Saint Louis MO
2901 Olive
Saint Louis, MO 63103
Ph: (314)531-5355
Fax: (314)533-2796
URL: http://www2.va.gov

Springfield

52008 ■ **Vet Center**
Springfield MO
3616 S Campbell
Springfield, MO 65807
Ph: (417)881-4197
Fax: (417)881-4932
URL: http://www2.va.gov

MONTANA

Billings

52009 ■ **Vet Center**
Billings MT
2795 Enterprise Ave., Ste. 1
Billings, MT 59102

Ph: (406)657-6071
Fax: (406)657-6603
URL: http://www2.va.gov
Program(s): Counseling; Benefits Assistance and
Referral; Alcohol/Drug Assessment; Community
Education.

Great Falls

52010 ■ Great Falls Vet Center
615 2nd Ave. N
Great Falls, MT 59401
Ph: (406)452-9048
Fax: (406)452-9053
URL: http://www2.va.gov

Kalispell

52011 ■ Kalispell Vet Center
690 N Meridian Rd., Ste. 101
Kalispell, MT 59901
Ph: (406)257-7308
Fax: (406)257-7312
URL: http://www2.va.gov

Missoula

52012 ■ Vet Center
Missoula MT
500 N Higgins Ave., Se. 202
Missoula, MT 59802
Ph: (406)721-4918
Fax: (406)329-3006
URL: http://www2.va.gov

NEBRASKA

Lincoln

52013 ■ Vet Center
Lincoln NE
3119 O St., Ste. A
Lincoln, NE 68510
Ph: (402)476-9736
Fax: (401)476-2431
URL: http://www2.va.gov

Omaha

52014 ■ Vet Center
Omaha NE
2428 Cuming St.
Omaha, NE 68131-1600
Ph: (402)346-6735
Fax: (402)346-6020
URL: http://www2.va.gov

NEVADA

Henderson

52015 ■ Vet Center
Henderson NV
400 N Stephanie, Ste. 180
Henderson, NV 89014
Ph: (702)791-9100
Fax: (702)433-5713
URL: http://www2.va.gov

Las Vegas

52016 ■ Vet Center
Las Vegas NV
1919 S Jones Blvd., Ste. A
Las Vegas, NV 89146
Ph: (702)251-7873
Fax: (702)251-7812
URL: http://www2.va.gov

Reno

52017 ■ Vet Center
Reno NV
5580 Mill St., Ste. 600
Reno, NV 89502

Ph: (775)323-1294
Fax: (775)322-8123
URL: http://www2.va.gov

NEW HAMPSHIRE

Auburn

52018 ■ 1A RCS Northeast Vet Center
15 Dartmouth Dr., Ste. 202
Auburn, NH 03032
Ph: (603)623-4204
Fax: (603)623-5541
URL: http://www2.va.gov

Gorham

52019 ■ Berlin Vet Center
515 Main St.
Gorham, NH 03581
Ph: (603)752-2571
Fax: (603)752-3618
URL: http://www2.va.gov

Manchester

52020 ■ Vet Center
Manchester NH
103 Liberty St.
Manchester, NH 03104
Ph: (603)668-7060
Fax: (603)666-7404
URL: http://www2.va.gov

NEW JERSEY

Bloomfield

52021 ■ Vet Center
Bloomfield NJ
2 Broad St., Ste. 703
Bloomfield, NJ 07003
Ph: (973)748-0980
Fax: (973)748-0380
URL: http://www2.va.gov

Ewing

52022 ■ Trenton Vet Center
934 Parkway Ave., Ste. 201
Ewing, NJ 08611
Ph: (609)882-5744
Fax: (609)882-5743
URL: http://www2.va.gov

Lakewood

52023 ■ Vet Center
Lakewood NJ
Parkway 70 Plaza, Unit 32N
1255 Rte. 70
Lakewood, NJ 08701
Ph: (732)905-0327
Fax: (732)905-0329
URL: http://www2.va.gov

Secaucus

52024 ■ Jersey City Vet Center
110A Meadowlands Pkwy., Ste. 102
Secaucus, NJ 07094
Ph: (201)223-7787
Fax: (201)223-7707
URL: http://www2.va.gov

Ventnor

52025 ■ Vet Center
Ventnor NJ
Ventnor Bldg., Ste. 105
6601 Ventnor Ave.
Ventnor, NJ 08406
Ph: (609)487-8387
Fax: (609)487-8910
URL: http://www2.va.gov

NEW MEXICO

Albuquerque

52026 ■ Vet Center
Albuquerque NM
1600 Mountain Rd. NW
Albuquerque, NM 87104
Ph: (505)346-6562
Fax: (505)346-6572
URL: http://www2.va.gov

Farmington

52027 ■ Vet Center
Farmington NM
4251 E Main St., Ste. C
Farmington, NM 87402
Ph: (505)327-9684
Fax: (505)327-9519
URL: http://www2.va.gov

Las Cruces

52028 ■ Las Cruces Mobile Vet Center
1300 W Brown Rd.
Las Cruces, NM 88053
Ph: (575)523-9826
Fax: (575)523-9827
URL: http://www2.va.gov

52029 ■ Vet Center
Las Cruces NM
230 S Water St.
Las Cruces, NM 88007
Ph: (575)523-9826
URL: http://www2.va.gov

Santa Fe

52030 ■ Santa Fe Mobile Vet Center
1 Batman Blvd.
Santa Fe, NM 87508
Ph: (505)988-6562
Fax: (505)988-6564
URL: http://www2.va.gov

52031 ■ Vet Center
Santa Fe NM
2209 Brothers Rd., Ste. 110
Santa Fe, NM 87505
Ph: (505)988-6562
Fax: (505)988-6564
URL: http://www2.va.gov

NEW YORK

Albany

52032 ■ Vet Center
Albany NY
17 Computer Dr. W
Albany, NY 12205
Ph: (518)626-5130
Fax: (518)458-8613
URL: http://www2.va.gov

Babylon

52033 ■ Vet Center
Babylon NY
116 W Main St.
Babylon, NY 11702
Ph: (631)661-3930
Fax: (631)422-5677
URL: http://www2.va.gov

Binghamtom

52034 ■ Vet Center
Binghamton NY
53 Chenango St.
Binghamtom, NY 13901
Free: 866-722-2393
Fax: (607)722-0143
URL: http://www2.va.gov

Bronx

52035 ■ Vet Center
Bronx NY
2471 Morris Ave., Ste. 1A
Bronx, NY 10468
Ph: (718)367-3500
Fax: (718)364-6867
URL: http://www2.va.gov

Brooklyn

52036 ■ Vet Center
Brooklyn NY
25 Chapel St., Ste. 604
Brooklyn, NY 11201
Ph: (718)630-2830
Fax: (718)624-3323
URL: http://www2.va.gov

Buffalo

52037 ■ Vet Center
Buffalo NY
2372 Sweet Home Rd., Ste. 1
Buffalo, NY 14228
Ph: (716)862-7350
Fax: (716)691-6450
URL: http://www2.va.gov

Hicksville

52038 ■ Nassau Vet Center
970 S Broadway
Hicksville, NY 11801
Ph: (516)348-0088
Fax: (516)348-0266
URL: http://www2.va.gov

Middletown

52039 ■ Vet Center
Middletown NY
726 E Main St., Ste. 203
Middletown, NY 10940
Ph: (845)342-9917
Fax: (845)343-8655
URL: http://www2.va.gov

New York

52040 ■ Harlem Vet Center
2279 3rd Ave., 2nd Fl.
New York, NY 10035
Ph: (212)426-2200
Fax: (212)426-8273
URL: http://www2.va.gov

52041 ■ Manhattan Vet Center
32 Broadway
Ste. 200
New York, NY 10004
Ph: (212)742-9591
Fax: (212)742-9593
URL: http://www2.va.gov

Rochester

52042 ■ Vet Center
Rochester NY
Bldg. 5, Ste. 201
2000 S. Winton Rd.
Rochester, NY 14618
Ph: (585)232-5040
Fax: (585)232-5072
URL: http://www2.va.gov

Staten Island

52043 ■ Vet Center
Staten Island NY
150 Richmond Terr.
Staten Island, NY 10301
Ph: (718)816-4499
Fax: (718)816-6899
URL: http://www2.va.gov

Syracuse

52044 ■ Vet Center
Syracuse NY
109 Pine St.
Syracuse, NY 13210
Ph: (315)478-7127
Fax: (315)478-7209
URL: http://www2.va.gov

Watertown

52045 ■ Vet Center
Watertown NY
210 Court St.
Watertown, NY 13601
Free: 866-610-0358
Fax: (315)782-0491
URL: http://www2.va.gov

White Plains

52046 ■ Vet Center
White Plains NY
300 Hamilton Ave., 1st Fl.
White Plains, NY 10601
Ph: (914)682-6250
Fax: (914)682-6263
URL: http://www2.va.gov

Woodhaven

52047 ■ Queens Vet Center
75-10B 91st Ave.
Woodhaven, NY 11421
Ph: (718)296-2871
Fax: (718)296-4660
URL: http://www2.va.gov

NORTH CAROLINA

Charlotte

52048 ■ Vet Center
Charlotte NC
2114 Ben Craig Dr., Ste. 300
Charlotte, NC 28262
Ph: (704)549-8025
Fax: (704)549-8261
URL: http://www2.va.gov

Fayetteville

52049 ■ Vet Center
Fayetteville NC
4140 Ramsey St., Ste. 110
Fayetteville, NC 28311
Ph: (910)488-6252
Fax: (910)488-5589
URL: http://www2.va.gov

Greensboro

52050 ■ Vet Center
Greensboro NC
2009 Elm-Eugene St.
Greensboro, NC 27406
Ph: (336)333-5366
Fax: (336)333-5046
URL: http://www2.va.gov
Remarks: Ongoing services are available for all Veterans of the Vietnam era, and Veterans of conflicts in Lebanon, Panama, Granada, the Persian Gulf, WWII, Korea, and Veterans who experienced sexual abuse/harassment, any era. There is no fee or charge for the services.

Greenville

52051 ■ Vet Center
Greenville NC
1021 W.H. Smith Blvd., Ste. A100
Greenville, NC 27834
Ph: (252)355-7920
Fax: (252)756-7045
URL: http://www2.va.gov

Raleigh

52052 ■ Vet Center
Raleigh NC
1649 Old Louisburg Rd.
Raleigh, NC 27604
Ph: (919)856-4616
Fax: (919)856-4617
URL: http://www2.va.gov

NORTH DAKOTA

Bismarck

52053 ■ Vet Center Outstation
Bismark ND
619 Riverwood Dr., Ste. 105
Bismarck, ND 58705
Ph: (701)224-9751
Fax: (701)223-5150
URL: http://www2.va.gov

Fargo

52054 ■ Vet Center
Fargo ND
3310 Fiechtner Dr.
Ste. 100
Fargo, ND 58103
Ph: (701)237-0942
Fax: (701)237-5734
URL: http://www2.va.gov

Minot

52055 ■ Vet Center
Minot ND
1400 20th Ave. SW, Ste. 2
Minot, ND 58701
Ph: (701)852-0177
Fax: (701)852-5225
URL: http://www2.va.gov

OHIO

Cincinnati

52056 ■ Vet Center
Cincinnati OH
801B W 8th St.
Ste. 126
Cincinnati, OH 45203
Ph: (513)763-3500
Fax: (513)763-3505
URL: http://www2.va.gov

Cleveland

52057 ■ McCafferty Vet Center Outstation
4242 Lorain Ave, Ste. 203
Cleveland, OH 44113
Ph: (216)939-0784
Fax: (216)939-0276
URL: http://www2.va.gov

Columbus

52058 ■ Vet Center
Columbus OH
30 Spruce St.
Columbus, OH 43215
Ph: (614)257-5550
Fax: (614)257-5551
URL: http://www2.va.gov

Dayton

52059 ■ Dayton Mobile Vet Center
4100 W 3rd St.
Dayton, OH 45428
Ph: (937)461-9150
Fax: (937)461-4574
URL: http://www2.va.gov

52060 ■ Vet Center
Dayton OH
East Medical Plaza, 6th Fl.
627 Edwin C. Moses Blvd.
Dayton, OH 45408
Ph: (937)461-9150
Fax: (937)461-4574
URL: http://www2.va.gov

Maple Heights
52061 ■ Cleveland Heights Vet Center
5310 1/2 Warrensville Center Rd.
Maple Heights, OH 44137
Ph: (216)707-7901
Fax: (216)707-7902
URL: http://www2.va.gov

Parma
52062 ■ Vet Center
Parma OH
5700 Pearl Rd., Ste. 102
Parma, OH 44129
Ph: (440)845-5023
Fax: (440)845-5024
URL: http://www2.va.gov

Toledo
52063 ■ Vet Center
Toledo OH
1565 S Byrne Rd., Ste. 104
Toledo, OH 43614
Ph: (419)213-7533
Fax: (419)380-9583
URL: http://www2.va.gov

OKLAHOMA

Lawton
52064 ■ Vet Center
Lawton OK
1016 SW C Ave., Ste B
Lawton, OK 73501
Ph: (580)585-5880
Fax: (580)585-5890
URL: http://www2.va.gov

Oklahoma City
52065 ■ Vet Center
Oklahoma City OK
1024 NW 47th St., Ste. B
Oklahoma City, OK 73118
Ph: (405)456-5184
Fax: (405)521-1794
URL: http://www2.va.gov

Tulsa
52066 ■ Vet Center
Tusla OK
14002 E 21st St., Ste. 200
Tulsa, OK 74112
Ph: (918)628-2760
Fax: (918)439-7424
URL: http://www2.va.gov

OREGON

Bend
52067 ■ Central Oregon Vet Center
1645 NE Forbes Rd., Ste. 105
Bend, OR 97701
Ph: (541)749-2112
Fax: (541)647-5282
URL: http://www2.va.gov

Eugene
52068 ■ Vet Center
Eugene OR
1255 Pearl St., Ste. 200
Eugene, OR 97401

Ph: (541)465-6918
Fax: (541)465-6656
URL: http://www2.va.gov

Grants Pass
52069 ■ Vet Center
Grants Pass
211 SE 10th St.
Grants Pass, OR 97526
Ph: (541)479-6912
Fax: (541)474-4589
URL: http://www2.va.gov

Portland
52070 ■ Vet Center
Portland OR
1505 NE 122nd Ave., Ste. 110
Portland, OR 97220
Ph: (503)688-5361
Fax: (503)688-5364
URL: http://www2.va.gov
Program(s): Counseling; Information and Referral.
Remarks: Services are free to eligible veterans.

Salem
52071 ■ Vet Center
Salem OR
2645 Portland Rd., Ste. 250
Salem, OR 97301
Ph: (503)362-9911
Fax: (503)364-2534
URL: http://www2.va.gov

PENNSYLVANIA

Bristol
52072 ■ Bucks County Vet Center
2 Canal's End Plz., Ste. 201B
Bristol, PA 19007
Ph: (215)823-4590
URL: http://www2.va.gov

DuBois
52073 ■ Vet Center
DuBois PA
100 Meadow Ln., Ste. 8
DuBois, PA 15801
Ph: (814)372-2095
Fax: (814)940-6511
URL: http://www2.va.gov

Erie
52074 ■ Vet Center
Erie PA
Erie Metro Center, Ste. 105
240 W 11th St.
Erie, PA 16501
Ph: (814)453-7955
Fax: (814)456-5464
URL: http://www2.va.gov

Harrisburg
52075 ■ Vet Center
Harrisburg PA
1500 N 2nd St., Ste. 2
Harrisburg, PA 17102
Ph: (717)782-3954
Fax: (717)782-3791
URL: http://www2.va.gov

Lancaster
52076 ■ Lancaster Vet Center
1817 Olde Homestead Ln.
Lancaster, PA 17601
Ph: (717)283-0735
URL: http://www2.va.gov

McKeesport
52077 ■ Vet Center
McKeesport PA
2001 Lincoln Way, Ste. 21
McKeesport, PA 15131
Ph: (412)678-7704
Fax: (412)678-7780
URL: http://www2.va.gov

Norristown
52078 ■ Vet Center
Norristown PA
320 E Johnson Hwy., Ste. 201
Norristown, PA 19401
Ph: (215)283-5245
Fax: (610)272-2198
URL: http://www2.va.gov

Philadelphia
52079 ■ Vet Center Northeast
Philadelphia PA
101 E Olney Ave., Ste. C-7
Philadelphia, PA 19120
Ph: (215)924-4670
Fax: (215)224-4105
URL: http://www2.va.gov

52080 ■ Vet Center
Philadelphia PA
801 Arch St., Ste. 502
Philadelphia, PA 19107
Ph: (215)627-0238
Fax: (215)597-6362
URL: http://www2.va.gov

Pittsburgh
52081 ■ Vet Center
Pittsburgh PA
2500 Baldwick Rd., Ste. 15
Pittsburgh, PA 15205
Ph: (412)920-1765
Fax: (412)920-1769
URL: http://www2.va.gov
Remarks: Provides personalized, informal, and cost free counseling to eligible veterans.

Scranton
52082 ■ Vet Center
Scranton PA
1002 Pittston Ave.
Scranton, PA 18505
Ph: (570)344-2676
Fax: (570)344-6794
URL: http://www2.va.gov

Williamsport
52083 ■ Vet Center
Williamsport PA
49 E 4th St., Ste. 104
Williamsport, PA 17701
Ph: (570)327-5281
Fax: (570)322-4542
URL: http://www2.va.gov

PUERTO RICO

Arecibo
52084 ■ Vet Center
Arecibo PR
50 Gonzalo Marin St.
Arecibo, PR 00612
Ph: (787)879-4510
Fax: (787)879-4944
URL: http://www2.va.gov

Ponce
52085 ■ Vet Center
Ponce PR
35 Mayor St., Ste. 1
Ponce, PR 00730

Ph: (787)841-3260
Fax: (787)841-3165
URL: http://www2.va.gov

Rio Piedras

52086 ■ San Juan/Rio Pedros Vet Center
Condomino Medical Center Plz., LC Ste. 8-11
La Riviera
Rio Piedras, PR 00921
Ph: (787)749-4409
Fax: (787)749-4416
URL: http://www2.va.gov

RHODE ISLAND

Warwick

52087 ■ Vet Center
Warwick RI
2038 Warwick Ave.
Warwick, RI 02889
Ph: (401)739-0167
Fax: (401)739-7705
URL: http://www2.va.gov

SOUTH CAROLINA

Columbia

52088 ■ Vet Center
Columbia SC
1710 Richland St., Ste. A
Columbia, SC 29201
Ph: (803)765-9944
Fax: (803)799-6267
URL: http://www2.va.gov

Greenville

52089 ■ Vet Center
Greenville SC
14 Lavinia Ave.
Greenville, SC 29601
Ph: (864)271-2711
Fax: (864)370-3655
URL: http://www2.va.gov

North Charleston

52090 ■ Vet Center
North Charleston SC
5603A Rivers Ave.
North Charleston, SC 29406
Ph: (843)789-7000
Fax: (843)566-0232
URL: http://www2.va.gov

SOUTH DAKOTA

Martin

52091 ■ Pine Ridge Vet Center Outstation
105 E Hwy. 18
Martin, SD 57747
Ph: (605)685-1300
Fax: (605)685-1406
URL: http://www2.va.gov

Rapid City

52092 ■ Rapid City Mobile Vet Center
14930 Aviation Rd.
Rapid City, SD 57703
Ph: (605)348-0077
Fax: (605)348-0878
URL: http://www2.va.gov

52093 ■ Vet Center
Rapid City SD
621 6th St., Ste. 101
Rapid City, SD 57701
Ph: (605)348-0077
Fax: (605)348-0878
URL: http://www2.va.gov

Sioux Falls

52094 ■ Vet Center
Sioux Falls SD
601 S Cliff Ave., Ste. C
Sioux Falls, SD 57104
Ph: (605)330-4552
Fax: (605)330-4554
URL: http://www2.va.gov
Program(s): Individual Counseling, Referral for Benefits Assistance, Community Education, Job Counseling and Placement. **Remarks:** Services are free to eligible veterans and their families.

TENNESSEE

Chattanooga

52095 ■ Vet Center
Chattanooga TN
Bldg. 5700, Ste. 300
951 Eastgate Loop Rd.
Chattanooga, TN 37411
Ph: (423)855-6570
Fax: (423)855-6575
URL: http://www2.va.gov

Johnson City

52096 ■ Vet Center
Johnson City TN
2203 McKinley Rd.
Johnson City, TN 37604
Ph: (423)928-8387
Fax: (423)928-6320
URL: http://www2.va.gov

Knoxville

52097 ■ Vet Center
Knoxville TN
2817 E Magnolia Ave.
Knoxville, TN 37914
Ph: (865)545-4680
Fax: (865)545-4198
URL: http://www2.va.gov

Memphis

52098 ■ Vet Center
Memphis TN
1407 Union Ave., Ste. 410
Memphis, TN 38104
Ph: (901)544-0173
Fax: (901)544-0179
URL: http://www2.va.gov

Nashville

52099 ■ Vet Center
Nashville TN
1420 Donelson Pke., Ste. A-5
Nashville, TN 37217
Ph: (615)366-1220
Fax: (615)366-1351
URL: http://www2.va.gov

TEXAS

Abilene

52100 ■ Taylor County Vet Center
400 Oak St.
Abilene, TX 79602
Ph: (325)674-1328
URL: http://www2.va.gov

Amarillo

52101 ■ Vet Center
Amarillo TX
3414 Olsen Blvd., Ste. E
Amarillo, TX 79109
Ph: (806)354-9779
Fax: (806)351-1104
URL: http://www2.va.gov

Austin

52102 ■ Vet Center
Austin TX
Southcliff Bldg.
2015 S Industrial Hwy. 35, Ste. 101
Austin, TX 78741
Ph: (512)416-1314
Fax: (512)416-7019
URL: http://www2.va.gov

Corpus Christi

52103 ■ Vet Center
Corpus Christi TX
4646 Corona, Ste. 250
Corpus Christi, TX 78411
Ph: (361)854-9961
Fax: (361)854-4730
URL: http://www2.va.gov

Dallas

52104 ■ South Central Vet Center
Bldg. 69
4500 S Lancaster Rd.
Dallas, TX 75216
Ph: (214)857-1254
Fax: (214)462-4944
URL: http://www2.va.gov

52105 ■ Vet Center
Dallas TX
10501 N Central, Ste. 213
Dallas, TX 75231
Ph: (214)361-5896
Fax: (214)361-0981
URL: http://www2.va.gov

El Paso

52106 ■ Vet Center
El Paso TX
1155 Westmoreland, Ste. 121
El Paso, TX 79925
Ph: (915)772-0013
Fax: (915)772-3983
URL: http://www2.va.gov

Fort Worth

52107 ■ Vet Center
Fort Worth TX
1305 W Magnolia St., Ste. B
Fort Worth, TX 76104
Ph: (817)921-9095
Fax: (817)921-9438
URL: http://www2.va.gov

Harker Heights

52108 ■ Killeen Heights Vet Center
302 Millers Crossing, Ste. 4
Harker Heights, TX 76548
Ph: (254)953-7100
Fax: (254)953-7120
URL: http://www2.va.gov

Houston

52109 ■ Harris County Vet Center
14300 Corner Stone Village Dr., Ste. 110
Houston, TX 77014
Ph: (713)578-4002
Fax: (281)583-8800
URL: http://www2.va.gov

52110 ■ Vet Center
Houston TX
2990 Richmond, Ste. 325
Houston, TX 77006
Ph: (713)523-0884
Fax: (713)523-4513
URL: http://www2.va.gov

Laredo

52111 ■ Vet Center
Laredo TX
6999 McPherson Rd., Ste. 102
Laredo, TX 78041
Ph: (956)723-4680
Fax: (956)723-9144
URL: http://www2.va.gov

Lubbock

52112 ■ Vet Center
Lubbock TX
3106 50th St., Ste. 400
Lubbock, TX 79413
Ph: (806)792-9782
Fax: (806)792-9785
URL: http://www2.va.gov

McAllen

52113 ■ Vet Center
McAllen TX
801 Nolana Loop, Ste. 140
McAllen, TX 78504
Ph: (956)631-2147
Fax: (956)631-2430
URL: http://www2.va.gov

Mesquite

52114 ■ Dallas County Vet Center
502 W Kearney, Ste. 300
Mesquite, TX 75149
Ph: (972)288-8030
Fax: (972)288-8051
URL: http://www2.va.gov

Midland

52115 ■ Vet Center
Midland TX
2817 W Loop 250 N, Ste. E
Midland, TX 79701
Ph: (432)697-8222
Fax: (432)697-0561
URL: http://www2.va.gov

Pantego

52116 ■ Tarrant County Vet Center
Northlake Center
3337 W Pioneer Pkwy.
Pantego, TX 76013
Ph: (817)274-0981
Fax: (817)274-9712
URL: http://www2.va.gov

San Antonio

52117 ■ Vet Center
San Antonio TX
9504 Industrial Hwy. 35 N, Ste. 214 & 219
San Antonio, TX 78233
Ph: (210)650-0422
Fax: (210)650-0169
URL: http://www2.va.gov

UTAH

Provo

52118 ■ Vet Center
Provo UT
1807 No. 1120W
Provo, UT 84604
Ph: (801)377-1117
Fax: (801)377-0227
URL: http://www2.va.gov

Salt Lake City

52119 ■ Vet Center
Salt Lake City UT
1354 E 3300 South, Ste. C-105
Salt Lake City, UT 84106

Ph: (801)584-1294
Fax: (801)487-6243
URL: http://www2.va.gov

VERMONT

South Burlington

52120 ■ Vet Center
South Burlington VT
359 Dorset St.
South Burlington, VT 05403
Ph: (802)862-1806
Fax: (802)865-3319
URL: http://www2.va.gov

White River Junction

52121 ■ Vet Center
White River Junction VT
222 Holiday Inn Dr.
Gilman Office Center, Bldg. 2
White River Junction, VT 05001
Ph: (802)295-2908
Fax: (802)296-3653
URL: http://www2.va.gov

VIRGIN ISLANDS

Saint Croix

52122 ■ Vet Center Outstation
Saint Croix VI
RR2 Box 10553, Kingshill
Village Mall
Saint Croix, VI 00850
Ph: (340)778-5553
Fax: (340)778-5545
URL: http://www2.va.gov

Saint Thomas

52123 ■ Vet Center Outstation
Saint Thomas VI
Medical Foundation Bldg., Ste. 101
50 Estate Thomas
Saint Thomas, VI 00802
Ph: (340)774-5017
Fax: (340)774-5384
URL: http://www2.va.gov

VIRGINIA

Alexandria

52124 ■ Vet Center
Alexandria VA
6940 S Kings Hwy., Ste. 204
Alexandria, VA 22309
Ph: (703)360-8633
Fax: (703)360-2935
URL: http://www2.va.gov

Norfolk

52125 ■ Vet Center
Norfolk VA
1711 Church St., Ste. A & B
Norfolk, VA 23504
Ph: (757)623-7584
Fax: (757)441-6621
URL: http://www2.va.gov

Richmond

52126 ■ Vet Center
Richmond VA
4902 Fitzhugh Ave.
Richmond, VA 23230
Ph: (804)353-8958
Fax: (804)353-0837
URL: http://www2.va.gov

Roanoke

52127 ■ Vet Center
Roanoke VA
350 Albemarle Ave. SW
Roanoke, VA 24016

Ph: (540)342-9726
Fax: (540)857-2405
URL: http://www2.va.gov

Virginia Beach

52128 ■ Vet Center
Virginia Beach VA
324 Southport Cir., Ste. 102
Virginia Beach, VA 23452
Ph: (757)248-3665
Fax: (757)248-3667
URL: http://www2.va.gov

WASHINGTON

Bellingham

52129 ■ Vet Center
Bellingham WA
3800 Byron, Ste. 124
Bellingham, WA 98229
Ph: (360)733-9226
Fax: (360)733-9117
URL: http://www2.va.gov

Everett

52130 ■ Vet Center
Everett WA
3311 Wetmore Ave.
Everett, WA 98201
Ph: (425)252-9701
Fax: (425)252-9728
URL: http://www2.va.gov

Federal Way

52131 ■ Federal Way Vet Center
32020 32nd Ave. S, Ste. 110
Federal Way, WA 98001
Ph: (253)838-3909
Fax: (253)874-5083
URL: http://www2.va.gov

Seattle

52132 ■ Vet Center
Seattle WA
2030 - 9th Ave.
Ste. 210
Seattle, WA 98121
Ph: (206)553-2706
Fax: (206)553-0380
URL: http://www2.va.gov

Spokane

52133 ■ Vet Center
Spokane WA
100 N Mullan Rd., Ste. 102
Spokane, WA 99206
Ph: (509)444-8387
Fax: (509)444-8388
URL: http://www2.va.gov

Tacoma

52134 ■ Vet Center
Tacoma WA
4916 Center St., Ste. E
Tacoma, WA 98409
Ph: (253)565-7038
Fax: (253)565-4981
URL: http://www2.va.gov

Yakima

52135 ■ Vet Center
Yakima WA
2119 W Lincoln Ave.
Yakima, WA 98902
Ph: (509)457-2736
Fax: (509)457-1822
URL: http://www2.va.gov

WEST VIRGINIA

Beckley

52136 ■ Vet Center
Beckley WV
1000 Johnstown Rd.
Beckley, WV 25801
Ph: (304)252-8220
Fax: (304)254-8711
URL: http://www2.va.gov

Charleston

52137 ■ Vet Center
Charleston WV
521 Central Ave.
Charleston, WV 25302
Ph: (304)343-3825
Fax: (304)347-5303
URL: http://www2.va.gov

Glen Jean

52138 ■ Buckley Mobile Vet Center
409 Wood Mountain Rd.
Glen Jean, WV 25846
Ph: (304)252-8220
Fax: (304)254-8711
URL: http://www2.va.gov

Henlawson

52139 ■ Logan Vet Center Outstation
21 Veterans Ave.
Henlawson, WV 25624
Ph: (304)752-4453
Fax: (304)752-6910
URL: http://www2.va.gov

Huntington

52140 ■ Vet Center
Huntington WV
3135 16th St., Ste. 11
Huntington, WV 25701
Ph: (304)523-8387
Fax: (304)529-5910
URL: http://www2.va.gov

Martinsburg

52141 ■ Vet Center
Martinsburg WV
900 Winchester Ave.
Martinsburg, WV 25401

Ph: (304)263-6776
Fax: (304)262-7448
URL: http://www2.va.gov

Morgantown

52142 ■ Morgantown Mobile Vet Center
228 Comfort Inn Rd.
Morgantown, WV 26501
Ph: (304)291-4303
Fax: (304)291-4251
URL: http://www2.va.gov

52143 ■ Vet Center
Morgantown WV
34 Commerce Dr., Ste. 101
Morgantown, WV 26501
Ph: (304)291-4303
Fax: (304)291-4251
URL: http://www2.va.gov

Parkersburg

52144 ■ Vet Center Outstation
Parkersburg WV
2311 Ohio Ave., Ste. D
Parkersburg, WV 26101
Ph: (304)485-1599
Fax: (304)485-4212
URL: http://www2.va.gov

Princeton

52145 ■ Vet Center
Princeton WV
905 Mercer St.
Princeton, WV 24740
Ph: (304)425-5653
Fax: (304)425-2837
URL: http://www2.va.gov

Wheeling

52146 ■ Vet Center
Wheeling WV
1508 Bethlehem Blvd.
Wheeling, WV 26003
Ph: (304)232-0587
Fax: (304)232-1031
URL: http://www2.va.gov

WISCONSIN

Green Bay

52147 ■ Vet Center
Green Bay WI
1600 S Ashland Ave.
Green Bay, WI 54304

Ph: (920)435-5650
Fax: (920)435-5086
URL: http://www2.va.gov

La Crosse

52148 ■ La Crosse Vet Center
20 Copeland Ave.
La Crosse, WI 54601
Ph: (608)782-4403
Fax: (608)782-4423
URL: http://www2.va.gov

Madison

52149 ■ Vet Center
Madison WI
706 Williamson St.
Madison, WI 53703
Ph: (608)264-5342
Fax: (608)264-5344
URL: http://www2.va.gov

Milwaukee

52150 ■ Vet Center
Milwaukee WI
5401 N 76th St., Ste. 100
Milwaukee, WI 53218
Ph: (414)536-1301
Fax: (414)536-1568
URL: http://www2.va.gov

WYOMING

Casper

52151 ■ Casper Vet Center - Satellite
1030 N Poplar
Casper, WY 82601
Ph: (307)261-5355
Fax: (307)261-5439
URL: http://www2.va.gov

Cheyenne

52152 ■ Vet Center
Cheyenne WY
3219 E Pershing Blvd.
Cheyenne, WY 82001
Ph: (307)778-7370
Fax: (307)638-8923
URL: http://www2.va.gov

This is an alphabetical listing of all resources included in this directory as well as former or alternate names of the resources. Index references are to entry numbers rather than page numbers. Entry numbers appear in lightface type if the reference is to a former or alternate name; otherwise, entry numbers appear in boldface type. Consult the "User's Guide" at the beginning of this directory for more detailed information about the index.

A

A--1 Healthcare Center [13431]
A-1 International Homecare, Inc. [15770]
A-1 Solutions Counseling Service [50197]
A 1 Solutions Counseling Service • Everett [49946]
A1 Premier Home Care Agency, Inc. [13889]
AA Alternatives of Minnesota Inc [45299]
AA and Associates [43553]
AA and Associates Approved Alcohol/Drug • Programs CRS Inc [43641], [43673], [43769]
AA Hearing Aid Center [1448]
AA Hearing Assistance Center [2256]
A.A. Pain Clinic [35276]
AAA Health Inc • Chemical Dependency Outpatient Program [46469]
AAA Healthcare Services, Inc.--Houston [17948]
AAA Home Health Care Inc.--Simi Valley [13350]
AAA Home Health and Hospice [19866]
AAA Home Healthcare, Inc.--Dallas [17856]
AAA Homecare, Inc.--Glendale [13015]
AAA Medical & Oxygen Supply--Austin [17809]
AAA Medical & Oxygen Supply--Corpus Christi [17848]
AAA Medical & Oxygen Supply--Harker Heights [17940]
AAA Medical & Oxygen Supply--Kingsland [18028]
AAA Medical & Oxygen Supply--Lockhart [18047]
AAA Medical & Oxygen Supply--McAllen [18067]
AAA Medical & Oxygen Supply--Rockdale [18123]
AAA Medical & Oxygen Supply--Round Rock [18126]
AAA Medical & Oxygen Supply--San Antonio [18135]
AAA Medical & Oxygen Supply--San Marcos [18154]
AAA Treatment Center [41047]
AACS [49998]
Aaction Home Health Care [13719]
Aadi Home Health [17849]
AAE Crosby Center [40544]
AAMA
    AMISTAD Programs [49312]
    Concilio Hispano Libre [49437]
    Ganadores [49313]
    Judith Zaffirini Residential Center [49314]
    Selena Outpatient [49510]
A&A Staffing Health Care Services [16665]
A&S Home Health Care [17857]
AAR Counseling Services
    Fort Myers [41659]
    Main Office North Naples [41810]
Aaron E. Henry Community Health Services Center, Inc. [6880]
ABA Home Care Providers [13890]
Abacus Program [42654]
Abana Health Care [13891]
ABARIS Behavioral Health • Sober Living [44986]
Abate Abuse Counseling [49880], [50071]
ABBCON Counseling [42454]
    Douglas Treatment Center [42935]
    Edgar Treatment Center [42848]
Abbe Center for Community Mental Health [29844]
Abbeville Area Medical Center--Abbeville • Health Related Home Care [17561]
Abbeville Area Medical Center • Health Related Home Care - Greenwood Office [17599]

Abbeville Family Health Center [6181]
Abbeville Mental Health Clinic--Commercial Drive [32186]
Abbeville Mental Health Clinic--E Vermilion Street [30124]
Abbey Hospice [19420]
Abbis Care Team, LLC [17949]
Abbore Care [15797]
Abbotsford Hearing Clinic [1045]
Abbott and Burkhart Therapy [1355]
Abbott House, Inc. [34436]
Abbott Northwestern Hospital [2708]
    Center for Reproductive Medicine [22134]
    Sleep Disorders Center [37212]
    Virginia Piper Cancer Institute [5410]
Abbott Northwestern Transplant • Allina Hospitals & Clinics [25041]
Abby's Home Health Agency Corporation [14197]
ABC Counseling Center [41184]
ABC DUI Services [42794], [42899]
ABC Health Group/Matrix Center/Wichita [43474]
ABC Health Service Registry, Inc. [16459]
ABC Home Health Care [16894]
ABC Home Health--Las Vegas [16141]
ABC Home Health--Scottsdale [12815]
ABC Hospice [18756]
ABC Medical Supply [15882]
ABC Pediatric Therapy LLC [2088]
ABC Recovery Center Inc [39935]
ABC Sober Living • Soledad House [40545]
ABC Speech and Language Services [3253]
ABC Speech and Language Therapists [2932]
ABC Therapies of Florida Inc. [1801]
ABC Therapy [45830], [45834]
ABC Therapy Inc. [1565]
Abcare's HomeHealth Exchange [15798]
ABCD Inc. [3635]
A.Bel Audiology Associates [1716]
Abercorn Dialysis • DaVita • Dialysis Center [23783]
Aberdeen Area Youth Regional Treatment Center • Chief Gall Treatment Center [49004]
Aberdeen Behavioral Health Clinic [32800]
Aberdeen Clinic [6630]
Aberdeen Counseling Center [31099]
Aberdeen Public Schools • Aberdeen SD [741]
Abet Universal Services, Inc. [16629]
ABG Therapy and Wellness Center [1435]
Abiding Care Services, Inc. [17785]
Abilene RDSPD [764]
Abilene State School [8526]
Abilities in Action [2938]
Abilities Center [2661]
Abilities Rehabilitation Center [38709]
Abilities Services [7985]
Abilities for Speech and Language [2300]
A-Ability Medical Equipment, Inc. [14404]
Ability Building Center Inc. [2728]
Abington Dialysis • Dialysis Center & At Home • DaVita [26611]
Abington Hospice at Warminster-Hospice Volunteer Office [21166]
Abington Memorial Health Center [17511]
Abington Memorial Hospital [17230]
    Rosenfeld Cancer Center [5809]
    Sleep Disorders Center [37635]

Abington Reproductive Medicine [22224]
Able Care Home Health Products [16020]
Able to Change Recovery Inc [39968], [40668], [40669]
Able Hands Inc. [13432]
Able Health Care Services--Elmhurst [16441]
Able Health Care Services--Hicksville [16484]
Able Health Care Services--Islandia [16494]
Able Health Care Services--Merrick [16521]
Able Health Care Services--White Plains [16666]
Able Health Products [16191]
Able Home Care [12628]
Able Talk, Speech & Language Services Inc. [3288]
Abling Hands Home Health Care [16895]
ABODE Treatment Inc
    Counseling Center [49328]
    Residential/Outpatient Program [49584]
Aborn Dialysis Center • DaVita [22967]
About An Alternative Counseling Services [41048], [41270]
About Families CEDARR Center--Pawtucket [51308]
About Families CEDARR Center--Woonsocket [51314]
Above and Beyond Counseling [43674]
Above and Beyond Counseling - Valley [43675]
Above & Beyond Home Health Care [19714]
Above the Water House [44781]
ABQ Health Partners • New Mexico Center for Sleep Medicine [37368]
ABR Counseling Associates Kent County • Margaret Leister LCDP [41501]
ABR Counseling Associates • Sussex County [41515]
Abracadabra Recovery Center/Spanaway • Branch of Doorway to Recovery Inc [50159]
Abraham Home Health Care [13892]
Abraham Lincoln Center [29578]
Abraham Lincoln Memorial Hospital [2063]
Abrams and Associates • Center for Family Psychotherapy [11077]
ABRAXAS Youth and Family Services
    Life Works Interventions [42714]
    Southwood Interventions [42461]
Abriendo Puertas [9009]
ABS Lincs • DBA Cumberland Hall [43628]
Absher Neurology • Multiple Sclerosis Center [34705]
Absolut Home Care Inc. [13443]
Absolute Caregivers Home Health Agency [14450]
Absolute Control Transitional • Counseling Center Inc [40361]
Absolute Home Health Agency [13117]
Absolute Home Health Care--Grand Blanc [15671]
Absolute Performance Physical Therapy Center [38558]
Absolute Rehabilitation Center Inc • DBA LA County Outpatient Program [39933]
Abstemious Outpatient Clinic Inc [50162], [50163]
Abstinent Living at the Turning Point [48670]
Abstinent Living Turning Point • Washington Women with Children [48671]
Abundant Home Health Care--South Holland [14935]
Abundant Life Hospice [21240]
Abuse Alternatives, Inc. [10392]
Abuse Counseling and Treatment, Inc. [9050]

Abuse and Dependency Services [45693]
Abuse Network [10294]
Abuse and Rape Crisis Center [10319]
Abuse and Rape Crisis Shelter of Warren County [10155]
Abuse Resource Network [10115]
Abused Adult Resource Center [10108]
Abused Deaf Women's Advocacy Services [10640]
Abused Persons Outreach Center, Inc. [10117]
Abused Women's Advocacy Project/Safe Voices [9426]
Abused Women's Aid in Crisis, Inc. [8654]
Abusive Partners Program of Palm Beach [41562]
A.C. Home Health Agency, Inc. [13118]
Acacia Clinic, Inc. [32966]
Acacia Counseling Inc [41026], [41088], [41322]
Academic Guidance Services [7788]
Academy CareGivers [16351]
Academy Diagnostics Sleep Center [37796]
Academy Home Care [15831]
Academy Medical Center • United States Sports Academy [38002]
Academy Orthopaedic Clinic [38770]
Academy School District Number 20 [321]
Acadia Family Center [44066]
Acadia Hawaii - Pu'ukamalu [33395]
Acadia Hearing Center [2346]
Acadia Home Care--Fort Kent [15390]
Acadia Home Care--Hermon [15391]
Acadia Home Care--Portland [15396]
Acadia Home Care--Presque Isle [15398]
Acadia Hospital [43922]
The Acadia Hospital [33551]
Acadia Hospital Blue Hill Clinic [33553]
Acadia Hospital Pittsfield Clinic [33554]
Acadia, Inc. [4383]
Acadia Northwest [48176], [48177]
Acadia Vermilion [30148]
Acadia Vermilion Hospital [43838]
Acadian Hearing and Speech Services [2322]
Acadian Home Care of Abbeville [15261]
Acadian Home Care--Acadia Parish [15283]
Acadian Home Care--Church Point • Saint Landry Home Health [15278]
Acadian Home Care--Kaplan • Kaplan Home Care [15305]
Acadian Home Care of New Iberia [15338]
Acadian Home Care Services
    Jeff Davis Home Health [15302]
    Welsh Home Care [15379]
Acadian Home Care • Ville Platte Home Health Agency [15377]
Acadian HomeCare, Inc.--Lafayette [15307]
Acadiana Addiction Center [43839]
Acadiana Recovery Center [43840]
ACCEL [7738]
Accelerated Home Care [14787]
Accelerated Homecare Services [15777]
Accelerated Rehab--Brighton [38581]
Accelerated Rehab--Farmington Hills [38587]
Accelerated Rehab--Royal Oak [38603]
Accent Audiology [1585]
Accent Care of New York [16667]
Accent on Communication--Castro Valley [1078]
Accent on Communication--Sparta [2948]
Accent Modification Center [3584]
Accent On Business [2131]
Accent On Communication--Stamford [1492]
Accent On Speech--Silver Spring [2434]
Accent Reduction Clinic [1776]
Accent and Speech Consulting [2442]
Accent on Speech--San Diego [1253]
Accent and Speech Solutions [3141]
AccentCare-Windsor [19134]
AccentMarq Communication [2407]
Accents Away [1751]
Access Behavioral Healthcare [30621]
Access Behavioral Healthcare LLC [44959]
Access Behavioral Services Inc [42462]
Access to Better Communication [2301]
Access to Care, LLC [15031]
Access Center [28879]
Access Community Health Center--New York [7026]
Access Community Health Centers--Madison [7429]
ACCESS Family Care at the Ozark Center [6907]
Access Family Health Services, Inc. • Access Family Medical Clinic [6897]
Access Health Systems, inc. [13893]

Access Home Care and Hospice--Chubbuck [19454]
Access Home Care and Hospice--Garden City [21605]
Access Home Care and Hospice--Logan [21615]
Access Home Care and Hospice--Sandy [21655]
Access Home Health Care--Dearborn [15616]
Access Home Health Care Inc.--Walnut [13433]
Access Hospice Care [20283]
ACCESS Inc [50437], [50528], [50530]
Access Medical South, LC [13696]
Access Nursing Services--Manhattan [16515]
Access Nursing Services of Maryland [15452]
Access Nursing Services of New Jersey [16226]
ACCESS Nursing Services--New York [16546]
Access Plus Home Health Services, Inc. [18128]
Access Recovery Solutions LLC [41881]
Access Rehabilitation Centers LLC [1498]
Access Sports Medicine and Orthopaedics [38705]
Access Therapy [3289]
accessAbilities Foundation, Inc. [8461]
Accessible Home Health of Broward [13686]
Accessible Home Health Care--Ocala [14275]
Accessible Home Health Care of South Miami-Dade [13894]
Acclaim Counseling Center LLC [41323]
Acclaim Home Health Services, Inc. [20863]
Acclaim Home Healthcare [13895]
Acclaim Hospice and Palliative Care [20826]
Accolade Chiropractic Care [38134]
Accolade Hospice-Burleson [21413]
Accolade Hospice-Lubbock [21520]
Accolade Hospice--Yoakum [21594]
ACCORD Corp. • Open Door [9898]
Accord Home Health Services--Cerritos [12935]
Accord Home Health Services--Granada Hills [13063]
Accredited Addiction Recovery Services [43407]
Accredited Aides-Plus, Inc. [16532]
Accredited Home Care, Inc. [15868]
Accredo Health Group--Chesterfield, MO [15992]
Accredo Health Group--Elmhurst, IL [14782]
Accredo Health Group--Fort Lauderdale, FL [13687]
Accredo Health Group--Greensboro, NC [16730]
Accredo Health Group, Inc.--Chantilly, VA [18253]
Accredo Health Group Inc.--Corona, CA [12955]
Accredo Health Group Inc.--Eagan [15938]
Accredo Health Group Inc.--Englewood [13485]
Accredo Health Group, Inc.--Houston, TX [17950]
Accredo Health Group, Inc.--Irving, TX [18018]
Accredo Health Group, Inc.--Kent, Washington [18434]
Accredo Health Group Inc.--Las Vegas, NV [16142]
Accredo Health Group Inc.--Lenexa, KS [15138]
Accredo Health Group Inc.--Little Rock [12863]
Accredo Health Group, Inc.--Memphis, TN [17730]
Accredo Health Group, Inc.--Nashville, TN [17750]
Accredo Health Group Inc.--Norcross, GA [14562]
Accredo Health Group Inc.--Novi, MI [15759]
Accredo Health Group, Inc.--Oklahoma City, OK [17141]
Accredo Health Group Inc.--Phoenix, AZ [12800]
Accredo Health Group Inc.--Richmond [13263]
Accredo Health Group, Inc., --Salt Lake City, UT [18218]
Accredo Health Group, Inc.--Virginia Beach, VA [18399]
Accredo Health Group, Inc.--Warrendale, PA [17500]
Accredo Health Group--Iowa City, IA [15089]
Accredo Health Group--Jacksonville, FL [13806]
Accredo Health Group--Louisville, KY [15215]
Accredo Health Group--Marlboro, MA [15514]
Accredo Health Group--McPherson, KS [15142]
Accredo Health Group of New York-- [16447], [16462], [16471]
Accredo Health Group--Omaha, NE [16116]
Accredo Health Group--Overland Park,KS [15146]
Accredo Health Group--Pine Brook, NJ [16255]
Accredo Health Group--Tampa, FL [14405]
Accredo Health Group--Totowa, NJ [16277]
AccuHear [1759]
Accurate Care Pain Relief Center [35285]
Accurate Evaluations [42440], [42705]
Accurate Health Services Corp. [14406]
Accurate Home Care [15799]
Accurite Health Services, Inc. [13059]
Ace Addiction Recovery Inc [48033]
Ace-ellent Healthcare Services, Inc. [18163]
Ace Health Services [13896]

A.C.E. Home Health Care [15686]
Ace Home Health Corp. [14231]
Ace Home Health Services Corp. [13897]
Ace Medical Inc. [14645]
ACE Speech and Language Clinic LLC [2737]
AceraCare Hospice-Richmond [19645]
ACES [3952]
ACES Community Services • Pioneer Health Resources [42306]
Aces Community Services • Pioneer Health Resources [42354]
ACES, Inc. [1254]
A.C.G. Therapy Center [1586]
ACH Child and Family Services • Runaway and Homeless Youth Program [36209]
Achieve Center [3643]
Achieve Home Health Care, LLC [15667]
Achieve Speech and Language Clinic [3186]
Achievekids [7803], [28691]
Achievement Center [8595]
The Achievement Center [8456]
Achievement Center for Children [8413]
Achievement Centers [7959]
Achievement Through Counseling and Treatment
    ACT I [48494]
    ACT II [48495]
Ackerman Institute for the Family [31405]
ACL Dialysis • Dialysis Clinic Inc. [25560]
ACME Counseling [48087]
ACMI House [10189]
Acosta-Rua Center for Caring [19237]
ACP Health Care Resources, Inc. [18159]
Acredo Health Group Inc. [12678]
ACS Crisis Residential [47552]
ACT Big Pine [29138]
ACT Center Inc [41558], [41846], [41847], [41980], [42004]
    La Mirada Plaza [41718]
ACT Corporation [29139], [50754]
ACT Corporation - Flagler Center [29123]
ACT Home Health Services, Inc. [17402]
Act II Counseling Services Inc [44304]
ACT Main Center [29140]
ACT • New Smyrna Beach Center [29235]
ACT Ocean Breeze [29141]
ACT Pine Grove Beach House [29142]
ACTION Associates, Inc. [10194]
Action for a Better Community • New Directions CD Outpatient Clinic [47024]
Action Consultants/Therapy [39745]
Action Counseling [50061]
Action Counseling Clinic Inc • Substance Abuse Services [44705]
Action Counseling and Consulting [49058], [49192]
Action Counseling Dependency Center [49977]
Action Family Counseling Inc [40362], [40800]
    Action Family Center [40830]
    Adolescent IOP Program [40741]
    Adult IOP Program [40258]
    Intensive Outpatient Program [40904]
Action For Kids [2074], [2106]
Action Home Health Care [13119]
Action Net Psychological Services PLLC [44776]
Action Now • Chemical Dependency Treatment Services [43254]
Action Physical Medicine and Rehabilitation--Naperville [38392]
Action Physical Medicine and Rehabilitation--Shorewood [38411]
Action Physical Therapy [39140]
Action Steps Counseling Inc [48034]
Action Substance Abuse Recovery [40981], [40985], [41089]
Activa Home Health--Boynton Beach, FL [13597]
Activa Home Health--Coral Springs, FL [13626]
Activa Home Health--Delray Beach, FL [13646]
Active Healthcare, Inc.--Cary [37452]
Active Healthcare, Inc.--Clayton [37453]
Active Healthcare, Inc.--Durham [37454]
Active Healthcare, Inc.--Raleigh [37455]
Active Home Health Services Inc.--Madison Hieghts, MI [13012]
Active Infusion Saginaw [15733]
Active Infusion-Troy [15734]
Active Sports Medicine Foot and Ankle [38721]
ACTS for Children [33163]
ACTS Helpline [51419]
ACTS Home Health Care [15297]

ACTS Hospice [21048]
ACTS Inc • Horton Lee E [47529]
ACTS • Turning Points [10563]
Actual Care Home Health [18317]
Acu-Ear Audiology and Hearing Aid Associates [2181]
Acupuncture and Sports Clinic [39144]
Acupuncture Treatment Concepts II [44723]
Acute Care, Inc. [18486]
Acute and Chronic Pain and Spine Center [35680]
Acute Home Health Care--Troy [15857]
Acute Home Healthcare--Altamonte Springs [13578]
Acute Treatment Unit [28911], [28942]
Ada Area Chemical Dependency Center Inc [47899]
Ada County Juvenile Court Services [42307]
Ada Dialysis Center • Renal Advantage Inc. [26245]
Ada S. McKinley Community Services, Inc. [29579]
Adair Eldercare [29994]
Adam Wells Crisis Center [9271]
Adams and Associates [43569]
Adams Cnty Community Counseling Services [50046]
Adams County Family Health Center [6893]
Adams County Health and Human Services [32973]
Adams County Memorial Hospital [14974]
Adams County Regional Medical Center [17036]
Adams County School District Number 12 [319]
Adams/Hanover Counsel Service--Hanover • Crisis Intervention Program [51282]
Adams Hanover Counseling Services Inc [48380], [48386], [48643], [48707]
Adams Hanover Counseling Services, Inc. [32022]
Adams/Hanover Counseling Services, Inc.-- Gettysburg • Crisis Intervention Program [51281]
Adams Memorial Hospital • Behavioral Health Resource Center [42991]
Adams Nursing Home [27821]
Adams Physical Therapy Services Inc. [38919]
Adan Home Health [13898]
Adanta Behavioral Health Services
	Albany Clinic [43520]
	Burkesville Clinic [43546]
	Campbellsville Clinic [43549]
	Columbia Clinic [43557]
	Greensburg Clinic [43609]
	Jamestown Clinic [43640]
	Liberty Clinic [43671]
	Somerset Clinic Hardin Lane [43782]
	Wayne County Clinic [43716]
	Whitley City Clinic [43797]
Adanta Group [30113]
Adanta Group - Clinton County Mental Health Center [29964]
Adanta Group • Russell County Mental Health Center [30038]
ADAP Counseling Services [41940]
ADAPT Aware Zone Inc [40950]
ADAPT Cares [44100]
ADAPT Clinic [33002]
ADAPT/Corrections [48228]
ADAPT Counseling Associates [43029], [43624]
ADAPT/Crossroads [48229]
ADAPT/Deer Creek • Adolescent Treatment Center [48230]
ADAPT/Grants Pass [48118]
ADAPT Inc [47553]
ADAPT/Jackson [48231]
ADAPT of Minnesota [45090]
Adapt of Missouri, Inc. [30894]
ADAPT North Bend [48159]
ADAPT Program • 10 MDOS/SGOW [41332]
Adapt Psychotherapy [10925]
ADAPT and Recover [46287]
Adaptive Group Residence [29426]
ADC Sleep Disorders Center [37797]
ADCARE Hospital • Outpatient [44403]
Adcare Hospital • Satellite [44527], [44544], [44597]
AdCare Hospital
	Warwick [48885]
	Worcester [44607]
ADCI LLC [47249]
Addcare Counseling Inc [48940]
Addicare Group of Texas • The Zenith Program [49349]
Addiction Alternatives • A Division of Life Management Skills [39658]
Addiction Awareness LLC [45606]

Addiction/Behavior Counseling Services [43151]
Addiction Center of Broome County Inc • CD Outpatient Rehabilitation Program [46379]
Addiction Counseling Associates [49277]
Addiction Counseling and Educational • Resources [43851], [43902]
Addiction and Counseling Services [47586]
Addiction Counseling Services LLC [43475]
Addiction Family Resources [48991]
Addiction Institute of NY OTP • Saint Lukes Roosevelt Hospital [46804]
Addiction Medicine and Health • Advocates Inc [48496]
Addiction Pain Associates • Behavioral Health Services [46161]
Addiction and Psychological Services [49652]
Addiction Recover Center • Greenwich Hospital [41386]
Addiction Recovery Care Association [47534]
Addiction Recovery Care of Tampa • (ARC) [41952]
Addiction Recovery Center for Men [47371]
Addiction Recovery Institute [48864]
	South [48886]
Addiction Recovery Resources Inc [43858]
Addiction Recovery Services [44224], [45595]
	Univ Hosp of Cleveland/Dept of Psych [47676]
Addiction Recovery Systems [45955], [46165], [48425]
Addiction Recovery Systems LLC • ARS Pantops Clinic [49772]
Addiction Recovery Technologies [45192]
Addiction Research and Consulting Corp [41991]
Addiction Research and Treatment Corp • REACH Program [46805]
Addiction Research and Treatment Inc [39604], [39839], [40053], [40054], [40287], [40447]
	Bay Area Addiction Research and Treatment [39840], [40186]
	BBHS [39841]
Addiction Resources Inc [39416]
Addiction Solutions Counseling Center [44633], [44928]
Addiction Solutions Inc [47515]
Addiction Specialists [48663]
Addiction Specialists of Kansas Inc • Postive Adjustments [43476]
Addiction Specialists LLC • John F Natale LCADC [46213]
Addiction Stress Center • Kansas City [43373]
Addiction Treatment Center of New England [44426]
Addiction Treatment Outpatient Services [41090], [41223], [41285]
Addiction Treatment Resources • Texas Counseling/ Professional Services [49463]
Addiction Treatment Serv of Marysville • (ATS) [40207]
Addiction Treatment Services [44101]
	BBRC Johns Hopkins Bayview Medical Center [44102]
Addiction Treatment Services Inc [45034]
	Dakoske and Phoenix Hall [45035]
Addiction Treatment Services • Merriam [43430]
Addiction Treatment Strategies [42647]
Addictions Associates [44343]
Addictions Associates Therapy Inc [42747]
Addictions Care Center of Albany Inc [46324]
	Intensive Day Rehab [46325]
	Outpatient Rehab [46326]
Addictions Center of Broome County Inc • CD Intensive Outpatient Program [46380]
Addictions Counseling Service [44103]
Addictions Counseling Treatment Services [45159]
Addictions and Family Care Inc [43077]
Addictions Recovery Center Inc [48148]
Addictions Recovery Centers Inc [43008], [43022], [43066], [43200], [43226]
	Cornerstone of Recovery [43130]
Addictions Rehabilitation Association • (ARA) [42335]
Addictive Behaviors Counseling [41192], [41193]
Addicts Rehabilitation Center Fund Inc
	Drug Free Residential/Homeless [46806]
	Residence I [46807]
Addis-Genkin Speech and Language Associates [3351]
Addison Behavioral Care Inc [48581]
Adelante Familia/Saint Vincent de Paul of Baltimore [9441]

Adelante Healthcare Avondale Obstetrics and Gynecology [6224]
Adelante Healthcare Buckeye [6225]
Adelante, Inc. [10174]
Adelphi University
	Eating Disorder Treatment Center [11152]
	Hy Weinberg Center for Communication Disorders [3023]
Adena Health System • Cancer Program [5689]
Adena Home Care [16869]
ADEPT Assessment Center/Colville [49930]
Adept Assessment Center • DBA ADEPT [50164]
ADEPT Assessment Center/Deer Park [49935]
ADF Counseling [44777]
ADHD Mood and Behavior Center • Eating Disorder Center [11140]
Adirondack Medical Center ESRD • Dialysis Center [25773]
Adirondack Sports Medicine and Physical Therapy Center [38822]
Adler School of Professional Psychology [29580]
Adlerian Center for • Therapy Consultation and Education [45781]
Adm Servicios Salud Mental y Contra • Adiccion Centro de Tratamiento Menores [48741]
Admiral Hospice Care [18955]
Adolescent Chemical Dependency Program [49034]
Adolescent Counseling Exchange [41091]
Adolescent Counseling Services • Adolescent Substance Abuse Treatment Prog [40354]
Adolescent Day Treatment West • Land O'Lakes High School [29200]
Adolescent and Family Institute of Colorado Inc [41344]
Adolescent Substance Abuse Program [46005]
Adolescent Substance Abuse Programs [47647]
Adolescent Treatment Center of • Winnebago Inpatient and Extended Care [45349]
Adolescent Treatment Centers Inc • Thunder Road [40288]
Adonai Home Healthcare, LLC [18023]
Adoni Home Health, Inc. [18136]
ADORAY Home Health and Hospice [21784]
ADOSA Counseling [43775]
Adriel School [8433]
Adrina Home Health Care [13899]
Adult Addiction Clinic [44280]
Adult Adolescent Alcohol Treatment • (AAAT) [41204]
Adult and Child Development Center • Infant Toddler Program [7925]
Adult & Child Mental Health Center [29729]
Adult and Child Rehabilitation Center [7978]
Adult Community Connections • Allegan County Community Mental Health Service Program [30498]
Adult Counseling Center Inc • Outpatient Services [42386]
Adult Counseling and Educational Services [42715]
Adult Crisis Stabilization Unit [29230]
Adult Day Treatment [29358]
Adult Education Associates [42627]
Adult Extended Care Services [32836]
Adult Outpatient • Alta Pointe Health Systems, Inc. [27975]
Adult Outpatient Services Pembroke 6 • Outpatient Program [49851]
Adult Rehab Program--Salvation Army [6207]
Adult Rehabilitation Center [6704]
Adult Rehabilitation Services Inc [49359]
Adult Services Harvest House/ACT [29014]
Adult Well Being Services [44724], [44991]
Adult Well-Being Services [30536]
Adult and Youth Counseling Services Inc [41030]
Adult/Youth Counseling Services Inc [41289], [41336]
AdvaCare Home Services, Inc.--Beaver [17250]
AdvaCare Home Services, Inc.--Bridgeville [17264]
AdvaCare Home Services, Inc.--Pittsburgh [17430]
Advacare Medical Corp. [15144]
AdvaCare Systems [14718]
AdvanCare Healthcare Services [14936]
Advance Care Home Health Agency [13608]
Advance Counseling Services Inc [42463]
Advance Healthlink Home Healthcare [13190]
Advance Home Care, Inc. [12916]
Advance Home Health [14802]
Advance Home Health Care Services [15599]

Advance Home Health Corporation [14198]
Advance Home Health of Tampa [14407]
Advance Home Oxygen and Medical Supply, Inc. [15406]
Advance Neurology and Pain • Multiple Sclerosis Center [34662]
Advance Speech Expert Services [1136]
Advance Speech Therapies [1373]
Advance Therapy Associates LLC [1502]
Advanced Addiction Treatment Center • The Phoenix Group [41606], [41887]
Advanced Audiology [1453]
Advanced Audiology LLC [2568]
Advanced Back & Neck Pain Center [38204]
Advanced Behavioral Consultants [43772]
Advanced Biohealing Inc. [34931]
Advanced Care Hospice-Houston • Q-Staff [21479]
Advanced Care Inc.--Albany [16331]
Advanced Care, Inc.--Farmingdale [16454]
Advanced Center for Sleep Disorders [37752]
Advanced Choices [49897]
Advanced Comprehensive Treatment [49938]
Advanced Counseling Services PC [44677], [44687], [44699], [45016]
Advanced Counseling Services, PC--Brighton [30517]
Advanced Counseling Services, PC--Canton [30520]
Advanced Counseling Services PC--Clarkston [30529]
Advanced Counseling Services, PC--Saint Clair Shores [30630]
Advanced Counseling Services, PC--Southfield [30636]
Advanced Counseling Services, PC--Taylor [30643]
Advanced Dialysis Center--Baldwin Park [22599]
Advanced Dialysis Center--Easton [24679]
Advanced Dialysis Center of Ft. Lauderdale [23434]
Advanced Dialysis Center--Potomac [27459]
Advanced Dialysis Center--Randallstown [24716]
Advanced Dialysis Center--Rockville [24718]
Advanced Dialysis Institute, Inc. [23317]
Advanced Dialysis LLC [26188]
Advanced Dialysis of Parma [26182]
Advanced DUI School [45864]
Advanced Fertility Associates [21905]
Advanced Fertility Care--Scottsdale [21890]
Advanced Fertility Care--Tempe [21891]
Advanced Fertility Center of Chicago [22031]
Advanced Fertility Group [22054]
Advanced Fertility and Reproductive Endocrinology Institute [22242]
Advanced Fertility Services [22176]
Advanced Health Services, Inc. [17339]
Advanced Healthcare [40546]
Advanced Hearing and Balance Center [1840]
Advanced Hearing Solutions [1447], [1507]
Advanced Home Care [15858]
Advanced Home Medical Inc. [13434]
Advanced Homecare, Inc.--Sarasota [14372]
Advanced Homecare LLC--Bradenton [13600]
Advanced Human Services Inc • Chemical Dependence Outpatient Program [46641]
Advanced Infusion Solutions [15955]
Advanced Medical Equipment, Inc. [15306]
Advanced Medical Solutions, Inc. [15687]
Advanced Neurodiagnostic Center, Inc. • Advanced Sleep Center [37058]
Advanced Neurosciences Institute • Multiple Sclerosis Center [34712]
Advanced Nu Med Technologies, Inc. [35168]
Advanced Orthopaedic Centers [39130]
Advanced Orthopaedic Sports Medicine & Arthritis Center [38228]
Advanced Orthopaedic & Sports Physical Therapy [38295]
Advanced Orthopaedic Surgery Center [38147]
Advanced Orthopaedics Sports [38199]
Advanced Orthopedic and Sports Medicine Specialists--Denver [38170]
Advanced Orthopedic and Sports Medicine Specialists--Parker [38180]
Advanced Orthopedics--Boynton Beach [38220]
Advanced Orthopedics--Hollywood [38232]
Advanced Orthopedics--Orlando [38262]
Advanced Orthopedics--Palm Beach Gardens [38272]
Advanced Orthopedics--Port Saint Lucie [38278]
Advanced Orthopedics--Sarasota [38285]

Advanced Orthopedics and Sports Medicine Institute [38724]
Advanced Orthopedics and Sports Medicine--Las Vegas [38698]
Advanced Orthopedics and Sports Medicine--Saint Louis [38663]
Advanced Pain Management Institute [35426]
Advanced Physical Therapy [38929]
Advanced Physical Therapy of Alaska--Anchorage [38015]
Advanced Physical Therapy of Alaska--Fairbanks [38020]
Advanced Physical Therapy of Alaska--Wasilla [38026]
Advanced Professionals Healthcare [14693]
Advanced Pulmonary and Sleep Solutions, PA • Sleep Disorders Center [37798]
Advanced Recovery Rehabilitation Center [1316]
Advanced Renal Care [23527]
Advanced Reproductive Center of Hawaii [22024]
Advanced Reproductive Concepts [22198]
Advanced Reproductive Health Center [22032]
Advanced Research Systems/Pioneer Valley Hospital • Sleep Disorders Center [37868]
Advanced Sleep and Breathing Disorders Laboratory [37375]
Advanced Sleep Neurodiagnostics PC [37143]
Advanced Solutions • Addiction Management [43330]
Advanced Speech and Language Associates [2874]
Advanced Speech Therapy [1384]
Advanced Speech and Therapy Services Inc. [1736]
Advanced Therapy and Learning Center Inc. [1599]
Advanced Therapy Solutions [940], [39017]
Advancing Communication and Learning Inc. [3499]
Advancing at Home Health Care, LLC [17947]
Advanta Care--Capitola [12931]
Advanta Care--Sunnyvale [13375]
AdvantaCare--Monterey [13186]
Advantage Behavioral Health System--Dainelsville [29403]
Advantage Behavioral Health Systems [42095]
    Child and Adolescent Services [29339]
    Crisis Stabilization Program [29340]
    Greene County Mental Health Center [29434]
    Jackson County Clinic [42111]
    Jackson County Service Center [29395]
    Miles Street Clinic [42022]
    Oglethorpe Mental Health Clinic [29399]
    Walton County Mental Health Center [42136]
    Women's Day Service [29341]
Advantage Counseling/Education Services [43150]
Advantage Counseling and Fitness Services [43177]
Advantage Family Health Center [6862]
Advantage Group Foundation Ltd [42605]
Advantage Hand Center [38491]
Advantage Health Care [17648]
Advantage Health Systems [13291]
Advantage Home Care [15885]
Advantage Home Health Care, Inc. [14714]
Advantage Home Health Care Services [15479]
Advantage Home Health & Hospice [20970]
Advantage Hospice and Home Care--Clinton [20637]
Advantage Hospice and Home Care-Fayetteville [20658]
Advantage Orthopaedics, PC [38812]
Advantage Physical Therapy--Boutte [38489]
Advantage Physical Therapy--Destrehan [38490]
Advantage Physical Therapy & Hand Specialty Center--Harahan [38493]
Advantage Physical Therapy and Hand Specialty Center--Metairie [38499]
Advantage Sleep Centers [37334]
Advantage Speech Therapy LLC [3187]
AdvantageHEALTH Sports Medicine and Physical Therapy [38571]
Advantages Counseling Services • Bremerton [49911]
Advantis Home Care, Inc. [13900]
Advent Group Ministries [40650]
    Gateway [40677]
    Genesis [39886]
    Laurel Home [40246]
    South Valley [40651]
    Summit Ranch [40247]
Advent Healthcare Services Inc. [13439]
Advent Home Health Agency [16143]
Advent Home Medical [15735]

Adventist Behavioral Health [44330]
Adventist Dialysis Services • Fresenius Medical Care [24727]
Adventist Gordon Hospital • Cancer Program [5017]
Adventist Health Home Care and Hospice Services--Hanford [13069]
Adventist Health Home Care and Hospice Services--Willits [13450]
Adventist Health Home Care and Personal Care Services [18479]
Adventist Health and Home Care Services [12898]
Adventist Health Home Care Services--Chula Vista [12943]
Adventist Health Home Care Services--Tillamook [17228]
Adventist Health Hospice--Portland [21019]
Adventist Health/Hospice--Tillamook [21037]
Adventist Hinsdale Hospital
    New Day Center [42961]
    Sleep Disorders Center [36888]
Adventist Home Care [17212]
Adventist La Grange Memorial Hospital • Cancer Program [5104]
Adventist Medical Center [3317]
    Cancer Program [5798]
    Sleep Disorders Center [37609]
Adventist Rehab Silver Spring [4087]
Adventist Rehab Takoma Park [4088]
Adventist Rehabilitation Hospital of Maryland [4089]
Advocacy and Resource Center [10764]
Advocare Home Health [15869]
Advocate Addiction Treatment Program [42623]
Advocate Christ Medical Center [33435]
Advocate Christ Medical Center - Cancer Program [5116]
Advocate Christ Medical Center--Palos Heights • Sleep Disorders Center [36889]
Advocate Christ Medical Center • Substance Abuse Services [42820]
Advocate Christ Medical Center--Tinley Park • Sleep Disorders Center [36890]
Advocate Condell Medical Center [2059]
    Cancer Program [5106]
Advocate Counseling Center Inc [42958]
Advocate Counseling Services [41645]
Advocate Good Samaritan Hospital [2019]
Advocate Good Samaritan Hospital - Cancer Program [5086]
Advocate--Good Samaritan Sleep Center [36891]
Advocate Good Shepherd Hospital--Barrington [1960]
Advocate Good Shepherd Hospital--Lake Zurich [2056]
Advocate Good Shepherd Hospital - Oncology Services [5062]
Advocate Good Shepherd Rehabilitation Services--Crystal Lake [2010]
Advocate Healthcare • Clean Start [42464]
Advocate Home Care, Inc. [15870]
Advocate Home Care Services [14884]
Advocate Home Health Services--Crystal Lake [14759]
Advocate Home Health Services--Downers Grove [14769]
Advocate Home Health Services--Hazel Crest [14814]
Advocate Home Health Services and Hospice [14831]
Advocate Home Health Services--Park Ridge [14901]
Advocate Home Health Services--Worth [14960]
Advocate Hope Children's Hospital • Pediatric Cystic Fibrosis Center [7525]
Advocate Hospice-Danville [19591]
Advocate Hospice--Downers Grove [19515]
Advocate Hospice-Park Ridge [19556]
Advocate Illinois Masonic Medical Center • Creticos Cancer Center [5067]
Advocate Lutheran Children's Hospital • Down Syndrome Clinic [10792]
Advocate Lutheran General Hospital
    Adult Down Syndrome Center [10793]
    Cancer Program [5119]
    Sleep Disorders Center [36892]
Advocate Program [41640], [41762]
Advocate Safehouse Project [8966]
Advocate South Suburban Hospital • Cancer Program [5096]

Advocates Against Domestic Abuse [9580]
Advocates Against Domestic Assault [9581]
Advocates for Bartow's Children • Runaway and
   Homeless Youth Program [35904]
Advocates Building Peaceful Communities [8984]
Advocates Community Counseling [44469], [44511]
   Satellite [44399]
Advocates--Crisis Support Services [8944]
Advocates to End Domestic Violence [9787]
Advocates for Family Peace [9599]
Advocates For A Violence Free Community [8971]
Advocates, Inc.--Acton [30316]
Advocates, Inc. • Advocates Community Counseling
   Center [30379]
Advocates, Inc.--Bellingham [30329]
Advocates, Inc.--Blackstone [30339]
Advocates, Inc.
   Community Counseling [30415]
   Day Habilitation Services [30322]
Advocates, Inc.--Framingham [30380]
Advocates, Inc.--Natick [30421]
Advocates, Inc.--Newton [30427]
Advocates, Inc.--Walpole [30473]
Advocates, Inc.--West Goylston [30475]
Advocates, Inc. -Windward Program [30414]
Advocates of Lake County [8974]
Advocates of Ozaukee [10734]
Advocates for Survivors of Domestic Violence/
   Sexual Assault [9173]
Advocates for Victims of Abuse in Langlade County,
   Inc. [10687]
Advocates for Victims of Assault--Frisco [8964]
Advocates for Victims of Assault--Silverthorne [8983]
Advocates for Victims of Violence [8675]
Advocates for Wellness LLC [49978]
AdvoSERV [7862]
AdvoSERVE, Carlton Palms [7898]
Aegis Battered Women's Program [9902]
Aegis Institute Inc [39626]
Aegis Medical Systems Inc [39614], [39627],
   [39698], [39778], [39805], [39842], [39928],
   [39938], [40208], [40213], [40225], [40317],
   [40337], [40363], [40399], [40770], [40801],
   [40822], [40941], [40958]
   La Mirada Methadone Treatment Program
      [39960]
   Roseville [40473]
   Santa Barbara [40724]
   Santa Maria Unit [40755]
Aeratech Home Medical, LLC [16988]
Aeschbach and Associates • DBA Addictions and
   Psychotherapy Services [49218]
Affable Home Care--New York, NY [16547]
Affable Home Care--Plantation, FL [14340]
Affable Home Healthcare Network [15800]
Affectionate Home Health Care, Inc.--Homewood
   [14822]
Affectionate Home Health Care--Oak Forest [14886]
Affiliate Speech Pathology Inc. [1061]
Affiliated Counseling Center LLC [50388]
Affiliated Home Dialysis--Elk Grove [23984]
Affiliated Home Dialysis, LLC--East Peoria [23980]
Affiliated Hospital Dialysis Center--West County • St.
   John's Mercy Health Care [25190]
Affiliated Sports Physicians • Family Medicine of
   South Bend [38447]
Affiliates for Consultation and Psychotherapy
   [41429]
Affinity Behavioral Health • Mercy Counseling
   Service [50499]
Affinity Counseling and Treatment [50092]
Affinity Health Services LLC [1978]
Affinity Home Care [15787]
Affinity Home Care Agency [15614]
Affinity Home Health [13444]
Affinity-Hospice of Life--Aurora [19085]
Affinity-Hospice of Life--Las Vegas [20412]
Affinity - Hospice of Life--Phoenix [18802]
Affinity Hospice of Life--Salt Lake City [21640]
Affinity-Hospice of Life--Southgate [20126]
Affinity Hospice Of Life--Bedford [19947]
Affinity Plus [18605]
Affinity Therapy [11058]
Affinity Visiting Nurses [18606]
Affirmation Counseling Services [50198]
Affordable Chiropractic • Pain Clinic [35300]
Affordable Nursing Services [14273]
Affordable Treatment Program • Lenexa [43391]

African American Family Services [9611], [45202],
   [45300]
After Care Home Health, Inc. [14874]
Against Abuse, Inc. • La Casa de Paz [8679]
Agape Christian Counseling [43431]
Agape Community Health Center--Jacksonville
   [6480]
Agape Community Health Center--Washington
   [7062]
Agape Counseling Center LLC [45348]
AGAPE Counseling Services [43535], [43773]
Agape Counseling Services [46032]
Agape Family Ministries [41763]
Agape Home Care services, LLC [18057]
Agape Hospice Care of Shreveport, LLC [19874]
Agape Hospice Group-Ruston [19873]
Agape Hospice Group-West Monroe [19881]
Agape Hospice Services [19111]
Agape House of Mountain View [9705]
Agape Inc [49100], [49101], [49102]
Agape Northwest Hospice Group-Minden [19862]
Agape Unlimited [49912]
Agassiz Associates PLLC [47579]
Agates Home Health Agency, Inc. [18040]
Agawam Counseling Center [30376]
Agency for Community Treatment Services
   Adult Addict Receiving Facility [41953]
   Adult Outpatient [41954]
   Drew Park Transitional Housing [41955]
   Juvenile Addict Receiving Fac [41956]
   Residential II/New Horizons Group Home
      [41809]
   Tarpon Springs Site [41976]
   Thonotosassa Youth Residential [41979]
Agility Center Sports Medicine [38061]
Aging Paradise, Inc. [14318]
AGM Home Health Care Inc. [13412]
Agnesian Healthcare • Central Wisconsin Cancer
   Program [6150]
Agnesian Healthcare-Hospice Home of Hope
   [21832]
Agnesian HealthCare, Inc. [18567]
Agnews Developmental Center [7818]
Agramonte Home Care Corporation [13901]
Ahava Care of Florida Corporation [13651]
Ahlbin Center [1449]
Ahlfeld Sports Medicine Orthopaedic Center [38431]
Ahni Health Services, Inc. [17122]
Ahoskie Dialysis • DaVita [25813]
AHRC Health Care Inc • Outpatient Chemical
   Dependency Program [46808]
Ahwatukee Sports & Spine [38041]
Al DuPont Hospital for Children • Pediatric
   Headache Program [12395]
AICS Dental Clinic [6219]
AID--Assistance Information Direction Center
   [50908]
AID Behavioral Health Services [42392]
Aid in Dover • Runaway and Homeless Youth
   Program [35868]
Aid to Victims of Domestic Abuse--Houston [10472]
Aid to Victims of Domestic Abuse, Inc.--Delray
   Beach [9047]
AIDB--Alabama School for the Deaf • Residential/
   Boarding/Day Programs [210]
AIDB--E.H. Gentry Facility • Residential/Boarding/
   Day Programs [211]
AIDB--Talladega Regional Center [209]
Aides at Home--Bay Shore [16345]
Aides at Home--Elmhurst [16442]
Aides at Home--Hempstead [16477]
Aides at Home, Inc.--Hicksville [16485]
Aides at Home--Patchogue [16587]
Aides at Home--Staten Island [16633]
Aiding Women in Abuse and Rape Emergencies,
   Inc. [8663]
AIDS Research Alliance: Chicago • Community
   Program for Clinical Research on AIDS [50]
AIDS Research Alliance, HIV Vaccine Trials Unit [78]
AIDS Research Consortium of Atlanta • Community
   Program for Clinical Research on AIDS [48]
Aiken--Barnwell Mental Health Center [51315]
Aiken Center [48899]
Aiken County Help Line, Inc. [51316]
Aiken Dialysis & At Home • DaVita [26674]
Aiken Treatment Specialists [48900]
AIM for the Handicapped Inc. [3235]
AIM Hospice [21547]

Aim Target Programs Inc [41660]
AIM for The Handicapped [8410]
Aim Therapy Inc. [1752]
Ain Dah Yung Shelter • Runaway and Homeless
   Youth Program [36029]
Air Force Village Home Health & Hospice [21550]
AirCare Medical Supply, Inc. [13413]
Airmid Counseling Services [45969]
Airport Dialysis • DaVita [22729]
AIRS/Empire Homes of Maryland • Runaway and
   Homeless Youth Program [35991]
Airway Breathing Company, Inc.--Chesapeake
   [18265]
Airway Breathing Company, Inc.--Hampton [18309]
Aitru Health Institute • Speech/Language Pathology
   [3205]
AKC of Deerfield Beach • DaVita [23286]
Akeela Inc • Akeela House [39303]
Akiak Native Community Suicide Prevention [50625]
Akron/Canton Kidney Center • Fresenius Medical
   Care [26221]
Akron Children's Hospital NeuroDevelopmental
   Center • Down Syndrome Clinic [10843]
Akron Children's Hospital - Ohio Region VI Sickle
   Cell Program [36409]
Akron Children's Hospital Sports Medicine Center •
   Center for Orthopedics and Sports Medicine
   [38848]
Akron City Hospital [16823]
   Hemodialysis Center [26001]
Akron Community Based Outpatient Clinic • Louis
   Stokes Cleveland VA Medical Center [4360]
Akron Community Health Resources, Inc. [7075]
Akron General Edwin Shaw Rehab Inst • The
   Dobkin Recovery Center [47735]
Akron General Hospital • Edwin Shaw Rehabilita-
   tion, LLC [4361]
Akron General Medical Center
   Cancer Program [5675]
   Sleep Disorders Center [37503]
Akron Public Schools [644]
Akron Urban Minority Alcohol/Drug Abuse •
   Outreach Prog Inc/Addiction Treatment Services
   [47601]
Akron Veterans Affairs Clinic [31642]
AKT Enterprise [14262]
Al Con Counseling [47335]
Al ta Counseling [50199]
Al Dupont Hospital for Children [1517]
Al Tech Services Inc • Drug/Alcohol Outpatient
   Treatment [42885]
Alabama Abuse Counseling Center [39213]
Alabama Clinical Schools [27843]
Alabama Department of Public Health • Child Death
   Review System [36444]
Alabama Eye Bank [34915]
Alabama Fertility Specialists [21883]
Alabama Institute for the Deaf and Blind •
   Birmingham Regional Center [186]
Alabama Institute for Deaf and Blind • Library and
   Resource Center for the Blind and Physically
   Handicapped [3745]
Alabama Institute for the Deaf and Blind • Talladega
   [212]
Alabama Organ Center [34916]
Alabama Orthopaedic and Sports Medicine Clinic
   [38009]
Alabama Orthopedics and Spine Center [37990]
Alabama Recovery Center [39258]
Alabama Regional Hospice Care [18767]
Alabama Regional Library for the Blind and Physi-
   cally Handicapped [3746]
Alabama School of the Deaf and the Blind • Dothan
   Regional Center [192]
Alabama School for the Deaf and Blind
   Huntsville Regional Center [196]
   Mobile Regional Center [200]
   Montgomery Regional Center [204]
   Shoals Regional Center [216]
   Tuscaloosa Regional Center [215]
Alachua County Crisis Center [50761]
Alakanuk Clinic [6205]
Alakanuk Suicide Prevention [50626]
Alamance Health Services • Speech Language
   Pathology Department [3160]
Alamance Regional Medical Center • Cancer Center
   [5629]
Alamance Regional Medical Center Inc • Behavioral

Medicine Div/Inpt Psych/CD [47233]
Alameda Community Support Center and Children's Outpatient Services [28365]
Alameda County Behavioral Health Care Services • Guidance Clinic [28784]
Alameda County Behavioral Health • Mental Health Division [28666]
Alameda County Health Care Services [6333]
Alameda County Medical Center [40289]
Alameda Family Services [28366], [35805], [39585]
Alameda Hospital [1050]
Alameda Unified School District [261]
Alamo Area Resource Center Inc • Positive Recovery [49511]
Alamo City Dialysis • Fresenius Medical Care [27313]
Alamo City Treatment Services [49512]
Alamo Hospice [21551]
Alamo Sleep Disorders Center [37799]
Alamo Tissue Service, Ltd. [35219]
Alamogordo Dialysis • Fresenius Medical Care • Dialysis Facility [25530]
Alamogordo Veterans Affairs Clinic [31180]
Alamosa Dialysis • DaVita [23087]
Alarys Home Health [12816]
Alaska Addiction Rehab Services • Nugens Ranch [39357]
Alaska Childrens Service Inc [39304]
Alaska Department of Health and Social Services - Family Health Section • Maternal Infant Mortality Review Project [36446]
Alaska Family Services [8676], [39358]
Alaska Family Services - Support Services [8670]
Alaska Human Services Inc/Outpatient • Alcohol/ Substance Abuse Treatment Prog [39305]
Alaska Island Community Services [28126]
    Church Street [6220]
    TideLine Clinic [6221]
Alaska Islands Community Services [39360]
Alaska Psychiatric Institute [33105]
Alaska Regional Hospital
    Cancer Center [4656]
    Neurology Center [34751]
Alaska Sleep Clinic--Anchorage • Sleep Disorders Center [36618]
Alaska Sleep Clinic--Fairbanks [36619]
Alaska Sleep Clinic--Soldotna [36620]
Alaska Sleep Clinic--Wasilla [36621]
Alaska Speech and Hearing Clinic [929]
Alaska Speech and Language Depot [930]
Alaska Sports Medicine Clinic [38016]
Alaska State Library • Talking Book Center [3749]
Alaska State School for the Deaf and Hard of Hear- ing • Anchorage [218]
Alaska VA Healthcare Sys/Reg Office • Social and Behavioral Health Service [39306]
Alaska VA Healthcare System and Regional Office [12737]
Alaska Veterans Affairs Health Care System
    Kenai Veterans Affairs Community Based Outpatient Clinic [28104]
    PTSD Clinical Team Outpatient [51683]
Alaska Veterans Affairs Healthcare System [51531]
Alaska Veterans Affairs Healthcare System & Regional Office [28070]
Alaska Youth & Parent Foundation [33958]
Alaska Youth and Parent Foundation • Runaway and Homeless Youth Program [35785]
Alaskan Aquatic Therapy Inc. [38024]
Alatna Health Clinic [6206]
Albany Addiction Associates • DBA Private Clinic Albany [42017]
Albany Area Community Service Board--Albany [29327]
Albany Area Community Service Board
    Early County Mental Health Center [29369]
    Early-Miller Mental Retardation Service Center [29370]
Albany Area Hospice [20138]
Albany Citizens Council on Alcohol and Other Chem Dep Inc • Supportive Living [46327]
The Albany Clinic [27894]
Albany Community Hospice [19339]
Albany County Crime Victim and Sexual Violence Center [9891]
Albany County Mental Health Center [31223]
Albany County Substance Abuse Clinic • CD Outpatient [46328]

Albany Dialysis Center [25566]
Albany Medical Center
    Cancer Center [5555]
    Children's Hospital • Comprehensive Sickle Cell Treatment Center [36388]
Albany Medical Center Hospital
    Department of Pediatrics • Division of Clinical Genetics [12281]
    MDA Clinic [34832]
Albany Medical College
    Adult Cystic Fibrosis Center [7610]
    Center for Multiple Sclerosis [34641]
    Pediatric Pulmonary and Cystic Fibrosis Center [7611]
    Regional Comprehensive Hemophilia and von Willebrand Treatment Center [12560]
Albany Regional Kidney Center [25567]
Albany Veterans Affairs Medical Center [31224]
Albemarle Adult Activity Center--Chowan County [31529]
Albemarle Hopeline [10035]
Albemarle Hospice [20652]
Albemarle Mental Health Center--Camden [31513]
Albemarle Mental Health Center • Currituck Unit [31535]
Albemarle Mental Health Center--Manteo [31558]
Albemarle Mental Health Center • Martin County Office • Early Intervention Program [31610]
Albemarle Mental Health Center--Nags Head [31568]
Albemarle Mental Health Center--Plymouth [31579]
Albemarle Mental Health Center--Swan Quarter [31596]
Albert Einstein College of Medicine
    Centers for AIDS Research [59]
    Div of SA/Wellness Center at Port Morris [46396]
    Div of Substance Abuse/Med Maint Prog [46397]
    Division of Subst Abuse/Melrose Clinic [46398]
    Division of Substance Abuse [46399]
    Division of Substance Abuse/Melrose 9 [46400]
    DOSA Next Steps Chem Dep Services South [46401]
    Next Steps Wellness Center [46402]
Albert Einstein Medical Center [5850], [17403]
    Transplant/Dialysis Center [26501]
Albert Gallatin Home Care and Hospice Services-- Butler [21062]
Albert Gallatin Home Care and Hospice Services-- Canonsburg [21066]
Albert Gallatin Home Care and Hospice Services-- Masontown • Amedisys Home Health Services [21112]
Albert Gallatin Home Care and Hospice Services-- Monogahela • Amedisys Home Health Services [21114]
Albert Gallatin Home Care and Hospice Services-- Scottdale • Amedisys Home Health Services [21153]
Albert Gallatin Home Care and Hospice--Uniontown [21165]
Albert Galvan Health Clinic [7290]
Albert Lea Medical Center-Mayo Health System [15889]
Albert O Nichols House [46693]
Albert Pujols Wellness Center • Adults with Down Syndrome [10819]
Alberta Children's Hospital Burn Unit [4505]
Alberta Children's Hospital • Calgary Eating Disorder Program [10885]
Alberta School for the Deaf [224]
Albertina Kerr Centers [31954]
Albertville Nursing Home [27819]
Albia Health Center [6701]
Albion Fellows Bacon Center, Inc. [9273]
Albuquerque Dialysis • Dialysis Clinic Inc. [25531]
Albuquerque Family Health Centers, Inc. [6989]
Albuquerque Girls Community Residential Center [34304]
Albuquerque Healthcare • For the Homeless Inc/ Behavioral Health [46227]
Albuquerque Kidney Center • Fresenius Medical Care [25532]
Albuquerque Speech, Language, Hearing Center [2960]
Alburg Health Center [7330]
Alc and Drug Council of Tompkins Cnty • Outpatient

Clinic [46717]
Alcala Counseling Services [43462]
Alchemy [29471]
Alcocare Inc • The River Commons [50416]
Alcohol and Addictions Outpatient Center [42914]
Alcohol/Behavior Information [40986], [41092], [41259]
Alcohol and Chemical Abuse Consultants (ACAC), Inc [44802], [44934]
Alcohol/Chemical Evaluation Services • DBA ACES Ltd [42610]
Alcohol Counseling and • Guidance Services LLC [41172]
Alcohol Drug Abuse Center [39983]
Alcohol/Drug Abuse Council
    Concho Valley/Outpatient [49505]
    Concho Valley/Saras House [49506]
    Concho Valley/Williams House [49507]
Alcohol and Drug Abuse Council of Deep • East Texas [49469]
Alcohol and Drug Abuse Education • Prevention and Treatment/The Horizons [44322]
Alcohol and Drug Abuse Program [44104]
Alcohol and Drug Abuse Services Inc [48355], [48616], [48617]
    Bradford Unit [48301]
    Kane Unit [48421]
    Saint Marys Unit [48634]
Alcohol and Drug Abuse • Treatment Centers Inc/ Pearson Hall [39215]
Alcohol and Drug Care Services Inc [39816]
    Bonnie Brown Program [39817]
    J Street Program [39818]
    Lee Brown Program [39819]
Alcohol Drug Council • High Gain Project [40765]
Alcohol Drug Dependency Service • Ellensburg [49943]
Alcohol Drug Dependency Services [50022]
Alcohol and Drug Dependency Services
    Casa Di Vita Community Residence [46544]
    CD Inpatient Rehabilitation Unit [46545]
    Drug Abuse Inpatient Unit/Youth/LT Boy [47177]
    Family Addiction Outpatient Clinic [46546]
Alcohol and Drug Dependency Services Inc [46547]
Alcohol and Drug Dependency Services
    Ivy House Community Residence [46548]
    Renaissance House [47178]
Alcohol and Drug Dependency Services of Southeast Iowa [43240], [43284], [43290], [43310]
Alcohol and Drug Dependency Services
    Stepping Stones [47179]
    Supportive Living [46549]
Alcohol and Drug Education Clinic Inc [42881]
Alcohol/Drug Evaluations and Treatment [42882]
Alcohol and Drug Freedom Center of • Knox County [47822]
Alcohol and Drug Intervention Inc [44281]
Alcohol and Drug Professionals of Fulton County [42853]
Alcohol and Drug Professionals of • Fulton County [42434]
Alcohol and Drug Recov Centers Inc
    Alternate Living Center [41392]
    Coventry House Pregnant Womens Program [41393]
    Detoxification Center [41394]
    Latino Outpatient [41395]
    Outpatient Counseling Center [41396]
    Residential Program/Intensive [41397]
    Residential Program/Intermediate [41398]
Alcohol and Drug Recovery [44095], [44263], [44282], [44378]
Alcohol and Drug Services [47205], [47234]
    ADS East [47336]
    ADS West [47385]
Alcohol and Drug Services of
    Gallatin County [45688]
    Guernsey County [47632]
Alcohol and Drug Services of the • Fairfax Falls Church Comm Services Board [49779]
Alcohol and Drug Services of Tulare • Alternative Services [40410]
Alcohol and Drug Unit [43852]
Alcohol Education and Counseling Services [43676]
Alcohol Information and Counseling Center • Lapeer County Health Department [44894]
Alcohol Safety Action Project • Kansas [43374]
Alcohol Services Center Inc [45385]

Alcohol Services Inc • Alcoholism Outpatient Clinic [46773]
Alcohol Services of Kentucky [43590]
Alcohol and Substance Abuse Programs [39587]
Alcoholic Recovery Center [49204]
Alcoholic Rehab Community Home [42690]
Alcoholic Rehab Services of Hawaii Inc
    DBA Hina Mauka Adult Continuum [42242]
    Hina Mauka/IHS [42203]
    Hina Mauka/Waipahu Site [42297]
Alcoholic Services of Texoma Inc • House of Hope [49537]
Alcoholics Home Inc • House of Prayer [47398]
Alcoholics Resocialization Counseling
    Help (ARCH) Inc [45782]
    Help (ARCH) Inc/OHanlon House [45783]
Alcoholism Center for Women Inc
    Miracle House Residential [40055]
    Outpatient Services [40056]
Alcoholism Council of Cincinnati Area
    Mount Airy Shelter [47648]
    NCADD Outpatient [47649]
    Womens Program [47650]
Alcoholism Council of Cochise County • Verhelst Recovery House [39365]
Alcoholism Intervention Services [42308]
Alcon Research Ltd. [35220]
Alcona Health Center--Alpena Services [6832]
Alcott Center for Cognitive Enhancement LLC [2638]
Alcott Center for Mental Health Services [28578]
The Alcove, Inc. [29476]
The Alcove • Runaway and Homeless Youth Program [35905]
Aldea Children and Family Services [7795]
Aldea Children and Family Services--Napa [33164]
Aldea Children and Family Services • Supported Living Program [33165]
Aldea Children and Family Services--Vallejo [33205]
Aldea Children and Family Services • Wolfe Center [33166]
Alderman Speech Pathology Services LLC [2368]
Alderwood Recovery LLC [50027]
Aldie Counseling Center [48339], [48435]
Aleda E. Lutz VA Medical Ctr. [15792]
Aleda E. Lutz Veterans Affairs Medical Center [51590]
    Oscoda Clinic [30616]
    PTSD Clinical Team [51756]
Aleda E. Lutz Veterans Affairs Medical Center--Saginaw [30627]
Aledo Kidney Center, LLC [23890]
Alegent Health Behavioral Services [29848]
Alegent Health Bergan Mercy Health Center Health at Home [16117]
Alegent Health Bergan Mercy Medical Center • Bergan Mercy Cancer Center [5479]
Alegent Health Hospice [20396]
Alegent Health Immanuel Medical Center • Immanuel Cancer Center [5480]
Alegent Health Immanuel Rehabilitation Center [4259]
Alegent Health
    Immanuel Rehabilitation Center [8226]
    Immanuel Sleep Disorders Center [37308]
Alegent Health Lakeside Hospital • Midwest Cancer Center [5481]
Alegent Health • Lakeside Hospital Sleep Disorders Center [37309]
Alegent Health Mercy Hospital
    Cancer Center [5183]
    Mercy Sleep Disorders Center [36973]
Alegent Health Midlands Community Center • Sleep Disorders Center [37310]
Alegent Health Midlands Community Hospital • Cancer Program [5485]
Alegent Health Psychiatric Associates [45727]
    Immanuel Clinic [45784]
Alegre's Home Health Care, Inc. [13720]
Alera Health, LLC [16896]
Alere Women's and Children's Health--Albany, NY [16332]
Alere Women's and Children's Health--Chanhassen, MN [15893]
Alere Women's and Children's Health--Charlotte, NC [16706]
Alere Women's and Children's Health--Clearwater, FL [13614]

Alere Women's and Children's Health--Creve Coeur, MO [16004]
Alere Women's and Children's Health--Des Plaines, IL [14764]
Alere Women's and Children's Health--Harahan, LA [15299]
Alere Women's and Children's Health--Indianapolis, IN [14992]
Alere Women's and Children's Health--Lenexa, KS [15139]
Alere Women's and Children's Health, LLC--Broken Arrow, OK [17106]
Alere Women's and Children's Health, LLC--Chattanooga, TN [17649]
Alere Women's and Children's Health, LLC--Columbia, SC [17570]
Alere Women's and Children's Health LLC--Concord, CA [12952]
Alere Women's and Children's Health, LLC--Dallas, TX [17858]
Alere Women's and Children's Health, LLC--Fort Lauderdale, FL [13688]
Alere Women's and Children's Health, LLC--Greenville, SC [17592]
Alere Women's and Children's Health, LLC--Houston, TX [17951]
Alere Women's and Children's Health LLC--Irvine, CA [13081]
Alere Women's and Children's Health, LLC--Knoxville, TN [17697]
Alere Women's and Children's Health, LLC--Memphis, TN [17731]
Alere Women's and Children's Health, LLC--Nashville, TN [17751]
Alere Women's and Children's Health, LLC--Plymouth Meeting, PA [17452]
Alere Women's and Children's Health, LLC--Richmond, VA [18359]
Alere Women's and Children's Health, LLC--Round Rock, TX [18127]
Alere Women's and Children's Health LLC--Scottsdale, AZ [12817]
Alere Women's and Children's Health LLC--Washington, DC [13570]
Alere Women's and Children's Health--Marietta, GA [14547]
Alere Women's and Children's Health--Nashua, NH [16176]
Alere Women's and Children's Health--Omaha, NE [16118]
Alere Women's and Children's Health--Orange Park, FL [14288]
Alere Women's and Children's Health--Ridgeland, MS [15978]
Alere Women's and Children's Health--Sunrise, FL [14393]
Alere Women's and Children's Health--Towson, MD [15466]
Alere Women's and Children's Health--Westbury, NY [16661]
Alere Women's and Children's Health--Whitestone, NY [16676]
Alere Women's and Children's Health--Woodbridge, NJ [16296]
Alert Respiratory Services [14251]
Aletheia House [39216]
    Women Only [39217]
Alexa Home Health Care [13902]
Alexander Center [2690]
Alexander Cohen Hospice House [18942]
Alexander G. Bell Montessori and AEHI [415]
Alexander Group Home [31597]
Alexander Hearing Services [1338]
Alexander Human Development Center [7752]
Alexander Infusion, LLC [16538]
Alexander Nininger State Veterans Nursing Home [14319]
Alexander Opportunities [31598]
Alexander PSR Program [31599]
Alexander Youth Network [34362]
Alexander Youth Network--Charlotte [31516]
Alexander Youth Network, Charlotte • Runaway and Homeless Youth Services [36128]
Alexander Youth Network • Children and Family Services Center [31517]
Alexander Youth Network--Lenoir Regional Office [31555]

Alexander Youth Nerwork--The Relatives, Inc. [51161]
Alexander Zubenko and Associates [42751]
Alexandra House, Inc. [9585]
Alexandra Marine and General Hospital of Goderich--Clinton • Eating Disorders Outreach Program [11204]
Alexandra Marine and General Hospital of Goderich • Eating Disorders Outreach Program for Youth [11205]
Alexandra Marine and General Hospital of Goderich--Exeter • Eating Disorder Outreach Program for Youth [11206]
Alexandra Marine and General Hospital of Goderich--Goderich • Eating Disorder Program [11207]
Alexandra Marine and General Hospital of Goderich--Wingham • Youth Eating Disorders Program [11208]
Alexandria Community Services Board [32694]
    Substance Abuse Services [49754]
Alexandria Detention Center [32695]
Alexandria Domestic Violence Program [10552]
Alexandria Health Department • Casey Health Center [7344]
Alexandria Kidney Center • Fresenius Medical Care [27451]
Alexandria Library-Beatley Central • Talking Book Service [3843]
Alexandria Mental Health Center • Community Support Program [32696]
Alexandria Orthopaedic Associates PA [38612]
Alexandria VA Medical Center • Chemical Dependency Program [43882]
Alexandria Veterans Affairs Medical Center [30169]
    Multiple Sclerosis Center [34587]
Alexandria Wellness Center [30125]
Alexian Brothers Behavioral Health Hospital [33421]
Alexian Brothers • Behavioral Health Hospital [42709]
Alexian Brothers Behavioral Health Hospital • Center for Eating Disorders [11043]
Alexian Brothers • Bonaventure House [42465]
Alexian Brothers Home Health [14810]
Alexian Brothers Hospice [19527]
Alexian Brothers Medical Center [14777]
Alexian Brother's Medical Center • Cancer Program [5090]
Alexian Brothers Medical Center • Sleep Health Center [36893]
Alexian Center for Mental Health [29560]
Alexian Health Clinic [40652]
Alexis Dialysis Center • Innovative Dialysis Centers [26208]
Alfred F. Zampella Public School 27 [547]
Alfred I. DuPont Hospital for Children • Cystic Fibrosis Center [7495]
Alfred I. DuPont Hospital for Children's Dialysis Center • Transplant/Dialysis Center [23202]
Alfred I. DuPont Institute • Department of Medical Genetics [12175]
Algen Health and Dialysis at Home [17952]
Algonac Community Counseling Center [44629]
Algonquins Road Elementary School [2038]
Alhambra Community Dialysis Unit [22581]
Alhambra Deaf and Hard of Hearing Program [262]
Alhambra Dialysis Center • DaVita [22914]
Alhambra Hospital [33176]
Alianza Dominicana Inc • CREO Program/DF Outpatient [46809]
Alianza of New Mexico [46298]
Alice Counseling Center [49202]
Alice G. Ransdell Community Mental Health Center [30027]
Alice Logan Home • JBS Mental Health Authority [27844]
Alice Paul House [10284]
Alice Renal Center • Diversified Specialty Institutes [26933]
Alice's Place, an Empowerment Center [8743]
Alicia Roberts Medical Center [6213]
Aliton's Pharmacy Home Healthcare Centers [16598]
Alive Hospice, Inc. [21356]
Alive Hospice - Murfreesboro Office [21354]
Alive Hospice at St. Thomas Hospital [21357]
ALIVE, Inc. [10173]
Aliviane NO/AD Inc [49317]

Aliviane Family Recovery Center [49318]
Alpine Outpatient Clinic [49203]
Inner Resources Recovery Center/Men [49319]
Methadone Clinic [49320]
Outpatient Clinic/Adults [49321]
Van Horn Outpatient Clinic [49567]
Alivio Medical Center [6651]
All 1 Star Home Health Care, Inc. [13903]
All 4 Home Care, LLC [16824]
All 4 Kids Therapy Services [1141]
All Aboard Therapy of the Treasure Coast [1787]
All About Care, LLC [18360]
All About Choices LLC [49881]
All About Healthcare, LLC [13715]
All About Recovery [49360], [49477]
All About You Home Health Agency [13586]
All-Access Home Health, Inc. [13016]
All American Health Care, Inc. [13017]
All Around Home Health Agency [13904]
All At Home Health Care [12818]
All Brothers Inc. [13721]
All Care Enterprises Inc. [13014]
All Care Health Services of Miami Corporation
   [13905]
All Care Home Care, Inc. [17338]
All Care Home Health, Alhambra [13273]
All Care Home Health Provider [13018]
All Caring Health Provider [16144]
All Children's Hospital • Clinical Genetics [12180]
All Children's Hospital - Cystic Fibrosis Center
   [7498]
All Children's Hospital Dialysis • Dialysis Center
   [23502]
All Children's Hospital
   Hemophilia Treatment Center [12502]
   Sickle Cell Disease Center [36317]
All Children's Therapy [3150]
All County Home Care, LLC [17829]
All Florida Home Health Services [13906]
All For Kids Pediatric Therapy [931]
All by Grace Home Health Care, inc. [17859]
All Health Medical Equipment, Inc. [15444]
All--Med Services of Florida, Jupiter [13824]
All--Med Services of Florida, Orlando [14289]
All N One Home Health Agency [12801]
All Nursing Home Health Services, Inc. [17953]
All Saint's Healthcare System, Inc. • SE Wisconsin
   Regional Cancer Center [6173]
All Smiles Home Health [12989]
All Solutions Healthcare, Inc. [14778]
All Speech and Language Inc. [3356]
All Star Home Health Care Corporation [14907]
All Types Counseling Services LLC [42673], [42844]
All--Ways Home Care [13907]
All for You Counseling [50200]
Allan D Wright Addiction Counselor [45938]
AllCare Medical [16264]
ALLCARE Therapy Services [2921]
Alle--Kiski Area HOPE Center [10317]
Alle-Kiski Medical Center/Allegheny Valley Hospital •
   Cancer Program [5845]
Alleanza Health Care Associates [13908]
Allegan County Community Mental Health Services
   [30499]
Allegan General Hospital Home Care [15570]
Allegany Co Health Dept Addictions Ser • Lois E
   Jackson Unit [44236]
Allegany Council on Alcohol/Subst Abuse
   Allegany Council CD Outpatient Clinic [47170]
   Trapping Brook House/Prevention [47171]
   Trapping Brook House Supportive Living [47172]
Allegany County Addictions Services
   Alcohol and Drug Outpatient [44237]
   Joseph S Massie Unit [44238]
Allegany County Health Department • Intensive
   Outpatient Addictions Prog [44239]
Allegany Rehabilitation Associates Inc • Wyoming
   Cnty Chem Abuse Treatment Prog [47161]
Alleghany Highlands Community Services • Guinan
   Center [49777]
Alleghenies United Cerebral Palsy [8467]
Allegheny General Hospital Cancer Center [4701]
Allegheny General Hospital Home Care [17431]
Allegheny General Hospital • Sleep Disorders
   Center [37636]
Allegheny General Hospital - Transplant Services
   [26542]
Allegheny House [34421]

Allegheny Intermediate Unit Number 3 [702]
Allegheny Neurological Associates • ALS Center
   [141]
Allegheny University • Multiple Sclerosis Treatment
   Center [34686]
Allegheny Valley Dialysis Center • Davita [26490]
Allegheny Valley School [8454]
Allegiance Addiction Recover Center [44860]
Allegiance Health [30577]
   Cancer Center [5381]
Allegiance Health Home Care [15700]
Allegiance Home Health Care Services [15859]
Allegiance Home Health, Inc. [12888]
Allegiance Hospice Care Agency [18797]
Allegiance Hospice Group, Inc. [19973]
Allegiance Hospice Home [20074]
Allegiance Substance Abuse Services • (formerly
   Bridgeway Center of Foote Hospital) [44861]
Allen Care, Inc. [17954]
Allen County Community • Corrections Day Report-
   ing Center [43041]
Allen County Health Partners [7090]
Allen County Hospice • Allen County Hospital
   [19758]
Allen County Hospital Home Health [15130]
Allen Health Care Services--Hempstead [16478]
Allen HealthCare Services--Jamaica [16496]
Allen Hospital [15109]
Allen Memorial Hospital Satellite • Grundy County
   Public Health [15085]
Allen Mental Health Center [30167]
Allen Parish Hospital • Recovery Unit [43835]
Allen Sports and Spine Care [39043]
Allen Women's Resource Center [9933]
Allendale Association [34112]
   Bradley Outpatient Clinic [34113]
Allendale County Dialysis • DaVita [26709]
Allentown State Hospital [33794]
Allentown Veterans Affairs Outpatient Clinic [17232]
Allergy Alliance of the Permian Basin • Pediatric
   Cystic Fibrosis Center [7668]
Alleve Hospice [20951]
Alliance [30256]
Alliance Against Domestic Abuse [8982]
Alliance Against Family Violence--Bakersfield [8791]
Alliance Against Family Violence--Leavenworth
   [9368]
Alliance Against Violence and Abuse, Inc. [9535]
Alliance Area Domestic Violence Shelter [10121]
Alliance Behavioral Services Inc [42466]
Alliance Clinic [45203]
Alliance Clinical Services [49593]
Alliance for Community Care [28773]
Alliance Community Hospital • Cancer Program
   [5678]
Alliance Consultants [46055]
Alliance Counseling Associates [43604], [45433],
   [45441]
Alliance Counseling Center • Eating Disorder
   Program [11247]
Alliance Family Services Inc [42321], [42328],
   [42351], [42371], [42373]
Alliance Family Services Inc/North [42374]
Alliance for Health [16372]
Alliance Health Center [30791]
   DBA Laurel Wood Center Inc [45403]
Alliance Home Care Services, Inc. [15801]
Alliance Home Health Services [13019], [15703]
Alliance Hospice [19356], [21267]
Alliance Hospice-Woodbury [20513]
Alliance House [32617]
Alliance House Social Club [31342]
Alliance Inc • MISA Day Program [44105]
Alliance, Inc.--Aberdeen [30253]
Alliance, Inc.--Bel Air [30266]
Alliance, Inc.--Belcamp [30267]
Alliance, Inc.--Dundalk [30280]
Alliance, Inc.--Howard County [30276]
Alliance Institute for the • Treatment of Chemical
   Dependency [42748]
Alliance Medical Center--Windsor [6379]
Alliance Medical Services Inc
   Ensign II [48582]
   Johnstown [48415]
   Pittsburgh [48583]
Alliance Orthopaedics & Sports Medicine [38318]
Alliance Recovery Center [42076]
Alliance Recovery Center Conyers [42062]

Alliance Treatment Center [41426]
Alliance Veterans Affairs Clinic [30971]
Alliance Visiting Nurse Association & Hospice
   [16835]
Alliant Health Systems, Inc. [13440]
Allied Behavioral Management Inc [47512]
Allied Counseling Group [44315]
   Drug and Alcohol Treatment [44264]
Allied Counseling Resources Ltd [42414], [42641]
Allied Drug and Alcohol • Treatment Center [40861]
Allied Foot Clinic [38177]
Allied Health Care Services [16251]
Allied Health Professionals [2048]
Allied Health Services Beaverton [48072]
Allied Health Services East [48178]
Allied Health Services, Inc. [16352]
Allied Medical [18442]
Allied Preferred Care [17860]
Allied Professionals Health Care, LLC [14803]
Allied Services Health Care Services [17284]
Allied Services Home Health [17503]
Allied Services Institute of Rehabilitation Medicine •
   Spinal Cord Injury Services [4384]
Allied Services Speech and Audiology Department
   [3377]
AlliedCare Home Health of Illinois, Inc. [14765]
Allina Homecare, Hospice & Palliative Care--
   Homestead House [20190]
Allina Homecare, Hospice and Palliative Care-New
   Ulm [20183]
Allina Hospice and Palliative Care [20206]
Allina Medical Clinic [2683]
Allograft Innovations LLC [34980]
Allosource--Buffalo [35125]
AlloSource--California [34932]
Allosource--Chicago [35020]
AlloSource--Colorado [34970]
Allosource--Minneapolis [35080]
Allosource--Ohio [35154]
Allosource--Saint Louis [35090]
Allosource--San Diego [34933]
Allotech LLC [35221]
Allstate Home Health Services [16145]
Alltime Home Health Providers [16146]
Almity International Home Health [12946]
Almond Healthcare Services [17796]
Aloha Home Health services, Inc. [13722]
Aloha House Inc
   Adult Residential Treatment [42269]
   IOP/OP For Lanai [42263]
   Outpatient Services. [42293]
Aloha Medical Supplies and Services, Inc. [14634]
Aloha Respiratory Services [14609]
Alpar Human Development Services • Alcohol
   Outpatient Treatment [41093]
Alpena Dialysis Services [24828]
Alpena General Hospital
   Cancer Center [5364]
   Rehabilitation/Speech Pathology Services [2551]
Alpena Regional Medical Center Home Care [15574]
Alpenglow Hospice, Inc. [19047]
ALPHA Audiology Hearing Health Services Inc.
   [1710]
ALPHA Center [48907]
Alpha Center [48915]
Alpha Center Psychological Services [41205]
Alpha Center for Treatment Inc [49907], [50018]
Alpha Cord Inc. [35009]
Alpha Counseling Center Inc [42800]
ALPHA Counseling and DWI Services [47449]
Alpha Home Health Agency [13909]
Alpha Home Health Solutions [14290]
Alpha Home Healthcare [15627]
Alpha Home Healthcare Services, Inc.--Canton
   [15600]
Alpha Home Healthcare Services--Taylor [15844]
Alpha Home Inc [49513]
   Residential/Outpatient [49514], [49515]
Alpha Homecare and Therapy Agency [13879]
Alpha House Inc [48584]
Alpha II Inc [48030]
Alpha Neurology PC • Comprehensive Multiple
   Sclerosis Center of Staten Island [34642]
Alpha Omega Home Health Care [17821]
Alpha-Omega Hospice [21457]
Alpha Plus Home Health Services [13104]
Alpha Project • Casa Raphael [40925]
Alpha Project for the Homeless [40926]

Alpha Recovery Centers Inc [42026]
Alpha Recovery LLC • Lawrence [43385]
Alpha Rehabilitation [2846]
Alpha Resources Inc [43083], [43084], [43085]
Alpha School Center/Progressive Living • Chemical Dependency Outpatient Program [46470]
AlphaSleep Diagnostic Centers--Aurora [36719]
AlphaSleep Diagnostic Centers--Lone Tree [36720]
AlphaSleep Diagnostic Centers--Thornton [36721]
Alphonsa Home Health Care, Inc. [14783]
Alpine Center Counseling and Recovery [39659]
Alpine Center for Personal Growth • Substance Abuse Outpatient Treatment [49678]
Alpine Clinic [38708]
Alpine Counseling Center [43131]
Alpine County • Behavioral Health Services [40203]
Alpine Family Medicine [6284]
Alpine Hospice-Brigham City [21599]
Alpine Hospice-Heber [21607]
Alpine Hospice - Logan [21633]
Alpine Hospice--Murray [21619]
Alpine Hospice - Orem [21631]
Alpine Orthopaedics and Sports [38175]
Alpine Recovery Services Inc [49879], [50010]
Alpine Springs Counseling PC [41082], [41160], [41162]
Alpine Treatment • Chateau [49632]
Alsip Dialysis Center • Fresenius Medical Care [23891]
ALSO--Cornerstone, Inc.
    Dwight House [29020]
    Orange Street, New Haven [29021]
    West Village [29022]
Alsobrook Counseling Center [50624]
Alta Bates Adult Sickle Cell Disease Center [36292]
Alta Bates In Vitro Fertilization Program [21906]
Alta Bates Medical Center
    Acute Rehabilitation Program [3887]
    Alta Bates Campus [3888]
Alta Bates Medical Center, Ashby Ave. • Behavioral Health [28409]
Alta Bates Medical Center, Dwight Way • Behavioral Health [28410]
Alta Bates Medical Center
    Small Voice Program [7764]
    Summit Campus [3889]
Alta Bates Summit Medical Center
    Center for Anorexia and Blumia at Herrick [10926]
    Comprehensive Cancer Program [4813]
Alta California Regional Center • Down Syndrome Clinic [10774]
Alta Institute Inc • Chemical Dependency Intervention Prog [39872]
Alta Mira Recovery [10927]
Alta Services [42309]
Alta View Hospital • Cancer Program [6045]
Alta View Sports Medicine Center [39110]
Alta Vista Healthcare, LP [35681]
AltaMed Health Services • Boyle Heights Zonal [40057]
AltaMed Health Services Corp. [6312]
AltaPointe Health Systems Inc • AltaPointe Medication Assisted Treatment [39270]
AltaPointe Health Systems, Inc.- BayPointe [27976]
AltaPointe Health Systems, Inc.--Mobile [27977]
AltaPointe Health Systems, Inc. • Washington County Mental Health [27884]
Altavista Group Home [32701]
Alterna-Care, Inc.--Springfield [14941]
Alterna--Care, Jacksonville [14826]
Alterna--Care, Litchfield [14842]
Alternacare--Muskogee [17132]
Alternate Family Care, Inc. [34084]
Alternate Family Care Inc.
    Jupiter Office [33311]
    Melbourne Office [33317]
Alternate Staffing, Inc. [16373]
Alternative Action Program [40338]
Alternative Behavior Consultation [42467]
Alternative Behavior Consultations Inc [42468]
Alternative Behavior Treatment Centers [34116]
Alternative Behavioral Care [45634]
    Eating Disorders Program [11116]
Alternative Behaviors Counseling Inc [41232]
Alternative Care Providers Inc. [15528]
Alternative Care Treatment Systems [47303]
Alternative Center for Behavioral Hlth [49322]

Alternative Counseling Associates [48619]
Alternative Counseling
    Edmonds [49939]
    Kent [49981]
Alternative Counseling Service [39379]
Alternative Counseling Service Inc [39476]
Alternative Counseling • Spanaway [50160]
Alternative Drug and Alcohol • Counseling ADAC [44290], [44308]
Alternative Family Care Inc. [33323]
Alternative Healthcare Inc. of South Florida [13910]
Alternative Home Care [13343]
Alternative Horizons [8958]
Alternative Hospice [20297]
Alternative House [9488]
    Runaway and Homeless Youth Program [36242]
Alternative Integrated Methods Health • Services/ AIM Health Services [47283]
Alternative Medical Healthcare Services [13911]
Alternative Opportunites Inc [39558], [39561]
Alternative Opportunities Inc • Carol Jones Recovery Center [45643]
Alternative Options Counseling Center Inc [39697], [40391]
Alternative Outpatient Services [43841]
Alternative Paths, Inc. [31805], [51226]
Alternative Services Inc [40862], [40918]
Alternative Sleep Disorders Center [36894]
Alternative • Soul Sobriety [41764]
Alternative Treatment International Inc [41589]
Alternative Youth Care [45704]
Alternatives [45644]
Alternatives for Battered Women [9981]
Alternatives in Behavioral Health Inc [41739]
Alternatives for Better Living [40252]
Alternatives Counseling Outpatient Service [47018]
Alternatives to Dependency [44260], [44369]
Alternatives to Domestic Violence--Hackensack [9828]
Alternatives to Domestic Violence--Riverside [8876]
Alternatives to Domestic Violence--Streator [9252]
Alternatives East End Counseling Proj • Alternatives Counseling/DF Outpatient [47086]
Alternatives for Girls • Runaway and Homeless Youth Program [36006]
Alternatives Inc [42469], [50093]
Alternatives Inc. of Madison County--Anderson [9262]
Alternatives Inc. of Madison County--Greenfield [9279]
Alternatives to Living In Violent Environments--Saint Louis [9715]
Alternatives to Living in Violent Environments-- Yerington [9803]
Alternatives Professional Counseling [50037], [50038]
Alternatives in Treatment Inc [41563]
Alternatives to Violence [9878]
Alternatives to Violence, Inc.--Loveland [8976]
Alternatives to Violence of the Palouse, Inc.-- Moscow [9180]
Alternatives to Violence of the Palouse--Pullman [10638]
Altheimer Clinic [6256]
Altimate Care LLC [16897]
Alton Dialysis • DaVita [23892]
Alton Memorial Hospital • Cancer Program [5057]
Alton Mental Health Center [33404]
Altona Brown Clinic [6216]
Altoona Center [8449]
Altoona Community Health Center [7152]
Altoona Hospital • Cancer Program [5812]
Altoona Hospital Center for Mental Health Services [51271]
Altoona Regional Health System • Dialysis Center [26368]
Altoona Regional Mental Health and • Drug and Alcohol Services [48272]
ALTR of Jackson LLC [45386]
Altru Clinic and Home Services [16808]
Altru Dialysis Satellite • Mercy Hospital [25988]
Altru Health Institute • Pediatric Therapy Services [8393]
Altru Health System
    Cancer Center [5673]
    Rehabilitation Center [35598]
    Sports Medicine Department [38844]

Altru Home Services/First Care Health Center [16821]
Altru Home Services--Karlstad [15908]
Altru Home Services-McVille [20789]
Altru Home Services--North Valley [15947]
Altru Home Services and Outreach Therapy--Nelson County [16819]
Altru Home Services-Park River [20791]
Altru Home Services of Unity Medical Center - Grafton [20781]
Altru Hospice-Cavalier [20777]
Altru Hospice--Grand Forks [20782]
Altru Hospice--Warren [20215]
Altru Hospital • Renal Dialysis Center [25994]
Altru Rehabilitation Center • Audiology and Hearing Aid Center [3206]
Altruist Home Health Care, Inc. [17861]
Altu Clinic Family Medical [16814]
Altus Healthcare and Hospice, Inc. [19346]
Altus Home Health Services, LLC [13801]
Alvarado Hospital and Medical Center [1255]
    Cancer Program [4833]
Alvarado Parkway Institute Behavioral Health System [33151]
Alvarado Parkway Institute • Behavioral Health System [28547]
Alvarado Parkway Institute BHS [39957]
Alvin C. York Veterans Affairs Medical Center [17745]
Alvin Dialysis Center • Fresenius Medical Care [26936]
Always Health Services, Inc. [17862]
Always Hope Adult Homecare [14232]
Always There Home Health Services [16135]
Always There Respiratory Home Care, Inc. [16634]
Ama Doo Alchini Bighan, Inc. [8683]
Amalthea Home Health Agency, Corp. [13723]
Amanecer Home Care Services, Inc. [13724]
Amanecer Inc [42443]
Amarillo Council on Alcoholism and • Drug Abuse [49205]
Amarillo Kidney Specialists, LLC [26937]
Amarillo Regional Education Program for the Deaf [765]
Amarillo VA Healthcare System [49206]
Amarillo Veterans Affairs Health Care System [17790]
Amarillo Veterans Affairs Health Care System - Cancer Program [5956]
Amazing Angels Home Health & Hospice, LLC [16119]
Amazing Care Home Health Agency, Inc. [14233]
Amazing Medical Care, Inc. [14885]
Amazing Miracles LLC [44850]
Amazing Treatment [48239]
AMB Healthcare [15654]
Amber Home Health Care, Inc. [15617]
Amber Ridge [28172]
Ambercare Hospice Inc-LasCruces [20538]
Ambercare Hospice, Inc.--Albuquerque [20515]
Ambercare Hospice Inc.--Belen [20527]
Ambercare Hospice-Santa Fe [20544]
Amberly's Place [8745]
Ambi Lingual Associates Inc. [1595]
Ambiance Home Health [12917]
Ambis Home Health Care, LLC [16128]
Ambler Clinic [6214]
Ambrosia Treatment Center [41907]
Ambulatory Infusion Care, Inc. [15754]
Ambulatory Pharmaceutical Services [16448]
AMC Hospice of the Shenandoah [21694]
A+Medics Services, Inc. [17955]
Amedisys Home Health of Tennessee [17691]
Amedisys Hospice of Anchorage [18775]
Amedisys Hospice of Baton Rouge [19834]
Amedisys Hospice-Burlington [20628]
Amedisys Hospice Care-Anmoore [21782]
Amedisys Hospice Care of Birmingham [18721]
Amedisys Hospice Care-Bluefield [21788]
Amedisys Hospice Care of Brownsboro [18691]
Amedisys Hospice Care of Cartersville [19370]
Amedisys Hospice Care of Foley [18713]
Amedisys Hospice Care of Newnan [19409]
Amedisys Hospice Care of Parkersburg [21809]
Amedisys Hospice Care of Plains [21145]
Amedisys Hospice-El Dorado [19750]
Amedisys Hospice of Garner [20666]
Amedisys Hospice-Gonzales [19843]

Amedisys Hospice of Greater Chesapeake [19910]
Amedisys Hospice of Greenville [21336]
Amedisys Hospice-Houma [19846]
Amedisys Hospice, Inc.--Chattanooga [21313]
Amedisys Hospice, Inc.--Elizabethtown [21330]
Amedisys Hospice, Inc.--Knoxville [21341]
Amedisys Hospice, Inc.--Salem [21733]
Amedisys Hospice-Kennesaw [19395]
Amedisys Hospice-Kokomo [19620]
Amedisys Hospice-Lawrenceville [19399]
Amedisys Hospice of Londonderry [20442]
Amedisys Hospice of Memphis [21346]
Amedisys Hospice-Metairie [19858]
Amedisys Hospice of Montgomery [18742]
Amedisys Hospice--Morristown [21352]
Amedisys Hospice of Omak [21764]
Amedisys Hospice-Portsmouth [20454]
Amedisys Hospice-Rainbow City [18755]
Amedisys Hospice of Roseburg [21029]
Amedisys Hospice Services--Athens [21309]
Amedisys Hospice Services--Baltimore • Upper
  Chesapeake/Saint Joseph Home Care [19911]
Amedisys Hospice Services--Dalton [19377]
Amedisys Hospice Services--Homewood [18722]
Amedisys Hospice Services-Indianapolis [19607]
Amedisys Hospice Services-Wichita [19784]
Amedisys Hospice of South Pittsburg [21351]
Amedisys Hospice-Tupelo [20266]
Amedisys Hospice of Tuscaloosa [18768]
Amedisys-Sweetwater [21368]
Amego [8134]
Amelia Center [32702]
The Amelia Center [36445]
Amelia Island Dialysis • DaVita [23296]
Amenity Home Health Care [15835]
Amenity Hospice, Inc. [21561]
Ameri-Tech Kidney Center [26943]
Ameri-Tech Kidney Center--HEB [26968]
Ameribest Office [17404]
America Home Care [13912]
America Home Health Care [13725]
American Behavioral Clinic [50468], [50469]
American Behavioral Health Systems • Mission
  [50189]
American Care Home Health, Inc. [13020]
American Care Quest, Inc. [13306]
American CareQuest, Inc. [19022]
American College of Acupuncture and Oriental
  Medicine [35682]
American Community Home Care Services [15871]
American Critical Care Services [18361]
American Donor Services [35081]
American Dream Home Health Care, Inc. [13446]
American Drug Recovery Program Inc [40058]
American Eldercare Inc.--Clearwater [13615]
American Eldercare, Inc.--Delray Beach [13647]
American Eldercare Inc.--Doral [13652]
American Eldercare Inc.--Fort Lauderdale [13689]
American Eldercare Inc.--Fort Myers [13697]
American Eldercare Inc.--Jacksonville [13807]
American Eldercare Inc.--Lake Worth [13834]
American Eldercare Inc.--Melbourne [13880]
American Eldercare Inc.--Orlando [14291]
American Eldercare Inc.--Ormond Beach [14302]
American Eldercare Inc.--Tampa [14408]
American Eldercare--Ocala [14276]
American Eldercare--Pensacola [14331]
American Family Counseling Inc [41646]
  Deerfield Office [41619]
American Family Institute, Inc. [32952]
American Fork Dialysis Center [27399]
American Foundation for Suicide Prevention [50984]
American Generations Home Health [13913]
American Habitare [46085]
American Health Care Agency [13914]
American Health Home Care Group, Inc. [18397]
American Health Services at • Bakersfield Health
  Services [39628]
American Health Services--Charlotte, NC [16707]
American Health Services--Florence, SC [17584]
American Health Services--Greenville, SC [17593]
American Health Services • Hollywood Medical
  Mental Health Services [40059]
American Health Services LLC • Venice Medical and
  Mental Health Services [40900]
American Health Services--Murrells Inlet, SC
  [17606]

American Health Services--North Charleston, SC
  [17612]
American Health Services
  Palmdale Medical [40351]
  Van Nuys [40888]
American Hearing Aids [2540]
American Home Health Care, Corp. [13915]
American Home Health and Hospice-Cumberland
  [19590]
American Home Health, Inc.--Aurora, IL [14682]
American Home Health Inc.--Glendale, CA [13021]
American Home Health, LLC--Columbus, OH
  [16898]
American Home Health Providers Corp. [14199]
A American HomeCare & Community Services, LLC
  [18058]
American HomeCare Hospice [18762]
American HomeCare, Inc. [18362]
American Homecare Services [15628]
American Indian Changing Spirits [40011]
American Indian Health and • Family Services of SE
  Michigan [44725]
American Indian Health Service Chicago [42470]
American Indian Health Services • Counsel Lodge
  [40725]
American Institute for Stuttering [3054]
American Medical Supply Inc. [16374]
American Nursing Care--Cincinnati, OH [16872]
American Nursing Care--Columbus, IN [14971]
American Nursing care--Evansville, IN [14975]
American Nursing Care, Inc.--AThens, OH [16841]
American Nursing Care, Inc. --Columbus East
  [16899]
American Nursing Care, Inc.--Dayton, OH [16923]
American Nursing Care Inc.--Indianapolis, IN
  [14993]
American Nursing Care, Inc.--Kettering, OH [16952]
American Nursing Care Inc.--Lexington, KY [15201]
American Nursing Care, Inc.--Lima, OH [16962]
American Nursing Care, Inc.--Marion, OH [16979]
American Nursing Care, Inc.--Springfield, OH •
  Community Mercy Home Care [17043]
American Nursing Care, Inc.--Troy, OH [17059]
American Nursing Care, Inc.--Waverly, OH [17067]
American Nursing Care, Inc.--Worthington, OH
  [17082]
American Nursing Care, Inc.--Zanesville, OH [17091]
American Nursing Care--Milford, OH [16999]
American Nursing care--Mishawaka, IN [15029]
American Nursing Care--Petersburg, IN [15040]
American Oxygen Home Care--LaFollette [17714]
American Oxygen Home Care--Morristown [17740]
American Oxygen Home Care--Tazewell [17776]
American Quality Home Services [13916]
American Red Cross--Des Moines • Community
  Telephone Service Crisis Line [50902]
American Red Cross--Hilo [50813]
American Red Cross--Lihue [50816]
American Red Cross - Mile High Chapter [50715]
American Red Cross--Wailuku [50817]
American Renal Associates [23239]
American Renal Associates--Adelphi [24621]
American Renal Associates--Augusta, LLC [23609]
American Renal Associates • Fairfield Kidney Center
  [26145]
American Renal Associates--Jacksonville [23335]
American Renal Associates--Ohio Valley Hospital
  [26473]
American Renal Associates--South Augusta Clinic
  [23610]
American Renal Associates - South Boca Raton
  Dialysis LLC [23240]
American Renal Associates • Vidalia Clinic LLC
  [23824]
American Renal Associates--West Jacksonville
  [23336]
American River College • Disabled Student Services
  • Deaf Services [296]
American School for the Deaf [336]
American Sleep Diagnostics, Long Beach, LLC •
  Sleep Disorders Center [37241]
American Sleep Medicine--Birmingham [36562]
American Sleep Medicine--Brentwood [37753]
American Sleep Medicine Center • St. Louis Sleep
  Center, LLC [37271]
American Sleep Medicine of Chicago [36895]
American Sleep Medicine--Crestview Hills [37016]
American Sleep Medicine--Indianapolis [36938]

American Sleep Medicine--Jacksonville [36766]
American Sleep Medicine--Leawood [36989]
American Sleep Medicine--Livingston [37335]
American Sleep Medicine of Louisville, Kentucky
  [37017]
American Sleep Medicine--Memphis [37754]
American Sleep Medicine--Newark [36758]
American Sleep Medicine--Orange [36657]
American Sleep Medicine--Rockville [37094]
American Sleep Medicine--San Diego [36658]
American Sleep Medicine--Saratoga [36659]
American Sleep Medicine--Towson [37095]
American Sleep Medicine--Vienna [37881]
American Sleep Medicine--Webster [37800]
American Sports Medicine Association [38073]
American Surgeons Group [38383]
American Therapy Group Inc. [2154]
American Tissue Services Foundation [35169]
Americare Home Health Care Services, Inc. [13917]
Americare Hospice [19602]
Americare Hospice-Mooresville [19635]
Americare In-Home Care, Inc. [18137]
Americare, Inc. [16375]
America's HealthCare at Home [15449]
Americas Keswick • Colony of Mercy [46219]
Americord Registry LLC [35126]
Americus Area Mental Health/Mental Retardation
  Program--Buena Vista, Georgia [29374]
Americus Area Mental Health/Mental Retardation
  Program • Taylor County Clinic [29375]
Americus Dialysis • DaVita • Dialysis Center [23576]
AmeriHealth Home Care Agency, LLC [13918]
AmeriMed [17068]
Ameriprime Home Health Providers Inc. [13265]
Amerst H. Wilder Foundation [34254]
Amesbury Renal Center • Diversified Specialty
  Institutes [24741]
Amethyst Counseling Services • Outpatient Chem
  Dep Treatment Services [45247]
Amethyst House Inc [42993], [42994], [42995]
  Addiction Services [43030]
  CD Community Residence [47088]
Amethyst Inc [47708]
Amethyst Personal Growth and • Counseling LLC
  [46166]
AMHC-Crisis Stabilization Unit [30202]
AMHC--Grand Isle Family Treatment [30214]
AMHC--Helpline/ACSU [30233]
AMHC Skyhaven [30234]
AMHC-Vickers Hope [30203]
Amherst Counseling Center [32703]
Amherst Group Home [32704]
Amherst Therapy Connections [2875]
Amicus Counseling Service [40400]
Amicus House [40653]
Amigenics [12270]
Amistad Crisis Shelter [34305]
Amistad Family Violence and Rape Crisis Center
  [10456]
Amite County Medical Services, Inc. [6888]
Amity Center [32925]
Amity Community Health Center [6257]
Amity Foundation [46228]
Amity Foundation at Circle Tree Ranch [39485]
Amity Home Health, Inc. [13207]
Amity House • Glynn Community Crisis Center
  [9093]
Ammonoosuc Community Health Services, Inc. •
  Ammonoosuc Community Health Center [6960]
AMNA Healthcare Services--Miami Lakes [14200]
AMNA Healthcare Services--Miramar [14234]
Ampla Health [6381]
Amsterdam Dialysis Center • Fresenius Medical
  Care [25569]
Amy's House • Lincoln County Coalition Against
  Domestic Violence [10055]
Anaconda Pintler Hospice [20348]
Anaconda VA Community Based Outpatient Clinic •
  VA Montana Health Care System [4243]
Anaconda Veterans Affairs Clinic [30917]
Anacortes Speech, Language and Hearing Therapy
  [3618]
Anacupa Hospital • Stanislaus County Behavioral
  Health and Recovery Center [50686]
Anagram Premier • Division of ResCare Premier
  [4379]
Anaheim Dialysis • DaVita [22584]
Anaheim Health Medical Center [1054]

Anaheim Hills Dialysis Center [22585]
Anaheim Hills Speech and Language Center [1055]
Anaheim Memorial Medical Center
    Cancer Program [4755]
    Pain Management Center [35301]
Analenisgi • Recovery Services Center [47268]
Anamika Recovery Center [39600]
Anandale Fluency Clinic [3575]
Anchor Counseling Inc [40987], [41072]
Anchor Healthcare Services [18398]
Anchor Hospital [33369]
Anchor House [33400]
    Mens Facility [46471]
Anchor House--People Incorporated [30696]
Anchor House • Runaway and Homeless Youth
    Services [36073]
Anchor Point Counseling Center [49887]
Anchor of Walden Sierra [44215]
Anchorage [45239]
Anchorage Children's Home • Runaway and Home-
    less Youth Program [35874]
Anchorage Community Mental Health Services
    [28071]
Anchorage Foot and Ankle Clinic [38017]
Anchorage Inc [42123]
Ancora Psychiatric Hospital [33658]
A and A Health Services [13726]
A & C Home Health Care, Inc. [13919]
A and E Behavioral Healthcare [42617]
A and E Home Health Services Inc. [13404]
A and E Hospice, Inc. • aka Unity Hospice Care,
    LLC-Olive Branch [20254]
A and G Love 'N Care Inc. [13920]
A & J Health Associates [17142]
A and K Home Service Inc. [14201]
A and L Counseling Services PC [42451]
A & M Recovery LLC [45645]
A and O Recovery Services Inc [48497]
A & P Home Health, Inc. [13238]
A and T Healthcare [16212]
A & T Healthcare--Kingston [16505]
A & T Healthcare, LLC--New City [16535]
A & T Healthcare--New York [16548]
A & T Healthcare--Newburgh [16571]
Andalusia Regional Hospital • Sleep Related Breath-
    ing Disorders Center [36563]
Andalusia Regional Physical Therapy and Sports
    Medicine [37989]
Anderson Area Medical Center, Radiologic Technol-
    ogy Program [5899]
Anderson County Veterans Affairs Hospital [29925]
Anderson Dialysis • DaVita [26010]
Anderson Hospital [14852]
Anderson House [28449], [46218]
Anderson/Oconee • Behavioral Health Services
    [48975]
Anderson/Oconee Counties • Behavioral Health
    Services [48902]
Anderson-Oconee-Pickens Mental Health Center •
    Teen Suicide Prevention [51318]
Anderson Oconee Speech and Hearing Services
    [3394]
Anderson Regional Medical Center • Sleep
    Disorders Center [37242]
Anderson School [8356]
Anderson Substance Abuse Treatment Center
    [44803]
Anderson Valley Health Center [6293]
Anderson's Institute for Rehabilitative Medicine
    [2768]
Andiv Health Care Corporation [13921]
Andover Dialysis • DaVita [26011]
Andover Orthopaedic Surgery & Sports Medicine
    Group, PA [38748]
Andrew Brown's Home HealthCare Center [17470]
Andrew McFarland Mental Health Center [33439]
Andrews Center--Athens [32406]
Andrews Center--Canton [32424]
Andrews Center--Mineola [32515]
Andrews Center--Tyler [32562]
Andrews County Mental Health Center [32402]
Andrew's Sports Medicine [37991]
Andromeda Transcultural Health Center [29082]
Andromeda Transcultural Health • Decatur Center
    [41524]
Androscoggin Home Care & Hospice--Auburn
    [19882]

Androscoggin Home Care and Hospice--Bridgton
    [15387]
Androscoggin Home Care & Hospice--Lewiston
    [15394], [19895]
Androscoggin Home Care and Hospice--Norway
    [15395]
Androscoggin Home Care and Hospice--Wilton
    [15403]
Androscoggin Kidney Center • Fresenius Medical
    Care • Dialysis Facility [24602]
Androscoggin Valley Hospital Home Health &
    Hospice [20431]
Androscoggin Valley Mental Health Clinic • Berlin
    Emergency Service [51079]
Andy Boyd's Inhome Medical--Elkview [18511]
Andy Boyd's Inhome Medical--Huntington [18516]
Andy Boyd's Inhome Medical--Parkersburg [18531]
Aneway [45187], [45324]
Angel of Caring Health & Staffing Services, LLC
    [13727]
Angel City Family Care Services, Inc. [12936]
Angel Eyes SIDS Program [36458]
Angel Heart Hospice, LLC [21385]
Angel Home Health Care, LLC [18094]
Angel Kidney Care of Inglewood, Inc. [22730]
Angel Medical Center Home Care & Hospice
    [16727]
Angel River Health and Rehabilitation [2174]
Angel of Shavano Hospice [19126]
Angel Watch Inc. of Amelia Island [13684]
Angel Wings Outreach Center [9653]
Angela Hospice Home Care Inc. • Angela Hospice
    Care Center [20087]
Angeles Home Health Agency, Inc. [13802]
Angelic Hospice-Broken Arrow [20926]
Angelo J Melillo Center for Mental Health Inc •
    Chemical Dependency Services [46652]
Angelo Kidney Connection [27310]
Angel's Care, LLC [16252]
Angels on Earth Home Health Inc. [13181]
Angels of Grace [8764]
Angel's Health Care, Inc. [14202]
Angels Recovery LLC [41988]
Angels Solutions Home Health Care [14235]
Angel's Touch Home Care Services [13922]
Angels Touch Home Health [13923]
Angelus House [28969]
Angleton Kidney Center [26941]
Anglican Social Services [43152]
Anisa Counseling Group • Lisa B Werth [43230]
Anishinaabe Miikana • Gidamaajitaamin Bois Forte
    [45245]
Anishinaabe Miikana Tower • Gidamaajitaamin Bois
    Forte [45331]
Anita Jackson House [32153]
Anita Stoudymire • DBA Recovery Counseling
    [46363]
Anixter Center [29581]
    Addiction Recovery of the Deaf [42471]
    Schwab Rehabilitation Center [42472]
Anka Behavioral Health • Concord Day Treatment
    [28450]
Anka Behavioral Health Inc • Central County MSC
    [39734]
Anka Behavioral Health Inc East County • MSC and
    Don Brown Shelter [39605]
Anka Behavioral Health Inc
    Hope Program [40875]
    West County MSC [40686]
Anka Behavioral Health--Nevin House [28719]
Anka Behavioral Health • Nierika House [28451]
Anka Behavioral Health--SouthPoint [28531]
Anka Behavioral Health--Willow Pass Road [28452]
Ankod Home Health Care [13855]
AnMed Health - Home Health Agency [17562]
AnMed Health Lund and Sleep Center [37730]
Ann Arbor Consultation Services Inc [44636],
    [44678]
Ann Arbor Consultation Services, Inc. [30503]
Ann Arbor Rehabilitation Centers Inc. [4154]
Ann E. Gordon Associates [3126]
Ann M. Kiley Developmental Center [7975]
Ann Martin Children's Center [28702]
Ann Whitehill Down Syndrome Program [7994]
Anna Bixby Women's Center [9233]
Anna Home Health Agency, Corp. [13808]
Anna Hospital Corp. [14679]
Anna Marie's Alliance [9634]

Anna Nursing Services Corporation [13924]
Annandale Fluency Clinic Inc. [2404]
Annandale Village [7919]
Annapolis Junction HME [15409]
Anna's Place [8765]
Anne Arundel Counseling Inc [44283]
Anne Arundel County Health Department • Addic-
    tions Services/Adolescent/Family [44284]
Anne Arundel County Mental Health Clinic •
    Adolescent and Family Services [8092]
Anne Arundel Home Care [15436]
Anne Arundel Medical Center • Oncology Program
    [5281]
Anne Carlsen Center for Children [8394]
Anne and Donald McGraw Center for Caring [19238]
Anne Molini Fitch Memorial Domestic Violence
    Shelter [9669]
Annette M Wellington-Hall, Inc. [14236]
Annie B Jones Community Services Inc [42473]
Anniston Fellowship House Inc [39205]
Anodyne Pain Care [12466]
Anorexia and Bulimia Center of Hawaii • Ai Pono
    Hawaii [11040]
Another Chance Counseling [48441]
Another Chance Counseling Center Inc [42005]
Another Choice Another Chance [40478]
Another Way Addiction Svc [45678]
Another Way, Inc. [9059]
ANOVA Hospice and Palliative Care Services LLC
    [21050]
Anson Community Hospice [20755]
Anson Community Hospital [16791]
Anson County Domestic Violence Coalition [10092]
Anson Regional Medical Services, Inc. [7061]
Antelope Dialysis Center • DaVita [22637]
Antelope Valley Council on Alcoholism and Drug
    Dependency [39984], [40352]
Antelope Valley Home Care [13098]
Antelope Valley Mental Health [28557]
Antelope Valley Rehabilitation Centers • Warm
    Springs Rehabilitation Center [39583]
Anthem Village Dialysis • DaVita [25354]
Anthony House [6575]
Anthony Louis Center [45098]
    Blaine [45087]
    Woodbury/Outpatient [45354]
Anti Aging and Longevity Center of • Texas PA
    [49278]
Antioch Substance Abuse Programs [39843]
Antlers Inc [45750]
Anuvia Prevention and Recovery Center [47250]
ANX Home Healthcare [12972]
The Anxiety & Stress Management Institute [29344]
Any--Time Home Care Inc.-- Albany [16333]
Any--Time Home Care Inc.--Hudson [16492]
Any--Time Home Care Inc.--Jamaica [16497]
Any--Time Home Care Inc.--Kingston [16506]
Any--Time Home Care Inc.--Middletown [16522]
Any--Time Home Care Inc.--Newburgh [16572]
Any-Time Home Care, Inc.--Nyack [16578]
Any--Time Home Care Inc.--Poughkeepsie [16599]
Any--Time Home Care Inc.--White Plains [16668]
Apac Centers for Pain Management [35440]
Apache Behavioral Health Services [8742]
Apalachee Center [6552]
Apalachee Center, Inc. • Gadsden County Clinic
    [29274]
Apalachee Center, Inc.--Monticello [29228]
Apalachee Center, Inc.--Tallahassee [29294]
Apalachee Center, Inc. • Wakulla County Clinic
    [29130]
AP&S Clinic [2188]
APC Home Health Service, Inc./Nurse Placement
    Service, Inc. [17941]
Apex Behavioral Health PLLC [44716]
    Brownstown [44683]
    Westland [45059]
Apex Foundation [40060]
Apex Home Health Care Inc.--Glendale [13022]
Apex Home Healthcare--Southfield, MI [15802]
Apex Speech Therapy Inc. [1711]
Apex Support Services [41049]
APG Center for Sleep Disorders [36831]
APG Homecare, Inc. [17919]
Apguard Medical, Inc. [13454]
Aphasia Center of California [1204]
Apna Ghar [9201]
Apnix Sleep Diagnostics [37801]

Apogee Health Care [13648]
Apollo Home Care, Inc. [14719]
APOLLO Resource Center--People Incorporated [30720]
Apopka Artificial Kidney Center • Fresenius Medical Care [23232]
Apopka Children's Health Center [6434]
Apopka Dialysis • DaVita [23233]
Apopka Family Health Center [6435]
Appalachia Family Health Center [7346]
Appalachia Intermediate Unit 8 Hearing Impaired Program [698]
Appalachian Community Health Center--Bellington [32887]
Appalachian Community Health Center--Elkins [32898]
Appalachian Community Health Center Inc
  Barbour County Office Adult Services [50285]
  Randolph County Office Adult Services [50298]
  Tucker County Substance AbuseServices [50337]
  Upshur County Office Adult Services [50288]
Appalachian Community Services [47431]
  The Balsam Center [47509]
Appalachian Counseling Services [43619]
Appalachian Dialysis Center [26914]
Appalachian Mental Health Center--Buckhannon [32890]
Appalachian Mental Health Center--Parsons [32927]
Appalachian Psychiatric Healthcare System
  Athens [33749]
  Cambridge Campus [33750]
Appalachian Regional Healthcare, Inc.--Hazard [15190]
Appalachian Regional Healthcare, Inc.--McDowell [15232]
Appalachian Regional Healthcare Inc.--Pikeville [15245]
Appalachian Regional Healthcare, Inc.--West Liberty • DBA ARH Home Health [15256]
Appalachian Regional Hospital, Inc. Home Health--Whitesburg [15257]
Appalachian Regional Medical Center [2269]
Appalachian State University • Communication Disorders Clinic [3157]
Apple Behavioral Counseling [42407]
Apple Creek Developmental Center [8398]
Apple Health Care Services [13728]
Apple HomeCare Associates, Inc. [15550]
Apple Valley Counseling Services [50263]
AppleCore Outpatient Treatment/Olathe [43419]
Applegate HomeCare and Hospice-American Fork [21595]
Applegate Homecare and Hospice-Bountiful [21597]
Applegate HomeCare and Hospice--Coeur D Alene [19455]
Applegate HomeCare and Hospice--Heber City [21608]
Applegate HomeCare and Hospice--Ogden [21625]
Applegate HomeCare and Hospice-St. George [21636]
Applegate HomeCare and Hospice-Salt Lake City [21641]
Appleseed Community Mental Health Center [31654]
  Rape Crisis and Domestic Violence Shelter [10122]
Appleton Medical Center • ThedaCare Sleep Disorders Center [37962]
Appleton Psychiatric/Counseling Center [50358]
Applewood Center [31761]
Applewood Centers Inc.--Children's Aid Society Campus [31700]
Applewood Centers Inc.--Eleanor Gerson Alternative High School [31701]
Applewood Centers Inc.--Jones Campus [31702]
Applewood Centers Inc.--Richard Paulson Center [31703]
Applied DBT Clinicians [10928]
Appomattox Dialysis Center • DaVita [27534]
Apria Health Care Inc. [12629]
Apria Healthcare--Cromwell, CT [13520]
Apria Healthcare, Inc.--Afton, WY [18644]
Apria Healthcare Inc.--Alamosa, CO [13459]
Apria Healthcare Inc.--Albany, NY [16334]
Apria Healthcare Inc.--Albuquerque, NM [16299]
  Coram Specialty Infusion Services [16300]
Apria Healthcare, Inc.--Alexandria, VA [18244]
Apria Healthcare Inc.--Alliance, NE [16094]

Apria Healthcare, Inc.--Altoona, PA [17238]
Apria Healthcare, Inc.--Amarillo, TX [17791]
Apria Healthcare, Inc.--Amherst, OH [16837]
Apria Healthcare Inc.--Anchorage, AK [12738]
Apria Healthcare Inc.--Ann Arbor, MI [15576]
Apria Healthcare Inc.--Arco, ID [14646]
Apria Healthcare Inc.--Arden, NC [16688]
Apria Healthcare Inc.--Asheville, NC • Coram Specialty Infusion Services [16691]
Apria Healthcare Inc.--Athens, GA [14475]
Apria Healthcare Inc.--Augusta, GA [14484]
Apria Healthcare Inc.--Aurora, IN [14961]
Apria Healthcare Inc.--Austin, TX [17810]
Apria Healthcare Inc.--Austin, TX • Coram Specialty Infusion Services [17811]
Apria Healthcare Inc.--Bakersfield, CA [12899]
  Coram Specialty Infusion Services [12900]
Apria Healthcare Inc.--Baltimore, MD [15411]
Apria Healthcare Inc.--Bangor, ME [15384]
Apria Healthcare Inc.--Baton Rouge, LA [15267]
Apria Healthcare, Inc.--Beaumont, TX [17822]
Apria Healthcare Inc.--Beckley, WV [18494]
Apria Healthcare, Inc.--Belgrade, MT [16083]
Apria Healthcare, Inc.--Bellingham, WA [18417]
Apria Healthcare, Inc.--Beltsville, MD [15425]
Apria Healthcare, Inc.--Bend, OR [17178]
Apria Healthcare Inc.--Bethlehem, PA [17257]
Apria Healthcare Inc.--Beverly Hills, FL [13585]
Apria Healthcare Inc.--Biloxi, MS [15953]
Apria Healthcare Inc.--Birmingham, AL • Coram Specialty Infusion Healthcare Company [12630]
Apria Healthcare Inc.--Bloomington, IL [14691]
Apria Healthcare Inc.--Bloomington, IN [14966]
Apria Healthcare, Inc.--Boardman, OH [16854]
Apria Healthcare Inc.--Boise, ID [14647]
Apria Healthcare Inc.--Bowling Green, KY [15165]
Apria Healthcare Inc.--Bradford, PA [17262]
Apria Healthcare, Inc.--Bradley, IL [14697]
Apria Healthcare, Inc.--Brea, CA [12912]
Apria Healthcare, Inc.--Bridgeport, WV [18499]
Apria Healthcare, Inc.--Brooklyn Heights, OH [16856]
Apria Healthcare Inc.--Brooklyn, NY [16376]
Apria Healthcare Inc.--Bullhead City, AZ [12782]
Apria Healthcare, Inc.--Butler, PA [17269]
Apria Healthcare Inc.--Cadillac, MI [15598]
Apria Healthcare Inc.--Camden, ME [15389]
Apria Healthcare, Inc.--Cameron, MO [15987]
Apria Healthcare, Inc.--Camp Hill, PA [17275]
Apria Healthcare Inc.--Canon City, CO [13460]
Apria Healthcare Inc.--Cape Girardeau, MO [15988]
Apria Healthcare Inc.--Carroll, IA [15065]
Apria Healthcare Inc.--Carson City, NV [16133]
Apria Healthcare Inc.--Carthage, MO [15991]
Apria Healthcare Inc.--Casa Grande, AZ [12784]
Apria Healthcare Inc.--Centennial, CO [13462]
  Coram Specialty Infusion Services [13463]
Apria Healthcare, Inc.--Champaign, IL [14710]
  Coram Specialty Infusion Services [14711]
Apria Healthcare Inc.--Chantilly, VA • Coram Specialty Infusion Services [18254]
Apria Healthcare, Inc.--Charlotte Ave., Nashville, TN [17752]
Apria Healthcare Inc.--Charlotte, NC [16708]
  Coram Specialty Infusion Services [16709]
Apria Healthcare, Inc.--Charlottesville, VA [18257]
Apria Healthcare, Inc.--Chattanooga, TN [17650]
Apria Healthcare, Inc.--Cheyenne, WY [18647]
Apria Healthcare, Inc.--Chicago, IL [14720]
Apria Healthcare Inc.--Chico, CA [12941]
Apria Healthcare Inc.--Chillicothe, MO [15996]
Apria Healthcare, Inc.--Chubbuck, ID [14655]
Apria Healthcare, Inc.--Clare, MI [15610]
Apria Healthcare, Inc.--Clarksville, TN [17653]
Apria Healthcare Inc.--Clearlake, CA [12949]
Apria Healthcare Inc.--Clinton, MO [15998]
Apria Healthcare Inc.--Clovis, NM [16307]
Apria Healthcare Inc.--Coeur D Alene, ID [14656]
Apria Healthcare, Inc.--Colby, KS [15117]
Apria Healthcare, Inc.--Collinsville, IL [14756]
Apria Healthcare Inc.--Colorado Springs, CO [13464]
Apria Healthcare Inc.--Columbia, MD • Coram Specialty Infusion Services [15431]
Apria Healthcare Inc.--Columbia, MO [16000]
Apria Healthcare Inc.--Columbia, SC [17571]
Apria Healthcare Inc.--Columbia, SC • Coram Specialty Infusion Services [17572]
Apria Healthcare Inc.--Columbus, GA [14503]

Apria Healthcare, Inc.--Columbus, OH [16900]
Apria Healthcare, Inc.--Colville, WA [18425]
Apria Healthcare Inc.--Concord, CA [12953]
Apria Healthcare, Inc.--Conover, NC [16716]
Apria Healthcare, Inc.--Conyers, GA [14508]
Apria Healthcare, Inc.--Cookeville, TN [17657]
Apria Healthcare, Inc.--Coos Bay, OR [17184]
Apria Healthcare Inc.--Corpus Christi, TX [17850]
Apria Healthcare Inc.--Cranberry Township, PA • Coram Specialty Infusion Services [17293]
Apria Healthcare Inc.--Crescent City, CA [12966]
Apria Healthcare, Inc.--Creston, IA [15072]
Apria Healthcare, Inc.--Crestwood, MO [14757]
Apria Healthcare Inc.--Crown Point, IN • Coram Specialty Infusion Services [14973]
Apria Healthcare Inc.--Dahlonega, GA [14514]
Apria Healthcare Inc.--Dallas, TX • Coram Specialty Infusion Services [17863]
Apria Healthcare, Inc.--Danville, PA [17294]
Apria Healthcare, Inc.--Davenport, IA [15073]
  Coram Specialty Infusion Services [15074]
Apria Healthcare Inc.--Daytona Beach, FL [13641]
Apria Healthcare, Inc.--Decatur, IL [14761]
Apria Healthcare, Inc.--Dekalb, IL [14763]
Apria Healthcare, Inc.--Denver, CO [13472]
Apria Healthcare Inc.--Des Moines, IA [15076]
Apria Healthcare, Inc.--Dickson City, PA [17295]
Apria Healthcare, Inc.--Dodge City, KS [15118]
Apria Healthcare, Inc.--Duluth, FA [14524]
Apria Healthcare, Inc.--Duluth, MN [15897]
Apria Healthcare, Inc.--Duncan, SC [17582]
Apria Healthcare, Inc.--Durango, CO [13481]
Apria Healthcare Inc.--Earth City, MS • Coram Specialty Infusion Services [16005]
Apria Healthcare, Inc.--East Providence, RI [17537]
Apria Healthcare Inc.--East Providence, RI • Coram Specialty Infusion Services [17538]
Apria Healthcare Inc.--East Syracuse, NY [16438]
Apria Healthcare, Inc.--Easton, MD [15433]
Apria Healthcare, Inc.--Eau Claire, WI [18566]
Apria Healthcare, Inc.--Effingham, IL [14772]
Apria Healthcare, Inc.--Egg Harbor Township, NJ [16205]
Apria Healthcare Inc.--El Centro, CA [12981]
Apria Healthcare, Inc.--El Paso, TX [17906]
Apria Healthcare Inc.--El Paso, TX • Coram Specialty Infusion Services [17907]
Apria Healthcare, Inc.--El Segundo, CA [12986]
Apria Healthcare, Inc.--Elmira, NY [16444]
Apria Healthcare, Inc.--Elmsford, NY [16449]
Apria Healthcare, Inc.--Endwell, NY [16452]
Apria Healthcare, Inc.--Erie, PA [17311]
Apria Healthcare, Inc.--Escanaba, MI [15647]
Apria Healthcare, Inc.--Eureka, CA [12995]
Apria Healthcare, Inc.--Evansville, IN [14976]
Apria Healthcare, Inc.--Everett, WA [18428]
Apria Healthcare, Inc.--Fairbanks, AK [12750]
Apria Healthcare, Inc.--Fairfield, CA [12997]
Apria Healthcare, Inc.--Farmington, MO [16008]
Apria Healthcare, Inc.--Farmington, NM [16312]
Apria Healthcare, Inc.--Fayetteville, NC [16722]
Apria Healthcare, Inc.--Fenton, MO [16011]
Apria Healthcare, Inc.--Fife, WA [18430]
Apria Healthcare, Inc.--Florence, SC [17585]
Apria Healthcare, Inc.--Flowood, MS • Coram Specialty Infusion Services [15959]
Apria Healthcare, Inc.--Folcroft, PA [17324]
Apria Healthcare, Inc.--Fort Bragg, CA [13001]
Apria Healthcare, Inc.--Fort Myers, FL [13698]
Apria Healthcare, Inc.--Fort Scott, KS [15120]
Apria Healthcare, Inc.--Fort Washington, PA [17327]
Apria Healthcare, Inc.--Fort Wayne, IN [14980]
  Coram Specialty Infusion Services [14981]
Apria Healthcare, Inc.--Franklin, CT [13526]
Apria Healthcare, Inc.--Freeport, IL [14796]
Apria Healthcare, Inc.--Fresno, CA [13006]
Apria Healthcare, Inc.--Gainesville, FL [13707], [14531]
Apria Healthcare Inc.--Gilbert, AZ [12788]
Apria Healthcare, Inc.--Golden, CO [13490]
Apria Healthcare Inc.--Goleta, CA • Coram Specialty Infusion Services [13062]
Apria Healthcare Inc.--Grand Island, NE [16099]
Apria Healthcare, Inc.--Grand Junction, CO [13491]
Apria Healthcare Inc.--Grand Rapids, MI [15673]
Apria Healthcare, Inc.--Grants Pass, OR [17192]
Apria Healthcare Inc.--Grass Valley, CA [13066]
Apria Healthcare Inc.--Grayling, MI [15679]

Apria Healthcare Inc.--Great Falls, MT [16088]
Apria Healthcare Inc.--Greeley, CO [13494]
Apria Healthcare, Inc.--Green Bay, WI [18569]
Apria Healthcare, Inc.--Greensboro, NC [16731]
Apria Healthcare, Inc.--Greensburg, PA [17328]
Apria Healthcare, Inc.--Greenville, NC [16734]
Apria Healthcare, Inc.--Greenville, SC [17594]
Apria Healthcare, Inc.--Hagerstown, MD [15445]
Apria Healthcare, Inc.--Hanover Township, PA [17331]
Apria Healthcare, Inc.--Harlingen, TX [17942]
Apria Healthcare, Inc.--Harriman, TN [17675]
Apria Healthcare, Inc.--Hattiesburg, MS [15964]
Apria Healthcare Inc.--Hays, KS [15126]
Apria Healthcare Inc.--Hayward, CA • Coram Specialty Infusion Services [13073]
Apria Healthcare Inc.--Henderson, NV [16136]
Coram Specialty Infusion Services [16137]
Apria Healthcare, Inc.--Hershey, PA [17343]
Apria Healthcare Inc.--Hilo, HI [14611]
Apria Healthcare Inc.--Hobbs, NM [16319]
Apria Healthcare Inc.--Hot Springs, AR [12853]
Apria Healthcare Inc.--Houghton, MI [15685]
Apria Healthcare Inc.--Houlton, ME [15392]
Apria Healthcare Inc.--Houston, TX • Coram Specialty Infusion Services [17956]
Apria Healthcare Inc.--Hudson, FL [13804]
Apria Healthcare Inc.--Huntersville, NC [16741]
Apria Healthcare Inc.--Huntsville, AL [12680]
Apria Healthcare Inc.--Idaho Falls, ID [14660]
Apria Healthcare Inc.--Independence, KS [15128]
Apria Healthcare Inc.--Indianapolis, IN [14994]
Coram Specialty Infusion Services [14995]
Apria Healthcare Inc.--Iowa City, IA [15090]
Apria Healthcare Inc.--Iron Mountain, MI [15694]
Apria Healthcare Inc.--Irvine, CA [13082]
Apria Healthcare, Inc.--Irving, TX [18019]
Apria Healthcare Inc.--Jackson, CA [13086]
Apria Healthcare, Inc.--Jackson, TN [17681]
Apria Healthcare Inc.--Jacksonville, FL [13809]
Coram Specialty Infusion Services [13810]
Apria Healthcare Inc.--Jefferson City, MO [16015]
Apria Healthcare, Inc.--Jefferson City, TN [17687]
Apria Healthcare Inc.--Joplin, MO [16017]
Apria Healthcare Inc.--Kahului, HI [14627]
Apria Healthcare Inc.--Kalamazoo, MI [15704]
Coram Specialty Infusion Services [15705]
Apria Healthcare Inc.--Kansas City, KS [15132]
Apria Healthcare Inc.--Kearney, NE [16105]
Apria Healthcare, Inc.--Keene, NH [16172]
Apria Healthcare, Inc.--Kennewick, WA [18432]
Apria Healthcare, Inc.--Kentwood, MI • Coram Specialty Infusion Services [15708]
Apria Healthcare, Inc.--Kingsport, TN [17695]
Apria Healthcare Inc.--Kingston, NY [16507]
Apria Healthcare, Inc.--Kirby Dr., Houston, TX [17957]
Apria Healthcare, Inc.--Klamath Falls, OR [17197]
Apria Healthcare, Inc.--Knoxville, TN [17698]
Apria Healthcare, Inc.--Knoxville, TN • Coram Specialty Infusion Services [17699]
Apria Healthcare Inc.--Kokomo, IN [15014]
Apria Healthcare Inc.--La Junta, CO [13496]
Apria Healthcare Inc.--Lafayette, IN [15020]
Apria Healthcare Inc.--Lafayette, LA [15308]
Apria Healthcare Inc.--Lake City, FL [13831]
Apria Healthcare, Inc.--Lake Forest, CA [13096]
Apria Healthcare Inc.--Lakeland, FL [13838]
Apria Healthcare Inc.--Lakewood, NJ [16229]
Apria Healthcare Inc.--Lancaster, CA [13099]
Apria Healthcare Inc.--Lansing, MI • Coram Specialty Infusion Services [15710]
Apria Healthcare Inc.--Las Cruces, NM [16320]
Apria Healthcare Inc.--Lawrence, KS [15133]
Apria Healthcare, Inc.--Layton, UT [18199]
Apria Healthcare Inc.--League City, TX [18039]
Apria Healthcare Inc.--Lees Summit, MO [16025]
Apria Healthcare Inc.--Lenexa, KS [15140]
Apria Healthcare, Inc.--Lexington, KY [15202]
Apria Healthcare, Inc.--Lexington, OH [16961]
Apria Healthcare, Inc.--Lima, OH [16963]
Apria Healthcare Inc.--Linbar Dr., Nashville, TN [17753]
Apria Healthcare Inc.--Lincoln, NE [16107]
Apria Healthcare Inc.--Lincoln Park, NJ [16233]
Apria Healthcare Inc.--Little Rock, AR [12864]
Apria Healthcare Inc.--Littleton, CO [13500]
Apria Healthcare Inc.--Littleton, NH [16173]

Apria Healthcare Inc.--Livermore, CA [13105]
Apria Healthcare, Inc.--Longview, TX [18048]
Apria Healthcare, Inc.--Los Angeles, CA • Coram Specialty Infusion Services [13120]
Apria Healthcare Inc.--Louisville, CO [13501]
Apria Healthcare Inc.--Louisville, KY [15216]
Apria Healthcare Inc.--Loveland, CO [13503]
Apria Healthcare, Inc.--Lowell, AR [12872]
Apria Healthcare, Inc.--Lubbock, TX [18053]
Apria Healthcare Inc.--Ludington, MI [15731]
Apria Healthcare Inc.--Macon, GA [14540]
Apria Healthcare Inc.--Madison Heights, MI [15736]
Apria Healthcare, Inc.--Malvern, PA • Coram Specialty Infusion Services [17381]
Apria Healthcare Inc.--Marietta, GA [14548]
Coram Specialty Infusion Services [14549]
Apria Healthcare Inc.--Marion, IA [15094]
Apria Healthcare, Inc.--Marion, IL [14850]
Apria Healthcare, Inc.--Marquette, MI [15744]
Apria Healthcare, Inc.--Marshfield, WI [18584]
Apria Healthcare, Inc.--Martinsville, VA [18328]
Apria Healthcare, Inc.--Maumee, OH [16984]
Apria Healthcare, Inc.--McAllen, TX [18068]
Apria Healthcare, Inc.--McCook, NE [16111]
Apria Healthcare, Inc.--Medford, OR [17203]
Apria Healthcare, Inc.--Melbourne, FL [13881]
Apria Healthcare, Inc.--Memphis, TN [17732]
Apria Healthcare, Inc.--Memphis, TN • Coram Specialty Infusion Services [17733]
Apria Healthcare Inc.--Mendota Heights, MN [15912]
Apria Healthcare, Inc.--Menlo Park, CA [13170]
Apria Healthcare, Inc.--Menominee, MI [15748]
Apria Healthcare, Inc.--Merced, CA [13171]
Apria Healthcare, Inc.--Meridian, MS [15972]
Apria Healthcare, Inc.--Merrillville, IN [15026]
Apria Healthcare, Inc.--Miami, FL [13925]
Apria Healthcare, Inc.--Miamisburg, OH [16991]
Apria Healthcare, Inc.--Middletown, NY [16523]
Apria Healthcare, Inc.--Midland, TX [18087]
Apria Healthcare, Inc.--Milford, CT [13531]
Apria Healthcare, Inc.--Minnetonka, MN [15917]
Apria Healthcare, Inc.--Minocqua, WI [18602]
Apria Healthcare, Inc.--Minster, OH [17002]
Apria Healthcare, Inc.--Miramar, FL [14237]
Coram Specialty Infusion Services [14238]
Apria Healthcare, Inc.--Missoula, MT [16092]
Apria Healthcare Inc.--Mobile, AL [12691]
Apria Healthcare, Inc.--Modesto, CA [13175]
Apria Healthcare, Inc.--Monona, WI [18603]
Apria Healthcare, Inc.--Monroe, LA [15334]
Apria Healthcare, Inc.--Monroeville, PA [17390]
Apria Healthcare, Inc.--Monterey, CA [13187]
Apria Healthcare, Inc.--Moorhead, MN • Coram Specialty Infusion Services [15919]
Apria Healthcare, Inc.--Morrisville, NC [16758]
Coram Specialty Infusion Services [16759]
Apria Healthcare, Inc.--Morton Grove, IL [14864]
Apria Healthcare, Inc.--Mount Prospect, IL • Coram Specialty Infusion Services [14867]
Apria Healthcare, Inc.--Mount Shasta, CA [13193]
Apria Healthcare, Inc.--Mountville, PA [17393]
Apria Healthcare, Inc.--Mountville, PA • Coram Specialty Infusion Services [17394]
Apria Healthcare Inc.--Muncie, IN [15032]
Apria Healthcare, Inc.--Murfreesboro, TN [17746]
Apria Healthcare, Inc.--Murrells Inlet, SC [17607]
Apria Healthcare, Inc.--Muskegon, MI [15755]
Apria Healthcare, Inc.--Nacogdoches, TX [18097]
Apria Healthcare, Inc.--Naperville, IL [14875]
Apria Healthcare, Inc.--Nashville, TN • Coram Specialty Infusion Services [17754]
Apria Healthcare, Inc.--Neenah, WI [18607]
Apria Healthcare, Inc.--New Berlin, WI [18609]
Apria Healthcare, Inc.--New Berlin, WI • Coram Specialty Infusion Services [18610]
Apria Healthcare, Inc.--New Orleans, LA [15341]
Apria Healthcare Inc.--Newark, DE [13564]
Apria Healthcare Inc.--Newnan, GA [14560]
Apria Healthcare, Inc.--Newton, KS [15143]
Apria Healthcare, Inc.--Nitro, WV [18530]
Apria Healthcare, Inc.--Norfolk, VA [18338]
Apria Healthcare, Inc.--North Charleston, SC [17613]
Apria Healthcare Inc.--North Platte, NE [16114]
Apria Healthcare Inc.--Northfield, NH [16181]
Apria Healthcare Inc.--Norwood, MA [15531]
Coram Specialty Infusion Services [15532]
Apria Healthcare Inc.--Novato, CA [13218]
Apria Healthcare Inc.--Novi, MI • Coram Specialty

Infusion Services [15760]
Apria Healthcare, Inc.--NW 56th St., Oklahoma City, OK [17143]
Apria Healthcare, Inc.--Oak Ridge, TN [17765]
Apria Healthcare, Inc.--Ocala, FL [14277]
Apria Healthcare, Inc.--Oceanside, CA [13221]
Apria Healthcare, Inc.--Oklahoma City, OK • Coram Specialty Infusion Services [17144]
Apria Healthcare, Inc.--Olympia, WA [18441]
Apria Healthcare Inc.--Omaha, NE [16120]
Coram Specialty Infusion Services [16121]
Apria Healthcare, Inc.--Onalaska, WI [18614]
Apria Healthcare Inc.--Ontario, CA • Coram Specialty Infusion Services [13223]
Apria Healthcare, Inc.--Oregon, OH [17014]
Apria Healthcare, Inc.--Orlando, FL [14292]
Apria Healthcare, Inc.--Ormand Beach, FL [14303]
Apria Healthcare, Inc.--Osage Beach, MO [16035]
Apria Healthcare, Inc.--Ottumwa, IA [15099]
Apria Healthcare, Inc.--Oxford, CT [13539]
Apria Healthcare, Inc.--Oxnard, CA [13228]
Apria Healthcare, Inc.--Palm Desert, CA [13230]
Apria Healthcare, Inc.--Panama City, FL [14312]
Apria Healthcare, Inc.--Pearl City, HI [14643]
Apria Healthcare, Inc.--Pennbright, Houston, TX [17958]
Apria Healthcare, Inc.--Pensacola, FL [14332]
Apria Healthcare, Inc.--Peoria, AZ [12798]
Apria Healthcare, Inc.--Peoria, IL [14903]
Apria Healthcare, Inc.--Phoenix, AZ [12802]
Coram Specialty Infusion Services [12803]
Apria Healthcare, Inc.--Piscataway, NJ [16256]
Apria Healthcare, Inc.--Plainview, NY [16594]
Apria Healthcare, Inc.--Pleasant Valley, MO [16040]
Apria Healthcare, Inc.--Poplar Bluff, MO [16041]
Apria Healthcare, Inc.--Port Angeles, WA [18443]
Apria Healthcare, Inc.--Port Huron, MI [15778]
Apria Healthcare, Inc.--Portland, OR [17213]
Apria Healthcare, Inc.--Portland, OR • Coram Specialty Infusion Services [17214]
Apria Healthcare, Inc.--Pottsville, PA [17456]
Apria Healthcare Inc.--Pueblo, CO [13505]
Apria Healthcare Inc.--Rancho Cucamonga, CA [13249]
Apria Healthcare, Inc.--Rapid City, SD [17634]
Apria Healthcare, Inc.--Red Oak, IA [15102]
Apria Healthcare, Inc.--Redding, CA [13253]
Apria Healthcare, Inc.--Redmond, WA [18447]
Apria Healthcare, Inc.--Redmond, WA • Coram Specialty Infusion Services [18448]
Apria Healthcare Inc.--Reno, NV • Coram Specialty Infusion Services [16162]
Apria Healthcare, Inc.--Rice Lake, WI [18623]
Apria Healthcare, Inc.--Richland, MS [15977]
Apria Healthcare, Inc.--Richmond, VA [18363]
Apria Healthcare, Inc.--Riverside, CA [13266]
Apria Healthcare, Inc.--Roanoke, VA [18374]
Apria Healthcare, Inc.--Rochester, IN [15047]
Apria Healthcare, Inc.--Rochester, MN [15930]
Apria Healthcare, Inc.--Rochester, NY [16613]
Apria Healthcare, Inc.--Rockford, IL [14913]
Apria Healthcare, Inc.--Rocky Mount, NC [16774]
Apria Healthcare Inc.--Rolla, MO [16045]
Apria Healthcare Inc.--Rome, GA [14575]
Apria Healthcare Inc.--Roswell, NM [16324]
Apria Healthcare, Inc.--Rothschild, WI [18625]
Apria Healthcare, Inc.--Sacramento, CA [13279]
Coram Specialty Infusion Services [13280]
Apria Healthcare Inc.--Safford, AZ [12813]
Apria Healthcare, Inc.--Saginaw, MI [15793]
Apria Healthcare, Inc.--Saint Augustine, FL [14362]
Apria Healthcare, Inc.--Saint Cloud, MN [15934]
Apria Healthcare, Inc.--Saint Joseph, MI [15795]
Apria Healthcare, Inc.--Saint Joseph, MO [16048]
Apria Healthcare, Inc.--Saint Louis, MO [16050]
Apria Healthcare, Inc.--Saint Paul, MN [15939]
Apria Healthcare, Inc.--Saint Peters, MO [16064]
Apria Healthcare, Inc.--Saint Rose, LA • Coram Specialty Infusion Services [15356]
Apria Healthcare, Inc.--Salem, OR [17222]
Apria Healthcare, Inc.--Salina, KS [15150]
Apria Healthcare, Inc.--Salisbury, MD [15463]
Apria Healthcare, Inc.--Salmon, ID [14672]
Apria Healthcare, Inc.--Salt Lake City, UT [18219]
Apria Healthcare, Inc.--Salt Lake City, UT • Coram Specialty Infusion Services [18220]
Apria Healthcare, Inc.--San Antonio, TX [18138]
Apria Healthcare Inc.--San Antonio, TX • Coram

Specialty Infusion Services [18139]
Apria Healthcare Inc.--San Diego, CA [13292]
 Coram Specialty Infusion Services [13293]
Apria Healthcare Inc.--San Jose, CA [13314]
Apria Healthcare Inc.--San Leandro, CA [13321]
Apria Healthcare Inc.--San Luis Obispo, CA [13322]
Apria Healthcare Inc.--Sanford, ME [15399]
Apria Healthcare Inc.--Santa Fe, NM [16325]
Apria Healthcare Inc.--Santa Fe Springs, CA [13334]
Apria Healthcare Inc.--Santa Rosa, CA [13339]
Apria Healthcare Inc.--Sarasota, FL [14373]
Apria Healthcare Inc.--Savannah, GA [14580]
Apria Healthcare Inc.--Savannah, MO [16065]
Apria Healthcare, Inc.--Schaumburg, IL [14920]
Apria Healthcare Inc.--Scottsbluff, NE [16130]
Apria Healthcare Inc.--Scottsdale, AZ [12819]
Apria Healthcare, Inc.--Sewickley, PA [17476]
Apria Healthcare Inc.--Sharon Hill, PA [17479]
Apria Healthcare Inc.--Sharonville, OH [17037]
Apria Healthcare Inc.--Shingle Springs, CA [13348]
Apria Healthcare Inc.--Show Low, AZ [12821]
Apria Healthcare Inc.--Shreveport, LA [15358]
Apria Healthcare Inc.--Sidney, NE [16132]
Apria Healthcare Inc.--Sierra Vista, AZ [12822]
Apria Healthcare Inc.--Silverdale, WA [18458]
Apria Healthcare Inc.--Sioux City, IA [15103]
Apria Healthcare, Inc.--Sioux Falls, SD [17638]
Apria Healthcare, Inc.--Smock, PA [17482]
Apria Healthcare, Inc.--Soldotna, AK [12774]
Apria Healthcare Inc.--Solon, OH [17040]
Apria Healthcare Inc.--South Bend, IN [15051]
Apria Healthcare Inc.--South Burlington, VT [18237]
Apria Healthcare Inc.--South San Francisco, CA
 [13364]
Apria Healthcare, Inc.--South Zanesville, OH [17042]
Apria Healthcare Inc.--Southern Pines, NC [16782]
Apria Healthcare Inc.--Southfield, MI [15803]
Apria Healthcare, Inc.--Sparks, NV [16167]
Apria Healthcare, Inc.--Spearfish, SD [17641]
Apria Healthcare, Inc.--Spokane, WA [18460]
Apria Healthcare, Inc.--Spokane, WA • Coram
 Specialty Infusion Services [18461]
Apria Healthcare, Inc.--Springfield, IL [14942]
Apria Healthcare, Inc.--Springfield, MA [15545]
Apria Healthcare, Inc.--Springfield, MO [16069]
Apria Healthcare Inc.--Springfield, OR [17225]
Apria Healthcare Inc.--Stockton, CA [13367]
Apria Healthcare, Inc.--Storm Lake, IA [15106]
Apria Healthcare, Inc.--Streator, IL [14947]
Apria Healthcare, Inc.--Suwanee, GA [14589]
Apria Healthcare, Inc.--Tacoma, WA [18468]
Apria Healthcare, Inc.--Tallahassee, FL [14397]
Apria Healthcare, Inc.--Tampa, FL [14409]
Apria Healthcare Inc.--Tampa, FL • Coram Specialty
 Infusion Services [14410]
Apria Healthcare Inc.--Temecula, CA [13379]
Apria Healthcare Inc.--Tempe, AZ [12824]
Apria Healthcare Inc.--Terre Haute, IN [15054]
Apria Healthcare Inc.--Thibodaux, LA [15373]
Apria Healthcare Inc.--Tifton, GA [14595]
Apria Healthcare, Inc.--Tilton, IL [14950]
Apria Healthcare, Inc.--Toledo, OH [17053]
Apria Healthcare Inc.--Topeka, KS [15152]
Apria Healthcare Inc.--Totowa, NJ • Coram Specialty
 Infusion Services [16278]
Apria Healthcare Inc.--Triadelphia, WV [18542]
Apria Healthcare Inc.--Tucson, AZ [12828]
 Coram Specialty Infusion Services [12829]
Apria Healthcare, Inc.--Tullahoma, TN [17780]
Apria Healthcare, Inc.--Tulsa, OK [17163]
Apria Healthcare Inc.--Tustin, CA • Coram Specialty
 Infusion Services [13400]
Apria Healthcare Inc.--Ukiah, CA [13402]
Apria Healthcare Inc.--Van Nuys, CA [13414]
Apria Healthcare Inc.--Victorville, CA [13424]
Apria Healthcare Inc.--Vienna, WV [18554]
Apria Healthcare, Inc.--Visalia, CA [13427]
Apria Healthcare, Inc.--W Memorial Dr., Oklahoma
 City, OK [17145]
Apria Healthcare, Inc.--W Reno Ave., Oklahoma City,
 OK [17146]
Apria Healthcare, Inc.--Wallingford, CT • Coram
 Specialty Infusion Services [13548]
Apria Healthcare, Inc.--Warren, PA [17499]
Apria Healthcare Inc.--Warrensburg, MO [16081]
Apria Healthcare Inc.--Wasilla, AK [12780]
Apria Healthcare Inc.--Waterloo, IA [15110]
Apria Healthcare Inc.--Waterville, ME [15402]

Apria Healthcare, Inc.--Waukegan, IL [14954]
Apria Healthcare Inc.--Webster, MA [15557]
Apria Healthcare Inc.--Wenatchee, WA [18483]
Apria Healthcare Inc.--West Palm Beach, FL [14451]
Apria Healthcare Inc.--Westhampton, NJ [16290]
Apria Healthcare Inc.--Wichita, KS [15156]
Apria Healthcare, Inc.--Williamsport, PA [17509]
Apria Healthcare Inc.--Williamsville, NY [16677]
Apria Healthcare Inc.--Wilmington, MA [15562]
Apria Healthcare Inc.--Wilmington, NC [16798]
Apria Healthcare Inc.--Winston Salem, NC [16803]
Apria Healthcare, Inc.--Wintersville, OH [17075]
Apria Healthcare Inc.--Woodland, CA [13452]
Apria Healthcare, Inc.--Wray, CO [13512]
Apria Healthcare, Inc.--Yakima, WA [18487]
Apria Healthcare Inc.--Yarmouth, ME [15404]
 Coram Specialty Infusion Services [15405]
Apria Healthcare, Inc.--York, PA [17515]
Apria Healthcare Inc.--Yuba City, CA [13457]
Apria Healthcare Inc.--Yuma, AZ [12837]
Apria Healthcare Inc.i--Bellevue, WA • Coram
 Specialty Infusion Services [18415]
Apria Healthcare, Inc.Wisconsin Rapids, WI [18643]
APT Foundation Inc
 Access and Treatment Services [41430]
 APT Meth Main Prog/APT Legion Clinic [41431]
 Orchard Clinic [41432]
 Park Hill Clinic [41433]
 Residential Services Division [41361]
 Women in Treatment [41434]
Aquatic Rehabilitation Sport Medicine & Hand
 Center [38160]
Aquila of Delaware [41516]
Aquila of Delaware/Georgetown [41505]
AR Home Health [17959]
ARA--Naples Dialysis Center LLC [23418]
Arapahoe/Douglas Mental Health [28868]
Arapahoe/Douglas Mental Health Center • Santa Fe
 House [28932]
Arapahoe Douglas Mental Health Network [28933],
 [41250], [41251]
Arapahoe/Douglas Mental Health Network •
 Administrative Office [28869]
Arapahoe Douglas Mental Health Network •
 Adolescent Day Resource Center [28898]
Arapahoe/Douglas Mental Health--Parker Office
 [28941]
Arapahoe Hearing Associates Inc. [1383]
Arapahoe House [40988], [41073], [41233], [41324],
 [41325]
 Adolescent/Adult Outpatient [41094]
 Aspen Center [41326]
 Aurora Outpatient [40989]
 Detox West/STIRRT Cont Care/Female [41345]
 New Directions for Families [41252]
 School Based Services [41095]
 The Wright Center [41346]
Ararat Home Health Care Inc. [13415]
Arbor Circle Corporation [44804]
 The Bridge for Runaways • Runaway and
 Homeless Youth Program [36007]
Arbor Circle Counseling Services • Newaygo County
 [44942]
Arbor Counseling [47450]
Arbor Court • Mobile Community Mental Health
 Center [27978]
Arbor Family Counseling Associates inc [45785]
Arbor Hospice and Home Care--Ann Arbor [20028]
Arbor Hospice-Western Wayne [20105]
Arbor Medical [44902]
Arbor Place Dialysis • DaVita [23683]
Arbor Place Inc • Alcohol and Other Drug Abuse
 [50464]
Arbor Woods Home Healthcare [15601]
Arbors Center--Olney [29658]
Arbors North [29671]
Arbour Counseling Services [44395], [44533]
 Structured Outpatient Addictions Prog [44509]
 Substance Recovery Program [44606]
Arbour Fuller EATS [44566]
Arbour Fuller Hospital [33570], [44567]
Arbour Fuller Partial Hospital [44568]
Arbour Hospital [33578]
Arbour - HRI Hospital [33575]
Arbour Substance Abuse Treatment Program •
 Detox [44488]
Arbuckle Life Solutions Inc [47908]
Arc of Bergen and Passaic Counties [31132]

ARC Clinic [1333]
ARC Community Services Inc
 ARC Center for Women and Children [50441]
 ARC House [50442]
 Healthy Beginnings [50443]
 Substance Abuse Services for Women [50389]
ARC/Later Life Domestic Violence Services [8734]
ARC of Madison County • Infant and Toddler
 Program [7715]
ARC Manor • Addiction Recovery Center [48325]
Arc of Monmouth [8273]
The ARC • Oneida-Lewis Chapter [8361]
ARC Opportunities [7992]
A.R.C. Professional Services, Inc. [13926]
ARC Riverside [7810]
Arc of Somerset County • Jerry Davis Center for
 Children and Families [8257]
Arc of the Virginia Peninsula, Inc. [8587]
Arcadia Dialysis Center • Davita [23234]
Arcadia Hospice [21040]
Arcadia Mental Health [28378]
ARCare [6271]
ARcare--85 [6269]
ARcare--93 [6261]
Archangel Home Health, Inc. [12974]
Archbishop Ryan School for Deaf and Hard of Hear-
 ing [706]
Archbold Health Services--Georgia [14594]
Archbold Home Health Services--Camilla [14497]
Archbold Home Health Services--Monticello [14250]
Archbold Home Health Services--Quitman [14573]
Archbold Northside [42167]
Archstone Recovery Center Inc [41738]
Archuleta County Victim Assistance Program [8979]
Archway Counseling [47482]
Archway Programs [8242]
Archway Recovery Center [49429]
Archway Youth Service Center • Runaway and
 Homeless Youth Program [36236]
Archways Inc [41647]
Arctic Women in Crisis [8656]
Ardent Hospice [21456]
Area Agency on Aging [18849]
Area Agency on Aging, Region One [8708]
Area Community Hospice, Inc. [21546]
Area Education Agency 4 [2209]
Area Mental Health Center
 Community Support Services, Dodge City
 [29916]
 Community Support Services, Garden City
 [29923]
Area Mental Health Center--Dodge City [50913]
Area Mental Health Center • Dodge City Branch Of-
 fice [29917]
Area Mental Health Center--Garden City [50916]
Area Mental Health Center • Garden City Branch
 Office [29924]
Area Mental Health Center--Scott City [50924]
Area Mental Health Center
 Scott City Branch Office [29953]
 Ulysses [43471]
 Ulysses Branch Office [29959]
Area Residential Care, Inc. [8015]
Area Substance Abuse Council [43243]
Area Youth Shelter Inc [47900]
AREBA Casriel Inc
 Chemical Dependence Outpatient Service
 [46810]
 Inpatient Rehabilitation Program [46811]
 Medically Supervised Withdrawal [46812]
Arecibo Norte Dialicentro • Fresenius Medical Care
 [26622]
Areta Crowell Center [28746]
ARFC • Saint Clares Social Services [46086]
Argus Community Inc
 Argus IV Mens Residential Program [46403]
 Elizabeth L Sturz Outpatient Center [46404]
 Harbor House MICA Treatment Program [46405]
ARH Psychiatric Center [43620]
ARH Recovery Homes Inc • House on the Hill
 [40654]
Aria Health [17405]
Aria Health, Bucks County Campus • Sleep
 Diagnostic Center [37637]
Aria Health - Home Health [17406]
Ariamni Home Health, Corp. [13927]
Ariel Amana Health Care, Inc. [17797]
Arise Counseling Center • Courtland Center [32756]

Arise Home Care [12947]
ARIZA Resource Center [42413]
Arizona Addiction Treatment Prog Inc [39402]
Arizona Advanced Therapy [941]
Arizona Associates for Reproductive Health [21892]
Arizona Baptist Children's Services [33968]
Arizona Bone and Joint Specialists [38047]
Arizona Burn Center at Maricopa Medical Center • Burn Center [4508]
Arizona Center for Fertility Studies [21893]
Arizona Center for Physical Therapy and Rehab [38051]
Arizona Center for Reproductive Endocrinology and Infertility [21894]
Arizona Children' Association - Yuma Office [33973]
Arizona Children's Association - Bisbee Office [33964]
Arizona Children's Association - Regional Office [33971]
Arizona Coast Ear, Nose and Throat LTD [945]
Arizona Commission for the Deaf and the Hard of Hearing [962]
Arizona Department of Health Services • Child Fatality Review Program [36447]
Arizona Genetics and Fetal Medicine [12144]
Arizona Hearing Specialists [987]
Arizona Institute for Communicative Cognitive Disorders [963]
Arizona Literacy and Learning Center [964]
Arizona Otolaryngology Center [978]
Arizona Otologic Associates, Ltd. [965]
Arizona Physical Therapy & Sports Rehabilitation, PC [38040]
Arizona Sports and Spine Physicians [38037]
Arizona State Braille and Talking Book Library [3750]
Arizona State Hospital [33108]
Arizona State School for the Deaf and the Blind [3698]
Arizona State Schools for the Deaf and Blind
 Desert Valleys Regional Cooperative [231]
 Eastern Highlands Regional Cooperative [230]
 North Central Regional Cooperative [229]
Arizona State Schools for the Deaf and the Blind • Phoenix Day School for the Deaf [232]
Arizona State Schools for the Deaf and Blind
 Southeast Regional Cooperative [237]
 Southwest Regional Cooperative [242]
Arizona State Schools for the Deaf and the Blind--Tucson [238]
Arizona State Schools for the Deaf and the Blind • Tucson AZ [239]
Arizona State University • Disability Resource Center [236]
Arizona Teen Crisis Solutions [50646]
Arizona Total Hearing Care [988]
Arizona West Valley Wellness and Rehabilitation [38042]
Arizona Youth Partnership • Runaway and Homeless Youth Program [35793]
Arizona's Children Association--Phoenix [7739]
Arizona's Children Association--Prescott [7744]
Arizonas Children Association • Substance Abuse Treatment Program [39519]
Arizona's Children Association--Tucson [7749]
ARJ Home Health Care, Inc. [16147]
Ark [45387]
The Ark [10448]
Ark Counseling [45262]
Ark of Little Cottonwood [32582], [49703]
The Ark of Little Cottonwood [32625]
Arkadelphia Human Development Center [7753]
Arkadelphia Physical Therapy Center [38059]
Arkansas Center for Ear, Nose, Throat and Allergy [1013]
Arkansas Center for Sleep Medicine [36642]
Arkansas Children's Hospital • Arkansas Center for Bleeding Disorders [12484]
Arkansas Children's Hospital Burn Center [4510]
Arkansas Children's Hospital
 Center for Cancer and Blood Diseases [36290]
 Headache Clinic [12383]
 Outpatient Dialysis Clinic [22549]
 Pediatric Sleep Disorders Center [36643]
 Transplant Center [22550]
Arkansas Children's Hospital/University of Arkansas for Medical Sciences • Arkansas Cystic Fibrosis Center [7464]

Arkansas Department of Health Area III Hospice [18844]
Arkansas Department of Health - Child and Adolescent Health Division • Arkansas SIDS Information and Counseling Program [36448]
Arkansas Department of Health - Forrest City [18847]
Arkansas Department of Health Hospice 9 - East Crittenden County HU [18882]
Arkansas Department of Health Hospice iV-Mtount Ida [18867]
Arkansas Department of Health Hospice-Little Rock [18860]
Arkansas Department of Health Hospice--Malvern [18865]
Arkansas Department of Health Hospice-Russellville [18875]
Arkansas Department of Health Hospice-Texarkana [18880]
Arkansas Department of Health Hospice VI [18863]
Arkansas Department of Health Hospice X [18871]
Arkansas Fertility and Gynecology Associates [21903]
Arkansas Headache Clinic [12384]
Arkansas Hospice - Cabot [18840]
Arkansas Hospice Conway [18843]
Arkansas Hospice Hot Springs Unit [18857]
Arkansas Hospice, Inc-Pine Bluff [18873]
Arkansas Hospice Little Rock Inpatient Center [18861]
Arkansas Hospice North Little Rock [18872]
Arkansas Hospice Russellville [18876]
Arkansas Methodist Medical Center [12879]
Arkansas Nephrology Services
 Ashley Kidney Center • Dialysis Facility [22535]
 Hot Springs Dialysis [22543]
 Ouachita Regional Dialysis Center [22544]
 Ouachita Valley Kidney Center [22532]
 River Valley Dialysis Center • Dialysis Facility [22571]
 South Arkansas Kidney Center--El Dorado • Dialysis Facility [22536]
 Springhill Dialysis Center [22565]
Arkansas Orthopedics and Sports [38064]
Arkansas Otolaryngology [1020]
Arkansas Pediatric Therapy [1043]
Arkansas Rehab Services • Learning and Evaluation Center [1021]
Arkansas Renal Systems • Nephrology Associates, P.A. [22526], [22533]
Arkansas School for the Blind and Visually Impaired [3699]
Arkansas School for the Deaf [246]
Arkansas Sports Performance [38065]
Arkansas State Hospital [33121]
Arkansas State University Speech & Hearing Center [1017]
Arkansas Valley Hospice [19114]
Arkansas Valley Regional Medical Center [1422]
Arkansas Valley Resource Center [8972]
Arken Healthcare Services, Inc. [13196]
Arlanza Family Medical/Dental Clinic [6345]
Arle Home Care Agency [13928]
Arlington Center for Recovery LLC [42387], [42655]
Arlington County Behavioral Health Services Division [7347]
Arlington County Behavioral Healthcare • Alcohol and Drug Program [49759]
Arlington County Community Services • Aging and Disability Services [32706]
Arlington Developmental Center [8512]
Arlington Dialysis • DaVita [26944]
Arlington Memorial Hospital [3456]
Arlington Pediatric Therapy Management Services [1956]
Arlington Public Library • Talking Book Service [3844]
Arlington RDSPD/Arlington Intermediate School District [766]
Arlington Sleep Disorder Center [37802]
Arlington Sleep Medicine, Ltd. [37882]
Arms Acres [31300]
Arms Acres Inc
 Alcoholism Outpatient Clinic [46982]
 CD Inpatient Rehabilitation [46581]
 CD Primary Care Program [46582]
 CD for Youth Residential [46583]
 Chemical Dependency Outpatient Clinic [46584]

 Outpatient Clinic [46406], [46739]
Arms of Grace Humanitarian Srvs ADP [40061]
Arms of Love Home Health Agency [13929]
ArmsCare, Inc. [17362]
Armstrong Alcohol and Drug Recovery [50228]
Armstrong County Council on Alcohol and Other Drugs • ARC Manor [48423]
Armstrong County Memorial Hospital • Laube Cancer Center [5835]
Armstrong Speech and Hearing Aid Center [3342]
Army Substance Abuse Program [45482], [45994]
 Building 201-A [42100]
 CDR USA Aeromedical Center [39247]
 CDR USAG [42284]
 CDR USAMEDDAC [43345]
Army Substance Abuse Program/KAHC • CDR Kenner USAHC [49785]
Army Substance Abuse Program • SARD [49974]
Army Substance Abuse Services • CDR USAMEDDAC [49327]
Arnette House • Runaway and Homeless Youth Program [35875]
Arnold and Cox Knee and Shoulder Ctr. [38063]
Arnold Palmer Hospital • Specialty Practice [7499]
Arnot Health Schuyler Dialysis • Schuyler Dialysis [25706]
Arnot-Odgen Medical Center--Elmira • Hemodialysis Unit [25655]
Arnot Ogden Medical Center [3014]
Arnot Ogden Medical Center--Corning • Dialysis Unit [25645]
Arnot Ogden Medical Center • Falck Cancer Center [5576]
ARO Behavioral Healthcare Inc [50562]
ARO Counseling Centers Inc [50406], [50470], [50494], [50504], [50546]
Aroostook Medical Center • Sleep Disorders Center [37088]
Aroostook Mental Health Center--Caribou [30204]
Aroostook Mental Health Center--Fort Kent [30212]
Aroostook Mental Health Center--Houlton [30215]
Aroostook Mental Health Center--Limestone • Residential Treatment Facility [30223]
Aroostook Mental Health Center--Madawaska [30227]
Aroostook Mental Health Center
 Outpatient Substance Abuse Services [43978], [43986], [44013], [44042]
 Residential Treatment Facility [44004]
 Washington County [43955], [44009]
Aroostook Mental Health Services
 AMHC [43960]
 Center for Integrated Neuro-Rehabilitation [4070]
Around the Clock Home Care [12901]
ARP Addiction Recovery and Prevention • Formerly ARP/Phoenix [47207]
ARP/Crossroads [47378]
ARROW • Wichita [43477]
Arrowhead Behavioral Health [47808]
Arrowhead Center Inc [45334]
Arrowhead Dialysis Center • Fresenius Medical Care [26160]
Arrowhead Health Center and Medical • Arrowhead Sleep Center [36624]
Arrowhead Home Health [12790]
Arrowhead Regional Medical Center [22641]
 Cancer Program [4766]
 Edward G. Hirschman Burn Center [4514]
Arrowhead West Child Services [8022]
Arroyo Grande Clinic [28381]
Arroyo Grande Community Hospital
 Coastal Cancer Care and Diagnostic Center [4758]
 Pain Management Clinic [35302]
Arroyo Vista Family Health Center, El Sereno [6313]
ARS New Castle LLC [41510]
ARSI-Care Group, LLC [13930]
ART Fertility Program of Alabama [21884]
Art Home Health Care Inc. [13102]
ART Institute of Washington, Inc. [21980]
ART Reproductive Center [21907]
Art Smart [32272]
ARTC
 Brooklyn Clinic 11/Fort Greene [46472]
 Brooklyn Clinic 13/Bushwick [46473]
 East NY MMTP [46474]
ARTC Manhattan

Clinic 21/Starting Point MMTP [46813]
Clinic 22/Kaleidoscope [46814]
Clinic 23/Third Horizon [46815]
Highbridge [46816]
Artemis Center for Alternatives to Domestic Violence [10143]
Artemis House • Victims of Violence Intervention Program [10386]
Artemis--Lead Satellite Office [10373]
Artesia Counseling and Resource Center [31185]
Artesia Dialysis • DaVita [25539]
Arthritis and Orthopedic Medical Clinic [38099]
Arthur B. and Ethel V. Horton VNA Hospice Center [19656]
Arthur Center [30874]
Arthur Flaxs • Comprehensive Psychosocial Services [44106]
Artificial Kidney Center--Broward • DaVita [23485]
Artificial Kidney Center--Suffolk • Fresenius Medical Care [27573]
Artist of Therapy Inc. [1646]
Artreach, Inc. [29034]
ARTS Counseling Agency [41680]
ARTS/ Univ of CO De Health Science Center • Peer I Motivation House [41096]
ARTS Univ of CO Health Science Center
ARTS Crosspoint Clinic [41097]
ARTS Parkside Clinic [41098]
First Arts Outpatient Program [41099]
Outpatient Womens Treatment Services [41100]
PEER I Dedication House [41101]
Peer I Inspiration House [41102]
Potomac Street Center [40990]
Special Services Clinic [41103]
Synergy Outpatient [41104]
Westside Center for Change [41234]
ARTS University of CO Denver
The Haven [41105]
The Haven Mothers House I [41106]
ARTS University of Colorado Denver • Synergy Residential [41107]
Artz Center Audiology • Hearing and Speech Institute [687]
Arvada Clinic [6383]
Arvada Counseling Center Inc [40982]
Arvada Dialysis Center • DaVita [23088]
Asante Home Care and Hospice • dba Rogue Valley Medical Center • Home Health Agency [21016]
ASAP Consulting Plus [43756]
ASAP Counseling Center • HQ US Army Alaska [39332]
ASAP Home Care, Inc.--Wadsworth [17062]
ASAP Homecare, Inc.--Canton [16863]
ASAP Homecare, Inc.--Millersburg [17001]
ASAP Homecare, Inc.--Wooster [17078]
ASAP Program [43712]
ASAP Residential Treatment Youth Focus [47337]
Ascend Recovery [49614]
Lake House [49594]
Ascendi Home Health Agency, Inc. [13931]
Ascension Counseling and • Transformation LLC [40976], [41226]
Ascension Parish Schools [452]
Ascent Behavioral Health Services [42348], [42353]
Reentry Center [42310]
Ascent Children's Health Services, Arkadelphia [28231]
Ascent Children's Health Services, Batesville [28237]
Ascent children's Health Services, Benton [28240]
Ascent Children's Health Services, Blytheville [28247]
Ascent Children's Health Services, Glendale St. [28291]
Ascent Children's Health Services, North Little Rock [28332]
Ascent Children's Health Services, Paragould [28336]
Ascent Children's Health Services, Turman Dr. [28292]
Ascent Children's Health Services, West Memphis [28362]
Ascent Counseling and DUI Services [42415], [42915]
Ascention Home Health Services [15618]
Asepsis Infusion, Inc. [17504]
Asera Care Home Health--Lakeland [13839]
Asera Care Home Health--Largo [13846]

Asera Care Home Health--New Port Richey [14258]
Asera Care Home Health--Ocala [14278]
AseraCare Home Health--Largo [13847]
AseraCare Hospice-Akron [20840]
AseraCare Hospice-Allentown [21041]
AseraCare Hospice-Altoona [21046]
AseraCare Hospice-Atlanta [19347]
AseraCare Hospice-Bastrop [21395]
AseraCare Hospice-Beatrice [20376]
AseraCare Hospice - Bloomington [20147]
AseraCare Hospice-Brookville [21061]
AseraCare Hospice Care of Nebraska [20406]
AseraCare Hospice-Clarks Summit [21073]
AseraCare Hospice-Clarksville [21316]
Aseracare Hospice--Concord [18910]
AseraCare Hospice-Corinth [20230]
AseraCare Hospice--Council Bluffs [19677]
Aseracare Hospice--Decatur [18700]
AseraCare Hospice-Dexter [20293]
AseraCare Hospice--Erie [21082]
AseraCare Hospice-Evansville [19640]
AseraCare Hospice-Foley [18714]
AseraCare Hospice-Fresno [18928]
AseraCare Hospice-Grand Island [20382]
AseraCare Hospice - Green Bay [21837]
AseraCare Hospice-Hamilton [18720]
AseraCare Hospice - Harrisburg [21092]
AseraCare Hospice--Houston [21480]
AseraCare Hospice--Indianapolis [19608]
AseraCare Hospice - Jackson [18729]
AseraCare Hospice-Jackson [21338]
AseraCare Hospice--Johnstown [21100]
AseraCare Hospice--Kansas City [20306]
AseraCare Hospice-Kearney [20385]
AseraCare Hospice--Lincoln [20388]
AseraCare Hospice-McKenzie [21345]
AseraCare Hospice-Memphis [21324]
AseraCare Hospice-Mid Valley Hospital [21126]
AseraCare Hospice--Mountville [21117]
AseraCare Hospice - Nashville [21358]
AseraCare Hospice-Norfolk [20393]
AseraCare Hospice-Northport--Tuscaloosa [18769]
AseraCare Hospice--Omaha [20397]
AseraCare Hospice--Pittsburgh [21134]
AseraCare Hospice-Richmond [21720]
AseraCare/Hospice Senatobia [20261]
AseraCare Hospice-Sioux Falls [21299]
AseraCare/Hospice South Jackson [18730]
AseraCare/Hospice South of Mobile, LLC [18736]
AseraCare/Hospice South of Philadelphia LLC [20258]
AseraCare Hospice - Tullahoma [21370]
AseraCare Hospice-Tupelo [20267]
AseraCare Hospice-Valparaiso [19657]
AseraCare Hospice-Wellesley Hills [20010]
AseraCare Hospice-Wichita [19751]
AseraCare Hospice-Winterville [20772]
AseraCare Hospice--Worcester [20013]
AseraCare Hospice--York [21179]
AseraCare-Monroeville [18741]
AserCare Home Health--Leesburg [13862]
Asercare Hospice [19054]
AserCare Hospice-O'Neil [20395]
Ash Tree Dialysis • DaVita [22693]
Asha Family Services, Inc. [10721]
Ashanti Hospice and Palliative Care • Sunset Retirement Communities [20898]
Ashby House [43451]
Asher Clinic [38093]
Asher Community Health Center [7129]
Asherah Home Health Services, Inc. [12918]
Asheville Regional Resource Center for the Deaf and Hard of Hearing • Division of Services for the Deaf and Hard of Hearing [3155]
Ashland Area Council on Alcoholism and Other Drug Abuse Inc [50363]
Ashland Community Health Center [6922]
Ashland Community Hospital [17175]
Ashland Community Hospital Hospice & Palliative Care Services [20984]
Ashland County Council on Alcoholism and Drug Abuse Inc [47614]
Ashland Health Resources, LLC [17960]
Ashley County Medical Center • Behavioral Health [28260]
Ashley House Inc • DBA Road to Recovery [45180]
Ashley Inc • Outpatient Program [44090]
Ashley Medical Center Hospice [20774]

Ashtabula County Medical Center [16840]
Cancer Program [5679]
Ashtabula Dialysis • DaVita [26013]
Ashuelot Valley Counseling Center [31097]
ASI of Cortland LLC [46601]
Asian American Chemical Dependency Treatment Services (ACTS)/Kent [49982]
Treatment Services/Lynnwood [50011]
Asian American Drug Abuse Program Inc [39939], [40062]
Olympia Academy for Youth [40063]
Therapeutic Community [40064]
Youth Outpatient Treatment [39883]
Asian American Recovery Services Inc [39774], [40655]
Project Oasis [40816]
Asian American • Residential Recovery Services [40593]
Asian Americans for Community Involvement [40656]
Asian Association of Utah [49679]
Asian Community Mental Health Services [40290]
Asian Counseling and Referral Service [50094]
Asian Counseling Treatment Services • Tacoma Branch [50201]
Asian Health Services [6334]
Asian Network Hospice [18981]
Asian Pacific Counseling and Treatment Center [28429]
Asian Pacific Counseling and Treatment Center, Lafayette Park [28579]
Asian Pacific Counseling and Treatment Center, Wilshire [28580]
Asian Pacific Health Care Venture, Inc. [6314]
Asian Pacific Islander Domestic Violence Resource Project [9014]
Asian Pacific Psychological Services [28667]
Asian Pacific Women's Center [8835]
Asian Rehabilitation Services [3890]
Asian Task Force Against Domestic Violence [9468]
Asian Women's Shelter [8885]
Askia Academy at Dimock [44551]
Asociacion Puertorriquenos en • Marcha Inc [48498]
Aspell Recovery Center [49088]
ASPEN/Central Washington Comprehensive Mental Health [10618]
Aspen Counseling and Education [41354]
Aspen Family Counseling [33007]
Aspen Home Health and Rehab [12937]
Aspen House [29795]
Aspen House of Montana [20374]
Aspen Institute for Behavioral Assessment [32626]
Aspen Treatment Services [41229]
Aspire Behavioral Health System [29703]
Aspire Home Healthcare [14890]
Aspire Hospice [21598]
Aspire IN [42978], [43086]
Aspire IN Inc [43003], [43140]
Aspire Indiana
Deaf Group Home [2155]
Deaf Services [2156], [43087]
Aspirus Comfort Care and Hospice Services [21870]
Aspirus Hospital • Dialysis Center [27800]
Aspirus Superior Home Health Hospice--Hancock [20066]
Aspirus Superior Home Health & Hospice-Lanse [20082]
Aspirus Superior Home Health Hospice-Ontonagon [20102]
Assault Care Center Extending Shelter and Support [9316]
Assault Crisis Center [30656]
Assential Therapies Inc. [2081]
Assertive Community Treatment [30633], [33256]
Assertive Community Treatment Team [31406]
Assessmennt Solutions of Charlotte LLC [47251]
Assessment Counseling and • Educational Services [49680]
Assessment and Counseling Solutions [45477], [45478]
Festus - WIP [45479]
Kirkwood - WIP [45546]
Saint Louis Site [45612]
Assessment for Direction LLC [43463]
Assessment Referral Counceling [41173]
Assessment and Treatment Associates • Franklin County [50047]
Assessment/Treatment Associates Inc [49888]

Auburn [49882]
Assessment and Treatment Associates • Snohomish County [50028]
Assessment and Treatment Association • ATA Port Townsend [50064]
Assets, Inc. [28072]
ASSETS Program • Community Outreach Inc [48088]
Assets School [7921]
Assis Professional Home Health [13932]
Assisi Bridge House [43890]
Assisted Daily Living, Inc. [17555]
Assisted Fertility Program [22279]
Assisted Fertility Program of North Florida [21986]
Assisted Recovery Center of GA Inc [42152]
Assisted Recovery Centers of America [39417], [45613]
Assisted Recovery Centers of • America-Mid Atlantic [44091]
AssistedCare Home Health--Elizabethtown [16719]
AssistedCare Home Health--Leland [16744]
AssistedCare Home Health--Supply [16786]
AssistedCare Home Health--Whiteville [16795]
AssistedCare Home Health--Wilmington [16799]
ASSMCA Centre de Serviceos con Metedona [48792]
Associate Behavioral Services [47412]
Associated Audiologists Inc. [2234]
Associated Behavioral Healthcare Inc
    Bellevue [49889]
    North Seattle Facility [50095]
    West Seattle Branch [50096]
Associated Centers for Therapy [31915]
Associated Fertility and Gynecology [22055]
Associated Healthcare Systems Inc. [16339]
Associated Learning and Language Specialists [1240]
Associated Rehab Program for Women Inc
    Alpha Oaks [39685]
    Cornerstone [39686], [39687]
Associated Speech and Language Services [2435]
Associated Speech and Language Specialists--Arden Hills [2672]
Associated Speech and Language Specialists--Maplewood [2707]
Associated Speech and Language Specialists--Plymouth [2726]
Associated Speech and Language Specialists--Saint Paul [2738]
Associated Speech Pathologists [1299]
Associated Stuttering Treatment Clinics [1380]
Associated Therapeutic Services PC [47930]
Associated Word of Life Counselors [43478]
Associated Youth Services • Kansas City ADAPT [43375]
Associates in Alcohol and • Drug Counseling Inc [42716], [42821], [42833], [42962]
Associates in Behavioral • Health and Recovery Inc [41957]
Associates in Behavioral Healthcare • ABC DUI Century Plaza [42955]
Associates in Communication Therapies [3421]
Associates in Counseling and Mediation • ACM Recovery Services Inc [40319]
Associates Home Care [13781]
Associates at Hope Harbor Outpatient [43432]
Associates In Counseling and Mediation • ACM Recovery Services Inc [39971]
Associates for Life Enhancement Inc [46104]
Associates in Neurology of Pittsburgh • Multiple Sclerosis Center [34687]
Associates in Pediatric Therapy [2297]
Associates in Pediatrics [38550]
Associates in Professional Counseling and Coaching [42801], [42840], [42868]
Associates for Psychological Services
    Davie Substance Abuse Services [41610]
    Hollywood Substance Abuse Services [41688]
    Homestead Substance Abuse Program [41693]
Associates for Psychotherapy and • Education PC [41290]
Associates in Rehabilitation Medicine [38743]
Associates in Speech, Language and Learning Inc. [3500]
Associates for Speech and Language Pathology [3338]
Association for the Adv of Mexican Amer Inc
    Casa Phoenix Outpatient [49361]

Casa Phoenix Resid Youth Treatment [49362]
    Selena Youth Residential Treatment [49516]
Association to Aid Victims of Domestic Violence [8854]
Association on Battered Women of Clayton County • Securus House [9120]
The Association for Community Living [8147]
Association for the Help of Retarded Children, New York City [8331]
Association House [29582]
Association House of Chicago [42474]
Association for Indian Development • Crisis Line of the Fox Valley [50828]
Association for Individual Development [29562]
Association for Prevention of Family Violence [10701]
Association of Professionals Treating Eating Disorders [10929]
Association for Retarded Citizens, Alameda County [7820]
Assumption Home Care Inc. [13267]
Assurance Home [34315]
Assured & Associates Personal Care of Georgia [14521]
Assured Care Home Health Services, Inc. [15804]
Assured Health Care [16953]
Assured Home Health & Hospice • Visiting Nurse Associations of America [21749]
AssureImmune LLC [34981]
Asterand [35075]
Asthma and Allergy Specialists, PA • Pediatric Cystic Fibrosis Center [7628]
Aston Home Health Inc. [13566]
ASTOP Inc • The Maslow Center [47788]
The Astor Child Guidance Center [34328]
The Astor Counseling Center [34346]
The Astor Day Treatment Program [34329]
Astor Gillis LADC [43967]
Astor Home for Children [8346]
Astor Services for Children [34348]
Astoria Dialysis Center [25571]
Astoria Pointe [48065]
Asuncion Home Healthcare Corporation [13933]
At Home Health Care, LLC [17902]
At Home Health Services [16148]
At Home, Ltd. [16533]
At Home Rehab, LLC [17297]
At Home Solutions [16609]
AT HomeHealth [14721]
At Peace Hospice Care [19368]
ATA - Clallam County [50147]
Atascadero State Hospital [33127]
Atascosa Medical Associates, LLP [39093]
ATC Home Health, LLC [18114]
ATECH Services [2877]
Atencion Medica en el Hogar, Inc. [17524]
Athena Home Health Agency, LLC [14239]
Athens Area • Commencement Center [42023]
Athens Center [32949]
Athens Center for Sleep Disorders [37803]
Athens--Clarke County Regional Library • Northeast Georgia Talking Book Center [3770]
Athens Dialysis • DaVita [22307]
Athens East Dialysis • DaVita [23578]
Athens Kidney Center • Dialysis Facility [23579]
Athens-Limestone Counseling Center [27834]
Athens - Limestone Hospital [12624]
Athens Limestone Sleep Center • Sleep Disorders Center [36564]
Athens Regional Medical Center [1806]
Athens Regional Medical Center, Inc. [14476]
Athens Regional Medical Center
    Sleep Disorders Center [36832]
    Winship Institute [5006]
Athens Sleep Center [36939]
Athens Sports Medicine Clinic, Inc. [38306]
Athens VA Community Based Outpatient clinic [16842]
Athens West Dialysis • DaVita [23580]
Athletic Center of Excellence and Sports Medicine--Hoboken [38730]
Athletic Center of Excellence and Sports Medicine--Paramus [38751]
Athletic Conditioning and Injury Center--Irvine [38089]
Athletic Conditioning and Injury Center--Mission Viejo [38104]

Athletic Conditioning and Injury Center--Tustin [38154]
Athletic Medicine and Performance [38674]
Athletic Physical Therapy, Inc.--Los Angeles [38096]
Athletic Physical Therapy, Inc.--Westlake Village [38159]
Athleticare Amherst [38775]
Athleticare • Catholic Health System [38809]
Athleticare Kenmore [38789]
AthletiCare/Rehabilitation South • Saint John's Hospital [38412]
AthleticCo Sports Medicine and Physical Therapy Center • N Clark Street, Chicago [38354]
AthletiCo Sports Medicine and Physical Therapy Center
    Bannockburn [38345]
    East Bank Club [38355]
    Glenview [38377]
    LaGrange Park [38385]
    Lemont [38388]
    Lisle [38389]
    N Michigan Avenue, Chicago [38356]
    Oak Brook [38398]
    River Grove [38407]
    Schaumburg [38410]
    Sportsplex/St. Charles [38409]
    Tinley Park [38413]
    W Diversey Parkway, Chicago [38357]
    W Irving Park, Chicago [38358]
    Willowbrook [38420]
AtHome Medical, Inc. [16242]
Atishwin Institute [43479]
Atkinson Visiting Nurses Service [14570]
Atlanta Area School for the Deaf [367]
Atlanta Area Stuttering Specialists [1811]
Atlanta Back Pain Clinic [35401]
Atlanta Center for Eating Disorders [11036]
Atlanta Center for Reproductive Medicine [22013]
Atlanta Center for Sleep Disorders [36833]
Atlanta ENT, Sinus, and Allergy Associates, PC [1892]
Atlanta Falcons Physical Therapy Centers - Dacula [38316]
Atlanta Falcons Physical Therapy Centers - Marietta East [38323]
Atlanta Falcons Physical Therapy Centers - Su-wanee [38330]
Atlanta Family Counseling Center Inc [42119]
Atlanta Intervention Network Inc [42063]
Atlanta Medical Center • Behavioral Health Services [29345]
Atlanta Metro Speech Center, Inc. [1921]
Atlanta Metro Subregional Library [3771]
Atlanta Metro Treatment Center [42139]
Atlanta Orthopaedics Specialists [38324]
Atlanta Pain Relief Center [35402]
Atlanta Sleep Medicine Clinic, LLC [36834]
Atlanta South Dialysis • DaVita • Dialysis Facility [23690]
Atlanta Speech School, Inc. [362]
Atlanta Speech School • Speech-Language Pathology and Audiology Clinics [1812]
Atlanta Speech School/Wardlaw School [7909]
Atlanta Sports Medicine [38307]
Atlanta VA Medical Center • Audiology and Speech Pathology Clinic [1852]
Atlanta Veterans Affairs Medical Center [51559]
    Lawrenceville Clinic [29455]
    Oakwood Clinic [29484]
    PTSD Clinical Team [51715]
Atlantic Audiology, Inc. [2530]
Atlantic Behavioral Health Morristown • Memorial Hosp Outpatient Addictive Service [46068]
Atlantic CAPD and Home Training [25601]
Atlantic Care Health Services • Mission Healthcare [45925]
Atlantic City Medical Center
    Dialysis Unit [25400]
    Psychiatric Intervention Program [51091]
Atlantic Counseling Services [41568]
Atlantic County Division of Intergenerational Youth Shelter • Runaway and Homeless Youth Shelter [36074]
Atlantic County Women's Center [9834]
Atlantic Dialysis • DaVita [24250]
Atlantic Health System
    Eating Disorders Program [11141]

Goryeb Children's Hospital • Pediatric Cystic Fibrosis Center [7600]
Morristown Memorial Hospital • Adult Cystic Fibrosis Center [7601]
Atlantic Health Systems • Overlook Hospital [46179]
Atlantic Hemodialysis Center [25602]
Atlantic Hemodialysis at Cobble Hill Nursing Home • Dialysis Facility [25603]
Atlantic Home Care and Hospice [16241]
Atlantic Home Health Agency of South Florida [13587]
Atlantic Home Health Care, LLC [12804]
Atlantic Homecare and Hospice [20480]
Atlantic Kidney Center • Dialysis Center & At Home • DaVita [25425]
Atlantic Kidney Centers KKC • American Renal Associates [23551]
Atlantic Medical Supply, inc. [13934]
Atlantic Prevention Resources Inc [46140]
Outpatient Services [46141]
Atlantic Provinces Special Education Authority [643], [3729]
Atlantic Recovery Services
Antelope Valley Community Day School [39985]
Atlantic Recovery Services Charter XII [40065]
Bell Gardens High School [39648]
Boys and Girls Club [39649]
Compton [39724]
Corporate [40012]
Crenshaw [40066]
East LA [40067]
Estrada Court School [40068]
Firestone [40069]
Girls Academy [40070]
Harding [40237]
Highland Park [40071]
Hollywood [40072]
Huntington Park College Ready Academy [39934]
Lakewood High School [39979]
Long Beach SEA [40013], [40014]
Manchester School [40073]
Montebello Intermediate [40238]
MUSD [40239]
North Facility [40015]
North Hills [40266]
Norwalk [40281]
Odyssey [40806]
Pacoima School [40285]
Pacoima SEA [40344]
Paramount High School [40358]
South Central [40074]
South Office [40016]
Atlantic Shores Hospital [33302]
Atlantic Sleep Center [37456]
Atlantic Sleep Disorders Center [36767]
Atlantic Speech Therapy LLC [1601]
Atlanticare Behavioral Health [45979]
AtlantiCare Behavioral Health--Atlantic City [31101]
Atlanticare Behavioral Health--Galloway [31130]
Atlanticare Behavioral Health--Hammonton [31138]
Atlanticare Behavioral Health • OASIS [46052]
Atlanticare Health Services [6967]
Atlanticare Hospice [20490]
AtlantiCare Regional Medical Center • Cancer Care Institute [5510]
Atlantis/Aguadilla • Dialysis Center [26620]
Atlantis Caguas Dialysis Clinic [26626]
Atlantis Carolina Dialysis Center [26629]
Atlantis Fajardo Renal Center [26631]
Atlantis Home Care Group [13729]
Atlantis HRG Guaynabo Dialysis Center [26634]
Atlantis Isabela Dialysis Center [26636]
Atlantis Lares • Atlantis Healthcare Group of Puerto Rico Inc [26637]
Atlantis Manati Dialysis Center [26639]
Atlantis Mayaguez Dialysis Center [26640]
Atlantis Ponce CNDS [26643]
Atlantis San Sebastian • Dialysis Center [26656]
Atlantis Toa Baja • Dialysis Center [26638]
Atlas Home Health [13620]
Atmautluak Community Health Clinic [12741]
Atrium Medical Center
Compton Cancer Center [5741]
Outpatient Services [26165]
ATS of North Carolina Inc • Carolina Treatment Center/Goldsboro [47329]
ATS Wheelchair and Medical [14648]

Attalia Health Care, Inc. [27835]
Attention Homes • Runaway and Homeless Youth Program [36278]
Attention Plus Care [14616]
Attleboro Area Medical Equipment Co. [15472]
Atwood House [32148]
Auberle [48458]
Auburn Clinic • Sierra Family Services, Inc. [28384]
Auburn Counseling Associates [44782]
Auburn Family Institute [8108]
Auburn Gresham Veterans Affairs Clinic [29583]
Auburn Hearing and Speech [1060]
Auburn Kidney Center • Northwest Kidney Center [27593]
Auburn Regional Medical Center
Cancer Program [6092]
Sleep Disorders Center [37907]
Auburn University, Montgomery • Speech & Hearing Clinic [917]
Auburn University • Speech and Hearing Clinic [900]
Auburn Veterans Affairs Medical Center [31230]
Auburn Youth Resource [32802]
Auburn Youth Resources • Runaway and Homeless Youth Program [36249]
Audibel Hearing and Audiology [1679]
Audibel Hearing Center [2591]
Audie L. Murphy Veterans Affairs Hospital [32544]
Audio Hearing Center--Andover [2441]
Audio Hearing Center--Lowell [2491]
Audio--Logic Hearing Services [2022]
Audio-Logic PC [2840]
Audiological Services [1950]
Audiological Services of Cadillac Inc. [2563]
Audiology Associates [1352]
Audiology Associates of Georgia [1878]
Audiology Associates of Greeley Inc. [1416]
Audiology Associates of Hammond [2316]
Audiology Associates Hawaii [1932]
Audiology Associates Inc. [2626]
Audiology Associates • Manhattan Medical Center [2230]
Audiology Associates of Marquette • Hearing Health Clinic [2622]
Audiology Associates of North Florida [1768]
Audiology Associates PC--Irvine [1132]
Audiology Associates PC--Mill Valley [1179]
Audiology Associates Professional Hearing Services [2329]
Audiology Associates of Worcester [2541]
Audiology and Balance Centers of America [2298]
Audiology Center of the Black Hills [3413]
Audiology Center of Merrimack Valley Inc. [2496]
Audiology Clinic--Emporia [2215]
Audiology Clinic--Ottawa [2233]
Audiology Consultants of Boynton Beach [1545]
Audiology Consultants of Panama City [1712]
Audiology Consultants of Southwest Florida [1553], [1574]
Audiology HEARS, PC [1850]
Audiology Professionals [2592]
Audiology Research Associates [1945]
Audiology Services Inc. [2448]
Audiology and Speech Pathology Service • VA Medical Center [1541]
Audioscope Audiology Group APC [1256]
Auditory Learning Center [629]
Auditory Oral School of New York [2986]
Auditory Processing Center of Pasadena [1219]
Auditory Verbal Center [1813]
Auditory--Verbal Services [1346]
Audrain County Crisis Intervention Services [9703]
Audrain Medical Center • Cancer Program [5454]
Audrey Kazmierczak Counseling Service [47554]
Auglaize County Crisis Center [10180]
Augusta Behavioral Health • Recovery Choice [49784]
Augusta Community Care [18298]
Augusta Medical Center • Cancer Program [6060]
Augusta Mental Health Institute [33549]
Augusta Metro Treatment Center [42040]
Augusta Multiple Sclerosis Center • Department of Neurology [34563]
Augusta Orthopaedic Associates • MaineGeneral Musculoskeletal Center [38504]
Augusta Steppingstones to Recovery Inc • DBA Awakening Center [42041]
Augusta Veterans Affairs Medical Center • Athens Clinic [29342]

Augustana Therapy Services [2709]
Augustin Nerva [47304]
Augustus F. Hawkins Comprehensive Community Mental Health Center [28581]
Aultman Dialysis Center of Canton [26029]
Aultman Health Foundation • Cancer Center [5686]
Aultman Hospice Program [20808]
Aultman Hospital - Dialysis Unit [26030]
Aultman Woodlawn [16864]
Aunt Marthas Outpatient Adult/Adolescent [42729]
Aunt Martha's Women's Health Center [6667]
Aunt Martha's Youth Service Center [33418]
Aunt Martha's Youth Service Center, Inc. • Runaway and Homeless Youth Program [35922]
Aurora Audiology and Speech Inc. [3009]
Aurora Bay Care Medical Center • Multiple Sclerosis Center [34741]
Aurora Baycare Medical Center • Vince Lombardi Cancer Center [6151]
Aurora BayCare • Sleep Wake Center [37963]
Aurora Behavioral Health Center [32971], [33922]
Aurora Behavioral Health Center--Airport [33947]
Aurora Behavioral Health Center
Aurora Medical Center Oshkosh [33945]
Behavioral Health Services [33921], [33923], [33929], [33931]
Aurora Behavioral Health Center--Fond Du Lac [33924]
Aurora Behavioral Health Center--Franklin [33925]
Aurora Behavioral Health Center--Germantown [33926]
Aurora Behavioral Health Center--Manitowoc [33933]
Aurora Behavioral Health Center--New Berlin [33943]
Aurora Behavioral Health Center--North Shore [33935]
Aurora Behavioral Health Center--Racine [33946]
Aurora Behavioral Health Center--Waukesha [33949]
Aurora Behavioral Health System [28149], [39390]
Aurora Behavioral Healthcare • Charter Oak [39760]
Aurora Behavioral Healthcare/San Diego [33185]
Aurora Behavioral Healthcare • San Diego [40547]
Aurora Center for Treatment Inc [40991]
Aurora of Central New York Inc. • Deaf Services [3129]
Aurora Charter Oak Hospital [33139]
Aurora Charter Oak Hospital--Behavioral Health [28463]
Aurora Community Mental Health Center [28853]
Aurora Counseling Services Inc [47971]
Aurora Dialysis Center • Fresenius Medical Care [23895]
Aurora Dialysis
DaVita [23090]
Fresenius Medical Care [23091]
Aurora Family Counseling [47507]
Aurora Family Service [51511]
Aurora Health Care-Milwaukee [21855]
The Aurora House [32822]
Aurora Lakeland Medical Center • Cancer Care Program [6149]
Aurora Medical Center • Cancer Program [6155]
Aurora Medical Center Manitowoc • Vince Lombardi Cancer Center [6176]
Aurora Medical Center Oshkosh • Vince Lombardi Cancer Center [6170]
Aurora Medical Center of Washington County • Cancer Program [6153]
Aurora Medical Group
Brown County Dialysis • DaVita [27719]
DaVita • Marinette Dialysis [27736]
Aurora Medical Group Dialysis Unit • Aurora Health Care [27714]
Aurora Medical Group - Manitowoc Dialysis • DaVita [27734]
Aurora Medical Group--Oshkosh West • Dialysis Unit • DaVita [27768]
Aurora Medical Group--Sheboygan • DaVita [27783]
Aurora Medical Group • Sturgeon Bay Dialysis • DaVita [27789]
Aurora Medical Group--Wautoma Dialysis • DaVita [27802]
Aurora Memorial Hospital of Burlington • Cancer Care Program [6147]
Aurora Mental Health Center
Offenders Group [40992]
Substance Abuse Treatment Services [40993]

Aurora Pavilion Behavioral Hlth Services [48901]
Aurora Psychiatric Hospital [11306]
    Chemical Dependency Services [50559]
Aurora Psychiatric Hospital Inc. [33951]
Aurora Public Schools • Deaf and Hard of Hearing Program [317]
Aurora Rehabilitation Center [3664]
Aurora Sheboygan Memorial Medical Center [33013]
    Behavioral Health Services [50523]
    Regional Oncology Center [6174]
Aurora Sinai Medical Center • Cancer Program [6162]
Aurora Sports Medicine Institute [39183]
Aurora Strategies Inc. [1922]
Aurora Visiting Nurse Association Hospice • Green Bay Branch [21838]
Aurora Vista del Mar Hospital [33209]
Aurora VNA Hospice Jackson Branch [21840]
Aurora VNA Hospice-Lake Geneva [21847]
Austell Day Supports and Peer Supports [29361]
Austen Riggs Center [33582]
Austin Community Kidney Center • Fresenius Medical Care [23914]
Austin Drug and Alcohol Abuse Program [49219]
Austin Medical Center • Chemical Dependency Services [45080]
Austin Medical Center Homecare and Hospice [20142]
Austin Medical Center- Mayo Health System [15890]
Austin Pain Associates [35683]
Austin Recovery Inc
    Detox/Edith Royal Campus [49220]
    Family House [49221]
    Hicks Family Mens Recovery Ranch [49259]
    Outpatient Program [49222]
    Womens Program/Edith Royal Campus [49223]
Austin Sleep Disorders Center [37804]
Austin State Hospital [33857]
Austin State Hospital Center for the Deaf • Texas Mental Health/Mental Retardation Department [3457]
Austin State School [8528]
Austin-Travis Counties Mental Health Center • Hotline to Help [51372]
Austin-Travis County Integral Care • Autism Center [32407]
Austin/Travis County Integral Care • CARE Program Journey OTP [49224]
Austin Travis County Integral Care • Narcotic Treatment Program [49225]
Austin/Travis County Integral Care • Oak Springs Treatment Center [49226]
Austin Veterans Affairs Clinic [32408]
Austin Waterloo Dialysis • DaVita [26949]
Authentic Home Health, LLC [13716]
Autism Matters Inc. [2716]
Autistic Treatment Center [8541]
Autumn Bridge Hospice [20952]
Autumn Home Health [17838]
Autumn House [32635]
Autumn Journey Hospice [21428]
Autumn Woods Hospice Care • Country Trails Hospice [21474]
Autumn Woods at Vesta, Inc. [30315]
Autumnleaf Group, Inc. [32718]
Auxiew Adult Day Habilitation Center [30100]
Auxilio Mutuo Hospital TX • Dialysis Center [26649]
AV Pain Medical Clinic [35303]
Avada Audiology and Hearing Care Centers--Elizabethtown [2266]
Avada Audiology and Hearing Care Centers--Louisville [2278]
Avada Audiology and Hearing Care Centers--New Albany [2173]
AVALON [10599]
Avalon Carver Community Center [40075]
Avalon Center • Domestic Violence and Sexual Assault Program [10399]
Avalon Center Inc [50097]
Avalon Center of Lakeview [33325]
Avalon Correctional Services • Carver Transitional Center [47972]
Avalon • Eagan [45137]
Avalon Eating Disorder Center [11153]
Avalon Hills [32605], [32608]
Avalon Hills Residential Eating Disorders Program [11289]
Avalon Hospice [20055]

Avalon Hospice of Athens [21310]
Avalon Hospice-Dickson [21328]
Avalon Hospice-Joplin [20304]
Avalon Hospice-Nashville [21359]
Avalon Hospice and Palliative Care [19015]
Avalon • Midway Womens Program [45301]
Avalon in Pine City [45260]
Avalon Programs • Cottage Grove [45116]
Avalon Prospect Park [45204]
Avalon • Stillwater/Outpatient Program [45326]
Avance Inc [42475]
Avanti Home Health Care [15715]
Avatar Home Health Care Agency, LLC [18158]
Ave Maria Dialysis • DaVita [23236]
Aven Home Health Services [13344]
Avenal Community Health Center [6286]
Aventura Dialysis Center • American Renal Associates [23387]
Aventura Hospital and Medical Center • Cancer Care Program [4928]
Aventura Kidney Center • DaVita [23315]
Aventura Medical Center [19254]
A Avenue of Recovery [50202]
Avenues [9682]
Avenues Crisis Program [28761]
Avenues for Homeless Youth • Runaway and Homeless Youth Program [36030]
Avenues to Recovery Inc [49836]
Avenues to Recovery • Olathe [43420]
Avera Behavioral Health Center [51347]
Avera Gregory Healthcare Dialysis Unit [26787]
Avera McKennan Branch Hospice and Palliative Care [19730]
Avera McKennan Hospice and Palliative Care [21300]
Avera McKennan Hospice and Palliative Care-Flandreau [21291]
Avera McKennan Hospice and Palliative Care-Sioux Falls [21301]
Avera McKennan Hospital • Addiction Recovery Program [49014]
Avera McKennan Hospital/University Health Center [4428]
Avera McKennan Hospital and University Health Center • Avera Cancer Institute [5918]
Avera McKennan Hospital/University Health Center • Avera McKennan Sleep Diagnostic Center [37748]
Avera McKennan Hospital and University • Health Center • Burn Unit [4633]
Avera Neuroscience Institute • ALS Clinic [149]
Avera Queen of Peace • Cancer Center [5917]
Avera Queen of Peace Hospital [17631]
Avera Sacred Heart Home Care [16101]
Avera Sacred Heart Hospice [21307]
Avera Sacred Heart Hospital • Cancer Program [5920]
Avera Sacred Heart--Yankton • Dialysis Center [26803]
Avera Saint Anthony's Hospital • ESRD [25336]
Avera Saint Luke's Hospital
    Cancer Program [5916]
    Dialysis Facility [26784]
Avera St. Luke's North Plains Hospice [21289]
Avera Saint Luke's • Pain Management Center [35668]
Avera Saint Lukes • Worthmore Addiction Services [48989]
Avera Transplant Institute [26797]
Avers Group Home [34100]
Avery Counseling [41185]
Avery House • Halfway House for Women and Children [44331]
Avery Road Combined Care [44332]
Avery Road Treatment Center • Intermediate Care Facility [44333]
Avida Health Care, Inc. [17908]
Avis Goodwin Community Health Center [6957]
Avista Rehabilitation • Avista Hospital • Avista Therapy Clinic [38179]
Avita Community Partners [29409]
    Adult Behavioral Health Services [29424]
    Ambulatory Detox [42102]
    Child and Adolescent Day Services [33381]
    Child & Adolescent Services [29431]
Avita Community Partners--Flowery Branch [33380]
Avita Community Partners
    Forsyth County Mental Health [42071]

    Forsyth County Mental Health/Substance Abuse and Psychiatric Rehabilitation [33375]
Avita Community Partners--Gainesville [33382]
Avita Community Partners
    Habersham County Mental Health/Substance Abuse [34091]
    Hart County Mental Health/Substance Abuse and Psychiatric Rehabilitation [33383]
    LARC--Lumpkin County [33376]
    Lumpkin County [42073]
    Stephens County Mental Health--North Star Ventures [33394]
    Union County [42051]
    Union Mental Health/Substance Abuse Clinic [33373]
Aviva Family and Children's Services--Franklin Avenue [28582]
Aviva Family and Children's Services--Wilshire Boulevard [28583]
Avon Chiropractic Health Center [38186]
Avon Manor Group Home [29153]
Avon Township Offices [29673]
Avondale House [8549]
Avondale Medical Services [6386]
Avow Hospice [19265]
Avoyelles Addictive Disorders Clinic [43855]
Avoyelles Mental Health Center [30157]
AVP Counseling and DUI Services Inc [42809]
Awakened Alternatives, Inc.--Flossmoor [14792]
Awakened Alternatives, Inc.--Olympia Fields [14893]
Awakenings [49975]
Awakenings By the Sea [48248]
Awakenings LLC [43153]
Aware [44370]
AWARE--Hardwick [10543]
AWARE, Inc.--Hermitage [10282]
AWARE, Inc.--Jackson [9548]
AWARE--Lakeport [8827]
AWARE--SaintLouis [9716]
Awareness Addiction Center [41108]
Awareness Counseling Consulting Inc [43599], [43753], [43792]
Awareness Institute Inc [41291]
Awfod Home Healthcare Services--Houston [17961]
Awfod Home Healthcare Services--Missouri City [18095]
AxelaCare Health Solutions--Detroit [15630]
AxelaCare Health Solutions--Richmond [15785]
Axiom Home Health, Inc. [18140]
Axis Community Health [6342], [40396]
Axis Community Health Inc • Axis Community Health Drug and Alcohol [40001]
Axis Health System [41079], [41156]
    Detox Unit [41157]
    New Day Counseling [41158]
Axis Health Systems, LLC [13730]
Axis Home Health Care, Inc. [14996]
Axis I Center of Barnwell [48904]
AxoGen Inc. [34982]
Ayer Outreach Site [30326]
Ayuda [41050]
Ayudantes, Inc.--Espanola [31191]
Ayudantes, Inc.--Sante Fe [31217]
AZ Home Health, LLC--Phoenix [12805]
AZHomeHealth--Fountain Hills [12787]
Azleway Inc • Substance Abuse [49246]
AZOR Homecare, Inc. [16528]
Aztec Counseling Agency Inc [42717]
Aztec Counseling Services Inc [39486]
Azure Acres/CRC Health [40793]
Azure Acres Recovery Center [40479]
Azusa Dialysis Center, LLC [22592]
A--Cure Healthcare Solutions [14717]
A. Holly Patterson Extended Care Facility • North Shore/LIJ Health System [25792]
A-Med Health Care Center [3886]
A-Med Supply [13480]
A-One Hospice, Inc. [20086]
A Place to Remember [36494]
A-Superior Home Health Agency, Inc. [14196]
A--V First Therapy Services LLC [1775]

B

B & B Care Services [14598]
B & B Home Health Services, Inc.--Hollywood, FL [13791]
B & B Medical Services--Houston, TX [17962]

B & B Medical Services, Inc.--Oklahoma City, OK [17147]
A B Consulting Associates [3138]
B & F Home Health, Inc. [13110]
B Friends Home Health, Inc. [13935]
B & K Home Medical Services, Inc. [17049]
B Plus H Care [13936]
BAART [45786]
BAART Bay Area Addict Research Treatment
    Addiction Research and Treatment Inc [39962]
    Behavioral Health Services Inc [39963]
BAART Behavioral Health Services [49721],
    [49740], [49744]
BAART Behavioral Health Services Inc [39373],
    [39606], [40076], [40077], [40187], [40291],
    [40448]
        Detox Program [39844], [39845]
        Market Street Clinic [40594]
BAART Community Healthcare [47284]
BAART Programs • Addiction Research and Treat-
    ment Inc [40919]
BAART Turk Street Clinic • FACET [40595]
Baby Love Case Management Inc • Pregnant
    Women Program [49132]
Bach Medical Supply [16070]
Bacharach Institute for Rehabilitation [4271], [35557]
Back to Health Physical Therapy, LLC [38745]
Back In Action [38197]
Back On Track • Intensive Outpatient Treatment
    [47372]
Back Rehabilitation Institute, Hamilton [35558]
Back on Track Physical Therapy [38538]
Backus Children's Hospital • Hemophilia Treatment
    Center [12506]
Bacon Street Inc [49864]
Bacterin International, Inc. • Biologics Division
    [35099]
Bad River AODA [50497]
The Baddour Center [8192]
Baden Street Counseling Center [47025]
Badlands Human Service Center [51187]
    Chemical Dependency Program [47565]
Bailey Speech and Language Services [1874]
Bainbridge Treatment Center [42048]
Bainbridge Veterans Affairs Clinic [31233]
Baio Enterprises, Developmental Therapies [947]
Bair Counseling Center [41190]
The Baird Center [34211]
Baird Center for Children and Families [32647]
Baitul Salaam Network, Inc. [9087]
Baker Clincal Office [30919]
Baker Clinic [2238]
Baker Clinic, Fort Scott [2217]
Baker Community Counseling Services Inc (BCCS)
    Inc [41752]
Baker County Medical Services • Ed Fraser Hospital
    • Sleep Center [36768]
Baker County Mental Health Center [29482]
Baker Healthcare--Jonesboro [12860]
Baker Healthcare--Mountain Home [12876]
Baker House [48068]
Baker Places Inc
    Acceptance Place [40596]
    Ferguson Place [40597]
Baker Victory Services [31375]
Bakers Ferry Dialysis • DaVita [23583]
Bakersfield Dialysis Center • DaVita [22593]
Bakersfield Recovery Services
    Capistrano Community for Women [39629]
    DBA Jasons Retreat Intensive Outpatient
        [39630]
    Lincoln Street Retreat [39631]
Bakersfield Vet Center [51872]
BALANCE: Eating Disorder Treatment Center
    [11154]
Balance Orthopaedic Foot and Ankle Center [38094]
Balanced Ear [998]
Balanced Life Solutions [43647], [43648]
Balanced Living, A Home Health Agency Inc.
    [12892]
Balanced Perspectives Inc [50231]
Bald Knob Medical Clinic [6259]
Baldpate Hospital [33577]
    Outpatient Substance Abuse Services [44478]
Baldwin Bone & Joint, P.C. [38003]
Baldwin County Community Mental Health Center
    Axalea Manor [27838]

Bradford Place Therapeutic Group Home
    [28029]
Baldwin County Community Mental Health Center--E
    Laurel Avenue [27925]
Baldwin County Community Mental Health Center--
    Medical Center Drive [27839]
Baldwin County Community Mental Health Center •
    Rockstall House [27926]
Baldwin County Community Mental Health Center--S
    Green Road [27912]
Baldwin County Service Center [29472]
Baldwin Family Health Care--Foley [6187]
Baldwin Family Health Care, Inc.--Baldwin • Family
    Health Care [6833]
Baldwin Hills Dialysis Center [22768]
Baldwin Park Medical Center • Peritoneal Dialysis
    Unit • Kaiser Permanente [22600]
Baldwin Schools [569]
Baldwins Counseling/Consulting Services [47451]
Ball Acute Muncie • Renal Advantage Inc. [24207]
Ball Dialysis--Daleville • Renal Advantage Inc.
    [24129]
Ball Dialysis--Renaissance [24208]
Ball Memorial Hospice [19636]
Ball Memorial Hospital • Division of Cardinal Health
    System • Cancer Program [5169]
Ball State University • Disabled Student Develop-
    ment [426]
Balm of Gilead Home Health Agency [16353]
The Balsam Center for Hope and Recovery [31605]
Baltic Street Community Health Center [31258]
Baltimore Behavioral Health Inc [44107]
Baltimore Cares Inc [44108]
Baltimore Community Resource Center [44109]
    Courage House [44110]
    Serenity House [44111]
Baltimore County Dialysis Facility • DaVita [24717]
Baltimore County Maryland Department of Health •
    Liberty Family Resource Center • Division of
    Speech, Language and Hearing [2425]
Baltimore County Public Schools [464]
Baltimore Crisis Response Inc [44112]
Baltimore Crisis Response, Inc. [50967]
Baltimore Geriatric • DaVita [24626]
Baltimore Station [44113]
Baltimore VA Medical Center [4090]
Baltimore Veterans Affairs Medical Center [30257]
    Veterans Affairs Maryland Health Care System
        [51579]
Baltimore Washington Medical Center [2413]
    Tate Cancer Center [5304]
BAM Recovery House [42946]
Bama Equine Assisted Therapy [925]
Bamberg Dialysis • Renal Advantage Inc. [26678]
Ban-Nix Home Medical Equipment, Inc. [14635]
Bancroft-Brick Campus [4272]
Bancroft-Judith B. Flicker Residences [4273]
Bancroft-Mullica Hill [4274]
Bancroft NeuroHealth [8253]
Bancroft NeuroHealth Preschool • Early Intervention
    Program [4275]
Bancroft--Plainsboro [4276]
Bandon Veterans Affairs Clinic [31930]
Bangor Area Visiting Nurses [15385], [19884]
Bangor Regional Program for Deaf and Hard of
    Hearing [456]
Bangor Veterans Affairs Clinic [30192]
Banks County Mental Health [50805]
Banner Baywood Medical Center • Banner Baywood
    Sleep Disorders Center [36625]
Banner Behavioral Health Hospital [39465]
    Scottsdale [33109]
Banner Boswell Medical Center • Cancer Program
    [4747]
Banner Boswell Pain Center [35286]
Banner Del E Webb Medical Center [39479]
Banner Desert Medical Center • Banner Desert
    Sleep Disorders Center [36626]
Banner Good Samaritan Regional Medical Center •
    Cancer Center [4742]
Banner Good Samaritan Transplant Services • Ban-
    ner Health [22466]
Banner Medical Sleep Institute • Arizona Medical
    Sleep Institute [36627]
Banner Mesa Medical Center [948]
Banner Thunderbird Behavioral Health [39391]
Banner Thunderbird Medical Center [28150]
Banning Dialysis • DaVita [22601]

Banning Mental Health Services [28398]
Bannock Youth Foundation • Runaway and Home-
    less Youth Program [35919]
Baptist Children's Services, Collegeville • Runaway
    and Homeless Youth Program [36176]
Baptist East Sleep Disorders Center [36565]
Baptist Health Center • Cancer Center [6024]
Baptist Health Centers • Shelby Baptist Sports
    Medicine [38012]
Baptist Health Home Infusion [12870]
Baptist Health Med. Ctr. • Dialysis Center [22551]
Baptist Health Medical Center
    Behavioral Health [28297]
    Dialysis Facility [22552]
Baptist Health Medical Center-Little Rock • Sleep
    Disorders Center [36644]
Baptist Health Rehabilitation Institute [1022], [3883]
Baptist Home Care and Hospice--North Mississippi
    [15951]
Baptist Home Care and Hospice-Tipton [21325]
Baptist Home Care and Hospice--Union City [21372]
Baptist Home Health Agency--Metropolis [14861]
Baptist Home Health Agency--Paducah [15242]
Baptist Home Health Care--Miami [13937]
Baptist Home Health Care--Pensacola [14333]
Baptist Home Health Network--Arkadelphia [12838]
Baptist Home Health Network--Herber Springs
    [12852]
Baptist Home Health Network--Little Rock [12865]
Baptist Home Healthcare [13811]
Baptist Home Medical Equipment [17734]
Baptist Homecare and Hospice-North Mississippi
    [20219]
Baptist Hospice [18743]
Baptist Hospital • Adolescent Stress Treatment
    Program [50778]
Baptist Hospital East
    Cancer Center [5222]
    Chemical Dependency Program [43677]
Baptist Hospital East Home Health Agency [2279],
    [15217]
Baptist Hospital East
    MDA Clinic [34801]
    Sleep Disorders Center [37018]
Baptist Hospital Inc.-Pensacola • Kugelman Cancer
    Center [4981]
Baptist Hospital of Miami • Cancer Program [4962]
Baptist Hospital--Nashville • Cancer Program [5946]
Baptist memorial Hospital - North Mississippi
    [15973]
Baptist Hospital • Sleep Disorders Center [36769]
Baptist Hospital Speech and Hearing Clinic [1718]
Baptist Medical Center [1602]
    Baptist Regional Cancer Institute [4949]
    Integris Sleep Disorders Center of Oklahoma
        [37599]
Baptist Medical Center, Nassau • Sleep Disorders
    Center [36770]
Baptist Medical Center - Princeton • Behavioral
    Health [27845]
Baptist Medical Center Princeton • Sleep/Wake
    Disorders Center [36566]
Baptist Medical Center • Sleep Disorders Center
    [36771]
Baptist Medical Center South [12700]
Baptist Medical Center South--Jacksonville •
    Beaches Sleep Disorders Center [36772]
Baptist Medical Center South--Montgomery • Sleep
    Disorders Center [36567]
Baptist Medical Center • Wake Forest University •
    Dialysis Center [25977]
Baptist Medical Center/Wake Forest University
    School of Medicine • Sleep Disorders Center
    [37457]
Baptist Memorial Homecare & Hospice [21337]
Baptist Memorial Hospice - Columbus [20229]
Baptist Memorial Hospital
    Behavioral Healthcare [49196]
    Chemical Dependency Unit [45369]
Baptist Memorial Hospital, Collierville • Baptist Sleep
    Disorders Center [37755]
Baptist Memorial Hospital--Golden Triangle • Sleep
    Laboratory [37243]
Baptist Memorial Hospital-Huntingdon [17680]
Baptist Memorial Hospital--Memphis
    Regional Cancer Center [5941]
    Sleep Disorders Center [17700], [37756]
Baptist Memorial Hospital-North Mississippi • Sleep

Disorder Center [37244]
Baptist Memorial Hospital - North MS • Cancer Center [5432]
Baptist Memorial Hospital-Tipton [17661]
Baptist Memorial Hospital-Union City [17781]
Baptist Rehabilitation Germantown [4431]
Baptist Saint Anthony Health System • Cancer Program [5957]
Baptist Saint Anthony's Home Care [17792]
Baptist Sleep Institute West [37757]
Baptist--South Miami Regional Cancer Program [4963]
Baptist Sports Medicine [39037]
Baptist Trinity Home Care & Hospice [17735]
Baptist Trinity Homecare and Hospice [21347]
Baraga County Memorial Hospital [15709]
Baraga County Shelter Home • Women's Center [9550]
Baraton Health Care Services, LLC [17963]
Barbara Ann Karmanos Cancer Institute Hospice [20117]
Barbara Ann Karmanos Cancer Institute • J.P. Mc-Carthy Cord Stem Cell Bank [35076]
Barbara B Fuller LCSW PA [41884]
Barbara E. Cheung Memorial Hospice [20467]
Barbara Kettle Gundlach Shelter • Home for Abused Women [9524]
Barber National Institute [700]
Barberton Hospice and Palliative Care [20802]
BARBS Place • Babies Adults Recovery Based Services [39541]
Barceloneta Primary Health Services, Inc. [7193]
Bardstown Dialysis • DaVita [24362]
Bardstown Therapeutic Rehabilitation Programs [29968]
Barium Springs Home for Children [47315]
Barker Sleep Institute [37758]
Barkley Memorial Speech Language and Hearing Clinic [2848]
Barksdale Management Corp. [16593]
Barlite Southwest Kidney Center • Innovative Dialysis Systems [27314]
Barnes Health Care Services [14600]
Barnes Jewish Dialysis Center [25264]
Barnes-Jewish Hospital • Siteman Cancer Center [5459]
Barnes Jewish Hospital Sports Medicine [38664]
Barnes Jewish Hospital--Transplant [25265]
Barnes Jewish Hospital • Washington University Medical Center [4575]
Barnes Jewish West County Hospital • Sports Therapy and Rehabilitation Center [38655]
Barnes Jewish West County • Sleep Disorders/EEG Center [37272]
Barnesville Dialysis [23624]
Barnesville Family Health Center [7076]
Barnsville Hospital Association, Inc. [16846]
Baron Speech-Language Therapy [1471], [1511]
Barren River Area Safe Space, Inc. • Spouse Abuse Center [9385]
Barrett Effective Speech Therapy Inc. [3353]
Barrett Hospital and Healthcare [20357]
Barrett Outpatient Center [1557]
Barrier Free Living [9947]
Barrington Health Center [6688]
Barrington House [32138]
Barrio Family Health Center [7310]
Barrow County Dialysis Center [23836]
Barrow County Mental Health Center [29508]
Barrow Neurological Institute/Saint Joseph Hospital [3859]
Barrow Neurology Clinic • Multiple Sclerosis and Related Diseases Clinic [34513]
Barry County • Community Mental Health Authority [44835]
Barry Eaton District Health Department • Eaton Behavioral Health [44696]
Bartels Counseling Services Inc [49015]
Barth and Associates • Barth Clinic [50264]
Barth Clinic [50280]
    Barth and Associates [49944]
Bartholomew County Public Library [3790]
Bartholomew Educational Services [7983]
Bartlett Counseling Services LLC [43221]
Bartlett Regional Hospital- Mental Health Unit [28097]
Barton Healthcare System [13362]
Barton Hospice [19053]

Barton Memorial Hospital [1325]
Barton Memorial Hospital Home Health and Hospice [13363]
Bartow Dialysis • DaVita [23237]
Bashor Children's Home [34127]
BASIC [45614]
Basic Concepts [2427]
Basic Home Infusion [16213]
BASICS Inc Bronx Addiction Services • BASICS/Franklin House [46407]
BASICS Inc • CD Outpatient Program [46408]
Basin Alcohol and Drug Services [47600]
Basin Coordinated Health Care, Inc. [16313]
Basin Home Health and Hospice [20535]
Basin Home Health, Inc. [16314]
Bassett Healthcare [3007]
    Bassett Cancer Institute [5574]
    Renal Dialysis Facility [25750]
    Sleep Disorders Center [37376]
Bassi and Gartner Speech--Language Services [3055]
Bastrop Behavioral Health Clinic • Addictive Disorders [43805]
Batavia Dialysis • DaVita [26016]
Batavia Veterans Affairs Medical Center [31234]
Batesville Behavioral Health Clinic [28238]
Batesville Counseling Center • Community Mental Health Center Inc [42988]
Batesville Office [29697]
Bath County Community Hospital [18312]
Bath VAMC [46370]
Bath Veterans Affairs Medical Center [31235]
Bathfol Health Services, Inc.--Houston [17964]
Bathfol Health Services, Inc.--Missouri City [18096]
Baton Rouge Area • Alcohol and Drug Center Inc [43806]
Baton Rouge Clinic, AMC • MDA Clinic [34802]
Baton Rouge Crisis Intervention Center, Inc. [50942]
Baton Rouge General Medical Center
    Burn Center [4553]
    Regional Cancer Center [5241]
Baton Rouge HomeCare [15268]
Baton Rouge Regional Eye Bank [35055]
Baton Rouge Renal Center & At Home • DaVita [24459]
Baton Rouge Speech and Hearing Foundation [2302]
Baton Rouge Treatment Center Inc [43807]
Baton Rouge Veterans Affairs Clinic [30126]
Battered Families Services, Inc. [9870]
Battered Service Action Center [8836]
Battered Women's Justice Project [9612]
Battered Women's Project [9429]
Battered Women's Resources, Inc. [9487]
Battered Women's Services of Hubbard County, Inc. • Headwaters Intervention Center [9628]
Battered Women's Shelter [10120]
Battin Clinic Inc. [3501]
Battle Creek Health System
    Cancer Program [5367]
    Sleep Center [37144]
Battle Creek VA Medical Center [4155], [20031]
Battle Creek Veterans Affairs Medical Center [30509]
Battle Mountain Mental Health Center [31019]
Batzofin Fertility Services [22177]
Baxley Dialysis • DaVita [23625]
Baxter Regional Medical Center
    Behavioral Health [28326]
    Center for Individual and Family Development [28277]
Baxter and Sheeren Inc [42845]
Bay Area Communication Access [1277]
Bay Area Community Resources Inc
    Marin County DUI Program [40698]
    Youth Substance Abuse Program [40699]
Bay Area Community Services, Inc.--Oakport Street [28668]
Bay Area Community Services--Oakland Avenue [28669]
Bay Area Foot Clinic [39173]
Bay Area Hearing Services [3488]
Bay Area Hospital • Cancer Program [5788]
Bay Area Hospital Home Health Agency [17209]
Bay Area Medical Center • Dialysis Facility [27737]
Bay Area Nutrition [10930]
Bay Area Pain and Wellness Center [35304]

Bay Area Recovery Center [49309], [49310], [49311]
    Outpatient [49582]
Bay Area Regional Dialysis Center--Saginaw • Fresenius Medical Care [24965]
Bay Area Regional Dialysis Center--Saginaw Riverside • Fresenius Medical Care [24966]
Bay Area Regional Dialysis--Essexville • Fresenius Medical Care [24893]
Bay Area Substance Education Services Inc • (BASES) [44694]
Bay Area Treatment Center [41895]
Bay Area Turning Point, Inc. [10519]
Bay Area Women's Center [9518]
Bay-Arenac Behavioral Health Authority [30511]
Bay Breeze Dialysis Clinic Inc • DaVita [23366]
Bay Care Home Care--Bradenton [13601]
Bay Care Home Care--Crystal River [13632]
Bay Care Home Care--Dunedin [13682]
Bay Care Home Care--Fruitland Park [13706]
Bay Care Home Care--Lakeland [13840]
Bay Care Home Care--Largo [13848]
Bay Care Home Care--New Port Richey [14259]
Bay Care Home Care--Ocala [14279]
Bay Care Home Care--Saint Petersburg [14365]
Bay Care Home Care--Sarasota [14374]
Bay Care Home Care--Spring Hill [14389]
Bay Care Home Care--Tampa [14411]
Bay Care Home Care--Zephyrhills [14464]
Bay Cove Human Services
    Andrew House Detoxification Center [44545]
    Chelsea ASAP Substance Abuse Programs [44440]
Bay Cove Human Services, Inc. [30340]
    Center House [30341]
Bay Cove Human Services
    Methadone Services [44404]
    New Hope Transition Support Program [44572]
Bay Manor Health Care Center • Mobile Community Mental Health Center [27979]
Bay Medical Center [1713]
    Cancer Program [4978]
Bay Mills Health Center • Substance Abuse Program [44682]
Bay Mills Indian Community Victim Assistance Program [9522]
Bay Pines VA Healthcare System [14366], [19195]
Bay Pines Veterans Affairs Health Care System [51551]
    Fort Myers Outpatient Clinic [3953]
Bay Pines Veterans Affairs Healthcare System • Fort Myers Outpatient Clinic [29159]
Bay Pines Veterans Affairs Medical Center • Cancer Program [4929]
Bay Psychological Associates PC [44658]
Bay Regional Medical Center [2560]
    Cancer Program [5368]
    Sleep Disorders Center [37145]
Bay Shore Dialysis Center • Good Samaritan Hospital • Chronic Dialysis Center [25575]
Bay Shore Dialysis • DaVita [27718]
Bay Shore Home Nursing/LMAS District Health Department [20100]
Bay Springs Dialysis Unit [25101]
Bay State Community Services Inc [44546]
Bay State Community Services, Inc. [30449]
Bay View Homecare, Inc. [15412]
Bayada Hospice [21665]
Bayada Nurses [15918]
Bayamon Dialysis Center • Fresenius Medical Care [26624]
Bayberry House [30373]
BayCare Behavioral Health
    The Academy [41817]
    Brooksville [41578]
Bayfront Medical Center [38281]
    Cancer Care Center [4990]
Bayfront Medical Center Rehabilitation Services [3954]
Bayhealth Home Health Care--Dover [13558]
Bayhealth Home Health Care--Milford [13560]
Bayhealth Medical Center--Front Street, Milford [1514]
Bayhealth Medical Center--Kent General Campus [23187]
Bayhealth Medical Center-Kent General Hospital • Cancer Center [4913]
Bayhealth Medical Center-Milford Memorial Hospital

• Cancer Center [4915]
Bayhealth Medical Center • Sleep Disorders Center [36759]
Bayhealth Medical Center--W Clarke Avenue, Milford [1515]
Bayhealth SleepCare Centers of Wilmington [36760]
BayHouse [29237]
Baylife Services [29300]
Baylor All Saints Medical Center [3493], [49329]
Cancer Center [4708]
Baylor All Saints Medical Center Transplant Center [27083]
Baylor All Saints Medical Centers [17920]
Baylor Center for Pain Management •
Comprehensive Outpatient Program [35684]
Baylor College of Medicine
Department of Molecular and Human Genetics [12344]
Cardiovascular Genetics Clinic [12345]
Neurofibromatosis Clinic [12346]
Prenatal Genetics Clinic [12347]
Skeletal Dysplasia Clinic [12348]
Baylor College of Medicine - Department of
Molecular Virology and Microbiology • Centers for
AIDS Research [73]
Baylor College of Medicine
Department of Pediatrics • Pediatric Cystic
Fibrosis Center [7669]
Methodist Hospital • Adult Cystic Fibrosis Center [7670]
Sickle Cell Disease Center [36434]
Baylor College of Medicine Sleep Center [37805]
Baylor College of Medicine • Texas Center for
Reproductive Health [22249]
Baylor College of Medicine/Texas Children's Hospital
• Center for AIDS Research [33]
Baylor College of Medicine/The Methodist Hospital •
Multiple Sclerosis Center [34715]
Baylor College of Medicine - Transition Medicine
Clinic [10865]
Baylor Health Care System • Outpatient Therapy
and Sports Medicine Clinic at Frisco [39065]
Baylor Institute for Rehab at Gaston Episcopal
Hospital [17864]
Baylor Rehabilitation System [39080]
Baylor Research Institute • Institute for Immunology
Research • Center of Research Translation •
Center for Lupus Research [181]
Baylor Speech and Hearing Clinic [3546]
Baylor University Medical Center • Baylor-Sammons
Cancer Center [5973]
Baylor University Medical Center, ESRD Transplant [27016]
Bayonet Point Health & Rehabilitation Center [1598]
Bayonet Point--Hudson Kidney Center • DaVita [23332]
Bayonne Hospital Renal Center • Dialysis Unit [25402]
Bayonne Medical Center • Center for Cancer Treat-
ment [5501]
Bayonne Visiting Nurse Association and Hospice [20458]
Bayou City Dialysis • DaVita [27126]
Bayou City Speech and Language [3502]
Bayou Region Supports and Services Center [8078]
Bayridge Sunset Park Dialysis Center [25604]
Bayshore Community Hospital [2920]
Cancer Center [5517]
Bayshore Counseling Services Inc
Erie County Outpatient Office [47851]
Ottawa County Outpatient Office [47838]
Bayshore Counseling Services, Inc. [31831]
Bayshore Dialysis Center • Fresenius Medical Care [27284]
Bayshore Medical Center • Cancer Program [6016]
Bayshore Podiatry Center [38290]
Bayside Dialysis Center [25576]
Bayside Health Center [6836]
Bayside Marin [40700]
Bayside NeuroRehabilitation Services [4071]
Bayside Orthopaedic, Sports Medicine and
Rehabilitation Center [38005]
Bayside Orthopaedics--C. Faunce Corner Road,
North Dartmouth [38562]
Bayside Orthopaedics--Pequot Bldg., North Dart-
mouth [38563]
Bayside and Special Services Library • Department
of Public Libraries [3845]

Bayside Therapy [11078]
Baystate Brightwood Health Center [6827]
Baystate Children's Hospital • Baystate Pediatric
Genetics [12236]
Baystate Community Services • Satellite [44573]
Baystate Franklin Medical Center
Oncology Program [5336]
Rehabilitation Center [2482]
Baystate Home Infusion and Respiratory Service--
Springfield [15546]
Baystate Home Infusion and Respiratory Services--
Greenfield [15497]
Baystate Medical Associates [38569]
Baystate Medical Center
Cystic Fibrosis Center [7565]
D'Amour Cancer Center [5356]
MDA Clinic [34810]
Neurodiagnostics and Sleep Center [37113]
Baystate Medical Center--Transplant [24801]
Baystate Reproductive Medicine [22098]
Baystate Visiting Nurse Association and Hospice--
Springfield [15547]
Baystate Visiting Nurse Association and Hospice--
Ware [15555]
Baytown Dialysis • DaVita [26963]
Baytown Dialysis Facility • Fresenius Medical Care [26964]
Baytown Opportunity Center [8532]
Bayview Behavioral Health Campus [28439]
Bayview Center for Mental Health [29227]
Broward Case Management [29136]
Crisis Stabilization Unit [29213]
Bayview Center for Mental Health--DART Program [29257]
Bayview Center for Mental Health--Fastrack [29258]
Bayview Center for Mental Health Inc [41765]
Bayview Center for Mental Health--START Program [29259]
Bayview Hunters Point Foundation
Substance Abuse Programs [40598]
Youth Services [40599]
BayView Professional Associates [27980]
BC Aphasia Centre [1049]
BCD Hoover Treatment Center [39543]
B.C.I. Greenleaf Day Program [29131]
B.C.I. Satellite Apartments [29168]
B.C.I. Supervised Apartments [29169]
BD Health Services [44114]
Be-Da-Bin Behavioral Health Program [44908]
BE Gentle Home Health, Inc. [17865]
BE Good HealthCare, Inc. [17866]
Be Well Now Institute Inc • Reeducation and
Rehabilitation Center [39689]
Beachcomber Family • Treatment Center [41625]
Beachcomber Retreat LLC • DBA As Bridging the
Gap Recovery [41886]
Beaches Ear, Nose and Throat [1603]
Beachway Therapy Center [41626]
Beachway Therapy Center LLC [41627]
Beacon Center
Daybreak Girls' Home [34040]
Daybreak Girls' Home--Princeton [34041]
Englewood [34046]
Marilee Center [34042]
Outpatient Chemical Dependency [46694]
Outpatient Chemical Dependency Program
[46349], [46550], [46754], [46945]
Beacon Children's Hospital [27967]
Beacon Community Residence [31240]
Beacon Counseling LLC [41109]
Beacon Healthcare Services, Inc. [18333]
Beacon Home Care, LLC [15779]
Beacon of Hope Hospice Inc.--Davenport [19681]
Beacon Hospice [19153]
Beacon Hospice-East Providence [21190]
Beacon Hospice, Inc-Augusta [19883]
Beacon Hospice, Inc-Charlestown [19951]
Beacon Hospice, Inc.--South Portland [19904]
Beacon Hospice-Keene [20436]
Beacon Hospice-Lewiston [19896]
Beacon Hospice-Longview [21516]
Beacon Hospice and Palliative Care-Fall River [19960]
Beacon Hospice & Palliative Care-Haverhill [19967]
Beacon Hospice and Palliative Care-Hyannis Office [20020]
Beacon Hospice-York [19908]
Beacon House [40342], [50390]

Beacon House Aftercare Program Inc [43678]
Beacon House Association of San Pedro [40688]
Channel View House [40689]
Lighthouse [40690]
Palos Verdes House [40691]
Beacon of the North [4156]
Beacon Orthopaedics and Sports Medicine [38893]
Beacon Place [20672], [30309]
Beacon Therapeutic Diagnostic and Treatment
Center [7936]
Beal Counseling and Consulting [48645]
The Beaman Home [9313]
Bear Creek Dialysis • DaVita [27127]
Bear Creek Speech Therapy LLC [3649]
Bear Lake Community Health Center, Inc. [7322]
Bear Lake Dialysis Center [23878]
Bear Paw Hospice • Hospice Program [20360]
Bear River Health Department
Division of Substance Abuse [49628]
Substance Abuse Treatment [49601]
Bear River Mental Health Center
Brigham City House [32576]
Group Home [32588]
Bear River Mental Health Center--Tremonton [32628]
Bear River Mental Health Services--Brigham City [32577]
Bear River Mental Health Services, Inc.--Logan [32589]
Bear River Mental Health Services--Randolph [32612]
Bear Valley Family Counseling [28414]
Beartooth Hospice [20371]
Beary Good Speech Services [1867]
Beatrice Community Hospital and Health Center, Inc. [16095]
Beatriz Home Health Care [13938]
Beau Cote • Eating Disorders Program [10910]
Beaufort County • Alcohol and Drug Abuse Depart-
ment [48905]
Beaufort County Hospital Association, Inc. Home
Health [16793]
Beaufort-Jasper-Hampton Comprehensive Health
Services, Inc. [7241]
Beaumont Dialysis Services--Berkley [24839]
Beaumont Home Health Service [17823]
Beaumont Hospital Dialysis--Hazel Park [24915]
Beaumont Kidney Center • American Renal Associ-
ates [26965]
Beaumont Sleep Evaluation Services • Macomb
Center [37146]
Beauregard De Ridder Community Help Line [50943]
Beauregard Memorial Hospital [15288]
Beauregard Mental Health Center [30137]
Beauregard Parish Schools [451]
Beaver Dam Dialysis Center [27701]
Becker Program [28813]
Beckley Speech Therapy Inc. [3651]
Beckley Treatment Center Inc [50282]
Beckley Veterans Affairs Medical Center [4488], [32885]
Beckman Center--Crisis Intervention [51332]
Bedford Counseling Center [32709]
Bedford Domestic Violence Services [10556]
Bedford Hospice Care [21676]
Bedford Park Dialysis Center • DaVita [25581]
Bedford Regional Medical Center [14963]
Cancer Program [5137]
Bedford Somerset Mental Health/Mental Retardation
Program [32121]
Bedford/Stuyvesant Alcohol Treatment Center
Holoman Halfway House [46475]
Outpatient Rehab [46476]
Bedford Stuyvesant Family Health Center [7015]
Beebe Home Health Agency [13559]
Beebe Medical Center [1513]
Dialysis Center [23191]
Robert and Eolyne Tunnell Cancer Center [4914]
Beech Brook--Cleveland [34374]
Beech Brook--Pepper Pike [34383]
Beechnut Dialysis Center [27128]
Beechwood Rehabilitation Services • Woods
Services [4385]
Beeler Street House [28854]
Beeville Dialysis & At Home • DaVita [26970]
Beeville Renal Center • Diversified Specialty

Institutes [26971]
Behavior Management Systems [32244]
    Crisis Intervention and Suicide Stabilization
        [51346]
    Full Circle [49006]
    Mainstream and IMPACT West [32245]
Behavior Management Systems - Northern Hills
    [32257]
Behavior Management Systems - Southern Hills
    [32227]
Behavior Services Center [42910]
Behavior Services Institute • CCESJ [41110]
Behavioral Awareness Center Inc [39487]
Behavioral Connections of Wood County [47837]
Behavioral Connections of Wood County, Inc.--
    Gypsy Lane [31663]
Behavioral Connections of Wood County, Inc.--North
    Prospect [31664]
Behavioral Connections of Wood County • Womens
    Residential Program [47626]
Behavioral Consultants • Wichita [43480]
Behavioral Counseling Associates [45995]
Behavioral Crossroads Recov Services LLC [45980]
Behavioral Health Adams County • Memorial
    Hospital Inc [43017]
Behavioral Health Alternative, Inc. of Madison
    County [50881]
Behavioral Health Alternatives, Inc. [29686]
Behavioral Health Branch • Substance Abuse
    Program [48969]
Behavioral Health Center [47338]
The Behavioral Health Crisis Team [50704]
Behavioral Health and Developmental Services •
    Rochester Clinic [31093]
Behavioral Health and Developmental Services of
    Strafford County [31068]
Behavioral Health Network Inc
    ADS Carlson Recovery Center [44577]
    My Sisters House [44578]
Behavioral Health Network, Inc. [30463]
Behavioral Health of the Palm Beaches [41728]
    [41729]
    Eating Disorders Program [11011]
Behavioral Health Resources [6706]
Behavioral Health Response--Maryland Heights
    [51058]
Behavioral Health Response--Saint Louis [51061]
Behavioral Health Service and Community Health
    Center [29638]
Behavioral Health Services [6309], [45821], [50265]
    American Recovery Center [40401]
    Feather River Tribal Health Center [40331]
Behavioral Health Services Inc [40078]
    Boyle Heights Family Recovery Center [40079]
Behavioral Health Services • Inglewood Community
    Recovery Center [39940]
Behavioral Health Services of the Lake County
    [29685]
Behavioral Health Services North [8342]
Behavioral Health Services North Inc • Twin Oaks
    Community Residence [46978]
Behavioral Health Services North, Inc. [31448]
Behavioral Health Services North • STOP Domestic
    Violence [9975]
Behavioral Health Services of
    Central DuPage Hospital [42967]
    Lake Norman [47422]
    Shenandoah Valley Medical Systems [50325]
Behavioral Health Services Outpatient • Campbell
    County Memorial Hospital [50583]
Behavioral Health Services
    Pacifica House [39907]
    Patterns [39908]
Behavioral Health Services of Pickens County
    [48970]
Behavioral Health Services
    Redgate Memorial Recovery Center [40017]
    South Bay Family Recovery Center [39884]
Behavioral Health Services of South GA [42170]
    Romer Jackson [42015]
Behavioral Health Services of South Georgia
    Ben Hill Mental Health Center [29423]
    Cook County Mental Health [29326]
    Turner Alternative Service Center [29338]
Behavioral Health Services • Wilmington Community
    Recovery Center [40959]
Behavioral Health Specialists Inc [45773]
    Sunrise Place [45774]

Behavioral Health Specialists, Inc. [31002]
Behavioral Health and Wellness Center • Copley
    Professional Services Group [49739]
Behavioral Healthcare Associates Ltd • Substance
    Abuse Services [42901]
Behavioral HealthCare Columbus [33448]
Behavioral Healthcare/Fauquier [49861]
Behavioral Medicine Center [50547]
    Brookfield [50373]
    Mukwonago [50490]
    New Berlin [50493]
Behavioral Mental Health Services • DBA
    Comprehensive Treatment Line [49629]
Behavioral Resources Inc [43704]
Behavioral Services Center [42411], [42749]
Behavioral Support Services Inc [42006]
Behavioral VA Healthcare Line [46576]
BehaviorCorp [29740], [29767]
BehaviorCorp Deaf Services [29741]
BehaviorCorp, Inc. [29742]
BehaviorCorp--Noblesville [29794]
BehaviorCorp • Outpatient Services [29743]
BeHome [17521]
Beier and Associates, LLC [17845]
Beit T Shuvah [40080]
Belair Clinic [49898]
Belcaro Dialysis • Davita [23108]
Belden Community Dialysis • DaVita [26031]
Belen Home Care Corporation [13939]
Belgrade Regional Health Center [6769]
Bell Center • Africenter Therapeutic Community
    [47709]
Bell Chem Dependency Counseling Inc [42360]
    Caldwell [42322]
    Harmony House [42349]
    Linden House [42323]
Bell Hill Recovery Center [45338]
Bell School Program for Deaf and Hard of Hearing
    Students [393]
Bell Socialization Services [32135]
Bell Therapy • Florist House [34485]
Bell Therapy--North 35th Street [32993]
Bell Therapy • Silver Lawn [32994]
Bella Vida Hospice [18909]
The Bella Vita • A Beautiful Life Psychology Group,
    Inc. [10931]
Bella Vita, Los Angeles [10932]
Bellaire Home Health Care, LLC [17965]
Bellaire Neurology [12467]
Belle Fourche Outreach [10365]
Belle Plaine Group Home [29584]
Belleair Dialysis Center • Fresenius Medical Care
    [23265]
Bellefaire JCB • Runaway and Homeless Youth
    Program [36140]
Bellefaire and Jewish Children's Bureau [34384]
Bellefaire Jewish Childrens Bureau • Substance
    Abuse Treatment Programs [47853]
Bellefontaine Habilitation Center [8208]
Bellefonte Home Health Care Agency--Greenup
    [15183]
Bellefonte Home Health Care Agency--Ironton
    [16948]
Belleview Orthopaedic Center [38217]
Belleville Veterans Affairs Clinic [29564]
Bellevue Behavioral Health Clinic [32806]
Bellevue Dialysis Center • DaVita [27594]
Bellevue Drug Co., Inc. [16221]
Bellevue Healthcare [18416]
The Bellevue Hospital [16850]
Bellevue Hospital • Cancer Care Center [5683]
Bellevue Hospital Center • Detox Unit [46817]
Bellevue Hospital • Dialysis Unit [25713]
The Bellevue Hospital home Health Agency [16891]
Bellevue Veterans Affairs Community Based
    Outpatient Clinic [29974]
Bellflower Dialysis Center • DaVita [22604]
Bellin Health System Hospital Center • Bellin Sleep
    Center [37964]
Bellin Home Health Agency [18570]
Bellin Psychiatric Center [33927], [50397]
Bellingham Behavioral Health Clinic [32809]
Bellingham IVF and Fertility Care [22294]
Bellmead Kidney Disease Center • Dialysis Facility •
    Fresenius Medical Care [26972]
BellMont Speech--Language Partners [2396]
Bellwood Health Services Inc. [11209]
Belmont Behavioral Health Center for

Comprehensive Treatment [33815]
Belmont Court Dialysis Center Inc. [26414], [26461]
Belmont Court Dialysis Center--Northeast Campus •
    Dialysis Facility [26502]
Belmont Court Dialysis Center--Roosevelt Campus
    [26503]
Belmont Court Dialysis Center--Warminster Campus
    [26595]
Belmont Court Dialysis--Fairless Hills Campus
    [26462]
Belmont Court Dialysis--Torresdale Campus [26376]
Belmont Dialysis Center • Fresenius Medical Care
    [25819]
Belmont Dialysis--Crestview [26190]
Belmont Pines Hospital [33762]
Beloit Area Community Health Center [7420]
Beloit Domestic Violence Center [10693]
Beloit Memorial Hospital
    Counseling Care [50368]
    Dialysis Center [27702]
Beloit Memorial hospital, Inc. [18558]
Beloit Regional Hospice [21824]
Belor Home Health, Inc. [17966]
Beloved Community Family Wellness [6652]
Belpre Dialysis & At Home • DaVita [26019]
Belton Police Department Victim Services Unit
    [9661]
Belton Veterans Affairs Clinic [30829]
Belvedere of Albany LLC • Specialized OP Services
    TBI Program [46752]
Belvedere CD Outpatient [46329]
Bemidji Area Program for Recovery [45083]
Bemidji Veterans Affairs Clinic [30661]
Ben Archer Health Center [6996]
Ben Atchley State Veterans Home [17701]
Ben El Child and Family Center [31661]
    Day Treatment [31662]
Ben Gordon Center [42616], [50838]
Benchmark Behavioral Health System [32630]
Bend Language and Learning [3304]
Bend Memorial Clinic • Sleep Center [37610]
Bend Orthopedic and Fracture • Orthopaedic Center
    of the Cascades [38915]
Bend Veterans Affairs Community Based Outpatient
    Clinic [17179]
Benedictine Hospital
    Cancer Program [5587]
    Chemical Dependency Inpatient Rehab [46740]
Benedictine School [8097]
Beneficial Hearing Center [1680]
Beneficial Home Health Services, Inc. [12913]
Benefis Dialysis Center [25308]
Benefis Health Care East • Pain Clinic [35534]
Benefis Health System [2834], [16089]
    Sletten Cancer Institute [5469]
Benefis Healthcare [45698]
Benefis Healthcare System • Sports Medicine
    [38681]
Benefis Peace Hospice of Montana [20358]
Benewah Medical Wellness Center [6641]
Benicia Dialysis Center • DaVita [22606]
Benilde Hall Program [45513]
Bennettsville Dialysis Center • Fresenius Medical
    Care [26682]
Bennington School [34460]
Bensalem Dialysis Center • American Renal Associ-
    ates [26377]
Bensalem House • Saint Joseph Children's Home
    [34406]
Bensonhurst Community Mental Health Center
    [31259]
Bentleyville Clinic [31993]
Benton Community Health Center [7125]
Benton County Dialysis Center [22528]
Benton County Dialysis & PD Center [22529]
Benton County Mental Health--Crisis Line [51250]
Benton Dialysis • DaVita [23898]
Benton and Franklin Counties Crisis Response Unit
    [51445]
Benton Hospice Service [20996]
Berea Primary Care Clinic [6724]
Berea Veterans Affairs Outpatient Clinic [29977]
Bereaved Parents of the USA [36476]
Bergen Care Home Health--Fort Lee [16217]
Bergen Care Home Health--Westwood [16292]
Bergen County Community Action Partner • Ladder
    Project [46006]
Bergen County Dept of Health Services • Addiction

Recovery Program [46007]
Bergen County Special Services • SHIP/HIP at
Midland [549]
Bergen County Speech and Language Associates
[2937]
Bergen RCC • Dialysis Center [25514]
Berger Hospice Care [20820]
Bering Sea Women's Group [8669]
Berkeley Addiction Treatment Services [39654]
Berkeley Adult Day Health Center [6289]
Berkeley Advanced Biomaterials Inc. [34934]
Berkeley Audiology Services [1065]
Berkeley City Mental Health--Adelene Street • Fam-
ily, Youth, & Children's Clinic [28404]
Berkeley City Mental Health--Center Street [28405]
Berkeley Community Mental Health Center [51335]
Berkeley Cottage [33199]
Berkeley County School District [733]
Berkeley County Schools • Hearing Impaired
Program [876]
Berkeley Dialysis Center • DaVita [22607]
Berkeley Drop-In Center [28406]
Berkeley Lodge [33200]
Berks Counseling Center Inc [48627]
Berks County Intermediate Unit [712]
Berks Deaf and Hard of Hearing Services [3375]
Berks Women in Crisis [10313]
Berkshire Farm Center and Services for Youth--
Binghamton [31243]
Berkshire Farm Center and Services for Youth--
Canaan [31296]
Berkshire Farm Center and Services for Youth--
Madison [34342]
Berkshire Farm Center and Services for Youth •
Outpatient Dept [46575]
Berkshire Farm Center and Services for Youth--
Plattsburgh [34345]
Berkshire Farm Center and Services for Youth •
Runaway and Homeless Youth Program [36089]
Berkshire Farm Center and Services for Youth--
Schenectady • Community Services Office [34355]
Berkshire Farm Center & Services for Youth--
Syracuse • Community Service Office [34357]
Berkshire Farm Center and Services for Youth--
Valatie [31482]
Berkshire Farms Services for Youth--Rochester
[34349]
Berkshire Meadows [8130]
Berkshire Medical Center
Cancer Program [5351]
Dialysis Unit [24793]
Berkshire Orthopedics Associates, Inc. [38993]
Berkshire Sleep Disorders Center [37114]
Berlin House [31103]
Berlin Vet Center [52019]
Berlin VNA [13513]
Bernalillo County • Metropolitan Assessment and
Treatment [46229]
Bernie Lorenz Recovery Inc [43260]
Bernies Lil Women Center [39725], [40081]
Bernstein House [31331]
Berrien County Health Department • Substance
Abuse Treatment Services [44664]
Berrien Springs Public School System • Special
Education Hearing Impaired Program [2561]
Bert Fish Medical Center [1676]
Bert Nash Community Mental Health Center [8028]
Bertha Sirk Dialysis Center • DaVita [24627]
Berwick Hospice [21053]
Bessa, Inc. • Mountain View Dialysis Center [27433]
Best Care Agency [14458]
Best Care Agency of Dade County [14263]
Best Care Health Systems Inc. [13294]
Best Care Home Health Agency Inc.--Torrance
[13386]
Best Care Home Health Agency, LLC--Glendale
[13023]
Best Care Home Health Services [15716]
Best Care, Inc.--Englewood, CO [13486]
Best Care, Inc.--Levittown, NY [16509]
Best Care Nursing & Residential Sources, Inc.
[15458]
Best Choice Home Care [16873]
Best Choice Home Health Care--Bronx [16354]
Best Choice Home Health Care--Brooklyn [16377]
Best and Dependable Home Health Care, Inc.
[18400]
Best Home Health Care, Inc. [17943]

Best Medical Services, Inc. [14191]
Best Recovery Healthcare Inc [49363], [49493],
[49569]
Best Solution Home Health Care [13940]
Bestcare Home Health Services [16280]
Bestcare Inc.--Bay Shore [16346]
Bestcare Inc.--Bronx [16355]
Bestcare Inc.--Brooklyn [16378]
Bestcare Inc.--Forest Hills [16463]
Bestcare Inc.--New York [16549]
Bestcare Inc.--Staten Island [16635]
Bestcare Inc.--Yonkers [16680]
BestCare • Programa de Recuperacion de Madras
[48145]
BestCare Treatment Services [48077], [48225]
BestCare Treatment Services--Madras [31950]
BestCare Treatment Services--Redmond [31966]
BestCare Treatment Services • Visions of Hope
[48226]
Betancourt Stuttering [1647]
Beth Israel Deaconess Hospital • Cancer Program
[5346]
Beth Israel Deaconess Hospital - Plymouth • Cancer
Program [5352]
Beth Israel Deaconess Medical Center - ALS Center
[120]
Beth Israel Deaconess Medical Center - Cancer
Program [5320]
Beth Israel Deaconess Medical Center - Critical
Care and Pain Medicine [35487]
Beth Israel Deaconess Medical Center--Transplant
[24743]
Beth Israel Hospital • Audiology Department [2452]
Beth Israel Medical Center
Albert Einstein College of Medicine • Pain
Management [35575]
Cancer Center [5594]
Department of Pediatrics [12282]
Division of Medical Genetics [12283]
Domestic Violence Department [9948]
Marie Nyswander Clinic [46818]
Methadone Clinic/Billies Place [46819]
MMTP Avenue A Clinic [46820]
MMTP Clinic 1 [46821]
MMTP Clinic 1E [46822]
MMTP Clinic 2 [46823]
MMTP Clinic 2C [46824]
MMTP Clinic 2F [46825]
MMTP Clinic 3 [46826]
MMTP Clinic 3C [46827]
MMTP Clinic 3G [46828]
MMTP Clinic 6/7 [46829]
MMTP Clinic 8 [46830]
MMTP Clinic 8D [46831]
MMTP Cumberland Clinic [46477]
MMTP Gouverneur Clinic [46832]
MMTP Saint Vincents Clinic [46833]
Speech and Hearing Program [3056]
Stuyvesant Square Chem Depend Treatment
Prog [46834]
Upper Manhattan Dialysis Center • Renal
Research Institute [25714]
Vincent Dole Clinic [46478]
Bethany for Children & Families • Runaway and
Homeless Youth Program [35923]
Bethany Christian Services
[36008]
Substance Abuse Counseling Program [44805]
Bethany Hall Inc • Recovery Home for Chemically
Dependent Women [49837]
Bethany Hospice Services [21135]
Bethany House [10175]
Bethany House Abuse Shelter, Inc. [9400]
Bethany House • Catholic Charities of Terre Haute
[9309]
Bethany House of East Alabama Medical Center
[18677]
Bethany Ranch Home [7740]
Bethel Colony of Mercy [47404]
Bethel Counseling Services [46087]
Bethel Family Counseling/Outreach Center [41944]
Bethel Licensed Home Care Agency [16583]
Bethel Outpatient Services [45127]
Bethel Port Rehabilitation Center [45128]
Bethesda Alcohol and Drug Treatment Program
[47651]
Bethesda Blue Ash Treatment Program [47652]
Bethesda Care/dba Keston Care [16704]

Bethesda Center for Reproductive Health and Fertil-
ity [22208]
Bethesda Centre for Speech & Hearing • Bethesda
Memorial Hospital [1546]
Bethesda Children's Home [34418]
Bethesda Hospital • Brain Injury Care [4218]
Bethesda, Inc. [18041]
Bethesda Lutheran Home [8630]
Bethesda Memorial Hospital • Comprehensive
Cancer Center [4931]
Bethesda North Hospital
Cancer Program [5690]
Sleep Center [37504]
Bethesda Recovery Center • Choices in Recovery/
Plumosa [40927]
Bethesda Rehabilitation Hospital [2739]
Bethlehem House [43088]
Bethpage Adolescent Development • Association Inc
[46377]
Beths Place • Branch of Triumph Treatment
Services [50266]
Bettendorf Veterans Affairs Clinic [29840]
Better Alternatives Counseling [43679]
Better At Home, Home Health [13588]
The Better Brain Center--Alexandria [12473]
The Better Brain Center--Washington [12396]
Better Choices Counseling Services [48146]
A Better Community Counseling Program [39742]
Better Hearing Center of San Leandro [1295]
Better Home Care, LLC--Feasterville Trevose
[17318]
Better Home Care, LLC--Huntingdon Valley [17347]
Better Home Health Care Agency, Inc.--Rockville
Centre [16618]
A Better Home Health Care--Akron [16825]
Better Home Health Care--Forest Hills [16464]
A Better Home Health Care, Inc.--Massillon [16983]
A Better Home Health Care--New Philadelphia
[17008]
Better Life Home Health [13941]
Better Living Now, Inc. [16474]
A Better Today Inc [48401], [48635], [48657]
A Better Tomorrow [40249]
A Better Way Counseling Center • Eating Disorder
Program [11248]
Better Way Counseling Services [44225]
Better Way of Greater Miami [6497]
A Better Way Home [19447]
Better Way of Miami Inc [41766]
Better Way Program [41525]
A Better Way Services [9300]
Betty Carter Home [27991]
Betty Clooney Foundation [3891]
Betty Ford Center at Eisenhower [40422]
Betty Griffin House [9077]
Betty Hardwick Center: A Community Mental Health
Resource [51368]
Betty Hardwick Center • Adult & Youth Outpatient/
Crisis Services [32397]
Betty Jane Memorial Rehabilitation Center [8429]
Between Friends [9202]
Beverly Dialysis • DaVita [23915]
Beverly Farm Foundation [7956]
Beverly Health & Rehabilitation Center of Searcy
[1038]
Beverly Healthcare [1918]
Beverly Hills Center for Domestic Conflict [8795]
Beverly Hills Dialysis Center • DaVita [22609]
Beverly Hills Speech and Language Center [1066]
Beverly Hospital • Cancer Program [5319]
Beverly Manor [1833]
Beverly Press Annex [6512]
Beverly Press Health Center [6513]
Beverly Rehabilitation & Healthcare Center [27840]
Beverly School for the Deaf [467]
Beverly Therapists [1979]
Bexar County Board of Trustees • Center for Health-
care Services [49517]
Beyamar Home Health Care, Inc. [17903]
Beyond Boundaries Speech Language Therapy
[3203]
Beyond Milestone Counseling [41051]
Beyond Play Therapy Group [2415]
Beyond Survival [10603]
Beyond Therapy Pediatric Group [2770]
BG Home Health Providers--Buffalo Grove [14701]
BG Home Health Providers--Northbrook [14883]

B.G. Tricounty Neurology and Sleep Clinic, PC [37147]
BGR Services CD Outpatient • DBA The PAC Program of Brooklyn [46479]
BH Health Services Inc [44383]
BHC Alhambra Hospital [28725]
BHC Alhambra Hospital Inc [40472]
BHC Alhambra Hospital • Reasons Eating Disorder Center [10933]
BHC Fairfax Hospital [33912]
BHC First Step [47417]
BHC Heritage Oaks Hospital Inc • Heritage Oaks Hospital Substance AbuseOutpatient Services [40480]
BHS- Broad Human Services • Counseling Center [46088]
Bi Bett Corp
    DAWN Center [40387]
    East County Community Womens Center [40388]
    East County Wollam House/Perinatal [40389]
    East Oakland Recovery Center [40292]
    Frederic Ozanam Center [39735]
    Frederic Ozanam Center/Crystal Palace [39736]
    Orchids Women Recovey Center [40293]
    Pueblos del Sol [39737]
    Shamia Recovery Center [40876]
    Southern Solano Alcohol Council [40877]
Bi Bett • Sunrise House Program [40204]
Bi--County Speech Language Pathology [1717]
BI Incorporated
    BI Day Reporting Center Colorado [40994], [41235]
    Denver Day Reporting Center [41111]
    Northglenn Day Reporting Center [41276]
BI-LINGUA Therapy Services [1596]
Bi Valley Medical Clinic
    Carmichael [39688]
    Norwood [40481]
Bibb County Board of Education [375]
Bida HHI California Health [12961]
Bienvenidos Childrens Center Inc • Institute for Womens Health [40082]
Bienvenidos Home Health Care, LLC [18078]
Bienville Dialysis Center North [24548]
Big Bend Hospice, Inc. • Carrabelle Office [19204]
Big Bend Hospice Inc • Madison Office [19250]
Big Bend Hospice, Inc.
    Monticello Office [19264]
    Perry Office [19299]
    Quincy Office [19306]
    Tallahassee Office [19318]
    Wakulla Office [19208]
Big Horn Basin Counseling [50568]
Big Horn Basin Counseling Services [50590]
Big Horn Counseling Center [33054]
Big Horn County Counseling Services [33031]
Big Horn Mountain Recovery Center LLC [50598]
Big Horn Mountain Recovery Center • Residential [50599]
Big Horn Regional Dialysis Center [27812]
Big Island Substance Abuse Council [42193]
    Kapolei Program Office [42252]
    North Hawaii Facility [42240]
    Oahu IOP/OP [42288]
    Outpatient Treatment Kealakekua Office [42261]
    Program Office [42194]
    School Based Program/Hilo Interm School [42195]
    School Based Program/Honokaa High School [42200]
    School Based Program/Honokaa Middle School [42201]
    School Based Program/Kalanianaole Elem and Inter [42281]
    School Based Program/Kau High School [42277]
    School Based Program/Keaau High School [42258]
    School Based Program/Keaau Middle School [42259]
    School Based Program/Kealakehe High School [42236]
    School Based Program/Kealakehe Inter School [42237]
    School Based Program/Kohala High School [42249]
    School Based Program/Kohala Middle School [42250]
    School Based Program/Konawaena High School [42262]
    School Based Program/Laupahoehoe High School [42264]
    School Based Program/Naalehu Inter School [42275]
    School Based Program/PaAuilo Elem and Inter [42276]
    School Based Program/Pahala Inter School [42278]
    School Based Program/Pahoa High School [42279]
    School Based Program/Pahoa Interm School [42280]
    School Based Program/Waiakea High School [42196]
    School Based Program/Waimea Middle School [42241]
    Waiakea Intermediate School [42197]
Big Oaks Dialysis • DaVita [24050]
Big Spring State Hospital [33862]
Big Springs Ranch for Children • Runaway and Homeless Youth Program [36210]
Big Stone Therapies [2723]
Big Timber Mental Health Center [30920]
Bilingual Counseling Center [44391]
Bilingual DUI Counseling and Clinical Services Inc [42476]
Bilingual Evaluation and Therapy Services [3188]
Bilingual Family Counseling Services • Center for Recovery [40318]
Bilingual Speech--Language Pathology Center Inc. [1575]
Bilingual Therapy Associates Inc. [1794]
Bilingual Therapy Center [1554]
Bill Brady Healing Center [39351]
Bill Willis Community Mental Health Center--Sallisaw [31914]
Bill Willis Community Mental Health Center--Tahlequah [31920]
Bill Willis Community Mental Health Center--Wagoner [31925]
Bill Willis Community Mental Hlth and • Substance Abuse Center/Adair County Satellite [48022]
Bill Wilson Counseling Center • Runaway and Homeless Youth Services [35806]
Billings Clinic [6923]
    Behavioral Health Clinic [30921]
    Dialysis Center [25303]
    Miles City Sleep Study [37296]
Billings Clinic Orthopedics and Sports Medicine [38675]
Billings VA Community Based Outpatient clinic • VA Montana Health Care System [4244]
Billings Veterans Affairs Clinic [30922]
Biloxi Public Schools Special Services [519]
Bimini Recovery Center • Mary Lind Recovery Centers [40083]
Bingham Behavioral Health [43527]
Bingham Child Guidance Center [8051]
Bingham Crisis Center [9158]
Binghamton Psychiatric Center • Community Treatment and Rehabilitation Center [33677]
Binghamton Veterans Affairs Clinic [31244]
Bio Dynamic Technologies [16202]
Bio-Medical Applications of Leawood • Fresenius Medical Care • Dialysis Facility [24333]
Bio Medical Behavioral Healthcare Inc [44706], [45046]
BioBank USA [34935]
Biogenetics Corp. [35113]
BioScrip Infusion Services--Elmsford [16450]
BioScrip Infusion Services--Morris Plains [16243]
Biotronics Kidney Center of Orange • Dialysis Facility [27279]
Birch House [29875]
Birch Tree Communities, Inc.
    AHC Campus [28241]
    Benton [28242]
    Benton Town Center [28243]
    Clarksville [28252]
    Clinton [28256]
    Conway [28256]
    Hope House [28244]
    Malvern [28312]
Birch Tree Communities, Inc., Melbourne, AR [28319]
Birch Tree Communities, Inc., Mountain View, AR [28327]
Birch Tree Communities, Inc.
    Newport [28330]
    Russellville [28344]
Birchwood Center [32954]
Bird and Bear Medical, Inc. [12866]
Birdville Regional Day School for the Deaf [795]
Birmingham Bloomfield Audiology [2562]
Birmingham Healthcare [39218]
Birmingham Metro Treatment Center [39219]
Birmingham Pain Center [35269]
Birmingham Veterans Affairs Medical Center [27846]
    Madison/Decatur Clinic [27971]
Biscayne Institutes of Health and Living, Inc. [3955]
Biscayne Milieu Health Center Inc [41767]
Biscayne Milieu Health Center Inc. [29238]
Bishop Hospice [21496]
Bismarck Public Schools [638]
Bismarck VA Outpatient Clinic [4350]
Bismarck Veterans Affairs Clinic [31621]
Bissonnet Dialysis Center [27129]
Bixby Knolls Dialysis • DaVita [22759]
Bixby Medical Center
    Hickman Cancer Center [5363]
    ProMedica Home Health Care [15569]
BJC Home Care Services--Alton, IL [14677]
BJC Home Care Services--Clayton Rd., Saint Louis, MO [16051]
BJC Home Care Services--Eager Rd., Saint Louis, MO [16052]
BJC Home Care Services--N Washington, Farmington, MO [16009]
BJC Home Care Services--Overland MO [16037]
BJC Home Care Services--Sullivan, MO [16076]
BJC Home Care Services--Weber Rd., Farmington, MO [16010]
BJC Hospice at Alton [19482]
BJC Hospice at Parkland [20294]
BJC Hospice at Sullivan [20344]
BJM Hospice, LLC/dba St. Jude Hospice [20186]
Black Alcohol/Drug Service Information Center • Charlotte Merrits Ottley Trans Women [45615]
Black Bear [1980]
Black Family Development Inc • Substance Abuse Services [44837]
Black Hawk Dialysis • DaVita [24305]
Black Hawk-Grundy Mental Health Center, Inc. [29901]
Black Hills Chronic Spine Pain [35669]
Black Hills Dialysis--Eagle Butte [26786]
Black Hills Dialysis--Pine Ridge [26793]
Black Hills Orthopedic and Spine Center [39022]
Black Hills Rehabilitation Hospital • Speech-Language Pathology Department [3414]
Black Hills Special Services Cooperative [8511]
Black Mountain Center [8368]
Black River Healthcare, Inc. [7238]
Black River Hospice [21825]
Black River Memorial Hospital, Inc. [18561]
Black Rock Dialysis • DaVita [23155]
Blackstone Adolescent Counseling Center • Community Counseling Center [32162]
Blackstone Valley Advocacy Center [10336]
Blackstone Valley Community Health Care Center, Inc. • Blackstone Valley Community Health Center [7221]
Blackwood Medical, Inc. [16187]
Blair House [31988]
Blairs Dialysis • Fresenius Medical Care [27465]
Blake Medical Center [1547]
    Cancer Care Center [4932]
Blanca Tavera Defensa de Mujeres [8924]
Blanchard Valley Dialysis Services • Innovative Dialysis Systems [26117]
Blanchard Valley Health System • Cancer Center [5722]
Blanchard Valley Sleep Disorders Center [37505]
Blanchard Valley Sports Medicine [38878]
Bland County Medical Clinic [7349]
Blandine House Inc [50391]
Blanding Family Practice Community Health Center [7319]
Blank Children's Hospital • Children's Health Center • Cystic Fibrosis Center [7543]
Bleeding and Clotting Disorders Institute •

Hemophilia Treatment Center [12515]
Blessed Drug and Alcohol Treatment and •
   Research Program Inc [40084]
Blessed Touch Home Health Agency, Inc. [17798]
Blessing Home Care [16038]
The Blessing Hospice-Greene County [19496]
The Blessing Hospice-Hancock County [19497]
The Blessing Hospice - Hannibal [20299]
The Blessing Hospice-Pike County [19564]
The Blessing Hospice--Quincy [19566]
Blessing Hospital [14909]
   Cancer Program [5122]
Bleuler Psychotherapy Center [31326]
Blick Clinic [8397], [10844], [31643]
Bliss Poston the Second Wind • Chemical
   Dependency Outpatient [46835]
Bliss Speech and Hearing Services Inc. [3478]
Block Institute [8302]
Blood and Tissue Center of Central Texas--Austin
   [35222]
Blood and Tissue Center of Central Texas--Bldg. L,
   Austin [35223]
Blood and Tissue Center of Central Texas--Cedar
   Park [35224]
Blood and Tissue Center of Central Texas--
   Georgetown [35225]
Bloomfield Dialysis • DaVita [23147]
Bloomfield Hills Deaf and Hard of Hearing Center
   Program [483]
Bloomfield-Pittsburgh Dialysis • DaVita [26543]
Bloomington Dialysis • Fresenius Medical Care
   [24117]
Bloomington Hospital • Cancer Center [5138]
Bloomington Hospital Home Health [14967]
Bloomington Hospital Home Health and Hospice
   [19587]
Bloomington Hospital
   Rebound Sports Medicine Center [38423]
   Rebound Sports Medicine Center, East [38424]
Bloomington Meadows GP [42996]
Bloomington Normal Audiology [1965]
Bloomington Veterans Affairs Outpatient Clinic
   [29699]
Bloomsburg University • Speech, Language, and
   Hearing Clinic [3324]
Blossburg Laurel Health Center [7153]
Blossom Home Health Care Agency, Inc. [15602]
Blossom Ridge Speech and Myofunctional Center,
   Inc. [1286]
Blossomland Learning Center [8165]
Blount Dialysis Center [26879]
Blount Memorial Hospital [17725]
   Cancer Program [5940]
   Emotional Health and Recovery Center [49128]
Blount Memorial Hospital Hospice [21344]
Blowing Rock Hospital/Davant Extended Care Facil-
   ity Home Health [16695]
Blue Ash Dialysis • Dialysis Center • DaVita [26037]
Blue Care Home Health Services, Inc. [13942]
Blue Dove Rehabilitation Inc. [1131]
Blue Earth County Violence Intervention Program •
   Committee Against Domestic Abuse [9608]
Blue Grass Community Hospital • Sleep Laboratory
   [37019]
Blue-Gray Community Hospice [19387]
Blue Horizon Eating Disorder Services • Eating
   Disorders Program [11012]
Blue Island Dialysis Center • Fresenius Medical
   Care [23902]
Blue Mountain Counseling of Columbia County
   [49934], [51436]
Blue Mountain Home Health Care [17377]
Blue Mountain Hospice [21008]
Blue Mountain Hospital Dialysis [27401]
Blue Mountain Kidney Center • DaVita [26337]
Blue Ridge Behavioral Health Care • Assesment
   Center [32782]
Blue Ridge Community Health Services [7052]
Blue Ridge Community Mental Health Center •
   Mitchell County Center [31594]
Blue Ridge Community Services [32783]
Blue Ridge Health Center, Inc. • Blue Ridge Medical
   Center [7348]
Blue Ridge Home Care--Asheville [16692]
Blue Ridge Home Care--Boone [16696]
Blue Ridge Home Care--Brevard [16699]
Blue Ridge Home Care--Marion [16751]
Blue Ridge Home Healthcare--Morganton • Grace

Hospital [16757]
Blue Ridge Hospice [21745]
Blue Ridge Hospital Systems, Inc. [16784]
Blue Ridge Medical [6586]
Blue Ridge Orthopaedics [39004]
The Blue Ridge PHP [33243]
Blue Ridge Speech and Hearing Center [3589]
Blue Skies Hospice, Inc. [19605]
Blue Skies Recovery Center [49643]
Blue Sky Bridge [8937]
Blue Sky Home Health Care, Inc. [13208]
Blue Sky Home Health Inc. [13198]
Blue Sky Orthopedics and Sports Medicine [38166]
Blue Springs Behavioral Health Clinic [33628]
Blue Star Home Health Agency [13943]
Blue Star Home Health, Inc. [12939]
Blue Valley Behavioral Health [45725], [45726],
   [45734], [45735], [45736], [45813], [45819]
Blue Valley Behavioral Health--Auburn [30973]
Blue Valley Behavioral Health--Crete [30980]
Blue Valley Behavioral Health--David City [30981]
Blue Valley Behavioral Health--Fairbury [30982]
Blue Valley Behavioral Health--Falls City [30983]
Blue Valley Behavioral Health--Geneva [30984]
Blue Valley Behavioral Health--Hebron [30990]
Blue Valley Behavioral Health--Nebraska City
   [31001]
Blue Valley Behavioral Health--Pawnee City [31011]
Blue Valley Behavioral Health--Seward [31012]
Blue Valley Behavioral Health • Substance Abuse
   Program [45817]
Blue Valley Behavioral Health--Tecumseh [31013]
Blue Valley Behavioral Health--Wahoo [31014]
Blue Valley Behavioral Health--York [31018]
Blue Valley Behaviorall Health [45771]
Blue Vista Home Health, Inc. [14240]
Blue Water Center for Independent Living [44895],
   [44974]
Blue Water Clinic [11097]
Blue Water Home Health Care [15668]
Blue Water Home Health care, Inc. [15788]
Blue Water Hospice [20106]
Blue Water Mental Health Clinic [51017]
Bluebonnet Trails Community Services [32541]
Bluegrass Comprehensive Center [30047]
Bluegrass Comprehensive Care Center • Nicholas
   County Comprehensive Care [43552]
Bluegrass Counseling Services [43649]
Bluegrass Domestic Violence Program [9391]
Bluegrass East Comprehensive Care Center
   Powell County Comprehensive Care [43788]
   Transitions [43650]
Bluegrass Education and • Treatment for Addiction
   [43595]
Bluegrass Farmworker Health Center [6731]
Bluegrass Impact--Frankfort [30016]
Bluegrass Impact--Lexington [30048]
Bluegrass Nutrition Counseling [11066]
Bluegrass Oxygen [15203]
Bluegrass Personal Care Home [30049]
Bluegrass Regional Mental Health [50935]
Bluegrass Regional MH/MR Board Inc
   Bourbon County Comprehensive Care [43754]
   Clark County Comprehensive Care [43802]
   Harrison County Comprehensive Care Center
   [43570]
Bluegrass South Comprehensive Care Center • The
   Recovery Center [43572]
Blueprint for Change [29518]
Blues Management Inc • DAPA Family Recovery
   Programs [49364], [49365]
Bluff City Dialysis & At Home • DaVita [25255]
Bluffton Counseling Services • Park Center Inc
   [42999]
Bluffton Regional Medical Center [14968]
Blum and Associates LLC [46066]
Blythe Mental Health and Substance Abuse [28417]
Blythedale Children's Hospital • Speech Pathology
   and Audiology Department [3139]
BMA--Avon Park • Fresenius Medical Care [23513]
BMA--Boynton Beach • Fresenius Medical Care
   [23247]
BMA--Clearwater • Fresenius Medical Care [23266]
BMA--Columbia Heights • Fresenius Medical Care
   [23209]
BMA--Cutler Ridge • Fresenius Medical Care
   [23388]
BMA--Deltona • Fresenius Medical Care [23292]

BMA Dupont Circle • Fresenius Medical Care
   [23210]
BMA Eureka • Fresenius Medical Care [22682]
BMA--Gainesville East • Fresenius Medical Care
   [23310]
BMA--Gainesville • Fresenius Medical Care [23311]
BMA--Hialeah • Fresenius Medical Care [23318]
BMA--Jacksonville • Fresenius Medical Care
   [23337]
BMA--Kendall • Fresenius Medical Care [23389]
BMA--Lake City • Fresenius Medical Care [23359]
BMA--Metropolitan Miami • Fresenius Medical Care
   [23390]
BMA--North Orlando • Fresenius Medical Care •
   Dialysis Facility [23231]
BMA--Palatka • Fresenius Medical Care • Dialysis
   Facility [23459]
BMA--Plantation • Fresenius Medical Care • Dialysis
   Facility [23481]
BMA--Port Saint Lucie • Fresenius Medical Care
   [23490]
BMA--Saint Johns • Fresenius Medical Care [23338]
BMA Santa Rosa • Fresenius Medical Care [23007]
BMA--South Collier • Fresenius Medical Care
   [23419]
BMA--South Ft. Myers • Fresenius Medical Care •
   Dialysis Facility [23303]
BMA--South Miami • Fresenius Medical Care
   [23391]
BMA--Tampa • Fresenius Medical Care • Dialysis
   Facility [23528]
BMA--West Date • Fresenius Medical Care [23392]
BMA--West Orlando • Fresenius Medical Care •
   Dialysis Facility [23444]
BMA--Ybor City • Fresenius Medical Care [23529]
BMRHC--Clinton Clinic [6263]
BNJ Health Services LLC [44285]
BNM Professional Consulting Services [2067]
BNV Home Care [16605]
Board of Education and Services for the Blind
   Adult Services [1508]
   Children's Services [1509]
Board Of Education City Of Birmingham Alabama
   [187]
Boardman Dialysis Center, LLC [26021]
Bob & Merle Scolnick Hospice House [20097]
Bob Michel Veterans Affairs Outpatient Clinic
   [29660]
Bob Stump Northern Veterans Affairs Medical Center
   • Multiple Sclerosis Center [34514]
Bobby Benson Center [42228]
Bobby Buonauro Clinic Inc [42662]
Bobby E Wright CBHC • Addictions Program
   [42477]
Bobby E. Wright Comprehensive Behavioral Health
   Center, Inc. [29585]
Boca Counseling Center [41564]
Boca Fertility [21987]
Boca Raton Artificial Kidney Center • DaVita [23241]
Boca Raton Community Based Outpatient Clinic
   [29112]
Boca Raton Community Hospital
   Home Health Services [13589]
   Lynn Regional Cancer Institute [4930]
Boca Raton Sleep Disorders Center [36773]
Boca Raton Speech and Rehabilitation Center Inc.
   [1542]
Body Dynamics Physical Therapy [38146]
The Body Image Therapy Center [11079]
Body, Mind, Therapy [11183]
Body Positive [10934]
Body Pros Physical Therapy--Alpharette [38304]
Body Pros Physical Therapy--Atlanta [38308]
Boerne Dialysis Center • DaVita [26974]
Bogalusa Mental Health Center [30133]
Boise Clinic [6631]
Boise Family Counseling [11041]
Boise Memorial Hospice [19456]
Boise State University • Women's Center [9159]
Boise Veterans Affairs Medical Center [29539]
Boise Veterans Center [29540]
Bolesta Center, Inc. [356]
Boley Centers for Behav Healthcare Inc [41740]
Boley Centers for Behavioral Healthcare, Inc.
   [29277]
Bolinas Community Health Center [6292]
Bolingbrook Dialysis • Fresenius Medical Care
   [23903]

Bolivar Dialysis • DaVita [26806]
Bollman Behavior and Speech Services Inc. [3363]
Bolton Family and Sports [38188]
Bolton Refuge House [10700]
Bon Homme School District [746]
Bon Secours Community Hospital [3099]
    Cancer Program [5619]
    New Directions [46987]
Bon Secours • Community Institute of Behavioral
    Health [30258]
Bon Secours DePaul Medical Center • Cancer
    Program [6072]
Bon Secours Home Care--Newport News [18334]
Bon Secours Home Care--Norfolk [18339]
Bon Secours Home Care--Portsmouth [18349]
Bon Secours Home Care--Richmond [18364]
Bon Secours Hospice--Portsmouth [21715]
Bon Secours Hospice--Richmond [21721]
Bon Secours Hospital Dialysis • Altoona Regional
    Health System [26369]
Bon Secours Hospital
    New Hope Treatment Center [44115]
    Renal Dialysis Unit [24628]
Bon Secours Maryview Medical Center • Cancer
    Program [6075]
Bon Secours Memorial Regional Medical Center •
    Cancer Program [6069]
Bon Secours Next Passage • Substance Abuse
    Program [44116]
Bon Secours Physical Therapy Sports Medicine
    [39127]
Bon Secours Saint Francis Health System • Cancer
    Program [5907]
Bon Secours Saint Mary's Hospital • Cancer Care
    Center [6079]
Bona Vista Comprehensive Rehabilitation Center
    [8002]
Bona Vista Rehabilitation Center [7997]
Bonaventura Reproductive Medicine [22056]
Bond Community Health Center, Inc. [6553]
Bond County Health Department • Prairie Counsel-
    ing Center [42692]
Bond County Hospice [19526]
Bondage Breaker Recovery Service Inc [40423]
Bone Bank Allografts [35226]
Bonfils Blood Center [34971]
Bonham Dialysis • DaVita [26976]
Bonita House--Berkeley [28407]
Bonita House--HOST [28670]
Bonita House--Oakland [28671]
Bonita Springs Dialysis • DaVita [23245]
Bonne Sante • Chemical Health and Wellness
    Center [43875]
Bonner Community Hospice [19479]
Bonner County Homeless Task Force • Domestic
    Violence Program [9188]
Bonner General Hospital [14673]
Bonneville Dialysis Center [27409]
Bonnie Brae [46036]
Bonnie Brae Educational Center [34301]
Bonnie House [34007]
Bonnie Mucklow • Families at Five [41039]
BonSecours Memorial Regional Medical Center
    [18331]
Bonutti Orthopaedic Services/Biomax Physical
    Therapy [38373]
Bookcliff Family Hearing Center [1415]
Boone County Domestic Violence Program [9295]
Boone County Hospital [2197], [15064]
Boone Hospital Center • Oncology Program [5440]
Boone Hospital Center Visiting Nurses Inc. [16001]
Boone Hospital Home Care [20290]
Boone Memorial Home Care [18510]
Booneville Human Development Center [7754]
Booth Memorial • Youth and Family Services
    [39307]
Border Area Mental Health Services--Deming
    [31190]
Border Area Mental Health Services--E 32nd Street,
    Silver City • Transitional Living [31218]
Border Area Mental Health Services Inc [46260],
    [46286], [46296], [46309], [46311]
    Substance Abuse Services [46310]
Border Area Mental Health Services Inc. [51128]
Border Area Mental Health Services--Lordsburg
    [31205]
Border Area Mental Health Services--N Silver Street,
    Silver City [31219]

Border Area Mental Health Services--Reserve
    [31212]
Border Area Mental Health Services--S Hudson
    Street, Silver City [31220]
Border Region Mental Health/Mental Retardation
    Center • Hebbronville [32476]
Border Region Mental Health/Mental Retardation •
    Rio Grande [32537]
Border Region MHMR Community Center • Laredo
    [32496]
Borger Family Service Center [32415]
Borgess Medical Center • Sleep Disorders Center
    [37148]
Borgess Visiting Nurse & Hospice [20076]
Borgess VNA Home Health & Hospice [15706]
Boriken Neighborhood Health Centers [7027]
Borinquen Behavioral Health • Resource Center
    [41768]
Borinquen Health Care Center, Inc. [6498]
Borinquen West Dade Health Care Center [6499]
Born2Win Ministries • Runaway and Homeless
    Youth Program [36129]
Borrego Community Health Foundation [6294]
Bossier Parish School District [448]
Bossier Regional Dialysis Center • Fresenius Medi-
    cal Care [24471]
Boston Alcohol and Substance Abuse Programs Inc
    [44405]
Boston Area Rape Crisis Center [9473]
Boston City Hospital • Comprehensive Sickle Cell
    Center [36356]
Boston College Campus School [8119]
Boston Dialysis Center • Fresenius Medical Care
    [24763]
Boston Dialysis • DaVita [24744]
Boston Hamilton House Inc • Hamilton Recovery
    Home [44445]
Boston Hearing Services [2468], [2538]
Boston Home Infusion, Inc. [15489]
Boston IVF • Bangor Women's HealthCare [22082]
Boston IVF--Brookline [22099]
Boston IVF, Inc • Central Maine Medical Center
    [22083]
Boston IVF - Metro West [22100]
Boston IVF
    Mount Auburn Hospital [22101]
    South Shore Center [22102]
    Waltham Center [22103]
Boston IVF--Worcester [22104]
Boston Medical Center [2453], [15474]
Boston Medical Center Family Medicine [38540]
Boston Medical Center
    Massachusetts Center for Sudden Infant Death
      Syndrome • Infant and Child Death Bereave-
      ment Program [36490]
    New England Regional Spinal Care Injury
      Center [4132]
    Pediatric Hematology/Oncology [36357]
    Psychiatric Services [50999]
Boston Medical Center--Transplant Surgery • Boston
    University School of Medicine [24745]
Boston Medical Center • University Hospital •
    Cancer Program [5321]
Boston Mountain Rural Health Center--Huntsville
    [6270]
Boston Mountain Rural Health Center, Inc.--Marshall
    [6275]
Boston Public Health Commission
    Addiction Services/Acupuncture Clinic [44406]
    Addiction Services/Outpt Counseling [44407]
    Entre Familia [44624]
    Narcotic Addiction Clinic Meth Services [44408]
    Transitions [44409]
Boston University
    Center for Anxiety and Related Disorders • Eat-
      ing Disorders Program [11086]
    Disability Services [468]
    Health Science Fitness Evaluation Center • Sar-
      gent College of Health & Rehabilitation Sci-
      ences [38541]
Boston University Medical Center • Genetics Clinic
    [12237]
Boston University School of Medicine • Arthritis
    Center • Multidisciplinary Clinical Research Center
    [166]
Boston Veterans Affairs Health Care System •
    Cancer Program [5322]
Boswell Center for Life Enrichment [11013]

Boswell Regional Center [8189]
Bothwell Regional Health Center [2823]
Bothwell Regional Health Center Home Health &
    Hospice [16066]
Botsford General Hospital [2582]
Botsford Hospital • Sleep Disorder Center [37149]
Boulder Alcohol Education Center [41013]
Boulder Center for Sports Medicine [38176]
Boulder Clinic [41014]
Boulder Community Hospital [41015]
    Behavioral Health [28858]
Boulder Community Hospital Behavioral Health
    Services [1381]
Boulder Community Hospital • Cancer Program
    [4869]
Boulder Community Sleep Disorders Center [36722]
Boulder County Public Health
    Addiction Recovery Center [41230], [41260]
    Addiction Recovery Center Broadway [41016]
    Addiction Recovery Center Valmont [41017]
Boulder County Safehouse [8938]
Boulder Dialysis • DaVita [23095]
Boulder Mountain Therapy [949]
Boulware Mission Inc • DUI Services [43733]
Boundary County Youth Crisis and Domestic
    Violence Hotline [50820]
Boundary County Youth Crisis Line and Domestic
    Violence Hotline [9165]
Boundary Regional Community Health Center
    Kaniska Health Services [6633]
    Sandpoint [6645]
Bountiful Treatment Center [49598]
Bourbon Community Hospital
    The Sleep Lab [37020]
    Stoner Creek Behavioral Health Centre [43755]
Bourbon County Dialysis • DaVita [24436]
Bournewood Health Systems • Bournewood Hospital
    [33576]
Bournewood Hospital [44442]
Bow Creek Recovery Center [42324]
Bowen Center • Otis R Services [43042]
Bowen Recovery Center [50012]
Bowers Hospice House • Hospice of Southern West
    Virginia [21785]
Bowery Residents Committee Inc
    Chemical Dependency Crisis Center [46836]
    Chemical Dependency Outpatient [46837]
Bowery Residents Committee, Inc. [31407]
Bowling Green CORPCARE Veterans Affairs Clinic
    [29979]
Bowling Green Inn • Brandywine [48422]
Bowling Green Kidney Center [24364]
Bowman's Home Care [16949]
Box Butte Dialysis Unit/Box Butte General Hospital
    [25315]
Box Elder School District [835]
Boyd Andrew Community Services [45685], [45703]
    Transitional Living Facility/Men [45686]
Boydton Community Health Facility, Inc. • Boydton
    Medical Center [7350]
Boyer Children's Clinic [8602]
Boynton Beach Dialysis Center • Fresenius Medical
    Care [23248]
Boynton/North Delray Dialysis • Davita [23289]
Boynton Speech Language Institute [1706]
Boys and Girls Aid Society of Oregon [31955]
The Boys and Girls Aid Society, Portland • Runaway
    and Homeless Youth Program [36166]
Boys and Girls Home of Alaska, Inc. [28087]
Boys and Girls Home and Family Services [33503]
Boys and Girls Home of Nebraska [34287]
Boys and Girls Republic [34222]
Boys and Girls Town of Missouri [30842]
    Columbia Center • Runaway and Homeless
      Youth Program [36045]
    Edgewood Children's Center • Runaway and
      Homeless Youth Program [36046]
    Great Circle • Runaway and Homeless Youth
      Program [36047]
Boys and Girls Town of Missouri, Saint James
    [30891]
Boys and Girls Town of Missouri, Saint Louis
    [30895]
Boys and Girls Town of Missouri • Springfield Center
    • Runaway and Homeless Youth Program [36048]
Boys Recovery Lodge • Phoenix Houses of the Mid-
    Atlantic [49760]
Boys Town Broward County • Runaway and Home-

less Youth Program [35876]
Boys Town Central Florida • Runaway and Home-
less Youth Program [35877]
Boys Town Chicago • Intervention and Assessment
Homes • Runaway and Homeless Youth Program
[35924]
Boys Town Home Campus • Runaway and Home-
less Youth Program [36064]
Boys Town National Research Hospital • Speech--
Language Pathology and Audiology Programs
[2854]
Boys Town Nevada • Assessment and Short-Term
Residential Program • Runaway and Homeless
Youth Program [36068]
Boys Town New England • Runaway and Homeless
Youth Program [36190]
Boys Town New York • Assessment and Short-Term
Residential Program • Runaway and Homeless
Youth Program [36090]
Boys Town North Florida • Intervention and Assess-
ment Services • Runaway and Homeless Youth
Program [35878]
Boys Town South Florida • Intervention and Assess-
ment Services • Runaway and Homeless Youth
Program [35879]
Boys Town Texas • Runaway and Homeless Youth
Program [36211]
Boys Town Washington DC • Assessment and
Short-Term Residential Program • Runaway and
Homeless Youth Program [35870]
Boys Village Youth and Family Services [29010]
Boystown Treatment Group Home [34282]
Bozeman Deaconess Cancer Center • Cancer
Program [5468]
Bozeman Deaconess Hospital [2831]
    Sleep Disorders Center [37297]
Bozeman Dialysis Center [25305]
Bozeman Help Center [9739], [51070]
Bozeman VA Community Based Outpatient Clinic •
VA Montana Health Care System [4245]
Bozeman Veterans Affairs Clinic [30928]
BPHC Substance Abuse Prevention and • Treatment
Services Satellite [44410]
BPX2 Inc./dba Bright Star Healthcare [14360]
BQC Home Health Agency, Inc. [18129]
Braddock Hospital • Cancer Care Program [5299]
Braden Counseling Center PC [42878], [42931]
Bradenton Artificial Kidney Center • Fresenius Medi-
cal Care [23252]
Bradenton Dialysis Center LLC • American Renal
Associates [23253]
Bradenton Dialysis • DaVita [23254]
Bradford County Clinic [29292]
Bradford Dialysis • DaVita • Dialysis Center & At
Home [26384]
Bradford Family Center [31996]
Bradford Health Center [7332]
Bradford Health Services [28064], [49103]
    Anniston Regional Office [39206]
    Augusta Regional Office [42042]
    Birmingham Regional Office/Jefferson [39220]
    Boaz Regional Office [39231]
    Chattanooga Regional Office [49047]
    Clarksville Regional Office [49056]
    Columbus Regional Office [42057]
    Cookeville Regional Office [49063]
    Dothan Outreach [39240]
    Florence Outreach [39243]
    Franklin Regional Office [49074]
    Huntsville Madison Inpt and Outpatient [39268]
    Huntsville Regional Office [39259]
    Manchester Outreach/Coffee [49126]
    Mobile Regional Facility [39271]
    Montgomery Regional Office [39278]
    Nashville Outreach [49153]
    Tuscaloosa Regional Office [39283]
    Warrior Lodge/Jefferson [39301]
Bradford Recovery Systems • Bradford Regional
Medical Center [48302]
Bradley - Angle House, Inc. [10245]
Bradley Center of Saint Francis Hospital [42058]
Bradley Dialysis Clinic • Fresenius Medical Care
[26820]
Bradley Health Care Center [17755]
Bradley Hospital [33829]
Bradley Manor [31704]
Braille Institute • Library Services [3752]
Brain Focus LLC [10884]

Brain Injury Day Treatment Program [3892]
Brainerd Regional Human Services Center [33605]
Brainerd Veterans Affairs Clinic [30664]
Braintree Rehabilitation Hospital [2464]
Branch County Coalition Against Domestic Violence
[9527]
Branch County Home Health and Hospice • Com-
munity Health Center [20050]
Branches [10675]
Brandon Artificial Kidney Center • Fresenius Medical
Care [23256]
Brandon Dialysis Center • Diversified Specialty
Institutes [23257]
Brandon East Dialysis • DaVita [23258]
Brandon Internal Medicine [7333]
Brandon Residential School and Treatment Center
[30422]
Brandon Residential Treatment Center, Inc. [34202]
Brandon Valley School District 49--2 [742]
Brandywine Center, LLC [11009]
Brandywine Counseling and Community Services
[41517]
Brandywine Counseling • South Chapel [41512]
Brandywine Hospital • Cancer Program [5818]
Brandywine River Valley Hospice [21125]
Branford Counseling Center [28972], [41359]
Branford Dialysis • DaVita [23148]
Branford Public Schools [328]
Brannon and Brannon
    Psych Services /Jefferson Cnty Probation
    [42370]
    Psychological Services [42369]
Branson Dialysis, LLC [25176]
Brantley Center, Inc. [29517]
Brantly Behavioral Health [29480]
Brattleboro Area Hospice [21661]
Brattleboro Memorial Hospital [3561]
The Brattleboro Retreat [33896]
Brattleboro Retreat
    Adult Alcohol Abuse Program [49725]
    Ambulatory Services [49726]
    Starting Now [49727]
Braxton County Fellowship Home [50344]
Brazoria--Fort Bend RDSPD [826]
Brazos Dialysis Center [27304]
Brazos Kidney Disease Center - Waco • Fresenius
Medical Care [27387]
Brazos Place [49347]
Brazos Valley Council on Alcohol and Drug •
(BVCASA) [49257]
Brazos Valley Council on Alcohol and SA [49258]
Brazos Valley Regional Day School for the Deaf
[777]
Brazosport Memorial Hospital
    Cancer Program [6008]
    Southwest SIDS Research Institute [36544]
Brazosport Regional Home Health [18032]
Brea Canyon Pain Relief and Rehabilitation Medical
Center [38077]
Brea Dialysis Center • DaVita [22613]
Break the Cycle [8837]
Break the Cycle Inc [41580]
Breakaway Health Corporation • Breakaway [39746]
Breaking Free, Alternatives to Domestic Violence
[9283]
Breaking Free Inc [42393]
Breakthrough [31956]
Breakthrough Clinic [11184]
Breakthrough Recovery Services Inc [41668],
[41839], [41933], [41986]
Breakthroughs Counseling and Recovery [41698]
Breakthru House Inc [42077]
Breath of Life Counseling Services LLC [46167]
Breatheasy Respiratory Services, Inc. [16246]
Breckenridge County Industries [30025]
Breckinridge Health, Inc. [15185]
Breese Dialysis • Renal Advantage Inc. [23905]
Breeze Health Care, Inc.--Dania [13635]
Breeze Health Care, Inc.--North Miami Beach
[14267]
Breeze Home Health Agency [13944]
Brehm Preparatory School [7931]
Brehm Prepatory School [1973]
Brema Healthcare, Inc. [17867]
Bremen Youth Services [42819]
Bremerton School District [859]
Brenford Place Residential Treatment Center
[34058]

Brenham State School [8537]
Brennan Speech Services Ltd. [1981]
Brentwood Clinic South [49330]
Brentwood Hospital [43891]
Brentwood Hospital--Jackson • Brentwood
Behavioral Healthcare of Mississippi [33616]
Brentwood Hospital--Shreveport [33548]
Brentwood Laboratory • Lifeline Sleep Disorders
Center [37638]
Brentwood Meadows [43168]
Brentwood Treatment Services [49331]
Brevard Best Care, Inc. [14307]
Brevard Counseling Center [47230]
Brevard County Exceptional Education [358]
Brevard County Libraries • Talking Books Library
[3759]
Brevard Learning Clinic [7892]
Brevard Outpatient Alternative Treatment • (BOAT)
[41932]
Brewer Rehab and Living Center [4072]
The Brewster Center • Domestic Violence Services
[8735]
Brewster Group--Hollywood [13792]
Brewster Group--Miami [13945]
Brewton Satellite Office [27874]
Brickell Home Health Services [13621]
Bridge to Awareness Counseling Center Inc [41052],
[41053], [41292]
Bridge Back of the Kingston Hospital
    Chemical Dependency Outpatient [46741]
    Methadone Maintenance [46742]
Bridge Back to Life Center Inc [46480], [46481],
[47089]
    Chemical Dependence Outpatient [46378]
    Chemical Dependence Outpatient Rehab
    [46482]
    Outpatient Services [46838]
Bridge Center of Schenectady Inc • Residential
Treatment Program [47071]
The Bridge of Central Massachusetts
    Northborough Community Residence [30437]
    Southboro Program [34196]
Bridge Clinic Antigo [7419]
Bridge Counseling Associates [45835]
The Bridge Family Center, Inc. • Runaway and
Homeless Youth Program [35862]
Bridge Health Recovery Center • Pain Center
[35742]
Bridge Home Health and Hospice [20804], [20841]
Bridge Home Health and Hospice--Bowling Green
[16855]
Bridge Home Health and Hospice--Findlay [16938]
Bridge Home Health and Hospice--Tiffin [17050]
Bridge Home Healthcare, Inc. [15717]
Bridge to Hope [10698]
Bridge House Inc [43867], [44117]
Bridge Inc [39248], [45743], [45950], [46017]
    Fort Payne Recovery Center [39245]
Bridge Inc/OASAS Program • Outpatient/Intensive
Outpatient [46839]
Bridge Inc
    Recovery Center for Teens [39272]
    Recovery Center for Teens/Ashville [39208]
    Recovery Center for Teens/Cullman [39234]
    Recovery Center for Teens/Tuscaloosa [39295]
    Westwood [39273]
Bridge Mental Health Continuum--Norman [33778]
Bridge Mental Health Continuum--Oklahoma City
[33780]
Bridge Over Troubled Waters Inc [44411]
Bridge Over Troubled Waters, Inc. [10497]
The Bridge Over Troubled Waters, Inc. • Runaway
and Homeless Youth Program [35996]
A Bridge to Recovery [11111]
Bridge to Recovery [45417], [45419]
Bridge for Runaway Youth • Runaway and Home-
less Youth Program [36031]
Bridge Way Recovery • Overland Park [43433]
A Bridge to Well Being PC [41221]
Bridge Youth and Family Services [42838]
BridgeCross Treatment Centre for Eating Disorders
[11210]
Bridgemark Inc [48887]
BridgePoint Center for Eating Disorders [11267]
Bridgepoint Rehabilitation Center [2135]
Bridgepointe Services and Goodwill of Southern
Indiana [7982]
Bridgeport Community Health Center, Inc. [6418]

Bridgeport Dialysis • DaVita [23150]
Bridgeport Home Health Care [13699]
Bridgeport Hospital
    Center for Sleep Medicine [36736]
    Norma F. Pfriem Cancer Institute [4888]
    Panetierri Burn Center [4530]
Bridgeport Public Schools SLH [329]
Bridger Health Center [6951]
Bridgerland Dialysis Facility [27407]
Bridges--A Community Support System [29011],
    [50732]
Bridges Against Domestic Violence [10378]
Bridges of America • Orlando Bridge [41849]
Bridges • A Community Support System Inc [41425]
Bridges Counseling and DUI Services [42383]
Bridges: Domestic Violence and Sexual Violence
    Support [9813]
Bridges Forensic Counseling Services [49605]
Bridges Inc • Outpatient Services [40482]
Bridges--Orange Family Counseling [29041]
Bridges Treatment and Recovery [49899], [49963]
BRIDGES of Williamson County [10402]
BridgesHome Health Care [16989]
Bridgeton South Jersey Hospital • Dialysis Unit
    [25411]
Bridgewater Dialysis Center • DaVita [25407]
Bridgewater State Hospital [33573]
BridgeWay [39563]
Bridgeway Behavioral Health [45671]
Bridgeway Behavioral Health Inc [45601], [45661],
    [45665]
Bridgeway Behavioral Health
    Montgomery City [45572]
    Saint Charles Center [45602]
Bridgeway Center Inc
    Addictions/Substance Abuse Program [41676]
    CASA [41677]
Bridgeway Center, Inc. [29132]
Bridgeway Center, Inc.--Day Services [29170]
Bridgeway Center, Inc. • Geriatric Residential Treat-
    ment System [29133]
Bridgeway Counseling Services • Women's Center
    [9713]
Bridgeway Hospice [21458]
Bridgeway Hospital [33124]
Bridgeway Inc [42682], [42731], [42784], [45981],
    [48007]
Bridgeway, Inc. • Administrative Office [31705]
Bridgeway, Inc.--Cleveland [31706]
Bridgeway, Inc.--Galesburg [29623], [50847]
Bridgeway, Inc.--West Side [31707]
Bridgeway--Keokuk [50906]
Bridgeway--Kewanee [50853]
Bridgeway--Macomb [50857]
Bridgeway--North Pekin [50862]
Bridgeway Psychiatric Center [30151]
Bridgeway Rehabilitation Services, Inc. [31126]
Bridgeway Robertson Center [9732]
Bridgeway/The Lodge [29624]
Bridging the Gaps Inc
    Drayton House [49867]
    Substance Abuse and Outpatient Services
        [49868]
Bridging the Tys to Jordan Inc [42478]
Brief Intensive Treatment Home • JBS Mental Health
    Authority [27847]
The Brien Center [30441]
The Brien Center - Brenton Group Home [30442]
The Brien Center - Central - Child and Adolescents
    [30443]
The Brien Center - Elm Group Home [30444]
The Brien Center - Forensic Services [30445]
Brien Center • Keenan House [44537]
Brien Center for Mental Health and Substance
    Abuse • Satellite [44538]
Brien Center • Mental Health/Substance Abuse
    Services [44539]
The Brien Center - Transitions [30446]
Brigham and Women's Hospital
    Adult Sickle Cell Program [36358]
    Boston Hemophilia Center [12529]
    Burn Center [4560]
    Center for Assisted Reproductive Medicine
        [22105]
    Department of Medicine, Rheumatology, and
        Immunology • Multidisciplinary Clinical
        Research Center [167]
    Dialysis Center [24746]

Brigham and Women's Hospital Dialysis Unit
    [24747]
Brigham and Women's Hospital
    HIV Vaccine Trials Unit [84]
    John R. Graham Headache Clinic [12431]
    Pain Management [35488]
    Renal Genetics Center [12238]
Brigham Young University • Human Performance
    Research Center [39105]
Bright Care Home Health Inc. [13381]
Bright Care Home Health Provider [13224]
Bright Dialysis • DaVita [23306]
Bright Future Foundation [8935]
Bright Horizon Home Health Services, Inc. [13121]
Bright Horizons [9778]
Bright Kavannagh House [19742]
Bright Path Counseling Center • Chemical
    Dependence Outpatient [47112]
Bright Path Speech Therapy [1883]
Bright Point Therapies, Inc. [2134]
The Bright School for the Deaf [455]
Bright Star--Brighton [15593]
Bright Star Care--Cincinnati [16874]
Bright Star--Novi [15761]
Bright Stars Speech Therapy [2289]
Bright Start Children's Rehabilitation Center [3473]
Bright Start Pediatric Services [3016]
Bright Start Therapies--Cirby Way, Sacramento
    [1245]
Bright Start Therapies--Watt Avenue, Sacramento
    [1246]
Brighter Tomorrows--Grand Prairie [10467]
Brighter Tomorrows Inc [43179]
Brighter Tomorrows, Inc.--Shirley [9986]
Brightmoor Hospice, Inc. [19390]
Brighton Bridge Hospice, LLC [19869]
Brighton Center, Inc. • Runaway and Homeless
    Youth Program [35965]
Brighton Hospital • Chemical Dependency Treatment
    Programs [44679]
Brighton Medical Center • Paincare Center [35473]
Brighton Salud Family Health Center [6389]
Brightside for Families and Children [8157]
BrightStar Care--Jupiter, FL [13825]
Brightstar Care of Northern Michigan [15855]
BrightStar--Miami, FL [13946]
Brimhall Dialysis • DaVita [22594]
Brimm Intensive Residential Program [31109]
Bringas Home Health, LLC [13947]
Brislain Learning Center [7769]
Bristlecone Family Resources [45865]
    Outpatient Services [45866]
Bristlecone Health Services Inc.--Frisco [13489]
Bristol Bay Area Health Corporation • Behavioral
    Health - Jakes Place [39323]
Bristol Bay Counseling Center [28085], [50632]
    Our House Crisis Respite Home [28086]
Bristol Hospice - California LLC [18966]
Bristol Hospice, Hawaii LLC [19437]
Bristol Hospice Sacramento [19004]
Bristol Hospice-Salt Lake City [21642]
Bristol Hospital [41370]
    Cancer Care Center [4890]
Bristol Hospital Counseling Center • Outpatient
    Program [41371]
Bristol Hospital, Inc. Home Health [13515]
Bristol Regional Counseling Center [32273]
Bristol Speech and Hearing Center [3574]
Bristol Youth Academy Residential Treatment
    [34065]
British Columbia Children's Hospital
    Burn Program [4511]
    Eating Disorders Program [10911]
British Columbia Provincial School for the Deaf [249]
British Columbia School for the Deaf [250]
Broad Horizons [34012]
Broad Reach Hospice and Palliative Care [19986]
Broadalbin--Perth Central School [567]
Broader Horizons Counseling Services [41112]
Broadlawns Medical Center • Addiction Treatment
    Services [43261]
Broadview Emergency Shelter [10641]
Broadway Counseling Services Inc [41166]
Broadway Counseling Services LLC [41113]
Broadway Dialysis Center • Elmhurst Hospital
    [25660]
Broadway Home Health Services, Inc. [13024]
Broadway House Inc [47909]

Broadway, Inc. • K Bar B Youth Ranch [34160]
Broadway Kidney Disease Center • Dialysis Center
    • Fresenius Medical Care [27315]
Broadway Medical Office [6463]
Broadway Respite and Home Care [16214]
Brockton Addiction Treatment Center [44428]
Brockton Area Multi-Services [30350]
Brockton Dialysis Center • Fresenius Medical Care
    [24753]
Brockton Helpline [50986]
Brockton Multi-Service Center [30351]
Brockton Neighborhood Health Center [6810]
Brockton Regional Kidney Center [24754]
Brockton Visiting Nurse [2465]
Brockton Visiting Nurse Association [15480]
Broe Rehabilitation Services, Inc. [4157]
Bromenn Home Health Services [14880]
BroMenn Hospice [19547]
BroMenn Regional Medical Center • Cancer Care
    Program [5115]
Bronson Methodist Hospital [4564]
Bronson Methodist Hospital Home Health Care
    [15707]
Bronx Addiction Treatment Center • CD Inpatient
    Rehab Program [46409]
Bronx Community Home Care [16356]
Bronx Comprehensive Sickle Cell Center [36389]
Bronx Dialysis Center & At Home • DaVita [25582]
Bronx Lebanon Hospital Center • Alcoholism
    Halfway House [46410]
Bronx-Lebanon Hospital Center • Bronx AIDS
    Research Consortium • Community Program for
    Clinical Research on Aids [60]
Bronx Lebanon Hospital Center
    Community Residential Program [46411]
    Department of Pediatrics • Pediatric AIDS Clini-
        cal Trials Unit [17]
    Detoxification Unit [46412]
Bronx-Lebanon Hospital Center • Inpatient
    Rehabilitation Program [46413]
Bronx Lebanon Hospital Center • MMTP [46414]
Bronx--Lebanon Hospital • Multiple Sclerosis Center
    [34643]
Bronx Psychiatric Center [33679]
Bronx Pulmonary Center for Pulmonary, Asthma and
    Sleep Disorders [37377]
Bronx River Nephro Care Inc. • Dialysis Facility
    [25583]
Bronx River Nephrology Care/Jewish Home and
    Hospital Life Care System [25584]
The Brook Hospital-Dupont [43680]
Brook Hospital • KMI/Substance Abuse Services
    [43681]
Brook Lane Health Services [33563]
Brookdale Hospital Medical Center [16498]
    Department of Pediatrics • Division of Genetics
        [12284]
Brookdale University Hospital and Medical Center
    Comprehensive Pediatric Sickle Cell Program •
    Community-Based Sickle Cell Project [36390]
    Dialysis Center [25605]
Brooke Army Medical Center • Cancer Program
    [5988]
Brooke Glen Behavioral Hospital [33804]
Brookhaven Home for Boys Inc. [34461]
Brookhaven Hospice, LLC-Framingham [19962]
Brookhaven Hospital [33785]
    Rader Programs [11201]
Brookhaven Memorial Hospital
    Acute Unit [25753]
    Dialysis Satellite [25648]
Brookhaven Memorial Hospital Med Center •
    Outpatient Behavioral Health Services [46973]
Brookhaven Memorial Hospital Medical Center
    [3092], [16588]
Brookhaven Memorial Hospital Medical Center
    Hospice [20595]
Brookhaven Retreat [49187]
Brookhollow Dialysis • DaVita [27130]
Brookings Hospital Hospice [21290]
Brookline Community Mental Health Center [30354]
    Runaway and Homeless Youth Program [35997]
Brookline Dialysis • DaVita • Dialysis Center [24755]
Brooklyn AIDS Task Force • Outpatient Drug Abuse
    Clinic [46483]
Brooklyn Campus of the Veterans Affairs • New York
    Harbor Healthcare System [51611]
Brooklyn Children's Psychiatric Center [33681]

Brooklyn Developmental Disabilities Services Office--
  Brooklyn [8303]
Brooklyn Hospital Center • 9B Detox Unit [46484]
The Brooklyn Hospital Center • Cancer Resource
  Center [5564]
Brooklyn Hospital Center
    Department of Obstetrics/Gynecology and
      Pediatrics
        Pediatric Genetics [12285]
        Reproductive Genetics [12286]
    Dialysis Unit [25606]
The Brooklyn Hospital Center Home Health Services
  [16379]
Brooklyn Hospital Center--II • Dialysis Unit [25607]
Brooklyn Kidney Center [25608]
Brooklyn Plaza Medical Center, Inc. [7016]
Brooklyn/Westside Fertility Center • Fertility Center
  [22178]
Brookriver Dialysis & At Home • DaVita [27017]
Brooks Counseling LLC [41011], [41078]
Brooks County Dialysis Facility [23772]
Brooks Memorial Hospital • Dialysis Unit [25649]
Brooks Rehabilitation Healthcare Plaza [3956]
Brooks Rehabilitation at Healthcare Plaza--
  Outpatient 1 • Pain and Spinal Rehabilitation
  Center [35378]
Brooks Rehabilitation Hospital [1604], [3957],
  [35379]
Brooks Rehabilitation-Ponte Vedra Beach [3958]
Brookside Community Health Center [6362], [44489]
Brookwood Dialysis Clinic • DaVita [22438]
Brookwood Florida - Central, Inc. [34083]
Brookwood Florida - East, Inc. [34068]
Brookwood Medical Center [27848]
    Brookwood Sleep Disorders Center [36568]
    Cancer Program [4723]
Brookwood Outpatient Rehabilitation for Women
  [37992]
Broome Developmental Disabilities Service Office--
  Binghamton [8298]
Broomfield Mental Health Center • Emergency
  Psychiatric Service [50711]
Brothers Home Health Care [13653]
Broughton Hospital [33740]
Broward Addiction Recovery Center • BARC -
  Central [41648]
Broward Adolescent Therapeutic Community [29266]
Broward Community and Family Health Center
  [6570]
Broward County Elderly and Veteran Services
  [29154]
Broward County Talking Book Library [3760]
Broward Dialysis • DaVita [23297]
Broward Fluency Clinic [1566]
Broward General Medical Center
    Cancer Program [4940]
    MDA Clinic [34777]
    Sleep Disorders Center [36774]
Broward Hearing and Balance Center [1725]
Broward Home Health Care Services Corporation
  [14320]
Broward House Inc • Substance Abuse Treatment
  Program [41649]
Broward Nursing Care [14345]
Broward Partnership for Homeless [6461]
Broward Treatment Center [41689]
Brown Baptist Youth Ranch [34152]
Brown Cancer Center • Hemophilia Treatment
  Center [12523]
Brown County Counseling [31771]
Brown County General Hospital [16943]
Brown County Human Services [33928]
Brown County Human Services Department • IV
  Drug Abuse Treatment [50398]
Brown County Victim Services [9627]
Brown University • Centers for AIDS Research [70]
Brownfield Dialysis • AccessCare [27233]
Brownsville Community Development Corp. •
  Brownsville Multi-Service Family Health Center
  [7017]
Brownsville Community Health Center [7279]
Brownsville Community Residential Center [46485]
Brownsville Dialysis • DaVita [26808]
Brownsville Kidney Center • Dialysis Facility •
  Diversified Specialty Institutes [26979]
Brownsville RDSPD [775]
Brownwood Intermediate School District [776]

Brownwood Renal Care Center • Dialysis Facility
  [26982]
Bruce Hall [48930]
Bruce W. Carter Department of Veterans Affairs
  Medical Center [3959]
Brunswick Dialysis Center • Fresenius Medical Care
  [26134]
Brunswick-Glynn County Regional Library • Three
  Rivers Regional Library [3772]
Brunswick Hospital Center [33673]
Brushton-Moira Central School [31282]
Bryan Dialysis • Fresenius Medical Care [26983]
Bryan Granelli PhD [46150]
Bryan LGH • Center for Sleep Medicine [37311]
Bryan LGH Medical Center • Cancer Program
  [5476]
Bryan LGH Medical Center West • Independence
  Center [45751]
Bryan W. Whitfield Memorial Hospital [12647]
    Sleep Disorders Center [36569]
BryanLGH Medical Center [16108]
Bryant Community Health Center [7244]
Bryant School District [243]
Bryce Hospital [33100]
BryLin Hospital [33690]
BryLin Hospitals • Williamsville Outpatient Clinic
  [47192]
Bryn Mawr College • Child Study Institute [8451]
Bryn Mawr Dialysis Services • Fresenius Medical
  Care [26388]
Bryn Mawr Hospital/Main Line Health • Bryn Mawr
  Hospital Sleep Medicine Services [37639]
Bryn Mawr Hospital • Main Line Health Hospitals •
  Comprehensive Cancer Care Center [5815]
Bryn Mawr Rehabilitation Hospital [4386]
BSA Hospice [21378]
    Baptist St. Anthony's Health System [21543]
BSLP [40600]
BT Healthcare Services [15430]
Buchanan General Hospital [18306]
Buchanan General Hospital Home Health Agency
  [18307]
Buckeye Counseling Center [47784]
Buckeye Ranch [47710], [47769]
    Deaf Srevices [3239]
The Buckeye Ranch--Grove City [31774]
The Buckeye Ranch, Inc.--Worthington [31861]
Buckeye Region Anti-Violence Organization [10140]
Buckeye VA Health Care Clinic • Division of Prescott
  VAMC [3860]
Buckhalter Recovery Center [43892]
Buckhead Dialysis [23584]
Buckhorn Children and Family Services • Runaway
  and Homeless Youth Program [35966]
Buckhorn Children's Foundation--Ohio [34373]
Buckley Mobile Vet Center [52138]
Buckner Family Medical Clinic/dba Family Physical
  Therapy and Rehabilitation [35685]
Buckner Hospice Houston [21481]
Bucks County Counseling [48625]
Bucks County School, Intermediate Unit 22 [697]
Bucks County Vet Center [52072]
Bucksport Regional Health Center • Bucksport
  Integrated Service Network [6770]
Buechler & Associates Speech Therapy Services
  [2183]
Buena Vista Hospice [19079]
Buena Vista Regional Medical Center--North
  Campus [15107]
Buffalo Beacon Corporation [47144]
Buffalo Federation of Neighborhood Centers, Inc.
  [31283]
Buffalo General Hospital
    Outpatient Chemical Dependency Clinic [46551],
      [46748]
    Transplant/Dialysis Center [25632]
Buffalo General Hospital--Transplant • Kaleida
  Health [25633]
Buffalo Grove Dialysis • Diversified Specialty
  Institutes [23906]
Buffalo Hearing and Speech Center [2998]
Buffalo Hospital • Sleep Center [37213]
Buffalo Psychiatric Center [31284]
    Cudmore Heights Residence [33691]
Buffalo Public Schools [576]
Buffalo Sleep Medicine [37378]
Buffalo State College • Speech-Language-Hearing
  Clinic [2999]

Buffalo Therapy Services [3090]
Buffalo Valley Inc [49083], [49084], [49085]
    Outpatient [49086]
Buffalo Veterans Affairs Medical Center [31285]
Buford Dialysis & At Home • DaVita [23631]
Building Blocks Comprehensive Services [3004]
Building Blocks Inc. [1671]
Building Blocks Therapy 2 [1522]
Building Bridges Camp [1129]
Building the Bridges Organization [50203]
Building Bridges Speech and Language Therapy
  LLC [2695]
Building Bridges Therapy Center [2633]
Building Futures with Women and Children [8894]
Bullard Community Health Center [6302]
Bullhook Community Health Center [6931]
Bulloch Recovery Resources [42156]
Bullock County Satellite [28059]
Bunkie Home Care [15277]
Burbank Home Care Inc. [13372]
Burbank Home Health Care Inc. [12919]
Burbank Unified School District [267]
Burdette and Doss • Psychological Services LC
  [45017]
Bureau of Vocational Rehabilitation [663]
Burell - Cox North • Center for Addictions [30905]
Burgess Hospice [19709], [19719]
Burke Center [32549]
Burke Center Family Counseling Center [32500]
Burke Center • Houston County Mental Health
  Center [32436]
Burke Center--Jasper [32489]
Burke Center--Lufkin [32503]
Burke Center for Mental Health • County Mental
  Health Center [32504]
Burke Center
    Nacogdoches Mental Health Center [32518]
    Substance Abuse Services [49459]
Burke Hospice and Palliative Care, Inc. [20754]
Burkwood Treatment Center [50413]
Burley Dialysis Center • DaVita [23869]
Burlingame Dialysis Center [22617]
Burlington Comp Counseling Inc [46073]
Burlington Comprehensive Counseling • Drug and
  Alcohol Treatment for the Deaf and Hard of Hear-
  ing [2934]
Burlington County Rape Care Program [9836]
Burlington Dialysis • DaVita [25824]
Burlington North Dialysis Center • DaVita [25412]
Burlington Regional Dialysis • DaVita [24756]
Burlington United Methodist Family Services--
  Beckley [34476]
Burlington United Methodist Family Services--
  Burlington [34477]
Burlington United Methodist Family Services--
  Grafton [34478]
Burlington United Methodist Family Services--Keyser
  [34480]
Burlington United Methodist Family Services--
  Morgantown [34481]
Burnaby Hospital • Multiple Sclerosis Center [34519]
Burncoat Family Center • Community Healthlink, Inc.
  [30481]
Burney Satellite [28422]
Burning Tree Recovery Ranch [49428]
Burns Paiute Reservation Health Program • Suicide
  Prevention Service [51257]
Burnsville Sleep Disorders Center [37214]
Burrell Adult Crisis Stabilization Unit [30906]
Burrell Behavioral Health • Adult Clinic [45458]
Burrell Behavioral Health--Branson Outpatient Satel-
  lite [30832]
Burrell Behavioral Health--Carrollton [30839]
Burrell Behavioral Health--Springfield • CSTAR
  Program [30907]
Burrell Behavioral Health • Transitions [45646]
Burrell Behavioral Health - Wilkinson [30908]
Burrell Behavioral Outpatient Satellite [30834]
Burrell Center, Inc. • Crisis Assist Team [51067]
Burrell Monett Outpatient Satellite [30878]
Burrell Transitions Program [30909]
Burt Center [33187]
Burtis & Noel Speech-Language Center Inc. [3479]
Business Speech Improvement [3422]
Bussenger Chiropractic Clinic [39029]
Butler Activity and Training Center [27937]
Butler County Dialysis Center • American Renal As-
  sociates [26389]

Butler County Mental Health Clinic [27938]
Butler County Sleep Center [37506]
Butler County Southwest Ohio Dialysis • DaVita [26122]
Butler Farm Dialysis Center & At Home • DaVita [27500]
Butler Hospital [33825]
  Alcohol and Drug Treatment Services [48870]
Butler Memorial Hospital • Cancer Care Program [5816]
Butler Regional Recovery Program
  Butler Memorial Hospital [48308]
  Family Resource Center [48309]
Butler Renal Center • Diversified Specialty Institutes [25179]
Butte Community Health Center • Dental Clinic [6927]
Butte County Behavioral Health Department • Runaway and Homeless Youth Program [35807]
Butte County Department of Behavioral Health-- Gridley [28524]
Butte County Department of Behavioral Health-- Oroville [28689]
Butte County Department of Behavioral Health-- Paradise [28693]
Butte County Department of Behavioral Health
  Paradise Treatment Center [28694]
  Special Services Division [28432]
Butte County Dept of Behavioral Health
  Access [39699]
  Adult Treatment Court Chico [39700]
  Chico Adult Outpatient Services [39701]
  Treatment Courts Oroville [40332]
Butte County Hearing Impaired Program [287]
Butte County Psychiatric Health [28433]
Butte Home Health and Hospice [18903]
Butte/Silver Bow • Chemical Dependency Services [45690]
Butterfield Youth Services • Child and Family Therapy Center [34272]
Butterfly Center • The Recovery Corporation [44983]
Buttonwood Hospital of Burlington County [33660]
Buttonwoods Group Home • The Kent Center [32181]
Butts County Counseling Center [29443], [42109]
By Grace Inc • Counseling Services [44118]
BZ Kids Inc. [2052]

C

C A Mayo and Associates Inc [44314]
C & C Homecare, Inc. [16595]
C and G Home Health Corporation [13948]
C Line Community Outreach Services [46021]
C and O Home Health Care Corporation [13731]
C. Paul Perry Pelvic Pain Center [35270]
C & S Home Health Care Services [15571]
CA Diversion Intervention Foundation [39590], [39894], [39909], [40240], [40320], [40951]
CA Hispanic Commission Alcohol/Drug Abuse
  Casa Elena [39591]
  La Familia Drug Abuse Services [40712]
  San Gabriel Valley Center [39806]
  Unidos Recovery Home [39880]
CAAP Inc. • Domestic Violence Program [10419]
CAB Boston Treatment Center [44412]
Cabarrus Baptist Association Inc [47275]
Cabarrus County Schools [613]
Cabell County Public Library • Services for the Blind and Physically Handicapped [3852]
Cabell County Schools [875]
Cabell Huntington Burn Center [4651]
Cabell Huntington Hospital [35767]
  Edwards Comprehensive Cancer Center [6136]
Cabell Huntington Hospital, Inc. [18517]
Cabell Huntington Hospital
  Sleep Disorders Center [37948]
  Speech Therapy Department [3655]
The Cabin [11059]
Cabin Creek Health Center, Inc. [7403]
Cabun Rural Health Services, Inc. • Hampton Clinic [6268]
Cache Creek Lodge [40962]
Cactus Counseling Associates PLLC [39488]
Caddo and Bossier Center [43893]
Caddo School for Exceptional Children [8075]
CADES [8487]
Cadillac Area OASIS/Family Rescue Center [9523]

Cadmus Lifesharing Association [8125]
Cadwalader Behavioral Clinics [11274]
Caguas Dialysis Center • Fresenius Medical Care [26627]
Caguas Dialysis & Nephrology Center [26650]
Cahaba Center [28060]
Cahaba Center for • Substance Abuse Services [39291]
Cahaba Center for Mental Health/Mental Retardation Services [28037]
  Cahaba Place [28038]
  Hilltop Home [28039]
  McDowell House [28040]
  Reynolds Building [28041]
  Wilcox County Satellite [27880]
Cahaba Center for Mental Health • Perry County Satellite [27972]
Cahaba Early Intervention Program • Mental Health/ Mental Retardation Center [7726]
Cahaba Hospice Inc. [18760]
Cairo Crisis Line • Mental Health Center [50833]
Cairo Home Care, Inc. [13835]
Cairo Women's Shelter, Inc. [9196]
Calais Veterans Affairs Clinic [30201]
Calavera Women's Crisis Line [8880]
Calaveras County Behavioral Hlth Services • Substance Abuse Programs [40519]
Calcare Home Health Inc. [12906]
Calcare Home Health, Inc. [12938]
Calcasieu Women's Shelter [9412]
Calcutta Veterans Affairs Clinic [31671]
Caldwell County Dialysis • Renal Advantage Inc. [24440]
Caldwell County Hospital, Inc. • Home Health Agency [15248]
Caldwell Dialysis Center • DaVita [23870]
Caldwell Hospice and Palliative Care, Inc. [20693]
Caldwell House [29706]
Caldwell Memorial Hospital • Cancer Center [5649]
Caldwell Veterans Affairs Clinic [29543]
Caledonia Home Health Care and Hospice • Northern Counties Health Care [21667]
Caleo Center [31355]
Calgary Board of Education • Deaf/Hard of Hearing Program [223]
Calgary Counseling Centre • Eating Disorder Program [10886]
Calgary Eating Disorder Program [10887]
Calhoun Cleburne Mental Health Board [27829]
Calhoun Cleburne Mental Health Center [27830]
  New Directions [39207]
Calhoun - Cleburne Mental Health • Day Treatment Outpatient Satellite [27949]
Calhoun County Mental Health Center [29477]
Calhoun Treatment Center Inc [39285]
California Care Corporation [39888]
California Caresource LLC [12910]
California Center for Reproductive Health [21908]
California Center for Sleep Disorders [36660]
California Cryobank, Inc., Cambridge [35066]
California Cryobank, Inc., Los Angeles [34936]
California Cryobank, Inc., New York [35127]
California Cryobank, Inc., Palo Alto [34937]
California Cryobank, Inc., Westwood [34938]
California Daily Comfort, Inc. [13165]
California Department of Education • State Special Schools and Services Division [1247]
California Diversion Programs Inc [39679]
California Drug Treatment Program Inc [40085]
California Ear Institute--East Palo Alto [1098]
California Ear Institute--San Ramon [1305]
California Elwyn [7778]
California Fertility Partners [21909]
California Foot and Ankle [38122]
California Healthcare Services, LLC [13072]
California Human Development Corp
  Athena House [40772], [40773], [40774]
  CHDCs Early Intervention Educ OTP [40775]
California Inst of Health and Social • Services Enlightenment Chem Dep Prog [40086]
California IVF: Davis Fertility Center, Inc. [21910]
California Kidney Care Center [22769]
California Medical Clinic for Headache [12386]
California Mental Health Connection [28584]
California Pacific MC Dialysis [22953]
California Pacific Medical Center, California Campus • Cancer Program [4841]
California Pacific Medical Center • Child Develop-

ment Center [7816]
California Pacific Medical Center - Cystic Fibrosis Center [7466]
California Pacific Medical Center • Forbes Norris MDA/ALS Research & Treatment Center [98], [34757]
California Pacific Medical Center Prenatal Diagnosis Center [12150]
California Pacific Regional Rehabilitation Center [3893]
California People Counseling Center [40269]
California School for the Blind [3700]
California School for the Deaf: Fremont [275]
California School for the Deaf: Riverside [295]
California SIDS Foundation [36450]
California SIDS Program [36451]
California Specialty Hospital [33206]
California Speech and Rehabilitation Inc. [1334]
California State University, Fresno • Speech and Hearing Clinic [1113]
California State University, Fullerton • Center for Children Who Stutter [1118]
California State University, Hayward • Speech, Language and Hearing Center [1128]
California State University, Northridge • National Center on Deafness [286]
California Transplant Services [34939]
California Treatment Services • DBA Recovery Solu- tions of Santa Ana [40713]
California's Best Home Health Services Inc. [12890]
Calipso Home Health Care Inc. [13345]
Call for Help, Inc. [29613]
  Runaway and Homeless Youth Program [35925]
Call for Help
  Sexual Assault Victim Care Unit [9223]
  Suicide and Crisis Intervention [50841]
Callaghan Road Dialysis • DaVita • Dialysis Center [27316]
Callahan County Behavioral Health [32409]
Callam County Public Hospital District No. 2 [18444]
Calle Real Mental Health Clinic [28799]
Callowhill Dialysis Center • DaVita [26504]
Calox, Inc. [13122]
Calumet Counseling and DUI Services • A Behavioral Health Agency [42430]
Calumet County Department of Human Services [32959]
Calumet County Department of • Health and Human Services [50375]
Calumet County Health Department • Hospice Program [21827]
Calumet Hearing Service [1982]
Calvary Center [39418]
Calvary Hill Health Services, LLC [17799]
Calvary Hospital [16357]
Calvary Hospital Hospice [20555]
Calvary Women's Services [9015]
Calvert Hospice [19937]
Calvert Memorial Hospital • Cancer Program [5310]
Calvert Substance Abuse Services
  Captains Quarters [44216]
  CCHD [44326]
  South Maryland Community Center [44312]
Calvert Treatment Facility • The Carol M Porto Treatment Center [44327]
Calverton Dialysis • DaVita [24657]
Camai Community Health Center [6215]
Camarillo Hospice [18896]
Camarillo Skilled Home Health, LLC [12928]
Cambodian Association of America [40018]
Cambria Medical Supply [17239], [17350]
Cambridge Developmental Center [8401]
Cambridge Dialysis Center • DaVita [24663]
Cambridge Eating Disorder Center [11087]
Cambridge Family Health Center [6952]
Cambridge Health Alliance
  Cancer Center [5328]
  Outpatient Addiction Service [44560]
Cambridge Home Health Care, Inc. [16826]
Cambridge Home Health Care, Inc. - Akron Branch [16937]
Cambridge Home Health Care, Inc. - Alliance Branch [16836]
Cambridge Home Health Care, Inc. - Ashland Branch [16838]
Cambridge Home Health Care, Inc. - Athens Branch [16843]
Cambridge Home Health Care, Inc. - Beachwood

Branch [16847]

Cambridge Home Health Care, Inc. - Bucyrus Branch [16858]

Cambridge Home Health Care, Inc. - Butler Branch [17270]

Cambridge Home Health Care, Inc. - Cambridge Branch [16860]

Cambridge Home Health Care, Inc. - Canton Branch [16865]

Cambridge Home Health Care, Inc. - Cincinnati Branch [16853]

Cambridge Home Health Care, Inc. - Columbus Branch [16901]

Cambridge Home Health Care, Inc. - Dayton Branch [16946]

Cambridge Home Health Care, Inc. - Elyria Branch [16934]

Cambridge Home Health Care, Inc. - Findlay Branch [16939]

Cambridge Home Health Care, Inc. - Hermitage Branch [17340]

Cambridge Home Health Care, Inc. - Mansfield Branch [16970]

Cambridge Home Health Care, Inc. - Marietta Branch [16978]

Cambridge Home Health Care, Inc. - Medina Branch [16990]

Cambridge Home Health Care, Inc. - Middleburg Heights Branch [16994]

Cambridge Home Health Care, Inc. - Mount Vernon Branch [17005]

Cambridge Home Health Care, Inc. - New Castle Branch [17007]

Cambridge Home Health Care, Inc. - New Philadelphia Branch [17009]

Cambridge Home Health Care, Inc. - Ravenna Branch [17025]

Cambridge Home Health Care, Inc. - Salem Branch [17030]

Cambridge Home Health Care, Inc. - Sandusky Branch [17033]

Cambridge Home Health Care, Inc. - Springfield Branch [17044]

Cambridge Home Health Care, Inc. - Steubenville Branch [17047]

Cambridge Home Health Care, Inc. - Toledo Branch [16985]

Cambridge Home Health Care, Inc. - Twinsburg Branch [17061]

Cambridge Home Health Care, Inc. - Warren Branch [17064]

Cambridge Home Health Care, Inc. - Wooster Branch [17079]

Cambridge Home Health Care, Inc. - Youngstown Branch [16844]

Cambridge Home Health Care, Inc. - Zanesville Branch [17092]

Cambridge Montessori School [8117]

Cambridge VA Outpatient Clinic [4091]

Cambridge Veterans Affairs Outpatient Clinic [30269]

Camcare Health Corp. [6969]

Camden-Clark Memorial Hospital [18532]
    Community Comprehensive Cancer Center [6140]

Camden Community Crisis Center [9122]

Camden County College • Mid-Atlantic Postsecondary Center for Deaf/Hard of Hearing [544]

Camden County Health Services Center • Psychiatric Division [33655]

Camden County Women's Center [9818]

Camden Dialysis • DaVita [26809]

Camden on Gauley Medical Center [7399]

Camelback Dialysis Center • DaVita [22493]

Camellia Home Health and Hospice--Bogalusa [19840]

Camellia Home Health and Hospice--Columbia [20228]

Camellia Home Health and Hospice--Hattiesburg [20242]

Camellia Home Health and Hospice--Jackson [20246]

Camelot Community Care--Green Acres [29175]

Camelot Community Care, Inc.--Bradenton [29117]

Camelot Community Care, Inc.--Clearwater [29124]

Camelot Community Care--Ocala [29241]

Camelot Community Care--Tallahassee [29295]

Camelot Community Care--Tampa [29301]

Camelot Home Health [12968]

Camelot Schools LLC • Palatine Campus [33436]

Camelot of Staten Island Inc
    Adolescent Day Program/CD Outpatient [47090]
    CD Outpatient Prog 2 Intensive Outpatient [47091]
    Drug Free Residential [47092]
    Outpatient Adult Program [47093]

CAMEO House [44291]

Cameron Counseling Center • Cameron Memorial Community Hospital [42982]

Cameron County Health Center [7160]

Cameron Dialysis • DaVita [25180]

Cameron Home Health Care and Hospice [19585]

Cameron Memorial Community Hospital • Cameron Sleep Center [36940]

Cameron Regional Medical Center • Renal Dialysis Center [25181]

Cameron Veterans Affairs Clinic [30836]

Caminiti Exceptional Center [7904]

Cammack Children's Center [34479]

Camp Hill Dialysis Center & At Home • DaVita [26390]

Camp Hill Veterans Affairs Outpatient Clinic [17276]

C.A.M.P. Home Health Services [15836]

Camp Recovery Centers • Outpatient Services [39677]

Camp Tokalot • Sondra Folley and Associates, Inc. [1548]

Campbell Chiropractic Wellness Center [39082]

Campbell County Adult Unit • Northern Kentucky Community Care [30088]

Campbell County Children's Unit • NorthKey Community Care [30015]

Campbell County Counseling Center [32786]

Campbell County Home Health Hospice [18651]

Campbell County Memorial Hospital
    Behavioral Health [33041]
    Dialysis Unit [27815]

Campbell County Memorial Hospital Hospice [21878]

Campbell County Outpatient Center [49115]

Camphill Special School [8460]

Campo Speech and Voice Improvement [1558]

Campobello Chemical Dependency
    Outpatient [40776]
    Recovery Center [40777]

Campy & Son Medical Equipment, Inc. [13949]

CAN/AM Youth Services Inc • Rose Hill Treatment Center [46775]

Can Do • Multiple Sclerosis Center [34541]

Canadian County Health Department • Speech and Hearing Clinic [3268]

Canal Dialysis • Fresenius Medical Care [24217]

Canandaigua Veterans Affairs Medical Center [31297]

Cancer Center/Radiation Oncology Services at UWMC [6112]

Cancer Institute of New Jersey • Institute for Children with Cancer and Blood Disorders • Sickle Cell Disease Center [36376]

Cancer Treatment Centers of America • Midwestern Regional Medical Center • Cancer Treatment Center [5133]

Candace Boltuch Fagan [45996]

Candler County Dialysis • DaVita [23756]

Candler Hospital [1906]

Cangleska Inc. [10380]

Cangleska, Inc. [10371]

Cangleska Inc. Outreach [10375]

Canku Luta Inc [45787]

Cannulif Healthcare Services, Inc. [17868]

Canon City Counseling Inc [41031]

Canon City Dialysis • Fresenius Medical Care [23097]

Canon Human Services Center • Brown Scapular Program [40087]

Cantalician Center for Learning [8308]

Canterbury Place [2191]

Canton City Schools [645]

Canton Community Clinic, Inc. [7077]

Canton/Postdam Hospital • Chemical Dependence Outpatient Clinic [47016]

Canton--Potsdam Hospital [3100]

Canton/Potsdam Hospital
    Chemical Dependency Services/Detox Unit [46992]
    Rehabilitation Unit [46993]

Canton Veterans Affairs Clinic [31674]

Canyon Acres [33980]

Canyon Acres Children and Family Services--Anaheim [28370]

Canyon Acres Children and Family Services--Orange [28687]

Canyon Country Dialysis Center, LLC [22621]

Canyon Creek Women's Crisis Center [10523]

Canyon Crisis Center [10240]

Canyon Park Treatment Solutions • Branch of WCHS Inc/CRC Health Corp [42378]

Canyon at Peace Park [40192], [40193]

The Canyon at Peace Park [28619]

Canyon Ridge Hospital [33133]

Canyon Springs [7768]

Canyon View Psychiatric and Addiction • Services of SLMVMC [42378]

Canyonlands Community Health Care [6241]

CAO/Drug Abuse Research and Treatment Prog [46552]

CAP of Downers Grove [42630]

Cap Quality Care Inc [44082]

Cape Ann Early Intervention [2449]

Cape Canaveral Hospital • Cancer Program [4936]

Cape Cod Artificial Kidney Center • Fresenius Medical Care [24823]

Cape Cod Center for Women [9496]

Cape Cod Hospital • Davenport-Muyar Cancer Center [5338]

Cape Cod Human Services [30374]

Cape Cod and Islands Community Mental Health Center--Hyannis [30398]

Cape Cod and Islands Community Mental Health Center--Pocasset [30450]

Cape Cod Rehabilitation Orthopedic & Sports Physical Therapy--Hyannis [38554]

Cape Cod Rehabilitation Orthopedic & Sports Physical Therapy--Mashpee [38559]

Cape Cod Speech and Language [2512]

Cape Community Health Center [6970]

Cape Coral Medical Office [6450]

Cape Coral South Dialysis • DaVita [23259]

Cape Counseling Services [31114]

Cape Fear Valley Health System • Cancer Center [5639]

Cape Fear Valley Home Care [16723]

Cape Girardeau Public Schools [524]

Cape Girardeau Veterans Affairs Clinic [30837]

Cape May Courthouse • Fresenius Medical Care [25415]

Cape May Health Department • Speech Therapy Program [2897]

Cape May Veterans Affairs Clinic [31113]

Cape Medical Supply, Inc. [15539]

Cape Regional Medical Center [51094]
    Brodessor Cancer Center [5506]

Cape Speech Therapy LLC [1555]

Capehart Community Clinic [6766]

Capelville Dialysis Center • DaVita [26883]

Capital Area Center for Adult Behav Hlth [43808]

Capital Area Center for Adult Behavioral Health Services [30127]

Capital Area Counseling Service [32240], [51345]

Capital Area Counseling Services
    Betty's Place [32241]
    Bridgeway [32242]
    The Care Center [32243]

Capital Area Counseling Services Inc [49005]

Capital Area Family Violence Intervention Center [9403]

Capital Area Human Services District • Child/Adolescent Services [30128]

Capital Area Recovery Program [43809]

Capital Area Speech [3458]

Capital City Dialysis & At Home • DaVita [25326]

Capital City Youth Services • Runaway and Homeless Youth Program [35880]

Capital District Beginnings [3136]

Capital District Dialysis Center [25775]

Capital District Psychiatric Center [33672], [51132]
    Schenectady County Clinic Treatment [31472]

Capital Health Eating Disorder Clinic [11185]

Capital Health Services [13950]

Capital Health System [20508]

Capital Health System at Mercer • Regional Cancer Center [5545]

Capital Health System
    Sleep Disorders Center [37336]
    Snoring and Sleep Apnea Center [37337]

Capital Home Health Care--Falls Church [18289]
Capital Home Health Care--Leesburg [18318]
Capital Home Infusion [18255]
Capital Hospice--Alexandria [21672]
Capital Hospice--Arlington • Halquist Memorial Inpatient Center [21675]
Capital Hospice--Falls Church [21690]
Capital Hospice-Largo [19932]
Capital Hospice--Leesburg [21703]
Capital Hospice--Manassas [21706]
Capital Hospices--Washington DC [19187]
Capital Neurological Associates • Multiple Sclerosis Center [34644]
Capital Region Medical Center [2793]
Capital Region Southwest Campus [16016]
Capital Regional Medical Center • Pediatric Therapy [8196]
Capital Speech & Learning [3632]
Capital Therapy, PA [1769]
Capitol Care [46176]
Capitol City Family Health Center, Inc. [6743]
Capitol Clubhouse [30180]
Capitol Community Health Center [6678]
Capitol Dialysis • American Renal Associates [23211]
Capitol District Developmental Disabilities Service Office [8352]
Capitol Hill Group Ministry • Families First [9016]
Capitol Hill Health Care Center, Inc. [27992]
Capitol Hill ILT and CTT [28880]
Capitol Home Program of DaVita--PD Unit • DaVita [25079]
Capitol Rehabilitation Inc.--Annandale [39117]
Capitol Rehabilitation Inc.--Arlington [39118]
Capitol Sleep Center [37507]
Capitol Sleep Medicine [37508]
Capitol Sports Medicine [38211]
Capland Center for Communication Disorders [3531]
Capper Center [2795]
The Capper Foundation [8035]
    Speech Language Pathology Department [2242]
Caprice of the Christian Appalachian Project [2272]
CAPS Educational Collaborative • Deaf and Hard of Hearing Program [2479]
Capstone Behavioral Healthcare Inc • Substance Abuse Division [43293]
Capstone Behavioral Healthcare, Inc.--Knoxville [29878]
Capstone Behavioral Healthcare, Inc.--Newton [29888]
Capstone Rural Health Center [6197]
Capstone Treatment Center [39574]
Captain James A Lovell Federal Health • Care Center [42815]
Captain James A. Lovell Federal Health Care Center • PTSD Residential Rehabilitation Program [51726]
Captain of Shenendehow, Inc. • Runaway and Homeless Youth Program [36091]
Caravan House • Adolescent Counseling Services [34006]
Carbon County Counseling Center [33061], [50594]
Carbon County COVE [10760]
Carbon Medical Service Assoc., Inc. • East Carbon Community Health Center [7320]
Carbon/Monroe/Pike Drug and Alcohol Commission, Inc • Carbon County Clinic [48446]
Carbondale DUI and Counseling Program [42437]
Cardeza Foundation Hemophilia Center • Thomas Jefferson University Hospital [12584]
Cardiac Rehabilitation Program [39111]
Cardinal Clinic [47305]
Cardinal Cushing Center [8113]
Cardinal Cushing School and Training Center [8127]
Cardinal Glennon Children's Hospital
    Department of Pediatrics • Medical Genetics Clinic [12262]
    Knights of Columbus Developmental Center [8209]
    Renal Dialysis Unit [25266]
Cardinal Glennon Children's Hospital/Saint Louis University Medical Center • Pediatric Cystic Fibrosis Center [7585]
Cardinal Glennon Children's Medical Center/Saint Louis University Medical Center • Adult Cystic Fibrosis Center [7586]
Cardinal Health Care Pharmacy [15036]
Cardinal Hill of Northern Kentucky [2268], [8042]

Cardinal Hill Rehabilitation Center [8052]
Cardinal Hill Rehabilitation Hospital [8048]
    Spinal Cord Injury Program [4058]
Cardinal House [30105]
Cardiopulmonary Medical Equipment Corp. [17523]
Cardiopulmonary Sleep and Ventilatory Disorders Center • Columbia University [37379]
CardioVascular Home Care [17921]
Cardiovascular Medical Associates • Center for Sleep Medicine [37380]
Cardone Reproductive Medicine and Infertility [22106]
Care for All Health Services, Inc. [13025]
Care Alternatives--Fort Washington [21087]
Care Alternatives Hospice--Riverside [19001]
Care Alternatives of Kansas [19767]
Care Alternatives--Marlborough [19977]
Care Alternatives of Missouri LLC [20307]
Care Alternatives of Virginia, LLC [21722]
Care At Home--Diocese of Brooklyn, Inc. [16380]
CARE CD Outpatient Services [46715]
Care Center • Family Domestic Violence Program [10036]
Care Center Inc [48672]
CARE Center--McAlester [10202]
Care Center Rehabilitation and Pain Management [35305]
Care Centers of Virginia • Renal Advantage Inc. [27501]
Care for Change Inc [47973]
Care Clinics Inc [42394]
Care Clinics of Naperville Inc [42802]
Care & Comfort [30251]
CARE Consultants Treatment Center [44221]
CARE Counseling Centers [40714]
Care Counseling Services [43216]
Care First Home Care [16149]
Care First Home Health [13782]
Care First Homecare [15845]
Care First Hospice [18680]
Care Force [14203]
Care Hawaii • Ala Nui Adolescent IOP/OP [42204]
Care Hawaii Inc • Adolescent IOP/OP [42243]
Care in the Home Health Services [14959]
Care Initiative Hospice-Waterloo [19670]
Care Initiatives Hospice-Albia [19660]
Care Initiatives Hospice-Cedar Rapids [19671]
Care Initiatives Hospice--Greenfield [19695]
Care Initiatives Hospice-Sioux City [19732]
Care for Life [18475]
Care Link Community Support Services [32016]
Care Lodge Domestic Violence Shelter, Inc. [9654]
Care Medical Equipment, Inc. [17215]
Care Net Robeson Family Counsel [47413]
Care One Home Health Inc.--El Monte [12983]
Care One Home Health--Miami [13951]
Care One Home Health Services [15674]
Care OPTIONS at Home [14891]
Care Partners [7440]
Care Partners Hospice and Palliative Care [20621]
Care Plus--Groton [28998]
Care Plus New Jersey--Fairlawn [31128]
Care Plus New Jersey Inc [46111]
Care Plus New Jersey, Inc.--Paramus [31159]
Care Provider Home Health Inc. [13351]
Care Regional Medical Center Hospital • Care Medical Detox [49212]
CARE Resource [41769]
Care of Savannah Inc
    Jack Gean Shelter for Men [49179]
    Jack Gean Shelter for Women [49180]
Care Source Hospice [21643]
Care Source, Inc. [15586]
Care South/Crisp Regional Hospital [14510]
Care South--Enterprise, AL [12653]
Care South--Eufaula, AL [12656]
Care South--Nashville, TN [17756]
Care South--Thomaston, GA [14592]
Care South--Winchester, TN [17782]
Care Specialist, Inc. [14722]
Care Time Home Health Services [13952]
Care We Love [16248]
Care4Life Home Health Agency [16150]
Career and Recovery Resources Inc [49251], [49357]
    Drug Abuse Treatment Program [49366]
    Jackson Hinds [49367]

Carefirst Medical Associates and Pain Rehabilitation [35686]
Caregivers Home Health Service [18290]
Careline Healthcare Inc. [13416]
Carelink Community Support Services [32035]
    Mobile Psychiatric Rehabilitation [32036]
Carelink Home Health Inc.--Thousand Oaks [13383]
Carelink Home Health, LLC--South Barrington [14934]
Carelink, Inc. [16456]
CareLink--Quincy [14910]
CareLink--Springfield [14943]
Caremark, Inc.--Mount Prospect [14868]
Caremark, Inc.--Redlands [13257]
Caremed [17692]
CareNet Homecare Services [15805]
Carenet, Inc. [17967]
CarePartners, Inc. [18526]
Carepoint Health, Inc. [17968]
Carepoint Home Health Services, Inc. [13071]
CarePointe Partners--Canfield [16862]
CarePointe Partners--North Canton [17011]
CareResource Hawaii--Hilo [14612]
CareResource Hawaii--Honolulu [14617]
CareResource Hawaii--Kahului [14628]
CareResource Hawaii--Kailua Kona [14632]
CareResource Hawaii--Kaunakakai [14638]
CareResource Hawaii--Lihue [14639]
CARES--Basin [10746]
Cares Center [30776]
Cares Home Healthcare [14355]
CARES--Lovell [10756]
CareSouth--Athens [14477]
CareSouth--Brunswick [14494]
CareSouth Carolina, Inc. [7234]
CareSouth--Dothan, AL [12648]
CareSouth--Hinesville [14537]
CareSouth Homecare Professionals--Greensboro [16732]
CareSouth Homecare Professionals--Lexington [16745]
CareSouth Homecare Professionals omec--Asheboro [16689]
CareSouth--Washington, GA [14605]
Caress Home Health Providers, Inc. [12929]
Caretenders--Akron [16827]
Caretenders--Beachwood [16848]
Caretenders--Breese [14699]
Caretenders--Columbus [16902]
Caretenders--Godfrey [14807]
Caretenders--Middleburg Heights [16995]
Caretenders--Mount Vernon [14871]
Caretenders--O Fallon [16034]
Caretenders--Saint Louis [16053]
Caretenders--Sullivan [16077]
Caretenders Visiting Services--Braintree [15476]
Caretenders Visiting Services--Columbus [16903]
Caretenders Visiting Services--Edgewood [15170]
Caretenders Visiting Services--Elizabethtown [15173]
Caretenders Visiting Services--Frankfort [15178]
Caretenders Visiting Services--Jeffersonville [15008]
Caretenders Visiting Services--LaGrange [15196]
Caretenders Visiting Services--Lancaster [16956]
Caretenders Visiting Services--Lexington [15204]
Caretenders Visiting Services--Louisville [15218]
Caretenders Visiting Services--New Albany [16534]
Caretenders Visiting Services--Newton [15525]
Caretenders Visiting Services--North Andover [15527]
Caretenders Visiting Services of Orlando [13869]
Caretenders Visiting Services--Owensboro [15238]
Caretenders Visiting Services of Saint Augustine [14363]
Caretenders Visiting Services--Saint Louis [16054]
Caretenders Visiting Services--Shelbyville [15252]
Caretenders Visiting Services--Sullivan [16078]
Caretenders VS of Central Kentucky [15179], [15205]
Caretenders VS of Louisville [15174], [15219], [15253]
Caretenders VS of Northern Kentucky [15171]
Caretenders VS of Western Kentucky [15239]
Caretenders--Youngstown [17086]
Carey Counseling Center--Camden [32276]
Carey Counseling Center Inc
    Paris Site [49175]
    Trenton Site [49194]

Union City Site [49197]
Carey Counseling Center--Paris [32372]
Carey Counseling Center--Trenton [32387]
Carey Counseling Center--Union City [32393]
Carey Counseling at Huntington [32318]
Carey Services, Inc. [8001]
Caribbean Kidney Center [27447]
Carilion Franklin Memorial Hospital [18379]
Carilion Home Care Services [18352]
Carilion Hospice Service, NRV [21717]
Carilion Hospice Services of Franklin County [21731]
Carilion Medical Center • Cancer Center of Western Virginia [6084]
Carilion New River Valley Medical Center [18353]
Carilion Saint Alban's Psychiatric Hospital [33900]
Carilion Sleep Center [37883]
Carilion Stonewall Jackson Hospital [18319]
Carillion Clinic Home Care Services [18250], [18375]
Carillion Home Care Services - Radford [18354]
Carillon Dialysis LLC [25683]
Caring [16628]
Caring About People Inc • Counseling Services [43043]
A Caring Alternative Home Health Care [16882]
Caring Alternatives, Inc.--Monore [15750]
Caring Alternatives, Inc.--Temperance [15853]
Caring Associates, Inc. [14268]
Caring At Home Health Care, LLC [14341]
Caring for Children • Trinity Place • Runaway and Homeless Youth Program [36130]
Caring Choice Network [15806]
Caring Communication Speech and Language Services [1108]
Caring Community Hospice of Cortland [20566]
Caring Hands Hospice--Batesville [18838]
Caring Hands Hospice--Cherokee Village [18842]
Caring Hands Pediatric Therapy Inc. [3199]
A Caring Heart Hospice [21210]
Caring Hearts Counseling Services LLC [47439]
Caring Hearts Home Health [17893]
Caring Hearts Hospice--Gun Barrel City [21477]
Caring Home Health [15699]
Caring Hospice Services of New York, LLC [20557]
Caring House, Inc. [9546]
Caring Nurses, Inc. [14723]
The Caring Place/Advocate House [8700]
The Caring Place, Inc.--Lebanon [9390]
The Caring Place, Inc.--Valparaiso [9311]
Caring Professional Services [13953]
Caring Professionals [16465]
Caring Services Inc [47386]
A Caring Solution Home Health Care Services, LLC [17844]
Caring Together Addictions and Mental Health Program for Women [48499]
A Caring Touch Home Health Services [18059]
Caring Touch Home Healthcare [16766]
Caring Unlimited [9438]
Caris Health Care, LP--Milan [21350]
Caris Healthcare--Algood [21308]
Caris HealthCare-Bristol [21677]
Caris Healthcare--Chattanooga [21314]
Caris Healthcare-Dickson [21329]
Caris Healthcare-Greenville [21335]
Caris Healthcare, LP--Columbia [21321]
Caris HealthCare, LP-Crossville [21326]
Caris Healthcare, LP--Murfreesboro [21355]
Caris Healthcare, LP--Nashville [21360]
Caris Healthcare, LP--Somerville [21365]
Caris Healthcare--Sevierville [21363]
Caris Healthcare-Springfield [21366]
Caritas Carney Hospital • Cancer Program [5331]
Caritas Good Samaritan Hospice [19949], [19991]
Caritas Good Samaritan Medical Center • Cancer Program [5325]
Caritas Home Care--Fall River [15490]
Caritas Home Care--Methuen [15516]
Caritas Home Care--Norwood [15533]
Caritas Home Care--Waltham [15553]
Caritas Home Health Providers, Inc. [12930]
Caritas Inc [48865]
  Caritas House [48845]
  Corkery House Boys Program [48897]
  Eastman House [48866]
Caritas Norwood Hospital [2509]

Caritas Norwood Hospital, Inc. • Cancer Program [5350]
Caritas Saint Elizabeth's Medical Center [5324]
  Pain Management Center [35489]
Caritas Sports Medicine & Rehabilitation [38481]
Carizzo Springs Kidney Disease Clinic • Fresenius Medical Care [26987]
Carl Albert Community Mental Health Center [8436], [33784]
Carl Albert Community Mental Health Center--Heavener [33769]
Carl Albert Community Mental Health Center--Hughes County [33770]
Carl Albert Community Mental Health Center--Hugo [33771]
Carl Albert Community Mental Health Center--McAlester [33775]
Carl Albert Community Mental Health Center--McCurtain County [33772]
Carl R. Darnall Army Medical Center • Cancer Program [5987]
Carl T. Curtis Health Education Center Dialysis [25332]
Carl T. Hayden VA Medical Center [3861]
Carl T Hayden VA Medical Center • SARRTP and Aftercare [39419]
Carl T. Hayden VA Medical Ctr. [12806]
Carl T. Hayden Veterans Affairs Medical Center
  Cancer Program [4743]
  Mental Hygiene [28173]
  Multiple Sclerosis Center [34515]
  PTSD Clinical Team [51684]
  Substance Abuse PTSD Clinical Team [51685]
Carl Vinson VA Medical Center [3999]
Carl Vinson Veterans Affairs Medical Center [51560]
  PTSD Clinical Team [51717]
Carle Addictions Recovery Center [42936]
Carle Clinic Association [34790]
  Child Diagnostic Clinic [7934]
Carle Clinic Association - Cystic Fibrosis Center [7526]
Carle Echo Program • Carle Foundation [2115]
Carle Foundation Hospital
  Cancer Center [5129]
  Carle Regional Sleep Disorders Center [36896]
Carle Home Care [14715]
Carle Home Care/Hospice--Champaign [14712]
Carle Home Care & Hospice-Danville [19509]
Carle Home Care/Hospice--Urbana [14951]
Carle Hospice [19499]
Carlinville Area Hospital Association [14706]
Carlisle Regional Medical Center • Capital Region Sleep Disorders Center of Carlisle [37640]
Carlos and Mary Jones Center • Shelter for Children [31708]
Carls Speech and Hearing Clinic [2647]
Carlsbad Battered Family Shelter [9863]
Carlsbad Dialysis • Dialysis Clinic, Inc. [25540]
Carlsbad Mental Health Association [31187], [46251]
  Crossroads [46252]
Carlsbad Mental Health Center [46253]
  Villa de Esperanza [46254]
Carlsbad Municipal Schools [556]
Carlson ENT Associates [989]
Carlton County Sexual and Domestic Abuse Program [9591]
Carlton G Wood PhD and • Deborah S Wood LA-DAC [49117]
Carmel Dialysis • DaVita [24120]
Carmel Home Health Services, Inc. [13329]
Carmel Physical Therapy and Rehabilitation [38432]
Carmelite Home for Boys [34495]
Carnales Unidos Reformando Adictos • CURA Inc [39835]
Carnegie Hill Institute Inc • Methadone Clinic [46840]
Carnegie Library of Pittsburgh • Library for the Blind and Physically Handicapped [3832]
Caro Center [8166], [33590]
Caro Dialysis • Fresenius Medical Care [24846]
Carobell [8382]
Carobell, Inc. [31550]
Carol A Goulette LCPC CCS [43940]
Carol Fischbach LCSW [45963]
Carol K. Crider Home • JBS Health Authority [27849]

Carol Molinaro Dialysis Center • Dialysis Clinic Inc. [25778]
Carol S. Roberson Hospice Center [20659]
Carolina Behavioral Care--Burlington [31509]
Carolina Behavioral Care--Durham [31523]
Carolina Behavioral Care--Henderson [31542]
Carolina Behavioral Care--Hillsboro [31548]
Carolina Behavioral Care--Louisburg [31557]
Carolina Behavioral Care--Pinehurst [31577]
Carolina Behavioral Care--Raleigh [31581]
Carolina Behavioral Care--Roanoke Rapids [31584]
Carolina Behavioral Care--Rockingham [31585]
Carolina Behavioral Care--Roxboro [31589]
Carolina Center for Behavioral Health [32203], [48952]
Carolina Compreh Psychiatric Services [47355]
Carolina Counseling and • Consultation Services PA [47495]
Carolina Counseling Services [47484]
Carolina Dialysis--Carrboro • Dialysis Center • Renal Research Institute [25826]
Carolina Dialysis LLC • American Renal Associates [26770]
Carolina Dialysis--Pittsboro • Renal Research Institute [25924]
Carolina Dialysis--Sanford • Renal Research Institute [25944]
Carolina Dialysis--Siler City • Renal Research Institute [25950]
Carolina East Home Care and Hospice/Duplin Home Care and Hospice [20687]
Carolina East Home Care and Hospice--Seven Springs [20731]
Carolina East Medical Center Home Care [16763]
Carolina Family Health Centers [7064]
Carolina Health Centers, Inc. [7233]
Carolina Home Care, Inc. [17586]
Carolina Hospice Care, Inc. [21260]
Carolina House • North Carolina Eating Disorder Treatment [11171]
Carolina Neurology • Multiple Sclerosis Center [34706]
Carolina Performance [47452]
Carolina Psychological Association [3179]
Carolina Pulmonary and Comprehensive Sleep Center [37458]
Carolina Speech Services Inc. [3165]
Carolina Sports Medicine and Joint Replacement [38837]
Carolina Treatment Center • Fayetteville [47306]
Carolina Treatment Center of Pinehurst [47443]
Carolina Youth Development Center [34433]
Carolinas Cord Blood Bank [35145]
Carolinas Counseling and Consulting [47220]
Carolinas Health System • Behavioral Health Center CMC--Randolph [33736]
Carolinas Healthcare System • Multiple Sclerosis Center [34663]
Carolinas Hospice [21233]
Carolinas Medical Center
  Blumenthal Cancer Center [5631]
  Carolinas Neuromuscular/ALS-MDA Center [34846]
Carolinas Medical Center--Charlotte [16710]
Carolinas Medical Center • Department of Pediatrics • Clinical Genetics Program [12306]
Carolinas Medical Center Dialysis Unit [25831]
Carolinas Medical Center • Dialysis Unit [25830]
Carolinas Medical Center--Lincoln [16748]
Carolinas Medical Center--Mercy • Cancer Center [5632]
Carolinas Medical Center • Mercy Horizons [47252]
Carolinas Medical Center - Pineville • Cancer Center [5633]
Carolinas Medical Center Union • Cancer Care Program [5651]
Carolinas Medical Center--Union Home Care [16754]
Carolinas Medical Center - University • Cancer Center [5634]
Carolinas Psychiatric Associates • Christian Counseling Clinic [47319]
Carolinas Rehabilitation [4325]
  Pediatric Outpatient Brain Injury Program [4326]
Carolinas Sleep Services--Pineville [37459]
Carolinas Sleep Services--University [37460]
Caroline County Health Department • Caroline Counseling Center [44243]

Carolyn Croxton Slane Residence [21161]
Carolyn E Wylie Center for Children, Youth and Families [40454]
Carolyn E. Wylie Center for Children, Youth and Families [7811]
Carolyn H. Overbay & Associates, Speech-Language Pathology [3429]
CaroMont Pediatric Therapy Services [3177]
Caron Counseling Services [48704]
Caron Renaissance [41565]
Caron Treatment Centers
    Adolescent Treatment Center [48684]
    Adult Primary Care Services [48685]
Carondelet Home Care Services [16026]
Carondelet Home Care Services, Inc. [15147]
Carondelet Hospice and Palliative Care [18825]
Carondelet St. Joseph's Hospital • Speech Language Hearing [990]
Carondelet Saint Mary's Hospital • Burn and Wound Care Center [4509]
Carousel [10935]
Carousel Live LLC • Client Centered Counseling [43403]
Carpenter House [31724]
Carquinez Dialysis Center • DaVita [23051]
Carrboro Community Health Center [7047]
Carriage Dialysis • DaVita [26848]
Carriage House [6387]
Carrie Gray Home [27887]
Carrie Knause Elementary School [502]
Carrier Clinic [33653]
    Blake Recovery Center [45931]
Carroll County • Alcohol and Addiction Program [47641]
Carroll County Board of Education [465]
Carroll County Branch Office • Northkey Community Care [29989]
Carroll County Dialysis • Fresenius Medical Care [23637]
Carroll County Emergency Shelter, Inc. [9095]
Carroll County Health Department • Outpatient Addictions Treatment Services [44384]
Carroll County Long Term Treatment Program [44362]
Carroll County Mental Health Services--Conway [31063]
Carroll County Mental Health Services--Wolfeboro [31098]
Carroll Home Care [15469]
Carroll Hospice [19943]
Carroll Hospital Center • Behavioral Health Services IOP Program [44385]
Carroll Hospital Center sleep and Breathing Disorders Center [37096]
Carroll Hospital Center • Cancer Center [5317]
Carroll Institute • Outpatient Alcohol and Drug Center [49016]
Carrollton Dialysis • DaVita [26988]
Carrollton Veterans Affairs Healthcare Center [29990]
Carrollwood Artificial Kidney Center • Fresenius Medical Care [23530]
Carson Artificial Kidney Center, LLC [22623]
Carson Center for Adults and Families [44601]
The Carson Center for Human Services, Inc. • Center for Children and Youth [30477]
Carson Center for Human Services • Westfield Clinic [30478]
Carson City Community Counseling Center [45822], [45823]
Carson City Dialysis Center • Dvita [25348]
Carson City Dialysis • Dialysis Clinic, Inc [25349]
Carson City School District [541]
Carson Mental Health Center [31020]
Carson Shelter/Employment Readiness Support Center [8801]
Carson Tahoe Regional Healthcare • Cancer Center [5487]
Carson Valley Childrens Aid [48332]
Carson Valley Medical Center • Speech and Language Therapy [2862]
Carter Behavioral Health Services [47356]
Carter Health Care and Hospice--Clinton [20929]
Carter Health Care and Hospice--Tulsa [20979]
Carter Health Care, Inc.--New Braunfels [18099]
Carter Healthcare and Hospice--Bartlesville [20921]
Carter Healthcare and Hospice--Enid [20933]
Carter Healthcare and Hospice--Norman [20948]

Carter Healthcare and Hospice--Tahlequah [20977]
Carter Healthcare, Inc.--Altus [17095]
Carter Healthcare, Inc.--Anadarko [17097]
Carter Healthcare, Inc.--Ardmore [17099]
Carter Healthcare, Inc.--Bartlesville [17102]
Carter Healthcare, Inc.--Chickasha [17109]
Carter Healthcare, Inc.--Clinton [17111]
Carter Healthcare, Inc.--Enid [17118]
Carter Healthcare, Inc.--Lawton [17124]
Carter Healthcare, Inc.--Muskogee [17133]
Carter Healthcare, Inc.--Norman [17137]
Carter Healthcare, Inc.--Oklahoma City [17148]
Carter Healthcare, Inc.--Okmulgee [17155]
Carter Healthcare, Inc.--Shawnee [17159]
Carter Healthcare, Inc.--Stillwater [17160]
Carter Healthcare, Inc.--Tahlequah [17162]
Carter Healthcare, Inc.--Tulsa [17164]
Carter Healthcare, Inc.--Vinita [17173]
Carter Healthcare--Irving [18020]
Carteret Counseling Services Inc [47424]
Carteret County Domestic Violence Program [10064]
Carteret General Hospital Home Health [16756]
Cartersville Medical Center [1845]
    Cancer Care Program [5018]
Carterville Family Practice [6648]
Carthage Area Hospital [3005]
Carthage Dialysis Center • Fresenius Medical Care [26990]
Carthage Veterans Affairs Outpatient Clinic [31301]
Carver Community Counseling Services • Drug Abuse Outpatient/Medically Supervised [47072]
Cary Kidney Center • Dialysis Facility • Fresenius Medical Care [25827]
Cary Neurology Disorders, Inc. [37461]
Cary Speech Services Inc. [3162]
Casa de Amigas [39420]
Casa de las Amigas
    Drug and Alcohol Rehab for Women [40364]
    Sober Living [40365]
Casa de la Bondad [10332]
Casa Calmecac [40778]
Casa Caribe Apartments [4442]
Casa Clare • A Divison of Mooring Programs Inc [50359]
Casa Colina Centers for Rehabilitation • Transitional Living Center [3894]
Casa Colina Comprehensive Out-Patient Rehabilitation Services Inc. [3895]
Casa Colina Multiple Sclerosis Centers [34523]
Casa de ConseJeria Drug and Alcohol Co [48500]
Casa De La Luz Hospice [18826]
Casa De La Luz Hospice--Tucson • Inpatient Unit [18827]
Casa Esperanza Inc
    Casa Esperanzas Mens Program [44552]
    Relapse Prevention and Outpatient Services [44553]
Casa de Esperanza--Saint Paul [9636]
Casa de Esperanza--Yuba City [8931]
Casa Grande Community Based Outpatient Clinic • Division of Prescott VAMC [3862]
Casa Grande Inpatient Unit [18783]
Casa Grande Regional Medical Center [28134]
Casa Grande Union High School [228]
Casa Guadalupe, Family Growth Center [9676]
Casa La Providencia [48811]
Casa Luz y Vida [48826]
Casa Maria • Transitional Housing Program [40366]
Casa Myrna Vazquez [9469]
Casa Norte [4262]
Casa Pacifica [28684], [33981]
Casa Palmera [10936]
Casa Protegida Julia de Burgos [10333]
Casa de San Bernardino [40520]
Casa Serena [40726]
    Casa Serena Graduate Recovery Program [40727]
Casa Serena/Concord Therapy Center for Eating Disorders [10937]
Casa Serena • Oliver House for Mothers and Children [40728]
Casa Solana [39899]
CASA - Women's Shelter [8781]
Casa Youth Shelter • Runaway and Homeless Youth Program [35808]
Cascade Child Treatment Center [31967]
Cascade Children's Therapy [3630]
Cascade City-County Health Department • Com-

munity Health Care Center [6930]
Cascade Health Solutions [20997]
Cascade Hemophilia Consortium [12532]
Cascade Mental Health Care
    Child & Adolescent Program [32813]
    Morton Site [32839]
Cascade Mental Health Center [32814]
Cascade Recovery Center • Silverdale [50157]
Cascade Recovery Resource Center [49945]
Cascade Regional Program [682]
Cascade RegionalLBL--ESD [680]
Cascadia Addiction • Bountiful Life Treatment Center PLLC [49913]
Cascadia Behavioral Healthcare [48179]
Cascadia Behavioral Healthcare, Inc. • Hillsboro Family Center [31943]
Cascadia Behavioral Healthcare, Inc.--Portland [31957]
Cascadia Behavioral Healthcare • Woodland Park [48180]
Cascadia Behavorial Healthcare • Garlington [48181]
Cascadia Multiple Sclerosis Center [34733]
Casco Bay Dialysis Facility • Fresenius Medical Care [24618]
Casco Bay • Substance Abuse Resource Center [44023]
CASCO Program [34161]
CASE Hearing/Speech/Language Program [472]
Case Management Services [31683]
Case Western Reserve University
    Department of Dermatology • Psoriasis Center of Research Translation [174]
    Department of Molecular Biology and Microbiology • Centers for AIDS Research [66]
    University Hospitals of Cleveland • Adult AIDS Clinical Trials Unit [26]
Case Western University • University Hospitals of Cleveland • Center for Human Genetics Clinic [12313]
Casey County Mental Health Center [30057]
Casey House • Montgomery Hospice Inpatient Facility [19939]
Casita • Branch of Triumph Treatment Services [50267]
Caspar House [44561]
Caspar Inc
    Mens Recovery Home [44562]
    New Day For Preg and Postpartum Women [44563]
    Womanplace [44436]
Casper Vet Center - Satellite [52151]
Casper Veterans Affairs Clinic [33033]
Cass County Community Mental Health • Woodlands Addictions Center [45040]
Cass Family Clinic OB/GYN [6854]
Cass Family Medicine [6945]
Cass Lake Dialysis • DaVita [25011]
Cass Regional Medical Center [16013]
Cass-Schuyler Area Hospice [19580]
Casselberry Dialysis • DaVita [23260]
Cassia Regional Medical Center [14653]
Castaner General Hospital • Castaner Health Care Center [7194]
Casteele Williams and Associates [50204]
Castle Medical Center [14631]
Castle Professional Center [14637]
Castleton State College • Fine Arts Performance Center [39112]
Castleview Dialysis [27413]
Castlewood Treatment Center [11117]
Caswell [8383]
Caswell Family Medical Center [7067]
Caswell Family Violence Prevention Program [10106]
CAT 5/Substance Abuse Services [50326]
Catahoula Parish Hospital District 3 • Medical Center [6764]
Catalyst Domestic Violence Services [8802]
Catar Clinic [39544]
Catawba Community Mental Health Center [32212]
Catawba Community Mental Health Center--Chester [32190]
Catawba Community Mental Health Center • York County Adult Services [32213]
Catawba Hospital [33899]
Catawba Rehabilitation Services, Inc. [39014]

Catawba Valley Behavior Healthcare • Burke County [31563]
Catawba Valley Behavioral Healthcare • Main Center [31544]
Catawba Valley Medical Center
  Cancer Program [5645]
  Sleep Disorders Center [37462]
Cathedral Canyon Mental Health and Substance Abuse Services [28427]
Cathedral Clinic [7294]
Cathedral Home for Children [3695], [34503]
Cathedral Shelter of Chicago • Adult Outpatient Program [42479]
Catherine Cobb Safe House and Domestic Violence Program [9510]
Catherine Freer • Wilderness Therapy Expeditions [48059]
Catherine Tanner-Harron [47387]
Cathleen Naughton Associates [17549]
Catholic Charites • Family Counseling and Guidance Center [44444]
Catholic Charities [41477], [45788]
Catholic Charities And Counseling Adop [48357]
Catholic Charities • Angels' Flight • Runaway and Homeless Youth Program [35809]
Catholic Charities Archdiocese of Boston • Runaway and Homeless Youth Program [35998]
Catholic Charities--Bay Shore • Mental Health Clinic [31237]
Catholic Charities--Brooklyn & Queens • Brooklyn West Family Center [31260]
Catholic Charities of Broome County [31245]
Catholic Charities • Bureau Arch Boston Genesis 11 [44524]
Catholic Charities Community Services
  Geauga County [47643]
  Monroe Clinic/Medically Supervised Outpatient [46787]
  Newburgh Clinic/Med Supervised Outpatient [46938]
Catholic Charities Community Services of Orange County [46778]
Catholic Charities Community Services • Walden Clinic [47157]
Catholic Charities of Cortland County
  The Charles Street Halfway House [46602]
  Supportive Living Facility [46603]
Catholic Charities • Crescent House Shelter [9419]
Catholic Charities Crime Victims/Domestic Violence [9969]
Catholic Charities • Crozier House [44608]
Catholic Charities of the Diocese of Albany • Runaway and Homeless Youth Program [36092]
Catholic Charities Diocese of Brooklyn • Deafness Services [2987]
Catholic Charities
  Diocese of Covington [43563]
  Diocese PGH Outpatient [48673]
Catholic Charities/Diocese of Syracuse • Mens Rutger House [47145]
Catholic Charities--Diocese of Trenton • Delaware House of Mental Health Services [31174]
Catholic Charities Family Services • Domestic Violence Services [9138]
Catholic Charities of Greater Nebraska [45732]
Catholic Charities Harbor House [9379]
Catholic Charities, Inc.--Fort Atkinson [32972]
Catholic Charities--Jackson [34260]
Catholic Charities, Jackson • Runaway and Homeless Youth Program [36041]
Catholic Charities Maine
  Counseling Services [44024]
  Saint Francis Halfway House [43911]
  Saint Francis House Extended Shelter [43912]
Catholic Charities--Medford • Mental Health Clinic [31387]
Catholic Charities Mental Health Center--Edison [31125]
Catholic Charities Mental Health Services--Freeport [31329]
Catholic Charities of Miami • Saint Lukes Center [41770]
Catholic Charities--Mineola • Mental Health Clinic [31392]
Catholic Charities of Montgomery County [9894]
Catholic Charities • Mount Carmel House for Women [9017]
Catholic Charities--New Haven • Family Service

Center [29023]
Catholic Charities of
  Monroe County [44923]
  Shiawassee and Genesee Counties [44783], [44951]
Catholic Charities/Omaha
  Campus for Hope [45789]
  Monsignor Kelligar Intermediate RTC [45790]
Catholic Charities--Racine [33009]
Catholic Charities of Rockville Centre
  Chemical Dependency Services [46674]
  Outpatient Alcohol Clinic/Commack [46597]
Catholic Charities • Saint Cloud Children's Home [34253]
Catholic Charities of Saint Paul and Minneapolis • Hope Street Shelter • Runaway and Homeless Youth Program [36032]
Catholic Charities Services
  Hispanic Program [47677]
  Midtown Youth Chemical Dependency [47678]
  Parmadale/Saint Augustine [47834]
Catholic Charities • Shelter for Battered Families [9651]
Catholic Charities/Somerset • Comprehensive Family Treatment of Addictions [45946]
Catholic Charities/Talbot House • Medically Monitored Withdrawal Services [46389]
Catholic Charities--The Shelter [9781]
Catholic Charities of Utica/Rome • Womens Halfway House [47146]
Catholic Charities West Michigan [44851], [44935]
  Crossroads [44842]
  Grand Rapids [44806]
Catholic Children's Home [29557]
Catholic Community Hospice--Overland Park [19768]
Catholic Community Hospice-Topeka [19779]
Catholic Community Services [50017]
Catholic Community Services--Cranford • Mount Carmel Guild Behavioral Healthcare [31121]
Catholic Community Services--Jersey City [31140]
  Mount Carmel Guild Project Home [31141]
Catholic Community Services • Recovery Center/Everett [49947]
Catholic Community Services of Seattle/King County [34468]
Catholic Community Services--Union City • Mount Carmel Guild Behavioral Healthcare • Hudson House [31169]
Catholic Community Services of Utah • Saint Marys Home for Men [49681]
Catholic Family Center
  CR Alexander Street [47026]
  CR Jones Avenue [47027]
  Restart Substance Abuse Services [47028]
  Restart Substance AbuseServices /Liberty Manor [47029]
  SLN Clinton [47030]
Catholic Family Service • Runaway and Homeless Youth Program [36212]
Catholic Family Services, Kalamazoo • Runaway and Homeless Youth Program [36009]
Catholic Family Services--New Britain [29015]
Catholic Family Services-Torrington [29045]
Catholic Family Services-Waterbury [29047]
Catholic Healthcare West [19055]
Catholic Home Care [16490]
Catholic Hospice--Fort Lauderdale [19217]
Catholic Hospice-Miami [19255]
Catholic Hospice--Miami Lakes [19261]
Catholic Human Services Inc [44634], [44666], [44684], [44695], [44909], [44989], [45036]
  Alcohol and Drug Services [44797]
Catholic Medical Center
  New England Sleep Center [37327]
  Oncology Services [5497]
  Rehabilitation Services [2884]
Catholic Memorial Home • Pain Management Program [35490]
Catholic Services of MaComb [44707]
Catholic Social Services [48470]
Catholic Social Services Diocese of Charlotte • Runaway and Homeless Youth Program [36131]
Catholic Social Services of the Diocese of Scranton • Runaway and Homeless Youth Program [36177]
Catholic Social Services Dodge City • Rural Family Addiction/Behav Health [43332]

Catholic Social Services of Lansing • Saint Vincent's Home, Inc. [34233]
Catholic Social Services of Oakland County [44993], [45047]
Catholic Social Services of
  Saint Clair County Inc/Substance Abuse Services [44975]
  The Upper Peninsula [44774]
  Wayne County [44726]
  Wayne County Substance Abuse Services [44720]
  Wayne County/Substance Abuse Services [44830]
Catholic Social Services of the UP • Iron Mountain Branch [44854]
Catoctin Counseling Center [44292], [44365]
Catoctin Summit • Adolescent Program [44341]
Caton Farm House [33425]
Catoosa County Schools [378]
Catskill Area Hospice and Palliative Care, Inc-Delhi [20567]
Catskill Area Hospice and Palliative Care, Inc.--Cobleskill [20564]
Catskill Area Hospice and Palliative Care Inc.--Oneonta [20593]
Catskill Dialysis Center • DaVita [25705]
Catskill Regional Medical Center
  Biochemical Dependency Unit [46678]
  Cancer Program [5581]
Catskill Veterans Affairs Clinic [31303]
Cattaraugus Community Action • Domestic Violence Program [9983]
Cattaraugus County Council on Alcohol and • Substance Abuse/Substance Abuse Clinic [46960]
Cattaraugus Indian Reservation Health
  Center [46712]
  System/Behavioral Health Unit [46713]
Cavalier Senior Care [16183]
Cavanaugh Treatment Center [43817]
Cawn Krantz and Associates [2084]
Cayce Family Health Center [7266]
Cayuga Addiction Recovery Services [47139]
  Outpatient Program [46718]
Cayuga County Action Agency • Battered Women's Program [9895]
Cayuga County Behavioral Health Unit [31231]
Cayuga County Mental Health Center [31232]
Cayuga Medical Center at Ithaca [3033]
  Cancer Program [5583]
Cayuga Medical Center • Sleep Disorders Center [37381]
Cazenovia Recovery Systems Inc
  Cazenovia Manor [46553]
  New Beginnings Community Residence [46554]
  Supportive Living Program [46555]
  Turning Point House [46618]
CBR YouthConnect • Denver Office [33223]
CBS House [30735]
CC/Rochester • Chemical Dependence Supportive Living [46598]
CC/Rochester/Kinship Community Res • CD Community Residence [46371]
CCD Counseling PA • Denton Recovery Options [49307]
Cchat Center [1231]
CCMH HomeCare/Hospice, Inc. [19665]
CCNS Flatbush Addiction • Treatment Center [46486]
CCS Recovery Center [49900]
CDHS Inc [49214]
A CDM Assesment and Counseling of Guilford [47339]
CDR USAMEDDAC • Army Substance Abuse Program [43593]
CDRP Clinic Veterans Administration • Bangor Clinic [43923]
CDS Family and Behavioral Health Services [35881]
CDS Family/Behavioral Health Services Inc [41678]
CDS Family/Behavioral Health Services • SAMH/East [41870]
Cease Addiction Now Inc [49235]
Cease Domestic Violence & Sexual Assault [10421]
Cecil Chiropractic [38933]
Cecil County Domestic Violence/Rape Crisis Center [9453]
Cecil County Health Department • Alcohol and Drug Recovery Center [44251]
CED

Cherokee County Office [27882]
Dekalb County Office [27927]
CED Fellowship House Inc [39249]
Cedar Community Health Center [6851]
Cedar Community Hospice [21873]
Cedar Creek Family Counseling Inc [50408]
Cedar Crest Hospital • Eating Disorders Program [11275]
Cedar Crest Hospital & Residential Treatment Center [33861]
Cedar Grove Counseling Inc [50054]
Aberdeen [49872]
Cedar Home Health, LLC [17534]
Cedar Lake Lodge [8053]
Cedar Lodge • A Program of MLBH [39255]
Cedar Mountain Center at • West Park Hospital [50579]
Cedar Mountain Center • Outpatient [50580]
Cedar Mountain Rehabilitative Day Services [28343]
Cedar Park Counseling Network [49976]
Cedar Park Dialysis Center and At Home • DaVita [26991]
Cedar Park Sleep Center [37806]
Cedar Rapids Counseling & Psychotherapy Group [29845]
Cedar Ridge Health Care [2058]
Cedar Springs Austin [11276]
Cedar Springs Hospital • Cedar Springs Behavioral Health [33214]
Cedar Street Training Program [27917]
CeDAR/University of Colorado Hospital [40995]
Cedar Valley Dialysis Center • DaVita [24306]
Cedar Valley Friends of the Family [9350]
Cedar Valley Hospice--Grundy Center [19697]
Cedar Valley Hospice--Independence [19699]
Cedar Valley Hospice-Waterloo [19739]
Cedar Valley Hospice-Waverly [19740]
Cedar Valley Medical Clinic • Pain Clinic [35449]
Cedar Valley Recovery Services [43242], [43288]
Cedarcrest [8237]
Cedarcrest Regional Hospital [33260]
Cedards Hospice Home [21116]
Cedars Hospital [33865]
Cedars-Sinai Center for ALS Care • ALS Center [99]
Cedars Sinai Medical Center • Pain Center [35306]
Cedars-Sinai Medical Center • Samuel Oschin Comprehensive Cancer Institute [4796]
Cedars Youth Service • Runaway and Homeless Youth Program [36065]
Cedartown Dialysis • DaVita • Dialysis Facility [23640]
CEI Community Mental Health [2615]
CeJa Counseling Service LLC [48492]
Celebrate Your Body [10938]
Celebration Dialysis • DaVita [23261]
Celia Dill Dialysis Center • DaVita [25640]
Cells for Life Limited--Calgary [34919]
Cells for Life Limited--Markham [35172]
Cells for Life Limited--Montreal [35197]
Cells for Life Limited--Toronto [35173]
Celtic Community Services of Northeast Ohio [17087]
Celtic Healthcare of Lawrence [21118]
Celtic Hospice and Palliative Care [21119]
Celtic Hospice and Palliative Care Services LLC [21111]
Cenikor Foundation [43810]
Cenikor Foundation Inc • North Texas Facility [49332]
Cenikor Foundation • Substance Abuse Program [49306]
Cenla Chemical Dependency Council
Adolescent Outpatient [43883]
Bridge House/Phase II [43884]
Gateway Adolescent Unit [43885]
Centegra Health Systems-Home Health services [14857]
Centegra Memorial Medical Center • Cancer Program [5132]
Centegra Northern Illinois Medical Center • Cancer Center [5110]
Centegra Outpatient Behavioral Health [42971]
Centennial Dialysis • Fresenius Medical Care [25358]
Centennial Dilaysis Center • DaVita [25359]
Centennial Medical Center and Parthenon Pavilion • Sarah Cannon Cancer Center [5947]

Centennial Medical Center • Sleep Disorders Center [37759]
Centennial Medical Center--Transplant [26902]
Centennial Mental Health Center--Akron [28851]
Centennial Mental Health Center--Burlington [28866]
Centennial Mental Health Center--Elizabeth [28897]
Centennial Mental Health Center--Fort Morgan [28904]
Centennial Mental Health Center • Fourth Street House [28954]
Centennial Mental Health Center--Holyoke [28915]
Centennial Mental Health Center Inc [40975], [41028], [41164], [41186], [41224], [41225], [41249], [41316], [41357]
Centennial Mental Health Center--Julesburg [28917]
Centennial Mental Health Center--Limon [28931]
Centennial Mental Health Center--Sterling [28955]
Centennial Mental Health Center--Wray [28966]
Centennial Mental Health Center--Yuma [28967]
Centennial Peaks Hospital [33232], [41263]
Center 4 Clean Start • Worcester County Health Department [44344]
Center for Abuse and Rape Emergencies, Inc. [9076]
Center for Abused Persons [50981], [50982]
Center Academy [7903]
Center for Addiction and Counseling [48240]
Center for Addiction Medicine [44119]
Center for Addictions • Cox Health [45647]
Center for Addictive Diseases [48370]
Main Line [48342]
Center for Addictive Problems [42480]
Center for Adult Services [43745]
Center for Advanced Reproductive Endocrinology [21988]
Center for Advanced Reproductive Services • Hartford Fertility and Reproductive Endocrinology Center [21967]
Center for Advanced Sports Medicing [38739]
Center for Advocacy and Personal Development [10655]
Center Against Domestic and Sexual Violence [10279]
Center Against Domestic Violence [9905]
Center Against Family Violence [10459]
Center Against Rape and Domestic Violence [10227]
Center Against Sexual and Domestic Abuse, Inc.--Superior [10739]
Center Against Sexual and Domestic Abuse--Solon Springs [10736]
Center for Alcohol and Drug Services
Country Oaks [43255]
East Locust Adolescent Facility [43256]
East Moline [42637], [42638]
Center for Alcohol and Drug Services Inc • Rock Island Office [42883]
Center for Alcohol and Drug Services • Intake Outpatient Administration [43257]
Center for Alcohol and Drug Treatment [45129], [50256]
Howard Friese House [45130]
Marty Mann House [45131]
Center for Alexandria's Children [32697]
Center for Assisted Reproduction [22250]
Center Associates [8018]
Center for Athletic Medicine [38584]
Center of Balance [11266]
Center for Behav Health Las Vegas Inc [45858]
Center for Behavioral Health [45836], [48889]
Center for Behavioral Health Idaho Inc [42311], [42350]
Center for Behavioral Health IN Inc • Outpatient Treatment [43044]
Center for Behavioral Health Iowa Inc [43262]
Center for Behavioral Health KY Inc [43682]
Center for Behavioral Health
Louisiana Inc [43894]
Nevada [45867]
Rhode Island Clinic [48853]
South Carolina Inc [48908]
Center for Behavioral Hlth Phoenix Inc [39421], [39480]
Center for Behavioral Hlth Tucson Inc [39489]
Center for Better Hearing LLC [1452]
The Center for Bilingual Speech and Language Dis-abilities, Inc. [1648]
Center for Bleeding and Thrombotic Disorders • Saint Louis University Hospital • Hemophilia Treat-

ment Center - Adult Program [12548]
Center for Change [11290], [41347], [43481]
Center for Change of Florida [11014]
Center for Change LLC [41236]
The Center for Change and Recovery LLC [46060]
Center for Chemical Addictions Treatment [47653]
Center for Child Development [1791]
Center for Child & Family Advocacy, Inc. [31754]
Center for Child and Family Health • Child Health Section [36533]
Center for Children's Services [29603]
Center for Children's Speech-Language Disorders [1425]
Center for Communication [2364]
Center for Communication Advancement [2905]
Center for Communication Care LLC [2974]
Center for Communication Disorders [1366], [1594], [7767]
Center for Communication and Learning Skills [3314]
Center for Communication Skills--Fresno [1114]
Center for Communication Skills--New Haven [1475]
Center for Community Resources Inc. [51275]
Center for Community Services [8809]
Center for Community Solutions [8883]
Center for Comp Health Practice Inc
ECP [46841]
MAP [46842]
MS [46843]
PAAM [46844]
Center for Comprehensive Services [3960]
Center for Congenital and Inherited Disorders • Genetics Clinic [12215]
Center for Consulting Services--South [30061]
Center for Consulting Services--West [30062]
Center for Counseling and • Health Resources Inc/Edmonds [49940]
The Center for Counseling & Consultation [29927]
Center for Counseling and Evaluation [47392]
Center for Counseling & Health Resources Inc. [11300]
Center for Craniofacial Disorders • Children's Hospital [1814]
Center for the Deaf and Hard of Hearing • Com-munication Link • Interpreter Coordination Services [3688]
The Center for Developmental Disabilities [8364]
Center for Dialysis Care--Canfield [26028]
Center for Dialysis Care--Cityview • Dialysis Facility [26059]
Center for Dialysis Care--Cleveland East [26060]
Center for Dialysis Care--Cleveland West [26061]
Center for Dialysis Care--Euclid [26110]
Center for Dialysis Care--Jefferson • Dialysis Center [26140]
Center for Dialysis Care--Shaker Heights [26198]
Center for Dialysis Care--Warrensville Heights [26227]
Center for Dialysis Carehealth:ther Hill [26132]
Center Dialysis • Fresenius Medical Care [26993]
Center for Disability Services [2969]
Multiple Sclerosis Clinic [34645]
Center for the Disabled [8292]
Center for Discovery Adolescent Residential Eating Disorders Menlo Park [10939]
Center for Discovery • Eating Disorders Program [10940]
Center for Domestic Violence Prevention [8898]
Center for Donation and Transplant [35128]
Center for Drug Free Living Inc
Addiction Receiving Facility [41850]
CENTAUR [41851]
Clarcona Pointe/Adolescence Subst Prog [41852]
Outpatient [41873]
William R Just Center [41853]
Womens Residential Program [41854]
Center for Dual Diagnosis Recovery • Columbia River Mental Health Services [50235]
The Center for Early Intervention on Deafness [265]
Center East • Sumner Branch [50193]
Center for Eating Disorder Recovery Associates - EDaR Associates [11155]
A Center for Eating Disorders [10881]
Center for Eating Disorders and Psychotherapy [11193]
Center for Elderly Suicide Prevention and Grief Related Services [50693]

Center for Emotional, Compulsive, and Binge Eating [11080]
Center for Expressive Wellbeing [1220]
Center for Families and Children [31709]
Center for Families Inc • Center for Addictive Disorders [43895]
Center for Family Counseling [28672]
Center for Family Development [44503], [48098]
Center for Family Living [34035]
Center for Family Practice and Sports Medicine [38246]
Center for Family Resources, Inc. [9697]
Center for Family Services [31110]
Center for Family Services of Palm Beach County [41992]
Center for Family Services
    Runaway and Homeless Youth Program [36075]
    Substance Abuse Treatment Services [46207], [46220]
Center for Fertility and Gynecology [21911]
Center for Fertility and Reproductive Endocrinology [22225]
Center for Fertility and Reproductive Endocrinology-- Butler [22226]
Center for Fertility and Reproductive Endocrinology-- Hermitage [22227]
Center for Fertility and Reproductive Endocrinology-- Johnstown [22228]
Center Glen Elementary School [406]
Center for Great Expectations [46168]
Center for Group Counseling [29113]
Center for Head and Facial Pain [38760]
The Center for Head Injury Services [4233]
The Center for Health Care Services [32545]
    Eastside Multiservice Unit [32546]
    Mental Retardation Clinical Services [8564]
    Psychiatric Emergency Services/Multi Service Center [32547]
    Westside Multiservice Center [32548]
Center for Health and Development, Inc. • Atlantic Clubhouse [30451]
Center for Health and Development, Inc.--Boston [30342]
Center for Health Promotion • Timken Mercy Medical Center [38857]
Center for Health and Rehabilitation [38510]
The Center for Health & Rehabilitation [29346]
Center for Health and Wellness [43482]
Center for Healthcare Services
    Criminal Justice Outpatient Unit [49518]
    Palo Alto [49519]
    Restoration Center [49520]
Center for Hearing and Communication [347], [3057]
Center for Hearing and Deaf Services--Greensburg [3333]
Center for Hearing and Deaf Services Inc.-- Pittsburgh [3364]
Center for Hearing Science [1057]
Center for Hearing and Speech [792]
The Center for Hearing Speech and Language [1390]
Center for Hearing and Speech--St. Louis/St. Charles [2813]
Center of Hope [41237]
Center for Hope Hospice and Palliative Care [20494]
Center of HOPE of Myrtle Beach LLC [48964]
Center for Hope of the Sierras [11132]
Center for Hospice and • Palliative Care, Inc. [19651]
Center for Hospice Care [19633]
Center for Hospice and Palliative Care-Cheektowaga [20563]
Center for Hospice and Palliative Care - Elkhart [19593]
Center for Hospice and Palliative Care - Plymouth [19642]
Center for Human Development [8164]
Center for Human Development Inc [43483]
    Alcohol and Drug Services [48140]
Center for Human Development, Inc. [30464]
    Connecticut Outreach [29001]
Center for Human Development • Runaway and Homeless Youth Program [35999]
The Center for Human Reproduction [22033]
Center for Human Resources [44976]
Center for Human Services [28626], [50154]
The Center for Human Services • Children's Therapy Center [8219]

Center for Human Services • Runaway and Homeless Youth Program [35810]
Center for Independent Learning • The Friendship Connection [45388]
Center for Independent Living • Youth Services Department [7765]
Center for Individual and • Family Services [47797]
The Center for Individual and Family Services [31797]
    Blymyer House [31798]
Center for Infant and Child Loss [36545]
The Center for Infant and Child Loss [36488]
Center for Information and Crisis Services • Crisis Line [50768]
Center for Integrative Manual Therapy and Diagnostics [38162]
Center for Kidney Disease • DaVita [23393]
Center for Language and Cognitive Rehabilitation [3215]
Center for Learning and Achievement [1287]
Center for Learning & Attention Disorder [31090]
Center for Life Management [8240], [51082]
    Beaver Lake Lodge [31066]
    Behavioral Health [31094]
Center for Life Management--Derry [31067]
Center for Life Resources • Substance Abuse and COPSD Services [49255]
Center for Life Solutions [45491]
Center Main Facility • Metropolitan Development Council [50205]
Center for Mental Health [48691]
The Center for Mental Health [29689], [29716]
Center for Mental Health
    Cut Bank Center for Mental Health [30932]
    Havre Center for Mental Health [30947]
The Center for Mental Health, Inc. [29690]
Center for Mental Health, Inc.
    Hudson Place [29691]
    McMahan House [29692]
Center for Mental Health LLC [44371]
Center for Mental Healthcare • Birdsboro Memorial Community Center [48297]
Center for Network Therapy LLP [46015]
Center for Neurological Rehabilitation Inc.-- Swarthmore • Down Syndrome Clinic [10851]
Center of Neurological Services Orlando • Multiple Sclerosis Care Center [34554]
Center for New Beginnings Shelter and Services • A Program of The Woodlands [10163]
Center for New Image Inc [40088]
Center for Nonviolence [9275]
Center for Optimal Health and Performance • San Diego State University [38123]
Center for Organ Recovery and Education [35184]
Center for Orthopaedic Care [38859]
Center for Orthopaedic and Sports Physical Therapy [39125]
Center of Orthopaedic and Sports Physical Therapy--Herndon [39126]
Center of Orthopaedic and Sports Physical Therapy--Vienna [39135]
Center for Orthopaedics [38498]
The Center for Orthopaedics and Sports Medicine [38325]
Center for Orthopedic Surgery and Sports Medicine [38879]
Center for Orthopedics and Sports Medicine [38520]
Center for Outpatient • Alcoholism Treatment [42665]
Center for the Pacific Asian Family, Inc. [8838]
Center for Pain Control [35687]
Center for Pain Management--Columbia, SC [35661]
Center for Pain Management--Indianapolis, IN [35441]
Center for Pain Medicine [35620]
Center for Pain Rehabilitation [35356]
Center for Pain Relief [35768]
Center for Pediatric Rehabilitation Inc. [1719]
Center for Pediatric Therapies [3611]
Center for Pediatric Therapies Inc. [3579]
Center for Pediatric Therapy Inc.--N Kendall Drive, Miami [1649]
Center for Pediatric Therapy Inc.--SW 37th Avenue, Miami [1650]
Center for Personal & Family Development [29260]
Center for Personal and Family Development--Gulf Breeze [33305]
Center for Personal and Family Development--

Pensacola [33338]
Center for Physical Medicine [38043]
Center Point Inc [48035]
    Lifelink Perinatal Serv/Women/Children [40701]
    Lifelink Program [40702]
    The Manor [40703]
    Non Residential Services [40704]
    Residential Program [40705]
Center Pointe of Saint Louis Hospital [33633]
Center for Positive Change Inc [48058]
Center for Positive Prevention Alternatives, Inc. [28821]
Center for Positive Prevention Alternatives • Runaway and Homeless Youth Program [35811]
Center for Prevention of Abuse [9242]
Center for Prevention and Counseling [46102]
Center for Problem Resolution Inc [43023], [43067]
Center for Psychiatric and Addiction Treatment [49809]
Center for Psychiatric and Chemical • Dependency Services WPIC [48585]
Center for Rapid Recovery Inc • Outpatient Drug Abuse Clinic [46688]
Center for Recovering Families at The Council on Alcohol Drugs Houston [49368]
Center for Recovery Inc [41114]
Center for Recovery • MSA Drug Program [46659]
Center for Rehabilitation and Development-- Blacksburg [3572]
Center for Rehabilitation and Development-- Lynchburg [3591]
Center for Rehabilitation Medicine • Emory University [1815]
Center for Renal Care--Shadyside [26544]
Center for Renal Replacement LLC [24022]
Center of Renewed Promises [42137]
Center for Reproduction and Women's Health Care [22251]
Center for Reproductive Health--Nashville [22247]
Center for Reproductive Health--Oklahoma City [22219]
Center of Reproductive Medicine [22252], [22253]
The Center for Reproductive Medicine [22067]
Center for Reproductive Medicine - Alabama [21885]
Center for Reproductive Medicine - Maryland [22085]
Center for Reproductive Medicine of New Mexico [22173]
Center for Reproductive Medicine--Orlando [21989]
Center for Reproductive Medicine and Surgery [22115]
Center for Reproductive Medicine--Webster [22254]
Center for Respiratory and Sleep Disorders [37150]
Center for the Retarded [8550]
Center of Revitalizing for Psychiatry • PC [46008]
Center for Sexual Assault and Domestic Violence Survivors [9767]
Center for Sexual Assault Survivors [10581]
Center for Sleep Disorders • Skagit Valley Hospital [37908]
Center for Sleep Medicine--Chicago [36897]
Center for Sleep Medicine--Lafayette Hill [37641]
Center for Sleep Medicine--Naperville [36898]
Center for Sleep Medicine--Orland Park [36899]
Center for Sleep Medicine--Oswego [36900]
Center for Sleep Medicine--Ridgewood • Valley Hospital [37338]
The Center for Sleep Medicine • Saint Joseph Hospital [37382]
The Center for Sleep & Wake Disorders [37097]
Center for Small Jewels Inc. [3053]
Center for Solutions [43045], [47562]
Center South Gravelly Lake • Lakewood Metropolitan Develop Council [49999]
Center for Speech and Language [2658]
Center for Speech and Language Disorders [7952]
Center for Speech and Language Disorders-- Elmhurst [2025]
Center for Speech and Language Disorders-- Naperville [2075]
Center for Speech & Language, Inc. [1691]
Center for Speech, Language and Learning-- Carrboro [3161]
Center for Speech, Language and Learning Inc.-- Oakdale [2722]
Center for Speech, Language and Occupational Therapy--Fremont [1112]
Center for Speech, Language and Occupational

Therapy--Los Altos [1158]
Center for Speech, Language and Occupational
Therapy--San Jose [1288]
Center for Speech and Language Pathology [913]
Center for Speech and Language TC, Inc. [1616]
Center for Speech and Learning [1476]
Center for Speech Pathology [1093]
The Center for Sports Medicine and Fitness [38578]
Center for Sports Medicine & Orthopaedics [39025]
Center for Sports Medicine--Phoenix [38044]
Center for Sports Medicine • Saint Francis Memorial
Hospital [38127]
Center for Sports Medicine--Schnectady [38820]
Center for Sports and Occupational Medicine
[38372]
Center for Sports and Osteopathic Medicine [38791]
Center for the Study of Anorexia and Bulimia [11156]
Center for Stuttering Therapy [2028]
Center for Substance Abuse [48459]
Center for Success and Independence [49369]
Center for Sucess [47563]
Center for Supported Living--Downtown [30063]
Center for Supported Living--East [30064]
Center for Supported Living--South [30065]
Center for Supported Living--West [30066]
Center for Therapeutic Interventions • PLLC [48036]
Center for the Treatment of Addiction [39931]
Center for Treatment of Addiction Inc [39881]
Center for Treatment and Recovery [48867]
Center at University of Arizona Health Sciences •
MDA Center [34752]
Center at the University of California, Irvine • MDA/
ALS Center [100], [34758]
Center at the University of Kansas Medical Center •
MDA/ALS Center [116], [34799]
Center at the University of New Mexico • Health Sci-
ences Center • MDA/ALS Center [34830]
Center at the University of Texas at San Antonio •
Health Science Center • MDA/ALS Center [34881]
Center for Violence Prevention [9658]
Center for Violence Protection--Monadnock [9809]
Center for Voice and Swallowing Services [1427]
Center for Women and Children in Crisis--Orem •
Outreach and Sexual Assault Services Office
[10527]
Center for Women and Children in Crisis--Provo
[10530]
Center for Women and Families [9393]
The Center for Women and Families--Bridgeport
[8990]
The Center for Women and Families--Sellersburg
[9307]
Center for Women and the Family [48168]
Center for Women and Family Health at Saint Cloud
[6544]
Center for Women and Family Health at Stadium
Place [6481]
Center for Women in Transition [9542]
Center for Women's Medicine • Fertility Clinic
[22255]
Center for Youth and Families • Therapeutic
Independent Living [28298]
Center for Youth and Family Services [30395]
The Center for Youth Services • Runaway and
Homeless Youth Program [36093]
CenterIMT Cherry Hill [38716]
Centerpoint • Adolescent Treatment Services
[49745]
Centerpoint Crisis Line [51259]
Centerpoint Health--College Hill [31684]
Centerpoint Health--Oakley [31685]
Centerpoint Health--Roselawn [31686]
Centerpoint Health--Victory Parkway, Cincinnati
[31687]
Centerpoint Health--Western Hills [31688]
CenterPoint Human Services • ADD Program
[31613]
CenterPoint Human Services--Davie County [31560]
CenterPoint Human Services
Partial Hospitalization Program [31614]
Services Office [31615]
CenterPoint Human Services--Winston Salem
[31616]
Centerpoint Medical Center [2791]
Cancer Center [5443]
CenterPointe • Adult Long Term Residential Prog
[45752]
CenterPointe Hospital [45603]

CenterPointe • Outpatient [45753]
Centers Against Abuse and Sexual Assault [9348]
Centers for Dialysis Care--Garfield [26126]
Centers for Dialysis Care--Harborside [26017]
Centers for Dialysis Care--Mentor [26163]
Centers for Dialysis Care--Oakwood [26179]
Centers for Dialysis Care--Warren [26226]
Centers For Youth & Families--Little Rock [33976]
Centers for Health Excellence, PC [38446]
Centers Inc
Adult Outpatient Services [41830]
Detoxification Unit [41831]
Substance Abuse Programs [41748]
The Centers • Martin Luther King Campus [29242]
Centers for Rehab Services [4387]
Centers for Youth and Families [7737]
Centers for Youth & Families
Adolescent Day Treatment Program [33979]
Elizabeth Mitchell Adolescent Center [33977]
Jacksonville Branch Office [33975]
Parent Center Programs [33978]
Centers for Youth and Families/Stepping Stones
Shelter • Runaway and Homeless Youth Program
[35800]
Centerston--LIFE Solutions Psychosocial [32295]
Centerstone [42997], [43010], [49070], [49124],
[49195]
Centerstone - Adolescent Residential • Dede Wal-
lace Center--Adolescent Residential Treatment
[32347]
Centerstone - Adult A and D Services [32348]
Centerstone Associates • Cumberland Associates
[32283]
Centerstone--Bedford [29698]
Centerstone - Bedford County [32376]
Highland Rim Mental Health Center [32377]
Centerstone • Between Friends Drop-In Center
[32310]
Centerstone--Brentwood [32271]
Centerstone
Brown County [43164]
Brown County Consulting Associates [29789]
Centerstone - Cheatham County • Harriett Cohn
Center of Cheatham County [32266]
Centerstone - Child and Youth Services - East
[32365]
Centerstone - Columbia Area [32296]
Centerstone Community Health Centers, Inc.
[51364]
Centerstone Community Living Center [32389]
Centerstone
Cumberland Associates [32297]
Cumberland Valley Group Home [32284]
Centerstone - Davidson Street • Highland Rim
Mental Health Center [32390]
Centerstone
DBA Center for Behavioral Health [29700]
Depression Treatment Clinic [29701]
Dickson Regional Intervention Program •
Regional Intervention Program [32303]
Do Drop In--Drop-In Center- [32285]
Centerstone - Estill Springs • Highland Rim Mental
Health Center [32309]
Centerstone • Fayette County [43011]
Centerstone - Fayetteville • Highland Rim Medical
Center [32311]
Centerstone - Frank Luton Center [32366]
Centerstone
Giles County Mental Health Center [32373]
Hand-In-Hand Drop-In Center [32339]
Centerstone - Harbor House [32367]
Centerstone - Harriet Cohn Center [34444]
Centerstone • Harriet Cohn Center [49057]
Centerstone - Harriett Cohn Center
Harriett Cohn Center--Craig Bldg. [32286]
Psychosocial Rehabilitation Enrichment Program
[32287]
Centerstone
Harriett Cohn Center • Regional Intervention
Program [32288]
Hickman County Health Department [32277]
Centerstone of IN Inc [43197]
Centerstone • Jackson Hall Residential Treatment
[32298]
Centerstone - Jackson Street [32391]
Centerstone - Lawrence County
Cumberland Associates [32340]
Lawrence County Counseling [32341]

Centerstone - Lewis County [32317]
Centerstone--Lewisburg [32343]
Centerstone • Luton Mental Health Services [49154]
Centerstone - Marshall County Mental Health Center
[32344]
Centerstone • Marshall County Mental Health Center
[49119]
Centerstone - Maury County Mental Health Center •
Maury County Mental Health Center [32299]
Centerstone at Maury Regional Hospital • Crisis
Center [32300]
Centerstone • My Place Drop-In Center [32392]
Centerstone--Nashville [32368]
Centerstone--North Vernon [29796]
Centerstone - Oak Hill Residential • Oak Hill
Residential [32289]
Centerstone • Randolph County [29835], [43232]
Centerstone - Ridgeview Residential • Ridgeview
Residential [32385]
Centerstone - Robertson • Harriett Cohn Center of
Springfield [32381]
Centerstone
Rush County [43193]
Samuel Gaar Resource Center [29808]
Centerstone--Seymour [29816]
Centerstone • Silver Linings Drop-In Center [32382]
Centerstone - Southridge • Southridge Psychological
Services [32304]
Centerstone • Stepping Stones Drop-In Center
[32305]
Centerstone - Sumner County • Sumner County
Family Services [32312]
Centerstone - The Lodge • The Lodge [32290]
Centerstone • Union City Children & Family Services
[29823]
Centerstone - Vivian House • Vivian House [32291]
Centerstone - Waverly • Harriett Cohn Center of
Humphreys County [32395]
Centerstone - Wayne County [32396]
Centerstone
Wayne County Mental Health Center [49199]
Wayne County Office [43186]
Wayne County OP [29809]
Weems Academy [32292]
Centra Health Hospice of the Hills [21705]
Centra Health, Inc. [18321]
Centra Health • Pearson Regional Cancer Center
[6066]
Centra Hospice of the Hills [21692]
Centra Sleep Disorders Center • Centra Health, Inc.
[37884]
Centra Wellness Network [44910]
Centracare Dialysis--Brainerd [25006]
Centracare Dialysis at Douglas County Hospital
[25000]
Centracare Dialysis at Lakewood Health System
[25089]
Centracare Dialysis at Monticello [25052]
Centracare Dialysis at Princeton [25063]
Centracare Dialysis/Saint Gabriel's Hospital [25034]
Centracare Kidney Program [25074]
Centracare Kidney Program at Big Lake [25003]
Centracare Kidney Program--Cabridge [25009]
Centracare Kidney Program--Litchfield [25033]
Central Adult Mental Health and Vocational Services
[28747]
Central Alabama Comprehensive Health, Inc. [6202]
Central Alabama Sleep Center • Sleep Disorders
Center [36570]
Central Alabama Veterans Affairs Health Care
System • PTSD Clinical Team [51682]
Central Alabama Veterans Health Care System •
East Campus [51530]
Central Alabama Veterans Health Care System--
Montgomery • West Campus [12701]
Central Alabama Veterans Health Care System--
Tuskegee [12732]
Central Alabama Veterans Health Care System •
West Campus [51528]
Central Alabama Veterans • Healthcare System
[39300]
Central Arkansas Dialysis--Jacksonville [22546]
Central Arkansas Dialysis--Searcy [22572]
Central Arkansas Health Center • Little Rock Health
Center [11334]
Central Arkansas Veterans Affairs Health Care
System • PTSD Program [51688]
Central Arkansas Veterans Healthcare

Substance Abuse Treatment [39545]
Substance Use Disorder/(SUD) Program [39564]
Central Arkansas Veterans Healthcare System
    Cancer Program [4754]
    Eugene J. Towbin Healthcare Center [51536]
    John L. McClellan Memorial Veterans Hospital [51535]
        Genetic Counseling Clinic [12146]
Central Arkansas Veterans Healthcare System--Little Rock [12867]
Central Atlanta Dialysis Center • Fresenius Medical Care [23585]
Central Bamberg Dialysis • DaVita [26679]
Central Baptist Hospital [19808]
    Cancer Care Center [5219]
Central Baptist Hospital Home Health [15206]
Central Baptist Hospital Sleep diagnostic Center [37021]
Central Basin Home Health & Hospice [21760]
Central Brooklyn Dialysis Center LLC [25609]
Central California Recovery Inc [39846]
Central City Community Health Center [6315]
Central City Health Center [6285]
Central City Home Health Office [15168]
Central City Mental Health Center [30163]
Central Coast Headway [40005]
    Drug and Alcohol Awareness Program [40756]
Central Coast Home Health Inc. [13323]
Central Coast Intensive Outpatient Eating Disorder Program [10941]
Central Coast Kidney Disease Center [23002]
Central Coast Language and Learning Center [1188]
Central Coast Pain Institute [35307]
Central Coast Sleep Disorders Center [36661]
Central Coast VNA and Hospice--Hollister [18941]
Central Coast VNA and Hospice--King City [18947]
Central Coast VNA and Hospice--Monterey [18970]
Central Coast VNA Hospice--Salinas [19009]
Central Columbia Dialysis & At Home • DaVita [26696]
Central Community Health Board • Drug Services Program [47654]
Central Connecticut Dialysis Center • Fresenius Medical Care [23163]
Central Counseling and • Education Services [39422]
Central Counties Center for Mental Health/Mental Retardation [32492], [32494], [32557]
    Hamilton [32472]
Central Counties Center for Mental Health/Mental Retardation Services • Milam County [32423]
Central Counties Services [49549]
Central Dallas Dialysis • DaVita [27018]
Central Denver Dialysis • Fresenius Medical Care [23109]
Central Des Moines Dialysis • DaVita [24264]
Central DuPage Hospital • Center for Sleep Health [36901]
Central Dupage Hospital--Crisis Stabilization Program [50880]
Central DuPage Hospital • Oncology Services [5131]
Central East Alcohol and Drug Council [42455]
    Adolescent Outpatient Services [42767]
    Adolescent Residential Treatment Program [42746]
    All Alcohol/Substance Abuse Progs on Site [42456]
    Charleston Primary Outpatient Services [42457]
    DHS/DCFS Initiative Program [42458]
    Outpatient Services [42768], [42908]
    Womens Recovery Home [42459]
Central Florida Behavioral Hospital • The Palms • Eating Disorders Program [11015]
Central Florida Community Center [6547]
Central Florida ENT Associates [1626]
Central Florida Family Health Center--Alafaya [6522]
Central Florida Family Health Center--Hoffner [6523]
Central Florida Health Care, Inc. • Central Florida Health Care - Avon Park [6436]
Central Florida Hearing Center [1799]
Central Florida Helpline [50772]
Central Florida Kidney Center [23445]
Central Florida Kidney Center--Longwood • Dialysis Facility [23374]
Central Florida Kidney Center--Osceola [23355]
Central Florida Kidney Center--Vineland [23446]

Central Florida Kidney Center--Winter Garden [23559]
Central Florida Pulmonary Group • Cystic Fibrosis Center [7500]
Central Florida Regional Hospital [1749]
Central Florida Sleep Centers, Osceola [36775]
Central Florida Sleep Centers, Polk [36776]
Central Florida Speech and Hearing Center [1627]
Central Florida Therapy Solutions Inc. [1637]
Central Florida Treatment Center [41602], [41730]
    Fort Pierce [41669]
        Outpatient Methadone Maintenance [41855]
    Palm Bay [41874]
Central Fort Wayne Dialysis Center • Diversified Specialty Institutes [24140]
Central Georgia Home Care [14541]
Central Georgia Home Health [14542]
Central Georgia Professional Hearing Aid Services [1925]
Central Harlem Alcohol Crisis Center [46845]
Central Health Care [12625]
Central Health Care--Huntsville [6190]
Central Health Center [7222]
Central Health Corporation [13954]
Central Home Health Agency [13026]
Central Home Health Care [15807]
Central Illinois Community Blood Bank--Edwardsville [35021]
Central Illinois Community Blood Bank--Springfield [35022]
Central Illinois Pain Center [35427]
Central Imaging of Arlington • Pain Management Services [35688]
Central Indiana Sports Medicine--Anderson [38422]
Central Indiana Sports Medicine--Muncie [38441]
Central Jersey Speech [2924]
Central Jersey Speech and Language [2907]
Central Jersey Sports Medicine and Orthopaedic Center [38732]
Central Juvenile Hall [28585]
Central Kansas Cooperative in Education [438]
Central Kansas Foundation
    Abilene [43316]
    Junction City [43370]
    McPherson [43404]
    Residential Services [43452]
Central Kansas Medical Center [15125]
Central Kansas Mental Health Center [29904]
Central Kentucky Psychiatry [43573]
Central Kittanning Dialysis Center, LLC • American Renal Associates [26457]
Central Los Angeles Continuing Care [28586]
Central Louisiana State Hospital [33547]
Central Main Family Counseling PA • Blue Willow Counseling [43994]
Central Maine Medical Center • Cancer Program [5271]
Central Maine Sleep Center [37089]
Central Maine Sports Medicine [38507]
Central Maryland Sleep Center [37098]
Central Michigan University
    Communication Disorders Department • Speech, Language, and Hearing Clinic [2628]
    DeafBlind Central: Michigan's Training and Resource Project [2629]
Central Minnesota Mental Health Center [45096]
    Detox [45289]
Central Minnesota Task Force on Battered Women [9635]
Central Mississippi Civic Improvement Assoc., Inc. [6883]
Central Mississippi Health Services, Inc. [6884]
Central Mississippi Medical Center • Cancer Program [5426]
Central Montgomery Mental Health and Mental Retardation Center [8472]
Central Montgomery MH/MR Center • Substance Abuse Services [48486]
Central Naples Pediatrics [6515]
Central Nassau Guidance and Counseling Services [31350]
Central Nassau Guidance and Counseling • Services Inc/Community Program [46695]
Central Naugatuck Valley Help Inc • Rev Edward Dempsey Drug Serv Program [41482]
Central Nebraska Orthopedics--Grand Island [38685]
Central Nebraska Orthopedics--Hastings [38686]
Central Nebraska Rehabilitation/Children's Rehab

Center • Speech Pathology Services [2842]
Central Nebraska Support Service Program [536]
Central New Hampshire Kidney Center [25390]
Central New Mexico Kidney Center • Fresenius Medical Care [25553]
Central New York Developmental Disabilities Services Office [8350]
Central New York Dialysis Center [25785]
Central New York Eye and Tissue Bank [35129]
Central New York Infusion Service, LLC [16436]
Central New York Psychiatric Center [33701]
Central New York Services Inc
    Dual Recovery Program [47113]
    Milestones Dual Recovery Program [47147]
Central North Alabama Health Services, Inc. [12681]
Central Ohio Lions Eye Bank, Inc. [35155]
Central Oklahoma Community Mental Health Center [31896]
    Youth Services [31897]
Central Oklahoma Family Medical Center, Inc. [7107], [17123]
Central Oregon Sleep Disorders Center [37611]
Central Oregon Vet Center [52067]
Central Orlando Dialysis • DaVita [23447]
Central Ozark Medical Center [6915]
Central Park of Lisle/Sanya Syrstad [42752]
Central Peninsula Counseling Services [28122], [50636]
Central Peninsula General Hospital • Serenity House Residential Treatment [39338]
Central Peninsula Health Centers
    Aspen Dental Center [6212]
    Cottonwood Health Center [6217]
Central Piedmont Community College • Disability Services [612]
Central Plains Center Crisis Hotline [51389]
Central Plains Center • Dimmitt Outpatient Clinic [32447]
Central Plains Center for Mental Health/Mental Retardation [32526]
    Children's Development Center [32527]
    New Horizons [32528]
    Plainview Outpatient Clinic [32529]
Central Plains Center
    Reed Adolescent Center [49485]
    Reed Adolescent Center Outpatient Prog [49486]
Central Plains Center - Tulia Satellite [32561]
Central Plains Early Childhood Intervention [8561]
Central Plains Hospice • Cozad Community Health System [20380]
Central Psychiatric Clinic [31689]
Central Rappahannock Regional Library • Fredericksburg Area Subregional Library [3846]
Central Recovery Treatment • Pain Clinic [35546]
Central Rehabilitation, Ltd. [2212]
Central Speech and Language Clinic Inc. [2065]
Central Sports Care Center [38786]
Central Star Multi Care Services, Inc. [16971]
Central State Hospital [7915]
    Dual Diagnosis Service [43683]
Central State Hospital--Louisville [33526]
Central State Hospital--Milledgeville [33386]
Central State Hospital--Petersburg [33905]
Central State Orthopedic Specialists • Sports Medicine Services [38904]
Central States Mental Health Consultants Inc • Lexington Site [45554]
Central States Mental Hlth Consultants
    Blue Springs - Hampton Inn WIP [45437]
    Knob Noster - Whiteman Inn WIP [45547]
    Lees Summit [45550]
    Warrensburg [45667]
Central Suffolk AKC [25758]
Central Tampa Hematology and Oncology • Adult Sickle Cell Center [36318]
Central Texas Medial Center Home Health [18155]
Central Texas Medical Center Hospice [21562]
Central Texas Mental Health/Mental Retardation Center
    Brady Work Activity Center [32418]
    The Center for Life Resources [32419]
    Comanche County [32429]
    Respite Care [32420]
    San Saba/Mills [32550]
    Supported Housing Program [32421]
Central Texas Speech Pathology Services Inc. [3459]

Central Texas VA Healthcare Services • Temple Substance Abuse Treatment/Employ Prog [49550]
Central Texas Veterans Affairs Health Care System [51662]
Central Texas Veterans Affairs Healthcare System • PTSD Clinical Team [51831]
Central Texas Veterans Health Care System [18170]
Waco Veterans Affairs Medical Center [51663]
Central Texas Veterans Healthcare System
Olin E. Teague Veterans' Center • Cancer Program [6029]
PTSD Clinical Team [51824]
Central Texas Youth Services Bureau • Runaway and Homeless Youth Program [36213]
Central Utah Clinic • Sleep Disorders Clinic [37869]
Central Utah Counseling Center [49608], [49611], [49612], [49642]
Central Utah Counseling Center--Delta [32579]
Central Utah Counseling Center--Richfield [32613]
Central Utah Counseling Center • Substance Abuse Center [49668]
Central Utah Mental Health Center--Nephi [32597]
Central Utah Mental Health Center--S State Street, Mount Pleasant [32594]
Central Utah Mental Health Center--W Main Street, Mount Pleasant [32595]
Central Utah Mental Health/Substance Abuse Center--Ephraim [32583]
Central Utah Mental Health/Substance Abuse Center--Junction [32586]
Central Valley Addiction Center [40214]
Central Valley Dialysis Center [27421]
Central Valley Hospice [21624]
Central Valley Indian Health Program • Subst Abuse Services /Outreach [39718]
Central Vermont Home Health and Hospice Inc. [18231], [21659]
Central Vermont Medical Center [18232]
Central Vermont • Substance Abuse Services [49722]
Central Vet Center [52006]
Central Virginia Community Services Board [32757]
Central Virginia Community Services • Courtland Center [49807]
Central Virginia Health Services, Inc. • Central Virginia Community Health Center [7358]
Central Virginia Task Force on Domestic Violence in Later Life [10588]
Central Virginia Training Center [8590]
Central Washington Comprehensive Center • Lower Valley Center [32868]
Central Washington Comprehensive Mental Health [51478]
Central Washington Comprehensive Mental Health Services [32883]
Central Washington Comprehensive MH [50268]
Central Washington Comprehensive MH and Dependency Health Services [49970]
Central Washington Comprehensive Services [32823]
Central Washington Comprisive MH and Dependency Health Services/Detox [50269]
Central Washington Family Medicine [7395]
Central Washington Hospital [18484]
Dialysis Center [27660]
Family Health Services • Central Washington Genetics Program [12364]
Central Washington Hospital Home Health and Hospice [21781]
Central Washington Orthopedic & Sports Medicine Clinic [39156]
Central West Eating Disorder Program Regional Office [11211]
Central Westchester Community Mental Health Center [31492]
Central Wisconsin Center for the Developmentally Disabled [8617]
Central Wyoming Counseling Center [34496]
Residential Facility [50570]
Central Wyoming Hospice Program/Cara Lou Chapman Hospice Home [21876]
Central Wyoming Neurology Clinic • MDA Clinic [34914]
Centralia Dialysis • DaVita [23911]
Centralia School District [266]
CentraState Healthcare System • Cancer Program [5514]
CentraState HealthCare System • Center for Sleep

Disorders [37339]
CentraState • Linda E. Cardinale Multiple Sclerosis Center [34632]
Centre Clinic • Georgetown University Hospital [29083]
Centre Counseling Associates [48649]
Centre County Women's Resource Center, Inc. [10316]
Centre County Youth Service - Stormbreak • Runaway and Homeless Youth Program [36178]
Centre Crossings Hospice [21159]
Centre Inc [47568], [47580], [47589]
Centre for Neuro Skills--Bakersfield, CA [3896]
Centre for Neuro Skills--Centre Village [3897]
Centre for Neuro Skills, Irving [4443]
Centre for Neurological Rehabilitation, Inc.--Laredo [10866]
Centre for Sleep and Human Performance [36623]
Centrec Care Inc [45616]
Centria - Brighton [15594]
Centro de Acogida [7201]
Centro de Amistad Inc [39423]
Mesa Office [39403]
Centro de Amor El Elion Inc [48747]
Centro Detox y Tratamiento Metadona SJ • Pabellon G [48801]
Centro Latinoamericano [48099]
Centro Madre Dominga Casa Belen Inc [48793]
Centro Ponce Tratamiento • Residencial Para Varones [48794]
Centro Pulmonar and Desordenes De Sueno [37717]
Centro de Quimioterapia de Bayamon [48727]
Centro Renacer Inc [48760]
Centro Renal Universitario [26651]
Centro de Salud Familiar Le Fe [7287]
Centro de Salud Mental de la Comunidad de May-aguez [48784]
Centro San Vicente [7288]
Centro de Servicios para Hispanos [32062]
Centro de Servicios a la Juventud • Runaway and Homeless Youth Program [36188]
Centro de Servicios Primarios de Salud [7207]
Centro de Transformacion Social • Cristiano Inc [48728]
Centro de Tratamiento Ambulatorios • Menores Ponce [48795]
Centro de Tratamiento Con Metadona • De Agua-dilla [48718]
Centro de Tratamiento con Metadona [48748]
Centro de Tratamiento Para • Adultos de Ponce/Outpatient Drug Court [48796]
Centro de Tratamiento Residential • De Varones San Juan [48812]
Centromed Santa Rosa Clinic [7311]
Centros Sor Isolina Ferre • Runaway and Homeless Youth Program [36189]
CentroTratamiento Ambulatorio Adultos • Drug Court Arecibo [48722]
Centura Health at Home [13473]
Centura Home Care [13465]
Centura Home Care and HME [13506]
Centura/Penrose-Saint Francis Health Services • Penrose Cancer Center [4870]
Century City Dialysis Center • DaVita [22770]
Century Clinic [33295]
Century Health--Adult Treatment Center [31767]
Century Health South Campus [47760]
Century Home Healthcare [17869], [18117]
Century Home Healthcare, Inc. [13064]
Century Hospice [21429]
Century House [50548]
Cerebral Palsy Association of the Rochester Area [8347]
Cerebral Palsy Center [8243]
Cerebral Palsy of Colorado • Creative Options Center for Early Education [7835]
Cerebral Palsy KIDS Center [2280]
Cerebral Palsy of Massachusetts [8142]
Cerebral Palsy of North Jersey • Horizon School [8255]
Cerritos Dialysis Center, LLC [22626]
Certified Addiction Treatment for • Substances [41213]
Certified Counseling Services Inc [44313]
Certified Counseling Services LLC [44213]
CESA Number 11 • Hearing Impaired Program [893]
CESA Number 5 [891]

CESA Number 6 • Deaf/Hard of Hearing and Vision Programs [890]
CETPA Inc [42140]
CFC/Restart Substance Abuse Services • Hannick Hall [46935]
CFHC Frostproof Clinic [6466]
CFHC Lakeland OB/GYN [6484]
CFHC Wauchula Clinic [6566]
CFMC Home Health Agency [18188]
CFMH Home Care [18380]
CGH Medical Center [14946]
CGH Sleep Center [36902]
Chabad Residential Treatment Center • For Men [40089]
Chad Youth Enhancement Center [34443]
Chaddock Center [34120]
Chadron Comm Hospital/Home Health Hospice [20378]
Chadron Community Hospital Dialysis [25318]
Chafee Community Health Center [7223]
CHAI/Jewish Community Resource on Domestic Violence [8945]
Challenge Behavioral Healthcare [42708]
Challenge Programs of New Jersey Inc [46121]
Challenges [41756]
Challenges Inc • Overland Park [43434]
Chalmers P. Wylie Veterans Affairs Ambulatory Care Center • PTSD Clinical Team [51798]
Chalmers P. Wylie Veterans Clinic [31725]
Chalmette Dialysis Center [24475]
Chamberlain Children's Center [33987]
Chamberlain's Acres [33988]
Chamberlain's Mental Health Services [28513]
Chambers and Associates Company [44703]
Chambers County Addictions Center [27963]
Chambers County Board of Education [199]
Chambersburg Hospital of Speech-Language Pathology [3326]
Chambersburg Hospital • Summit Cancer Services [5817]
Champaign Residential Services, Inc.--Lima [31788]
Champaign Residential Services, Inc.--London [31792]
Champaign Residential Services, Inc.--Springfield [31835]
Champaign Residential Services, Inc.--Troy [31848]
Champaign Residential Services, Inc.--Urbana [31849]
Champaign Residential Services, Inc.--Wapakoneta [31851]
Champaign--Urbana Dialysis Center • Fresenius Medical Care [24099]
Champion Health [38167]
Champions Recovery • Alternative Programs Inc [39901]
Champlain Valley Family Center • Drug Treatment Youth Services Inc/Outpt [46979]
Champlain Valley Physicians Hospital /Elizabethtown Community Hospital • Dialysis Facility [25652]
Champlain Valley Physicians Hospital --Freedman Renal Center • Dialysis Center [25755]
Champlain Valley Physicians Hospital Medical Center
FitzPatrick Cancer Center [5607]
Renal Center [25756]
Chance Center [44120]
A Chance to Change Foundation [47974]
Chance Program [32869]
Chances For Youth • Runaway and Homeless Youth Program [36243]
Chandler Family Health Center [6227]
Chandler Hall Health Services, Inc. [17397]
Chandler Regional Medical Center [18785]
Chandler Valley Hope Alcohol/Drug and • Related Treatment Services [39374]
Change [40483]
A Change Counseling Services Inc • Tacoma [50206]
Change Lanes • Change Lanes Youth Support Services [39986]
Change Your Life Enterprises Inc • ADAPT [43484]
ChangePoint Inc [48073], [48182]
Changes Behavioral Services Inc [42769]
Changes Counseling/Consultation LLC [49704]
Changes Counseling Services [49227]
Changes Place [42678], [42886]
Changes for Recovery [40715]
Changing Echoes [39603]

Changing Steps [40889]
Channel Marker, Inc.--Cambridge [30270]
Channel Marker, Inc.--Denton [30279]
Channel Marker, Inc.--Easton [30282]
Channelview Dialysis • DaVita [26994]
CHANS Home Health Care [15388]
Chans Hospice Care [19890]
Chapa de Indian Health Program Inc • Substance
  Abuse Services [39617]
Chapel Haven [7861]
Chapel Hill Fertility Center [22199]
Chapel Hill Pediatric Speech Pathology [3164]
Chapel Home Health [13606], [14465]
Chapman and Associates Therapy Solutions [1703]
Chapman House Inc [40321], [40455]
Chapman Nursing Home [27822]
Charak Center for Health and Wellness
  Rakesh Ranjan MD and Associates [47767]
  Rakesh Ranjan MD and Associates Inc [47811]
Charg Resource Center [28881]
Charing Cross Dialysis LLC [24665]
Charis Center for Eating Disorders [11060]
Charity Home Health Services, Inc. [12933]
Charity Hospice, Inc. [20911]
The Charity League Hearing & Speech Center •
  Children's Hospital of Alabama [901]
CHARLEE Homes for Children [34067]
Charleroi Medical and Dental Center [7157]
Charles B. Wang Community Health Center, Inc.
  [7028]
Charles Cole Memorial Hospital [17292]
Charles County Department of Health • Substance
  Abuse Services [44393]
Charles Drew Health Center [6943]
Charles F. Kettering Memorial Hospital • Cancer
  Care Program [5727]
Charles George VA Medical Center [4327]
Charles George VA Medical Center at Ashville
  [16693]
Charles George VAMC/Ashville • Substance Abuse
  Treatment Program [47208]
Charles Glodner Counseling Group [40757]
Charles I Schwartz • Chemical Dependency Treat-
  ment Center [43651]
Charles K Post Addiction Treatment Center
  Community Residence Program [46391]
  Inpatient Rehabilitation Program [46392]
Charles Norwood Veterans Affairs Medical Center •
  PTSD Clinical Team [51716]
Charles P. Wylie Veterans Affairs Ambulatory Care
  Center [16904]
Charles Pfeiffer, Inc. [16636]
Charles William Leighton, Jr. Hospice [18835]
Charles Wilson Veterans Affairs Outpatient Clinic
  [18060]
Charleston Area Medical Center
  Behavioral Health Services Unit [50289]
  Cancer Care Center-Chemotherapy [12612]
  David Lee Cancer Center [6133]
  Kidney Dialysis Unit [27667]
  Medical Rehabilitation Center [4489]
  Sleep Disorders Center [37949]
Charleston Center of Charleston County [48909]
Charleston Dorchester Mental Health Center • As-
  sessment/Mobile Crisis [51321]
Charleston Genetic Center • Down Syndrome Clinic
  [10858]
Charleston Orphan House • Runaway and Home-
  less Youth Program [36193]
Charleston Renal Care--Goose Creek • DaVita
  [26720]
Charleston Scottish Rite Center [3395]
Charleston Speech & Hearing Center Inc. [3408]
Charleston Treatment Center Inc [50290]
Charleston Veterans Affairs Medical Center--Bee
  Street [32189]
Charleston Veterans Affairs Medical Center • Savan-
  nah Clinic [29492]
Charleston Veterans Affairs Primary Care Clinic--
  Alex Lane [32891]
Charlevoix Area Hospital • Sleep Center [37151]
Charlie Major Foster Home • JBS Mental Health
  Authority [27850]
Charlie Norwood VA Medical Center [14485]
Charlie Norwood VA Medical Center--Downtown
  Division [14486]
Charlie Norwood Veterans Affairs Medical Center
  [29359], [51558]

Charlotte Behavioral Healthcare [41909]
Charlotte Center for Balanced Living • Eating
  Disorders Program [11172]
Charlotte Community Mental Health Services, Inc.
  [29269]
    Crisis Stabilization Unit [29270]
    Group Residential Treatment Systems [29271]
    Therapeutic Family Care [29272]
Charlotte Dialysis • DaVita [25832]
Charlotte Eye, Ear, Nose and Throat Associates, PA
  • Sleep Center at Southpark [37463]
Charlotte Hearing Center [1731]
Charlotte Hungerford Hospital • Comprehensive
  Cancer Center [4909]
Charlotte Regional Medical Center • Sleep Disorders
  Center [36777]
Charlotte Regional Medical Center, Speech Pathol-
  ogy [1738]
Charlotte Rescue Mission [47253]
Charlotte Speech and Hearing Center [3166]
Charlotte Veterans Affairs Clinic [31518]
Charlotte White Administration [30206]
Charlottesville North Dialysis & At Home • DaVita
  [27467]
Charlton Memorial Hospital [2476]
Charlton Visiting Nurses Service [14558]
Charlton Visiting Nurses Service--Greater Savannah
  Area [14571]
Charter Colony Dialysis Center • DaVita [27515]
Charter Cypress Behavioral Health System [50944]
Charter Home HealthCare [15689]
Charter Hospice/dba Reche Canyon Rehabilitation
  and Health Care Center [18908]
Charter Oak Health Center, Inc. [6421]
Chartiers Mental Health/Mental Retardation Center,
  Inc. [31999]
Chartres Pontchartrain Behav Hlth Center [43868]
Chartres Pontchartrain Behavioral Health Center
  [30164]
Chartwell Midwest Wisconsin [18591]
Chase Brexton Health Services • Department of
  Behavioral Health [44121]
Chase Brexton Health Services, Inc. [6787]
Chase Group Home [34101]
Chase Healthcare Services, Inc. [18160]
Chateau Dialysis • DVA Renal Healthcare • DaVita
  [24512]
Chatham Counseling of Freedom House [47446]
Chatham--Kent Mental Health and Addictions
  Program • Eating Disorders Program [11212]
Chattahoochee Hospice [18771]
Chattahoochee Valley Home Health [12712]
Chattanooga Hamilton County Health Department •
  Homeless Health Care Center [7254]
Chattanooga Kidney Center [26811]
Chattanooga Kidney Center North, LLC [26812]
Chattanooga State Technical Community College •
  Disabilities Support Services [747]
Chatterbox Inc. [1899]
Chatterboxes LLC [2502]
Chatterbug LLC [1429]
Chautauqua County Department of MH
  Alcohol Clinic [46610]
    Chemical Dependency Services [46734]
Chautauqua Opportunities • Runaway and Home-
  less Youth Program [36094]
Chaya [10642]
CHC Branch County Substance • Treatment and
  Referral Services [44714]
CHCCW Conwell Clinic [7444]
CHD, Inc. • Community Support Program [30396]
Cheaha Mental Health Center [28045]
Cheaha Regional Mental Health/Caradale • Lodge/
  Mental Retardation Board Inc [39293]
CHEARS Homehealth & Hospice [19731]
Chee Woy Na Zhee • Halfway House [45818]
CHEER Mental Health Center [49131]
Chehails Business Council [50034]
Chehalis Tribe Behavioral Heath • Tsapowum/
  Chemical Dependency Program [50035]
Chelan Douglas Behavioral Health Care [32882]
Chelan-Douglas Behavioral Health Clinic [51477]
Chelsea Community Hospital [30528]
    Head Pain Treatment Program [35498]
Chelsea Counseling Center [30359]
Chelsea Day Treatment [34162]
Chelsea Health Center [32652]
Chelsea's Home Health Care Inc. [13123]

Chem Depend Services Inpt/Outpatient • Kootenai
  Behav Hlth/Kootenai Med Center [42329]
Chem Rx [16511]
Chemeketa Community College • Services for the
  Deaf [691]
Chemical Abuse Services Agency Inc
  DBA MAAS [41435]
  Eugenio Maria de Hostos [41362]
Chemical Addictions Program Inc
  Adolescent Intensive Outpatient Prog [39279]
  Adult Outpatient Services [39269]
Chemical Addictions Recovery Effort
  AWARE [41882]
  Bay County Outpatient Office [41883]
  Jackson County Outpatient Office [41757]
  Starting Over Straight [41884]
Chemical Data Services Corporation • The Sequoia
  Center [40438]
Chemical Dependency Training • Evaluation and
  Guidance Inc [47393], [47400]
Chemik Healthcare Services, Inc. [17969]
Chenango Cnty Alcohol and Drug Abuse Services •
  Drug Abuse Treatment [46953]
Chenango Speech Therapy Service Inc. [3086]
Chenango Therapeutics [38808]
Cherish Hospice, Inc. [19060]
Cherokee County ARC [8504]
Cherokee County Commission on Alcohol and Drug
  Abuse [48936]
Cherokee County Health Department • Speech and
  Hearing Clinic [3286]
Cherokee County Nursing Home [27883]
Cherokee County Schools [190]
Cherokee County Schools Hearing Impaired
  Program [365]
Cherokee Dialysis Center • DaVita [25843]
Cherokee Etowah Dekalb Community Mental Health
  Center [27836]
    Copeland/Matthews Home [27932]
Cherokee/Etowah/DeKalb Mental Health Center •
  Substance Abuse Services Men/Women [39210]
Cherokee Family Violence Center, Inc. [9094]
Cherokee Health Systems [7273], [49039], [49040],
  [49104], [49130], [49148], [49166], [49167],
  [49177], [49188]
  Bean Station Office [32268]
  Blaine Office [32269]
  Cocke County Office [32371]
  Jefferson City Office [32320]
  Lenoir City Office [32342]
  Maryville Office [32350]
  Morristown Office [32362]
  New Tazewell Office [32370]
  North Knox Office [32332]
  Seymour Office [32375]
  Substance Abuse Treatment Program [49193]
  Talbott Office [32383]
  Union Grainer Primary Care [32352]
  Washburn Office [32394]
  West Knoxville Office [32333]
Cherokee Hospice [18692]
Cherokee Nation Youth Services • Runaway and
  Homeless Youth Program [36153]
Cherokee/Pickens Mental Health Center [29380]
Cherokee Restoration Fellowship • Cherokee House
  [40333]
Cherry County Hospital • Dialysis Unit [25346]
Cherry Hill Dialysis Center • DaVita [25416]
Cherry Hospital [33737]
Cherry Lane House [28552]
Cherry Street Services, Inc. • Cherry Street Health
  Services [6845]
Cherry Valley Dialysis • DaVita [26172]
Chesapeake Center Inc. [3612]
Chesapeake Community Services Board [32722]
Chesapeake General Hospital • Cancer Center
  [6056]
Chesapeake Regional Home Care Services [18266]
Chesapeake Speech Language Associates [2367]
Chesapeake Speech Therapy Services [2398]
Cheshire Center [3180]
Cheshire Medical Center • Kingsbury Center for
  Cancer Care [5496]
Chespenn Center for Family Health [7158]
Chest Pain Clinic [35308]
Chester Counseling Center [48578]
Chester County Hospital • Cancer Program [5877]
Chester County Intermediate Unit [696]

Chester County Mental Health • Crisis Intervention Services [51299]
Chester Dialysis • DaVita [27475]
Chester Mental Health Center [33409]
Chester River Home Care and Hospice [19920]
Chesterfield County Crisis Intervention [51417]
Chesterfield County Public Schools [856]
Chesterfield Department of Mental Health Support Services [49775]
Chesterfield Mental Health Clinic [32191]
Chestnut Health Systems Inc [42691], [42766]
    Adolescent Chemical Dependency Services [42416]
    Adult Chemical Dependency Services [42417]
Chestnut Health Systems • Psychosocial Rehabilitation [29565]
Chestnut Hill Health System • Cancer Center [5851]
Chestnut Hills Wellness Center [38890]
Chestnut Ridge Center • WVU Hospitals Inc [50330]
Chestnut Ridge Counseling Services, Inc. [32126]
Chestnut Ridge Hospital [33919]
Chestnut Square Dialysis Center • Independent Dialysis Foundation [24629]
Cheyenne Community Drug Abuse • Treatment Council Inc/Pathfinder [50574]
Cheyenne Crossroads Clinic [7448]
Cheyenne Health and Wellness Center [7449]
Cheyenne Helpline [51524]
Cheyenne Medical Specialists • Headache Center [12478]
Cheyenne Regional Medical Center [3690]
    Cancer Center [4720]
Cheyenne VA Medical Center • Substance Abuse Treatment Program [50575]
Cheyenne Veterans Affairs Medical Center [33034]
    Greeley Clinic [28912]
    Multiple Sclerosis Center [34747]
Chez Hope, Inc. [9406]
Chicago Association for Retarded Citizens • Lakeview Early Intervention [7937]
Chicago Center for Recovery and • Empowerment NFP [42481]
Chicago Center for Sports Medicine and Orthopedic Surgery [38359]
Chicago Dialysis Center • Fresenius Medical Care [23916]
Chicago Family Health Center, Inc. [6653]
Chicago Girls Program [42482]
Chicago Hearing Society [1983]
Chicago Heights Dialysis • DaVita [23966]
Chicago Lakeshore Hospital [33410]
    Chemical Dependence Program [42483]
Chicago Midwest Home Health [14926]
Chicago Public Library - Talking Book Center [3785]
Chicago--Read Mental Health Center [33411]
Chicago Treatment and
    Counseling Centers Inc [42599]
    Counseling Centers Inc I [42484]
    Counseling Centers Inc II [42485]
    Counseling Centers Inc III [42600]
Chicago Veterans Resource Center [51946]
Chicago Westside Dialysis • Fresenius Medical Care [23917]
Chicana Service Action Center • Free Spirit and Bilingual Shelters [8839]
Chicanos Por La Causa Inc • Centro de La Familia [39424]
Chickasaw Nation Office of Violence Prevention [10187]
Chickasha Dialysis Center • DaVita [26251]
Chico Dialysis Center • DaVita [22627]
Chico Family Health Center/Dental [6297]
Chico Recovery Center [39702]
The Chicsaw Nation • Runaway and Homeless Youth Program [36154]
Child Abuse Program [34164]
Child and Adolescent Center--Flint [30550]
Child and Adolescent Center--Montgomery [27993]
Child and Adolescent Mental Health [29412]
Child and Adolescent Outpatient Clinic • Piedmont Hall [29347]
Child, Adolescent & Parent Service [32497]
Child and Adolescent Service Center--Alliance [31650]
Child and Adolescent Service Center--Belden [31675]
Child and Adolescent Service Center--Canton [31676]

Child & Adolescent Services [29360]
Child & Adolescent Treatment Services, Inc. [31377]
Child-Adult Resource Services [8005]
Child Center for Developmental Services [8341]
Child Center of New York • Jamaica Family Center Subst Abuse Program [46721]
Child Center of NY Asian Outreach • Clinic Outpatient Chemical Dependency Unit [46623]
Child Development Center [8224]
Child Development Center of Colorado Springs Inc. [1385]
Child & Family [32168]
Child and Family Center [32758]
Child and Family Center, Newhall [28651]
Child and Family Center • Santa Clarita [40742]
Child and Family Development • Midtown [3167], [8372]
Child and Family Guidance Center, Mesquite [32513]
Child and Family Guidance Center--Northridge [28657]
Child and Family Guidance Center, Plano [32530]
Child and Family Guidance Center • Step One Chemical Dependency Outpatient [46697]
Child and Family • Psychological Services [44865]
Child and Family Service, Inc. [30424]
Child and Family Service--Kahului [9149]
Child and Family Services [45906]
Child and Family Services--Buffalo [31286]
Child and Family Services Capital Area [44878]
Child and Family Services--Ewa Beach [9132]
Child and Family Services--Hilo • Hale Ohana Shelter--East Hawaii [9133]
Child and Family Services, Knoxville • Runaway and Homeless Youth Program [36204]
Child and Family Services--Muskegon [9563]
Child and Family Services of New Hampshire • Runaway and Homeless Youth Program [36072]
Child and Family Services of Newport [32154]
    County Family Counseling Outpatient Dept [48855]
Child and Family Services of Southwestern Michigan • Runaway and Homeless Youth Program [36010]
Child and Family Tennessee • Great Starts [49105]
Child & Family Therapy Center • DC Department of Mental Health [29084]
Child Focus, Inc. [31690]
Child Guidance Center [28420]
Child Guidance Center & Family Solutions [31644]
Child Guidance Center of Greater Bridgeport, Inc. [28976], [28995]
Child Guidance Center of Mid-Fairfield County [7855]
Child Guidance Clinic of Greater Bridgeport [7845]
Child Guidance Clinic • Henrietta Weill Memorial [28474]
Child Guidance Clinic--New Britain [29016]
Child Guidance Clinic of Southern Connecticut [7857]
Child Guidance Clinic • Washington County Health Department [31873]
Child Guidance Resource Centers [8465], [48400]
Child Guidance Resource Centers--Coatesville [32005]
Child Guidance Resource Centers--Havertown [32025]
Child Guidance Resource Centers--Middletown [32045]
Child Guidance Resource Centers--Norristown [32059]
CHILD Inc. [9010]
Child, Inc. • Runaway and Homeless Youth Program [35869]
Child Mental Health Service • County of Orange Health Care Agency [28553]
Child Study Center [8547], [32459]
Childhelp USA [28401]
Childhood League Center [8408]
Children and Adolescent Mental Health Program • The Center for Healthcare Services [49521]
Children and Adult Therapy Services [1887]
Children and Families First--Baynard Boulevard, Wilmington [33277]
Children and Families First--Dover [33270]
Children & Families First--Georgetown [34059]
Children and Families First--Seaford • Seaford House Residential Treatment Center [33276]

Children and Families First--Tatnall Street, Wilmington [33278]
Children & Families First--Wilmington [34062]
Children & Family Center of Northwest Missouri [9702]
Children in Motion Therapy Services [2870]
Children in Need of Hugs [35812]
Children and Parents Program [44210]
Children, Youth and Family Services • Runaway and Homeless Youth Program [36244]
Children's Advisory Network [1421]
Children's Aid Home Programs of Somerset County, Inc. [34429]
Children's Aid Society [31408]
The Children's Aid Society • East Harlem Center [31409]
Children's Aid Society • Runaway and Homeless Youth Program [35779]
Children's Aid Society, Wichita Falls • Runaway and Homeless Youth Program [36214]
Children's Bureau • Runaway and Homeless Youth Program [35947]
Children's Cabinet, Inc. • Runaway and Homeless Youth Program [36069]
Children's Campus, Inc. [33482]
Children's Care Hospital and School [8508]
Children's Center for Behavioral Development [7933], [34099]
The Children's Center--Bethany [8434]
Children's Center for Cancer and Blood Disorders • Richland Memorial Hospital [12592]
The Children's Center, Galveston • Youth Shelter • Runaway and Homeless Youth Program [36215]
Children's Center of Hamden [33242]
The Childrens Center of Hamden • Outpatient and Short Term Residential [41391]
The Children's Center--Kearns [34458]
Children's Center of Monmouth County [8261]
Children's Center of Montgomery [7721]
Children's Center for Neurodevelopmental Studies [7734]
The Children's Center of Riverside [7812]
The Children's Center--Salt Lake City [34459]
The Children's Center--Winston Salem [8392]
Children's Choice for Hearing and Talking [290]
Children's Clinics for Rehabilitative Services • MDA Clinic [34753]
Children's Communication Center--Bethesda [2390]
Children's Communication Center, Inc.--Tallahassee [1770]
Children's Community Support Collaborative [34185]
Children's Creative Therapies [3044]
Children's Crisis Outreach Response System [51464]
Children's Crisis Stabilization Unit [29231]
The Children's Day School [8275]
Children's Dialysis Center • DaVita [23918]
Children's Dialysis Clinic of Central Texas • Dialysis Clinic Inc. [26950]
Children's Garden of California [34022]
Children's Guild [8086]
Children's Habilitation Center • ChildServe [8017]
Children's Health Council [7804]
Children's Health of Decatur [6183]
Children's Healthcare of Atlanta [1816]
Children's Healthcare or Atlanta [36835]
Children's Healthcare of Atlanta at Alpharetta Hwy. [1804]
Children's Healthcare of Atlanta • at Scottish Rite • Day Rehabilitation Program [4000]
Children's Healthcare of Atlanta--Egleston [23586]
Children's Healthcare of Atlanta/Egleston Dialysis Unit [23587]
Children's Healthcare of Atlanta at Hughes Spalding [4001]
Children's Healthcare of Atlanta at Scottish Rite
    Day Rehabilitation Program [4002]
    Hematology/Oncology Center [12507]
    MDA Clinic [34786]
Children's Healthcare of Atlanta • Sickle Cell Disease Program [36332]
Children's Healthcare • Pediatric Neurology • Down Syndrome Program [10852]
Children's Hearing and Speech Centre of British Columbia [257]
The Children's Home [30272]
Children's Home Academy [34118]
Children's Home and Aid Society [33412]

Children's Home and Aid Society--Chicago [34102]
Children's Home and Aid Society--Evanston • Rice
Child and Family Center [34110]
Children's Home and Aid Society--Rockford •
Northern Regional Office [34121]
Children's Home Care [13007]
Children's Home of Cromwell [7846], [34052]
Children's Home of Detroit--Grosse Pointe [34230]
Children's Home of Detroit--Warren [34237]
Children's Home Health [17669]
Children's Home Health Care [16122]
Children's Home Healthcare's World [16123]
Children's Home of Illinois • Boys Group Home
[34119]
Childrens Home Inc [47535]
The Children's Home--Mount Holly [34303]
Children's Home of Northern Kentucky [34151]
Maplewood Campus [33519]
The Children's Home • Runaway and Homeless
Youth Program [36132]
Children's Home Society [29155]
Children's Home Society Crisis Nursery [9637]
Children's Home Society of Florida
Brevard Division • Runaway and Homeless
Youth Program [35882]
Clair's House • Runaway and Homeless Youth
Program [35883]
Haven House • Runaway and Homeless Youth
Program [35884]
North Central Division • Runaway and Homeless
Youth Program • Tree House [35885]
North Coastal Division • Runaway and Home-
less Youth Program--South Daytona [35886]
South Coastal Division • Runaway and Home-
less Youth Program--West Palm Beach
[35887]
Treasure Coast Division • Runaway and Home-
less Youth Program--Port Saint Lucie [35888]
Children's Home Society of South Dakota
Black Hills Children's Home [34437]
Sioux Falls Children's Home [34439]
Children's Home Society of Washington [34475]
Children's Home Society of Washington--Seattle
[34469]
Children's Home Society of Washington--Spokane
[34474]
Children's Home Society of West Virginia • Runaway
and Homeless Youth Program [36261]
Children's Home of Stockton [34031]
The Children's Home--Tampa [34085]
Childrens Home of York • STRIVE [48708]
Childrens Hosp Martha Eliot Hlth Center •
Substance Abuse Services [44490]
Children's Hospital [8071]
Children's Hospital of Alabama • Dialysis Center/
Solid Organ Transplant Clinic [22312]
Children's Hospital of Alabama Medical Center •
Burn Care Unit [4500]
Children's Hospital of Alabama • UAB Cystic
Fibrosis Center [7457]
Children's Hospital--Aurora CO [1375]
Children's Hospital--Aurora • MDA Clinic [34770]
Children's Hospital--Birmingham
Down Syndrome Clinic [10770]
Hematology Clinic [36286]
Neurology Office • MDA Clinic [34748]
Sleep Disorders Center [36571]
Children's Hospital--Boston • Boston Hemophilia
Treatment Center [12530]
Children's Hospital Boston/Brigham and Women's
Hospital
Adult Cystic Fibrosis Center [7566]
Pediatric Cystic Fibrosis Center [7567]
Children's Hospital Boston
Department of Pediatric Medicine • Genetics
Clinic [12239]
Dialysis Unit, Farley Four [24748]
Children's Hospital-Boston • Down Syndrome
Program [10810]
Children's Hospital Boston at Lexington • Genetics
Clinic [12240]
Children's Hospital Boston
Neurology Department [34811]
Sickle Cell Program [36359]
Children's Hospital Boston at Waltham • Genetics
Clinic [12241]
Children's Hospital at Bronson • Comprehensive
Pediatric Sickle Cell Clinic [36361]

Children's Hospital of Buffalo
Children's Sickle Cell Clinic [36391]
Robert Warner Rehabilitation Center [8309]
The Children's Hospital • Burn Program [4527]
Children's Hospital • Center for Cancer & Blood
Disorders [5256]
Children's Hospital Central California [1174]
Children's Hospital of Central California • Hematol-
ogy/Oncology [12485]
Children's Hospital Central California • Pediatric
Cystic Fibrosis Center [7467]
Children's Hospital, Christus Santa Rosa • Sickle
Cell Center [36435]
Children's Hospital and Clinics • Home Care and
Hospice [20180]
Children's Hospital of Columbus • Comprehensive
Pediatric Sickle Cell Center [36410]
Children's Hospital--Columbus • MDA Clinic [34850]
Children's Hospital--Denver CO • Department of
Audiology/Speech Language Pathology and Learn-
ing [1391]
Children's Hospital of Denver/University of Colorado
Health Sciences Center • Pediatric Cystic Fibrosis
Center [7489]
Children's Hospital • Dialysis Center [24549]
Children's Hospital of Eastern Ontario • Burn Unit
[4613]
Children's Hospital • Genetics Clinic [12221]
Children's Hospital and Health Center
Developmental Services [7814]
Children's Hospital Home Care [17353]
Children's Hospital Home care Services [18419]
Children's Hospital, Inc. Home Care & Hospice
[16905]
Children's Hospital Kidney Center [23110]
The Children's Hospital Kidney Center [23092]
Children's Hospital of the Kings Daughter • Eastern
Virginia Medical School • Down Syndrome Clinic
[10876]
Children's Hospital of the King's Daughters • Bleed-
ing Disorders Center of Hampton Roads [12606]
Children's Hospital of the King's Daughters - Cystic
Fibrosis Center [7685]
Children's Hospital of the King's Daughters
Pediatric Dialysis Center [27523]
Pediatric Sickle Cell Center [36437]
Speech-Language Pathology Center [3599]
Children's Hospital--London • London Health Sci-
ences Centre • Eating Disorders Program [11213]
Childrens Hospital of Los Angeles DAM • Substance
Abuse Prevention/Treatment [40090]
Children's Hospital of Los Angeles
Department of Pediatrics Pulmonology [12151]
Dialysis and TX Program [22771]
Hematology/Oncology • Hemophilia Treatment
Center [12486]
Sickle Cell Disease Center [36293]
Children's Hospital of Los Angeles/University of
Southern California • Cystic Fibrosis
Comprehensive Center [7468]
Children's Hospital and Medical Center [20398]
Children's Hospital Medical Center of Akron [16828]
Cancer Program [5676]
Children's Hospital Medical Center of Akron - Cystic
Fibrosis Center [7637]
Children's Hospital and Medical Center--Akron •
Dialysis Center [26002]
Children's Hospital Medical Center of Akron
Genetics Center [12314]
Hemophilia Treatment Center [12573]
Paul and Carol David Foundation Burn Institute
[4603]
Children's Hospital Medical Center
Cancer Program [5691]
Division of Rheumatology • Rheumatic Diseases
Core Center [175]
MDA Clinic [34851]
Multipurpose Arthritis and Musculoskeletal
Diseases Center [176]
Pediatric Cystic Fibrosis Center [7638]
Sickle Cell Program [36315]
Children's Hospital and Medical Center • Transplant
Center [26038]
Children's Hospital of Michigan [4158]
Burn Center [4565]
Department of Neurology • MDA Clinic [34814]
Department of Pediatrics • Division of Genetics
and Metabolic Disorders [12247]

Children's Hospital of Michigan--Detroit • Marie
Carls Communication Disorders Center [2570]
Children's Hospital of Michigan • Hemostasis and
Thrombosis Center [12533]
Children's Hospital of Michigan--Novi • Rehabilitation
Center--Novi [2631]
Children's Hospital of Michigan
Transplant/Dialysis Center [24865]
Wayne State University/Harper University
Hospital
Adult Cystic Fibrosis Center [7572]
Pediatric Cystic Fibrosis Center [7573]
Children's Hospital Michigan/Wayne State University
School of Medicine • Sickle Cell Clinic [36362]
Children's Hospital at Montefiore • Division of
Genetics [12287]
Children's Hospital National Medical Center • MDA
Clinic [34775]
Children's Hospital
Neurology--Headache Clinic [12391]
Neurotrauma Rehabilitation Center [7836]
Children's Hospital, New Orleans • Down Syndrome
Clinic [10805]
Children's Hospital--New Orleans • Sickle Cell Clinic
[36348]
Children's Hospital--Oakland • Down Syndrome
Clinic [10775]
Children's Hospital of Oakland • Hemophilia Treat-
ment Center [12487]
Children's Hospital--Oakland • Medical Genetics
Clinic [12152]
Children's Hospital of Oakland • Sickle Cell Disease
Center [36294]
Childrens Hospital Of Eastern Ontario [11214]
Children's Hospital of Oklahoma
Burn Care Unit [4610]
University Hospital • Cystic Fibrosis Center
[7644]
Children's Hospital--Omaha • Eating Disorders
Program [11129]
Children's Hospital--Omaha NE • Audiology/Hearing
Clinic [2855]
Children's Hospital Orange County • Cord Blood
Bank [34940]
Children's Hospital of Orange County
Department of Hematology/Oncology •
Hemophilia Treatment Center [12488]
Down Syndrome Clinic [10776]
MDA Clinic [34759]
Sickle Cell Disease Center [36295]
Children's Hospital • Pain Clinic [35344]
Childrens Hospital Pediatric Assoc • Adolescent
Substance Abuse Program [44413]
Children's Hospital of Philadelphia [17407]
Adult Cystic Fibrosis Center [7648]
Clinical Genetics Center • 22q and You Center
[12324]
Dialysis Center [26505]
Hemophilia Program [12585]
Pediatric Cystic Fibrosis Center [7649]
Sleep Center [37642]
Specialty Care Center • Sickle Cell Disease
Center [36377]
Children's Hospital of Philadelphia Specialty Center
[12555]
Children's Hospital of Philadelphia • Trisomy 21
Program • Down Syndrome Clinic [10853]
Children's Hospital Physicians at Norwood Hospital •
Genetics Clinic [12242]
Children's Hospital Physicians at S Weymouth •
Genetics Clinic [12243]
Children's Hospital of Pittsburgh • Audiology and
Communication Disorders Department [3365]
Children's Hospital of Pittsburgh - Cystic Fibrosis
Center [7650]
Children's Hospital of Pittsburgh
Down Syndrome Center [10854]
MDA Clinic [34860]
Pediatric Sickle Cell Program [36417]
Children's Hospital of Pittsburgh of UPMC • Dialysis
Unit [26545]
Children's Hospital and Regional Medical Center
Cancer Program [6113]
Family Conversations [3636]
Genetics Clinic [12365]
Odessa Brown Children's Clinic • Sickle Cell
Disease Center [36443]
Speech and Language Services [3637]

Children's Hospital and Regional Medical Center/ University of Washington • Pulmonary Disease and Cystic Fibrosis Center [7691]
Children's Hospital Research Center Oakland/ California Pacific Medical Center • Cystic Fibrosis Center [7469]
Children's Hospital--Richmond • MDA Clinic [34897]
Children's Hospital at Scott and White • Cystic Fibrosis Center [7671]
Children's Hospital of Southwest Florida/Lee Memorial Health System • Sickle Cell Disease Center [36319]
Children's Hospital Specialty Pediatric Clinic [16109]
Children's Hospital • Sports Medicine Division [38542]
Children's Hospital at The Cleveland Clinic [8405]
Children's Hospital • Transfusion Service [35056]
Children's Hospital of Wisconsin
    Burn Program [4652]
    Dialysis Center [27744]
    Down Syndrome Clinic of Wisconsin [10878]
    Infant Death Center of Wisconsin [36558]
    Medical College of Wisconsin • MDA Clinic [34909]
    Sleep Center [37965]
    Speech and Hearing Center [3681]
Children's Hospitals and Clinics [15913]
Children's Hospitals and Clinics, Minneapolis
    Adult Cystic Fibrosis Center [7581]
    Sickle Cell Disease Center [36365]
Children's Hospitals and Clinics of Minnesota
    Children's Genetics Program [12257]
    Hemophilia Treatment Center [12544]
    Minnesota Sudden Infant Death Center [36495]
Children's Hospitals and Clinics, Saint Paul
    Pediatric Sleep Disorders Program [37215]
    Sickle Cell Disease Center [36366]
Children's Inn [10383]
Children's Institute, Inc.--Long Beach [28568]
Children's Institute, Inc.--Los Angeles [28587]
The Children's Institute of Pittsburgh [8478]
Children's Language Development Center [3528]
Children's Learning Connection Inc. [1110]
Children's Lung Specialists • University of Nevada School of Medicine • Cystic Fibrosis Center [7596]
Children's Medical Center--Augusta, GA • Pediatric Sickle Cell Service [36333]
Children's Medical Center • Cancer Program [5712]
Children's Medical Center of Dallas [34882]
Children's Medical Center of Dallas - Cystic Fibrosis Care, Teaching and Research Center [7672]
Children's Medical Center of Dallas
    Down Syndrome Clinic [10867]
    Sleep Disorders Center for Children [37807]
    Southwestern Comprehensive Sickle Cell Center [36436]
Children's Medical Center--Dayton
    Department of Developmental Pediatrics [10845]
    Pediatric Sleep Disorders Center [37509]
Children's Medical Center of Dayton • West Central Ohio Comprehensive Sickle Cell Center [36411]
The Children's Medical Center Home Care [16924]
Children's Medical Center-Minneapolis • Down Syndrome Clinic of Minnesota [10816]
Children's Medical Center Transplant Services • Dialysis Center [27019]
Children's Memorial Hospital
    Center for Cancer and Blood Disease [5068]
    Division of Genetics [12197]
    Hemophilia Treatment Center [12516]
Children's Memorial Hospital/Northwestern University • Pediatric Cystic Fibrosis Center [7527]
Children's Memorial Hospital
    Sickle Cell Disease Center [36339]
    Sleep Medicine Center [36903]
Childrens Memorial Hospital Transplant Program [23919]
Children's Mercy Hospital [15148], [36369]
    Burn Unit [4576]
    Cancer Program--Hematology/Oncology [5446]
    Developmental Medicine and Behavioral Sciences [8198]
    Down Syndrome Center [10820]
    Hearing and Speech Department [2796]
    Medical Genetics and Molecular Medicine [12263]
    Transplant/Dialysis Center [25220]

Children's Mercy Hospitals and Clinics Home Care [16021]
Children's National Medical Center
    Adult Cystic Fibrosis Center [7496]
    Burn Unit [4531]
    Dialysis Unit [23212]
    Division of Genetics and Metabolism [12176]
    Hemophilia Treatment Center [12500]
    Pediatric Cystic Fibrosis Center [7497]
Children's National Medical Center--Transplant [23213]
Children's Outpatient [28388]
Childrens Recovery Center of Oklahoma [47967]
Children's Regional Program [32899]
Children's Rehab Center • Speech Therapy Services [2843]
Children's Rehabilitation Center [8432]
Children's Rehabilitation Service [914]
Children's Rehabilitation Services--Birmingham • Hemophilia Treatment Center [12479]
Children's Rehabilitation Services--Mobile • Hemophilia Treatment Center [12480]
Children's Resource Center [34372]
    Mental Health Care [29302]
Children's Respiratory Center • Cystic Fibrosis Center [7658]
Children's Response Center [10604]
The Children's School for Early Development [8321]
Children's Service Center of Wyoming Valley, Inc. [32131]
Childrens Services of Roxbury • Substance Abuse Service [44554]
The Children's Sleep Laboratory [36778]
Children's Solana Beach Center [1324]
Children's Specialized Hospital [4277]
    Child Evaluation Center [8260]
Children's Specialized Hospital, Fanwood [4278]
Children's Specialized Hospital • Speech and Hearing Department [2935]
Children's Speech Care Center [1339]
Children's Speech and Language Center [1328]
Children's Speech and Language Discover Center [2951]
Children's Speech Language and Learning Services [2143]
Children's Speech and Language Services--Arlington VA [3570]
Children's Speech and Language Services--Lexington MA [2488]
Children's Speech and Language Services of Springfield [3613]
Children's Speech and Language Therapy Center Inc. [3587]
Children's Speech and Reading Center [1411]
Children's Speech Services [1735]
Children's Speech Services Inc. [2589]
Children's Study Home and Kathleen Thorton • Day Treatment School [34213]
Children's Study Home • Sharp I [34214]
Children's System of Care [28627]
Children's Therapies Inc. [1617]
Children's Therapy Associates [2498]
Children's Therapy Center [7766]
The Children's Therapy Center [8248]
Children's Therapy Center--Athens [1807]
Children's Therapy Center Inc.--Apple Valley [2671]
Children's Therapy Center Inc.--Eagan [2689]
Children's Therapy Center--Moline [2072]
Children's Therapy Center--Oakville [1487]
Children's Therapy Center--Roberts [3687]
Children's Therapy Group [2235]
Children's Therapy Place [1939]
Children's Therapy Plus [2137]
Children's Therapy and Rehabilitation Specialists [2023], [2064], [2083]
Children's Therapy Services [2236]
Children's Therapy Solutions [2590]
Children's TLC [8199]
Childrens Treatment Center • The Harbor Behavioral Healthcare Inst [41818]
The Children's Unit for Treatment and Evaluation [8299]
The Children's Village--Bayside [34326]
Children's Village • Child & Adolescent Crisis Intervention [51479]
The Children's Village--Dobbs Ferry [34336]
The Children's Village--Flushing [34338]
The Children's Village, Inc. [36095]

Children's Wellness Center [6500]
Childress Regional Medical Center Dialysis [26995]
Childs Dialysis • DaVita [26402]
Child's Voice School • Education/Auditory Oral Day School [2124]
Childserve Homecare Service [19703]
ChildWorks Therapy Center [2931]
Chileda [8615]
Chilicothe Regional Dialysis Center • American Renal Associates [26036]
Chillicothe Dialysis • DaVita [25185]
Chillicothe Veterans Affairs Medical Center [31681]
Chilton Memorial Hospital
    Cancer Program [5537]
    Sleep Health Institute [37340]
Chimes School [8087]
Chinatown Dialysis Center Inc. [25715]
Chinle Valley School for Exceptional Children [7733]
Chinny Home Health [14241]
The Chinook Clubhouse [28859]
Chinook Kidney Center • DaVita [27633]
Chipley Dialysis • DaVita [23263]
Chippenham Hospital • CJW Medical Center • Sports Medicine Center [39131]
Chippenham Medical Center/Johnston-Willis Hospital • Community Cancer Center [6080]
Chippenham Medical Center • Tucker Pavilion [49823]
Chippewa Dialysis Services [24972]
Chippewa Valley Veterans Affairs Clinic [32960]
CHIPS - Change is Possible [10401]
Chiricahua Community Health Centers, Inc. [6229]
ChiroSports USA - Sports Rehabilitation & Conditioning Specialists [38157]
Chisholm Trail Hospice/Svc of • Duncan Regional Hospital [20931]
Chittenden/North Addison Regional Consulting Services • Deaf and Hard of Hearing Program [846]
CHN Home Care [18560]
CHO Hospice-Ottawa [19553]
Choate Mental Health Center [33405]
Choate Mental Health and Developmental Center [7926]
Choctaw Nation • Chi Hullo Li [48028]
Choctaw Nation Health Care Center [3287]
Choctaw Nation • Recovery Center [48029]
Choice and Change [40890]
Choice Health Care, Ltd. [16925]
Choice Hospice [20953]
Choice One Home Health [13955]
Choice One Home Health Care [15846]
Choice One Renal Care of Newark [26173]
Choice Respiratory Care, Inc. [17278]
Choice Skyward • Mid Coast Mental Health Center [43942], [44045]
Choices [31726]
Choices Adolescent Treatment Center Inc [49460]
Choices Alcohol and Drug Assessments • Education and Counseling [43421]
Choices for Change Counseling [45721]
Choices and Changes Inc [50089]
CHOICES--Columbus [10141]
Choices Counseling Center [44992], [48119]
Choices Counseling Services [43217]
Choices DVIP [48183]
Choices Group Inc [45837]
Choices In Living Counseling Center [41115], [41197]
Choices in Living Counseling Center [41027], [41337], [41348]
Choices of Louisiana Inc [43803], [43836]
CHOICES of Manistee County, Inc. [9555]
Choices Program of Wyoming Valley • Wilkes-Barre Behavioral Hosp Co LLC [48694]
Choices Psychological Services [29921], [43346]
Choices in Recovery Center [40928]
    Bethesda Recovery Center/Humble House [40929]
    Bethesda Recovery Center/New House [40930]
    Foundation House [40931]
Choices Recovery Services
    Choices II Outpatient [40019]
    Choices of Long Beach Inc [40020]
    Choices VII [40021]
    Choices XIII [40022]
    Choices XIV [40023]
    Choices XV [40024]

Choices Recovery Services LLC [49017]
Choices • A Road to Recovery [39847]
Choices Substance Abuse/MH Inc [47357]
CHOICES Substance Abuse Services LLC [47485]
Choptank Community Health System, Inc.--Daffin Lane • Denton Medical Center [6793]
Choptank Community Health System, Inc.--Randolph Street • Denton Medical Center [6794]
Chota Community Health Services [7275]
Chowan Hospital [3176]
Chowchilla Counseling Center [28438]
Christ Child House [30537]
Christ Community Health Services, Inc. [7264]
Christ Hospital
    Cancer Center [5692]
    Department of Psychiatry [46022]
    Sleep Center [37341]
    Transplant/Dialysis Center [26039]
Christa Drab Speech and Language Therapy Services [2832]
Christamore Family Treatment Center [34142]
Christian Alcohol Awareness Program • Drugs (CAAPD)/True Vines Mens Home [40521]
Christian Care Counseling Center Inc [41856]
Christian Communication and Learning Center [3096]
Christian Community Health Center [42486], [42741]
Christian Counseling [44832]
Christian Counseling and Addiction Services Inc [43166]
Christian Counseling Center • Hutchinson [43364]
Christian County Dialysis • DaVita [24391]
Christian County Mental Health Association [29680]
Christian County Mental Health Center • Taylorville Helpline [50878]
Christian County Prosecuting Attorney's Victim Services [9707]
Christian Family Care Center [9246]
Christian Farms Treehouse Inc [49551]
Christian Home Health Care [15611]
Christian Hospital Northeast-Northwest • Cancer Program [5460]
Christian Hospital • Recovery Center [45617]
Christian League for Battered Women • Tranquility House [9096]
Christian Women of Elegance Inc • DBA Beatties Ford Rd Family Couns Center [47254]
Christiana Care Health Services • Christiana Hospital • Hemophilia Program [12499]
Christiana Care Health Services Inc. [29074]
Christiana Care Health Services • Speech and Hearing Center • Wilmington Hospital [1518]
Christiana Care Health System • Helen F. Graham Cancer Center [4917]
Christiana Care Health System Renal Transplant [23195]
Christiana Care Health Systems • Sleep Disorders Center [36761]
Christiana Care Visiting Nurse Association-HME [13562]
Christiana Hospital Hemodialysis Unit • Christiana Care Health System [23196]
Christie Clinic [38353]
Christie Clinic at C U Sleep • Sleep Disorders Center [36904]
Christina Brown and Associates Inc. [2961]
Christine Ann Domestic Abuse Services, Inc.--Fox Cities Office [10718]
Christine Ann Domestic Abuse Services, Inc.--Neenah [10726]
Christopher East Health Care Center • Pathways Brain Injury Program [4059]
Christopher Greater Area Rural Health Planning Corp. • Rea Clinic [6668]
Christos House [9736]
Christus Children's Kidney Center [27317]
Christus Health Northern Louisiana [15359]
Christus Saint Catherine Hosptial • Cancer Care Program [6006]
Christus Saint Elizabeth Hospital • Mamie McFaddin Ward Cancer Center [5969]
CHRISTUS St. Frances Cabrini Hospital [15262]
Christus Saint Frances Cabrini Hospital • Center for Cancer Care [5238]
Christus Saint Francis Cabrini Hospital • Sleep Center [37059]
Christus Saint John Hospital • Cancer Care Program [6014]

Christus Saint Michael Health System • W. Temple Webber Cancer Center [6031]
Christus Saint Patrick Hospital • Sisters of Charity • Regional Cancer Services [5251]
CHRISTUS Saint Patrick Hospital • Speech and Hearing Center [2323]
CHRISTUS Santa Rosa Center for Children and Families • Genetics Clinic [12349]
Christus Santa Rosa Children's Clinic • Children's Hospital • Center for Children and Family [10868]
Christus Santa Rosa Children's Hospital
    Adult Cystic Fibrosis Center [7673]
    Pediatric Cystic Fibrosis Center [7674]
Christus Schumpert Medical Center • Cancer Treatment Center [5262]
Christus Spohn Hospital Shoreline • Cancer Program [5972]
Chromalloy American Kidney Center [25267]
Chronic Pain Center [35660]
Chronic Pain Recovery Center [35689]
Chrysalis Apartment Community • Serenity Apartments [43652]
Chrysalis Center [48931]
Chrysalis Center for Change [41261]
    Sussex One Building [41018]
Chrysalis Center for Counseling and Eating Disorder Treatment [11173]
Chrysalis Counseling [40996], [41320]
Chrysalis House [50593]
Chrysalis House Inc
    Chrysalis Court Program [43653]
    Hill Rise Program [43654]
    Long Term [44232]
    Maxwell Program [43655]
    Scattered Site Apartment Program [43656]
Chrysalis Intensive Group Treatment for Eating Disorders [11277]
Chrysalis Non--Shelter Services [8709]
Chrysalis Shelter [8728]
Chrysalis Shelter for Victims of Domestic Violence [8710]
CHS Home Support services [16475]
Chuathbaluk Health clinic [12746]
Chula Vista Clinic • VA San Diego Healthcare System [28440]
Chula Vista Vet Center [51873]
Church Street Pavilion [32314]
Churchview Dialysis Center • DaVita [24073]
Ciales Primary Health Care Services, Inc. [7195]
Cibola Counseling [34312]
CIC/Fond du Lac County Health Center [51505]
CID--Central Institute for the Deaf [531]
Cielo House [10942]
Cielo Vista Dialysis • DaVita [27061]
Cierra Therapy LLC [1952]
Cigna Healthcare of Arizona [950]
CIGNA HealthCare • The Hearing Center [966]
CILA • Ecker Center for Mental Health--CILA [29616]
Cimmarron Basin Community Corrections [43396]
Cincinnati Center for Improved Communication [3216]
Cincinnati Children's Home Care [16875]
Cincinnati Children's Hospital • Division of Developmental Disabilities • Jane and Richard Thomas Center for Down Syndrome [10846]
Cincinnati Children's Hospital Medical Center
    Adult Cystic Fibrosis Center [7639]
    Adult Genetics Clinic [12315]
    Division of Developmental and Behavioral Pediatrics [8402]
    Hemophilia Treatment Center [12574]
    Sleep Disorders Center [37510]
Cincinnati Comprehensive Sickle Cell Center [36412]
Cincinnati Eye Bank [35156]
Cincinnati Occupational Therapy Institute [8403]
Cincinnati Public Schools • Student Services [646]
Cincinnati Speech Services [3217]
Cincinnati Speech Therapy [3218]
Cincinnati Sports Medicine and Orthopaedic Center [38860]
Cincinnati Sportsmedicine and Orthopaedic Center [38474]
    Deaconess Hospital [38861]
Cincinnati Sportsmedicine and Orthopaedic Center, Inc. [38862]
Cincinnati Teen Challenge [47818]

Cincinnati Veterans Affairs Medical Center • Cancer Care Program [5693]
Cincinnati Veterans Affairs Medical • Center/ Substance Dependency Program [47655]
Cindy Baird DUI Services LLC [43555], [43612]
Cinema Dialysis • DaVita [26273]
Cintra Health Care [14311]
CIRCLE [10537]
Circle Drive Clinic [32460]
Circle Family Ministries [29586]
Circle Family Health Care Network [6654]
Circle of Friends [40025]
Circle of Friends Outpatient Services Inc [40091]
Circle of Help Foundation [40092]
Circle of Hope [9101]
Circle of Hope--Brooklyn [31261]
Circle of Hope Hospice of VNA [21449]
Circle of Hope--Jamaica [31365]
Circle of Life Hospice--Chariton [19675]
Circle of Life Hospice Inc.--Reno [20427]
Circle of Life Hospice-Shreveport [19875]
Circle of Life Hospice--Springdale [18878]
Circle of Love Center [9111]
Circle Medical Management • Dialysis Facility [23920]
Circle Park Behavioral Health Services • Florence County Commission on AODA [48932]
Circle Treatment Center PC [44275]
Circles of Care [50784]
Circles of Care--E Sheridan Road, Melbourne [33318]
Circles of Care, Inc. [29212]
Circles of Care, Inc.--Commerce Drive, Melbourne [33319]
Circles of Care, Inc.--Titusville [33358]
Circles of Care--Rockledge [33351]
Circles of Hope Psychotherapy and Addictions Services [41526]
Circulo de Andromeda [41527]
Circulo de la Hispanidad • SALVA [9941]
Cirque Lodge [49709]
CIS Counseling Center Inc • Outpatient Drug Abuse Clinic [46846]
Citizen Advocates Inc • North Star Chemical Dependency Service [46769], [47065]
Citizen Potawatomi Nation • Family Violence Program [10212]
Citizens Acting Together Can Help, Inc.
    Day Treatment [32063]
    Elderly Day Treatment [32064]
Citizens Against Domestic and Sexual Assault Abuse [10631]
Citizens Against Domestic Violence • Sunshine House [9664]
Citizens Against Family Violence [10579]
Citizens Against PSE Abuse [10314]
Citizens Against Sexual Assault • Family Systems [10360]
Citizens Against Spouse Abuse, Inc.--Sedalia • CASA [9727]
Citizens Against Spouse Abuse--Myrtle Beach [10356]
Citizens Against Violence [9124]
Citizens Assisting and Sheltering the Abused [9455]
Citizens Baptist Medical Center [12726]
Citizens Health Center [6689]
Citizens of Lake County For Health Care, Inc. • Lake County Primary Care Center [7274]
Citizens Medical Center • Kathryn O'Connor Regional Cancer Center [6035]
Citizens Memorial Healthcare [2777]
Citizens Memorial Hospital Home Care [15985]
Citizens Opposed to Domestic Abuse [10343]
Citizens Services Department [16742]
Citrine Home Healthcare [14927]
Citronelle Convalescent Center • Mobile Community Mental Health Center [27886]
Citrus County Abuse Shelter Association, Inc. [9055]
Citrus Dialysis Center [22649]
Citrus Health Network [6470]
    Center for Adolescent Treatment Services [34072]
Citrus Health Network Inc • Kiva/Residential [41682]
Citrus Health Network
    Kiva Outreach Team and Residential Program [29176]
    Lou Panci Alternative Education Center [29177]
    Partial Hospital Program [29178]

Shaman Residential Program [29179]
Citrus Heights Vet Center [51876]
Citrus Maternal and Child Health Center [6471]
Citrus MED [6472]
Citrus Memorial Home Health Agency [13805]
Citrus Memorial Hospital [1600]
Citrus Valley Home Health [13441]
Citrus Valley Hospice [19076]
Citrus Valley Medical Center • Inter-Community/
    Queen of the Valley • Cancer Program [4768]
City of Angels Best Care Inc. [13124]
City of Angels Home Health Care, LLC [13956]
City of Berkeley • Domestic Violence Prevention
    Program [8793]
City Center Chiropractic and Rehabilitation [38360]
City Clinic [50991]
City-Country Communication Speech Language
    Pathology [3121]
City/County Alcohol and Drug Programs [49007]
City Dialysis Center Inc. • Renal Research Institute
    [25716]
City of Gary [419]
City on a Hill • Garden City [43350]
City Home Health Care, Inc. [17970]
City of Hope National Medical Center
    Cancer Research Center [4770]
    Comprehensive Cancer Center [4658]
    Department of Clinical Cancer Genetics [12153]
    Hemophilia Treatment Center [12489]
City Hospice [20954]
City Hospital • Cancer Program/H.I.S [6138]
City Hospital Center at Elmhurst • Elmhurst Com-
    munity Residence [46624]
City Hospital Inc. [3658]
City of Jacksonville • Florida Victim Services Center
    [9056]
City Medical Services, Inc. [13957]
City On A Hill [43401]
City of Portland/Portland Public Health • Homeless
    Health Clinic [44025]
City Pro Group [16381]
City Speech Inc. [2782]
City University of New York • New York City Techni-
    cal College • Student Support Services Programs
    [573]
City View Treatment Center Sheehan Mem Hospital
    • CD Inpatient Treatment Program [46556]
Cityline Dialysis • Fresenius Medical Care [26438]
Civista Medical Center • Cancer Program [5307]
Civitan Home [27888]
Civitan International Research Center • Sparks
    Clinic [902]
CKCC Gateway to Recovery [43356]
CKGG Healthcare Services and Medical Supplies
    [14563]
Clackamas County Behavioral Health [48165]
Clackamas County • Behavioral Health Division
    [48166]
Clackamas County Community Health MHC • Sandy
    Clinic [48246]
Clackamas County Public Health Division [7138]
Clackamas Kidney Center • Fresenius Medical Care
    [26316]
Clackamas Women's Services [10243]
Claiborne County Department of Special Education
    [763]
Claiborne County Family Health Center [6894]
Claiborne Home Health Care [21369]
Claiborne Home Health Care and Hospice [17777]
Claire House [43862]
Clara Felix Sickle Cell Clinic [36296]
Clara Maass Medical Center • Community Hospital
    Cancer Program [5502]
Clara Martin Center [49723]
Clara Martin Center--Bradford [32642]
Clara Martin Center
    Emergency Services [51409]
    Quitting Time [49750]
Clara Martin Center--Randolph [32674]
Clara Martin Center • Substance Abuse Treatment
    Unit [49741]
Clara Martin Center--Wilder [32688]
Claras House [45290]
CLARE Foundation Inc
    CLARE Drug Court Program [40766]
    Culver Vista Family Center [40093]
    Mens Recovery Home [40767]
    Santa Monica Recovery Detox/Primary [40768]

Womens Recovery Home [40769]
Clare Woods Academy [7928]
Claremont Academy [479]
Claremore Safenet Services [10193]
Clarendon Cty Commission on Alcohol/Treatment •
    DBA Clarendon Behavioral Health Serv [48960]
Clarendon House [32707]
Clarendon Memorial Home Health Services [17604]
Clarian Center--Methodist Campus • Indiana
    University Health [24167]
Clarian Health Partners [14997]
    Adult Dialysis Center [24168]
Clarian Health Partners Home Care, Inc --
    Indianapolis [14998]
Clarian Health Partners Home Care--Tipton [15055]
Clarian Health Partners, Inc. • Methodist Cancer Ctr.
    [5154]
Clarian Home Care at BRMC [14964]
Clarian Home Care at Lafayette [15021]
Clarian Home Dialysis • Indiana University Health
    [24169]
Clarian IU
    Dialysis Center [24170]
    Indianapolis University Hospital • Clarian Health
        Partners [24171]
Clarian West Medical Center [2127]
Clarina Howard Nichols Center [10545]
Clarinda Mental Health Institute [33498]
Clarion Forest VNA Hospice [21105]
Clarion Health Hospice [19609]
Clarion Psychiatric Center [33799]
Clarity Counseling PC [46265]
Clarity Hospice of Baton Rouge [19835]
Clarity Way Inc [48387]
Clark and Associates • Psychological Services
    [45018]
Clark and Clark Counseling Services [43657]
Clark Community Mental Health Center [30879],
    [45571]
Clark County Community Services • Substance
    Abuse Services [50492]
Clark County Dialysis Facility [26202]
Clark County School District • Low Incidence Dis-
    abilities Department [542]
Clark County Special Education Cooperative [423]
Clark Fork Valley Hospital-Hospice [20369]
Clark Home Respiratory Supply, Inc. [16433]
Clark Home Training Center • Dialysis Clinic Inc.
    [23571]
Clark Memorial Hospital [15009], [43121]
    Cancer Program [5160]
Clark Place [27940]
Clark Regional Medical Center [2299]
Clark Sports Medicine [38693]
Clarke County Arc [7717]
Clarke Jacksonville Auditory/Oral Center [349]
The Clarke School for the Deaf [476]
Clarke School for the Deaf • Clarke School East
    [471]
Clarke School for Hearing and Speech [693]
    Clarke New York City Auditory/Oral Center [592]
Clark's Summit State Hospital [33800]
Clarksburg Treatment Center [50293]
Clarksdale Speech and Hearing Center [2756]
Clarkston Dialysis • DaVita [24851]
Clarksville Dialysis • DaVita [26817]
Clarksville/Montgomery County Crisis Intervention
    Center [51353]
Clarksville North Dialysis • DaVita [26818]
Clarksville Sleep Disorders Center [37760]
Classic City Dialysis [23581]
Classic Home Care--Arlington [17800]
Classic Home Care--Livingston [15595]
Classic Home Care--Plymouth [15771]
Clatsop Behavioral Health Care [31929]
Clatsop Behavioral Healthcare [8441], [51247]
Clatsop County Women's Resource Center [10220]
Clausen House [7797]
Claxton Dialysis Center • Fresenius Medical Care •
    Dialysis Center [23643]
Claxton-Hepburn Medical Center • Winter Cancer
    Center [5605]
Clay-Battelle Health Services Assoc. • Clay-Battelle
    Community Health Center [7398]
Clay Behavioral Health Center [41807]
Clay County Behavioral Health Center [50776]
Clay County Counseling Services [42755]
Clay County Hospital Home Care [12623]

Clay County Hospital • Sleep Disorders Laboratory
    [36572]
Clay County Receiving Center • Detox [45240]
Clay Crossing Foundation Inc [47952]
Clay Wilson and Associates • DBA The Cognitive
    Connection [47380]
Claymont Treatment Center [41499]
Claystone Clinical Associates [11098]
Clayton Center Behavioral Health Services [29447]
Clayton Center--Behavioral Health Services [50801]
Clayton Center Community Services Board •
    Substance Abuse Program [42113]
Clayton Center--Community Support Services
    [50806]
Clayton Center--Flint River Center [50809]
Clayton Dialysis Center, Inc. [25844]
Clayton House [41384]
Clayton Mental Health Center [50807]
Clayton Psychotherapy Center [11118]
Clayton Sleep Institute [37273]
Clayton Taylor Dialysis Facility • Fresenius Medical
    Care--Ohio State University [26071]
Clean and Clear Evaluation [47270]
Clean on Green [47405], [47426]
Clean Investments Counseling Center [49228]
Clean and Sober Detox [39826]
Clean and Sober Recovery Services Inc [40327]
Clean and Sober Streets [41528]
Clear Brook Lodge [48641]
Clear Choice Home Medical Equipment, LLC
    [18141]
Clear Choice Home Medical Equipment and Supply
    [12645]
Clear Concepts Counseling [48286], [48452],
    [48469]
Clear Creek County Advocates [8965]
A Clear Direction • Wichita [43485]
Clear Lake Counseling Center • Taira Saint John
    PhD MFT [39977]
Clear Lake Kidney Center • Fresenius Medical Care
    [27392]
Clear Lake Sleep Center [37808]
Clearbrook Center East [7927]
Clearbrook Manor [48695]
Clearfield Dialysis • DaVita [26406]
Clearfield Hospital Hospice [21074]
Clearfield Hospital • Therapy Works [38935]
Clearfield-Jefferson Community Mental Health
    Center [32004]
Clearfield Jefferson Community Mental Health
    Center, Inc. [32014]
Clearfield Jefferson Community Mental Health
    Center • Punxsutawney Clinic [32113]
Clearfield Jefferson
    Community MH/Drug/Alc Optt Program [48343]
    Community MHI/Drug/Alc Otpt Program [48326]
Clearlake Dialysis Center • DaVita [22639]
Clearly Speaking Inc. [1858]
ClearView Center Apartment & Program [31225]
ClearView Center, Inc. [31226]
    Outpatient Services [31227]
Clearview Counseling Services LLC [41277]
Clearview Recovery Center of Pine Belt Mental
    Healthcare Resources [45407]
Clearview Recovery Inc [43297]
Clearview Treatment Programs [10943], [40901],
    [40902]
    Outpatient [40094]
Clearwater Counseling/Court Services [45662]
Clearwater Hospice [20143]
Cleary School for the Deaf [590]
Cleburne Dialysis Center • Fresenius Medical Care
    [26996]
Clelian Heights School for Exceptional Children
    [8462]
Clem Mar House Inc
    For Men [48349]
    For Women [48336]
Clement C. Van Wagoner Department of Veterans
    Affairs Clinic [30500]
Clement J. Zablocki VA Medical Center - Milwaukee
    [18592]
Clement J Zablocki Veterans Affairs Medical Center
    [51676]
Clement J. Zablocki Veterans Affairs Medical Center
    Cancer Program [6163]
    Multiple Sclerosis Center [34742]
    PTSD Clinical Team [51850]

PTSD Domiciliary [51851]
Spinal Cord Injury Center [4490]
Clermont Counseling Center--Amelia [31651]
Clermont Counseling Center--Milford [31811]
Clermont Inc. • DaVita [26166]
Clermont Recovery Center Inc [47618]
Clermont YWCA • House of Peace [10125]
Cleve-Hill Dialysis & At Home • Dialysis Center • DaVita [25634]
Cleveland Center [31591]
Cleveland Center for Eating Disorders [11194]
Cleveland Christian Home • Residential Treatment Center [34375]
Cleveland Clinic • Alcohol and Drug Recovery Center [47679]
Cleveland Clinic--Beachwood [22209]
Cleveland Clinic Brunswick Family Health Center [38856]
Cleveland Clinic Cancer Center • Western Region Cancer Program [5701]
Cleveland Clinic--Canfield [22210]
Cleveland Clinic • Children's Hospital for Rehabilitation [26062]
Cleveland Clinic Florida [38225]
Cleveland Clinic Foundation
Andrology Laboratory and Sperm Bank [35157]
Communication Disorders Section [3227]
Mellen Center for Multiple Sclerosis Treatment and Research [34670]
Pain Management [35604]
The Cleveland Clinic Foundation • Sleep Disorder Center [37511]
Cleveland Clinic • Headache Center [12457]
Cleveland Clinic Home Care [16947]
Cleveland Clinic Hospital
Cancer Care Program [5004]
Sleep Disorders Center [36779]
Transplant and Dialysis Center [26063]
Cleveland Clinic Musculoskeletal Core Center • Lerner Research Institute • Center of Research Translation [177]
Cleveland Clinic--Solon [22211]
Cleveland Clinic Sports Health--Florida Weston [38297]
Cleveland Clinic Sports Health - Garfield Heights [38880]
Cleveland Clinic Sports Health and Orthopaedic Rehabilitation - Beachwood JCC [38853]
Cleveland Clinic Sports Health and Orthopaedic Rehabilitation--Cleveland [38865]
Cleveland Clinic Sports Health and Orthopaedic Rehabilitation - Euclid [38877]
Cleveland Clinic Sports Health and Orthopaedic Rehabilitation Independence [38881]
Cleveland Clinic Sports Health and Orthopaedic Rehabilitation - Solon [38894]
Cleveland Clinic Sports Health and Orthopaedic Rehabilitation Strongsville [38897]
Cleveland Clinic Sports Health and Orthopaedic Rehabilitation - Westlake [38900]
Cleveland Clinic Sports Health and Orthopaedic Rehabilitation Willoughby Hills [38901]
Cleveland Clinic--Strongsville [22212]
Cleveland County Abuse Prevention Council [10082]
Cleveland County Health Department • Speech and Hearing Clinic [3275]
Cleveland Department of Health • CenterPoint Treatment Program [47680]
Cleveland Dialysis Center • DaVita [26998]
Cleveland Eye Bank • Vision Share [35158]
Cleveland Foot and Ankle Institute [38866]
Cleveland Free Clinic--Mental Health Services [31710]
Cleveland Health Care, LLC [18069]
Cleveland Hearing and Speech Center [3228]
Cleveland Heights Vet Center [52061]
Cleveland Home Health Agency, Inc. [16779]
Cleveland Municipal Schools • Deaf/Hard of Hearing Program [648]
Cleveland Public Library • Ohio Library for the Blind and Physically Disabled [3829]
Cleveland Regional Medical Center • Cancer Center [5659]
Cleveland State University • Speech and Hearing Clinic [3229]
Cleveland Treatment Center Inc [47681]
Cleveland VA Medical Center • Breckville Campus [4362]

Cleveland Veterans Affairs Clinic [32961]
Cleveland Veterans Affairs Medical Center
Brecksville Campus [31666]
Wade Park Campus [31711]
Client Home Healthcare, Inc. [14888]
Clifford W. Beers Guidance Clinic • CAMPES [50733]
Cliffside Nursing Home • CRD Associates LLC • Dialysis Center [25661]
Clifton Counseling Services [45961]
Clifton Hospice Services, LLC [20001]
Clifton Park Veterans Affairs Clinic [31305]
Clifton Springs Health Center [29405]
Clifton Springs Hospital and Clinic
Inpatient Addiction Rehab Program [46591]
Outpatient Substance Abuse Program [46592]
Clifton T. Perkins Hospital Center [33565]
Clincare Corporation/Wyalusing Academy [34493]
Clinch River Health Services [7354]
Clinch Valley Treatment Center [49770]
The Clinic in Altgeld, Inc. • Public Housing Program [6655]
Clinic for Metabolic and Genetic Disorders of Bone • Baylor Genetics Clinic [12350]
Clinica Adelante, Inc. [6250]
Clinica del Alma [6252]
Clinica Campesina Family Health Services--Denver [6394]
Clinica Campesina Family Health Services--Lafayette [6412]
Clinica De Salud Del Valle De Salinas [6350]
Clinica De Tratamiento • Psicoterapeutico [48729]
Clinica Monsenor Oscar A Romero [40095]
Clinica Monsenor Oscar Romero [6316]
Clinica de Patologia del Habla y Lenguaje [3386]
Clinica Sierra Vista [6287]
Delano Clinic [39779]
Clinical 1 Home Medical [15561]
Clinical Associates [43392]
Clinical Associates of the Finger Lakes [3142]
Clinical Communication Consultants [3503]
Clinical Consultants [49644]
Clinical Consultants LLC [49715]
Clinical Day Treatment Program [33269]
Clinical Medical Services, Inc. [17525]
Clinical Outcomes Group Inc [48623]
Clinical Professional Counselors LLP [43450]
Clinical Services of Rhode Island [48852]
Clinical Services for Youth [51307]
Clinical Solutions of Charleston PA [48910]
Clinical Speech and Hearing Services Inc. [2776]
Clinical Stabilization Services [44604]
Clinical and Support Options [8126]
Clinical Support and Options [30391]
Clinicas del Camino Real, Inc.--Oxnard [6337]
Clinicas del Camino Real--Ventura [6374]
Clinicas de Salud del Pueblo [6295]
Clinilabs, Inc. • Sleep Disorders Institute [37383]
Clinique des Troubles Alimentaires • BACA Eating Disorders Clinic [11264]
Clinton Counseling Center • Comprehensive Youth Services [44927]
Clinton County Addiction Services • Chemical Dependence Outpatient [46980]
Clinton County Counseling Center [30632]
Clinton County Women's Center [10295]
Clinton Dialysis Center [26821]
Clinton-Eaton-Ingham CMHSP [30585]
Clinton Family Health Center [7038]
Clinton Lodge [31712]
Clinton Memorial Hospital [15794]
Cancer Program [5763]
Clinton Memorial Hospital, Home Care Agency [17073]
Clinton Memorial Hospital Home Health [17074]
Clinton Middle Health Center [6744]
Clinton Outpatient Clinic [30361]
Clinton Shelby CMHC [28014]
Clinton Township Dialysis and At Home • DaVita [24852]
Clinton YWCA • Domestic Violence/Sexual Assault Resource Center [9323]
Clipper Lane Residence [30366]
CLM Behavioral Health Systems [51089]
Cloud County Health Center [2213]
Cloud Peak Counseling Center [33076]
Clover Bottom Development Center • Speech and Hearing Department [3445]

Clover Bottom Developmental Center [8522]
Clover Health, LLC [18079]
Clover House Inc • Mens Clover House TTC [49471]
Clovis Elementary School--Based • Fresno County Department of Children and Family Services [33134]
Clovis Municipal Schools [557]
CLP Home Health Services [13654]
CLT Home Care [13958]
Club House Program/Friendship Center [31617]
CLUB Inc [42336]
Club Recovery LLC [45144]
Clues Saint Paul [34255]
Clybourn Consulting Corporation [42911]
Clyde Cosper State Nursing Home [17830]
CMB Rehabilitation Inc. [3669]
CMC Hospice [18868]
CMH Community Hospice [21735]
CMSU Service System • Behavioral Health Base Service Unit [32009]
CNN Home Health Agency, Inc. [17971]
CNOS Sports Medicine [39021]
CNR Long Term Home Health Care Program--Bronx [16358]
CNR Long Term Home Health Care Program--Brooklyn [16382]
CNR Long Term Home Health Care Program--Far Rockaway [16453]
CNS Home Health and Hospice [14707]
CNS Hospice [19495]
CNS Sleep Disorders Center [37809]
CO Mental Health Institute at Pueblo • Circle Program [41293]
Co-occurring Residential Program [49983]
Coach House Rehabilitation Center, Inc. [4159]
Coal Country Community Health Center [7068]
Coal Country Substance Abuse Program [47551]
Coalinga Regional Center • Fresno County Department of Children and Family Services [33136]
Coalition Against Rape and Abuse [9821]
Coalition Against Rape and Domestic Violence [9681]
The Coalition to End Family Violence [8864]
Coalition for Family Peace [10083]
COARC • The Starting Place [8323]
Coast Mountain School District Number 82 • Deaf/Hard of Hearing Program [256]
Coast Physical Therapy and Sports Medicine [38090]
Coast Valley Worship Center • Coast Valley Substance Abuse Treatment Center [40006], [40758]
Coastal Asian-Pacific Mental Health Services [28511]
Coastal Behavioral Healthcare--Fort Myers [29160]
Coastal Behavioral Healthcare Inc [41910], [41983]
Coastal Behavioral Healthcare--North Fort Myers [29236]
Coastal Behavioral Healthcare--North Port [29240]
Coastal Behavioral Healthcare--Punta Gorda [29273]
Coastal Behavioral Healthcare--Sarasota [29288]
Coastal Behavioral Healthcare--Venice [29314]
Coastal Bend Alcohol/Drug Rehab Center • DBA Charlies Place [49270]
Coastal Carolina Hospital [51326]
Coastal Center SCDDSN Residential Facility [8506]
Coastal Dialysis Center • Fresenius Medical Care [23784], [24605]
Coastal Empire Community Mental Health Center--Allendale • Crisis Intervention Center [51317]
Coastal Empire Community Mental Health Center--Beaufort • Crisis Intervention Center [51320]
Coastal Empire Community Mental Health Center--Hilton Head • Crisis Intervention Center [51333]
Coastal Empire Community Mental Health Center--Ridgeland • Crisis Intervention Center [51337]
Coastal Empire Community Mental Health Center--Varnville • Crisis Intervention Center [51339]
Coastal Empire Community Mental Health Center--Walterboro • Crisis Intervention Center [51340]
Coastal Family Health Center, Inc. [6877]
Coastal Harbor Treatment Center [33390]
Coastal Horizons Center Inc [47232], [47516]
Coastal Horizons Center • Runaway and Homeless Youth Program [36133]
Coastal Hospice & Home Care [19942]
Coastal Interventional Pain Associates [35662]

Coastal Kidney Centers LLC • DaVita [23466]
Coastal Medical Services, Inc. [17972]
Coastal Orthopedics & Sports Medicine [38506]
Coastal Plain Hospital [33743]
Coastal Pulmonary Medicine/Sleepcare of Wilmington [37464]
Coastal Recovery Center [48965]
Coastal Sleep Lab [37731]
Coastal Therapy and Learning Center Inc. [1730]
Coastal Treatment Services [49890]
Coastal Women's Shelter Board, Inc. [10068]
Coastside Mental Health [28525]
Coatesville Treatment Center [48329]
Coatesville Veterans Affairs Medical Center [32006]
COBAP Substance Abuse Treatment and Prevention Program [44727]
Cobb County Dialysis Center • Diversified Specialty Institutes [23749]
Cobb Day and Residential Care [29466]
Cobb Dialysis • DaVita [23618]
Cobb/Douglas Cnty Comm Services Board
    Douglas Outpatient Services [42124]
    Mothers Making a Change [42130]
Cobb Douglas Community Services [29467]
Cobb and Douglas Counties Community Services Board--Austell [50797]
Cobb and Douglass Counties Community Service Board--Crisis Line--Marietta • Intake Information and Referral [50808]
Cobb Memorial School [8294]
Cobb Outpatient Services [29468]
Cobb Pediatric Therapy Services [3396]
Cobblestone Therapy Group [1900]
Cobbs Creek Dialysis • DaVita [26506]
Coburn Place Safe Haven [9284]
Cocaine and Alcohol Awareness Program • (CAAP) [49133]
Cochran Mens Halfway House [45170]
Cochran Recovery Program [45171]
CoCo Home Health Care, Inc. [13959]
Cocoon House Clinic, Outreach [7377]
Cocoon House • Runaway and Homeless Youth Program [36250]
CODA Inc
    Gresham Recovery Center [48184]
    Hillsboro Recovery Center [48128]
    Portland Recovery Center [48185]
CODAC Behavioral Health Services, Inc. [28208]
CODAC Behavioral Healthcare
    CODAC Newport [48858]
    East Bay [48849]
CODAC Behavioral Healthcare II • South County [48883]
CODAC Cranston • Outpatient Drug Free [48846]
CODAC Outpatient [28209]
CODAC Providence [48871]
Codman Square Health Center • Outpatient Substance Abuse Services [44446]
C.O.E. Home Health, LLC [18064]
Coeur d'Alene Tribal Victims of Crime Assistance [9182]
Coeur d'Alene Veterans Affairs Clinic [29544]
Coffee County Day Mental Health Clinic [27907]
Coffee House Teen Shelter • Runaway and Homeless Youth Program [35813]
Coffee Regional Medical Center [14520]
Coffeyville Regional Medical Center [15116]
    Cancer Program [5196]
Cognitive Consultants LLC [44879]
Cognitive Speech Rehabilitation, Inc. [1689]
Cohen Speech and Feeding Solutions LLC [1984]
Cohoes Community Residence • Clearview Center [31306]
Cold Creek Wellness Center [49617]
Cold Spring Dialysis • DaVita [24369]
Cole Speech and Language Center [3504]
Colebeck Lodge [27918]
Colegio San Gabriel para Ninos Sordos [715]
The Coleman Foundation [8173]
Coleman Professional Services [31852]
    The 227 Place [31827]
    Main Office [31781]
    Rhodes Road House Group Home [31782]
    Vocational Rehabilitation Services [31783]
Coles County Mental Health Center [50858]
Coliseum Medical Centers • Cancer Program [5030]
Collaborative Function • Speech & Occupational Therapy [1692]

Colleen Quigley Women's Center [10529]
College Community Services [40235]
    Ridgecrest [40451]
College Dialysis • DaVita [22933]
College Hospital Cerritos [33132]
College House Group Home [34105]
College of Lake County • Lake County Prevention Services Program [29628]
College of New Jersey • New Jersey Consortium on Deafblindness • Center for Assistive Technology and Inclusive Education Studies [2912]
College Point Dialysis Center [25662]
College of Saint Rose • Winkler Speech-Language-Hearing Clinic [2970]
College of the Sequoias • Disability Resource Center [312]
College of Southern Idaho • AA--American Sign Language Studies [392]
College Station Medical Center • Cancer Center [5971]
College View State School [8197]
Collegeville Speech and Hearing [3327]
Colleton Commission on Alcohol and Drug Abuse [48984]
Colleton County Deaf Education Program [740]
Collier Health Services, Inc. • Marion E. Fether Medical Center [6477]
Collierville Dialysis • DaVita [26822]
Collierville Orthopedics and Sports Medicine [39027]
Collin County Dialysis Center • Fresenius Medical Care [27290]
Collin Intervention to Youth • Runaway and Homeless Youth Services [36216]
Collins Dialysis Unit • Hattiesburg Clinic • Dialysis Unit [25128]
Collinsville Nursing Home, Inc. [27891]
Colmery O'Neil VA Medical Center [15153]
Colonia Dialysis Center • Fresenius Medical Care [25419]
Colonial Behavioral Health • Substance Abuse Services [49865]
Colonial Clinic [50165]
Colonial Counseling Associates Center • East Office/Main Office [41857]
Colonial Heights Counseling Services [32723]
Colonial House Inc [48709]
    Outpatient [48710]
    Residential Program [48711]
Colonial Services Board [32742], [32797]
Colonial Springs Dialysis • DaVita [23619]
Colorado Anti-Violence Program [8946]
Colorado Assessment and Treatment Center [41116]
Colorado Boys Ranch [34049]
Colorado Center for Reproductive Medicine--Denver [21954]
Colorado Center for Reproductive Medicine--Lone Tree [21955]
Colorado Center for Reproductive Medicine--Louisville [21956]
Colorado City Dialysis • AccessCare [27002]
Colorado Coalition for the Homeless [41117]
Colorado Community Hospice/Interlink Healthcare Services [19098]
Colorado Counseling • Men and Women Seeking Empowerment [41163]
Colorado Department of Education • Colorado Services for Children and Youth with Combined Vision and Hearing Loss • Exceptional Student Leadership Unit [1392]
Colorado Department of Human Services • Runaway and Homeless Youth Program [35852]
Colorado Mental Health Institute at Fort Logan [33216]
Colorado Mental Health Institute, Fort Logan • Deaf Services [1393]
Colorado Mental Health Institute of Pueblo [33234]
Colorado MOVES [8947], [41118]
Colorado Neuro & Headache Center [12392]
Colorado Neurological Institute
    CNI Cochlear Kids Camp [1407]
    Head Pain Center [12393]
    Multiple Sclerosis Services [34542]
Colorado Pain Specialists [35345]
Colorado Plains Medical Center [13488]
Colorado Reproductive Endocrinology [21957]
Colorado River Regional Crisis Shelter [8705]
Colorado School for the Deaf and the Blind [322], [3701]

Colorado School of Medicine • JFK Partners [1394]
Colorado Sports and Spine Centers • The Pain Center [35346]
Colorado Springs Interventional Pain Management [35347]
Colorado Springs Outpatient Clinic • Community Based Substance AbuseTreatment Program [41054]
Colorado State University • Center for Central Auditory Research [1412]
Colorado Talking Book Library [3755]
Colorado Treatment Services LLC [41055]
Colorado West Mental Health Center [50718]
Colorado West Mental Health, Inc.
    Alpine Center [28908]
    Aspen Counseling Center [28852]
    Child & Family Program [28909]
    Craig Mental Health [28877]
    Eagle Valley [28896]
    Grand Junction Adult Outpatient Cliic [28910]
    Rangely Outpatient Clinic [28950]
    Steamboat Center [28953]
    Summit Center [28905]
    Vail Outpatient Clinic [28958]
Colorado West Regional Mental Health [50721]
Colorado West Regional Mental Health Center • Administrative Office & Garfield Service [28906]
Colorado West Regional Mental Health, Inc. [28907]
Colorado West Regional Mental Health Inc.
    Alpine Center [33224]
    Aspen Outpatient Clinic [33212]
    Craig Outpatient Clinic [33215]
    Eagle Outpatient Clinic [33218]
    Frisco Outpatient Clinic [33221]
    Garfield Outpatient Clinic [33222]
    Grand Junction Child and Adult Outpatient Clinic [33225]
    Meeker Outpatient Clinic [33233]
    Rangely Outpatient Clinic [33235]
    Rifle Outpatient Clinic [33236]
    Steamboat Springs Outpatient Clinic [33237]
    Vail Outpatient Clinic [33238]
Colorado West Regional Mental Hlth Center [41161]
    Alpine Counseling Services [41202]
    Aspen Counseling Center [40984]
    Craig Mental Health [41083]
    Eagle Valley [41333]
    Recovery Center [41194]
    Residential Substance Abuse Treatment Serv [41206]
    Rifle Center [41309]
    Rio Blanco Center [41307]
    Steamboat Mental Health [41313]
    Summit Center [41191]
    Walden Center [41334]
Colorado Western Slope Counseling [41085], [41284]
Colquitt County Mental Health Center [29479]
Colquitt Regional Home Health [14591]
Colquitt Regional Medical Center [14557]
Colquitt Regional Medical Center Dialysis [23764]
Colton Clinical Services [39721]
Columbia Addictions Center [44226]
Columbia Area Mental Health Center--Columbia [32193]
Columbia Area Mental Health Center
    Fairfield County Clinic [32217]
    Independent House Clubhouse [32194]
    Network Program [32195]
    New Horizons Clubhouse [32196]
Columbia Area Mental Health Services • Adult Crisis Services [51322]
Columbia Basin Health Association [7381]
Columbia Community Mental Health [48247]
Columbia Community Mental Health and Alcohol and Drug [48256]
Columbia Community Mental Health • Alcohol and Drug Outpatient [48236]
Columbia Community Mental Health Center [31972]
Columbia Community Mental Health • Pathways Residential [48237]
Columbia Counseling [50257]
Columbia County Health Center [6483]
Columbia County Mental Health • Crisis Intervention [51265]
Columbia County Women's Resource Center [10257]
Columbia Developmental Center [8064]

Columbia Dialysis--Grove Street • DaVita [26824]
Columbia Dialysis • Hattiesburg Clinic [25113]
Columbia Fertility Associates [21981]
Columbia Green Dialysis Centers--Ghent [25672]
Columbia--Green Domestic Violence Program [9915]
Columbia Greene Dialysis Center [25641]
Columbia/HCA Valley Hospital • Parkridge Medical Center [33839]
Columbia Hearing Impaired Program [649]
Columbia Heart • Sleep Center [37732]
Columbia Hospital • Pain Center [35773]
Columbia IP-Portsbridge [21217]
Columbia Lutheran Charities Home Health/Hospice [17176]
Columbia Memorial Hospital [3030]
Columbia Metro Treatment Center [48985]
Columbia Montour Home Hospice [21054] Bloomburg Health System [21075]
Columbia, Montour, Snyder Union Counties of Central Pennsylvania Service System • Mental Health & Drug & Alcohol Referral Service [32010]
Columbia Northeast Dialysis • DaVita [26697]
Columbia Orthopaedic Group [38653]
Columbia Presbyterian Hospital • Dialysis Center • New York Presbyterian [25717]
Columbia Presbyterian-Saint Luke's Medical Center • Oncology Program [4872]
Columbia Regional Program, Deaf/Hard of Hearing [688]
Columbia River Community Health Services [7123], [7132]
Columbia River Mental Health [50236]
Columbia River Mental Health Services [32878]
Columbia Road Health Services [6432]
Columbia Saint Mary's Hospital--Columbia Campus • Cancer Center [6164]
Columbia Saint Mary's Hospital--Milwaukee Campus • Cancer Program [6165]
Columbia Saint Mary's Hospital Milwaukee, Inc. [18593]
Columbia Street Residence [31353]
Columbia Treatment Clinic [45459]
Columbia Treatment Services [50237]
Columbia University
    Adult Cystic Fibrosis Program [7612]
    The Center for Women's Reproductive Care [22179]
    Children's Hospital of New York • New York-Presbyterian • Pediatric Pulmonary [7613]
    College of Physicians and Surgeons
        Department of Pediatrics Pediatric AIDS Clinical Trials Unit [18]
        Eleanor and Lou Gehrig MDA/ALS Center [34833]
Columbia University Dialysis • DaVita [25718]
Columbia University
    Harlem Hospital • Comprehensive Sickle Cell Center [36392]
    Mailman School of Public Health • HIV Vaccine Trials Unit [87]
    Teachers College • Edward D. Mysak Speech-Language-Hearing Center [3058]
Columbia Valley Community Health Services • Dental/Medical Clinic/WIC Nutrition and Social Services [7394]
Columbia Vet Center [52004]
Columbia Wesley Medical Center [2246]
Columbiana County Educational Service Center [660]
Columbiana County Mental Health Center
    Chemical Dependency Program [47790]
    East Liverpool Unit [31760]
Columbiana County Mental Health Center--Lisbon [31791]
Columbiana County Mental Health Clinic • DBA The Counseling Center [47753]
Columbus Alliance for Battered Women [9099]
Columbus Area Community Mental Health Center [31727]
    Intermediate Care [31728]
Columbus Area Halfway House [31729]
Columbus Area Inc [47711], [47712]
Columbus Community Health • Regional Sleep Disorder Center [37512]
Columbus Community Hospital [16098], [20379]
Columbus Developmental Center [8409]
Columbus Dialysis--Bradley Park Drive • DaVita [23647]

Columbus Downtown Dialysis • DaVita [26072]
Columbus East Dialysis & At Home • DaVita [26073]
Columbus East Dialysis • DaVita [26074]
Columbus Health Department • Alcohol and Drug Treatment Program [47713]
Columbus Hospice of Alabama [19375]
Columbus Library for Accessible Services • Columbus Public Library [3773]
Columbus Mental Health Center [30931]
Columbus Northeast Health Center [7082]
Columbus Regional Healthcare System [16796]
Columbus Regional Hospital • Cancer Program [5139]
Columbus Speech and Hearing Center [1847]
Columbus Speech and Hearing Program • Comprehensive Program for the Deaf • Ohio Deaf--Blind Outreach Program [3231]
Columbus State Community College • Disability Services [650]
Columbus Veterans Affairs Clinic [30753]
Columbus West Home Dialysis and Training • DaVita [26075]
Colusa County Department of Behavioral Health [28445]
Colusa County • Dept of Behavioral Health/Sub Abuse [39723]
Colusa Indian Health Clinic Dialysis [22643]
Colusa Regional Medical Center [12951]
Colville Tribal Alcohol/Drug Program • Inchelium Branch [49972]
Comal County Women's Center [10494]
Comanche County Health Department • Speech and Hearing Clinic [3270]
Comanche County Memorial Hospital • Cancer Program [5772]
Comanche County Memorial Hospital Home Health Care [17125]
COMCARE • Addiction Treatment Services [43486]
Comcare Health Services, LLC [18164]
ComCare Home Health, Inc. [13088]
COMCARE of Sedgwick County • Wichita Crisis Intervention Services [50926]
Comcare of Sedgwick County [50927]
Comet Club [31958]
Comfort Care of Holy Spirit, Inc. [17277]
Comfort Care Home Health [15968]
Comfort Care Hospice [18672], [18751], [20286]
Comfort Care Hospice of Brewton [18689]
Comfort Care Hospice of Cullman [18693]
Comfort Care Hospice of Gadsden [18717]
Comfort Care Hospice of Greenville [18719]
Comfort Care Hospice LLC [18702], [18764]
Comfort Care Hospice of Moulton [18748]
Comfort Care Hospice of Scottsboro [18758]
Comfort Care Hospice-Wetumpka [18772]
Comfort Care, Inc. [18133]
Comfort Hospice Care-Las Vegas [20413]
Comfort Hospice Care-Layton [21613]
Comfort Zone Health Care [14403]
ComfortCare Hospice [20247]
Comforting Hands Hospice [20922]
Comgraph Inc [42850]
COMHAR • Community Living Room [32065]
COMHAR, Inc. [32066]
    Intensive Care Residence/Mental Health Center [32067]
    Latino Outpatient and HIV Program [32068]
    Long-Term Structured Residence • Independence House [32069]
    Maximum Care Community Residence [32070]
    Outpatient Services [32071]
    PACTS - Outpatient/TRIAD [32072]
    Supported Independent Living Program [32073]
COMHAR
    Open Door Clubhouse [32074]
    Speakeasy [32075]
Comitis Crisis Center [50710]
    Runaway and Homeless Youth Program [35853]
Comm Mental Health Consultants Inc [45575]
    Cass County Psychological Services [45487]
Commack Center for Speech and Hearing Disorders [3006]
Commerce City Dialysis • DaVita [23106]
Commerce Kidney Center [23656]
Commerce Township Dialysis • DaVita [24856]
Commission for Libraries • Idaho Talking Book Service [3784]
Committed Home Healthcare [15690]

Committed Home Healthcare, LLC [15808]
Committee to Aid Abused Women [9798]
Committee on Drug Abuse • Outpatient Medically Supervised [46750]
Common Bond Association Inc • Isiah House [45389]
Common Goals Inc [40256]
Common Ground [45273]
Common Ground Counseling LLC [43980], [44016], [44019]
Common Ground Crisis Services [51026]
Common Ground • Runaway and Homeless Youth Program [36011]
Common Ground Sanctuary [9521], [51009]
Commonwealth Center for Children and Adolescents [33908]
Commonwealth Home Health Care, Inc.--Danville [18282]
Commonwealth Home Health Care Inc.--Montgomery [12702]
Commonwealth Home Nursing and Hospice [18283]
Commonwealth Orthopaedics and Rehabilitation [39119], [39136]
Commonwealth Pharmacy [18284]
Commonwealth Speech Center [2273]
Commonwealth Substance Abuse • Specialists [43556], [43591], [43785]
Commonwealth Substance Abuse Specialists • Dougherty House [43564]
Communicare [45383]
CommuniCare Associates Inc. [3518]
Communicare • Calhoun County Office [45413]
Communicare Clinic [43529]
Communicare at Countryside [3961]
Communicare • Haven House [45409]
Communicare Health Centers [6299]
CommuniCare Health Centers
    Outpatient Substance Abuse Treatment Program [40946]
    Substance Abuse Program [40963]
Communicare - Hernando [30773]
Communicare Inc [43543], [43614], [43643], [43645], [43786]
    Elizabethtown Clinic [43577]
    Recovery Center [43578]
Communicare, Inc. [30003]
    Adult and Children's Crisis Stabilization [30004]
Communicare Inc.--Elizabethtown • Regional Administration [30005]
Communicare Ltd. [2892]
Communicare Outpatient Clinic--Bardstown [29969]
Communicare Outpatient Clinic--Brandenburg [29983]
Communicare Outpatient Clinic--Lebanon [30042]
Communicare Outpatient Clinic--Leitchfield [30045]
Communicare Outpatient Clinic--Radcliff [30104]
Communicare • Outpatient Treatment [45410]
Communicare--Oxford [30800]
Communicare at Poinciana Terrace [3962]
Communicare Recovery Center [30006]
Communicare--Sardis [30811]
Communicare--Senatobia [30812]
Communicare • Tate County Office [45418]
Communicare--Water Valley [30821]
Communicare at Whitney Acres [3963]
Communicare at Whitney Oaks [3964]
Communicare at Whitney Pines [3965]
Communicare • Yalobusha County Office [45427]
Communication Access Center for the Deaf and Hard of Hearing [2584]
Communication Associates--Albany CA [1051]
Communication Associates--Harleysville [3335]
Communication Associates--San Antonio [3535]
Communication Builders Inc.--Tulsa [3290]
Communication Care Center, Ltd. [2029]
Communication Clubhouse Inc. [1985]
Communication Connection [1144]
Communication Corner [2292], [2419]
Communication Disorders Center • Yale-New Haven Hospital [1477]
Communication Disorders, Ltd. [1329]
Communication Disorders Specialist [3197]
Communication Enhancement Center [3017]
Communication Enhancement, Inc. [1367]
Communication Essentials [1693]
Communication Imaging [3343]
Communication Improvement Services [3213]
Communication Innovations Inc. [3672]

Communication Journey [1651]
Communication Links LLC [2391]
Communication Matters--Bellevue [3619]
Communication Matters LLC--Butte [2833]
Communication Matters--Newbury Park [1195]
Communication Milestone [1911]
Communication Partners--Fayetteville [1006]
Communication Partners--Houston [3505]
Communication Partners Inc.--Carrolton [1844]
Communication Partners Inc.--Rogers [1034]
Communication Plus Inc. [3620]
Communication Power LLC [2887]
Communication and Reading Therapies [903]
Communication Service for the Deaf Inc. [3415]
Communication Skills Center [979]
Communication Specialists [3334]
Communication Therapies [1976]
Communication Therapy [2330]
Communication Therapy Associates--Arlington [2443]
Communication Therapy Associates--Northampton [2506]
Communication Therapy Services, Inc. [1958]
Communication Works [1205]
Communications Associates [2414]
Communications In-Roads [2369]
Communications Services for the Deaf and Hard of Hearing [3181]
Communicative Health Care Associates, Inc. [2532]
Communicative Solutions Group Inc. [1853]
Communicorp Speech & Language Services [2893]
Communities Against Domestic Violence [9410]
Communities Organized for Health Options [28083]
Community Abuse Prevention Services Agency [10524]
Community Access [31410]
Community Access Program of Rutland [32675]
Community Access Unlimited • Runaway and Home-less Youth Program [36076]
Community Action Against Addiction [47682]
Community Action Agency of Columbiana County, Inc. • Unity Health Center [7091]
Community Action Agency of Franklin County [9944]
Community Action Council Clinic [7307]
Community Action Council of South Texas [7308]
Community Action Health Center, Beeville [7278]
Community Action Stops Abuse [9078]
Community Action for Wyoming County [9974]
Community Actions Inc. • Crossroads Project [10312]
Community Addiction Recov Enterprise • Valley Lake Boys Home-site [45093]
Community Addiction Recovery Enterpris • Anoka/Hennepin [45205]
Community Addiction Recovery
    Enterprise (CARE)/Anoka [45073]
    Enterprise (CARE) Brainerd [45091]
    Enterprise (CARE)/Fergus Falls [45151]
    Enterprise (CARE)/Liberalis [45107]
    Enterprise (CARE)/Saint Peter [45316]
    Enterprise (CARE) Willmar [45344]
Community Addiction Treatment Services • CATS Substance Abuse Treatment Program [49333]
Community Against Violence [9889]
Community AIDS Resources [41650]
Community Alcohol/Drug Rehab and • Education Center [41119]
Community Alcohol and Drug Treatment Foundation • Van Nuys Treatment Center [40891]
Community Alliance Against Family Abuse [8677]
Community Alliance Home Health Care and Services [14683]
Community Alliance for Traffic Safety [49522]
Community Alternatives Inc • Community Choices Inc CASCADE [47255]
Community Anti-Violence Alliance [9263]
Community Assessment and Treatment Services [47683]
Community Based Outpatient Clinic--Alpena [15575]
Community Based Outpatient Clinic--Columbus [14504]
Community Based Outpatient Clinics • (CBOC) [47634]
Community Based Outreach Center for Homeless Veterans [31030]
Community Behavioral Health Inc • Horizon Services [47770], [47816]

Community Behavioral Health Services--Fredonia [28148]
Community Behavioral Health Services • Fredonia Location [39386]
Community Behavioral Health Services--Page [28169]
Community Behavioral Health Services • Page Outpatient [39413]
Community Blood Services [35114]
Community Bridges Inc
    Center for Hope [39404]
    Outpatient [39387]
Community Bridges/WORCcenter [4246]
Community Care Hospice [18935]
Community Care Hospice, Inc. [20910]
Community Care Hospice-Somerville [20497]
Community Care Organization, Inc. [16383]
Community Care Partners, Inc. [16694]
Community Care Providers [14321]
Community Care Services [44663]
    Attleboro Clinic [30323]
Community Care Services--Belleville [30514]
Community Care Services • Counseling and Resource Center [44900]
Community Care Services Hospice [21445]
Community Care Services, Inc.--Taunton [30470]
Community Care Services--Lincoln Park [30590]
Community Care Services
    Outpatient Substance Abuse Services [44398]
    Substance Abuse Service [45030]
    Taunton Outpatient Services [44588]
Community Care Services--Taylor [30644]
Community CarePartners--Hendersonville [16738]
Community CarePartners--Waynesville [16794]
Community Child Guidance Clinic [7851]
Community Clinic [6799]
Community Clinic of Maui--Kaahumanu Avenue, Kahului [6620]
Community Clinic of Maui--Lahaina • NHOW Satel-lite Clinic [6625]
Community Clinic of Maui--Lono Avenue, Kahului [6621]
Community Clinic of Maui--Wailuku [6628]
Community Clinic Rogers Medical [6278]
Community Clinic Siloam Springs [6280]
Community Clinical Counseling [43995]
Community Clinical Services [6778]
Community College of Aurora • Accessibility Services Office [318]
Community College of Denver • Accessibility Center [323]
Community College of Rhode Island Disability Services [723]
Community Concepts Inc • School Based Services [44061]
Community Connections--Craig [28084]
Community Connections, Inc. [29085]
Community Connections, Inc.--Washington DC • Day Services Program [29086]
Community Connections--Ketchikan [28105]
Community Consortium of San Francisco • Com-munity Program for Clinical Research on AIDS [39]
Community Corrections • 25th Judicial District [43351]
Community Council of Idaho [6634]
Community Council of Nashua, New Hampshire Inc. [31085]
Community Council of Nashua, New Hampshire, Inc • Child and Adolescent Services [31086]
Community Counseling--Arkadelphia [28232]
Community Counseling of Bristol County [30457], [30471]
    Behavioral Health Adult Counseling [44589]
Community Counseling Center [43629], [43732], [45450], [45838], [48258], [51053]
Community Counseling Center of Ashtabula County [31655]
Community Counseling Center of Bollinger County [30868], [51057]
Community Counseling Center, Cape Girardeau [30838]
Community Counseling Center
    Gateway Healthcare [32163]
    Greenville Satellite Office [32021]
Community Counseling Center of Madison County [30848], [51054]
Community Counseling Center of Mercer County [8466], [32027]

Community Counseling Center of North Madison [29558]
Community Counseling Center of Perry County [51059]
Community Counseling Center at Perryville [30885]
Community Counseling Center • Sainte Genevieve [30903]
Community Counseling Center of Sainte Genevieve County [51066]
Community Counseling Center--Sharon [32118]
Community Counseling Center South Mobile County [27954]
Community Counseling Centers of Chicago [9203], [50835]
Community Counseling Centers Inc
    at PineView Psychiatric Hospital [39401]
    Outpatient Clinic [39397], [39517]
    Outpatient Unit [39475]
Community Counseling Centers, Inc.--Holbrook [28157], [50644]
Community Counseling Centers, Inc.--Show Low [28200], [50651]
Community Counseling Centers, Inc.--Winslow [28228], [50657]
Community Counseling Clinic LLC [50234]
Community Counseling and Crisis Center [51232]
Community Counseling • Excel/Advantage Programs [28286]
Community Counseling Institute Inc [50207]
Community Counseling - Malvern [28313]
Community Counseling Mediation Service • Alcohol and Substance Abuse Program [46487]
Community Counseling Services [49001]
Community Counseling Services of Adams County--Othello [51456]
Community Counseling Services of Adams County--Ritzville [51463]
Community Counseling Services
    Alcohol and Drug Treatment Unit [48998]
    Alcohol/Subst Abuse Outpatient Clinic [46642]
    Arenac Center [30640]
    Bradfield Leary Center [32229]
Community Counseling Services--Care Program [51341], [51343]
Community Counseling Services/Chestnut Health Systems [50848]
Community Counseling Services • Choctaw County Office [45360]
Community Counseling Services--Eupora [30757]
Community Counseling Services--Hot Springs [50662]
Community Counseling Services--Huron [32230]
Community Counseling Services, Inc.--Bucyrus [31669]
Community Counseling Services, Inc.--Hot Springs [28287]
Community Counseling Services--Louisville [30784]
Community Counseling Services--Macon [30786]
Community Counseling Services of • Ronkonkoma/Alcoholism Outpatient Clinic [47059]
Community Counseling Services
    Outreach Program [32223], [32224], [32232]
    Outreach Program/Tri-County Clinic [32262]
    Outreach Services - Hand County Memorial [32234]
Community Counseling Services--Starkville • Contact Helpline [51051]
Community Counseling Solutions [31932], [48063], [48086], [48114], [48125], [48134]
    North Office [48083]
Community Countermeasures [46182]
Community for Creative Non-Violence [9018]
Community Crisis Center [50842]
Community Crisis Center--Elgin [9225]
Community Crisis Center--Miami [10203]
Community Crisis Services, Inc. [50976]
Community Dialysis Center [22694]
Community Dialysis Center--Clovis [22640]
Community Dialysis Center of Columbus, LLC [23648]
Community Dialysis Centers Inc.--Baltimore [24630]
Community Dialysis of Harvey [24004]
Community Dialysis Unit--Alliance • DaVita [26007]
Community Drug and Alcohol Services [45099], [45302]
Community Enterprises, Inc. [30433]
Community Entry Services [8634]
Community Family Center [7314]

Community/Family Counseling Programs [40096]
Community Family Guidance Center [28430]
Community and Family Resources [43233], [43239], [43248], [43272], [43273], [43277], [43296], [43299], [43314]
Community General Hospital • The Sleep Center [37384]
Community Healing Center--Niles [30613]
Community Healing Center--Sturgis [30642]
Community Healing Center--Three Rivers [30645]
Community Healing Centers [44943], [45029]
    Elizabeth Upjohn [44866]
    Jim Gilmore Jr [44867]
Community Health Action of • Staten Island [47094]
Community Health Alliance Dental of Pasadena [6339]
Community Health Association of Spokane [7391]
Community Health Awareness Council • Alcohol and Drug Treatment [40248]
Community Health Care, Corp. [14230]
Community Health Care, Inc.--Bridgeton [6968]
Community Health Care, Inc.--Davenport [6705]
Community Health Care Systems, Inc. • Johnson County Center for Community Health [6610]
Community Health Care--Tacoma [7392]
Community Health Care Women's Center [6987]
Community Health Center of the Black Hills [7250]
Community Health Center of Branch County [15612]
Community Health Center of Burlington [7334]
Community Health Center of Cape Cod [6820]
Community Health Center of Central Missouri, Pathways Location [6906]
Community Health Center of Central Wyoming [7445]
Community Health Center • Community Drug Board Inc [47602]
Community Health Center of Fort Dodge [6709]
Community Health Center, Inc. • Community Health Center of Middletown [6423]
Community Health Center, Inc.--Medford [7136]
Community Health Center La Clinica [7382]
Community Health Center of Lubbock [7301]
Community Health Center • RAMAR Residential Treatment Center [47603]
Community Health Center--Sierra [13008]
Community Health Center of Southeast Kansas/Dental Clinic [6719]
Community Health Center • Womens Recovery Program [47604]
Community Health Centers of Buffalo [7019]
Community Health Centers of the Central Coast, Inc. [6328]
Community Health Centers at Clearwater [6451]
Community Health Centers of Greater Dayton • Corwin M. Nixon Community Health Center [7084]
Community Health Centers at Largo [6489]
Community Health Centers of Pinellas, Inc. • Johnnie Ruth Clarke Health Center [6546]
Community Health Centers of Rutland Region, Inc. [7331]
Community Health Centers--Salt Lake City [7327]
Community Health Centers of South Central Texas, Inc. • Gonzales Community Health Center [7291]
Community Health Centers of Southern Iowa, Inc.--Lamoni [6710]
Community Health Centers of Southern Iowa, Inc.--Leon [6711]
Community Health Centers of Western Kentucky, Inc. [6729]
Community Health Centers--Winter Garden [6572]
Community Health Clinic--Dove Creek [6400]
Community Health Clinic--Elk Point [7245]
Community Health Clinic Ole [6327]
Community Health Connections, Inc. [6815]
Community Health and Counseling Services • Adult Mental Health Services [30208]
Community Health and Counseling Services--Bangor [19885], [30193]
Community Health and Counseling Services • Big Red Redemption Center [30194]
Community Health and Counseling Services-Dover [19892]
Community Health and Counseling Services--Dover Foxcroft [30207]
Community Health and Counseling Services-Lincoln [19897], [30224]
Community Health and Counseling Services-Machias [19898]

Community Health and Counseling Services • Runaway and Homeless Youth Program [35979]
Community Health Development [7315]
Community Health of East Tennessee Clinic [7259]
Community Health and Emergency Services [42428]
Community Health Foundation of Man, West Virginia • Community Health Foundation [7408]
Community Health and Hospice [20438]
Community Health Improvement Center [6669]
Community Health Net Dental [7161]
Community Health Net--Highpoint [7162]
Community Health Network • Regional Cancer Center [5155]
Community Health Partners Hospital • Comprehensive Cancer Center [5733]
Community Health Partners, Inc. [6935]
Community Health Partnership of Illinois [6656]
Community Health Services Inc • Department of Behavioral Health [41399]
Community Health Services, Inc. [6422]
Community Health and Social Services Center • CHASS Center [6840]
Community Health of South Florida [6501]
Community Health of South Florida Inc • Martin Luther King Clinic [41694]
Community HealthCare and Hospice--McCook [20392]
Community Healthcare Inc • Community Substance Abuse Centers [44443], [44479], [44528], [44602]
Community Healthcore [49555]
    Beginning [49443]
    The Beginning [49561]
    Kirkpatrick Family Center [49444]
    Oak Haven Recovery Center [49461]
Community Healthlink Inc [44609]
    Detoxification Program [44610]
    Highland Grace House [44611]
    Orchard Street Program [44502]
    Worcester Youth and Family Services [44612]
Community Healthlink, Inc. [30482]
    Outpatient Services [30483]
Community Home Care and Hospice-Asheboro [20725]
Community Home Care and Hospice-Chapel Hill [20632]
Community Home Care and Hospice-Clayton [20636]
Community Home Care and Hospice-Clinton [20638]
Community Home Care and Hospice--Dillon [21229]
Community Home Care and Hospice-Durham [20647]
Community Home Care and Hospice--Elizabeth City [20653]
Community Home Care and Hospice-Engelhard [20656]
Community Home Care and Hospice--Erwin [20657]
Community Home Care and Hospice--Fayetteville [20660]
Community Home Care and Hospice--Goldsboro [20670]
Community Home Care and Hospice-Greenville [20676]
Community Home Care and Hospice-Henderson [20678]
Community Home Care and Hospice--Kinston [20688]
Community Home Care and Hospice--Leland [20692]
Community Home Care Hospice-Louisburg [20697]
Community Home Care and Hospice-Lumberton [20698]
Community Home Care and Hospice--Monroe [20705]
Community Home Care and Hospice-Morehead City [20708]
Community Home Care and Hospice-New Bern [20711]
Community Home Care and Hospice-Raleigh [20718]
Community Home Care and Hospice-Roanoke Rapids [20722]
Community Home Care and Hospice-Rockingham [20723]
Community Home Care and Hospice--Rocky Mount [20726]
Community Home Care and Hospice--Sanford [20729]

Community Home Care and Hospice--Siler City [20734]
Community Home Care and Hospice-Statesville [20741]
Community Home Care and Hospice-Swansboro [20746]
Community Home Care and Hospice--Tarboro [20748]
Community Home Care and Hospice-Troy [20753]
Community Home Care and Hospice--Wallace [20758]
Community Home Care and Hospice--Washington [20760]
Community Home Care and Hospice--Whiteville [20762]
Community Home Care and Hospice-Wilson [20767]
Community Home Care Referral Service, Inc. [16384]
Community Home Care--Rock Springs [18658]
Community Home Care--Torrington [18663]
Community Home Health Care Services [13027]
Community Home Health & Hospice [21777]
Community Home Health and Hospice [18438]
Community Home Health & Hospice-Longview [21759]
Community Home Health, Inc. [13330]
Community Home Health--Lake Worth [13836]
Community Home Health of Maryland--Annapolis [15407]
Community Home Health of Maryland--Baltimore [15413]
Community Home Health of Maryland--Owings Mills [15454]
Community Home Health of Maryland--Upper Marlboro [15467]
Community Home Health of Maryland--Westminster [15470]
Community Home Health--Port Saint Lucie [14350]
Community Home Health Services [14979]
Community Home Healthcare, Inc. [14895]
Community Home Oxygen--Casper [18646]
Community Home Oxygen--Cheyenne [18648]
Community Home Oxygen, Inc.--Billings [16084]
Community Home Oxygen, Inc.--Bozeman [16085]
Community Home Oxygen--Laramie [18655]
Community Home Oxygen--Riverton [18657]
Community Home Oxygen--Saratoga [18659]
Community Home Oxygen--Sheridan [18660]
Community Home Oxygen--Torrington [18664]
Community Home Oxygen--Wheatland [18665]
Community of Hope [9019]
Community Hospice of Albany County [20549]
Community Hospice of Amsterdam [20552]
Community Hospice--Ashland [19790]
Community Hospice of Baldwin County [18715]
Community Hospice Care-Tallahassee [18765]
Community Hospice Care--Tiffin [20897]
Community Hospice of Columbia/Greene [20562]
Community Hospice House--Merrimack [20445]
Community Hospice Inc.--Westland [20135]
Community Hospice Inn [20550]
Community Hospice-Ironton [20849]
Community Hospice of Maryland [19944]
Community Hospice--Modesto [18968]
Community Hospice of Northeast Florida [19239]
Community Hospice of Oklahoma [20955]
Community Hospice-Paintsville [19826]
Community Hospice of Rensselaer County [20600]
Community Hospice of Saratoga [20605]
Community Hospice of Schenectady [20606]
Community Hospice of Texas [21418], [21430]
Community Hospice of Victor Valley [18886]
Community Hospice of Virginia [18291]
Community Hospital of Anderson [4033]
Community Hospital of Anderson and Madison County • Cancer Program [5134]
Community Hospital--Anderson • ProCare Rehab Services [2125]
Community Hospital • Cancer Program [5170]
Community Hospital East--Indianapolis [14999]
Community Hospital--Grand Junction [13492]
Community Hospital Home Health & Hospice [16112]
Community Hospital of the Monterey • Peninsula/Behavioral Health Services [40241]
Community Hospital of Monterey Peninsula • Cancer Program [4809]
Community Hospital Monterey Peninsula • Pain

Clinic [35309]
Community Hospital of the Monterey Peninsula •
Sleep Disorders Center [36662]
Community Hospital--Munster [2172]
Community Hospital of New Port Richey • Cancer
Center [4973]
Community Hospital North [4034]
Community Hospital North--Indianapolis [15000]
Community Hospital North--Psychiatric Pavilion
[50891]
Community Hospital of the Roanoke Valley • Medical
Center for Children • Sickle Cell Disease Center
[36438]
Community Hospital of San Bernardino [13288]
Community Hospital • Sleep Diagnostics Center
[36941]
Community Hospital South--Indianapolis [15001]
Community Hospital, Tallassee, FL [28050]
Community Hospital and Wellness Centers • Cancer
Program [5684]
Community Hospitals • Hook Rehabilitation Center •
Center for Neurological Rehabilitation [4035]
Community Hospitals of Indiana--Carmel • Sleep/
Wake Disorders Center [36942]
Community Hospitals of Indiana--Clearvista Drive,
Indianapolis • Sleep/Wake Disorders Center
[36943]
Community Hospitals of Indiana--Greenwood •
Sleep/Wake Disorders Center [36944]
Community Hospitals of Indiana Inc
Crestview Center [42979]
Gallahue Mental Health Center [43089]
Community Hospitals of Indiana--N Ritter Avenue,
Indianapolis • Sleep/Wake Disorders Center
[36945]
Community Hospitals of Williams County, Inc.
[16857]
Community Hospitals of Williams County, Inc. -
Montpelier Building [17003]
Community House Home Health/Hospice [18249]
Community Human Services
Genesis House [40792]
Off Main Clinic [40513]
Runaway and Homeless Youth Program [35814]
Community Institute for Psychotherapy [10944]
Community Justice Serv of Boulder Cnty [41019]
Community Kare [16230]
Community of Landmark [7900]
Community Links • Huron Behavioral Health [30506]
The Community Living Program [34207]
Community Loving Care Hospice, LLC [20281],
[20347]
Community Medical Center
Cancer Program [5544]
Center for Sleep Disorders [37342]
Community Rehabilitation Center [4247]
Community Medical Center Home Care [16274]
Community Medical Center of Manchester [6596]
Community Medical Center • Physical and Hand
Therapy Department [38163]
Community Medical Centers • California Cancer
Center [4778]
Community Medical Centers, Inc. [6369]
Community Medical Services
Alpha [39425]
Bullhead Drug Abuse Program [39367]
Flagstaff [39380]
Glendale [39392]
Larkspur [39426]
Missoula [45712]
Prescott [39460]
Tucson [39490]
Community Medicine Foundation, Inc. [7242]
Community Memorial Health Center • Dialysis
Center [27565]
Community Memorial Healthcenter [18386]
Community Memorial Hospital [2682]
Community Memorial Hospital--Menomonee Falls •
Cancer Program [6161]
Community Memorial Hospital • Regional Sleep
Disorders Center [37966]
Community Memorial Hospital--Ventura • Cancer
Care Program [4863]
Community Mental Health Affiliates • Child Guidance
Clinic [7852]
Community Mental Health Affiliates, Inc. [28979]
Family Counseling Center [29017]

Intensive Assertive Community Treatment
[29018]
Community Mental Health Center • Eastman Annex
[42093]
Community Mental Health Center Inc [42989],
[43135], [43136], [43137], [43189], [43229]
Dearborn County [43138]
Franklin County Office [43002]
Community Mental Health Center Inc. [43173]
Community Mental Health Center, Inc. [50885]
Community Mental Health Center, Inc.--Vevay
[29825]
Community Mental Health Center • Lawrenceburg
Crisis Line [50895]
Community Mental Health Center--Muskegon
[30608]
Community Mental Health for Central Michigan
[51023]
Gladwin County Mental Illness [30556]
Midland County Branch [30602]
Midland County/Developmentally Disabled
[30603]
Community Mental Health of Clinton • Eaton and
Ingham Counties [44916], [45007]
Community Mental Health Council Inc • MISA
Outpatient Services [42487]
Community Mental Health Council, Inc. [29587]
Community Mental Health of Ottawa County [30566]
Community Mental Health of Ottawa County--Grand
Haven [30557]
Community Mental Health of Ottawa County •
Robert S. Brown Center [30567]
Community Mental Health of Ottowa--Hudsonville
[30571]
Community Mental Health Services--Crisis Link
[51516]
Community Mental Health Services Inc. [51220]
Community Mental Health Services of Muskegon
County • ACT/Outpatient [44936]
Community Mental Health of St Joseph • Mental
Health and Substance Abuse [44693]
Community Mental Health and Substance Abuse
Services Board • Prevention Division [51427]
Community Mental Health and Wellness Clinic
[31015]
Community Mental Health of West Michigan [51025]
Community Mental Healthcare [31758]
Community Mental Healthcare Inc [47749]
Community Mental Healthcare, Inc.
Carrollton Office [51202]
Dover Office [51215]
New Philadelphia Office [51230]
Community Mercy Health Partners [17045]
Community Mercy Hospice • Community Mercy
Health Partners [20893]
Community MHC of Crawford County [43336],
[43347], [43444]
Co-Girard [43354]
Outpatient [43445]
Community Missions of the Niagara Frontier Inc.
[31436]
The Community Network--Fairborn [51218]
Community Network Services Inc [44778], [45048]
The Community Network--Xenia • Greene County
Crisis Services [51236]
Community Nurse and Hospice Care [19958]
Community Nurses, Inc. [21152]
Community Nursing Services-Corporate Office
[21644]
Community Nursing Services-Moab [21617]
Community Nursing Services--Murray [21620]
Community Nursing Services of Northeast [21122]
Community Nursing Services-Ogden [21626]
Community Partners • Behavioral Health and
Developmental Services of Strafford County [8235]
Community Personal Care, Inc. [18340]
Community Program Office • Wedgwood Christian
Services [34225]
Community Programs Inc [45049], [45050]
Community Psychiatric Clinic [50098]
Belltown Branch [50099]
Bridge Way Program [32851]
Bridgeway Branch [50100]
City Center [32852]
City Center Branch [50101]
Clean Start [32853]
North Gate [32854]
Northgate Branch [50102]

Stone Way [32855]
Wallingford Branch [50103]
Community Psychiatric Institute [45970]
Community Psychotherapy Associates [45928]
Community Re-Entry Program [30465]
Community Reach Center [41327], [41338]
Community Reach Center--Brighton Office [28864]
Community Reach Center
Child and Family Services [28939]
Commerce City Office [28875]
Community Reach Center Inc [41023]
Community Recovery Resources [39896], [40860]
Hope House [39897]
Community Recovery Services
Alto Counseling Center [28804], [28842]
Santa Cruz Residential Recovery [28805]
Si Se Puede [28843]
Community Referral Agency, Inc. [10720]
Community Regional Medical Center--Fresno
[13009]
Community Rehab Care Inc.--Centre Street, Newton
[4133]
Community Rehab Care, Inc.--Medford [4134]
Community Rehab Care, Inc.--Quincy [4135]
Community Rehab Care, Inc.--W Suburban YMCA,
Newton [4136]
Community Rehab Center • Speech--Language/
Audiology [2838]
Community Renewal Team
Adult Substance Abuse Outpatient [41400]
Transitional Case Management [41401]
Community Research Foundation [28748]
Community Research Foundation Inc
Areta Crowell Center [40548]
South Bay Guidance Center [39707]
Community Residence [31351]
Community Resource Center [42441], [42450],
[42900], [42939]
Community Resource Center--Carlyle [29571]
Community Resource Center--Centralia [29572]
Community Resource Center • Libre! Services for
Women and Children [8808]
Community Resource Center--Salem [29675]
Community Resource Center--Vandalia [29682]
Community Resource and Counseling Center
[50865]
Community and Rural Health Services, Inc. [7085]
Community Safety Network [10753]
Community Service Board of Middle Georgia--
Chauncey [29387]
Community Service Board of Middle Georgia--East
Dublin [29416]
Community Service Board of Middle Georgia •
Middle Georgia Alcohol & Drug Clinic [29413]
Community Service Foundation Inc [48372], [48638]
Buxmont Academy/Bethlehem [48291]
Buxmont Academy/Lansdale [48437]
Buxmont Academy/Upper Providence [48579]
Community Service Organization
Brotherhood Center [39632]
De Colores Center [39982]
Community Service Programs, Inc. [28794]
Runaway and Homeless Youth Program [35815]
Community Services Council of New Hampshire
[51080]
Community Services Counseling [42312], [42355]
Community Services for the Deaf [3236]
Community Services for the Developmentally
Disabled, Inc. [9908]
Community Services Group [32049]
Community Services of MO [45431], [45468],
[45618], [45635]
Dexter Site [45469]
Ellisville Site [45474]
Hazelwood Office [45492]
Hillsboro Site [45494]
Houston Site [45497]
Kennett Site [45540]
O Fallon Site [45578]
Rolla Office [45598]
Sunset Hills Office [45657]
Community Social Model Advocates Inc
Hobie House [40215]
Rose Julia Riordan Tranquility Village [39616]
Community Solutions--Gilroy [28514]
Community Solutions • La Casa Del Puente Treat-
ment Center [28643]
Community Solutions--Morgan Hill [28644]

Community Speech and Hearing Center [1332], [7830]
Community Speech, Language and Learning Center [2904]
Community Speech Therapy Inc. [3581]
Community Spine Center [4036]
Community Substance Abuse Centers [44441], [44535]
    Ambulatory Detox [41402]
    High Point Treatment Center [44515]
    Merrimack River Medical Services Inc [44026]
Community Substance Abuse Services Inc [44875]
Community Support Center [31332]
Community Support Network [28814]
Community Support Program
    Grant Blackford Mental Health Inc [43145]
    Psychosocial Rehabilitation [28943]
Community Support Services--Bend [31931]
Community Support Services • Community Counseling Center [32164]
Community Support Services, Inc.--Cross Street, Akron [31645]
Community Support Services
    Pioneer House [28806]
    The Providence Center [32169]
    The River Street Shelter [28807]
Community Support Services--Shawnee [29955]
Community Support Services • Transition House [28808]
Community Support Services--Wolf Ledges Parkway, Akron [31646]
Community Support Systems Team • Mental Health Center of Boulder County [28860]
Community Support and Treatment Services [44637]
    PORT/JPORT Teams [44638]
    Towner Site [45068]
Community Surgical Supply [16275]
Community Therapy Center [1039]
Community Ties - South [30611]
Community Tissue Services--Boise [35018]
Community Tissue Services, California [34941]
Community Tissue Services, Dayton [35159]
Community Tissue Services, Fort Worth [35227]
Community Tissue Services, Indiana [35029]
Community Tissue Services--Kettering • Center for Tissues Innovation and Research [35160]
Community Tissue Services--Medford [35180]
Community Tissue Services, Mid-South [35205]
Community Tissue Services, Pennsylvania [35185]
Community Tissue Services, Portland [35181]
Community Tissue Services, Toledo [35161]
Community Treatment Inc [45493], [45495], [45496]
Community Treatment Solutions [46067]
Community United Against Violence [8886]
Community United Methodist Hospital, Inc. [15191]
Community--University Health Care Center [6867]
Community Visiting Nurse Association Hospice [19597]
Community Works [34398]
    Dunn House [10239]
Community Works Help Line [51260]
Community Works • Runaway and Homeless Youth Program [36167]
Community YMCA Family Services [46050]
Community Youth Services, Olympia • Runaway and Homeless Youth Program [36251]
CommunityCare Austin [7277]
Communityworks LLC [47968]
CommWell Health [7055]
Como Pediatric Communication Center [2659]
Companion Home Health Inc. [13268]
Companion Hospice and Companion Home Health Care [13225]
Companion Hospice, LLC [20936]
The Compass Center [10384]
Compass Corporation for Recovery Srvs • (COMPASS) [47865]
Compass Development Inc [42718]
Compass Halfway House [44207]
Compass Health--Broadway, Everett [32824]
Compass Health Family and Children Clinic [32801]
Compass Health--Federal Avenue, Everett [32825]
Compass Health Lopez Island Office [32833]
Compass Health--Lynnwood [32834]
Compass Health--Monroe [10627]
Compass Health Orcas Island Office [32821]
Compass Health/San Juan [49967]
Compass Health San Juan Island Office [32828]

Compass Health Second Street Building [32841]
Compass Health--Snohomish [32863]
Compass Health Veteran's Services [32842]
Compass Healthcare Inc
    Detoxification [39491]
    Outpatient [39492]
    Vida Serena [39493]
Compass House • Runaway and Homeless Youth Program [36096]
Compass Pointe • Behavioral Health Services [43276], [43298], [43301], [43307], [43308]
Compass Recovery Center [47843]
Compassion Health Services, LLC [14878]
Compassionate Care Center [19828]
Compassionate Care Home Care Services, Inc. [15631]
Compassionate Care Home Health, LLC [15526]
Compassionate Care Hospice of Delaware [19183]
Compassionate Care Hospice of the MidWest [21302]
Compassionate Care Inc. [20560]
Compassionate Caring [14342]
Compassionate Hands Hospice [21498]
Compassionate Health Care Services, Inc. [17973]
Compassionate Healthcare Mgmt Group Inc/dba Compassionate Hospice of North GA [19348]
Compassioncare Hospice [20414]
COMPDRUG Corporation • Methadone Program/ Outpatient AOD Treatment [47714]
Complete Care Medical Supply, Inc. [12990]
Complete Counseling Center Inc [44849]
Complete Dialysis Care and At Home • Davita [23377]
Complete Dialysis Care • DaVita [23273]
Complete Health Network, Inc. [13876]
Complete • Home Care, Inc. [17359]
Complete Home Care Services, Inc. [16624]
Complete Homecare Services, Inc. [18022]
Complete Learning Center [7907]
Complete Sleep Solutions [36663]
Complete Therapy [38216]
CompleteSleep Management, Inc. [37810]
CompreCare [18518]
Comprehbsive Renal Care--Michigan City • DaVita [24203]
Comprehend Inc [43544], [43713]
Comprehend Inc/Fleming County CMHC [43589]
Comprehend Inc/Lewis County CMHC [43791]
Comprehend Inc • Substance Abuse Outpatieint Services [43723]
Comprehensive Addiction Programs Inc [39848]
Comprehensive Addiction Treatment Serv • (CATS) [41120]
Comprehensive Addictions Treatment Services (CATS) Inc [41832]
Comprehensive Alcohol Services [49984]
Comprehensive Athletic Treatment Center [38994]
Comprehensive Behavior Health Center • Saint Clair County Inc/Center for ARTS [42645]
Comprehensive Behavioral Health Center • Saint Clair County Inc/SMARTS [42646]
Comprehensive Behavioral Healthcare [46039]
Comprehensive Behavioral Healthcare, Inc. [51108]
Comprehensive Behavioral Healthcare, Inc.-- Hackensack [31133]
Comprehensive Behavioral Healthcare, Inc.-- Lyndhurst [31145]
Comprehensive Blood and Cancer Center • Pain Clinic [35310]
Comprehensive Care Center--Carlisle [29988]
Comprehensive Care Center, Cumberland River [50937]
Comprehensive Care Center--Frankfort [30017]
Comprehensive Care Center--Georgetown [30020]
Comprehensive Care Center--Lawrenceburg • Rainbow House/Afterschool [30041]
Comprehensive Care Center--Richmond [30106]
Comprehensive Care Center/Southwood Recovery [30001]
Comprehensive Care Center--Winchester [30123]
Comprehensive Center for Bleeding Disorders • Children's Hospital of Wisconsin [12614]
Comprehensive Center for Sleep Medicine • Mount Sinai Medical Center [37385]
Comprehensive Communication Center Inc. [3266]
Comprehensive Communication Specialists [3248]
Comprehensive Community Health and • Psychological Services LLC [41529]

Comprehensive Community Health Centers Inc. [6303]
Comprehensive Community Health Centers, Inc., North Hollywood [6329]
Comprehensive Community Services [49078]
    Outpatient Counseling Center/Johnson City Office [49095]
    Outpatient Treatment Center/Kingsport Office [49098]
    Probations/Bristol Office [49042]
    Residential Treatment Center [49099]
Comprehensive Counseling and Consultation [43453]
Comprehensive Counseling Services [31808], [47817]
Comprehensive Dialysis of Western New York [25805]
Comprehensive Education Solutions [939]
Comprehensive Health and Attitude • Management Program Inc [42205]
Comprehensive Home Care--Bronx [16359]
Comprehensive Home Care--Brooklyn [16385]
Comprehensive Home Care, Inc.--White Plains [16669]
Comprehensive Home Care--Poughkeepsie [16600]
Comprehensive Home Health, Inc. [14724]
Comprehensive Juvenile Services • Runaway and Homeless Youth Program [35801]
Comprehensive Medical Home Care, Inc. [17247]
Comprehensive Mental Health Center
    Pearl Street Center [32870]
    Proctor Street Center [32871]
Comprehensive Mental Health Services [45500]
    Adult Services [32872]
Comprehensive Mental Health Services, Inc.-- Independence [30853]
Comprehensive Mental Health Services, Inc. • Jay County Services Department [29805]
Comprehensive Multiple Sclerosis Center of Southern Vermont [34727]
Comprehensive Neurologics and Sleep Clinic [37060]
Comprehensive Neurology • Pain and Headache Treatment Center [12423]
Comprehensive Nursing Services [15414]
Comprehensive Outpatient Services--Hampton [32744]
Comprehensive Outpatient Services--Newport News [32768]
Comprehensive Pain Care [35403]
Comprehensive Pain Center [35538]
Comprehensive Pain and Headache Treatment Centers [35357]
Comprehensive Pain Management [35559]
Comprehensive Pain Medicine Inc. [35380]
Comprehensive Psychiatric Center [41771]
    North [41772]
    South [41773]
Comprehensive Psychiatric Emergency Program • Commission on Mental Health Services • Crisis Helpline [50747]
Comprehensive Psychiatric Resources • Dietary Alignment Program [11088]
Comprehensive Quality Care, Inc. [14725]
Comprehensive Rehabilitation Center [2769], [4306]
Comprehensive Renal Care--Munster • Davita [24212]
Comprehensive Services, Inc. • Mount Vernon Crisis Line [50860]
Comprehensive Sickle Cell Center--Boston [36360]
Comprehensive Sickle Cell Center of Manhattan [36393]
Comprehensive Sickle Cell Center--Philadelphia [36418]
Comprehensive Sleep Care Center [37885]
Comprehensive Sleep Center [37761]
Comprehensive Sleep Disorder Center [36780]
Comprehensive Sleep Disorder Institute [37386]
Comprehensive Sleep Disorders Center of Northwest Pennsylvania [37643]
Comprehensive Sleep Medicine [37811]
Comprehensive Sleep Medicine Center of the Gulf Coast [37061], [37062]
Comprehensive Speech and Language Center Inc. [2609]
Comprehensive Speech Therapy Services of Long Island PC [3031]
Comprehensive Systems Inc. [8011]

Comprehensive Therapy Center [2593]
Comprehensive Therapy Children's Center [1843]
Comprehensive Treatment Center [41683]
Comprehensive Treatment Center of Maryland [9458]
Comprehensive Youth Services, Mount Clemens • Family Youth Interventions • Runaway and Homeless Youth Program [36012]
Compton Mental Health Center [28447]
Comtrea Community Mental Health Center [30828]
A Safe Place Shelter [9677]
COMTREA Inc [45432], [45480]
Comunicear [3045]
Comunidades Latinas Unidas en Servicio [45206], [45303]
Concept: CARE, Inc. [16670]
Concept House Inc [41774]
Outpatient and Administration [41775]
Concept Medical, Inc. [17246]
Conceptions Reproductive Associates--Lafayette [21958]
Conceptions Reproductive Associates--Littleton [21959]
Concepts in Counseling LLC [44896]
Conceptual Counseling Inc [45304]
Concern Hotline, Inc. [51425]
Concern, Inc. [51397]
Concerned Citizens Inc/Mothers House [42488]
Concho Valley Crisis Hotline [51392]
Concierge Health Care Services [19028]
Concilio de Salud Integral de Loiza, Inc. [7203]
Concord Counseling Services [47883]
Concord Dialysis Center • DaVita [22645]
Concord Home Health Care Inc. [13239]
Concord Hospital [45889]
Payson Center for Cancer Care [5492]
Sleep Disorders Center [37328]
Speech and Language Therapy [2878]
Concord Metro Treatment Center [45890]
Concord Regional VNA Hospice Services [20432]
Condell Medical Center [14832]
Condell Medical Center Hospice [19535]
Condon Center [31936]
Conejo Valley Clinic [28827]
Conemaugh Home Health--Boswell [17261]
Conemaugh Home Health--Ebensburg [17306]
Conemaugh Home Health--Everett [17315]
Conemaugh Home Health--Hastings [17337]
Conemaugh Home Health--Johnstown [17351]
Conemaugh Home Health--Meyersdale [17386]
Conemaugh Home Health--Philipsburg [17429]
Conemaugh Home Health--Portage [17454]
Conemaugh Regional Hospice [21101]
Conemaugh's Memorial Medical Center • Laurel Highlands Cancer Program [5834]
Conewago Indiana [48412]
Conewago Place • Inpatient [48408]
Coney Island Hospital
Acute Care Addictions Program/3 East [46488]
Chemical Dependency Rehab Component [46489]
Inpatient Substance Abuse Detox Prog [46490]
Rehabilitation Medicine Department • Audiology [2988]
Confederated Salish and Kootenai • Tribes [45719]
Confident Voice Solution Inc. [3168]
Confidential DUI Services [42601], [42826]
Confidential Health Consultants PC [41056]
Confidential Help for Alcohol Drugs • Outpatient Clinic [46364]
Confidential Mental Health Substance Abuse • Consultation Service LLC [43435]
Confidential Treatment Options [49891]
Congreso de Latinos • Unidos/Programa Horizontes [48501]
Conifer Counseling Services • Outpatient Drug Abuse Clinic [47031]
Conifer Park Inc
Alcoholism Outpatient Clinic [46660]
Alcoholism and Substance Abuse Clinic [46981]
Chemical Dependency Outpatient Clinic [47132]
Crisis Services [46661]
Inpatient Rehabilitation [46662]
Outpatient Chemical Dependency Clinic [46753]
Outpatient Clinic [47073]
Residential Rehab Services for Youth [46663]
Conlin's Pharmacy, Inc. [15517]
Connect Care Hospice [20171]

Connect Society • Deaf/Hard of Hearing Program [225]
Connect Society: D.E.A.F. Services [226]
Connecticut Children's Medical Center [1465]
Central Connecticut Adult Cystic Fibrosis Center [7491]
Central Connecticut Pediatric Cystic Fibrosis Center [7492]
Division of Human Genetics • Down Syndrome Program [10783]
Hemoglobin Disorders Treatment Center [36313]
Speech Pathology and Audiology Department [1466]
Connecticut College • Program for Children with Special Needs [7854]
Connecticut Commission on the Deaf and Hearing Impaired [1467]
Connecticut Counseling Centers Inc [41374]
Methadone Maintenance/Treatment [41483]
Norwalk Methadone Program [41453]
Norwalk Outpatient Treatment Program [41454]
Waterbury Outpatient Program [41484]
Connecticut Eye Bank and Visual Research Foundation • Research Foundation Inc. [34977]
Connecticut Fertility Associates - Bridgeport [21968]
Connecticut Fertility Associates--New York [22180]
Connecticut Fertility Associates - Norwalk [21969]
Connecticut Junior Republic [34053], [41485]
Connecticut Junior Republic--Litchfield [33249]
Connecticut Junior Republic--Waterbury [33266]
Connecticut Mental Health Center [33257]
Acute Care Services [50734]
Hispanic Clinic [41436]
Connecticut Pain Care--Bridgeport [35358]
Connecticut Pain Care--Danbury [35359]
Connecticut Pain Care--Hartford [35360]
Connecticut Pain Care--Norwalk [35361]
Connecticut Pain Care--Trumbull [35362]
Connecticut Pain Care--Waterbury [35363]
Connecticut Renaissance Inc
Behavioral Healthcare Center [41455]
East Residential Treatment Facility [41486]
Connecticut Spine and Pain Center [35364]
Connecticut State Library • Library for the Blind and Physically Handicapped [3756]
Connecticut Valley Home Care [16180]
Connecticut Valley Home Care/Hospice [20450]
Connecticut Valley Hospital
Addiction Services Division [41418]
Blue Hills Substance Services [41403]
Page Hall [33252]
Connecticut Valley House [31052]
Connecting Point • Runaway and Homeless Youth Program [36141]
Connecting Pointe LLC • Alcohol and Drug Education [43422]
A Connecting Pointe LLC • Individual Group and Family Counseling [43393]
Connection Counseling Center • Middletown [41419]
Connection House Inc [41420]
Hallie House Women/Childrens Center [41421]
Connection Inc
Mothers Retreat [41388]
Recovery House [41437]
Connection Inc/ The Connection • Counseling Center in Groton [41389]
Connection Telephone • Crisis Intervention and Referral [50854]
The Connection Youth Services • Livingston Family Center • Runaway and Homeless Youth Program [36013]
Connections [10639], [30050]
Connections for Abused Women and Their Children [9204]
Connections Counseling [50444]
Connections CSP Inc
Cornerstone Residential [41500]
Drug and Alcohol Outpatient [41513]
Connections CSP, Inc.--Camden [29057]
Connections CSP, Inc.--New Castle [29069]
Connections CSP, Inc.--Supervised Apartments [29075]
Connections CSP, Inc.--Wilmington [29076]
Connections Family Centered Therapies [3130]
Connections Health Care for the Homeless [6962]
Connections Health Wellness and Advocacy [47619]
Connections Individual and Family Services • Runaway and Homeless Youth Program [36217]

Connections, Speech and Language [3622]
Conners Children's Center [34335]
ConRoc Inc • DBA Rockdale House for Women [42064]
Conroe Intermediate School District--RDSPD [778]
Conroe Treatment and Recovery Center [49269]
Conroy Orthopaedic and Sports Physical Therapy [38374]
Conscious Eating TM [10945]
Consecrated Care Inc [42114]
Consejo Counseling and • Referral Services/Tacoma Branch [50208]
Consejo Counseling and Referral Services [50104]
Consejo Counseling and Referral Services Domestic Violence Program [10643]
Consejo De Salud De La Comunidad De La Playa De Ponce, Inc. [7208]
Consejo Youth and Family Services [50105]
Consolidated Care Inc [47623], [47872]
Union County Office [47804]
Consolidated Tribal Health Project Inc [39674]
Consolidated Youth Services • Runaway and Homeless Youth Program [35802]
Consortium Inc
Drug Abuse Rehabilitation Program [48502]
Methadone Maintenance Program [48503]
Consortium, Inc. [32076]
University City Counseling Center [32077]
Constance Brown Hearing Centers [2612]
Constant Care Home Health Inc. [13028]
Consultants in Neurology Multiple Sclerosis Center, Northbrook [34567]
Consultants in Sleep and Pulmonary Medicine [37152]
Consumer Friends Inc [45971]
CONTACS [8711]
CONTACT Altoona [3321], [51272]
CONTACT Beaver Valley [51274]
Contact Bucks County [51295]
Contact Burlington County [51111]
Contact Cape Atlantic [51109]
Contact Care Center [50674]
Contact Careline for Greater Philadelphia [51273]
Contact-Cares Inc. of Northwest Indiana [50897]
CONTACT Chattahoochee Valley [50800]
Contact of Chattanooga [51352]
CONTACT Community Connection [51234]
Contact Community Services [51096], [51137]
CONTACT-CONCERN of Northeast Tennessee, Inc. [51357]
CONTACT Counseling and Crisis Line [51376]
CONTACT Crawford County [51198]
CONTACT Crisis Line [51049]
Contact Crisis Line of Danville/Pittsylvania County [51418]
CONTACT Delaware, Inc. [50744]
CONTACT EARS HELPLINE [3357], [51289]
CONTACT of Fayetteville, Inc. [51169]
Contact/Help [50883]
CONTACT Helpline--Columbus [51047]
CONTACT Helpline--Durham [51164]
CONTACT Helpline Hall County [50804]
Contact Helpline--Harrisburg [51283]
CONTACT Helpline, Inc. [51366]
Contact Helpline of the Triad [51182]
Contact Hotline [51120]
Contact Huntington, Inc. [51487]
Contact Johnston County [51178]
Contact Lancaster Helpline [51286]
Contact Lubbock [51386]
Contact Martinsville/Henry County [51421]
Contact of Mercer County, NJ Inc. [51100]
Contact Ministries [51355]
Contact Mobile Helpline, Inc. [50618]
Contact Pittsburgh, Inc. [51293]
Contact of Rockford [50873]
CONTACT, Serving Steele and Waseca Counties [51043]
Contact of Southeast Connecticut [50739]
Contact Stephenson County [50846]
Contact Telephone Helpline [51241]
Contact Telephone of Knoxville [51358]
CONTACT We Care [2956]
CONTACT We Care, Inc. [51125]
CONTACT York [51303]
Continental Dialysis Center • DaVita [27452], [27571]

Continental Dialysis Center--Springfield • DaVita [27566]
Continental Dialysis Center--Woodbridge • Dialysis Facility • DaVita [27588]
Continental Healthcare, Inc. [17812]
Continu-Care [16068]
Continu-Care of Gerber Memorial Health Services [15757]
Continua Hospice-Kansas [19762]
ContinueCare Home Health, LLC [13590]
Continued Care of L.I., Inc. [16455]
Continuing Community Care
    Central Services [28720]
    South Services [28721]
Continuing Recovery Center [42711]
Continuity Care Home Health Agency [18029]
Continuous Home Care, Inc. [17497]
The Continuum [2871]
Continuum Care Hospice [20880]
Continuum Health Partners • Network Cancer Program [5595]
Continuum Home Care and Hospice [20683]
Continuum Home Care & Hospice of Craven County [20712]
Continuum Home Care & Hospice of Lenior County [20689]
Continuum Home Health Care [18258]
Continuum Pediatric Nursing--Pittsburgh [17432]
Continuum Pediatric Nursing--Schaumburg [14921]
Continuum Pediatric Nursing Services--McLean [18330]
Continuum Pediatric Nursing Services--Virginia Beach [18401]
Continuum Pediatric Nursing Services--Zelienople [17522]
Contra Costa County Health Services [35816]
Contra Costa County Mental Health [28620]
Contra Costa County Public Health Department • State SIDS Advisory Council [36452]
Contra Costa Crisis Center [50706]
Contra Costa Regional Medical Center • Cancer Program [4804]
Contra Costa Sleep Center [36664]
Conventional Wellness Home Health, Inc.--Hialeah [13732]
Conventional Wellness Home Health--Miami [13960]
Conventions Psychiatry and Counseling [42803]
Converge Home Health Care--Des Plaines [14766]
Converge Home Health Care, LLC--Schaumburg [14922]
Conversation Critters [2157]
Converse County Coalition Against Family Violence and Sexual Assault [10750]
Conway Dialysis Center • Fresenius Medical Care [26703]
Conway Home Based Primary Care Clinic [17580]
Conway Human Development Center [1001]
Conway Orthopaedic and Sports [38062]
Conway Regional Home Care Services [12840]
Conway Regional Medical Center • Cancer Program [4748]
Conway Veterans Affairs Clinic [31064]
Conyers Dialysis • DaVita [23657]
Cook Children's Home Health [17922]
Cook Children's Medical Center
    Cystic Fibrosis Center [7675]
    Department of Hematology/Oncology • Fort Worth Comprehensive Hemophilia Center [12598]
    Transplant and Dialysis Center [27084]
Cook County Bureau of Health Services • The Core Center [42489]
Cook County Children's Hospital • Stroger Hospital • Adult Hematology [12517]
Cook County Hospital • John H. Stroger Hospital • Pain Management [35428]
Cook County Program for Exceptional Students [360]
Cook County • Wilderness Outpatient Treatment Services [45161]
Cook--Fort Worth Children's Medical Center • MDA Clinic [34883]
Cook Inlet Council on Alcohol and Drug Abuse [39339]
Cook Speech and Language [1248]
Cookeville Dialysis • DaVita • Dialysis Center & At Home [26826]
Cookeville Regional Medical Center [17658]

Cancer Center [5927]
Cooley Dickinson Hospital [15529]
    Cancer Care Program [5349]
The Cooley Dickinson Hospital Rehabilitation Services [2507]
Coon Rapids Dialysis • DaVita [25013]
Cooper and Associates Physical Therapy, PC [38588]
Cooper Center for In Vitro Fertilization [22159]
Cooper Clinic [39054]
Cooper Fellowship Inc [40716]
Cooper Institute for Advanced Reproductive Medicine [22256]
Cooper Institute for Reproductive Hormonal Disorders [22229]
Cooper University Hospital
    Cancer Program [5504]
    Children's Hospital • Southern New Jersey Regional Genetics Program [12275]
    Children's Regional Center-Moorestown • Genetics Clinic [12276]
    Children's Regional Center-Voorhees • Genetics Clinic [12277]
    Sleep Disorders Center [37343]
Cooper Village [34285]
Cooperative Home Health of Atlantic City [16206]
Cooperative Home Health of Southern New Jersey • New Jersey [16283]
Coopersville Community Based Services [30533]
Coor Intermediate School District [499]
Coos County Correctional • Treatment Center [48160]
Coos County Family Health Services, Inc. [6956]
Coosa Valley Hospice [18763]
Coosa Valley Medical Center [12724], [28046]
Coosa Valley Sleep Disorders Center [36573]
COPAC • Eating Disorders Program [11112]
COPAC Inc [45363]
COPAY Inc [46669]
COPE Center Beachside Counseling [29146], [50755]
Cope Center Inc [46063]
COPE Center • TASC [41622]
COPE Community Services Inc [39494]
    Substance Abuse Services [39495]
Cope Hotline Ozaukee County [51502]
Cope Inc [47975]
COPE, Inc.--Alamogordo [9852]
COPE--Lebanon [9695]
Copia Healthcare, LLC [14358]
Copper Canyon Academy [28194]
Copper Country Mental Community Mental Health Service Program [30569]
Copper County Mental Health Services--Calumet Office [30519]
Copper River Native Association--Behavioral Health Services [50661]
Copper River Native Association • Behavioral Health Services Department [39321]
Copperfield Dialysis • DaVita [25847]
Coppinger House [33339]
COPSD Unit • Dual Diagnosis Program [49571]
COR Enterprises [8221]
Cora Services Inc • Community Services Division [48504]
Coral Gables Kidney Center • DaVita [23272]
Coral Reef Addiction Svc [45679]
Coral Spring Medical Center • Sleep Disorders Center [36781]
Coral Springs Medical Center [1561]
Coram Center for Health and Healing [38455]
Coram Healthcare Corporation of Greater New York--Plainview [16596]
Coram Healthcare Corporation of Greater New York--Rego Park [16606]
Coram Healthcare Corporation of New York--Albany [16335]
Coram Healthcare Corporation of New York--Amherst [16340]
Coram Healthcare Corporation of New York--Syracuse [16646]
Coram Specialty Infusion Services, an Apria Healthcare Company--Fairfield [16936]
Coram Specialty Infusion Services, an Apria Healthcare Company--Solon [17041]
Corbin Professional Associates [43559]
CorCell [35103]
Cord Blood America [35104]

Cord Blood Registry [34942]
Cord Blood Solutions [35010]
CORD:USE Cord Blood Bank [34983]
Corda Centro Orientacion Rehab • Orientacion y Drogadictos Alcoholicos [48770]
CordBanc USA [34943]
Cordele Dialysis • DaVita • Dialysis Center and At Home [23659]
Cordilleras Mental Health Center [33174]
Cordova Counseling Center [41889]
Cordova Family Resource Center [8658]
Core Care Technologies, Inc. [16265]
Corinthian Health Care Services Inc. [13260]
Corinthian House [41506]
Corinthians of Nevada Health Care [16151]
Corliss Institute [3391]
Cornell Abraxas Group Inc [47854]
Cornell Abraxas Interventions [42945]
Cornell Center [44977]
Cornell Surgical Co. [16186]
Cornell University
    AIDS Clinical Trials Unit [19]
    MDA/ALS Clinic [133]
Cornell University Medical College
    The Center for Reproductive Medicine and Infertility [22181]
    Midtown Center for Treatment and Research [46847]
Cornell University
    Weill Cornell Medical College • Center for Sleep Medicine [37387]
    Weill Medical College
        Eating Disorder Program [11157]
        Regional Comprehensive Hemophilia Diagnostic and Treatment Center [12561]
The Corner Clubhouse [28749]
Corner Clubhouse • Community Care Services [30324]
Corner House [46143]
Corner House Inc [43342]
Cornerhouse Dialysis Center • DaVita [22968]
Cornerstone [43924], [48898], [48929], [48950], [48962]
Cornerstone Addiction Services [47590]
Cornerstone Adult Outpatient [40717]
Cornerstone Advocacy Service [9586]
Cornerstone Behavioral Health • Branson Club [29779]
Cornerstone BHC • Chellie Morrison PhD [44027]
Cornerstone Care [7165]
Cornerstone of Care • Ozanam [45514]
Cornerstone Care Waynesburg Health Center [7190]
Cornerstone Clinical Services Inc [47945]
Cornerstone Clinical Services LLC [49609]
Cornerstone Counseling and
    Consulting Inc [47976]
    Education Services [48388]
Cornerstone Counseling Service--Oconomowoc [33003]
Cornerstone Counseling Services--Brookfield [32956]
Cornerstone Counseling Services--Glendale [32975]
Cornerstone Counseling Services--Greenfield [32977]
Cornerstone Counseling Services--Jefferson [32981]
Cornerstone Counseling Services LLC [43790]
Cornerstone Counseling Services--Milwaukee [32995]
Cornerstone Counseling Services--Mukwonago [33000]
Cornerstone Counseling Services--Waukesha [33018]
Cornerstone Counseling Services--West Bend [33025]
Cornerstone Day School [11142], [30400]
Cornerstone Dialysis • DaVita [24975]
CornerStone Hearing Centers Inc. [1376]
Cornerstone Home Healthcare, LLC [14881]
Cornerstone Hospice Inc. [12950]
Cornerstone Hospice Inc.--Phoenix [18803]
Cornerstone Hospice & Palliative Care-Tavares [19322]
Cornerstone Hospice-Sebring [19311]
Cornerstone Hospice-Winter Haven [19335]
Cornerstone • Juneau Youth Services, Inc. [28098]
Cornerstone of Medical Arts Center [46645]
Cornerstone Medical, Inc. [14479]

Cornerstone Orthopaedics and Sports Medicine [38185]
Cornerstone Physical Therapy Center [38977]
Cornerstone Psychological Services [47340]
Cornerstone Recovering Community [42490], [42491], [42492]
Cornerstone Recovery Center [43236]
Cornerstone of Recovery Inc [49122]
Cornerstone Recovery Inc [49370]
Cornerstone Recovery Systems • Cornerstone Mens Program [39902]
Cornerstone of Rhinebeck [47007]
    Alcohol and Drug Addiction Treatment [47008]
Cornerstone Services, Inc. [29633]
Cornerstone of Southern California • Recovery Homes of America Inc [40867]
Cornerstone Speech, Language and Learning Center [1841]
Cornerstone Speech and Language Practices [911]
Cornerstone Support Services [51231]
Cornhusker Place Inc [45754]
Corning Area Healthcare, Inc. • Family Medical Center [6264]
Cornwall Community Hospital • Eating Disorders Services [11215]
Corona-Elmhurst Guidance Center [31363]
Corona Regional Medical Center [12956]
    Behavioral Health [28457]
Corporacion Las Vegar, Inc. • Programa de Salud en el Hogar [17527]
Corporate Health Resource Center [42969]
    All Alcohol/Substance Abuse Progs on Site [42823]
Corp. De Servicios De Salud y Medicina Avanzada [7196]
Corp. De Servicos Medicos Hatillo [7200]
Corpus Christi Renal Center • Diversified Specialty Institutes [27005]
Corpus Christi State School [8540]
Correction Services • Clinical Treatment Program OEP WIP [45648]
Corry Dialysis • DaVita • Dialysis Center [26408]
Corsicana Regional Day School for the Deaf [779]
Cortez Addiction Recovery Services Inc [41080]
Cortez Counseling Center • Southwest Colorado Mental Health Center, Inc. [28876]
Cortland Community Reentry Program, Inc. [4307]
Cortland House [32176]
Cortland Medical Office [7021]
Cortland Memorial Hospital Services, Inc. [16435]
Cortland Veterans Affairs Clinic [31311]
Cory Place • Runaway and Homeless Youth Program [36014]
Corydon Dialysis Center • DaVita [24125]
Coshocton Counseling Center [31745]
Coshocton Dialysis • DaVita [26092]
Cosmic Home Healthcare [17839]
CoSport Physical Therapy [38375]
Costa Mesa Dialysis • DaVita [22647]
Cottage Grove Audiology and Hearing Aids Inc. [1446]
Cottage Health Care Services Inc [47453]
Cottage HomeCare Services [16679]
Cottage of Hospice [20176]
Cottage Hospital Pain Clinic [35552]
Cottage Outpatient Center • San Luis Obispo [40671]
Cottage Rehabilitation Hospital [3898]
Cottage Rehabilitation and Sports Medicine [2041]
Cotting School [8132]
Cottman Kidney Center • DaVita [26507]
Cottonwood CBOC • Division of Prescott VAMC [3863]
Cottonwood Residential Treatment Center [34264]
Cottonwood de Tucson [39496]
Coulee Youth Centers Inc [50429]
Council on Addiction Recovery Serv Inc
    Subst Abuse/Alc Supportive Living Fac [46961]
    Substance Abuse/Substance Abuse Inc [47062]
    Westons Manor [47183]
Council Against Domestic Abuse and Sexual Assault [9322]
Council Against Domestic Violence--Huntington County [9282]
Council for Alcohol/DA Services Inc [49048]
    Family Way [49049]
    Scholze Center for Adolescents [49050]
Council on Alcohol and Drug Abuse [48263]

Council on Alcohol and Substance Abuse [46628]
Council on Alcohol and Substance Abuse of Livingston County Inc [46650]
Council on Alcoholism and Drug Abuse [40729]
Council on Alcoholism and Drug Abuse of Northwest Louisiana [43896]
Council on Alcoholism/Drug Abuse of Northwest Louisiana STEPS Detox [43897]
Council on Alcoholism/Drug Abuse of
    Sullivan County Inc/Halfway House [46789]
    Sullivan County Inc/MMW [46790]
    Sullivan County Inc/MSW [46791]
    Sullivan County Inc/Recovery Center [46792], [46793]
Council on Alcoholism and Drug Abuse
    Project Recovery [40730]
    Project Recovery Detox [40731]
Council on Alcoholism • Lord Fairfax Community Inc [49869]
Council Bluffs Community Health Centers [6703]
Council Bluffs Dialysis Center • DaVita [24259]
Council of Churches of Greater Bridgeport • Runaway and Homeless Youth Program [35863]
Council on Crime and Justice [9613]
Council for the Deaf and Hard of Hearing [1940]
Council on Domestic Abuse [9310]
Council on Domestic Violence for Page County, Inc. [10577]
Council on Domestic Violence and Sexual Assault [9557]
Council on Families in Crisis/Moss House [9706]
Council on Rural Services Programs • Runaway and Homeless Youth Services [36142]
Council on Sexual Assault and Domestic Violence [9347]
Counsel House LLC [43012]
Counseling/Assessment Associates LLC [44779]
Counseling Associates [42719], [43550]
Counseling Associates of Door County [50536]
Counseling Associates • Gateway Behavioral Health [44203], [44345]
Counseling Associates Inc [39526], [39527], [45055], [46299]
    Russellville [39573]
Counseling Associates, Inc.--Clarksville [50659]
Counseling Associates, Inc. • Clarksville Clinic [28253]
Counseling Associates Inc.--Conway [50660]
Counseling Associates Inc.--Morrilton [50663]
Counseling Associates, Inc.
    Morrilton Clinic [28324]
    Park Place Clinic [28257]
    Perryville Clinic [28340]
Counseling Associates Inc.--Russellville [50664]
Counseling Associates, Inc. • Russellville Clinic [28345]
Counseling Associates/Morrilton [39559]
Counseling Associates of Port Orange Inc [41904]
Counseling Associates of South Texas [11278]
Counseling Association of Lexington [43600], [43658]
A Counseling Center [41603]
Counseling Center [43536]
The Counseling Center [43534], [43575], [43728]
Counseling Center • Adams County Outpatient [47882]
Counseling Center of Georgetown Inc [48937]
Counseling Center of Illinois [42388], [42846]
Counseling Center of Illinois Inc [42493]
Counseling Center Inc [42740], [42947], [43610], [43720], [43734], [46301]
The Counseling Center Inc [42606], [42695], [42696], [42737]
Counseling Center Inc • Outpatient Services [46225]
Counseling Center of Iredell [47423], [51179]
Counseling Center • James K Marsh House [47840]
Counseling Center of Lake Geneva [32984]
Counseling Center of Lake View [42494]
Counseling Center • Marsh House II [47796]
The Counseling Center of Milwaukee [34486]
Counseling Center • Outpatient [47841]
Counseling Center of the Rockies/North [41339]
Counseling Center of the Rockies/South [41167]
Counseling Center/Stepping Stone House • Residential Treatment Prog for Women [47842]
Counseling Center of Wayne and Holmes Counties--Millersburg [31812]
Counseling Center of Wayne and Holmes Counties--

Orrville [31822]
Counseling Center of Wayne and Holmes Counties--Wooster [31859]
Counseling Center of Wayne and Holmes • Rittman Unit [31829]
Counseling for Change Inc [43031]
Counseling Clinic Inc • Outpatient Substance Abuse Program [39522]
Counseling Clinic, Inc. [28245]
Counseling Clinic • La Crescent [45181]
Counseling and Coaching Services [10946]
Counseling and Consulting Services • A Division of CPES Inc [39497]
Counseling and Development Center Inc • Mental Health AODA Treatment Program [50503]
Counseling Group [42183]
Counseling and Hlth Subst Abuse Services [44827]
Counseling Inc [43340]
Counseling and Mediation Center [43487]
Counseling Mediation/Forensic Services • Chemical Dependence Outpatient Services [46390]
Counseling and Mental Health Center [28399]
Counseling Place LLP [41169]
Counseling Plus Inc [44354]
Counseling Professionals Incorporated [44379]
Counseling and Psychological Services [43343]
Counseling and Recovery Center Inc [41670]
Counseling and Recovery Services [49559]
Counseling and Research Associates • Masada Homes [39885]
Counseling Resource Associates [44122]
Counseling Resources [44255], [45359], [49018]
Counseling Service of Addison County [32657], [49737]
Counseling Service of Addison County--Bristol [32646]
Counseling Service of Addison County • Community Support Services [32658]
Counseling Service • Addison County Group Home [32659]
Counseling Service of Addison • Family Advocate Project [32660]
Counseling Service of EDNY [46722]
    Dual Diagnosis Recovery Program [46689]
Counseling Services of Addison County • Mental Health Services [32661]
Counseling Services of Addison • Outpatient Mental Health Services [32662]
Counseling Services and Consulting LLC [43046]
Counseling Services of Eastern Arkansas [28284]
    Marianna Clinic [28315]
Counseling Services of Eastern Arkansas/West Memphis Clinic • Crittenden County [28363]
Counseling Services of EDNY [46415], [46491]
Counseling Services Inc
    CSI at Sherry Sabo Center [43946]
    CSI at Westbrook [44083]
Counseling Services, Inc.
    CSI at Beach St. [30240]
    CSI at Kittery [30216]
    CSI at Springvale Square [30248]
    CSI at Westbrook [30250]
    Sherry Sabo Center [30197]
Counseling Services of Lake Worth [41731]
Counseling Services of Lancaster [48955]
Counseling Services of Longmont Inc [41262]
Counseling Services of Northeast Pennsylvania--Tunkhannock [51297]
Counseling Services of Northeast Pennsylvania--Wilkes Barre [51300]
Counseling Services of • Hollywood [44299]
Counseling Services • The Providence Center [32170]
Counseling Services of Southern UT LLC [49671]
Counseling Solutions [45949]
Countering Domestic Violence • Neville House [9195]
Countermeasures Inc [42418], [42855]
Counterpoint Outpatient Program [31959]
Country Doctor Community Clinic [7385]
Countryside Hospice Care--Birmingham [18681]
Countryside Hospice Care-Jacksonville [18731]
Countryside Hospice Care--La Fayette [19397]
Countryside Hospice-Roanoke [18757]
County Community Hospice of Baldwin County [18679]
County Dialysis Center [24615]
County Healthcare Inc. [17974]

County Hearing and Balance [1501]
County of Marin Community Mental Health Services • Community Client Services [28523]
County of Orange Health Care Agency Mental Health Service [28460]
County of Oswego Council on Alcoholism and Addictions [46646], [46968]
Countywide Program, Deaf and Hard of Hearing Students [533]
Courage Center [2710], [8179]
Courage Center Site • Vinland National Center [45190]
Courage to Change of • Southern Maryland Inc [44328]
Courage to Change Recovery [50356]
Courage Health Care Services, Inc. [17870]
Courage House [8748]
Courage Saint Croix [2747]
Court Educational Program [41977]
Court Supportive Services [49658]
Couseling of Lenawee PC • Adrian Outreach Office [44625]
Couture Speech [2863]
The COVE Center [32171]
Cove Forge Behavioral Health System • Division of White Deer Run Inc [48358]
Cove Forge Behavorial Health System [48699]
Cove Forge Renewal Center at Johnstown [48416]
COVE/Region Four Community Services [9554]
Covenant Adolescent Chemical • Dependency Treatment and Prevention Center [47684]
Covenant Community Inc [42027]
Covenant HealthCare RehabCare Program [4160]
Covenant Healthcare Services & Staffing, Inc. [14726]
Covenant HealthCare • Sleep Center [37153]
Covenant Home Care-Berks County [21150]
Covenant Home Care--Bloomfield Hills [15590]
Covenant Home Care-Pottsville [17457], [21148]
Covenant Home Health Care [18054]
Covenant Home Health and Hospice, Inc. [18594]
Covenant Homecare/Hospice--Knoxville [21342]
Covenant Hospice [14228]
Covenant Hospice--Crestview [19209]
Covenant Hospice--Dothan [18703]
Covenant Hospice, Inc.--Brewton [18690]
Covenant Hospice Inc.--Daphne [18699]
Covenant Hospice, Inc.--Milton [19262]
Covenant Hospice, Inc.--Mobile [18737]
Covenant Hospice, Inc.--Niceville [19271]
Covenant Hospice, Inc.--Panama City [19293]
Covenant Hospice, Inc.--Pensacola [19296]
Covenant Hospice--New Castle [19639]
Covenant Hospice and Palliative Care--Fort Worth [21459]
Covenant Hospice--Tallahassee [19319]
Covenant House • Addictions Management Project [41651]
Covenant House Alaska • Runaway and Homeless Youth Program [35786]
Covenant House California • Runaway and Homeless Youth Program [35817], [35818]
Covenant House Community Services Center • Runaway and Homeless Youth Program [36049]
Covenant House Florida • Runaway and Homeless Youth Program [35889]
Covenant House, Inc. • Covenant House Health Services [7172]
Covenant House--Mena [8774]
Covenant House Michigan • Runaway and Homeless Youth Program [36015]
Covenant House Missouri • Runaway and Homeless Youth Program [36050]
Covenant House New Jersey
  Rights of Passage Program • Runaway and Homeless Youth Program [36077]
  Runaway and Homeless Youth Program [36078]
Covenant House New York/Bronx Resource Center • Runaway and Homeless Youth Program [36097]
Covenant House New York/Brooklyn Resource Center • Runaway and Homeless Youth Program [36098]
Covenant House New York/Queens Resource Center • Runaway and Homeless Youth Program [36099]
Covenant House of New York • Runaway and Homeless Youth Program [36100]
Covenant House New York/Staten Island Resource

Center • Runaway and Homeless Youth Program [36101]
Covenant House-NineLine [51145]
Covenant House--Orlando • Runaway and Homeless Youth Program [35890]
Covenant House of Pennsylvania [51291]
Covenant House Pennsylvania • Crisis Center and Outreach • Runaway and Homeless Youth Program [36179]
Covenant House Texas • Runaway and Homeless Youth Program [36218]
Covenant House--Washington [9020]
Covenant House Washington • Runaway and Homeless Youth Program [35871]
Covenant Medical Center Horizons • Family Centered Recovery Program [43311]
Covenant Medical Center--Lubbock • Joe Arrington Cancer Center [6010]
Covenant Medical Center
  Speech-Language Pathology Services [2210]
  Sports Injury Center [38457]
Covenant Medical Center--Waterloo • Cancer Treatment Center [5195]
Covenant--Mercycare Dialysis--Independence • Wheaton Franciscan Healthcare [24277]
Covenant School [2444]
Covenant Southwest Hospice [18804]
Covenant VNA Hospice [20109]
Covenant Waverly Dialysis Center [24307]
CovenantCare at Home-Skokie [19571]
Covina Valley Unified School District [269]
Covington County Hospital [15956]
Covington Dialysis • Dialysis Facility • DaVita [27476]
Covington Renal Center • Diversified Specialty Institutes [23661]
Covington Speech and Language Center [2311]
Cow Creek • Drug and Alcohol Treatment Program [48232]
Cowley Cnty MHC and Counseling Center [43516]
Cowley County Community Corr/Day Treatment [43517]
Cowley County Safe Homes, Inc. [9383]
Cowlitz Family Health Center [7378]
Cowlitz Tribal Treatment Program • Cowlitz Indian Tribe [50004]
Cox Health • Sports Medicine [38671]
Cox Home Support--Houston, MO [16014]
Cox Home Support--Springfield [16071]
Cox Medical Center North • Audiology Department [2824]
Cox Monett Hospital [16028]
CoxHealth • Cox Sleep Disorders Center [37274]
CP Rochester [3109]
CPC Behavioral Healthcare [46148]
  Freehold Counseling Center [31129]
  High Point Center [31149]
  Men's Residence [31119]
  Women's Residence [31120]
CPMC Davies Campus • Dialysis Unit [22954]
CPO2 [18523]
CPRx, Inc. [38095]
CQI Homecare, Inc. [13029]
Craig Home Care, Inc. [18177]
Craig Hospital • Rocky Mountain Regional Spinal Injury System [3936]
Cranberry Hospice [19996]
Cranbrook Counseling and Crisis Services [51031]
Crane Clinic Sports Medicine [38651]
Cranford Group LLC [48350]
Craniofacial Diagnostic Center [35348]
CRASH
  Bill Dawson Residential Recovery Prog [40549]
  Short Term I [40550]
  Short Term II [40551]
Crater Community Hospice, Inc [21714]
Crater Community Hospice Inc. [21684]
Craven Regional Medical Center [16764]
  Cancer Program [5653]
Crawford County Drug and Alcohol • Executive Commission Inc [48460]
Crawford County Home Health Hospice and Public Health [19685]
Crawford County Kidney Center • Fresenius Medical Care [26026]
Crawford County Mental Health Center [8033]
Crawford County Services [29717]
  Southern Hills Counseling Center Inc [43028]

Crawford House Inc [46164]
Crawford Memorial Hospital [14912]
Crawfordsville Audiology [2136]
CRC/Allied Health Services • Belmont [48186]
CRC Health • DBA Allied Health Services [48187]
CRC Health Group • Capalina Clinic [40674]
CRC Health Group Inc • Wheeling Treatment Center [50346]
CRC Health Tennessee Inc • DBA New Life Lodge [49045]
CRC Inc • HOW House [40952]
CRC Renton Clinic [50080]
CRC-tell City Dialysis Center • DaVita [24239]
Crdentia Corporation--Charlotte [16711]
Crdentia Corporation--Jacksonville [13812]
Crdentia Corporation--Phoenix [12807]
Crdentia Corporation--Tampa [14412]
Crdentia Corporation--Winter Park [14461]
Create Inc [45207]
  Medically Supervised Outpatient Treatment Center [46848]
Create Inc Residential Intensive • Chemical Dependence Services [46849]
Create Inc • South [45077]
Creative Alternatives [34034]
Creative Alternatives, Inc. [28831]
Creative Care Inc [40194]
Creative Change Counseling Center • Substance Recovery [50081]
Creative Choices Counseling and • Consulting [41012]
Creative Communication Counseling [1086]
Creative Communication for Kids [1073]
Creative Counseling Services [41174], [41214], [41266]
Creative Health Services [32111]
Creative Health Services Inc • Drug and Alcohol Outpatient [48620]
Creative Health Solutions [11133]
Creative Hospice Care [19414]
Creative Interactions Inc. [2975]
Creative Living Center [28408]
Creative Recovery • Counseling and Consulting Inc [40997]
Creative Services • Ocala Rape Crisis/Domestic Violence Center [9068]
Creative Therapy Solutions Inc. [1792]
Creative Treatment Options [40983]
CREC Soundbridge [338]
Credence Therapy Associates [50384]
Credo Community Center for the Treatment of Addictions Inc [46633]
  Community Residence [47163]
  DF Residential Treatment Unit [47164]
  Mens Residence [47165]
  Outpatient Substance Abuse Clinic [47166]
Creedmoor Addiction Treatment Center • Addiction Inpatient Rehab Program [47004]
Creedmoor Psychiatric Center [31458]
Creedmoor Psychiatric Center--Astoria • Steinway Community Services [33675]
Creedmoor Psychiatric Center--Queens Village [33717]
Creek County Guidance Clinic [31876]
Creek County Health Department • Speech and Hearing Clinic [3284]
Creek Nation Behavioral Health [47935]
Creek Nation Behavioral Health and • Substance Abuse Services [48005]
Creekside Dialysis Center • DaVita [23048]
Creekside Family Physicians [38636]
Creekside Hospice [20415]
Creekview Group Home [30007]
Creighton Dialysis Center • Blanchard Valley Health System [26118]
Creighton University Sleep Disorders Lab [37312]
Crenshaw Community Health Center [6317]
Crenshaw Community Hospital • Special Services Unit [27968]
Crenshaw County Mental Health Clinic • South Central Alabama CMHC [27969]
Creoks Behavioral Mental Health Services--Okemah [31900]
Creoks Behavioral Mental Health Services--Okmulgee [31907]
Creoks Behavioral Mental Health Services--Sapulpa [31916]

Creoks Behavioral Mental Health Services--Tulsa [31921]
Crescent Care Home Health, Inc. [14688]
Crescent City Dialysis Center • DaVita [24550]
Crescent Hill Academy [8266]
Crescent Valley Medical Clinic [6947]
Cresent Home Healthcare [14727]
CressCare Medical--Carlisle [17279]
CressCare Medical--Harrisburg [17333]
CressCare Medical--Wyomissing [17513]
Crestline Home 2 • JBS Mental Health Authority [28018]
Creston Dialysis • DaVita [24260]
Crestview Hills Dialysis • DaVita [24372]
Crestwood Behavior Health, Inc.--Stockton [28822]
Crestwood Behavioral Health--Angwin [28374]
Crestwood Behavioral Health, Inc.--Bakersfield [28389]
Crestwood Behavioral Health Inc. • Crestwood Center San Jose [33190]
Crestwood Behavioral Health, Inc. • Crestwood Manor [28501]
Crestwood Behavioral Health Inc.
    Crestwood Manor Sacramento [33178]
    Crestwood Manor Vallejo [33207]
    Crestwood Treatment Center [33173]
Crestwood Behavioral Health, Inc.--Eureka [28490]
Crestwood Behavioral Health, Inc.--Fremont [28502]
Crestwood Behavioral Health Inc. • Monaco Court, Stockton [33195]
Crestwood Behavioral Health, Inc.--Sacramento [28727]
Crestwood Behavioral Health Inc. • Shoreline Drive, Stockton [33196]
Crestwood Behavioral Health, Inc.--Vallejo [28836]
Crestwood Center for Sleep Disorders [36574]
Crestwood Children's Center [34350]
    Group Home--Mills House [34351]
Crestwood Dialysis • DaVita [25268]
Crestwood Medical Center • ALS Center [95]
Crestwood Medical Center of Huntsville • Behavioral Services [39260]
CREW Inc [42976]
Crew Speech and Language Group [1904]
Cri-Help Inc [40270], [40271]
    The George T Pfleger Center [40272]
    Pfleger Outpatient [40273]
    SOCORRO/Drug Free Outpatient Program [40097]
    SOCORRO/Residential Treatment [40098]
    SOCORRO/Substance Abuse Treatment [40099]
Crider Center for Mental Health Services--O'Fallon [30883]
Crider Center for Mental Health Services--Saint Charles [30889]
Crider Center for Mental Health Services--Wentzville [30915]
Crime Victims Assistance Center, Inc. [9899]
Crime Victims Compensation Program [9021]
Crime Victims Resource Center [9583], [51037]
Crime Victims Services [10165]
Crime Victims Treatment Center • Saint Lukes-Roosevelt Hospital Center [9949]
Criminal Justice Services [49682]
Crimson Phoenix Social Club [31383]
Crisis Call Center [51078]
Crisis Care Line [10179]
Crisis Care of Winchester Medical Center [51426]
The Crisis Center [10302], [51362]
Crisis Center of Anderson and Cherokee Counties [10478]
Crisis Center--Birmingham [50610]
Crisis Center--Bristol [10557], [51415]
Crisis Center of Clinton, Essex, and Franklin Counties, Inc. [51148]
Crisis Center of Dodge City, Inc. [9353]
Crisis Center for Domestic Abuse/Sexual Assault [9769]
Crisis Center for Domestic Violence and Sexual Assault [9760]
Crisis Center of East Alabama, Inc. [50609]
Crisis Center Foundation [9235]
Crisis Center--Grand Island [9771]
Crisis Center, Inc. [50922]
Crisis Center, Inc. Alternative House • Runaway and Homeless Youth Program [35948]
Crisis Center, Inc.--Manhattan [9370]
Crisis Center of the Magic Valley [9189]

Crisis Center North [10308]
Crisis Center of Northern New Mexico [9867], [51129]
Crisis Center of the Plains [10499]
Crisis Center-Rap Line [50888]
Crisis Center of Russell County [8650]
Crisis Center for South Suburbia [9254]
Crisis Center of Southeast Texas [51373]
Crisis Center of Tampa Bay [50789]
Crisis Center and Women's Shelter [9344]
Crisis Central/OPC Area Program [51160]
Crisis Clinic of King County [51465]
Crisis Clinic of Kitsap County [51429]
Crisis Clinic of Pierce County • Comprehensive Mental Health [51472]
Crisis Clinic of Thurston and Mason Counties [51453]
Crisis Connection [9290], [51044]
Crisis Control Center [10197]
Crisis Council, Inc. [10091]
Crisis and Counseling Centers [43914]
Crisis and Counseling Centers Inc [44058]
Crisis Hotline [9176]
Crisis House [50671]
Crisis Intervention and Advocacy Center [9314]
Crisis Intervention Center [51365]
Crisis Intervention Center--Fort Smith [8761]
Crisis Intervention Center--Prince Frederick [9460]
Crisis Intervention Center of Stark County [31677]
Crisis Intervention Center of Stark County, Inc. [51201]
Crisis Intervention of Houston, Inc. [51380]
Crisis Intervention of Lehigh County [51270]
Crisis Intervention/Recovery Center Inc [47635], [47636]
Crisis Intervention Service - Mason City [9341]
Crisis Intervention Service • Santa Cruz Mental Health Service [50699]
Crisis Intervention Service--Sturgis [10387]
Crisis Intervention Services--Cody [10749]
Crisis Intervention Services--Oskaloosa [9343]
Crisis Life and Safe House [9117]
Crisis Line [51071]
Crisis Line/Bridgeway Center, Inc. [50760]
Crisis Line of Central Virginia [51420]
Crisis Line of Kittitas County [51437]
Crisis Line and Referral Service [51038]
The Crisis Line of The Planning Counsel [51422]
Crisis Line of Will County [50851]
Crisis Ministries [51319]
Crisis Residential Center [31656]
Crisis Residential Program [33811]
Crisis Response Services [50956]
Crisis Services [31450]
Crisis Services, Inc. [51136]
Crisis Services of North Alabama [8643]
Crisis Services of North Alabama, Inc. [50616]
Crisis Stabilization Outpatient Office [29105]
Crisis Stabilization Unit [33340], [50963]
Crisis Support Network [10657]
Crisis Support Services of Alameda County [50683]
Crisp Regional Hospital • Dialysis Unit [23660]
Crisp Urgent Care and Medical Center [6589]
Cristo Rey Community Center • Substance Abuse Program [44880]
Critical Care Systems--Bedford [16170]
Critical Care Systems--Birmingham [12631]
Critical Care Systems--Boise [14649]
Critical Care Systems--Braintree [15477]
Critical Care Systems--Burlington [15481]
Critical Care Systems--Columbia [17573]
Critical Care Systems--Dallas [17871]
Critical Care Systems--Dublin [16932]
Critical Care Systems--East Providence [17539]
Critical Care Systems--East Syracuse [16439]
Critical Care Systems--Elmhurst [14784]
Critical Care Systems--Fort Wayne [14982]
Critical Care Systems--Glen Burnie [15443]
Critical Care Systems--Grand Rapids [15675]
Critical Care Systems--Greensboro [16733]
Critical Care Systems--Harrisburg [17334]
Critical Care Systems--Hayward [13074]
Critical Care Systems--Indianapolis [15002]
Critical Care Systems--Las Vegas [16152]
Critical Care Systems--Lenexa [15141]
Critical Care Systems--Linwood [17380]
Critical Care Systems--Mobile [12692]
Critical Care Systems--Norcross [14564]

Critical Care Systems--Pace [14305]
Critical Care Systems--Pittsburgh [17433]
Critical Care Systems--Redding [13254]
Critical Care Systems--Reno [16163]
Critical Care Systems--Richmond [18365]
Critical Care Systems--S Gessner, Houston [17975]
Critical Care Systems--S Loopo W, Houston [17976]
Critical Care Systems--Saint Louis [16055]
Critical Care Systems--Salt Lake City [18221]
Critical Care Systems--Shrewsbury [15541]
Critical Care Systems--Somerset [16269]
Critical Care Systems--South Portland [15400]
Critical Care Systems--State College [17488]
Critical Care Systems--Tempe [12825]
Critical Care Systems--Tucson [12830]
Critical Care Systems--Tustin [13401]
Critical Care Systems--Urbandale [15108]
Critical Care Systems--Wixom [15883]
Critical care Systems--Vernon [13547]
Crittenden Health Systems [15230]
Crittenden Memorial Hospital [12883]
Crittenden Regional Hospital Home Health--Forrest City Branch [12846]
Crittenden Regional Hospital Home Health--Marked Tree [12875]
Crittenden Regional Hospital Home Health--Osceola [12878]
Crittenden Regional Hospital Home Health--West Memphis [12884]
Crittenden Regional Hospital Sleep Center [36645]
Crittenton Children's Center [30859]
Crittenton Childrens Center
    Hosptial/ Residential [45515]
    Intensive Outpatient Program [45516]
Crittenton Hospital Medical Center • Cancer Program [5394]
Crittenton Hospital • Speech Pathology and Audiology Department [2639]
CRMT, Inc. Hospice and Home Healthcare of Saunders County [20405]
Crook County Family Violence and Sexual Assault Services [10765]
Crooked River Counseling PA [44062]
Crosby Dialysis Facility • Fresenius Medical Care [27014]
Crosby Intermediate School District [780]
Cross County Clinical and Educational Services [2923]
Cross Roads Counseling Center [49184]
Cross Timbers Family Services [10510]
Cross Timbers Health Clinics, Inc. • Cross Timbers Community Health Center [7285]
Cross Timbers Hospice [20919]
Cross Trails Medical Center [6900]
Crossing Jordan Counseling Service LLC [46202]
Crossings Treatment Center Inc. [41833]
Crossmont and Associates Inc [42822]
Crosspoint Day Treatment [29604]
Crosspoint Human Services--Community Support [29605]
Crosspoint--Your Family Resource Connection • Women's Shelter [9218]
Crossroad [34126]
Crossroad Regional Hospital [33534]
Crossroads [46230]
Crossroads Apartment Program [47032]
Crossroads Behavioral Healthcare--Mount Airy [31566]
Crossroads Behavioral Healthcare--Statesville [31595]
Crossroads Behavioral Healthcare--Yadkinville [31619]
Crossroads Center [47656]
Crossroads Centers [44123], [44394]
    Frederick [44265]
Crossroads Clubhouse [30651]
Crossroads Community Hospice [20139]
Crossroads Community Hospital [14872]
Crossroads Community, Inc.--Cambridge [30271]
Crossroads Community, Inc.--Centreville [30274]
Crossroads Counseling [43201]
Crossroads Counseling Center [50417]
Crossroads Counseling and Education services [32120]
Crossroads Counseling Inc [48700]
Crossroads Counseling Services [50531]
Crossroads Counseling Services Inc [47630], [47848]

Awakenings Womens Residential Treatment
   Center [47624]
   Chase Bank Building [47622]
   Monroe County Health Clinic [47887]
   New Outlook Halfway House [47625]
Crossroads Counseling Services LLC [42781]
Crossroads Crisis Center [10156]
Crossroads of Delaware Inc [41518]
Crossroads Family Center [28478]
Crossroads Hospice [21403]
Crossroads Inc
   Amethyst House [41438]
   Intensive Outpatient Substance Abuse [41439]
   Men [41440]
   Womens Unit [41441]
Crossroads Lake County • Adolescent Counseling
   Service [47813]
Crossroads • Mayas Place [46231]
Crossroads Mental Health Services [33024]
Crossroads Mission of Yuma [39520]
CrossRoads Psychological Health Center [50680]
Crossroads Recovery [49279]
Crossroads Recovery Center • Gulf Coast Mental
   Health Center [45380]
Crossroads Recovery Services Inc [47715]
Crossroads Rescue Mission [8746]
Crossroads • Runaway and Homeless Youth
   Services [36079]
Crossroads Safehouse [8962]
Crossroads Speech and Hearing Inc. [3350]
Crossroads Treatment Center [47209]
Crossroads Treatment Center of Columbia [48918]
Crossroads Treatment Center Inc • Lakewood Facil-
   ity [50000]
Crossroads Treatment Center of Northwest Georgia
   PC [42143]
Crossroads Treatment Center of • Greensboro
   [47341]
Crossroads Turning Points Inc [40977], [41271],
   [41294], [41295], [41296], [41297], [41331],
   [41335]
Crossroads for Women [44028], [44086]
   Kennebunk Counseling Center [43989]
Crossroads Youth and Family Services • Runaway
   and Homeless Youth Program [36219]
Crossville Dialysis Clinic • Renal Advantage Inc.
   [26829]
Crosswinds Youth Services, Inc. • Runaway and
   Homeless Youth Program [35891]
Crotched Mountain Rehabilitation Center [8236],
   [10824]
Crotched Mountain School and Rehabilitation Center
   [543]
Crouse Hospital • Alcoholism Acute Care Unit
   [47114]
Crouse Hospital/Commonwealth Place • Chemical
   Dependence IP Rehabilitation [47115]
Crouse Hospital
   Methadone Maintenance Treatment Prog
      [47116]
   Outpatient Chemical Dependency Clinic [47117]
   Sleep Services Department [37388]
   Substance Abuse Clinic [47118]
Crovetti Orthopaedics and Sports Medicine [38694]
Crow Victim's Assistance Program [9744]
Crowley Behavioral Health Clinic [43823]
Crowley Mental Health Center [30136]
Crowleys Ridge Development Council • Northeast
   Ark Regional Recovery Center [39542]
Crown Home Health Services, Inc. [14856]
Crown of Texas Kidney Center • Fresenius Medical
   Care [26938]
Crowne Health Care of Montgomery [27994]
Crowne Health of Greenville [27939]
Crowne Healthcare [27928]
Crownpoint Behavioral Health Services • DBHS
   Outpatient Treatment Center [46258]
Crozer-Chester Medical Center
   Nathan Speare Regional Burn Treatment Center
      [4620]
   Regional Cancer Center [5876]
Crozer-Keystone Home Care & Hospice [17299]
CRS Rehabilitation Specialists [2118]
The Crumm Lynne Residence • Carelink Community
   Support Services [32008]
Crusaders Central Clinic Assoc. • Crusader Clinic
   [6675]
C.R.U.T.C.H., Inc. [50621]

Cruz and Sanz Health Services [14413]
Cryo-Cell International Inc. [34984]
Cryobiology, Inc. [35162]
Cryogenic Laboratories, Inc. [35082]
CryoLife Inc. [35011]
Crystal City Dialysis Center • DaVita [25193]
Crystal Clear Hearing [3110]
Crystal Clear Home Health, Inc. [13030]
Crystal Cove Hospice [18980]
Crystal Creek Lodge Treatment Center • Blackfeet
   Indian Reservation [45689]
Crystal heart Home Health Care, Inc. [13961]
Crystal Home Health Care, LLC [14958]
Crystal Home Healthcare [15632]
Crystal Hope Medical Services Inc [40100]
Crystal Lake Dialysis Center • American Renal As-
   sociates [23969]
Crystal River Dialysis Center & At Home • DaVita
   [23276]
Crystal River Dialysis Center • DaVita [23277]
Crystal Run Healthcare • Sleep Center [37389]
CSAH/UHHS-Canton, Inc. [16866]
CSG Better Hearing Center [1357]
CSG Counsel House [31991]
CSI at Springvale Square [44067]
CSULB Speech, Language and Hearing Clinic
   [1152]
Ctr for Adol Sub Use Treatment • Duke Child Dev/
   Behav Health Clinic [47285]
Ctr at Advanced Behav Care Services LLC [46030]
Ctr for Marital and Family Therapy Inc • Chemical
   Dependency Outpatient [46492]
Ctr for the Treatment of Addiction Inc [39873]
Cuero Lakeview Dialysis • DaVita [27015]
Culebra Health Center [7197]
Cullman County Treatment Center [39235]
Cullman Regional Medical Center [12640]
   Sleep Disorders Center/Neurodiagnostic Lab
      [36575]
Cullman Regional Orthopedics and Sports Medicine
   [38001]
Culpeper Regional Hospital [18280]
Cumbee Center to Assist Abused Persons [10341]
Cumberland Associates Counseling Services
   [42934]
Cumberland County • Alcoholism and Drug Abuse
   Services [45943]
Cumberland County CommuniCare [47307]
Cumberland County Guidance Center • Crisis Hot-
   line [51092]
Cumberland County Mental Health Center [29986]
   Bradford Avenue Center [31531]
   Fuller Center [31532]
Cumberland County Schools [616]
Cumberland County Women's Center [9848]
Cumberland Diagnostic and Treatment Center
   Chemical Dependence Outpatient Program
      [46493]
   Division of Addiction Psychiatry [46494]
Cumberland Dialysis Center • Dialysis Clinic Inc.
   [26819]
Cumberland Dialysis • Dialysis Facility • DaVita
   [26874]
Cumberland Hall [30033]
Cumberland Heights • Alcohol and Drug Treatment
   [49155]
Cumberland Heights Outpatient
   Services of Hermitage [49082]
   Services of Jackson [49089]
Cumberland Hospital for Children and Adults [8591]
Cumberland Medical Center [37762]
   Regional Cancer Center [4705]
Cumberland Mental Health Services Inc [49077],
   [49081]
   Alcohol and Drug Program [49118]
Cumberland Mountain Comm Services Board •
   Substance Abuse Program [49771], [49797],
   [49850]
Cumberland River Comp Care Center [43528],
   [43560], [43616], [43708], [43714], [43715],
   [43726], [43761], [43762], [43799]
   Crossroads [43561]
   Independence House [43562]
   Tri Cities Center [43533]
Cumberland River Comprehensive Care Center
   [50939]
Cumberland River Comprehensive Care Center--
   Benham [29975]

Cumberland River Comprehensive Care Center--
   London [30058]
Cumberland River Comprehensive Care Center--
   McKee [30077]
Cumberland River Comprehensive Care Center--
   Middlesboro [30078]
Cumberland River Comprehensive Care Center--
   Mount Vernon [30086]
Cumberland River Comprehensive Care Center--
   Williamsburg [30121]
Cumberland River Comprehensive Mental Health
   Board • Corbin Emergency Services [50931]
Cumberland River Homecare [17647]
Cumberland River Regional Mental Health/Mental
   Retardation Board--Barbourville [29967]
Cumberland River Regional Mental Health/Mental
   Retardation Board--Corbin [29995]
Cumberland River Regional • Mental Health/Mental
   Retardation Board--Harlan [30026]
Cumberland Treatment Center [44309]
Cumberland Valley Orthopedic Associates [38934]
Cumberland Veterans Affairs Clinic [30278]
Cumming Dialysis • DaVita [23664]
Cummins Mental Health Center Inc. [50884]
Cummins Mental Health Center, Inc. [50889]
Cummins Mental Health Center, Inc.--Avon [29696]
Cummins Mental Health Center, Inc. • Greencastle
   Clinic [29733]
Cunningham Children's Home [34123]
CURA Inc
   Adult Residential Newark [46089]
   Long Term Residential [46158]
   Outpatient and Residential Short Term [46090]
   Residential [46091]
   Youth Residential [46159]
Curative Care Network [4491]
Curative Rehabilitation Services • Sports Rehabilita-
   tion Program [39184]
Curran Seeley Foundation [50586]
Curry County Home Health/Hospice [20992],
   [21001]
Curry County Human Services [48084]
   Addiction Program [48117]
Curry Senior Center • Senior Alcohol and Drug
   Programs [40601]
Curt DuBois and Associates PT [38807]
Curtis V. Cooper Primary Health Care [6602]
Cushing Memorial Hospital [15134]
Cushing Regional Hospital, Inc. [17113]
Cushing Valley Hope [47923]
Custer County Community Health Center, Inc. [6936]
Custer Network Against Domestic Abuse [9756]
Cutchins Programs for Children and Families, Inc.
   [34206]
Cuyahoga Community College • ACCESS/DSS/
   Vocational Education • ACCESS Office [659]
Cuyahoga County Board of Mental Retardation and
   Developmental Disabilities [8406]
Cuyuna Regional Medical Center [15894]
CV Counseling Services [41741]
CVAN Women's Program [10030]
CVC Group in Speech Language Pathology [3195]
CVH Home Health Services [12934]
C.W. Williams Community Health Center [7048]
Cyfair Dialysis Center • DaVita [27131]
Cypress Basin Hospice [21535]
Cypress Creek Dialysis Center • Fresenius Medical
   Care [27378]
Cypress Creek Hospital [33870], [51381]
Cypress Creek Hospital Inc • Outpatient
   Services/CD IOP [49371]
Cypress Place [27919]
Cypress Recovery Inc • Olathe [43423]

D

D and A Detox Center [40419]
D A Wynne and Associates Inc [44355]
D and B Health Care Professionals Burbank Inc.
   [12920]
D & B Homecare [14543]
D-Best Nursing Services, Inc. [17977]
D and D and D Home Health Care [13962]
A D Psychotherapy and Clinical Counseling [49705]
D R E A M S Treatment Services Inc [47342]
D S Communication Services Inc. [2989]
D & V Home Health Care, Inc. [13655]
D. W. McMillan Memorial Hospital [12637]

DAC, Inc. [29880]
Dade City Family Health and Dental Center [6454]
Dade County Nurses, Inc. [13963]
Dade County Public Schools, ESE [352]
Dade County Sickle Cell Foundation/Miami Sickle Cell Center [36320]
Dade Dialysis Center • Fresenius Medical Care [23394]
Dade Family Counseling Inc [41842]
　Administrative Unit [41684]
　Westchester Unit [41776]
Dade Home Health Services, Inc. [13964]
Dade Kendall Home Healthcare Services [13965]
Daily Home Health, Inc. [13966]
Dakota Boys and Girls Ranch • Fargo Youth Home [34369]
Dakota Boys and Girls Ranch--Minot [34370]
Dakota Clinic • Speech Therapy [3204]
Dakota Counseling Institute [32236]
　C.A.R.E. Services & Crisis Intervention [51344]
Dakota Counseling Institute--Pathway [32237]
Dakota County Crisis Response Unit [51036]
Dakota County Receiving Center Inc • Detox [45172]
Dakota Drug and Alcohol Prevention Inc • Prairie View Prevention Services [49019]
Dakota Physical Therapy of Montville [38740]
Dakota Treatment Center [45100]
Dale County Clinic [28013]
Dale County Coalition Prevention Services [33094]
Dale E Lolar LADC MHRT [44021]
Dale Hollow Mental Health Center [32346], [49121]
Dale Medical Center Home Health [12709]
Dale Rogers Training Center [8438]
Dalhousie University • Multiple Sclerosis Research Unit [34669]
Dallas fertility Associates [22257]
Dallas Bone & Joint Clinic--Forest Lane, Dallas [39055]
Dallas Bone & Joint Clinic--Poppy Drive, Dallas [39056]
Dallas Center for Sleep Disorders [37812]
Dallas Challenge Inc [49280]
Dallas County Juvenile Department • Substance Abuse Unit [49281]
Dallas County Vet Center [52114]
Dallas East Dialysis • DaVita [27020]
Dallas Metrocare
　Lancaster-Kiest Clinic [32437]
　　Special Needs Offender Program [32438]
Dallas Metrocare Services [32439]
Dallas Metrocare • Westmoreland Clinic [32440]
Dallas North Dialysis Center & At Home • DaVita [27021]
Dallas Regional Day School for the Deaf [781]
Dallas Spinal Rehabilitation Center, Inc. [35690]
Dallas Veterans Affairs Medical Center [32441]
The Dalles Veterans Affairs Outpatient Clinic [17226]
Daly City Dialysis Center • DaVita [22655]
Damariscotta Dialysis • Fresenius Medical Care [24608]
Damascas Road [10431]
Damascus House [44124]
Dameron Hospital Home Care Services [13368]
Damon House Inc [46080]
　Damon Outpatient [46122]
Damon House New York Inc • Bushwick Community Residence [46495]
Dan Home Health Care ,Inc. [12893]
Dana--Farber/Brigham and Women's Cancer Center/ Massachusetts General Hospital • Comprehensive Cancer Center [4677]
Danbury Hospital CARES Program-2 South [19139]
Danbury Hospital Center for Speech-Language Pathology [1454]
Danbury Hospital
　Danbury Hospital Sleep Disorders Center [36737]
　Nelson A. Gelfman Dialysis Unit [23152]
　Praxair Cancer Center [4891]
Danbury Vet Center [51908]
D&E Counseling Center--Austintown [31658]
D&E Counseling Center--Youngstown [31862]
Danen Counseling Services [43068]
Daniel Freeman Memorial Hospital • Rehabilitation Centers • Pain Management Program [35311]
Daniel, Inc. [29185]
Daniel Struble LCSW LCADC [46013]

Daniels Memorial HomeHealth/Hospice [20373]
Danville Dialysis Services, LLC [23970]
Danville Pittsylvania Community Services • Mental Health Division [32725]
Danville Pulmonary Sleep Center [37886]
Danville Regional Home Health [18285]
Danville Regional Medical Center
　Behavioral Health [32726]
　Cancer Program [6057]
Danville School District Number 118 [397]
Danville Speech and Hearing Center [3580]
Danville State Hospital [33801]
Danzig Counseling Services PA [44087]
Dare Home Health and Hospice [20701]
Dare U to Care [40101]
Darin M. Camarena Health Center [6324]
Darke County Mental Health Clinic [31773]
Darke County Recovery Services [47768]
Darlene Swift Potter LADC CCS • ACME Counseling Cooperative [44075]
Darlington County Mental Health Center [32204]
Darlington County School District [729]
Darlington Dialysis Center • Fresenius Medical Care [26705]
Darlington Oaks [20275]
Darlington Regional Clinic [7423]
Dartmouth College • Dartmouth-Hitchcock Medical Center - Department of Orthopaedic Surgery • Multidisciplinary Clinical Research Center [170]
Dartmouth-Hitchcock Hemophilia Center [12554]
Dartmouth-Hitchcock Manchester • Genetics Clinic [12272]
Dartmouth Hitchcock Medical Center [20440]
　Adult Cystic Fibrosis Center [7598]
　Dartmouth Center for Genetics and Child Development [10825]
Dartmouth-Hitchcock Medical Center • In Vitro Fertilization Program [22155]
Dartmouth--Hitchcock Medical Center
　Medical Genetics Clinic [12273]
　Pain Management [35553]
Dartmouth-Hitchcock Medical Center • Sleep Disorders Center [37329]
Dartmouth Hitchcock Medical Center--Transplant [25392]
Dartmouth Hitchcock Memorial Hospital • Pediatric Cystic Fibrosis Center [7599]
Dartmouth Hitchcock Psychiatric Assoc • Intensive Outpatient [45899]
Dartmouth Medical Equipment, Inc. [15522]
DAS Drug Diversion Program [39666]
DASCO Home Medical Equipment [17070]
Daughters of Charity Health Center, Causeway [6752]
Daughter's of Devine Love Home Healthcare [14728]
Daughters of Jacob • Dialysis Center [25585]
Dauphin County Crisis Intervention [51284]
Dauphin Way Lodge [39274]
Davenport Dialysis Center • DaVita [23278]
David E. Condon, DPM--Incline Village [38697]
David E. Condon, DPM--Truckee [38152]
David Fox Counseling Solutions [46056]
David Harmon and Associates [43684], [43685]
David and Ivory Ministries • Lieutenants House [49372]
David Lawrence Center [7899], [41696]
　Adult Community Services [33327]
　Children's Community Services [33328]
　Court Related and Substance Abuse Outpatient Services [41811]
David Lawrence Center and Foundation [33329]
David Lawrence Center
　Immokalee Satellite Center [33307]
　Naples [33330]
　Outpatient/Residential and Detox [41812]
David Lawrence LADC CCS [44076]
David and Margaret Home, Inc. [33989]
David and Margaret Home Inc. • La Casa [33186]
David N Barry [43990]
David Physical Therapy & Sports Medicine Center [38970]
David Raines Community Health Center [6763]
David W Earle LPC • Earle Company [43811]
Davidson County Schools [623]
Davidson School [699]
Davie County Emergency Health Corporation [16753]

Davie Domestic Violence Services and Rape Crisis Center [10061]
Daviess Community Hospital Home Health [15061]
Daviess County Dialysis • DaVita [24246]
Davila Day School [268]
Davis Behavioral Health
　Bountiful Clinic [33891]
　Clearfield [33892]
　Farmington [33893]
Davis Behavioral Health Inc
　Children and Youth [49619]
　Intensive Outpatient [49620]
　Mens Recovery Center [49621]
　Substance Abuse Outpatient [49622]
　Womens Recovery Center [49623]
Davis Behavioral Health
　Layton Clinic [33894]
　Layton Comprehensive Treatment Program [32587]
Davis Center [29841]
Davis Center for Rehabilitation • Baptist Hospital [3966]
Davis Community Clinic [6300]
Davis County Mental Health Center • Bountiful Mental Health Clinic [32575]
Davis Medical Center • University of California • Department of Physical Medicine & Rehabilitation [38120]
Davis Mental Health/A and D Services • Davis Behavioral Health [32585]
Davis Speech and Language [3627]
Davison Dialysis • DaVita [24859]
DaVita--42nd Street • Dialysis Services [26508]
DaVita • Aberdeen Dialysis [24620]
DaVita--Alameda County • Dialysis Center [22845]
DaVita--Alexandria • Dialysis Facility [27453]
DaVita • Almond Wood Dialysis Clinic [22799]
DaVita--Altus • Dialysis Center [26246]
DaVita--Amelia • Dialysis Facility & At Home [27457]
DaVita--Amery [27695]
DaVita--Anadarko [26247]
DaVita
　Antelope Valley Dialysis [22748]
　Antioch Dialysis Center [22587]
DaVita--Arden Hills Dialysis [25001]
DaVita--Arlington • Dialysis Facility [27460]
DaVita
　Arrowhead Lakes Dialysis Center [22439]
　Ash Tree Dialysis, PD & At Home [22695]
　Asheville Kidney Center & At Home [25817]
　Atmore Dialysis Center [22308]
DaVita--Atwater • Dialysis Center [22590]
DaVita--Auburn • Dialysis Facility [22591]
DaVita • Aurora Medical Group--Lake Geneva [27731]
DaVita--Ballenger Pointe Dialysis & At Home [24895]
DaVita--Batesville Dialysis [24115]
DaVita Battle Creek Dialysis [24835]
DaVita--Bedford • HEB Dialysis Center [26969]
DaVita--Bel Air • Dialysis Facility [24656]
DaVita--Bentonville [22530]
DaVita • Berlin • Dialysis Facility [24659]
DaVita--Bessemer [22311]
DaVita--Birmingham • Home Training Dialysis [22313]
DaVita--Birmingham North • Dialysis Facility [22314]
DaVita--Bloomington Dialysis [25004]
DaVita--Bluemound [27803]
DaVita--Boaz • Dialysis Facility [22318]
DaVita--Bogalusa Kidney Care [24470]
DaVita • Boston Post Road Dialysis Center [25586]
DaVita--Brenham • Dialysis Center [26977]
DaVita--Brentwood • Dialysis Facility [23214]
DaVita Brighton Dialysis [23096]
DaVita--Brighton Dialysis [24842]
DaVita--Buena Vista • Dialysis Facility [23630]
DaVita--Burbank • Dialysis Center [22615]
DaVita--Burnsville Dialysis [25008]
DaVita • Butler County Home Training Dialysis [26123]
DaVita--Cadieux [24866]
DaVita
　Canyon Springs Dialysis [22829]
　Capitol Centre Dialysis [26698]
DaVita--Capitol Drive • Dialysis Facility & At Home [27704]
DaVita

Carabello Dialysis Center [22772]
Carroll County Dialysis Facility [24736]
DaVita--Catonsville [24631]
DaVita--Cedar Lane • Dialysis Facility [24670]
DaVita--Cedarburg • Dialysis Facility [27706]
DaVita • Center Point Dialysis [22321]
DaVita--Central City Dialysis Center [27062]
DaVita • Central Mesa Dialysis Center [22453]
DaVita--Central Tampa [23531]
DaVita--Central Tulsa • Dialysis Facility [26299]
DaVita--Ceres [22625]
DaVita--Charlottesville • Dialysis Facility [27468]
DaVita--Chelsea [24849]
DaVita--Chesterton [24225]
DaVita--Chestertown • Dialysis Facility [24666]
DaVita--Chinle [22431]
DaVita--Chino • Dialysis Facility [22631]
DaVita • Citrus Valley Dialysis & At Home [22927]
DaVita--Claremore • Dialysis Facility [26252]
DaVita--Clinton • Dialysis Facility [26253]
DaVita--Conroe • Dialysis Center [27003]
DaVita • Continental Dialysis Center--Manassas [27509]
DaVita--Corona Dialysis Center [22646]
DaVita--Cottage Grove [25016]
DaVita--Covina Dialysis Center [23068]
DaVita--Crescent Heights Dialysis Center [22773]
DaVita - Crossroads Dialysis Center [22701]
DaVita--Crystal City • Dialysis Facility [25194]
DaVita--Culpeper • Dialysis Facility [27477]
DaVita • Cypress Woods Northwest Dialysis [27132]
DaVita--Dearborn [24861]
DaVita • Delano Dialysis [22657]
DaVita--Delran • Dialysis Facility [25420]
DaVita--Demopolis • Dialysis Facility [22328]
DaVita--Denham Springs [24486]
DaVita--Desert Mountain Dialysis [22494]
DaVita--Detroit Dialysis [24867]
DaVita of Detroit--Kresge • Dialysis Facility [24868]
DaVita--Dialysis Care of Rutherford County Inc. [25867]
DaVita--Dialysis Center of Camarillo [22619]
DaVita Dialysis of Chadbourn [25828]
DaVita Dialysis of Middle Georgia [23741]
DaVita--Diamond Valley Dialysis Center [22724]
DaVita • Doctors Dialysis of East Los Angeles [22664]
DaVita--Downey Dialysis Center [22660]
DaVita • Downey Landing Dialysis Center [22661]
DaVita/Downriver Kidney Center [24826]
DaVita--Dublin [26103]
DaVita--Duncan • Dialysis Facility [26254]
DaVita--Dundalk [24677]
DaVita • East Bay Peritoneal Dialysis [22980]
DaVita--East Chicago • Dialysis Facility [24133]
DaVita--East Dialysis [27063]
DaVita--East End • Dialysis Center [27546]
DaVita--East Los Angeles Plaza • Dialysis Facility [22774]
DaVita--East Orange • Dialysis Facility [25422]
DaVita • East Wichita Dialysis Center [24351]
DaVita--Easton • Dialysis Unit [24680]
DaVita--Eaton Canyon Dialysis [22876]
DaVita--Ebensburg [26424]
DaVita--Edison [25426]
DaVita--Eighth Street • Dialysis Facility [23215]
DaVita Ellijay Dialysis [23695]
DaVita--Escondido Home Training [22680]
DaVita--Estrella [22467]
DaVita--Eufaula [22334]
DaVita--Exeter • DaVita [22683]
DaVita • Fallon Dialysis [25352]
DaVita--Falls Road • Dialysis Facility [24705]
DaVita--Fayette/Tuscaloosa • Dialysis Center [22338]
DaVita - Fayetteville [22537]
DaVita • Flamingo Park Kidney Center • Dialysis Facility [23319]
DaVita--Florence Dialysis [22339]
DaVita • Forest Park Dialysis Center [23701]
DaVita--Fort Valley [23704]
DaVita • Fort Walton Beach Dialysis Center & At Home [33308]
DaVita--Fox River Dialysis & At Home [27720]
DaVita--Franklin Dialysis & At Home [24148]
DaVita • Frederick Dialysis & At Home [24685]
DaVita--Freehold • Dialysis Facility [25464]
DaVita • Fresno At Home and PD Center [22696]

DaVita--Gadsden • Dialysis Center [22344]
DaVita--Garden West • Dialysis Center [24992]
DaVita--Garfield Hemodialysis Center [22826]
DaVita--Gary • Comprehensive Renal Care [24150]
DaVita--George Washington Southeast • Dialysis Unit [23216]
DaVita--Gilbert [22436]
DaVita--Glen Burnie Dialysis • Dialysis Center [24690]
DaVita--Gonzales • Dialysis Facility [27108]
DaVita--Grand Rapids Dialysis & PDI [24907]
DaVita--Grand Rapids East PDI [24908]
DaVita--Greater El Monte Dialysis Center [23017]
DaVita--Greater Portsmouth • Dialysis Unit [27537]
DaVita--Greenbrier [27678]
DaVita--Greene County Dialysis [22335]
DaVita--Greenview [24976]
DaVita--Greenwood • Dialysis Center [26725]
DaVita Grovepark Dialysis Center [23723]
DaVita--Gulf Shores [22348]
DaVita--Hackettstown [25439]
DaVita--Hammond [24161]
DaVita--Harbor Park Dialysis • Dialysis Facility [24632]
DaVita--Harrisonburg • Dialysis Facility [27502]
DaVita--Hazelwood [25212]
DaVita--Hendersonville Dialysis Center [25883]
DaVita--Henrico County • Dialysis & At Home [27547]
DaVita--Highland Park PDI [24916]
DaVita--Hopewell • Dialysis Center [27503]
DaVita--Hopi Dialysis Center [22487]
DaVita • Houston Kidney Center--Southwest [27133]
DaVita • Howard County • Dialysis Facility [24671]
DaVita • Hudson Valley Dialysis Center [25790]
DaVita--Humboldt Ridge [27745]
DaVita--Imperial Care Dialysis Center [22797]
DaVita Inc./Griffin Dialysis Center [23712]
DaVita Inc.--Milledgeville [23757]
DaVita • Indy South Dialysis and At Home [24159]
DaVita--J. B. Zachary Dialysis & At Home [24633]
DaVita--Jacksonville • Dialysis Centers of Arkansas [22547]
DaVita • Jacksonville Dialysis • Dialysis Facility [24010]
DaVita--Janesville [27725]
DaVita--Johnstown Dialysis & At Home [26453]
DaVita--Jonesboro Dialysis Center [23725]
DaVita • Joy of Dixon Dialysis Center [22658]
DaVita--K Street Dialysis [23217]
DaVita--Kayenta [22446]
DaVita--Kenneth Hahn Plaza Dialysis Center [22775]
DaVita
    Kidney Center--Syosset [25784]
    Kidney Dialysis Care Unit [22798]
Davita--Lake Charles Southwest Dialysis • Dialysis Center [24523]
DaVita--Lake Elsinore Dialysis Center [22745]
DaVita • Lake Worth Dialysis and At Home [23464]
DaVita--Lakeside • Dialysis Center [24667]
DaVita • Lakewood Dialysis Center [22747]
DaVita Lakewood Dialysis Center • DaVita [23127]
DaVita--Landover [24701]
DaVita--Lawrenceburg Dialysis LLC [24193]
DaVita--Lee Street • Dialysis Facility [23218]
DaVita • Life Care Dialysis Center [25719]
DaVita - Little Rock Dialysis [22553]
DaVita--Livingston • Dialysis Center [27230]
DaVita--Long Beach [22760]
DaVita--Los Angeles Dialysis Center [22776]
DaVita--Los Angeles Downtown • Dialysis Facility [22777]
DaVita--Louisville Dialysis [24409]
DaVita--Ludington • Dialysis Facility [24939]
DaVita--Madison • Dialysis Facility [24197]
DaVita--Magnolia • Dialysis Facility [24497]
DaVita--Main Place Dialysis Center [22858]
DaVita--Mar Vista [23003]
DaVita--Market Street [26509]
DaVita--Marshall Dialysis [25040]
DaVita--Marshall • Dialysis Facility [27248]
DaVita--Martinsville • Dialysis Facility [27511]
DaVita--Maryland • Dialysis Center [24634]
DaVita • Maryvale Dialysis Center [22468]
DaVita--Mechanicsville [27513]
DaVita--Mercy • Dialysis Facility [24635]
DaVita - Merrillville Dialysis & PD [24201]

DaVita--Metairie [24534]
DaVita--Midwest City • Dialysis Center [26267]
DaVita--Millington [26895]
DaVita--Minneapolis Northeast Dialysis [25042]
DaVita--Montclair Dialysis Center [22820]
DaVita--Monterey Park Dialysis Center [22827]
DaVita • Mountain Vista Dialysis Center [22454]
DaVita--Murrieta • Dialysis Center [22833]
DaVita--Muskegon • Dialysis Facility & At Home [24950]
DaVita • Muskogee Community • Dialysis Center [26269]
DaVita--Neptune • Dialysis Facility [25475]
DaVita--New Hope [25057]
DaVita • New Port Richey Kidney Center & At Home [23426]
DaVita--Newaygo County [24902]
DaVita Newnan Dialysis [23766]
DaVita--Newport News • Dialysis Facility [27518]
DaVita--Nogales • Dialysis Center [22461]
DaVita--Norman • Dialysis Facility [26271]
DaVita • North Highlands Dialysis Center [22840]
DaVita--North Little Rock [22566]
DaVita
    North Shore Massachusetts Acutes [24814]
    Northeast Philadelphia Dialysis Center [26510]
DaVita--Northport • Dialysis Center [22381]
DaVita--Northwest Bethany • Dialysis Facility & At Home [26250]
DaVita • Northwest Medical Center Dialysis [27318]
DaVita--Northwest Tucson [22513]
DaVita--Norwalk Dialysis Center [22843]
DaVita • Ocean Springs Dialysis & At Home [25151]
DaVita--Okmulgee • Dialysis Facility [26286]
DaVita • Ontario Dialysis [22855]
DaVita • Opelika [22383]
DaVita • Orange City Dialysis • Dialysis Facility [23441]
DaVita--Owings Mills • Dialysis Facility [24708]
DaVita--Ozark • Dialysis Center [22386]
DaVita--Paintsville Dialysis [24387]
DaVita--Palm Brook Dialysis Center [22501]
DaVita--Papago Dialysis Center [22469]
DaVita--Papillion [25344]
DaVita--Paramount Dialysis Center [22875]
DaVita--Pasadena [24711]
DaVita--PDI Grand Haven [24906]
DaVita--PDI Walnut Towers [26511]
DaVita • PDI--Worcester Dialysis & At Home [24819]
DaVita--PDL Annex--PD [26459]
DaVita--Pearsall • Dialysis Center [27287]
DaVita
    Peoria At Home [24064]
    Physicians Choice Dialysis--Elmore County [22415]
DaVita Pittsfield II [24068]
DaVita--Point Place [26209]
DaVita--Premier Dialysis Center [22651]
DaVita--Pryor • Dialysis Center [26290]
DaVita • Queens Dialysis & At Home [25663]
DaVita--Rainbow City [22395]
DaVita • Raven Dialysis Center [22470]
DaVita--Redford • Dialysis Facility [24869]
DaVita--Renaissance [22340]
DaVita • Renal Treatment Centers--Winfield • Dialysis Facility [24359]
DaVita--Richfield [25069]
DaVita • Rim Country [22463]
DaVita--River Center Drive • Dialysis Center [27746]
DaVita--Riverside Dialysis Center [22903]
DaVita--Rock Prairie Road [26999]
DaVita--Rockville • Dialysis Facility [24719]
DaVita--Rolla • Dialysis Center [25260]
DaVita--Romulus [24962]
DaVita--Rosemead Springs Dialysis • DaVita [22673]
DaVita--Russellville • Dialysis Facility [22397]
DaVita
    Salem Dialysis Center [24230]
    San Antonio At Home [27319]
DaVita--San Diego South • Dialysis Center [22934]
DaVita--Santa Ana Dialysis Center [22991]
DaVita • Santa Rosa Dialysis Center [23414]
DaVita--Schaefer Drive • Dialysis Facility [24870]
DaVita--Scottsdale Dialysis Center [22495]
DaVita--Sells [22498]
DaVita--Shawnee • Dialysis Facility [26293]
DaVita--Sheffield • Dialysis Center [22403]

DaVita--Sherman • Dialysis Facility [27360]
DaVita
  Shrewsbury Dialysis [25269]
  Siena Henderson Dialysis Center [25355]
DaVita--Siloam Springs [22573]
DaVita--Silver Spring • Dialysis Facility [24728]
DaVita--Sioux Falls Dialysis [26798]
DaVita--Slidell Kidney Care • Dialysis Center & At Home [24589]
DaVita--Smyrna [26923]
DaVita
  Snake River Dialysis Center and PD [23866]
  Snapfinger Center [23670]
DaVita--Snellville [23789]
DaVita • South Baldwin Dialysis Center [22341]
DaVita--South Orangeburg • Dialysis Facility [26755]
DaVita--South Ridge • Commonwealth Dialysis Center [27723]
DaVita
  South Sacramento Dialysis Center [22915]
  South Williamson Dialysis [24446]
DaVita--South Yuma • Dialysis Center [22525]
DaVita--Southcrest [26300]
DaVita--Southeast--Northshore Kidney Center [24590]
DaVita--Southern Crescent Dialysis Center [23774]
DaVita--Southern Maryland • Dialysis Facility [24668]
DaVita--Southgate • Dialysis Center [24979]
DaVita--Southwest San Antonio • Dialysis Facility & At Home [27320]
DaVita - Springdale [22575]
DaVita--Staunton [27570]
DaVita--Stillwater • Dialysis Facility [26295]
DaVita • Stonegate PD Dialysis & At Home [26849]
DaVita--Sunrise Dialysis Center [22720]
DaVita--Surprise [22507]
DaVita--Sylacauga • Dialysis Facility [22404]
DaVita--Tahlequah • Dialysis Facility [26298]
DaVita--Talladega [22406]
DaVita--Temecula Dialysis Center [23030]
DaVita--Tempe [22509]
DaVita - Thornton [23141]
DaVita--Titletown • Dialysis Center [27721]
DaVita--TRC/Harbor, University of California, Los Angeles • Dialysis Facility & At Home [23035]
DaVita--TRC--USC Kidney Center [22778]
DaVita--Tuba City Dialysis Unit [22512]
DaVita • Tucson Central Dialysis [22514]
DaVita--Tucson South • Dialysis Center [22515]
DaVita--Tulsa • Dialysis Facility & At Home [26301]
DaVita • Turlock Dialysis Center [23042]
DaVita--Tuscaloosa • Dialysis Facility [22411]
DaVita--Tustin Dialysis Center [22992]
DaVita--Tysons Corner • Dialysis Facility & At Home [27577]
DaVita • University Dialysis Unit and At Home Riverside [25080]
DaVita--Uptown Dialysis [25043]
DaVita/Utah Valley Regional Dialysis Center [27414]
DaVita--Valley Dialysis Center [23054]
DaVita--Valley View Dialysis [22830]
DaVita--ValParaiso • Dialysis Facility [24243]
DaVita--Victoria • Dialysis Facility & At Home [27386]
DaVita--Virginia Beach • Dialysis Facility [27578]
DaVita--Warren • Dialysis Facility [26597]
DaVita--Washington Plaza Dialysis Center [22779]
DaVita--Waycross [23833]
DaVita--Wayne County [23993]
DaVita--West Appleton [27747]
DaVita--West Bountiful Dialysis & At Home [27435]
DaVita • West Des Moines Dialysis [24310]
DaVita--West Texas • Dialysis Center [27064]
DaVita • Westbrook Dialysis [22504]
DaVita--Westwood Hills [25076]
DaVita--Weymouth Dialysis & At Home [24815]
DaVita--White Square [24636]
DaVita - Whittier Dialysis Center [23075]
DaVita--Willingboro [25529]
DaVita • Wiregrass Kidney Center [22329]
DaVita--Wisconsin Avenue • Dialysis Center [27748]
DaVita--Wishard [24172]
DaVita--Woodburn • Dialysis Center [26362]
DaVita--Woodland Dialysis Center [24376]
DaVita Woodstock Dialysis [23837]
DaVita--Wyncote [26614]
Dawn Center of Hernando County [9080]

Dawn Farm [51005]
Dawn Inc
  Dawn Farm [45069]
  Dawn Farm Detox [44639]
  Dawn Farm Huron Street [44640]
  Outpatient Services [44641]
Dawson County Mental Health Center [32493]
Dawson Springs Health and Rehabilitation Center [2263]
Day By Day Hospice [19592]
Day By Day Treatment Center of • Johnston County Inc [47493]
Day by Day Recovery Center [45160]
Day Kimball Hospital [13540]
  Sleep Disorder Center [36738]
Day One [30245]
  Outpatient Office [44063]
Day Rehabilitation Center [4328]
Day Street Community Health Center [6426]
Daybreak [8644]
Daybreak Adult Day Center [28073]
Daybreak • Runaway and Homeless Youth Program [36143]
Daybreak/Vancouver [50238]
Daybreak Youth Services
  Intensive Inpatient Program for Youth [50166]
  Outpatient Treatment [50167]
  Valley Outpatient [50190]
DAYMARK Recovery Services • Anson County Center [47508]
Daymark Recovery Services
  Davidson Center [47407]
  Harnett [47231]
  Moore Unit [47444]
  Outpatient Treatment [47276]
  Richmond County [47474]
  Rowan Center [47486]
  Stanly Center [47204]
  Substance Abuse Services [47536]
  Union Center [47418]
Daymark • Runaway and Homeless Youth Program [36262]
DayMont Behavioral Healthcare Inc
  Focus Care [47736]
  Sojourner Program [47737]
  Substance Abuse Services [47738]
DayOne • Fletcher Allen Healthcare [49730]
Dayowl Counseling [44051]
Dayspring Hospice, LLC [18706]
DaySpring Villa [10210]
Dayspring Village [44125]
Daystar Center for Spiritual Recovery [48389]
Daystar Home Health Care, Inc. [13967]
Daystar, Inc. [10722]
Dayton Children's Medical Center • West Central Ohio Hemophilia Treatment Center [12575]
Dayton Mobile Vet Center [52059]
Dayton Regional Dialysis--North [26136]
Dayton Regional Dialysis--South [26034]
Dayton Sports Medicine Institute [38872]
Dayton VA Medical Center [47739]
Dayton Veterans Affairs Hospice and Palliative Care [20831]
Dayton Veterans Affairs Medical Center [31748]
Daytona Beach Dialysis • American Renal Associates [23282]
Daytona Methadone Treatment Center [41612]
Daytona South Dialysis • DaVita [23283]
Daytona South Dialysis--South Daytona • DaVita [23517]
Daytop Village Inc
  Brightside Manor House Resid Facility [47009]
  Bronx Outreach Center [46416]
  Drug Rehab Re-Entry Program [46850]
  Far Rockaway Entry and Re-Entry Unit [46635]
  Fox Run Adult Facility [47010]
  Hartsdale Outreach [46681]
  Huntington Station/Med Super Outpatient [46708]
  Manhattan Criminal Justice Services [46851]
  Manhattan Outreach AOS [46852]
  Outpatient Criminal Justice Services [46853]
  Parksville Adult Residential Facility [46972]
  Rockland Outreach [46388]
  Staten Island Outreach [47095]
  Substance Abuse Residential/Meadow Run [47011]

  Substance Abuse Womens Residential Meadow Run [47012]
  Suffolk Outreach [46709]
  Swan Lake Adult Residential Facility [47110]
DC Children's Advocacy Center [9022]
DC Coalition Against Domestic Violence Victim Advocacy Program [9023]
DC Department of Mental Health [29087]
DC Rape Crisis Center [9024]
DCA of Central Valdosta • Dialysis Corporation of America [23817]
DCA of Eastgate • Dialysis Corporation of America [26040]
DCA of South Georgia • Dialysis Corporation of America [23818]
DCCCA Inc
  First Step at Lakeview [43386]
  Lawrence [43387]
  Options Adult Services [43488]
DCCCA Inc Womens Recovery Center [43394]
DCCCA Inc
  Womens Recovery Center of Central Kansas [43489]
  Youth and Family Service [43446]
DCH Home Health Services [12730]
DCH Laboratory • Medical Tower • Sleep Disorders Center [36576]
DCH Regional Medical Center [926]
  Cancer Program [4739]
  DCH Sleep Laboratory [36577]
  Paincare Unit [35271]
DCH Sportsmedicine [38013]
DCI Donor Services [35206]
DCI--Grand Junction [23121]
DCI Madison Dialysis Clinic [22916]
DCI Rancho Dialysis Clinic [22917]
DCI Redding [22894]
DCI/University Dialysis Clinic [22918]
De Colores Shelter [8712]
de l'Epee Deaf Center Inc. [2759]
De Paul Center [34189]
De Paul School for Hearing and Speech [708]
De Paul Treatment Centers Inc [48129]
De Ruyter Medical Office [7022]
Deaconess Cross Pointe [43032]
Deaconess Cross Pointe Center [33454]
Deaconess CrossPointe Outpatient Serv • Deaconess Hospital [43033]
Deaconess Hospice-Hattiesburg [20243]
Deaconess Hospital [14977]
Deaconess Hospital, Inc. • Deaconess Sleep Center [36946]
Deaconess Hospital, Inc.-Evansville • Cancer Center [5144]
Deaconess Hospital--Oklahoma City • Cancer Program [5776]
Deaconess Hospital • Outreach Clinic • Cystic Fibrosis Center [7538]
Deaconess Medical Center
  Cancer Center [6120]
  Cystic Fibrosis Center [7692]
Deaconess Riley Children's Services • Down Syndrome Clinic [10798]
Deaconess Saint Joseph's Hospital [2153]
Deaf ACCESS • Rehabilitation Services [1023]
Deaf Action Center [3480]
Deaf Action Center of Greater New Orleans [2332]
Deaf Addiction Services at Maryland • Outpatient [44126]
Deaf Children's Society of British Columbia [251]
  Preschool [1046]
Deaf Community Advocacy Network [2653]
Deaf Community Services of San Diego Inc. [1257]
Deaf Connect of the Midsouth • Interpreting Services for the Deaf Inc. [3438]
Deaf CONTACT [3344]
Deaf Counseling, Advocacy and Referral Agency [1296]
Deaf and Hard of Hearing Center [3476]
Deaf and Hard of Hearing Community Counseling Services [3602]
Deaf and Hard of Hearing Outpatient Mental Health Program [1652]
Deaf/Hard of Hearing Program [489]
Deaf and Hard of Hearing Service Center Inc. [1115]
Deaf and Hard of Hearing Services [2702], [2719]
Deaf/Hard of Hearing Services [511]
Deaf and Hard of Hearing Services Division [2729]

Deaf and Hard of Hearing Services of Lancaster County [3345]
Deaf and Hard of Hearing Services--Metro [2740]
Deaf and Hard of Hearing Services--Northeast [2749]
DEAF Inc. [2439]
    Independent Living Services [2527]
Deaf Iowans Against Abuse [9317]
Deaf-REACH [1523]
Deaf Services Inc. [2171]
DeafHope [8857]
Deale One Step Recovery Services [44220]
Dean I. Clerc National Deaf Education Center [342]
Dean Sports Medical Clinic [39180]
Dearborn County Hospital • Home Health & Hospice [19625]
Dearborn Home Dialysis and At Home • DaVita [24862]
Dearborn Plaza [29766]
Dearborn Sleep Laboratory [37154]
Debaca Family Practice Clinic [46270]
Deborah Health and Lung Center • Institute for Sleep Medicine • Sleep Lab [37344]
Deborah Spicer LCSW CADC [43571]
Debra Bourgeois and Associates [1817]
Debra L Gainor MA LLP CAADC [45015]
Decatur Back and Neck Center [38371]
Decatur County Dialysis [23622]
Decatur County General Hospital [17769]
Decatur County Memorial Hospital • Cancer Program [5152]
Decatur County Mental Health Center [29363], [42049]
Decatur County Program for Exceptional Children [363]
Decatur Dialysis Center • DaVita [23671]
Decatur East Wood Dialysis & At Home • DaVita [23971]
Decatur General Hospital
    Behavioral Health Services [33080]
    Cancer Program [4730]
Decatur General Sleep Disorders Center [36578]
Decatur Medical Office [6592]
Decatur Memorial Hospice [19511]
Decatur Memorial Hospital • Cancer Care Institute [5085]
Decatur Memorial Hospital Home Health Services [14762]
Decatur/Seminole Adult Day Support [29364]
Decatur Veterans Affairs Outpatient Clinic [29607]
Decibel Hearing Services [1321], [1335]
Decision Point Center Inc [39456]
Decision Point Inc [39576]
Dedicated Caregivers, LLC [14343]
Dedicated Home Health Agency [13240]
Deer Lodge Centre • Department of Communication Disorders [2366]
Deer River HealthCare Center [2687]
Deerbrook Dialysis • DaVita [27189]
Deerfield Centers for Addictions Treatment [48654]
    Deerfield Behavioral Health Inc [48655]
    Deerfield Behavioral Health of Warren [48668]
    Drug and Alcohol Program/Marlenville [48456]
Deerfield Dialysis Center • Fresenius Medical Care [23974]
Deerfield Dual Diagnosis [48359]
Deers Head Center • Dialysis Center [24723]
DeFeliceCare, Inc. [18543], [18549]
Defiance Dialysis Center • Innovative Dialysis Centers [26099]
Defuniak Springs Dialysis • DaVita [23287]
Deilee Hit/Safe Harbor House [39352]
DeKalb Addiction Clinic [42078]
DeKalb Community Service [29406]
DeKalb Community Service Board--Choice Program [29460]
DeKalb Community Service Board • DeKalb Regional Crisis Center [42079]
DeKalb Community Services Board [29407]
DeKalb County Health Department [7272]
DeKalb County Hospice [19510]
DeKalb County Schools [207]
DeKalb Medical Center [1854]
DeKalb regional Medical Center [27929]
Dekalb Medical Center • Charles B. Eberhart Cancer Center [5022]
DeKalb Medical Center
    Outpatient Rehabilitation [1855]

Sleep Disorder Center [36836]
Del Amo Behavioral Health • Eating Disorders Program [10947]
Del Amo Hospital [33198]
Deland Dialysis • DaVita [23288]
DeLand Medical Center [6457]
Delaware Back Pain and Sports Rehabilitation Centers--Newark [38205]
Delaware Back Pain and Sports Rehabilitation Centers--Wilmington [38208]
Delaware Center for Justice [9011]
Delaware County Comm Services Board • DE County Alcohol/Drug Abuse Services /Hamden [46673]
Delaware County Crisis Intervention--West Side [51298]
Delaware County Intermediate Unit [705]
Delaware County Memorial Hospital
    Hearing and Speech Center [3329]
    Regional Cancer Center [5822]
Delaware Curative Workshop • Speech-Language Pathology Department [1519]
Delaware Dialysis • Fresenius Medical Care [26101]
Delaware Guidance Services for Children and Youth [7867], [29077]
Delaware Guidance Services • Dover Branch [29058]
Delaware Guidance Services--Lewes [29066]
Delaware Guidance Services • Newark Branch [29071]
Delaware Guidance Services--Seaford [29073]
Delaware Health and Social Services
    Division of Public Health • SIDS Information and Counseling Program [36462]
    Division of Substance Abuse and Mental Health • Crisis Intervention Service [50740]
Delaware Health and Social Services--Georgetown • Division of Substance Abuse and Mental Health • Crisis Intervention Service [50741]
Delaware Health and Social Services--New Castle • Division of Substance Abuse and Mental Health • Crisis Intervention Service [50743]
Delaware Hospice • Dover Office [19177]
Delaware Hospice, Inc.--Wilmington [19184]
Delaware Hospice-Milford [19178]
Delaware Institute for Reproductive Medicine [21979]
Delaware Library for the Blind and Physically Handicapped • Division of Libraries [3757]
Delaware Opportunities Safe Against Violence [9918]
Delaware Program for Deafblind Children [340]
Delaware Psychiatric Center [33273]
Delaware School for the Deaf [341]
Delaware Speech and Hearing Center [3237]
Delaware Valley Community Health, Inc. [7173]
Delaware Valley Dialysis Center • DaVita [26479]
Delaware Valley Hospital • Addiction Treatment Program [47158]
Delaware Valley Medical [46130]
Delaware Valley Rehab and Detox Center [48505]
Delhi Dialysis • DaVita [26041]
Delhi HomeCare [15286]
Dell Children's Medical Center of Central Texas
    Cystic Fibrosis Center [7676]
    Down Syndrome Clinic [10869]
    Pediatric Cancer Care Program [5960]
Dellwood Recovery Center [45242]
    Cambridge Medical Center [45103]
    Cambridge Medical Center/Adolescent [45104]
    Crossroads [45105]
    Outpatient [45106]
Delmar Gardens Home Care [15993]
Delmarva Counseling Center [44242]
Delmarva Family Resources [44208], [44346]
Delnor - Community Hospital [14800]
Delnor-Community Hospital • Cancer Program [5094]
Delnor Community Hospital Home Health Services [14918]
Delores Project [8948]
DeLozier Recovery Services LLC • Port Townsend Branch [50065]
Delphi Drug and Alcohol Council Inc • CD Outpatient [47033]
Delray Beach Dialysis Center LLC • American Renal Associates [23290]
Delray Beach Health Center [6458]

Delray Medical Center • Pinecrest Rehabilitation Hospital [3967]
Del's Comprehensive Health Care Registry Agency, Inc. [16460]
Delta Behavioral Health [47517]
Delta Care Inc [39849]
Delta Center Inc [42429]
Delta Center, Inc.--Commercial Avenue [29568]
Delta Center Inc. • Runaway and Homeless Youth Program [35926]
Delta Center, Inc.--Washington Avenue [29569]
Delta Community Action Association • Delta Recovery Center [43876], [43905]
Delta Counseling Associates--Crossett [28261]
Delta Counseling Associates, Inc.--Monticello [28323]
Delta Counseling Associates--Lake Village [28296]
Delta Counseling Associates--McGehee [28318]
Delta County Memorial Hospital [13471]
Delta Health Center, Inc. [6892]
Delta Home Health Care, LLC [15603]
Delta Medical Center [49134]
Delta Recovery Center [43847]
Delta Regional Medical Center [2758]
Delta Regional Medical Center Home Health [15961]
Delta Regional Medical Center
    Mississippi Firefighter's Memorial Burn Center [4574]
    Sleep Center [37245]
Delta School District • Deaf/Hard of Hearing Program [253]
Delta Schoolcraft Intermediate School District [486]
Delta Sierra Dialysis Center • DaVita [23022]
Delta State University Infirmary • Mississippi Sports Medicine and Orthopaedic Center [38641]
Delta Waves Sleep Disorders and Research Center [36723]
DeLugach Group [48188]
Demeter House • Phoenix Houses of the Mid-Atlantic [49761]
Demming Dialysis • Fresenius Medical Care • Dialysis Facility [25543]
Denali Family Services--Anchorage [28074]
Denali Family Services--Palmer [28113]
Denison Dialysis Center & At Home • DaVita [27048]
Dennis C Hill Harm Reduction Center [50471]
Dennis Wear Group Home [34276]
DENT Neurologic Institute--Amherst • The Headache Center [12447]
Dent Neurologic Institute • MDA Clinic [34834]
DENT Neurologic Institute--Orchard Park • The Headache Center [12448]
Dent Neurologic Institute • Sleep Disorders Center [37390]
Dental Clinic/Support Services/Administration [6395]
Dental Health Clinic [6391]
Dentistry for Eating Disorders [11301]
Denton County Friends of the Family [10457]
Denton County Mental Health/Mental Retardation Center--Denton [32444]
Denton County Mental Health/Mental Retardation Center--Lewisville [32499]
Denton Regional Day School Program for the Deaf [782]
Denton Regional Medical Center • Cancer Center [5981]
Denton State School [8544]
Denton Treatment Services • Opioid Treatment [49308]
Denver Adult Down Syndrome Clinic [10782]
Denver Center for Crime Victims [8949]
The Denver Children's Home [34043]
Denver Children's Hospital • Audiology, Speech Pathology, and Learning Services [7837]
Denver Dialysis • DaVita [23111]
Denver Ear Associates [1408]
Denver Family Therapy Center • Adolescent Substance Abuse Program [41349]
Denver Health Community Detox • Denver Health Behavioral Health Services [41121]
Denver Health and Hospital Authority
    Denver Community Health Services [6396]
    Outpatient Behavioral Health Services [41122]
Denver Health Medical Center [1395]
Denver Hospice [19099]
Denver Inner City Parish • Project Renew [41123]
Denver Pain Management [35349]

Denver Public Health Department • Denver Community Program for Clinical Research on AIDS [43]
Denver Public Health • Infectious Disease Research Division • AIDS Clinical Trials Unit [7]
Denver--Vail Orthopedics [38171]
Denver Veterans Affairs Medical Center
    Colorado Springs Clinic [28870]
        Women's Stress Disorder Treatment Team Outpatient [51700]
    La Junta Clinic [28918]
    Pueblo Clinic [28944]
Department of Assistive and Rehabilitation Services • Office for Deaf and Hard of Hearing Services [3460]
Department of Corrections • DART Cherry Facility [47330]
Department of Family Services • Billings Helpline [51068]
Department of Health and Family Services • Office for the Deaf and Hard of Hearing [3673]
Department of Health and Human Services
    Adams County [50395]
        Division of Services for the Deaf and Hard of Hearing [3189]
Department of Human Services
    Deaf and Hard of Hearing Services Division [2741]
    New Jersey Division of the Deaf and Hard of Hearing [2952]
    Northwest Deaf and Hard of Hearing Services Division [2674]
    Office of Mental Health • Statewide Program for Persons Who Are Deaf and Hard of Hearing Chicago Road Mental Health Center [1986]
Department of Labor and Economic Growth • Division on Deaf and Hard of Hearing [2616]
Department of Psychiatry • Northwestern Memorial Hospital [29588]
Department of Social & Health Services--Mental Health Division [51454]
Department of Veteran Affairs • Medical Center [44654]
Department of Veterans Administration • New York Harbor Healthcare System [46854]
Department of Veterans Affairs [1175]
    Eastern Colorado Healthcare System [41298]
    Long Beach Healthcare System [40026]
    Medical Center [39221]
Department of Veterans Affairs Medical Center • Cancer Program [4674]
Department of Veterans Affairs
    Miami Medical Center [41777]
    Orlando VA Medical Center [41858]
    Outpatient Substance Abuse Services [49448]
    Recovery Center [47685]
    Substance Abuse Treatment Program 116 [42206]
    VA Sierra Nevada Healthcare System [45868]
    Veterans Recovery Center [41467]
DePaul Center [33887]
    Chemical Dependency Program [49572]
DePaul Treatment Center Inc • Youth and Family Services [48189]
DePaul Treatment Centers Inc • Adult Services [48190]
DePaul Tulane Behavioral Health Center [33543]
Depelchin Children's Center • Main Campus [32479]
DePelchin children's Center--Richmond [32536]
DePelchin Children's Center • Runaway and Homeless Youth Program [36220]
Dependable Care Health Services [17929]
Dependable Home Care services [13352]
Dependable Home Health Inc. [13180]
Dependable Nursing Home Health Services [14834]
Dependency Hlth Services/White Salmon • Branch of Central WA Comprehension [50261]
Dependency Hlth Services/Yakima Outpatient • Central WA Comprehensive Mental Health [50270]
Dept of Behavioral Healthcare Service • Substance Abuse Outpatient Treatment Services [49819]
Dept of Veterans Affairs Akron • Community Based Outpatient Clinics [47605]
Dept of Veterans Affairs Medical Center [48330]
DeQueen--Mena Education Cooperative [245]
Derby Recovery Center Inc [43331]
Derenne Dialysis • DaVita [23785]
Dermagenesis Health Care [13733]

DeRousse Counseling and DUI Services [42408], [42648]
Des Arc Dental Clinic and Health Center [6265]
Des Moines Division • Veterans Affairs Central Iowa Health Care System [51569]
Des Moines Public Schools [431]
Deschutes County Mental Health
    Alcohol and Drug Program [48078]
    Annex [48079]
Deschutes County Mental Health--Crisis Line [51249]
Desert Cities Dialysis of Barstow [22602]
Desert Cities Dialysis Center [23058]
Desert Dialysis Services Inc.--Sun City [22502]
Desert Hills of New Mexico [34306]
Desert Hospital Hospice of the Desert Communities [18986]
Desert Inn Dialysis • Fresenius Medical Care [25360]
Desert Milagro Dialysis Center • Fresenius Medical Care [27276]
Desert Oasis Hospice [18805]
Desert Pulmonary Consultants • Sleep and Diagnostic Center [36628]
Desert Regional Center [8232]
Desert Regional Medical Center • Cancer Program [4817]
Desert Rose Transitional Shelter [9298]
Desert Sanctuary, Inc. • Haley House [8792]
Desert Senita Community Health Center [6222]
Desert Sounds [951]
Desert Sports Medicine and Shoulder Clinic • David P. Richards, MD, FRCS [38038]
Desert Springs Dialysis Center • DaVita [25361]
Desert Star Addiction Recovery Center [39498]
Desert Therapies Inc. [960]
Desert Treatment Center [40348]
Desert View Family Counseling Services [46266]
Desert Vista Behavioral Health Center [33107]
Desert West Counseling [10895]
Design for Living Recovery Services [39987]
Desoto Dialysis • Fresenius Medical Care [24529]
DeSoto Memorial Hospital, Inc. Home Health Care [13582]
Dessie Scott Children's Home [34157]
Destin Hearing Specialists [1668]
Destination Hope Counseling LLC [49627]
Destination Hope Inc [41652]
Destiny Care Home Health [17930]
Destiny Home Health services, Inc. [13079]
Destructive Behavioral Alternatives [43333]
Detroit Central City Community Mental Health [30538]
Detroit Central City • Community Mental Health Inc [44728]
Detroit Community Health Connection, Inc. • East Riverside Health Center [6841]
Detroit East Inc • Community Mental Health Center [44729]
The Detroit Institute for Children [2571], [8168]
Detroit Light House Program [44730]
Detroit Police Department • Victim Assistance Program [9528]
Detroit Receiving Hospital
    Burn Center [4566]
    Comprehensive Center for Bleeding Disorders and Thrombosis [12534]
    Sleep Disorders Center [37155]
Detroit Rescue Mission Ministries
    Christian Guidance Center [44838]
    Genesis House III [44731]
Detroit Road Dialysis • DaVita [26064]
Detroit Subregional Library for the Blind and Physically Handicapped • Detroit Public Library • Frederick Douglass Branch for Specialized Services [3804]
Dettmer Behavioral Health Services [33760]
Deus Dignitas, Inc. [13188]
DeVaughn Int Teach and Treat Options [44127]
Developing Apex Inc [48705]
Developing Options to Violence • Child and Family Services [9139]
Development Center of the Ozarks [8220]
Development Home Health Care Corporation [13968]
Developmental Counseling Center Inc [49229]
Developmental Disabilities Clinic [29448]
Developmental Disabilities Health Alliance • Down

Syndrome Clinic [10827]
Developmental Disabilities Institute [8355]
Developmental Evaluation Center [3182]
Developmental Evaluation Center, New Bern [8387]
Developmental Evaluation Center, Rocky Mount [8389]
Developmental Evaluation Center, Smokies [8390]
Developmental Evaluation Center, Wilmington [8391]
Developmental Evaluation Clinic • East Carolina University [8378]
Developmental Pediatrics [1386]
Developmental Services [7984]
Developmental Services Center • Family Development Center [7935]
Developmental Therapy Program [7822]
Devereaux Children's Center of Washington, DC [34063]
Devereux [8345]
Devereux Aquarius Group Home [34078]
Devereux Arizona [28197]
Devereux Arizona--Scottsdale [7745]
Devereux Arizona--Tucson [7750]
Devereux Beneto Center • Devereux Foundation [33822]
Devereux Colorado Westminster Campus [33213]
Devereux Deland Outpatient Center [34069]
Devereux Edgewater Outpatient Center [33334]
Devereux Flagler Day School [34066]
Devereux Florida [29252], [34087]
Devereux Florida Specialty Hospital [34088]
Devereux Georgia [33384]
Devereux Glenholme School [34057]
Devereux Massachusetts [30460]
Devereux Melbourne Outpatient Center [33320]
Devereux Metro [33969]
Devereux Pine Grove Day School [33321]
Devereux Residential Treatment Center [34076]
Devereux Rockledge Outpatient Center [33352]
Devereux--Rutland [34212]
Devereux Sanford Outpatient Center [33355]
Devereux Semoran Outpatient Center [34077]
Devereux Sweetwater [28198]
Devereux Texas Treatment Network [32564], [33877]
Devereux Therapeutic Foster Care [34089]
Devereux Therapeutic Foster Care--Brevard [34080]
Devereux Therapeutic Foster Care--Dade • Kroger Center [33324]
Devereux Therapeutic Foster Care--Polk [33368]
Devereux Therapeutic Foster Care Volusia [34070]
Devereux Titusville Outpatient Center [33359]
Devereux Transitional Living Center [33335]
Devereux--Tucson [33972]
Devereux Volusia Counseling Center • Therapeutic Foster Care [29148]
Devereux Whispering Hills Day School [33360]
Devmar Home Health Services--Elkins Park [17307]
Devmar Home Health Services--Philadelphia [17408]
DeVos Children's Hospital • Coagulation Disorders Program [12535]
Devoted Health Care [14917]
DeWitt County Human Resource Center [50837]
Dewitt County Human Resource Center • Substance Abuse Treatment Program [42603]
Dexter Dialysis • DaVita [25195]
DFD Russell Medical Center, Leeds [6777]
DFD Russell Medical Center, Turner [6785]
DHL Home Care, LLC [16906]
Diablo Valley Ranch [39716]
Diagnostic Assessment Service [31713]
Diagnostic Center for Sleep Health [37909]
Diagnostic Services of Houston/Houston Hearing [3506]
Diagnostic Speech and Hearing Clinic [3380]
Diakon Hospice Saint John--Allentown [21042]
Diakon Hospice Saint John-Hazle Twp. [21095]
Diakon Hospice Saint John-Honesdale [21097]
Diakon Hospice Saint John-Wyomissing [21177]
Dial Help [9543]
    Copper Country Mental Health Services [51019]
Dial/Self • Runaway and Homeless Youth Program [36000]
Dialysis Affiliates of South Alabama [22319]
Dialysis Associates of Northern New Jersey • Fresenius Medical Care [25494]
Dialysis Association of the Palm Beaches • DaVita [23552]
Dialysis Association of Smyrna • Fresenius Medical

Care [26924]
Dialysis Care of Anson County • DaVita [25965]
Dialysis Care Center of Daytona • American Renal Associates [23284]
Dialysis Care Center of Palm Coast • American Renal Associates [23462]
Dialysis Care of Edgecombe County • DaVita [25962]
Dialysis Care of Franklin County • DaVita [25903]
Dialysis Care of Hoke County & At Home • DaVita [25926]
Dialysis Care of Martin County • DaVita [25973]
Dialysis Care of Mecklenburg County Inc. • Renal Advantage Inc. [25833]
Dialysis Care of Moore County & At Home • DaVita [25923]
Dialysis Care of Richmond County • DaVita [25881]
Dialysis Care of Rockingham County • DaVita [25857]
Dialysis Care of Rowan County • DaVita [25943]
Dialysis Center of Beatrice [25316]
Dialysis Center of Bucks County • American Renal Associates [26385]
Dialysis Center of Columbus [25319]
Dialysis Center of Darke County LLC [26129]
Dialysis Center • DaVita [27470]
Dialysis Center of Dayton--North [26094]
Dialysis Center of East Providence • American Renal Associates [26659]
Dialysis Center of Erie • DaVita [26430]
Dialysis Center of Fall River • American Renal Associates [24765]
Dialysis Center of Hutchinson [24323]
Dialysis Center of Johnston • American Renal Associates [26660]
Dialysis Center of Lincoln [25327]
Dialysis Center of Lincoln--Home [25328]
Dialysis Center--Lincoln Northwest [25329]
Dialysis Center of Lincoln--Southwest [25330]
Dialysis Center of Lubbock • Fresenius Medical Care [27234]
Dialysis Center of Middle Georgia • DaVita [23829]
Dialysis Center of Newington • Fresenius Medical Care [23172]
Dialysis Center of Ontario • Renal Carepartners [22856]
Dialysis Center at Oxford Court • DaVita [26463]
Dialysis Center of Pawtucket • American Renal Associates [26662]
Dialysis Center of Providence • American Renal Associates [26664]
Dialysis Center of Shreveport • Fresenius Medical Care [24576]
Dialysis Center of Siloam Springs [22574]
Dialysis Center of Simi Valley, Inc. • DaVita [23013]
Dialysis Center of Tiverton • American Renal Associates [26668]
Dialysis Center--Venice • DaVita [23547]
Dialysis Center of Wakefield [26669]
Dialysis Center at Waltham • American Renal Associates [24809]
Dialysis Center of Warwick • American Renal Associates [26670]
Dialysis Center of Westerly • American Renal Associates [26672]
Dialysis Center of Western Massachusetts • American Renal Associates [24759]
Dialysis Center of Woonsocket • American Renal Associates [26673]
Dialysis Centers of Dayton East [26095]
Dialysis Centers of Dayton--South [26167]
Dialysis Centers of Warren County [26201]
Dialysis Clinic Inc--Gateway [23339]
Dialysis Clinic, Inc. [25317]
Dialysis Clinic, Inc.--Albany [23572]
Dialysis Clinic Inc.--Albany West Town [23573]
Dialysis Clinic Inc.--Albuquerque East [25533]
Dialysis Clinic, Inc.--Arlington [23577]
Dialysis Clinic, Inc. of Atlanta--Piedmont • Home Dialysis [23588]
Dialysis Clinic, Inc.--Auburn [25573]
Dialysis Clinic Inc.--Azalea Place [26685]
Dialysis Clinic Inc.--Ball Square [24800]
Dialysis Clinic, Inc. of Banksville [26546]
Dialysis Clinic, Inc.--Baptist [25221]
Dialysis Clinic, Inc.--Beaver Falls/Chippewa [26374]
Dialysis Clinic Inc.--Beech Lake [26871]
Dialysis Clinic Inc.--Belfast [24606]

Dialysis Clinic, Inc.--Belton [25172]
Dialysis Clinic Inc.--Billerica [24786]
Dialysis Clinic, Inc.--Billings [25304]
Dialysis Clinic, Inc.--Birmingham [22315]
Dialysis Clinic Inc.--Blackfeet [25306]
Dialysis Clinic, Inc.--Boonville [25175]
Dialysis Clinic, Inc.--Boston [24749]
Dialysis Clinic Inc.--Boxwood Place [23649]
Dialysis Clinic Inc.--Bradhurst [25679]
Dialysis Clinic, Inc.--Brigham/Faulkner [24772]
Dialysis Clinic, Inc.--Central State--Freehold [25436]
Dialysis Clinic, Inc.--Chattanooga [26813]
Dialysis Clinic, Inc.--Cincinnati [26042]
Dialysis Clinic, Inc. of Clarion [26404]
Dialysis Clinic, Inc.--Clarksville Highway [26903]
Dialysis Clinic, Inc.--Clinton [25186]
Dialysis Clinic, Inc.--Columbia [25187]
Dialysis Clinic, Inc.--Columbus [23650]
Dialysis Clinic, Inc.--Corbin [24370]
Dialysis Clinic Inc.--Crawford [23589]
Dialysis Clinic, Inc.--Crowley [24480]
Dialysis Clinic, Inc.--Cullman [22323]
Dialysis Clinic, Inc.--Danville [24374]
Dialysis Clinic, Inc.--Dawson [23669]
Dialysis Clinic Inc.--Dayton [26814]
Dialysis Clinic, Inc.--Decatur [22326]
Dialysis Clinic Inc.--Dekalb [23672]
Dialysis Clinic Inc.--Desert Dialysis Center [22516]
Dialysis Clinic, Inc.--Dialysis Care Services Inc. [27268]
Dialysis Clinic, Inc.--Dickson [26830]
Dialysis Clinic, Inc.--Dothan [22330]
    Dialysis Facility [22331]
Dialysis Clinic, Inc.--Douglas [22433]
Dialysis Clinic Inc.--East Albany [23574]
Dialysis Clinic, Inc.--East Cooper [26746]
Dialysis Clinic, Inc.--East Falls [26512]
Dialysis Clinic, Inc.--East Liverpool [26104]
Dialysis Clinic, Inc.--East Ridge [26833]
Dialysis Clinic Inc.--East Shreveport [24577]
Dialysis Clinic, Inc.--East Spartanburg [26771]
Dialysis Clinic, Inc.--Enterprise [22333]
Dialysis Clinic, Inc.--Eunice [24489]
Dialysis Clinic, Inc.--Fayetteville [23698]
Dialysis Clinic Inc. of Five Points [26481]
Dialysis Clinic Inc.--Forest Park [26119]
Dialysis Clinic Inc. • Fort Bragg Dialysis [22689]
Dialysis Clinic, Inc.--Fort Oglethorpe [23703]
Dialysis Clinic, Inc.--Frankfort [24380]
Dialysis Clinic Inc.--Gaffney [26717]
Dialysis Clinic Inc.--Georgiana [22346]
Dialysis Clinic, Inc.--Goose Creek [26721]
Dialysis Clinic, Inc. of Grove City [26437]
Dialysis Clinic Inc.--Harmar Village [26401]
Dialysis Clinic Inc.--Hastings [26442]
Dialysis Clinic, Inc.--Hillpointe [26393]
Dialysis Clinic, Inc.--Hixson [26845]
Dialysis Clinic Inc. Home Dialysis [23590]
Dialysis Clinic, Inc.--Humboldt [26846]
Dialysis Clinic, Inc. of Indiana • Indiana Ambulatory Surgical Center [26451]
Dialysis Clinic Inc.--Indianapolis [24173]
Dialysis Clinic, Inc.--Jackson [26850]
Dialysis Clinic Inc.--Jacksonville [23340]
Dialysis Clinic, Inc.--James Island [26686]
Dialysis Clinic, Inc.--Jasper [26851]
Dialysis Clinic, Inc.--Jeannette [26452]
Dialysis Clinic, Inc.--Jefferson City East [25216]
Dialysis Clinic, Inc.--Jefferson City West [25217]
Dialysis Clinic Inc.--Jennings [24510]
Dialysis Clinic Inc.--Kalispell [25311]
Dialysis Clinic Inc.--Kings Mountain [25947]
Dialysis Clinic Inc.--Knoxville [26857]
Dialysis Clinic Inc.--LaFayette [23728]
Dialysis Clinic, Inc.--Landrum [26737]
Dialysis Clinic, Inc.--Lebanon [26868]
Dialysis Clinic, Inc.--Lees Summit [25237]
Dialysis Clinic Inc.--Lexington [24399]
Dialysis Clinic Inc.--Libby [25312]
Dialysis Clinic, Inc.--Louisiana [25241]
Dialysis Clinic Inc.--Lyerly [26815]
Dialysis Clinic Inc.--Madison [26875]
Dialysis Clinic Inc.--Madison Center [25467]
Dialysis Clinic, Inc.--Magnolia Court [26687]
Dialysis Clinic, Inc.--Maryville [26880]
Dialysis Clinic Inc.--Maysville [24425]
Dialysis Clinic Inc.--McCrory [22559]
Dialysis Clinic, Inc.--Medical Center [26904]

Dialysis Clinic, Inc.--Mexico [25244]
Dialysis Clinic, Inc.--Moberly [25245]
Dialysis Clinic Inc.--Monroe [25469]
Dialysis Clinic, Inc. of Monroeville [26482]
Dialysis Clinic, Inc.--Montgomery [22374]
Dialysis Clinic, Inc.--Moulton [22379]
Dialysis Clinic, Inc. of Mount Pleasant [26487]
Dialysis Clinic, Inc.--Murfreesboro [26899]
Dialysis Clinic, Inc.--Nashville [26905]
Dialysis Clinic, Inc. of New Kensington [26493]
Dialysis Clinic Inc.--New Orleans [24551]
Dialysis Clinic Inc.--New Orleans East [24552]
Dialysis Clinic, Inc.--North Borough [26547]
Dialysis Clinic, Inc.--North Brunswick • Dialysis Center [25491]
Dialysis Clinic Inc.--North Columbus [23651]
Dialysis Clinic, Inc. of North Hills [26548]
Dialysis Clinic Inc.--North Shreveport [24578]
Dialysis Clinic Inc.--North Versailles [26496]
Dialysis Clinic Inc.--Northside [23591]
Dialysis Clinic, Inc. of Oakland [26549]
Dialysis Clinic, Inc.--Omaha [25337]
Dialysis Clinic, Inc.--Onawa [24293]
Dialysis Clinic, Inc.--Opelousas [24565]
Dialysis Clinic Inc.--Paris [26917]
Dialysis Clinic, Inc.--Parks Bend [26371]
Dialysis Clinic, Inc.--Pell City [26388]
Dialysis Clinic Inc.--Phenix City [22390]
Dialysis Clinic Inc.--Port Royal [26681]
Dialysis Clinic Inc.--Portsmouth [26186]
Dialysis Clinic Inc.--Punxsutawney [26571]
Dialysis Clinic Inc.--Richmond [24441]
Dialysis Clinic, Inc.--Saint Joseph [25222]
Dialysis Clinic Inc./Saint Peter University Hospital [25480]
Dialysis Clinic Inc.--Saluda [26765]
Dialysis Clinic Inc.--Seaman [26197]
Dialysis Clinic, Inc.--Sedalia [25289]
Dialysis Clinic, Inc. of Seven Fields [26582]
Dialysis Clinic, Inc.--Sevierville [26921]
Dialysis Clinic, Inc.--Shelby [25948]
Dialysis Clinic, Inc.--Shelbyville [26922]
Dialysis Clinic, Inc.--Shenango Valley [26445]
Dialysis Clinic, Inc.--Shreveport [24579]
Dialysis Clinic Inc.--Skowhegan [24616]
Dialysis Clinic Inc.--South Shelby [25949]
Dialysis Clinic, Inc.--Southern Hills [26906]
Dialysis Clinic Inc.--Southland [24400]
Dialysis Clinic, Inc. of Southpoint [23341]
Dialysis Clinic, Inc.--Spartanburg [26772]
Dialysis Clinic Inc.--Staten Island [25779]
Dialysis Clinic Inc.--Steubenville [26204]
Dialysis Clinic, Inc.--Summit [26844]
Dialysis Clinic, Inc.--Sylvester [23805]
Dialysis Clinic, Inc.--Syracuse [25786]
Dialysis Clinic, Inc.--Union [26778]
Dialysis Clinic, Inc.--Walden Pond [24761]
Dialysis Clinic, Inc.--Warrensburg [25298]
Dialysis Clinic, Inc. of Washington [26599]
Dialysis Clinic, Inc.--West Ashley [26688]
Dialysis Clinic, Inc.--West Omaha [25338]
Dialysis Clinic, Inc.--West Plains [25302]
Dialysis Clinic, Inc.--West Spartanburg [26773]
Dialysis Clinic, Inc.--Westbank--Gretna [24499]
Dialysis Clinic Inc.--Westchester [26232]
Dialysis Clinic Inc.--Western Hills [26043]
Dialysis Clinic, Inc. of Wilkinsburg [26550]
Dialysis Clinics, Inc.--Kirksville [25234]
Dialysis Clinics, Inc.--Osage Beach [25253]
Dialysis Corporation of America of Adel [23570]
Dialysis Corporation of America of Aiken II [26675]
Dialysis Corporation of America--Ashland [27462]
Dialysis Corporation of America--Baltimore [24637]
Dialysis Corporation of America of Barnwell [26680]
Dialysis Corporation of America of Bedford [26432]
Dialysis Corporation of America of Calhoun [23633]
Dialysis Corporation of America of Camp Hill [26391]
Dialysis Corporation of America of Carlisle [26395]
Dialysis Corporation of America--Central Valdosta [23819]
Dialysis Corporation of America--Chambersburg [26398]
Dialysis Corporation of America--Chesapeake [24624]
Dialysis Corp. of America--Chevy Chase [24660]
Dialysis Corporation of America of Cincinnati [26168]
Dialysis Corporation of America of Columbus [26076]

Dialysis Corporation of America of Delaware County [26102]
Dialysis Corporation of America--Edgefield [26708]
Dialysis Corporation of America--Fitzgerald [23700]
Dialysis Corporation of America of Hawkinsville [23717]
Dialysis Corporation of America of Huntingdon • Dialysis Facility [26449]
Dialysis Corporation of America of Manahawkin [25462]
Dialysis Corporation of America--Mechanicsburg [26476]
Dialysis Corporation of America of North Baltimore [24638]
Dialysis Corporation of America of Pottstown [26568]
Dialysis Corporation of America--Royston [23780]
Dialysis Corporation of America--Selinsgrove [26579]
Dialysis Corporation of America--South Georgia • Dialysis Facility [23820]
Dialysis Corporation of America--Vineland [25523]
Dialysis Corporation of America of Warsaw [27584]
Dialysis Corporation of America of Wellsboro [26604]
Dialysis Corporation of America--York [26618]
Dialysis Corporation of AmericaA--Rockville [24720]
The Dialysis Cottage [27099]
Dialysis Facilities Inc.--Waycross [23834]
Dialysis Facility of Alma, Inc. [23575]
Dialysis of Huntington • Diversified Specialty Institutes [24165]
Dialysis Institute of Indiana • Fresenius Medical Care [24174]
Dialysis of Kannapolis & At Home • DaVita [25891]
Dialysis and Kidney Center of North Brevard [23543]
Dialysis of Lithonia • DaVita [23673]
Dialysis Partners--Maumee Bay [26180]
Dialysis Partners of Northwest Ohio--Glendale [26210]
Dialysis Service of Murrysville Inc. • Fresenius Medical Care [26433]
Dialysis Services of Abilene South • Fresenius Medical Care [26930]
Dialysis Services--Andrews • Fresenius Medical Care [26677]
Dialysis Services of Belpre [26020]
Dialysis Services of Briggs Avenue • Fresenius Medical Care [25852]
Dialysis Services of Central Philadelphia • Fresenius Medical Care [26513]
Dialysis Services of Congress Parkway • Fresenius Medical Care [23921]
Dialysis Services of Deer Park • Fresenius Medical Care [27045]
Dialysis Services Des Moines South • Fresenius Medical Care [24265]
Dialysis Services--East Georgia • Fresenius Medical Care [23738]
Dialysis Services of Exeter • Fresenius Medical Care [25388]
Dialysis Services Fort Lauderdale • Fresenius Medical Care [23298]
Dialysis Services of Gaylord [24903]
Dialysis Services of Grapevine • Fresenius Medical Care [27363]
Dialysis Services of Greenwood • Renal Advantage Inc. [24160]
Dialysis Services of Hartsville • Fresenius Medical Care [26728]
Dialysis Services of Houston County • Fresenius Medical Care [23830]
Dialysis Services of Ingram • Fresenius Medical Care [27321]
Dialysis Services of Jones County • Fresenius Medical Care [25964]
Dialysis Services of Lincoln County • Fresenius Medical Care [25295]
Dialysis Services of London • Fresenius Medical Care [26152]
Dialysis Services of Mon Valley • Fresenius Medical Care [26400]
Dialysis Services of Mount Hood • Fresenius Medical Care [26322]
Dialysis Services Murrells Inlet • Fresenius Medical Care [26749]
Dialysis Services of North Brownsville • Fresenius Medical Care [26980]
Dialysis Services--North Ramsey • Fresenius Medical Care [25863]

Dialysis Services of Palmer • Fresenius Medical Care [24791]
Dialysis Services of Pearland • Fresenius Medical Care [27285]
Dialysis Services of Pearlridge • Fresenius Medical Care [23844]
Dialysis Services of Plainview • Fresenius Medical Care [27289]
Dialysis Services of Salem • Fresenius Medical Care [24231]
Dialysis Services of Southwest San Antonio • Fresenius Medical Care [27322]
Dialysis Services Southwestern • Fresenius Medical Care [27022]
Dialysis Services--Waco West • Fresenius Medical Care [27388]
Dialysis Services Waxahachie • Fresenius Medical Care [27389]
Dialysis Services of West Laredo • Fresenius Medical Care [27219]
Dialysis Services of West Texas • Yoakum County Hospital [27050]
Dialysis Specialists of Central City • Fresenius Medical Care [24368]
Dialysis Specialists of Columbus • Fresenius Medical Care [26077]
Dialysis Specialists of Coshocton [26093]
Dialysis Specialists of Fairfield • Fresenius Medical Care [26113]
Dialysis Specialists of Marietta • Fresenius Medical Care [26156]
Dialysis Specialists of Seminole [26292]
Dialysis Systems of Covington • DaVita [24478]
Dialysis Systems of Hammond • DaVita [24501]
Diamond Consulting Corp • The Fletcher Center [49778]
Diamond Headache Clinic [12420]
Diamond Home Health Care, Inc. [16907]
Diamond Home Health, Inc. [12889]
Diamond Institute for Infertility and Menopause [22160]
Diamond Medical Equipment and Supply, Inc. [12868]
Diane Peppler Resource Center [9574]
Diaspora Community Services • Runaway and Homeless Youth Program [36102]
Dickenson County Behavioral Services • Substance Abuse Services [49776]
Dickinson County Healthcare System [15695]
   Upper Peninsula Sleep Disorders Center [37156]
Dickinson Dialysis Facility • Saint Joseph's Hospital [25989]
Dickinson Home Health [15696]
Dickinson-Iron Dental Center [6839]
Dickinson Mental Health Center [32017], [32116]
   Day Treatment Program [31997]
Dickinson VA Outpatient Clinic [4351]
Dickinson Veterans Affairs Clinic [31625]
Dickson County Schools [751]
Dicta Health Services Inc • Dicta Substance Abuse Treatment Center [39941]
Didi Hirsch CMHC
   Via Avanta Program [40345]
   Youth Services [40102]
Didi Hirsch Community Mental Health Center
   Inglewood Center [28542]
   Mar Vista Center [28588]
   S. Mark Taper Foundation Center [28589]
   Suicide Prevention Center [50669]
Didi Hirsch MHS [40103]
Didi Hirsh Community Mental Health Center • c/o PMR Corporation [28466]
Diebold Behavioral Counseling [39466]
Diel Counseling Inc [42650]
Di'game Speech and Language Consultants [2959]
Diggs Kraus Sickle Cell Center [36427]
Dignity Hospice of Southern WV [21792]
Dignity Program V [8713]
Dillon Mental Health Center [32199]
Dilworth Center for Chemical Dependency [47256]
Dimension in Recovery [45195]
Dimensions in Awareness [41124]
Dimock Center • John Flowers Recovery Home [44555]
Dimock Community Health Center [6823]
   Alcohol and Drug Detoxification Prog [44556]
Dimock Community Health Center, Inc. • Behavioral

Health Services [30459]
Dimock CSS Womens Renewal at Dimock [44557]
Dinwiddie Counseling Services [32727]
Diogenes Youth Services • Runaway and Homeless Youth Program [35819]
Direct Counseling Inc [42972]
Direct Dialysis [23967]
Direct Home Health Care, Inc. [14729]
Direct Medical Equipment [15884]
Direct Nursing Services, Inc. [13031]
Direct RehabMed [35691]
Direct RehabMed--Longview [35692]
Directions for Mental Health [29125]
Directions for Mental Health Inc [41590]
Directions for Mental Health--Oakwoods Office [29201]
Directions Services Counseling Center [31940]
Directions for Youth • Alcohol and Drug Treatment Program [47716]
Directorate of Human Resources • Army Substance Abuse Program [42097]
Dirigo Counseling Clinic • Alan Algee [43968], [43982], [44005]
Dirne Community Health Center [6636]
DISC Sports and Spine Center [38103]
DISC Village Inc
   Adolescent Outpatient [41945]
   Adolescent Treatment Program [41946]
   Adult Outpatient [41947]
   Gadsden Adult Outpatient [41911]
   Wakulla Adult Outpatient [41607]
   Wakulla County Juvenille Outpatient [41608]
DISC Village, Inc. [29296]
Discovery Center [45791]
   Windows of Discovery [43783]
Discovery Counseling • Alcohol and Drug Services [50278]
Discovery Counseling Center Inc [41020], [41264]
Discovery Counseling Center of the San Ramon Valley, Inc. [28468]
Discovery Counseling Inc [48089], [48144], [48156], [48257]
Discovery House [33999], [40205], [43925], [44064], [48327], [48334], [48390], [48411]
Discovery House BC Inc [48344]
Discovery House LT Inc [49624]
Discovery House NC Inc [48480]
Discovery House NPA [48371]
Discovery House PA [48586]
Discovery House Providence [48872]
Discovery House UC Inc [49653]
Discovery House Utah [49683]
   Taylorsville Clinic [49710]
Discovery House of Washington County [43956]
Discovery House • Woonsocket [48891]
Discovery Institute for Addictive Disorders • Outpatient Program [46044]
Discovery Institute for • Addict Disorders/Long/Short Term Resid [46045]
Discovery Paths [10948]
Discovery Place Group Home [28044]
Discovery to Recovery Substance Abuse [42651]
Dist 19 MH/MR Subst Abuse Services • Surry Counseling Service [49849]
Distinct Health Care Services [14192]
Distinct Home Health Care, Inc. [18049]
Distinct Home Health Services, Inc. [14322]
Distinctive Therapy Solutions [1423]
District 19 Community Services [32773]
District 19 Crisis Intervention [32749]
District 19 Substance Abuse Services • Petersburg Outpatient Services [49818]
District of Columbia Department of Health • Maternal and Child Health Contact • SIDS Program [36463]
District of Columbia Department of Mental Health • ACT 4 Program [33279]
District of Columbia General Hospital • Health Services for Children with Special Needs [7871]
District of Columbia Mental Health Services • Hearing Impaired Services Division [1524]
District of Columbia Public Library • Adaptive Services Division [3758]
District Heights Dialysis • DaVita [24675]
District II • Alcohol and Drug Program [45697]
District IV Human Resources Development Council • Domestic Abuse Program [9749]
District Resource Program for Deaf/Hard of Hearing--Victoria BC [259]

District Resource Program for the Deaf/Hard of Hearing--Victoria BC [260]
Diversified Family Services [47929]
Diversified Health Management [16908]
Diversified Health Solutions, LLC [17978]
Diversified Hearing Services [3148]
Diversified Home Care [14804]
Diversified Home Services, Inc [15507]
Diversified Human Services [32046]
Diversified Services LLC [3041]
Diversified Specialty Institutes--Austell [23620]
Diversified Specialty Institutes • Avondale Dialysis Center [22424]
Diversified Specialty Institutes--Baton Rouge • Dialysis Facility [24460]
Diversified Specialty Institutes--Brandon • Dialysis Facility [25104]
Diversified Specialty Institutes--Canton [23635] Dialysis Facility [25107]
Diversified Specialty Institutes • Cartersville Dialysis Center, LLC [23638]
Diversified Specialty Institutes--Carthage • Dialysis Facility [25109]
Diversified Specialty Institutes Cottonwood Dialysis Center [22432] Edinburg Dialysis Center [27056]
Diversified Specialty Institutes--Galleria [26884]
Diversified Specialty Institutes--Greenville [26722]
Diversified Specialty Institutes--Hazelhurst • Dialysis Facility [25131]
Diversified Specialty Institutes--Houma • Dialysis Center [24506]
Diversified Specialty Institutes--Jackson Southwest [25135]
Diversified Specialty Institutes--Lee's Summit Renal Center [25238]
Diversified Specialty Institutes--Lexington [25142]
Diversified Specialty Institutes--Marion County [24175]
Diversified Specialty Institutes--Markham [24031]
Diversified Specialty Institutes • Mesa Dialysis Center [22455]
Diversified Specialty Institutes--Munroe Falls [26170]
Diversified Specialty Institutes Northeast Phoenix Dialysis Center [22471] Norwood Clinic Dialysis Unit [22316]
Diversified Specialty Institutes--Philadelphia [26514]
Diversified Specialty Institutes--Plainfield [24221]
Diversified Specialty Institutes--Powderhorn [26768]
Diversified Specialty Institutes--Prescott [22488]
Diversified Specialty Institutes--Scottsburg • Dialysis Facility [24232]
Diversified Specialty Institutes--Simpsonville [26769]
Diversified Specialty Institutes--South Holland [24088]
Diversified Specialty Institutes South Phoenix Dialysis Center [22472] Southwest Mesa Dialysis Center [22456]
Diversified Specialty Institutes--Spokane Valley [27648]
Diversified Specialty Institutes • Tempe Dialysis Center [22510]
Diversified Specialty Institutes--Walker County [22360]
Diversified Specialty Institutes--Waukegan Home Program [24103]
Diversified Specialty Institutes--Waukeka Renal Center [24104]
Diversified Specialty Institutes--White Pond [26003]
Divide Health Clinic [6399]
Divine Grace Home Health, Inc. [13032]
Divine Health Care Corporation [13969]
Divine Healthcare Services Inc • Behavioral Counseling Therapeutic Serv [39942]
Divine Hope Counseling [45345]
Divine Hospice Care [19374]
Divine Savior Healthcare [18618]
Divine Savior Healthcare Dialysis [27772]
Divine Savior Sports Medicine [39187]
Divine Speech/Language Services Inc. [1869]
Divine Touch Health Services [17872]
Division of Mental Health • Alcoholism and Drug Dependency Services [49751]
Division for the Treatment and Education of Autistic and Related [8370]
Dixie County Clinic [29134]
Dixie Dialysis Center [27419]
Dixie Regional Medical Center [32615]

Cancer Program [6041]
Dixon Dialysis Center--W 2nd Street [23975]
Dixon Dialysis Services--N Lincoln Street [22659]
Dixon Family Services [39784]
Dixon Kidney Center • DaVita [23976]
Dixon Recovery Institute Inc [40104]
Dixon Social Interactive Services [47358]
Diyor Home Care Services [13734]
DM and ADR Inc [42024]
DMJ Home Health Services [14892]
Do It Now Foundation of • Southern California [40105]
Doan Center for Counseling • El Dorado [43337]
Dockside Services Inc [43202]
Dr. Arenia C. Mallory Community Health Center, Inc. • Mallory Community Health Center [6887]
Doctor Donald MacLellan Tissue Bank [35111]
Doctor Everett Chalmers Hospital • Eating Disorders Program [11136]
Dr. Frank Bryant Health Center [7312]
Dr. Fred Brown Children's Health Center [6520]
Dr. Gertrude A. Barber Center [8457]
Dr. Gertrude A. Barber Center, Inc. • Down Syndrome Clinic [10855]
Dr. I. Gonzalez Martinez Oncologic Hospital • Puerto Rico Medical Center [5885]
Doctor John C. Corrigan Mental Health Center [30370]
Dr. Jose S. Belaval Community Health Center [7211]
Doctor Kate Home Health & Hospice [18557]
Dr. Matthew S. Shwartz Hospice and Palliative Care [19953]
Doctor P. Phillips Hospital [1694]
Doctor P. Phillips Hospital Outpatient Rehabilitation [1695]
Dr. Paul J. Marsh DC, QME [38124]
Dr. Ravinder N. Agarwal Renal Center [25746]
Dr. Robert L. Yeager Health Center • Rockland County Department of Mental Health [31451]
Doctor Solomon Carter Fuller Mental Health Center [33572]
Doctor's Choice Home Care--Bradenton [13602]
Doctor's Choice Home Care--Englewood [13683]
Doctor's Choice Home Care--Sarasota [14375]
Doctors Community Hospital • Sleep Disorders Center [37099]
Doctor's Dialysis Center of Montebello • DaVita [22821]
Doctors Hospital • Cancer Care [4667]
Doctors Hospital • Joseph M. Still Burn Center [4537]
Doctor's Hospital of Laredo • Cancer Program [6009]
Doctors' Hospital of Michigan Euro-Peds [10814]
Doctor's Hospital West • Cancer Center [5706]
Doctors Medical Center Burn Care Center [4515] Cancer Program [4807]
Doctors Medical Center--San Pablo Campus • Regional Cancer Center [4849]
Doctors Medical Center • Sleep Disorders Center [36665]
Doctors Pain Clinic--Farrell [35640]
Doctors Pain Clinic--Youngstown [35605]
Doctor's Park Rehabilitation Services [2581]
Dodge County Department of Human Services and Health Department [50423]
Dodge County Dialysis • DaVita [25320]
Dodson Avenue Community Health Center [7255]
Doernbecher Children's Hospital • Oregon Health & Science University • Down Syndrome Clinic [10850]
Dogwood Place Apartments [27820]
Doheny Eye and Tissue Transplant Bank [34944]
Dolminis [48273]
Domestic Abuse Center [8856]
Domestic Abuse Council, Inc. [9046]
Domestic Abuse Crisis Center [9765]
Domestic Abuse Family Shelter [9652]
Domestic Abuse Intervention Center [9890]
Domestic Abuse Intervention Project • Grayson Crisis Center [10508]
Domestic Abuse Intervention Services [10713]
Domestic Abuse is Not Acceptable [10085]
Domestic Abuse Prevention Center, Inc. [9320]
Domestic Abuse Project [9614]
Domestic Abuse Project of Delaware County, Inc. [10298]

Domestic Abuse and Rape Crisis Center [9817]
Domestic Abuse Resistance Team [9422]
Domestic Abuse and Sexual Assault Crisis Center [9849]
Domestic Abuse and Sexual Assault Intervention Services, Inc. [9842]
Domestic Abuse/Sexual Assault Services [9777]
Domestic Abuse Shelter, Inc. [9064]
Domestic Abuse Women's Network [10664]
Domestic Assault Shelter Coalition [9577]
Domestic Harmony [9541]
Domestic Older Victims Empowerment and Safety [8714]
Domestic Safety Resource Center [8973]
Domestic and Sexual Abuse Assault Resource Center [9327]
Domestic/Sexual Assault Outreach Center [9334]
Domestic and Sexual Violence Crisis Center of Chelan/Douglas [10667]
Domestic Unity [9879]
Domestic Violence Action Center [9140]
Domestic Violence Advocacy Program [9326]
Domestic Violence Alternatives • Sexual Assault Center [9340]
Domestic Violence Association of Central Kansas [9376]
Domestic Violence Center of Chester County--Coatesville [10270]
Domestic Violence Center of Chester County--Kennett Square [10287]
Domestic Violence Center of Chester County--Oxford [10303]
Domestic Violence Center--Cleveland [10135]
Domestic Violence Center of Grays Harbor [10623]
Domestic Violence Center of Howard County, Inc. [9450]
Domestic Violence Coalition, Inc. [9566]
Domestic Violence Crisis Center, Inc.--Minot [10116]
Domestic Violence Crisis Center--Lenoir City • Iva's Place [10416]
Domestic Violence Crisis Center--Norwalk [9003]
Domestic Violence Crisis Center--Stamford [9005]
Domestic Violence Education and Shelter [9345]
Domestic Violence Education and Support Groups [9417]
Domestic Violence Emergency Service--Morehead [9395]
Domestic Violence Emergency Services--Atchison [9351]
Domestic Violence Escape, Inc.--Hurley [10706]
Domestic Violence Escape, Inc.--Ironwood [9547]
Domestic Violence Initiative for Women with Disabilities [8950]
Domestic Violence Intervention Center--Auburn [8647]
Domestic Violence Intervention Center--Idaho Falls [9174]
Domestic Violence Intervention, Inc.--Fallon [9790]
Domestic Violence Intervention of Lebanon County [10291]
Domestic Violence Intervention Program [9336]
Domestic Violence Intervention Services/Call Rape, Inc. [10217]
Domestic Violence • Intervention Services Inc [48037]
Domestic Violence Network [9285]
Domestic Violence OASIS Program [9185]
Domestic Violence Prevention, Inc--Texarkana [10511]
Domestic Violence Program of Herkimer County [9929]
Domestic Violence Program, Inc.--Murfreesboro [10423]
Domestic Violence Program of North Central Oklahoma [10208]
Domestic Violence Project--Glens Falls [9925]
Domestic Violence Project, Inc.--Ann Arbor • Safe House [9513]
Domestic Violence Project, Inc.--Canton [10129]
Domestic Violence Project, Inc.--Oxford [9656]
Domestic Violence and Rape Crisis Center [10051], [10110]
Domestic Violence and Rape Crisis Services of Saratoga County [9984]
Domestic Violence Resource Center--Hillsboro [10234]
Domestic Violence Resource Center/Resources Inc.--Albuquerque [9853]

Domestic Violence Resource Center of South County [10339]
Domestic Violence Resource Center--Taylorsville [10090]
Domestic Violence Service Center [10325]
Domestic Violence Services of Benton/Franklin Counties [10625]
Domestic Violence Services of Cumberland and Perry Counties [10267]
Domestic Violence Services Network--Concord [9476]
Domestic Violence Services--New Haven [9000]
Domestic Violence Services--Pendleton [10244]
Domestic Violence Services--Uniontown [10322]
Domestic Violence Services--Winnemucca [9802]
Domestic Violence/Sexual Assault Association [9373]
Domestic Violence and Sexual Assault Coalition [8819]
Domestic Violence/Sexual Assault Program of Jefferson County [10637]
Domestic Violence and Sexual Assault Services [10606]
Domestic Violence/Sexual Assault Services of the San Juan Islands [10617]
The Domestic Violence Shelter, Inc. [10158]
Domestic Violence Shelter and Services, Inc. [10102]
Domestic Violence Shelter for Women/Children [8850]
Domestic Violence Solutions [8831]
Domestic Violence Task Force of Cass County [9296]
Dominican Home Health Care [13332]
Dominican Hospital • Cancer Center [4659]
Dominican Sisters Family Health Service--Bronx [16360]
Dominican Sisters Family Health Service--Hampton Bays [16473]
Dominican Sisters Family Health Service, Inc.--Ossining [16584]
Dominican Sisters Family Health Service--Medford [16518]
Dominican Sisters Family Health Service--Wainscott [16653]
Dominion Fertility--Arlington [22280]
Dominion Fertility--Loudon [22281]
Dominion Fertility--Reston [22282]
Dominion Fertility--Washington [21982]
Dominion Psychiatric Associates • Turning Point IOP [49852]
Domser and Plummer Physical Therapy [2420]
Don Foster and Associates Inc [48941], [48976]
Don Guanella School [8486]
Donald R. Reed Speech and Hearing Center [3119]
Donate Life Today [35100]
Donlin Group Inc [47502]
Donna M. Edgmon Speech Pathology Clinic [1042]
Donna Memorial Clinic [2103]
Donor Alliance, Inc. [34972]
Donor Network of Arizona [34923]
Donor Services of Indiana [35030]
Door County Department of Community Programs [50537]
Door County Memorial Home Health [18632]
Door to Hope
    Nueva Esperanza [40514]
    Womens Recovery Center [40515]
The Door • Runaway and Homeless Youth Program [36103]
Doors Into the Future Inc [46117]
Doorway to Recovery • Lakewood [50001]
Doorways LLC [10896]
Doorways for Women and Families [10554]
Dorcas House [8768]
Dorchester County Addictions Program [44209]
Dorchester County Commission on Alcohol and Drug Abuse [48980]
Dorchester House [44447]
Dorchester House Multi-Service [30367]
Doris A. Sanders Learning Center [7888]
Doris Cook Smith Counseling Center [29135]
Doris E. Reid Center [30527]
Doris Foster Independent Living Center [34036]
Doris Lasley and Associates • Substance Abuse Services [47435]
Dorminy Medical Center [1862]
Dorothea Dix Hospital [33741]

Dorothea Dix Psychiatric Center [30195]
Dorothea Leicher [48506]
Dorothy B. Mitchell Counseling Center [33965]
Dorothy Day House [9988]
Dorothy F. Kirby Mental Health Center [28590]
Dorothy Groce MFT [40007]
Dorothy Mitchell Residence [33966]
Dorothy Rose Psychotherapy Services [45929]
Dorothy's Star Home Health, LLC [18063]
Dorsey Hall Medical Center [4092]
Dorthea Dix Psychiatric Center [33552]
Dos Rios Counseling Inc • AACES [41207]
DOT Caring Centers Inc [44952], [44996]
Dothan City Schools [193]
Dothan Dialysis [22332]
Double Nine Home Health [13970]
Douglas County Day Services [29362]
Douglas County Family Support [9796]
Douglas County Hospital [2669]
    Mental Health Unit [31008]
Douglas County Mental Health Department • Community Support Program [31969]
Douglas County Mental Health Division--Canyonville [31935]
Douglas County Mental Health Division--Drain [31939]
Douglas County Mental Health Division--Reedsport [31968]
Douglas County Mental Health Division--Roseburg [31970]
Douglas County Public Health Services [6899]
Douglas Dialysis • DaVita [23682]
Douglas Gardens Community Mental Health Center [29224]
Douglas Gardens Hospice, Inc. [19256]
Douglas Hospital • Eating Disorder Unit [11265]
Douglas Mental Health Center [31025]
Douglas Place Inc [45138]
Douglas Speech Associates [1160]
Douglas Young Clinic [28750]
Douglas Young Youth and Family Services [28751]
Douglasville Dialysis • DaVita [23684]
Doug's House • Project Transitions, Inc. [21386]
Dove Center [10532]
Dove Counseling Inc [41125], [41198]
DOVE--Decatur [9219]
DOVE - Dewitt County Domestic Violence Program [9217]
Dove House, Inc. [8755]
DOVE, Inc.--Milton [9491]
DOVE, Inc.--Quincy [9500]
Dover Air Force Base [41504]
Dover Behavioral Health System [29059]
DOVES of Big Bear Valley, Inc. [8796]
DOVES--Chadron [9766]
DOVES--Gering [9770]
DOVES, Inc.--Danville [10562]
Dower and Associates Inc. [3593]
Down Syndrome Clinic
    Greenwood Genetic Center [10859]
    University of Maryland Department of Pediatrics and Genetics [10806]
Down Syndrome--Epilepsy Foundation • Down Syndrome Clinic [10777]
Downers Grove Dialysis Center • Fresenius Medical Care • Dialysis Center [23977]
Downey Community Mental Health Center [33140]
Downey Regional Dialysis Center, LLC [22662]
Downey Regional Medical Center [1094]
Downing Community Treatment Team • Mental Health Center of Denver [28882]
Downing House [3937]
Downriver Community Services, Inc. [6831]
Downriver Mental Health Clinic
    Advanced Counseling Services [45031]
    Advanced Counseling Services PC [45006]
Downstate Medical Center/State University of New York, Brooklyn • Dialysis Unit [25610]
Downstate Medical Center--SUNY [25611]
Downtown Dallas Dialysis • DaVita [27023]
Downtown Dialysis Center • DaVita [24639]
Downtown Emergency Service Center [32856], [50106]
Downtown Houston Dialysis Center • DaVita [27134]
Downtown Impact [40552]
Downtown Mental Health Center [28591]
Downtown San Antonio Dialysis & At Home • DaVita [27323]

Doylestown Dialysis Center • Fresenius Medical Care [26415]
Doylestown Hospital • Cancer Institute [5821]
Doylestown Hospital Home Care/Visiting Nurse Services [17298]
Doylestown Hospital Hospice [21077]
Doylestown Hospital • Penn Center for Sleep Disorders [37644]
DPPS Inc [47530]
Dr Carmine J Pecoraro Psy D and Assoc [42002]
Dr Donald T Stokes and Associates Inc [43686]
Dr Jerry Meints Family Counseling Inc • Breaking Free/Village Counseling [40346]
Dr Martin Luther King Jr Bronx Lebanon • Hospital/Chem Depend Outpatient Services [46417]
Dr Martin Luther King Jr Health Center • DWI Program [46418]
Dr Miriam/Sheldon G Adelson • Clinic for Drug Abuse Treatment Res Inc [45839]
Dr Sam Pirozzi LLC • Behavioral Health Counseling Therapy [46187]
Dr Suresh B Kodali and Associates • Chem Dep Treat w/ or w/o Adjunctive Me [43579]
Dr Warren E Smith Health Centers [48507]
Dracut Public Schools [2473]
Drake Center, Inc. [3219]
Drake Counseling [47581]
Drake Counseling Services Inc [45122], [47569]
Drake Residential Treatment Center [45123]
DRD Kansas City Medical Clinic [45517]
DRD Knoxville Medical Clinic [49106]
DRD New Orleans Medical Clinic Central [49107]
DRD New Orleans Medical Clinic [43869]
DRD Springfield Medical Clinic [45649]
Dream Care LLC [18070]
Dream Obtainers • Teens In Action Inc [43020]
The Dream Tree Project • Runaway and Homeless Youth Program [36084]
Dreams Inc [43357]
Drenk Center Children's Mobile Response and Stabilization System [31136]
Drenk Center Crisis House [31151]
Drenk Center Gateway Group Home [31144]
Drenk Center Outpatient Services [31152]
Drevets Counseling Services [43436]
Drexel Counseling Services Inc [42495]
Drexel Multiple Sclerosis Center [34688]
Drexel University • Center of Hope • MDA Clinic [34861]
Drexel University College of Medicine
    Drexel Sleep Center of Manayunk [37645]
    MDA/ALS Clinic [142], [34862]
    Saint Christopher's Hospital for Children • Marian Anderson Comprehensive Sickle Cell Center [36419]
Drexel University of Medicine
    Hahnemann University Hospital • Adult Cystic Fibrosis Center [7651]
    Saint Christopher's Hospital for Children • Pediatric Cystic Fibrosis Center [7652]
Drexler and Associates [2158]
DRG Fayette [25119]
DRH HomeCare, Hospice and Rehab [17114]
Drink/Link Moderate Drinking Progs and • Products [40779]
Driscoll Children's Hospital • Dialysis Unit [27006]
Driskill House [49560]
Driver Benefits Inc • Southwest Driver Benefits Program [40853]
Driver Safety Schools [40892]
    AM/PM Culver City Budget School [39771]
Drop Inn Center [47657]
Drug Abuse Alternatives Center
    Drug Court Counseling [40780]
    Outpatient [40781]
    Perinatal Day Treatment [40782]
    Redwood Empire Addictions Prog [40783]
    Turning Point [40784]
Drug Abuse Comprehensive Coordinating Office
    Brandon Outpatient Services [41574]
    Medication Assisted Treatment Prog [41958]
    Mens Residential Treatment Program [41959]
    Residential Treatment Facility II [41960]
    Tampa Outpatient [41961]
    Women Residential Treatment Program [41962]
    Womens Outpatient Services [41963]
Drug Abuse Foundation of Palm Bch Cnty
    Detox Program [41628]

Halfway House [41629]
Intensive Residential [41630]
Outpatient [41631]
Phoenix [41632]
Drug Abuse Prevention Center
Castle Rock [49921]
Womens Services/PPW STARS PCAP [50005]
Drug Abuse Treatment Association Inc
Data Outpatient Services [41671]
Outpatient [41754]
Residential [41672]
Walter D Kelly Treatment Center [41993]
Drug and Alcohol Rehab Service Inc • Manos House
[48426]
Drug and Alcohol Services of • Beaver Valley Inc
[48667]
Drug and Alcohol Treatment Service Inc • Outpatient
Services [48636]
Drug Alternative Program [39895]
Drug Recovery Inc • DBA Catalyst Behavioral
Services [47977]
Drug Rehabilitation Inc • Day One Residence
[43985]
Drug Testing and Counseling Services [41994]
Drugco Discount Pharmacy [16772]
Dry Creek Treatment Center [41126]
DSI--Blue River Valley • Dialysis Facility [24235]
DSI--Hazelcrest • Diversified Specialty Institutes
[24005]
DSI--Louisville • Dialysis Facility [24410]
Du Page County Health Department
Mental Health Division • Access and Crisis
Center [50856]
North Office Mental Health [29554]
Dual Solutions Continuum of Care [48120]
Duane Dean Behavioral Health Center [42730]
Duane R. Dornheim Transitional Living Facility
[31630]
Dubet Health Services [13971]
Dubin Learning Center [7825]
Dublin Counseling Center [31759], [47751]
Dublin Day Treatment Services [29414]
Dublin Veterans Affairs Medical Center [29415]
Albany Clinic [29328]
Dubnoff Center for Child Development & Educational
Therapy [34003]
Dubois Dialysis • DaVita • Dialysis Center [26416]
Dubois Medical Clinic [7451]
DuBois Regional Medical Center • Hahne Regional
Cancer Center [5823]
DuBois Regional Medical Center - Home Health
services [17301]
Dubois--Spencer--Perry Exceptional Children's
Cooperative [422]
Dubuque ENT Head and Neck Surgery [2204]
Dubuque Veterans Affairs Clinic [29861]
Duffy Health Center [6817]
Duffys Myrtledale Inc • Alcohol and Drug Recovery
Facility [39673]
Duhaney Home Health Care, Inc. [12987]
DUI and Addiction Counseling [42923]
DUI and Addiction Counseling Center [42797]
DUI Alternatives Treatment Center Inc [42496],
[42497]
DUI Assessments and Services Inc [42835]
DUI Community Counseling Inc [42498]
DUI Counseling Center
Bayrach Counseling Center [42965]
Bayrach Counseling Services [42499], [42932]
DUI Counseling Center/Carol Stream • Bayrach
Counseling Service [42444]
DUI Counseling Center • Cumberland Business
Center [42812]
DUI Counseling Center/Kendall Cnty • Bayrach
Counseling Services [42869]
DUI Counseling Center/Saint Charles • Bayrach
Counseling Services [42897]
DUI Counseling Center/Wilke Commons • Bayrach
Counseling Services [42389]
DUI Court Services by Comgraph [42674]
A DUI and Defensive Driving Schools [49037]
DUI Education and Prevention Group [43594]
DUI - Metropolitan Services Inc [42500]
DUI-Metropolitan Services Inc [42501]
DUI Professional Providers [42502]
DUI Resolutions [41778]
DUI Services • Family Counseling and Psychology
Center [42884]

Duke Community Hospice Services At the Meadow-
lands [20681]
Duke Family Care Program [47286]
Duke Fertility Center [22200]
Duke Health Community Care, Inc. [16717]
Duke Home Care and Hospice [20648]
Duke Home Care & Hospice-Hock Family Pavilion
[20649]
Duke Raleigh Hospital • Cancer Care Program
[5655]
Duke University Center for Palliative Care [20650]
Duke University • Eating Disorders Program [11174]
Duke University Health System, Inc. [16767]
Duke University Hospital
Cancer Center [5637]
Duke Center for Human Genetics [12307]
Duke University Medical Center
Adult Cystic Fibrosis Center [7629]
Centers for AIDS Research [64]
Dialysis Center [25853]
Division of Infectious Diseases • Adult AIDS
Clinical Trials Unit [23]
Division of Speech Pathology and Audiology
[3173]
Duke Comprehensive Cancer Center [4692]
In Vitro Fertilization Program [22201]
Lenox Baker Children's Hospital •
Comprehensive Chromosome Clinic [10839]
MDA Clinic [34847]
Pain Clinic [35589]
Pediatric Cystic Fibrosis Center [7630]
Sleep Disorders Center [37465]
Duke University Sports Medicine Center [38833]
Duke University/University of North Carolina • Sickle
Cell Center [36403]
Dulaney Towson Dialysis Center • DaVita [24734]
Dulce Esperanza Home Health Care, LLC [18091]
Duluth Clinic • MDA Clinic [34822]
Duluth Dialysis Center [23688]
Dumas Center [32448]
Dunamis Inc Group Home [39850]
Duncan Health Clinic [6228]
Duncan Regional Hospital Home Care & Hospice
[17115]
Duncanville Dialysis • DaVita [27052]
Duneland Dialysis--Knox • Liberty Dialysis [24185]
Duneland Dialysis--La Porte • Liberty Dialysis
[24188]
Dunkirk Veterans Affairs Clinic [31314]
Dunmore Dialysis • DaVita [26418]
Dunn Kidney Center Inc. • Fresenius Medical Care
[25851]
Dunn Memorial Hospital [14965]
DuPage County Psychological Services • Depart-
ment of Community Services [42963]
DuPage County Vet Center [51945]
DuPage Medical Group • Institute of Sleep Medicine
[36905]
Dupage Peritoneal Dialysis Services • Fresenius
Medical Care [23987]
DuPont Dialysis • Fresenius Medical Care [24141]
Dupont Veterans Affairs Healthcare Center [30067]
Duquesne University • Speech-Language-Hearing
Clinic [3366]
Dura Medical Equipment [14204]
Durango Counseling Center • Southwest Colorado
Mental Health Center, Inc. [28894]
Durango Dialysis Center • DaVita [23116]
Durango Orthopedic Associates • Pain Clinic
[35350]
Durant Dialysis • DaVita [26255]
The Durham Center [31524]
Adult Services [31525]
Crisis & Access Services [31526]
Durham Crisis Response Center [10033]
Durham Treatment Center [47287]
Durham VA Medical Center • VA Raleigh II Clinic
[47454]
Durham Veterans Affairs Medical Center [31527]
Durham West Dialysis & At Home • DaVita [25854]
Dusy Street Group Home [33082]
Dutchess County BOCES, Deaf/Hard of Hearing
[594]
The Dutchess County Department of Mental Hygiene
• Helpline [51150]
Dutchess Dialysis Center • Renal Research Institute
[25760]
Dutchess Intensive Day Treatment Program [31457]

Dutchess Speech Language Pathology Services
[3101]
Dutton House [28815]
Duval County Public Schools [350]
Duval Speech Services [1605]
The Duvall Home [7884]
DVA Renal Healthcare--DeRidder Dialysis • DaVita
[24483]
DVA Renal Healthcare--Donaldsonville Dialysis •
DaVita [24488]
DVA Renal Healthcare--New Orleans Uptown
Dialysis • DaVita [24553]
DVA Renal Healthcare--Sulphur • DaVita [24593]
D'Val Home Health Agency [13972]
DVSA Resource Center • Dove Center [9459]
DW Counseling Center LLC • DBA Desert Winds
Counseling [39405]
Dwayne A Hogan LADC LCSW [43926]
Dwayne M Cox LCDC [49562]
Dwight D. Eisenhower VA Medical Center [15135]
Dwight D. Eisenhower Veterans Affairs Medical
Center [29938]
Dwight David Eisenhower Army Medical Center •
Cancer Program [5025]
Dwight Orthopedic Rehabilitation Co. [38593]
Dyersburg Dialysis • DaVita [26832]
Dyersburg Hospital Corp. [17664]
Dyker Heights Dialysis Center • DaVita [25612]
Dykes Speech Associates [2766]
Dyna Care Northwest Indiana, Inc. [15033]
Dynamic Directions Counseling Inc [41036], [41253]
Dynamic Living Counseling Inc [39427]
Dynamic Speech and Language Communicators
[3555]
Dynamic Therapy Associates, Inc. [1870]
Dynamic Therapy Solutions [1198]
Dynamic Youth Community Inc
Daycare Unit [46496]
Outpatient Drug Clinic [46497]
Residence [46498]
Residential Drug Rehabilitation Prog [46634]
Dynasty Healthcare Services, Inc. [17979]

E

820 River Street Inc [46468]
Alcoholism Supportive Living Facility [46720]
Altamont House Inpatient Rehab Services
[46348]
CD Community Residence [46658]
CD Outpatient Clinic [47005]
CD Supportive Living [46322]
Community Residence [46667], [47130]
Eleanor Young Clinic [46323]
Halfway House for Women [46668]
Supportive Living Facility [47131]
E. Carlton Powell Hospice Center [20695]
E & L Health Services, Inc. [13973]
E M Jellinek Center [49108]
E Street House [28816]
E Town Addiction Solutions LCC [43580]
E.A. Hawse Health Center [7397]
EAC Inc • Outpatient Clinic [46690]
Eagan Dialysis • DaVita [25020]
Eagle Counseling Services Inc [40998], [41127],
[41340]
Eagle Health care Services [16768]
Eagle Health Services, Corp. [13877]
Eagle Home Medical Corp. [16773]
Eagle Lake Health Center [6773]
Eagle Pass Kidney Disease Clinic • Fresenius Medi-
cal Care [27054]
Eagle Recovery Services [43397]
Eagle Ridge Family Treatment Center [47939]
Eagle Ridge Institute • Alcohol and Drug Program
[48055]
Eagle's Gate Optimum Wellness and Physical
Therapy • Pain Clinic [35351]
Eagleville Hospital [48346]
Ear Laboratory--Mobile [915]
Ear Laboratory--Montrose [920]
Ear, Nose, and Throat Associates of Ashland [2253]
Ear, Nose and Throat Associates--Fort Myers [1576]
Ear, Nose and Throat Associates--Mountain Home
[1032]
Ear, Nose & Throat Associates, PC--Fort Wayne
[2144]
Ear, Nose and Throat Associates of Southeast Con-

Easter Seals Jolicolur School [34294]
Easter Seals of LaSalle and Bureau Counties [7962]
Easter Seals--Manchester, New Hampshire [8238]
Easter Seals McWhorter Family Children's Center [8523]
Easter Seals, Miami Dade [1653]
Easter Seals Miami-Dade - Child Development Center and Demonstration School [7894]
Easter Seals Pediatric Therapy [922]
Easter Seals Rehabilitation Center Northwest Alabama [921]
Easter Seals Rehabilitation Center--San Antonio [8565]
Easter Seals Rehabilitation Center--Wheeling [8610]
Easter Seals - Rio Grande Valley [8559]
Easter Seals--Rockford, Illinois • Children's Development Center [7968]
Easter Seals Society of Broward County, Inc. [1726]
Easter Seals Society of Central Illinois [7948]
Easter Seals Society of Volusia and Flagler Counties [1568]
Easter Seals South Florida [1766]
Easter Seals Stepping Stones Child Development Center [8623]
Easter Seals--UCP [1966]
Easter Seals UCP Center--Raleigh [8388]
Easter Seals UCP • NC and VA [47288]
Easter Seals-UCP--Peoria [7966]
Easter Seals--Villa Park, Illinois • DuPage Center [7974]
Easter Seals West Alabama [927]
Easter Seals West Kentucky [2294]
Eastern Aleutian Tribes Inc [39349]
Eastern Associates Speech & Language Services Inc. [3178]
Eastern Avenue Health Solutions Inc [44128]
Eastern Christian Children's Retreat [8285]
Eastern Colorado Veterans Affairs Healthcare System • PTSD Residential Rehabilitation Program [51701]
Eastern Connecticut Rehab Centers--Norwich [38198]
Eastern Connecticut Rehabilitation Center--Lisbon [38194]
Eastern Connecticut Rehabilitation Centers--Colchester [38189]
Eastern Connecticut Rehabilitation Centers--Dayville [38190]
Eastern ENT Sleep Diagnostics Centers [37466]
Eastern Home Health, Inc. [13387]
Eastern Idaho Regional Medical Center • Cancer Program [5053]
Eastern Iowa Sleep Center [36974]
Eastern Kansas HCS • Saint Joseph CBOC [45607]
Eastern Kansas VA Healthcare Systems • Substance Abuse Treatment Program [43389]
Eastern Kentucky Dialysis • DaVita [24437]
Eastern Long Island Hospital
    Quannacut Addiction Services [46670]
    Quannacut Alcoholism Detox Program [46671]
    Quannacut Outpatient Services [47019]
Eastern Maine Dialysis • ESRD Satellite Unit [24610]
Eastern Maine Medical Center • CancerCare of Maine [5269]
Eastern Maine Medical Center - Cystic Fibrosis Clinical Center [7558]
Eastern Maine Medical Center
    Dialysis Unit [24604]
    Genetics Program [12225]
Eastern Maine Medical Center/Maine Rehabilitation [2347]
Eastern Maine Medical Center
    MDA Clinic [34807]
    Sleep Center of Maine [37090]
Eastern Michigan Hemophilia Treatment Center • Hurley Medical Center [12536]
Eastern Michigan University • Speech and Hearing Clinic [2668]
Eastern Middlesex Alcoholism Services • Residential Rehab/Recovery House [44510]
Eastern MO Alt Sentencing Services Inc [45604], [45619]
        EMASS/Florissant CIP/Outpatient [45481]
        EMASS/Troy CIP/Outpatient [45659]
Eastern Montana CMHC • Substance Abuse [45696]
Eastern Montana Community Mental Health Center [30937]

Eastern Montana Community Mental Health Clinic
    Scobey Clinical Office [30964]
    Sidney Clinical Office [30966]
    Terry Clinical Office [30967]
    Wibaux Clinical Office [30970]
Eastern Montana Mental Health • Substance Abuse Dependency Services [45711]
Eastern Nebraska Community Action • Partnership Behavioral Health Services [45792]
Eastern Niagara Hospital • Lockport Site [46755]
Eastern North Carolina School for the Deaf [635]
Eastern Oklahoma Orthopedic Center [38913]
Eastern Oregon Alcoholism Foundation [48169]
Eastern Oregon Detoxification Center [48170]
Eastern Oregon Dialysis Clinic • Fresenius Medical Care [26328]
Eastern Oregon Psychiatric Center [33791]
Eastern Oregon Training Center [8443]
Eastern Oxygen and Medical Equipment, Inc. [18267]
Eastern Pennsylvania Down Syndrome Center [10856]
Eastern Regional Center [47549]
Eastern Shore Coalition Against Domestic Violence [10585]
Eastern Shore Community Services Board • Emergency Services [51413]
Eastern Shore Hospital Center [33558]
Eastern State Hospital [8049]
    Day Treatment Unit [30051]
Eastern State Hospital--Lexington [33524]
Eastern State Hospital--Medical Lake [33913]
Eastern State Hospital--Vinita [33789]
Eastern State Hospital--Williamsburg [33911]
Eastern Suffolk BOCES [583], [3093]
Eastern Virginia Medical School/Sentara Norfolk General Hospital • Sleep Disorders Center [37887]
Eastern Virginia Medical School • Speech and Hearing Clinic [3600]
Eastern Virginia Medical School/The Children's Hospital of the King's Daughters • Department of Pediatrics • Division of Medical Genetics [12360]
Eastern Wyoming Mental Health Center--Douglas [33038]
Eastern Wyoming Mental Health Center--Lusk [33055]
Eastfield Ming Quong [33997]
    Children's and Family Services [33982]
Easthaven Halfway House [45291]
Eastlake Dialysis • DaVita [23675]
Eastland Dialysis and At Home • DaVita [25213]
Eastman Day Treatment • Live Oak Day Treatment Center [29418]
Eastman Mental Health Center [29419]
Easton Hospital • Cancer Program [5825]
Easton Hospital Hospice [21080]
Eastover Psychological and • Psychiatric Group PA [47257]
Eastpointe Sampson County [51162]
Eastpointe Wayne County [51165]
Eastport Health Care, Inc. [6774]
Eastport Healthcare Inc [43957], [43966]
    Machias Center [44010]
Eastridge Health Systems • Berkeley County Office [50327]
EastRidge Health Systems • Jefferson County [32913]
EastRidge Health Systems--Martinsburg [32918]
EastRidge Health Systems • Morgan County [32888]
Eastside Center For Family • Former Eastside Addiction Professional [49892]
Eastside Community Mental Health Center [27851]
Eastside Domestic Violence Program [10605]
Eastside Health Services [40384]
Eastside Neighborhood Service • Family Violence Program [9615]
Eastside Sleep Diagnostic Center [37514]
Eastside Substance Abuse Clinic [44939]
Eastview Dialysis Inc. [25799]
Eastway Corporation • Family Center [47740]
Eastway Corporation of Greater Dayton • Adult Outpatient Services [31749]
Eastway Corporation
    Marshall House [31750]
    Shelby County Counseling Center [31834]
Eastway Corporation/Springfield Plaza • Eastco Production and Employment Services [31751]

Eastway Corporation/Twin Towers Plaza • Crisis Residential [31752]
Eastway Corporation • Webster Street Academy and Family Center [31753]
Eastwood Clinics [44708], [44717], [44732], [44733], [44773], [44987], [44994], [45005]
    Residential Substance Abuse Treatment Prog [44995]
Eastwood Day Treatment Center • Positive Education Program [31764]
Easy For You To Say [2898]
Eating Disorder Associates [11016]
Eating Disorder Center of California [10949]
Eating Disorder Center of Denver [10997]
Eating Disorder Center of Fresno [10950]
Eating Disorder Center of Missouri [11119]
Eating Disorder Clinic [11186]
Eating Disorder Counseling Services of the Greater Toronto Area [11216]
Eating Disorder Program [10912]
Eating Disorder Recovery Center [11120]
Eating Disorder Recovery Services [10951]
Eating Disorder Resource Center [11158]
Eating Disorders Action Group [11187]
Eating Disorders Anonymous [10897]
Eating Disorders Associates [10952]
Eating Disorders Center at San Antonio [11279]
Eating Disorders Counseling and Consulting Services [10953]
Eating Disorders Services [11217]
Eating Disorders Treatment Centers [11143]
Eating Disorders of York Region [11218]
Eating Dynamiks and Therapy [11219]
Eating Recovery Center [10998]
Eating Recovery and Wellness Center of Nevada [11134]
Eaton Canyon Recovery Services Inc • Eaton Canyon Treatment Center [40367]
Eaton Dialysis Center • DaVita [26105]
Eaton Street Center • The Providence Center [32172]
Eatonville Family Health Center [6524]
Eau Claire Academy [34483], [50379]
Eau Claire Behavioral Health [32968]
Eau Claire Metro Treatment Center [50380]
Eau Claire Psychiatry [32969]
Ebenezer Medical Services [13974]
Ebony Counseling Center [39633]
Ebony House Inc [39428]
Ecclesiastes Home Healthcare, Inc. [17980]
Echo Community Health Care, Inc. [6684]
Echo Horizon School [270]
Echo House Multi Service Center Inc [44129]
ECI-KEEP PACE [8551]
Ecker Center for Mental Health [50843]
Ecker Center for Mental Health--Elgin [29617]
Ecker Center for Mental Health • Psychiatric Emergency Program [29618]
Ecker Center for Mental Health--Saint Charles [29674]
Ecker Center for Mental Health--Streamwood [29679]
Eckerd Academy at Brooksville [29122]
Eckerd Camp E-Ku-Sumee [31514]
Eckerd Camp E-Ma-Henwu [31573]
Eckerd Youth Alternatives Inc • Eckerd Academy at Brooksville [41579]
Eclipse Home Health Care, Inc. [13417]
Economic Opportunity Family Health Center, Inc. • Family Health Center North, Inc. [6502]
Ed Medical [17677]
EDCO Program for the Deaf and Hard of Hearing [475]
Eddie Rochester Anderson Foundation • Rochester House [40107]
Edelman Westside Mental Health Center [28592]
Eden Hospital [1079]
Eden Institute [8268]
Eden Medical Center
    Behavioral Health [28426]
    Cancer Program [4764]
Eden Mens Program [45208]
Eden Prairie Dialysis • DaVita [25021]
Edenton Dialysis • DaVita • Dialysis Center [25858]
Edenwald--Gunn Hill Neighborhood Center [9903]
Edgebrook House--People Incorporated [30721]
Edgecombe HomeCare & Hospice [20749]
Edgefield Mental Health Center [32200]

Edgewater Systems for Balanced Living [33467]
New Life Center [29730]
Edgewood Center for Children and Families [34020]
Edgewood Cleveland Day Treatment [33188]
Edgewood Independent School District [816]
Edimar Home Health Care, Corp. [13975]
Edina Dialysis • DaVita [25022]
Edina Sleep Disorders Center [37216]
The Edinburg Center, Inc.--Arlington [30319]
The Edinburg Center, Inc.--Bedford [30327]
The Edinburg Center, Inc.--Lexington [30406]
The Edinburg Center, Inc.--Waltham [30474]
Edinburg Kidney Center • Fresenius Medical Care [27057]
Edinburg Regional Medical Center [32449]
Edison Clinic [6361]
Edith Nourse Rogers Memorial VA Hospital [15473]
Edith Nourse Rogers Memorial Veterans Hospital [30328], [51582]
EDM Treatment Center [44997]
Edmarc Hospice for Children [21716]
Edmond Dialysis Center • DaVita • Dialysis Facility [26256]
Edmond Family Counseling Inc • Outpatient Drug/ Alcohol Services [47927]
Edmonds School District • Deaf/Hard of Hearing Program [860]
Edmonson County Service Center [29985]
Edna Dialysis Center • DaVita [27059]
The Education Center at the Watson Institute [8485]
Education Play Station [1539]
Educational Alliance Inc
Pride Site I [46855]
Pride Site II/DA Inpt Rehab Prog [46856]
Project Contact/Outpatient Prog [46857]
Educational Resource Associates [8020]
Educational Resource Consultants [7773]
Educational Service [7868]
Educational Service Center of Central Ohio [651]
Educational Service District 112 • New Options Youth Recovery Program [50239]
Educational Service District 123 • Youth Recovery Program [50048]
Educational Service Unit Number 9 [2844]
Educational Services of Glen Ellyn [7955]
Educational Therapy [44659]
Educational and Treatment Council Inc. • Educational and Treatment Center • Runaway and Homeless Youth Program [35971]
Edunel Health Services [13976]
Edwain Fair Community Mental Health Center [3281]
Edward Health Services Corp. [14876]
Edward Hines Jr. VA Hospital [14819]
Edward Hines Jr. Veterans Affairs Hospital [51564]
Multiple Sclerosis Center [34568]
Edward Hines Junior Veterans Affairs Hospital • Spinal Care Center [4016]
Edward Hines Jr. Veterans Affairs Medical Center • PTSD Clinical Team [51724]
Edward Hospital [2076]
Cancer Program [5113]
Linden Oaks Eating Disorders Center [11044]
Edward Sleep Center [36906]
Edward W Sparrow Hospital • Substance Abuse Program [44881]
Edwards Assessments and • Counseling Inc [47473]
Edwards Speech Pathology Center [1124]
Edwardsville Dialysis • DaVita [23982]
Edwardsville Speech and Language Center [2021]
Edwin Fair Community Mental Health Center [8440]
Edwin Fair Community • Mental Health Center Inc [48008]
Edwin Fair Community Mental Health Center, Inc.-- Stillwater [31918]
Edwin Fair Community Mental Health Center-- Pawhuska [31909]
Edwin Fair Community Mental Health Center--Perry [31910]
Edwin Fair Community Mental Health Center--Ponca City [31911]
Edwin Fair Community Mental Health Center • Transitional Living Center [31912]
Edwin Shaw Hospital for Rehabilitation at Hudson [4363]
Edwin Shaw Hospital for Rehabilitation at White Pond [4364]

Edwina Daniels Home • JBS Mental Health Authority [27852]
Efe Healthcare Services, Inc. [17786]
Effective Living Center Inc [45184], [45292]
Effective Transitions Inc [47978]
Efficient Home Health Services Inc. [13197]
Effingham Dialysis • DaVita [23983]
Effingham North Dialysis • DaVita [23792]
Effingham Veterans Affairs Clinic [29614]
Effingham Victim Awareness Services [9224]
Effort Counseling Center [40484]
Effort Inc
Detoxification Program [40485]
Mental Health and Addiction Counseling [40486]
The Effort, Inc. [28728]
Egan Health Services--Bogalusa [15276]
Egan Health Services--Franklinton [15293]
Egan Health Services--Laplace [15319]
Egan Health Services--Terrytown [15372]
Egan Healthcare of the Northshore [15279]
Egan Healthcare Services [15328]
Egg Harbor Dialysis Center • Fresenius Medical Care [25427]
Egida Home Health Care Inc. [13033]
Egleston Children's Hospital Sports Medicine [38309]
Eglin Air Force Base/Alcohol and Drug Abuse Prevention and Treatment [41642]
Egyptian Public and Mental Health Dept [42442], [42653], [42694], [42876], [42907]
Eileen Nevers • Lenexa [43395]
Eisenhower Center [4161]
Eisenhower Memorial Hospital and Betty Ford Center • Cancer Data Systems [4824]
Eisenhower Memorial Hospital • Pain Management Clinic [35312]
EJAL Health Services Inc [44286]
El Bethel United Home Health Care Agency, LLC [18172]
El Cajon Treatment Center • East Office [39795]
El Camino Community College • Special Resource Center [306]
El Camino Dialysis Center [22831]
El Campo Dialysis [27060]
El Centro [9362]
El Centro de Amistad, Inc. [28423]
El Centro de Ayuda Corporation • Substance Abuse Treatment Center [40108]
El Centro del Pueblo [40109]
El Cerrito Dialysis Center • DaVita [22672]
El Dorado Audiology [991]
El Dorado Community Service Center
Inglewood Medical/Mental Health Services [39943]
Santa Clarita Med/Mental Health Services [40259]
El Dorado Council on Alcoholism • Lifeskills [40392]
El Dorado County Alcohol and Drug • Programs Tahoe Prevention Network [40808]
El Dorado County Community Health Center [6341]
El Dorado County Mental Health [28703]
Western Slope Day Rehabilitation [28704]
El Dorado House [40823]
El Dorado Texas Community Svc Center • Durham Street Clinic [49373]
El Dorado Women's Center [8869]
El Futuro Inc [47289]
El Hogar Community Services Inc [40487]
El Hogar Community Services, Inc. [28729]
Sierra Elder Wellness Program [28730]
El Milagro Dialysis Center • DaVita [26951]
El-Nido Residential [28369]
El Paso Center for Children [34450]
Runaway and Homeless Youth Services [36221]
El Paso Community College • Center for Students with Disabilities [784]
El Paso Community Mental Health/Mental Retarda- tion Center [32451]
El Paso County Division of • Detoxification and Substance Abuse [41057]
El Paso Kidney Center--East • Diversified Specialty Institutes [27065]
El Paso Kidney Center--West • Dialysis Facility • Diversified Specialty Institutes [27066]
El Paso Mental Health/Mental Retardation
Assertive Community Treatment [32452]
East Valley Outpatient Services [32453]
Mental Retardation Services [32454]

Solana Outpatient Services [32455]
El Paso Methadone Maintenance and • Detox Treat- ment Center [49323]
El Paso Prime Home Health, LLC [17909]
El Paso RDSPD [785]
El Paso Rehabilitation Center [8545]
El Paso Sleep Center [37814]
El Paso State Center [8546]
El Paso Veterans Affairs Health Care System [17910]
Multiple Sclerosis Center [34716]
El Paso Veterans Affairs Healthcare System [32456]
PTSD Clinical Team [51827]
El Primer Paso Counseling Services [45209]
El Proyecto del Barrio [40356]
El Pueblo Boys and Girls Ranch [41299]
El Pueblo Boys' and Girls' Ranch [34051]
El Puente del Socorro [9888]
El Refugio, Inc. [9887]
El Regreso Foundation Inc
Chemical Dependence Intensive Resid [46499]
Julio Martinez Ambulatory Care [46500]
Women Residential Drug Treatment Prog [46501]
EL Rincon Community Clinic [42503]
El Rio Santa Cruz Neighborhood Community Health Center, Inc. [6253]
El Shadai Home Health Care [13878]
El Tuque Primary Care Center [7209]
El Valor [7938]
Elaine Goodrich [44069]
Elaine Hopkins LCSW • Psychotherapy Services [45966]
Elan Home Health, Inc. [13125]
Elangeni [11061]
Elba House [39429]
Elbert County Mental Health Center [29420]
Elberton Dialysis Facility Inc. • DaVita [23694]
Eldercare Garfield Senior Activity Center [31131]
ElderCare Home Health Services [17736]
Eldorado Community Service Center • Euclid Medi- cal and Mental Health Services [40553]
Eldorado Texas Community Service Center [49483]
Eleanor Slater Hospital [33824]
Electric Mobility Corp. [16266]
Electrostim Medical Services, Inc. [14414]
Eleventh Hour • Rehabilitation Programs [39719], [39851]
Eleventh Judicial District ReEntry Inc [47496]
Elghammer Family Center Ltd [43014]
Elgin Mental Health Center [33419]
Eli Home Health Services, Inc. [18080]
Elijah Haven Crisis Intervention Center, Inc. [9293]
Elik Dialysis Home Therapy [27135]
Elim Christian School [7964]
Eliot Community Human Health Services [44455]
Eliot Community Human Services
Bedford Street [30407]
Bennett Street [30480]
Concord Road [30317]
Congregate Lodge [30412]
Northeastern Avenue [30355]
Old Concord Road [30362]
Princess Street [30472]
Satellite Residence [30418]
Willow Court [30320]
Wright Terrace [30318]
Elisabeth Ludeman Developmental Center [7965]
Elite Counseling • Deborah Judith Inc [49523]
Elite Healthcare Providers, LLC [14844]
Elite Home Care [12887]
Elite Home Care Services, Inc. [15604]
Elite Home Health Care, Inc.--Feasterville Trevose [17319]
Elite Home Health Care, Inc.--Warren [15872]
Elite Home Health, Inc. [13034]
Elite Homecare Services [15650]
Elite House of Sober Living Inc • Elite Treatment Center [42598]
Elite Physical Therapy and Sports Medicine [38659]
Elite Speech Therapy [1578]
Elite Sports Medicine Center [39102]
Eliza Coffee Memorial Hospital
Behavioral Health Center [27920]
Sleep Center [36580]
Elizabeth Anton [47244]
Elizabeth Buffman Chase House [10340]
Elizabeth City • Dialysis Center • DaVita [25859]

Elizabeth Dialysis & At Home • DaVita [26426]
Elizabeth Freeman Center [9498]
Elizabeth G. and Jennifer J. Hildebrant Hospice Care Center [20601]
The Elizabeth Hospice [18922]
Elizabeth House [29736]
Elizabeth Layton Center [43441], [43442]
Elizabeth Layton Center Ottawa [43428]
Elizabeth Levinson Center [8080]
Elizabeth Seton Pediatric Center [20584]
Elizabeth Stone House, Inc. [9483]
Elizabeth Straka Speech Associates [1387]
The Elizabeth Upjohn Community Healing Center [30579]
Elizabethtown Crisis Line [50932]
Elizabethtown Dialysis • DaVita • Dialysis Center [26428]
Elizabethtown Veterans Affairs Clinic [31316]
Elk City Dialysis • DaVita • Dialysis Facility [26258]
Elk Grove Dialysis • DaVita [22674]
Elk Grove Home Dialysis Center • Fresenius Medical Care [23985]
Elk Grove Speech--Language Solutions [1099]
Elkhart Clinic • MDA Clinic [34796]
Elkhart County Special Education Cooperative [420]
Elkhart County Women's Shelter [9272]
Elkhart General Hospital
    Cancer Program [5142]
    Center for Behavioral Medicine [43024]
Elkhorn Adolescent Treatment Center [48069]
Elkind Headache Clinic [12449]
Elko Dilaysis • Dialysis Clinic Inc. [25351]
Elko Family Medical and Dental Center [6948]
Elko Mental Health Center [31021]
Elko's Harbor House--Committee Against Domestic Violence [9788]
Elkton Treatment Center • CRC Healthgroup [44252]
Ellen O'Brien Gaiser Addiction Center [48310]
Ellensburg Crisis Line [51438]
Ellensburg Dialysis Center • DaVita [27602]
Ellenton GIP [19291]
Ellicott City Dialysis Center [24682]
Ellington Family Clinic [6903]
Elliot Health System • Elliot Regional Cancer Center [5498]
Elliot Hospital
    Center for Sleep Evaluation [37330]
    Pain Management Center [35554]
Elliot House [30428]
Elliott and Associates • Adolescent and Adult Outpatient Prog [41878]
Elliott Bay Kidney Center • Northwest Kidney Center [27635]
Ellis and Badenhausen Orthopaedics [38482]
Ellis Hospital Psychiatry [33724]
Ellis Medicine • Sleep Disorders Center [37391]
Ellisville Dialysis Center [25196]
Ellisville Hearing Center [2789]
Ellisville State School [8187]
Elm Avenue Health Center [7186]
Elm Lifelines [46057]
Elm Street Health Center [31691]
Elmbrook Family Counseling Center [32957]
Elmbrook Memorial Hospital
    Cancer Care Program [6146]
    Pain Rehabilitation Center [35774]
Elmcor Youth and Adult Activities Inc • Residential [46600]
Elmcrest Children's Center, Inc. [34358]
Elmer Platz Physical Therapy and Rehabilitation [38824]
Elmhurst College Speech--Language--Hearing Clinic [2026]
Elmhurst Home Inc [44734]
Elmhurst Hospital Center
    Alcoholism Outpatient Clinic [46625]
    Cancer Program [5575]
    Dialysis Unit [25653]
    Opiate Dependence Treatment Services [46626]
Elmhurst Memorial Home Health [14785]
Elmhurst Memorial Hospital
    Coordinated Oncology Program [5091]
    Department of Speech Pathology [2027]
    Guidance Services [42659]
Elmira Psychiatric Center [33693]
Elmira Veterans Affairs Clinic [31317]
Elmore Blackley Fellowship Home [47280]

Elmore County Domestic Violence Council [9181]
Elmshade [31361]
Elmwood Club Community Treatment Service [31484]
Eloise R. Johnston and Associates [1258]
Elsmar Home Health Care [15633]
Elwyn [8455]
Elwyn--Nevil Center for Deaf and Hearing Impaired [3359]
Ely Mental Health Center [31022]
Ely Veterans Affairs Clinic [31023]
Elyria Renal Care--Amherst • Fresenius Medical Care [26009]
Elysian Hospice, LLC [21440]
Emages Inc [42504]
Emal Home Health Care [13977]
Emanuel County Service Center [29493]
Emanuel Inpatient & Pediatric Dialysis • Fresenius Medical Care [26338]
Emanuel Medical Center • Cancer Center [4660]
Emanuel Services [16386]
Embassy Lakes Artificial Kidney Center • DaVita [23271], [23322]
EmberWood Center [43090]
Embrace Recovery [39972]
Embracing Hospice Care of New Jersey West, LLC [20465]
Embracing Hospice Inpatient Unit [19419]
Embracing Hospice-South Office [19408]
Embracing HospiceCare of New Jersey [20510]
Emerald City Shelters [9730]
Emerald Coast Center [1583]
Emerald Coast Hospice--Crestview [19210]
Emerald Coast Hospice-Pensacola [19297]
Emerald Dialysis • DaVita [23922]
Emerald Health Care Services [16286]
Emerald Sleep Disorders [37612]
Emerge! Center Against Domestic Abuse [8736]
Emerge! Center Against Domestic Abuse--Casa Amparo [8737]
Emerge! Center Against Domestic Abuse--Westhouse [8738]
Emergence [48060], [48090], [48095], [48100]
Emergence Addictions and • Behavioral Therapies [48101], [48250]
Emergency Battered Women's Shelter [8873]
Emergency Housing Consortium [35820]
Emergency Housing Group • Runaway and Homeless Youth Program [36104]
Emergency Mental Health Care • Grand Prairie Services [29629]
Emergency Mental Health Services [50794]
Emergency Psychiatric Services [51114]
Emergency Service Mental Health Center of Dane County [51509]
Emergency Shelter Program/Emergency Women's Shelter [8821]
Emergency Support Shelter [10624]
Emerson College • Thayer Lindsley Program [2454]
Emerson-Davis Family Development Center [31262]
Emerson Hospital [2472]
    Cancer Program [5330]
Emerson Hospital Home Care [15487]
Emery J. Lilge Hospice House [21414]
EMH Recovery Inc • Edwina Martin Recovery House [44429]
EMH Regional Healthcare System [16935]
EMH Regional Medical Center • Cancer Program [5719]
Emil Fries Piano and Training Center [3741]
Emily Home Care [13978]
Emily Program
    Anna Westin House [11102]
    Anna Westin House--Adolescent [11103]
Emily Program--Bandana Blvd., Saint Paul [11104]
Emily Program--Burnsville [11105]
Emily Program-- Como Avenue, Saint Paul [11106]
Emily Program--Duluth [11107]
Emily Program--Seattle [11302]
Emily Program--Stillwater [11108]
Eminence Healthcare Inc [39852], [39853], [39854], [39953], [40326], [40360], [40442], [40794]
Emmanuel Community Home Care [15895]
Emmanuel Counseling/Educational Services [50107]
Emmanuel House Inc • Recovery Program [44735]
Emmet County Office [29870]
Emmonak Women's Shelter [8660]
Emmorton Treatment Services [44093]

Emogene Dolin Jones Hospice House • Hospice of Huntington [21801]
Emory-Adventist Hospital [14585]
Emory Clinic of Otolaryngology [1818]
Emory Dialysis at Candler • Emory Healthcare [23676]
Emory Dialysis at Greenbriar [23593]
Emory Dialysis--Northside • Emory Healthcare [23594]
Emory Eastside Medical Center [1914]
    Cancer Program [5040]
Emory Health Enhancement Program [38310]
Emory Reproductive Center [22014]
Emory Sleep Center [36837]
Emory Tinnitus and Hyperacusis Center [1819]
Emory University
    Adult Cystic Fibrosis Center [7518]
    ALS Center [112]
    Grady Memorial Hospital • Burn Center [4538]
    Hemophilia Program Office [12508]
    Hope Clinic • HIV Vaccine Trials Unit [80]
Emory University Hospital [29348]
    Cancer Program [5007]
    Center for Rehabilitation Medicine [4003]
Emory University Hospital MidTown • Winship Cancer Institute [5008]
Emory University Hospital • Pain Management [35405]
Emory University
    Multiple Sclerosis Clinic [34564]
    Pediatric Cystic Fibrosis Center [7519]
    Rollins School of Public Health • Centers for AIDS Research [49]
    School of Medicine
        Department of Human Genetics Division of Medical Genetics [12189]
        Department of Neurology, MDA/ALS [34787]
Emory University School of Medicine
    Down Syndrome Center [10788]
    MDA/ALS Clinic [113]
Emory Valley Center Preschool [762]
Emotional Resource Center • Marlene Kastrinos PhD LCSW SAP [41779]
EMPACT Suicide Prevention Center [50653]
Empact • Suicide Prevention Center [8733]
Empi Inc. [15940]
Empire Home Health Agency [13979]
Empire Outpatient Services [40798]
Empire Recovery Center Inc [40425]
Empire State Hands-on Physical Therapy and Pain Center [38793]
Empire State Home Care Services [16387], [16550]
Employee Assistance Resource Services Inc • Drug Abuse Outpatient [47081]
Employee Counseling Associates Inc [47428]
Employee and Family Resources [2201]
Employment Resource Specialist [32119]
Emporia Veterans Affairs Community Based Outpatient Clinic [29918]
EmPower CTC [45274]
Empowerment Program [41128]
    It Takes a Village [40999]
EMQ Families First [28469]
Enable [3131], [8358]
Encinitas Dialysis • DaVita [22678]
Encinitas Learning Center [1100]
Encino Hospital Medical Center [28487]
Encino Tarzana Regional Medical Center [1103]
Endeavor House [46028]
Endeavor Place LLC [45333]
Energetics of Eating Associates [10954]
Enfield Dialysis Center • Fresenius Medical Care [23154]
England Counseling Services [51399]
England Health Center [6266]
Englewood Cliffs Physical Therapy [38722]
Englewood Dialysis Center • Fresenius Medical Care [25431]
Englewood Dialysis • DaVita [23117]
Englewood Health Systems--Arlington [14474]
Englewood Health Systems, Inc.--Albany [14469]
Englewood Hospice Care, Inc. [19340]
Englewood Hospital Home Health Services [16209]
Englewood Hospital and Medical Center • Dizzy Gillespie Cancer Institute [5512]
English Mountain Recovery [49185]
Enhanced Clinical Solutions Inc [42505]
    Eisenhower Tower [42770]

Sclerosis Center [34734]
Evergreen Pharmaceutical, Inc. [18462]
Evergreen Presbyterian Ministries, Inc. [8061]
Evergreen Satellite Office Outpatient Services [27910]
Evergreen Sleep Disorders Center [37910]
Evergreen Speech and Hearing Clinic Inc. [3628]
Evergreen Treatment Center [46112]
Evergreen Treatment Services
    Unit 1 [50109]
    Unit 2 [50110]
    Unit 3 [50111]
EverGreen Women's Health Care • Fertility Services [22156]
Every Woman's House [10183]
Every Woman's Place [9564]
    Runaway and Homeless Youth Services [36016]
Everywoman's Center • University of Massachusetts [9466]
Eve's Place [8732]
Evolution Group Inc [46232]
Ewing Residential Center [34300]
Exceed Home Health, Inc. [13373]
Exceed Home Health System [15597]
Excel Center of Fort Worth [49334]
Excel Group [50658]
Excel Home Health Plus, LLC [16929]
Excel Naturals [1729]
Excel Physical Therapy [38945]
Excel Primary Care & Sports Medicine [38350]
Excel Program [50654]
Excel Speech Therapy Center, APC [1259]
Excela Health Hospice [21091]
Excela Health • Latrobe Area Hospital • Pain Control Center [35641]
Excell Home Care [13111]
Excell Hospice [20956]
Excellence in Home Care [14415]
Excellence Home Health, Inc. [13981]
Excellent Healthcare Services, Inc. [17802]
Excellent Home Care Givers [13737]
Excellent Home care, Inc. [15837]
Excelsior House [28543]
Excelsior Springs Hospital [16007]
Excelsior Youth Center [34039]
Excelsior Youth Centers Inc [50168]
Excelth, Inc. • Excelth Primary Care Network [6756]
Exceptional Children's Foundation [7771]
Exclusive Home Health Services, Inc. [13656]
Executive Addictive Disease Progs Inc [41530]
Executive Voice Enterprises [955]
Exempla Behavioral Health Services at • West Pines [41350]
Exempla Lutheran Medical Center [19132]
    Comprehensive Cancer Program [4887]
    Sleep Disorders Laboratory [36724]
Exempla West Pines [33239]
Exercise Science Consultants [39161]
Exercise and Sport Research Institute • Department of Exercise Science and Physical Education • Arizona State University [38052]
Exeter Hospital [6958]
    Cancer Program [5495]
    Ears, Nose and Throat Otolaryngology and Audiology [2883]
Exodus Clinic LLC [46788]
Exodus Counseling and Treatment Services [50194]
Exodus Recovery Services [48124]
Exodus Transitional Care Facility Inc [50427]
Expert Home Care, Inc. [17320]
Experts Home Health [14323]
Experts Home Health Care [14206]
Exponents Inc • Outpatient Drug Abuse Clinic [46858]
Express Healthcare Inc. [12659]
Express Medical Equipment, Inc [16224]
Expressions Speech--Language Pathology Services, Inc. [1121]
Extant Counseling LLC [41278]
Extendacare Inc. [16597]
Extended Aftercare Inc [49374]
Extended Family Care of Lancaster [17363]
Extended Family Care of Pittsburgh [17435]
Extended Home Health Services, Inc. [13982]
Extended Nursing Personnel CHHA--Brooklyn [16388]
Extended Nursing Personnel CHHA--New York [16551]

Extendicare Home Health--Dyesburg [17665]
Extendicare Home Health--Henderson [17676]
Extendicare Home Health--Jackson [17682]
Extendicare Home Health--Martin [17724]
Extendicare Home Health--Paris [17767]
Exton Dialysis Center • DaVita [26434]
Extra Care Health Services [46051], [46146]
Extracare Home Health Services [15860]
Eye Bank Association of America [34979]
Eye Bank of British Columbia [34929]
Eye Bank of Canada--Ontario Division [35174]
Eye-Bank for Sight Restoration [35130]
Eyerly Ball Community Mental Health Center [29852]
Ezra Kreamer LCSW • Sojourn Float Center [43943]

F

1st Alternative Counseling [44319]
1st Choice Healthcare Services [13713]
1st Choice Hospice, LLC [21495]
1st Mending Point Inc [40886]
1st Northstar Home Health Service, Inc. [18116]
1st Star Counseling [41165]
1st Step Referral Services [45067]
4 Better Sleep [37795]
446 Scholl Home Health Care, Inc. [13411]
45th Street Medical Clinic [7384]
5 Star Home Care [13714]
59th Medical Wing Wilford Hall Medical Center [18031]
5th Street Medical Clinic [40821]
A F Whitsitt Center [44217]
Fabens Intermediate School District [786]
Faber Place Dialysis • DaVita [26689]
Face to Face Health and Counseling Services • Runaway and Homeless Youth Program [36034]
Face To Face Healthcare Services, LLC [17982]
Facing Change PA [43996]
FACT Team [33341]
FACTS/New Alternatives [47766]
Fagen Sports Medicine [37993]
Fahrman Center [50381]
Fair Haven Community Health Clinic, Inc. • Fair Haven Community Health Center [6424]
Fair Lawn Mental Health Center [51101]
Fair Oaks Dialysis & At Home • DaVita [27481]
Fair West Clinic [32461]
Fairbanks Community Behavior Health Center [28088]
Fairbanks Counseling and Adoption • Runaway and Homeless Youth Program [35787]
Fairbanks Crisis Line [50633]
Fairbanks Hospital [43091]
    Supportive Living Program 1st Step [43092]
Fairbanks Memorial Hospital
    Burn Care Unit [4503]
    Cancer Care Program [4741]
Fairbanks Memorial Hospital/Denali Center [12751]
Fairbanks Memorial Hospital • Home Health [12752]
Fairbanks Native Association • Ralph Perdue Center [39325]
Fairborn Dialysis • DaVita [26111]
Fairfax County Domestic Abuse Program • Fairfax County Artemis House [10553]
Fairfax County Health [3582]
Fairfax County Health Department • Joseph Willard Health Center • Pediatric Program [8582]
Fairfax County Office for Women • Domestic and Sexual Violence Services [10565]
Fairfax County Public Library • Access Services [3847]
Fairfax County Public Schools • Hearing/Visions Services [850]
Fairfax Cryobank [35252]
Fairfax Dialysis Center • Fresenius Medical Care [27482]
Fairfax-Falls Church Community Service Board • Woodburn Center for Community Mental Health [32705]
Fairfax/Falls Church Community Services Board [32730]
Fairfax-Falls Church Community Services Board • Crisis Care Facility/Gregory House [32698]
Fairfax-Falls Church Community Services Board • Crisis Care Facility/Leland House [32719]
Fairfax-Falls Church Community Services Board

Mount Vernon Center • Comprehensive Treatment and Recovery Program [32699]
    Northwest Center [32777]
    Springfield Outpatient Unit [32789]
Fairfax/Falls Church Community Services Board • Woodburn Center for Community Mental Health [32732]
Fairfax Hospital • Addictions Behavioral Health [49989]
Fairfax Hospital for Children • Pediatric Kidney Center [27483]
Fairfax Hospital Inova Transplant Center [27484]
Fairfax Methadone Treatment Center • (FMTC) [49756]
Fairfield Behavioral Health Services [48988]
Fairfield Center for Disabilities and Cerebral Palsy [8416]
Fairfield Counseling Services Inc [41383]
Fairfield County Community Health Center [7089]
Fairfield County Dialysis • Fresenius Medical Care [26782]
Fairfield County Sleep Center [36739]
Fairfield Dialysis Center • DaVita [22684]
Fairfield Home Dialysis • Dialysis Facility • DaVita [26114]
Fairfield Medical Center
    Cancer Program [5730]
    Southeast Ohio Sleep Disorders Center [37515]
Fairfield Memorial Hospital--Fairfield, IL [14791]
Fairfield Memorial Hospital--Winnsboro [17627]
Fairfield Visiting Nurse Association • Caretenders [16957]
Fairhill Community Office [31715]
FairHope Hospice and Palliative Care, Inc. [16958], [20852]
Fairland Institute [30755]
Fairland Institute--Adolescents [30756]
Fairlawn Rehabilitation Hospital [38576]
    Department of Communication Disorders [2542]
Fairleigh Dickinson University • Center for Psychological Services [8251]
Fairmont General Hospital • Cancer Program [6135]
Fairmont General Hospital Center for • Behavioral Health [50299]
Fairmont General Hospital, Inc. [18512]
Fairmont Medical Center [2693]
Fairmont Medical Center Hospice [20160]
Fairmont Medical Center-Mayo Health System [15904]
Fairmont Regional Sleep Disorders Laboratory [37950]
Fairmount Behavioral Health System [33816], [48508]
Fairveiw Health Services • MICD [45210]
Fairview Community Health Center [6725]
Fairview Developmental Center [7770]
Fairview Health Center [6208]
Fairview Heights Dialysis • Renal Advantage Inc. [23994]
Fairview Home Infusion [15914]
Fairview Homecare and Hospice [20181]
Fairview Homecare and Hospice-Princeton Area Hospice [20193]
Fairview Hospital Dialysis Center [24769]
Fairview Lakes Hospice [20194]
Fairview Lakes Medical Center [15949]
Fairview Medical Ctr. [8180]
Fairview Nursing Home • JBS Mental Health Authority [27855]
Fairview Recovery Services
    Adolescent/Adult Outpatient [45120]
    Adolescent Outpatient Program [45146]
    Adult Chemical Dependency Program [45145], [45211]
    Chisago Adolescent Chemical Dependancy [45112]
    Deaf and Hard of Hearing Program [45212]
Fairview Recovery Services Inc
    Addictions Crisis Center [46381]
    Fairview Community Residence [46382]
    Merrick Community Residence [46383]
    Supportive Living Residential [46384]
Fairview Recovery Services • Outpatient Program [45153]
Fairview Ridges • Adult Outpatient Program [45101]
Fairview Ridges Hospital • Oncology Services [5404]
Fairview Southdale Hospital

Cancer Center [5407]
Fairview Sleep Center [37218]
Fairview Treatment Center [43863]
Fairview University MC - Mesabi • Cancer Center [5409]
Fairview University Medical Center • Dialysis Unit [25044]
Fairview University Medical Center - Mesabi • Behavioral Health Services [30684]
Fairview University Medical Center • Riverside Campus Clinical Laboratory/Blood Bank [35083]
Fairweather Lodge--Greenland [31071]
Fairweather Lodge--Marquette [30596]
Fairwinds Treatment Center [11018], [29126]
Residential [41591]
Faith Community Hospice, LLC [21396]
Faith Family Recovery Center [45173]
Faith Farm Inc [45944]
Faith Home Care Services [15789]
Faith Home Healthcare [14956]
Faith Home Inc • Christian Alcohol and Drug Rehab [48951]
Faith Hospice--Grand Rapids [20061]
Faith Hospice, Inc.--Saint Louis [20333]
Faith Hospice--Irving [21499]
Faith Hospice of Oklahoma [20949]
Faith Hospice of Southern Oklahoma LLC [20920]
Faith Hospice of SW Oklahoma [20918]
Faith Hospice at Trillium Woods [20041]
Faith House/Dream House • Runaway and Home-less Youth Program [36053]
Faith House, Inc. [9411]
Faith House/New Leaf [8687]
Faith Mission • Crisis Center Inc [47085]
Faith Outreach Services [10368]
Faith Regional Health Services [16113]
Carson Cancer Center [4685]
Speech Language Pathology [2853]
Faithful Home Health Care [16225]
FaithTrust Institute [10644]
Falcon Ridge Ranch [49714]
Fall Mountain Counseling Center [31096]
Fallbrook Hospice [18926]
Fallcreek Counseling Services Inc [43093], [43094]
Falls Community Health [7252]
Falls County Kidney Center • Dialysis Facility [27247]
Falmouth Hospital • Cancer Program [5334]
Faltz Associates, Inc. Speech and Language Pathol-ogy [1206]
Familias Unidas [28418]
Familias Unidas Counseling Center [28419]
Families and Adolescents in Recovery [42902]
Families Against Battering [9916]
Families Against SIDS Tragedies [36561]
Families By Design [11019]
Families in Crisis, Inc.--McMinnville [10418]
Families in Crisis--Killeen [10481]
Families First--Campbell [33983]
Families First of Central Indiana • Substance Abuse Services [43095]
Families First--Davis [33985]
Families First of the Greater Seacoast [6966]
Families First, Inc. [10100], [29349]
Families First Inc.--Campbell [33130]
Families First Inc.--Dlayton Road, Concord [33137]
Families First Inc.--Fairfield [33143]
Families First Inc.--Fresno [33986]
Families First Inc.--Mount Diablo High School, Concord [33138]
Families First--Modesto [34000]
Families First--Oakland [34004]
Families First--Stockton [34032]
Families Living Violence Free [10070]
Families Matter LLC [46201]
Families in Transition [8787]
Families United [30199], [30226]
Families United of Maine [30209]
Families and Youth Inc. [31199]
Families and Youth, Inc. • Runaway and Homeless Youth Program [36085]
FamiliesFirst--Sacramento [34013]
Family Abuse Center [10517]
Family Abuse Services of Alamance County, Inc. [10020]
Family Abuse Services MHA of Westchester [9992]
Family Abuse Shelter of Miami County, Inc. [10178]
Family ACTS Incorporated [48373]

Family Addiction Community Treatment Services • DBA FACTS/New Alternatives [47781]
Family Advocacy Center [8715]
Family Advocates, Inc.--Iowa County Office [10697]
Family Advocates, Inc.--Platteville [10729]
Family Aides--Elmhurst [16443]
Family Aides, Inc.--Hicksville [16486]
Family Aides--Patchogue [16589]
Family Aides--Spring Valley [16630]
Family Assessment, Counseling, and Education Services--Fullerton [28509]
Family Assessment, Counseling, and Education Services--Santa Ana [28795]
Family Beginnings [22057]
Family Behavior Resources [8463]
Family Behavioral Center [11020]
Family Behavioral Center Inc [41633]
Family Behavioral Health PLLC [47537]
Family Care Center [30052]
Family Care Center/American Asian • Pacific Substance Abuse Program [40942]
Family Care Center of Carondelet [6916]
Family Care Certified Services of Brooklyn/Queens [16389]
Family Care Certified Services--Kew Gardens [16502]
Family Care Certified Services of Nassau [16487]
Family Care Choice and Services--Southfield [15809]
Family Care Connection LLC [46223]
Family Care Home Health [18595]
Family Care Home Health & Hospice Care [18281]
Family Care visiting Nurse and Homecare LLC--New Haven [13533]
Family Care Services, Inc. [13983]
Family Care Visiting Nurse and Home Care Agency LLC--Norwalk [13537]
Family Care Visiting Nurse and Home Care Agency, LLC--Stratford [13544]
Family Care Visiting Nurse and Homecare, LLC--Waterbury [13549]
Family Center [10745]
Family Center for Counseling and Educ [44590]
Family Center, Inc. [28996]
Family Center of Thomas Jefferson Univ • Special-ized Program for Preg Women [48509]
Family Centered Hospice [19481]
Family-Centered Services of Alaska [33960]
Family Centered Services of Alaska • Residential Diagnostic Treatment Center [28089]
Family Centers, Inc. [28987]
Family and Child Abuse Prevention Center--Port Clinton [10167]
Family and Child Abuse Prevention Center--Toledo [10176]
Family and Child Treatment of Southern NV • (FACT) [45840]
Family and Children First • DBA Georgia H O P E [42074]
Family and Children Services [40355]
Deaf and Hard of Hearing Program [1289]
Family & Children Services • Palo Alto Office [28692]
Family and Children Services • Substance Abuse Treatment Program [40657]
Family and Childrens Agency Inc • Project Reward [41456]
Family and Childrens Association
Hempstead Chemical Dependency Treatment Center [46691]
Hicksville Counseling Center [46696]
Family and Children's Association, Mineola • Runaway and Homeless Youth Program [36106]
Family & Children's Center [34484]
Family and Children's Center • The Children's Campus, Inc. • Runaway and Homeless Youth Program [35949]
Family and Childrens Center • Counseling and Development Services [43159]
Family & Children's Service, Altoona • Runaway and Homeless Youth Program [36105]
Family and Children's Service of the Capital Region • The Samaritans of The Capital District [51133]
Family & Children's Service of Midland [8176], [30604]
Family and Children's Service of Niagara • Runaway and Homeless Youth Program [36107]
Family and Childrens Services [48038]

Family & Children's Services Center [28006]
Family and Children's Services of Central Maryland
West Baltimore County Office [9442]
West End Place [9464]
Family and Childrens Services Inc [43047]
Family and Children's Services of Ithaca [31359]
Family and Childrens Services of Nantucket County Inc [44514]
Family and Children's Services • Passage Program [9967]
Family Circle Crisis Shelter [10374]
Family Comfort Hospice of Alabaster, LLC [18668]
Family Comfort Hospice-Fultondale [18716]
Family and Community Resources [9471]
Family and Community Service of Delaware County [32044]
Clifton Heights [48328]
Media [48464]
Family and Community Services of • Somerset County [45939]
Family Connection [42804]
Family Connection, Inc. • Runaway and Homeless Youth Program [35967]
Family Connections [46109]
Family Cord Blood Services [34945]
Family Counseling Associates--Lufkin [32505]
Family Counseling Associates--Nacogdoches [32519]
Family Counseling Center [45577], [45592], [49637]
Family Counseling Center of Brevard Inc [41913]
Family Counseling Center
DOC Outpatient/Charleston [45455]
DOC Outpatient/Steele [45654]
Family Counseling Center Inc [42942], [45436], [45489], [45498], [45641], [45675]
Adolescent CSTAR [45541]
Adolescent CSTAR Poplar Bluff [45587]
Ava Site [45434]
Cape Girardeau Office [45451]
CPRC [45542]
DOC Outpatient/Hayti [45490]
Family Counseling Center, Inc.--Elizabethtown • Har-din County Office [29619]
Family Counseling Center, Inc.--Golconda [29627]
Family Counseling Center, Inc.--Hayti • The Staple-ton [30852]
Family Counseling Center, Inc.--Kennett [30866]
Family Counseling Center, Inc.--Vienna [29683]
Family Counseling Center--Indiana, PA [32030]
Family Counseling Center • Malden [45562]
Family Counseling Center of Missouri [9671], [45483]
Family Counseling Center of Missouri Inc [45439], [45484]
Alcohol and Drug Treatment Services [45446]
Alcohol/Drug Treatment Services [45461]
Cedar Ridge Treatment Center [45560]
Daybreak Residential Treatment Center [45462]
Fayette Outpatient Clinic [45476]
Jefferson City Outpatient Clinic [45504]
McCambridge Center [45463]
Family Counseling Center for Recovery [49824]
Southlake [49825]
Family Counseling Center • Youth and Shelter Services Inc [43234]
Family Counseling of Occupations, Inc. [31435]
Family Counseling Recovery Centers [39546]
Family Counseling Service [10006]
Family Counseling Service of Aurora [42395]
Family Counseling Service of Northern Nevada Inc [45869], [45880]
Family Counseling Service of Orange County [9965]
Family Counseling Services [29214], [47078]
Family Counseling Services Cortland Cnty • Chemi-cal Dependence Outpatient Clinic [46604]
Family Counseling Services of the Finger Lakes Inc. [9924]
Family Counseling Services • Outpatient Drug Abuse Clinic [47181]
Family Counseling Services of Wausau [50555]
Family Counseling Services • West San Gabriel Val-ley [40647]
Family Counseling and Shelter Services [9558]
Family Crisis Center--Ada [10188]
Family Crisis Center of Baltimore County, Inc. [9443]
Family Crisis Center--Bastrop [10442]
Family Crisis Center of the Big Bend, Inc. [10437]
Family Crisis Center--Columbus [10451]

Family Crisis Center--Giddings [10466]
Family Crisis Center--Great Bend [9357]
Family Crisis Center, Inc.--Farmington [9868]
Family Crisis Center, Inc.--Harlingen [10469]
Family Crisis Center--Keyser [10676]
Family Crisis Center--Knoxville [10409]
Family Crisis Center--La Grange [10483]
Family Crisis Center of North Iowa, Inc. [9315]
Family Crisis Center of Prince George's County [9449]
Family Crisis Center--Stevens Point [10738]
Family Crisis Center of Walker, Dade, Catoosa, Chattooga Counties [9115]
Family Crisis Centers of Northwest Iowa [9346]
Family Crisis and Counseling Center [10191]
Family Crisis and Counseling Center Inc • DBA Turning Point Alcohol and Drug Center [47912]
Family Crisis Intervention Center [10680]
Family Crisis Network [10130]
Family Crisis Resource Center, Inc. [9451]
Family Crisis Service--Garden City • Domestic Violence Program [9356]
Family Crisis Services, Inc.--Canon City [8940]
Family Crisis Services--North Tazewell [10583]
Family Crisis Services--Portland [9434]
Family Crisis Shelter--Hilo [9134]
Family Crisis Shelter, Inc.--Crawfordsville [9268]
Family Crisis Shelter--Williston [10119]
Family Crisis Support Network [9318]
Family Crisis Support Services • HOPE House [10584]
Family Development/Intervention Srvs [47980]
Family of Ellenville [51138]
Family Fertility Center [22230]
Family First Counseling Center [45820]
Family First Home Health Care, Inc. [15832]
Family First Hospice [21453]
Family First Support Center [47272]
Family First Support Center Inc [47430]
Family Focus Counseling Service PC [49862]
Family Focus Home Health, LLC [16909]
Family Guidance Center [32115], [48706]
Family Guidance Center for Behav Hlthcare [45608] Maryville [45565]
Family Guidance Center for Behavioral Health Care [51060]
Family Guidance Center Corp • Substance Abuse Recovery Program [46012], [46188]
Family Guidance Center of Warren Cnty [46209]
Family Guidance Centers Inc [42396], [42506], [42624], [42697]
Family Guidance Services of Orange [32770]
Family Haven Crisis & Resource Center, Inc. [10496]
Family Health Care Clinic--Florence [6186]
Family Health Care Clinic, Inc.--Monticello [6891]
Family Health Care Clinic--Town Creek [6199]
Family Health Care Corporation [13738]
Family Health Center of Battle Creek [6835]
Family Health Center • Bayfront Outpatient Rehabilitation [3968]
Family Health Center--Bolton Village [6581]
Family Health Center of Boone County [6901]
Family Health Center--Cobb [6597]
Family Health Center, Fairdale [6728]
Family Health Center • Hamilton Medical Building [44382]
Family Health Center, Inc. [6850]
Family Health Center, Inc.--Laurel [6885]
Family Health Center--Louisville [6733]
Family Health Center of Marshfield • Marshfield Family Health Center [7431]
Family Health Center--Patagonia [6242]
Family Health Center • Psychological Services [44276]
Family Health Center--Salisbury [6921]
Family Health Center--Southwest [6734]
Family Health Center Taylorsville [6898]
Family Health Center--Waco [7316]
Family Health Center of Worcester, Inc. [6829]
Family Health Centers of Baltimore • Community Recovery Program [44131]
Family Health Centers, Inc.--Orangeburg [7240]
Family Health Centers--Okanogan [7380]
Family Health Centers of Southwest Florida, Inc. [6464]
Family Health Services Corporation • Twin Falls Clinic [6646]

Family Health Services of Coventry [7214]
Family Health Services--Cranston [7215]
Family Health Services of Darke County [7086]
Family Health Services--Jerome [6638]
Family Health Services--Twin Falls [6647]
Family Health and Sports Medicine [38996]
Family Health and Wellness Opportunity • Center [45964]
Family Healthcare [44651]
Family Healthcare Associates [39044]
Family Healthcare Center--Fargo • Homeless Health Services [7069]
Family Healthcare Center/Moorhead Dental [6870]
Family Healthcare--Chillicothe [7078]
Family Healthcare Network--Visalia [6375]
Family Hearing Center [1354]
Family Hearing Resource Centre/British Columbia Family Hearing Resource Centre [255]
Family Home Care and Hospice [21758]
Family Home Health Agency LLC [12894]
Family Home Health Care [2295]
Family Home Health Care Professionals [14731]
Family Home Health Care, SE [17778]
Family Home Hospice • UnitedHealthcare Nevada [20416]
Family Home Medical, Inc. [17392]
Family HomeCare and Hospice [21318]
Family Hospice--Belleville [19486]
Family Hospice--Boulder [19088]
Family Hospice Care [18987]
Family Hospice & Palliative Care [17436], [21136]
Family Hospice and Palliative Care [17341]
Family Hospice and Palliative Care - Anderson Manor [17437]
Family Hospice and Palliative Care-Berne [19586]
Family Hospice and Palliative Care - Forest Hills [17438]
Family Hospice and Palliative Care Service of the VNA Indiana County [21098]
Family Hospice of Punxsutawney • VNA of Indiana County [21149]
Family Hospice • Saint Joseph Regional Medical Center [19468]
Family House/Louisiana [43906]
Family House • Norristown [48487]
Family House Now [48510]
Family Institute of the Ozarks [30831]
Family Intervention Center [29048], [41487]
Family Life Abuse Center/Christian Appalachian Program [9396]
Family Life Center [9042], [39209], [39246], [39256], [39290]
The Family Life Center--SAFEHOUSE [9354]
Family Life Consultants [11045]
Family Life Mental Health Center [30672]
Family Lifeline • Oasis House • Runaway and Homeless Youth Program [36245]
Family Links [48587]
    Family Treatment Center [48588]
    Runaway and Homeless Youth Program [36181]
Family Matters of Greater Washington [9025]
Family Medical Center of Michigan [6860]
Family Medical Center of Michigan, Inc. [6838]
Family Medical Center at the Shores [6518]
Family and Medical Counseling Service [41531]
Family Medical and Dental Center [6532]
Family Medical Practice [6452]
Family Medicine Health Center [6632]
Family Mental Health Clinic of Westchester Jewish Community Services [31447]
Family Mental Health PA [47316]
Family Net of Catawba County [47381]
Family of New Paltz [51143]
Family Options Inc [43605]
Family Oriented Primary Health Care Clinic • Mobile County Health Department [6192]
Family Outreach Center • Outpatient Mental Health and Substance Use Disorder Prog [44807]
Family Outreach Program [31459]
Family Paths, Inc.--Fremont [28503]
Family Paths, Inc.--Hayward [28527]
Family Paths, Inc.--Oakland [28678]
Family Place [30539]
The Family Place [10453]
Family Planning Associates of San Antonio
    Ashby Family Planning Health Center [11947]
    Las Palmas Family Planning Health Center [11948]

    Marbach Sexual Health Center [11949]
    Southeast Sexual Health Center [11950]
Family Preservation Program [30053]
Family Preservation Services of North Carolina Inc [47373]
Family Prospective Resources, Inc. [30663]
Family Quality Home Health Care [13984]
Family Recovery Center
    Alcoholism Outpatient Clinic [46617]
    Fleming House [47791]
    Outpatient Program [47792]
Family in Recovery Program • Word 1 [48511]
Family Refuge Center [10677]
Family Renewal Shelter [10661]
Family Rescue [9205]
Family Resource Agency • Harbor Safe House [10396]
Family Resource Associates [41475]
Family Resource Center [45816], [50436]
Family Resource Center--Camden [10345]
Family Resource Center of Lincoln County [10616]
Family Resource Center of Seminole County [10211]
Family Resource Center of South FL Inc [41780]
Family Resource Center--Wytheville [10602]
Family Resource Centers [47761]
Family Resource Centers--Findlay [31768]
Family Resource Centers--Kenton [31785]
Family Resource Centers--Saint Marys [31830]
Family Resource Centers • We Care Center [47850]
Family Resource Counseling and • Learning Center Inc [44912]
Family Resources Associates Inc [50438]
Family Resources, Inc. [29886]
Family Resources, Inc.--Bradenton [50751]
Family Resources, Inc.--Pinellas Park [50781]
Family Resources, Inc.--Rock Island [9247]
Family Resources, Inc. • Runaway and Homeless Youth Program [35892]
Family Resources, Inc.: Sexual Assault/Domestic Abuse Advocacy [9342]
Family Resources of Rutherford County [10037]
Family Respiratory and Medical Supply Corp. [15415]
Family Restoration Services [45155]
Family Safety Network--Driggs [9171]
Family Safety Network--Walker [9643]
Family Self Help Center Inc • Lafayette House/Drug Court [45573]
Family Service [40027]
Family Service Agency [8780], [28162], [39406], [39430], [39431], [39565]
Family Service Agency of the Central Coast [50700]
Family Service Agency of Marin [50697]
Family Service Agency of Marin County • Substance Abuse Recovery Program [40706]
Family Service Agency • Runaway and Homeless Youth Program [36144]
Family Service Agency of San Bernardino [50690]
Family Service Assoc of Bucks County [48436]
    Georgetown Commons [48340]
Family Service Association [31100]
Family Service Association of Howard County, Inc. [9291]
Family Service Association of Santa Cruz • Suicide Prevention Service [50701]
Family Service Bureau of Newark • Gateway to Freedom Addiction Program [46092]
Family Service of Burlington County
    Florence Klemmer House [31153]
    Young Adult Services [31175]
Family Service and Children's Aid [30578]
Family Service and Childrens Aid [44626]
    Born Free [44862]
Family Service and Community • Mental Health Center for McHenry County [42773]
Family Service and Community Mental Health for McHenry County [29645]
Family Service Counseling of Wood County [31665]
Family Service of the Desert [28537]
Family Service of El Paso [32457]
Family Service Foundation Inc. • Outpatient Mental Health Clinic • Psychiatric Services for Deaf and Hard of Hearing Individuals [2417]
Family Service of Greater New Orleans [43870]
Family Service Inc
    Dearborn Office [44718]
    Downtown Detroit Office [44736]
    East District Office [44737]

Family Service, Inc.--Bagley, Detroit [30540]
Family Service, Inc.--Canton [30521]
Family Service, Inc.--Harper Avenue, Detroit [30541]
Family Service, Inc.--Southfield [30637]
Family Service, Inc.--Southgate [30638]
Family Service League [9349]
Family Service League Crisis Services [50909]
Family Service League
    Iovino South Shore Family Center [31238]
    Olsten Family Center [31357]
    Riverhead Family Center [31464]
Family Service League--Yaphank [31497]
Family Service of Long Beach [39651]
Family Service of Northwest Ohio [31844]
Family Service of the Piedmont [47343], [47388]
Family Service of the Piedmont, Inc. • Carpenter
    House [10047]
Family Service of Rhode Island [32173], [48873]
Family Service of Santa Monica [33193]
Family Service Thames Valley • Eating Disorders
    Program for Youth and Young Adults [11220]
Family Services Agency, Inc. [30288]
Family Services Alliance of Southeast Idaho [9183]
Family Services of Burlington County [31176]
Family Services Center [27950], [42325]
Family Services and Children's Aid, Inc. [30494]
Family Services and Childrens Aid Society [48376],
    [48491]
Family Services of the Cincinnati Area [47658]
Family Services of Davidson County [10053]
Family Services, Inc. [30534]
Family Services Inc.--Altoona [10263]
Family Services, Inc.--Poughkeepsie [9978]
Family Services League/Suffolk County Inc • Chemi-
    cal Dependency Outpatient [47020]
Family Services League of Suffolk County • Non
    Intensive Chemical Dep Prog [46374]
Family Services of McDowell County [10059]
Family Services of Montgomery County [32015]
Family Services of Napa Valley [28645]
Family Services of Northeast WI Inc [50462]
Family Services of Northeast Wisconsin [32976],
    [50399]
Family Services of Northeast Wisconsin, Inc.
    Crisis Center [51506]
    Runaway and Homeless Youth Program [36265]
Family Services of Northwest Ohio [31667]
Family Services of the Piedmont [10041]
Family Services Society of Yonkers [16681]
Family Services of Tulare County [8923]
Family Services of Westchester [31454]
Family Services of Western PA [48653]
Family Services of Western Pennsylvania [32056]
    Downtown Offices [32106]
    Family-Based Mental Health Services [32020]
    Maverick Drop In Center [32057]
Family Services--Winston Salem [10104]
Family Shelter Service [9258]
Family Shelter Services [9230]
Family Shelter of Southern Oklahoma for Victims of
    Domestic Violence [10190]
Family Speech Center [3018]
Family Speech and Therapy Services [2670]
Family Stress Center [28376]
Family Sunshine Center [8646]
Family Support Center--Chippewa Falls [10694]
Family Support Center--Colville [10614]
Family Support Services • Rape Crisis/Domestic
    Violence [10438]
Family Therapy Institute [47487]
Family Time Foundation, Inc. [10476]
Family Tree [8987]
Family Tree, Inc.--Gemini House • Runaway and
    Homeless Youth Program [35854]
Family Tree, Inc. • Runaway and Homeless Youth
    Program [35855]
Family United-N-New Beginnings Inc [39910]
Family Violence Center--Des Moines [9328]
Family Violence Center--Houston [10473]
Family Violence Center, Inc.--Green Bay • Golden
    House [10704]
Family Violence Center, Inc.--Springfield [9729]
Family Violence Coalition of Yancey County, Inc.
    [10021]
Family Violence Law Center [8858]
The Family Violence Prevention Center of Greene
    County [10184]
Family Violence Prevention Center of Orange

County [10023]
Family Violence Prevention, Inc. [8749]
Family Violence Prevention Program [10564]
Family Violence Prevention Project [9909]
Family Violence Prevention Services, Inc. [10504]
Family Violence Program, Inc. of Pitt County [10042]
Family Violence Program--Newark [9841]
Family Violence Project--Augusta [9427]
Family Violence Project--Gloversville [9926]
Family Violence Project--Van Nuys [8919]
Family Violence and Rape Crisis Services [10071]
Family Violence Task Force [10004]
Family of Woodstock [51155]
    Runaway and Homeless Youth Program [36108]
Family Works • Psychological Center [47331]
Family Works Psychological Center PLL [47518]
Family and Youth Alternative • A Program of Mental
    Health Systems Inc [39855]
Family and Youth Inc [46278]
    Stepping Stones Program [46279]
    Stepping Stones Programs [46280]
Family and Youth Intervention [28015]
FamilyCare HealthCenter--5th Avenue, Charleston
    [7400]
FamilyCare HealthCenter--Pennsylvania Avenue,
    Charleston [7401]
FamilyCord--Cambridge [35068]
FamilyCord--New York [35131]
FamilyCord--Palo Alto [34946]
FamilyCord--Southeast Region [35088]
Familylinks • Family Treatment Center [48589]
Farabaugh Chiropractic Clinic [38868]
Fargo Dialysis and At Home • DaVita [25990]
Fargo Veterans Affairs Medical Center [31627]
Faribault Area Hospice [20161]
Faribault Dialysis • DaVita [25025]
Farkas Associates [16227]
Farmers Branch Dialysis Center • Fresenius Medical
    Care [27080]
Farmington Bay Dialysis Center [27405]
Farmington Dialysis Clinic • Renal Advantage Inc.
    [25198]
Farmington Valley VNA Hospice Program [19164]
Farmington Veterans Affairs Clinic--C W Broadway
    [31194]
Farmington Veterans Affairs Clinic--W Columbia
    Street [30845]
Farmville Center [32733]
Farnham Family Services • Chemical Dependency
    Outpatient [46647], [46969]
Farnsworth Dialysis • Fresenius Medical Care
    [26065]
Farnum Center [45907]
Farrell Treatment Center [41427]
Farrington House • Mingus Mountain Academy
    [28143]
Farryl Dickter & Associates in Speech & Educational
    Therapy [1317]
Father Alfred Center • Saint Anthony Foundation
    [40604]
Father Ed Judy House [8951]
Father Flanagan's Boy's Home • Boys Town
    National Hotline [51074]
Father Flanagan's Boys Home of New Orleans •
    Runaway and Homeless Youth Program [35972]
Father Flanagan's Boys Town--Oviedo [33336]
Father Flanagan's Boys Town--Tallaahassee [33357]
Father Hudson House [20470]
Father Martins Ashley [44298]
Faulkner Hospital
    Addiction Recovery Program [44491]
    Audiology Service [2455]
    Cancer Program [5323]
    Sleep Health Center [37115]
The Fauquier Hospital, Inc. [18404]
Favor House of Northwest Florida, Inc. [9075]
Fawcett Memorial Hospital
    Cancer Program [4985]
    Chest Pain Center [35381]
Faxton Saint Luke's Healthcare • Audiology Services
    [3137]
Faxton St. Luke's Healthcare--Herkimer Satellite
    [25681]
Faxton--Saint Luke's Healthcare • Masonic Dialysis
    Unit [25793]
Faxton--Saint Lukes Healthcare • Oneida Dialysis
    Unit [25749]
Faxton-Saint Luke's Healthcare • Regional Cancer

Center [5622]
Faye Hogge Home [27956]
Fayette Cares Inc. [10433]
Fayette Counseling Center [29422]
Fayette County Board of Education [373]
Fayette County • Drug and Alcohol Commission Inc
    [48664]
Fayette County DUI Services [43659]
Fayette County Health Department Hospice-Vandalia
    [19579]
Fayette County Memorial Hospital [17066]
Fayette County School District [195]
Fayette Home Care and Hospice [17378], [21109]
Fayette Medical Center [12662]
Fayette Recovery Center [47877]
Fayetteville, Arkansas Veterans Affairs Medical
    Center [28268]
Fayetteville Dialysis • DaVita [23699]
Fayetteville Kidney Center • Fresenius Medical Care
    [25864]
Fayetteville VA Medical Center [4329]
Fayetteville VAMC [47308]
FDG Home Health Agency, Inc. [13985]
Feather River Home Health [13237]
Feather River Hospital • Cancer Center [4819]
Fedcap Home Care [16552]
Federal City Recovery Services [41532]
Federal Way Community Dialysis Center & At Home
    • DaVita [27605]
Federal Way Vet Center [52131]
Feeling Great
    Burlington Sleep Medical Center [37467]
    Jacksonville Sleep Medical Center [37468]
    North Durham Sleep Medical Center [37469]
The Felician School for Exceptional Children [8256]
Feliciana Center for Addictive Disorders [43819]
Feliciana Forensic Facility [33538]
Feliciana Home Health East [15269]
Feliciana Home Health South [15294]
Feliciana Home Health West [15352]
Felicianas Dialysis Center • Fresenius Medical Care
    [24509]
Fellowship Center • Alcohol and Other Drug
    Services [39810]
Fellowship Hall [47344]
Fellowship Health Resources Inc [47455]
Fellowship Health Resources, Inc.
    Community Continuum of Care Program [29062]
    Hope House Group Home [29067]
    Taton House Group Home [29068]
Fellowship House [41781]
    Detox/Rehab/OP/IOP/Prev/MISA/Gambling
    [42385]
Fellowship House Inc [39222]
    Fellowship House Supportive Living [46946]
Fellowship House Inc/Madonna House • Intensive
    Res Rehab for Woman w/Child [46756]
Fellowship House Inc
    Somerset House/Alcohol Halfway House
    [46361]
    Sundram Manor [46947]
Fellowship House, Inc.--Baltimore [30259]
Fellowship House--Miami [29215]
Fellowship of Lights, Inc. • Runaway and Homeless
    Youth Program [35992]
Fenix Outpatient Services [40936]
Fenton Dialysis Center • Affiliated Hospital Dialysis
    Center--Fenton [25200]
Fenton Dialysis • DaVita [24894]
Fenway Community Health Center [6802]
    Satellite [44414]
    Substance Abuse Treatment Program [44415]
Fenway Health • Fenway Institute • HIV Vaccine
    Trials Unit [85]
Fergus Falls Regional Treatment Center [33606]
Fergus Falls VA Outpatient Clinic [4219]
Fergus Falls Veterans Affairs Clinic [30677]
Fern Cottage [4073]
Fernandez Health Services [13986]
Fernandez Martin
    Gunsmoke [43458]
    Gunsmoke Dodge City [43334]
    Gunsmoke Garden City [43352]
Ferncliff Manor [8365]
Fernwood Counseling Center [32737]
Ferry County Community Services [51461]
Ferry Point Inc • Treatment Center [44317]

Fertility Center and Applied Genetics of Florida [21990]
Fertility Center of Assisted Reproduction and Endocrinology [21991]
Fertility Center of Colorado [21960]
The Fertility Center--Grand Rapids [22116]
The Fertility Center--Kalamazoo [22117]
The Fertility Center--Lansing [22118]
Fertility Center of Las Vegas [35105], [35106]
The Fertility Center--Las Vegas [22150]
Fertility Center of Maryland [22086], [22087]
Fertility Center of Northwest Ohio [22213]
Fertility Center of San Antonio [22258]
Fertility Centers of Illinois--River North IVF [22034]
Fertility Centers of Illinois, S.C. [22035]
Fertility Centers of New England [22157]
Fertility Centers of New England--Bedford [22158]
Fertility Centers of New England--Reading [22107]
Fertility and Endocrine Associates [22073]
The Fertility Experts [21992]
Fertility and Gynecology Center • IVF Clinic [21912]
Fertility Institute--Baton Rouge [22074]
Fertility Institute of Hawaii [22025]
    Hale Pawa'a [22026]
Fertility Institute--Metairie [22075]
Fertility Institute of New Orleans [22076]
Fertility & IVF Center of Miami [21993]
Fertility Physicians of Northern California [21913]
Fertility and Reproductive Medicine Center for Women [21994]
Fertility Resources Center • Appalachian Fertility and Endocrinology Center [22248]
Fertility Solutions--Cambridge [22108]
Fertility Solutions--Dedham [22109]
Fertility Solutions--Peabody [22110]
Fertility Solutions--Providence [22239]
Fertility Solutions--Woburn [22111]
Fertility Specialists of Houston [22259]
Fertility Treatment Center--Glendale • Northwest Valley Office [21895]
Fertility Treatment Center--Scottsdale [21896]
Fertility Treatment Center--Tempe [21897]
Fertility & Women's Health Center of Louisiana
    Lake Charles Memorial Hospital [22077]
    Rapides regional Medical Center [22078]
Fetal Diagnostic Institute of the Pacific [12192]
Few Steps [44738]
FHC Cumberland Hall--Chattanooga [33840]
FHC Cumberland Hall - Hopkinsville [33521]
FHCC • Substance Abuse Rehabilitation Program [42816]
FHN Family Counseling Center [42680]
FHN Hospice [19520]
FHN - Memorial Hospital [14797]
Fidelity Health Care [16926]
Fidelity Speech--Language Services LLC [2324]
FIEL Family and Sports Medicine [38053]
Fields and Fields Treatment Center [44244]
Fieldstone Center • Battle Creek Health Systems Department of Psychiatry and Behavioral Health [33589]
Fifth District Drug Court Inc [43877]
Fifth Generation Chem Dependency Prog [47550]
Fifth Street Counseling Center Inc • Outpatient [41897]
Fight Abuse in the Home [9098]
Filling Memorial Home of Mercy [8427]
Fillmore Family Resources [9631]
Findlay Hall Group Home • Oesterlen Services for Youth, Inc. [34386]
Findlay Program for the Hearing Impaired [656]
Fine Living Health Care Agency, Inc. [13657]
Finetech Home Health [13987]
FINEX House, Inc. [9484]
Finger Lakes Addictions Counseling and
    Referral Agency/Alc Crisis Center [46593]
    Referral Agency/Alc Outpatient Clinic [47168]
    Referral Agency/Alc Support Living Center [46594]
    Referral/Alc Outpatient Clinic [46651]
    Referral/Alcohol Outpatient Clinic [46936]
    Referral/Otte Hall [46937]
Finger Lakes Alcohol Counseling and • Referral Agency/Alcohol Outpatient Clinic [46595]
Finger Lakes Developmental Disabilities Service Office [8348]
Finger Lakes Migrant Health [7036]
Finley-Hartig Home Care [15079]

Finley Home Healthcare--Dubuque [15080]
Finley Home Healthcare--Galena [14798]
The Finley Hospital [2205]
Finley Hospital • Wendt Regional Cancer Center [5188]
Fircrest School--Shoreline [8605]
Fircrest School--Vancouver [8608]
Fire Mesa Dialysis • Fresenius Medical Care [25362]
Firefighters Regional Burn Center [4634]
Firelands Counseling/Recovery Services [47763], [47831], [47852]
Firelands Counseling & Recovery Services of Erie County [31653], [31832]
Firelands Counseling/Recovery Services • Seneca and Wyandot Counties [47864]
Firelands Dialysis Center--South • Firelands Regional Medical Center [26194]
Firelands Home Health Services [17034]
Firelands Regional Medical Center
    Cancer Centre/Main Campus [5748]
    Sleep Disorders Center [37516]
Firely Pediatric Home Care [17332]
First Accurate Home Healthcare Corporation [17983]
First at Blue Ridge Inc [47472]
First Call For Help--Alexandria [50941]
First Call For Help/Berkshire United Wayfield [50996]
First Call For Help--Des Moines [50903]
First Call For Help, Inc.--Kalispell • Help Net [51073]
First Call For Help--Itasca County [51039]
First Call For Help/United Way [50765]
First Call for Help [9900]
First Call for Help/Broward County [50756]
First Call for Help--Great Rivers 211 [51515]
First Call for Help, Inc.--Napoleon [51228]
First Call for Help--Pensacola [50779]
First Call for Help--Port Richey [50783]
First Call for Help--Victorville • Victor Valley Community Service Council [50705]
First Call Home Care & Hospice [18905]
First Care Health Services, Inc [18384]
First to Care Home Care, Inc. [16390]
First Care Home Health, Inc. [18322]
First Care Hospice-Fosston [20163]
First--Care of New York [16361]
First Choice Community Health Centers [7054]
First Choice DUI Services and • Evaluations [42913]
First Choice Health Centers [6420]
First Choice Healthcare [18071]
First Choice Healthcare Services, Inc. [17984]
First Choice Home Care [15774]
First Choice Home Care, Inc. [15737]
First Choice Hospice, Inc. [18705]
First Choice Primary Care Inc. [6595]
First Choice Recovery of Statesboro [42157]
First Coast Dialysis Center • Fresenius Medical Care [23342]
First Colonial--DaVita at Home • DaVita [27579]
First Colony Dialysis Center and At Home • DaVita [27367]
First Community Care [18238]
First Family HealthCare [39067]
First Home Health Care [13988]
First Home Health Care Services [14863]
First Hospital Panamericano [48750]
First Hospital Wyoming Valley [33806]
First Landing Dialysis Center • DaVita [27580]
First Light Counseling Services [43975], [43976]
First Nation Recovery Center [45213]
First Nations Community Healthsource [46233]
First Option Home Health [15309]
First Place [50006]
First Precision Healthcare Services [18103]
First Quality Healthcare [19349]
First Rapha Home Health, inc. [17931]
First Resources and Treatment - North [30530]
First Resources and Treatment - Southeast [30631]
First Resources and Treatment - Southwest [30652]
First Start Home Health Care [13989]
First Step [50968]
First Step: A Response to Domestic Violence, Inc. [10573]
First Step Adolescent Center [48154]
First Step Center • Crisis Center [46948]
First Step Comm Counseling Services LLC [49979]
First Step • A Community Counseling Resource Center [44223], [44329]

First Step--Coshocton • Family Violence Intervention Services, Inc. [10142]
First Step Counseling [46059]
First Step Counseling Center [49282], [49488]
    Midway Road Unit [49283]
First Step Counseling Inc [41286]
A First Step Counseling • Kopje [41819]
First Step Counseling Services /Brookings [48993]
First Step Counseling Services/SF [49020]
First Step Detoxification Unit [43842]
First Step Domestic Violence Services [10046]
First Step Farm of WNC Inc
    Mens Facility [47241]
    Womens Facility [47242]
First Step--Fostoria [10148]
First Step Home Inc • Residential [47659]
First Step House [49684]
First Step House of Orange County [39747]
First Step, Inc. [10520]
First Step Mercy Recovery Center • Mercy Franklin Center [43263]
First Step Perinatal Program [40226]
First Step--Plymouth [9568]
First Step Recovery [39949], [41029]
First Step Recovery Center Inc [44096]
First Step Recovery PLLP [47570]
First Step Recovery and Wellness Center [45755]
First Step of Sarasota Inc
    Detox Program [41926]
    Outpatient Program/Youth and Adult [41927]
    Outpatient Venice Office [41984]
    Residential Center [41928]
First Step Services LLC [47290], [47456]
First Steps [40971]
First Steps Detoxification Program [41363]
First Steps Pediatrics [2814]
First Steps to Recovery Inc
    CD Outpatient [46859]
    Outpatient Chemical Dependency Clinic [46502]
First Stop Home Care, Inc. [15634]
First Things First • Counseling and Consulting Ltd [50382]
First Things First Inc [47224]
    DWI Services of Wilkes [47514]
First Words Speech Services [1912]
First Words Speech Therapy Services [1948]
Firstat Nursing Services [16231]
FirstCall [15428]
Firstcare Home Health Services [13739]
FirstHealth Hospice and Palliative Care [20715]
FirstHealth Moore Regional Hospital • Cancer Program [5654]
Fisher Home for End-of-Life Care [19945]
Fisher-Titus Medical Center [17013]
    Cancer Program [5743]
Fit N Wise Rehabilitation Center [35694]
Fitchburg Veterans Affairs Clinic [30377]
Fitcorp Boston [38543]
Fite Center for Independent Living [400]
Fitness, Sports and Physical Therapy [38810]
Fitzgerald Physical Therapy Associates [38556]
Fitzgibbon - Mary Montgomery Hospice [20320]
Five Cities Speech and Language Therapy [1226]
Five County Mental Health Authority--Granville [31576]
Five County Mental Health Authority--Warren [31604]
Five Rivers Services, Inc. [32384]
Five Sandoval Indian Pueblos Inc • Behavioral Health Services Program [46249]
Five Star Dialysis Center and At Home • DaVita [25363]
Five Star Home Health Care, LLC [15619]
Five Stars Recovery Center [45111]
FLACRA Yates • CD Outpatient [46976]
Flagler Hearing Services [1744]
Flagler Hospital • Cancer Center [4989]
Flagler Institute for Rehabilitation [3969]
Flagler Outpatient Center • Oakwood Center of the Palm Beaches [33361]
Flagstaff Dialysis Center • Fresenius Medical Care [22434]
Flagstaff Medical Center Behavioral Health [28145]
Flagstaff Medical Center • Behavioral Health Services [39381]
Flagstar Home Health Services, Inc. [15873]
Flambeau Home Health & Hospice [21862]
Flanders Health Center [1456]

Flandreau Santee Sioux Tribe [48995]
Flatbush Surgical Supply [16446]
Flathead Community Health Center [6933]
Flathead Valley Chem Dependency Clinic [45705]
    Libby Office [45708]
    Thompson Falls Office Sanders County [45722]
Flatlands Guidance and Psychosocial Center [31263]
Fleming County Hospital [15176]
    Sleep Laboratory [37024]
Fletcher Allen Health Care [27440]
    Cancer Program [6047]
    Center for Disorders of Communication [3564]
Fletcher Allen Health Care Center • MDA Clinic [34896]
Fletcher Allen Health Care
    Children's Specialty Center
        Adult Cystic Fibrosis Center [7683]
        Cystic Fibrosis Center [7684]
        Multiple Sclerosis Center [34728]
        Vermont Regional Sleep Center [37877]
Fletcher Allen Healthcare--Chittenden County • Dialysis Unit [27446]
Fletcher Allen Healthcare--RRMC Satellite • Dialysis Unit [27443]
Fletcher Allen Healthcare Satellite--Barre • Renal Dialysis Facility [27438]
Fletcher Allen Healthcare Satellite--Saint Albans • Dialysis Unit [27444]
Fleur de Lis Dialysis • DaVita [24554]
Flint Community Schools [487]
Flint Dialysis • DaVita [24896]
Flint Odyssey House Inc [44784]
    Residential/Outpatient Program [44785]
Flint River Center [29487]
Flint Veterans Affairs Outpatient Clinic [30551]
Flo and Phil Jones Hospice House • St. Bernard's Development Foundation [18858]
Flordia Home Health Acquisition, LLC [13598]
The Florence Crittenton Agency, Inc. [32334]
Florence Crittenton Agency • Intensive Outpatient/ Pregnant [49109]
Florence Dialysis Center [22780]
Florence Dialysis Clinic • Fresenius Medical Care [26710]
Florence Genetic Center • Down Syndrome Clinic [10860]
Florence Veterans Affairs Clinic [30010]
Flores Home [31765]
Flores Home Health Care, Inc. [13990]
Floresville Dialysis • DaVita • Dialysis Facility [27081]
Florida Assertive Community Treatment Team [33290]
Florida Blood Services, Inc. [34985]
Florida Bureau of Braille and Talking Book Library Services [3761]
Florida Center for Addictions and Dual Disorders [29104]
Florida Center for Recovery Inc [41673]
Florida Centers of Sleep Medicine, LaVilla • Sleep Disorders Center [36782]
Florida Community Health Centers Corporate Office [6567]
Florida Department of Health • Family Health Services HSFFM • Florida SIDS Program [36464]
Florida Detox and Wellness Institute [41879]
Florida Ear and Balance Center [1556]
Florida Elite Home Care [14443]
Florida Family Home Health Care, Inc. [13991]
Florida First Health Services, Corp. [13992]
Florida Health Services [14264]
Florida Home Health [13603]
Florida Home Health Acquisition, LLC--Jupiter [13826]
Florida Home Health Acquisition, LLC--Orlando [14293]
Florida Home Health Acquisition, LLC--Sunrise [14394]
Florida Home Health Association [13993]
Florida Home Health Care Services, Inc. [13740]
Florida Home Medical Equipment [14294]
Florida Home Medical Equipment, Inc. [14242]
Florida Hospital Celebration • Sleep Disorders Center [36783]
Florida Hospital Deland [41623]
Florida Hospital • Dialysis Unit [23448]

Florida Hospital East Orlando • Sports Medicine-- Orthpedics [38263]
Florida Hospital Fish Memorial [14286]
Florida Hospital Flagler [14308]
Florida Hospital-Flagler • Flagler Cancer Center [4665]
Florida Hospital Heartland Medical Center [14384]
Florida Hospital Heartland Priority Health Care [14385]
Florida Hospital Home Care Services [14386]
Florida Hospital Memorial Hospice Care [19281]
Florida Hospital Memorial Systems • FHMMC Comprehensive Cancer Center [4937]
Florida Hospital North Pinellas [14432]
Florida Hospital Oceanside Inpatient Unit [19282]
Florida Hospital Rehabilitation and Sports Medicine [3970]
Florida Hospital Rehabilitation and Sports Medicine-- International Drive, Orlando [38264]
Florida Hospital Rehabilitation and Sports Medicine-- Lake Nona Road, Orlando [38265]
Florida Hospital • Sleep Disorders Center [36784]
Florida Hospital, South • Cancer Institute [4976]
Florida Hospital Tampa Bay Division • Tampa Sleep Center [36785]
Florida Hospital Volusia Home Care Services [14287]
Florida Hospital Waterman • Cancer Center [4999]
Florida Hospital Waterman Home Care Services [14433]
Florida Hospital Zephyrhills [14466]
Florida Institute for Neurologic Rehabilitation, Inc. [3971]
Florida Institute for Reproductive Medicine [21995]
Florida Institute for Reproductive Sciences and Technologies [21996]
Florida Institute of Sports Medicine [38275]
Florida Integrated Neurologic Group [3972]
Florida Keys Children's Shelter • Runaway and Homeless Youth Program [35893]
Florida Kidney Center • Fresenius Medical Care [23368]
Florida Lions Eye Bank Inc. [34986]
Florida Lung and Sleep Associates • Lehigh Pulmonary Associates [36786]
Florida Medical Associates--Daytona Beach [12398]
Florida Medical Associates--Orange City [12399]
Florida Medical Center • Hospice Inpatient Unit [19218]
Florida Nurses Home Health Agency [14265]
Florida Orthopaedic Institute [38291]
Florida Orthopedic Associates [38223]
Florida Parish Kidney Center • Fresenius Medical Care • Dialysis Services [24502]
Florida Pediatric Pulmonary Associates • Cystic Fibrosis Center [7501]
Florida Primary Health Center [7198]
Florida Renal Center • DaVita [23395]
Florida School for the Deaf and the Blind [355], [3702]
Florida Sheriffs Boys Ranch [34073]
Florida Sheriffs Youth Ranch • Safety Harbor [34081]
Florida Sheriffs Youth Ranches • Boys Ranch [33289]
Florida Sheriffs Youth Ranches--Bradenton/Sarasota [33291]
Florida Sheriffs Youth Ranches
    Caruth Camp [33309]
    Youth Camp [33287]
    Youth Villa--Bartow [33288]
Florida SIDS Alliance [36465]
Florida Sleep Institute • Sleep Disorders Center [36787]
Florida Sports Medicine Institute [38279]
Florida State Hospital [33296]
    Dual Purpose Facilities [7880]
Florida State University • L.L. Schendel Speech & Hearing Clinic [1771]
Florida Suicide Prevention Coalition [50766]
Florida Tissue Services [34987]
Florida Tropical Home Health Care, Inc. [13794]
Floridian Home Healthcare Corporation [13741]
Florin Dialysis Center • DaVita [22919]
Florissant Dialysis • DaVita • Dialysis Facility [25203]
Flossie Lewis Recovery Center • New Life Center [40028]

Flower Hospital • Northwest Ohio Sleep Disorders Center [37517]
Flower Hospital Rehabilitation Therapy Services • Speech/Audiology Services [3254]
Flowers Hospital [908]
    Cancer Program [4731]
    Sleep-Wake Disorders Center [36581]
Floyd Behavioral Health Center [42145]
Floyd Curl Dialysis • DaVita [27324]
Floyd and Floyd Associates [3403]
Floyd Heyman Hospice Care [19412]
Floyd Medical Center [1896], [14576]
    Cancer Program [5035]
    Pain Clinic [35406]
Floyd Memorial Hospital and Health Service • Cancer Program [5171]
Floyd Memorial Hospital and Health Services [15035]
Floyd Memorial Hospital • Sleep Laboratory [36947]
Floydada Outpatient Clinic [32458]
Flushing Dialysis • DaVita [24901]
Flushing Hospital and Medical Center
    Chemical Dependence Unit [46639]
    Reflections Outpatient Program [46640]
Flushing Hospital Medical Center • Renal Services • Outpatient Dialysis Facility [25664]
Flushing Manor Dialysis Center, LLC [25665]
Fluvanna Correctional Center for Women Dialysis Services [27576]
Flynn Fellowship Home of • Gastonia Inc [47320]
FM 1960 Speech, Language, and Myofunctional Therapy Center [3507]
F.M. Kirby Center • Summit Speech School [550]
FMC Balboa--Kearny Mesa Dialysis Center • Fresenius Medical Care [22935]
FMC--Belleair Home Therapies • Kidney Group of Clearwater LLC [23267]
FMCNA--Natchitoches DX • Dialysis Facility [24544]
F.M.R.S. Health System [32886]
FMRS Health Systems Inc [50303], [50306]
    Raleigh County Office [50283]
FMRS Health Systems, Inc. [32902], [32939]
FOCUS [10758], [28731]
Focus Care, Inc. [13126]
Focus Healthcare • Center for Eating Disorders [11270]
Focus Healthcare of Florida • High Point [41605]
Focus Healthcare of Tennessee [49051]
FOCUS House [29239]
Focus One Inc [41592]
Focus Physical Therapy, Inc. [38117]
Focus Psychological Associates Inc [48465]
Fola Community Action Services Inc [42507]
Foley Sleep Professionals [36582]
Follman Agency • Burlington [49920]
Fond Du Lac County • Department of Community Programs [50392]
Fond du Lac Dialysis Center [27715]
Fonda Veterans Affairs Clinic [31325]
Fontainebleau Treatment Center [43853]
Fontana Dialysis • DaVita [22686]
Food Addiction/Chemical Dependency [43997]
Food Addiction and Chemical Dependency Consultants LLC [44065]
Foot and Ankle Care of Boulder [38164]
Footco Orthopedic [38361]
Foothill AIDS Project [40522]
Foothill Family Service--El Monte [28486]
Foothill Family Service--Pasadena [28695]
Foothill Home Care, Inc. [13085]
Foothills Alliance [10342]
Foothills Family Service--Duarte [28477]
Foothills Hospital • Calgary Firefighters' Burn Treatment Centre [4506]
Foothills Mental Health Center of Alexander County [31600]
Foothills Neurology [12380]
Foothills Physical Therapy [38703]
Foothills Presbyterian Hospital • Citrus Valley Centers for Rehabilitation Services [1126]
Foothills Speech and Language [1107]
Footprints Beachside Recovery [41981]
For All Seasons, Inc.--Cambridge [50970]
For All Seasons, Inc.--Chestertown [50971]
For All Seasons, Inc.--Denton [50973]
For All Seasons, Inc.--Easton [50974]
Forbes Hospice [17439], [21137]
Forbes House [10166]

Forbes Norris ALS Research Center [1278]
Forbes Regional Hospital [17391]
Forbush School [30260]
Ford Factory Square Dialysis • DaVita [23595]
Henry Ford Hospital • Sladen Library K-17 [15635]
Ford Street Project Inc [40868]
Forensic Mental Health Services [30479]
Forensic Services [30054]
Forest City Medical Center • Behavioral Health [28271]
Forest Counseling Center [42728]
Forest County Potawatomi Domestic Abuse Program [10695]
Forest Fair Dialysis • DaVita [26120]
Forest Heights Lodge [7841]
Forest Heights Lodge School [34047]
Forest Hills Dialysis • DaVita [25975]
Forest Hills Hospital • Cancer Program [5578]
Forest Hills Speech Pathology Services PC [3022]
Forest Lake Dialysis • DaVita [25027]
Forest Oneida Vilas Counties Human • Services Center [50516]
Forest Park Dialysis Center • American Renal Associates [27548]
Forest Ridge Youth and Family Resource Services [33504]
Forest View Hospital [33595]
    Easting Disorders Program [11099]
Forest Warren Department of Human Services • People Place [32127]
Forever Caring Home Health and Companion Services [13127]
Forever Home Health Care, LLC [13658]
Forever Recovery [44655]
Forever Young Home Health Agency [13994]
Forgach House • Domestic Crisis Shelter [8731]
Forgey SportsMed & Rehabilitation Clinic [39154]
Forks Abuse Program [10621]
Forrest General Home Care--Hattiesburg [15965]
Forrest General Home Care--Lumberton [15970]
Forrest General Home Care--Prentiss [15976]
Forrest General Home Care--Tylertown [15981]
Forrest General Hospital [37246]
    Cancer Program [5425]
    Pine Grove Women's Center [11113]
Forsyth County Mental Health/Substance Abuse Outpatient Clinic [29400]
Forsyth Medical Center [16804]
    Cancer Program [5665]
Forsyth Sleep Center [37470]
Forsyth Sleep disorders Center • Northside Hospital [36838]
Forsyth Substance Abuse Services • Forsyth Medical Center [47538]
Forsythe County Family Haven [9102]
Fort Bayard Medical Center • Yucca Lodge [46302]
Fort Belknap • Chemical Dependency Program [45702]
Fort Bend County Sheriff's Office and Hearing Impaired Line • Communications Division [3534]
Fort Bend County Women's Center [10501], [51391]
Fort Bend Dialysis Center • Fresenius Medical Care [27265]
Fort Bend Family Health Center, Inc. [7306]
Fort Bend Regional Council on • Substance Abuse Inc [49503], [49544]
Fort Campbell Veterans Affairs Clinic [30013]
Fort Cobb Health Center [7105]
Fort Collins Salud Family Health Center [6404]
Fort Collins Vet Center [51905]
Fort Defiance Outpatient Treatment Center • Fort Defiance Agency Dawn of Recovery [39384]
Fort Dodge Veterans Affairs Clinic--2nd Avenue [29872]
Fort Dodge Veterans Affairs Clinic--Custer [29920]
Fort Duncan Home Health and Hospice Care [17901], [21447]
Fort Hamilton Hospital • Gebhart Center for Cancer Care [5726]
Fort Healthcare [18568]
    Behavioral Health [50394]
Fort Help LLC [40605]
Fort Help Mission Inc [40606]
Fort Howard VA Outpatient clinic [4093]
Fort Howard Veterans Affairs Clinic [30285]
Fort Lauderdale Artificial Kidney Center [23300]
Fort Lauderdale Hearing Center [1571]
Fort Lauderdale Hospital [33303], [41653]

Fort Lauderdale Renal Associates • DaVita [23301]
Fort Leonard Wood Veterans Affairs Clinic [30847]
Fort Lewis Army Community Services • Family Advocacy Program [10622]
Fort Logan Comprehensive Care [30117]
Fort Logan Comprehensive Care Center [43787]
Fort Madison Community Hospital [15084]
Fort McDowell Yavapai Nation • Wassaja Family Services [39385]
Fort Meyers South Dialysis • DaVita [23304]
Fort Mill Dialysis • DaVita [26714]
Fort Myers North Dialysis • DaVita [23305]
Fort Peck Tribal Dialysis Unit [25314]
Fort Sanders Dialysis • Fresenius Medical Care [26858]
Fort Sanders-Parkwest Medical Center • Cancer Program [5936]
Fort Sanders Regional Medical Center [17703]
    Sleep Disorders Center [37764]
    Thompson Cancer Survival Center [5937]
Fort Scott Veterans Affairs Community Based Outpatient Clinic [29922]
Fort Smith Public Schools--Hearing Impaired Program [244]
Fort Stockton Dialysis • AccessCare [27082]
Fort Walton Beach Medical Center • Cancer Program [4943]
Fort Wayne Neurological Center • Multiple Sclerosis Center [34577]
Fort Wayne State Developmental Center [7989]
Fort Wayne Womens Bureau Inc • Transitions [43048]
Fort Worth RDSPD [787]
Fort Yuma Alcohol and Drug Abuse • Prevention Program [40961]
Fortress Outreach [9678]
Fortuna Adventist Community Services • Humboldt Alcohol Recovery Treatment [39833]
Fortune Healthcare, Inc. [17985]
Fortune Society Inc [46762]
Fortwood Center, Inc. [32278]
    Adult Services [32279]
Forum Health Diagnostics - MRI [4365]
Forum Health
    Hillside Rehabilitation Hospital [35606]
        Department of Speech Pathology and Audiology [3257]
Forum Health Sickle Cell Program • Pediatric and Adult Sickle Cell Care [36413]
Forum Health Trumbull Memorial Hospital [4366]
Forum Health-Trumbull Memorial Hospital • Cancer Program [5756]
Forum Health • Youngstown Hemophilia Center • Regional Referral Center [12576]
The Forum School [8278]
Foster City Dialysis Center • DaVita [22690]
Foster Drive Dialysis Services • Fresenius Medical Care--West Baton Rouge [24461]
Foster Elementary School [7905]
Foster Home [27905]
Foster McGaw Hospital of Loyola--Transplant • Loyola University Health System [24036]
Fostoria Alcohol/Drug Center [47762]
Fostoria Community Dialysis Center [26121]
Fostoria Hospital Home Health Care [16941]
Foundation for Blood Research • Maine Institute for Human Genetics and Health [12226]
Foundation for Contemporary MH • The Next Step Program [41533]
Foundation for Exceptional Children [8172]
Foundation II Crisis Center [50901]
Foundation II • Youth Shelter • Runaway and Homeless Youth Program [35955]
Foundation for Living [47798]
Foundation for Multicultural Solutions • El Camino Program [50209]
Foundation Performance, Inc. [39000]
Foundation for the Retarded of the Desert [7802]
Foundations [48161]
Foundations Behavioral Health [32013]
Foundations Behavioral Health Services [31679]
Foundations Development House II [942]
Foundations LLC [50576]
Foundations Medical Services LLC [48311]
Foundations Recovery Center [31802], [47802]
Foundry Sports Medicine [39001]
Fountain Center of Fairmont [45148]
Fountain Center of Rochester [45275]

Fountain Center of Waseca [45340]
Fountain Centers [45070]
Fountain Dialysis Center • DaVita [23120]
Fountain Health Clinic [6406]
Fountain House [31412]
Fountain House Inc. [31413]
Fountain House North Supervised Residence [31414]
Fountain of Life Home Health [18105]
Fountain of Life Home Health LP [17904]
Fountain Recovery [40002]
Fountain Valley Regional Hospital and Medical Center • Orange County Regional Cancer Center [4775]
Four Bridges Creative Living Center [28367]
Four Circles Recovery Center [47390]
Four Corners Community Behav Hlth Inc [49660]
    Emery County Office [49602]
    MOAB Clinical Office [49635]
Four Corners Community Behavioral Health--Castle Dale [32578]
Four Corners Community Behavioral Health--Moab [32593]
Four Corners Community Behavioral Health--Price [32609]
Four Corners Community Mental Health Center [34456]
Four Corners Dialysis Center • DaVita [25545]
Four Corners Dialysis Clinic--Cortez • DaVita [23107]
Four Corners Home Health, Inc. [16315]
Four Corners Sleep Disorders Center [36725]
Four County Counseling Center [43141], [43190]
    Cass Satellite [29770]
    Center Cass County Office [29771]
    Four County Comprehensive Mental Hlth [43175]
    Fulton County Satellite [29812]
    Miami County Satellite [29799]
    North Street Office [29772]
    Pulaski County Satellite [29834], [43231]
    Residence [29773]
    Residence--Group Home [29774]
    Spear Street Office [29775]
    Stepping Stones [29776]
    Supported Employment [29777]
Four County Family Center--Defiance [31755]
Four County Family Center--Montpelier [31813]
Four County Family Center--Napoleon [31816]
Four County Family Center--Wauseon [31855]
Four County Mental Health Center [43368]
Four County Mental Health Center--Coffeyville [29914]
Four County Mental Health Center • Coffeyville [43325]
Four Freedoms Dialysis • DaVita [23376]
Four Oaks, Inc.--Cedar Rapids [29846]
Four Oaks, Inc.--Des Moines [29853]
Four Oaks, Inc.--Mason City [29882]
Four Oaks, Inc.--Monticello [29885]
Four Rivers Behavioral Health--Benton [29976]
Four Rivers Behavioral Health--Clinton [29993]
Four Rivers Behavioral Health--Fulton [30019]
Four Rivers Behavioral Health/Lakes • Center/Benton/Calloway/Marshall County [43729]
Four Rivers Behavioral Health--Mayfield [30075]
Four Rivers Behavioral Health--Murray [30087]
Four Rivers Behavioral Health--Paducah [30095]
Four Rivers Behavioral Health--Smithland [30112]
Four Rivers Behavioral Health • William H Fuller Memorial Substance AbuseCenter [43709]
Four Rivers Dialysis Center & At Home • DaVita [26335]
Four Rivers Home Health Care, Inc. [16079]
Four Rivers Hospice [19448]
Four Rivers Resource Services [7998]
Four Rivers Special Education District [401]
Four Seasons Hospice and Palliative Care [20662]
    Elizabeth House [20663]
Four Seasons Rehabilitation Inc. [3573]
Four Winds Family Recovery LLC • Topeka [43464]
Four Winds Hospital--Saratoga [33723]
Four Winds Hospital--Westchester [33698]
Four Winds Ranch Recovery Center for Adolescent Females LLC [47940]
Four Winds Recovery Center Inc [46267]
Fourth Street Dialysis Center • DaVita [27231]

Fowler House • North Central Mental Health/Satellite [47717]
Fowler Sports Medicine and Orthopaedics [38014]
Fox Chase Cancer Center [5849], [17409], [21127]
Fox Home Care Services [15810]
Fox Home Medical [17726]
Fox Run Hospital [33758]
Fox Valley Dialysis [23896]
Fox Valley Hospice [19522]
Fox Valley Orthopaedic Institute [38376]
Fox Valley Pastoral Counseling Center [32946]
Fox Valley Speech and Swallowing Center [1959]
Framingham Veterans Affairs Clinic [30381]
Framingham Wellness Center [44470]
Frances Haddon Morgan Center [8597]
Frances Mahon Deaconess Hospital [16087]
      Pain Management Program [35535]
Frances Nelson Health Center [6650]
Frances Schervier Home and Hospital LTHHCP [16362]
Francis Allen School for Exceptional Children [1024]
Francis X. Gallagher Services [8105]
Franciscan Children's Hospital and Rehabilitation Center
      Kennedy Day School [8115]
      Pediatric Rehabilitation Program [8116]
Franciscan Health Support, Inc [16510]
Franciscan Health System [18469]
Franciscan Hospice [21776]
Franciscan Hospice Care [19149]
Franciscan Occupational Health • Outpatient Physical Therapy and Sports Rehabilitation [39151]
Franciscan Saint Anthony Health [2138]
Franciscan Skemp Behavioral Health • Villa Success [50507]
Franciscan Skemp Healthcare [32982]
      Cancer Program [6156]
      Womens LAAR House [50430]
Franciscan Skemp Hospice • Mayo Health Clinic [21845]
Franciscan Sports Medicine Center • Dayton Campus [38873]
Franconia Dialysis Center • DaVita [27454]
Frank & Helen DeScipio Hospice House-Tavares [19323]
Frank Murano LCSW LCADC [46043]
Frank R. Howard Memorial Hospital [13451]
Frankford Avenue Health Center [7175]
Frankfort Habilitation [8044]
Frankfort Hearing Impaired Program [418]
Frankfort Regional Medical Center • Central Kentucky Sleep Center [37025]
Franklin C. Fetter Family Health Center [7225]
Franklin Commons Dialysis • DaVita [26596]
Franklin County Board of Education [208]
Franklin County Family Resource Center [10594]
Franklin County Home Health Agency [21663]
Franklin County Schools [624]
Franklin Dialysis Centers & At Home • DaVita [26515]
Franklin Home Care [15292]
Franklin Hospital Medical Center • Cancer Program [5623]
Franklin Hospital Medical Center--Lynbrook • Home Health Agency [16514]
Franklin Memorial Center Speech and Hearing Center [2483]
Franklin Memorial Primary Health Center, Inc. [6193]
Franklin Primary Health Center [39275]
Franklin Regional Medical Center--Louisburg [16749]
Franklin Square Hospital Center [2673]
      Cancer Program [5282]
Franklin Square Hospital • Sleep Disorders Center [37100]
Franklin Veterans Affairs Clinic [31533]
Franklin VNA & Hospice [20435]
Fraser Center [42108]
Fraser Health Authority--Delta • Eating Disorders Program [10913]
Fraser Health Authority--Port Coquitlam • Eating Disorders Program [10914]
Fraser School [8181]
Frazer Center • Child Development Program [7910]
Frazier Rehab Institute [4060]
Frazier Rehab Institute--Springhurst [38483]
Fred Brown Recovery Services Inc [40692], [40693]
      19th Street Services [40694]
Fred E. McGilberry & Associates, Inc. [17831]

Fred Hutchinson Cancer Research Center • Comprehensive Cancer Center [4716]
Frederick County Health Department • Substance Abuse Services [44266], [44267]
Frederick House [29788]
Frederick Institute [44268]
Frederick Memorial Healthcare System • Regional Cancer Therapy Center [5303]
Frederick Memorial Hospital Home Health [15438]
Frederick Memorial Hospital
      Mount Airy Rehabilitation Services [2421]
      Rose Hill Rehabilitation [2411]
Frederick Renal Care [24686]
Frederick Sport and Spine Clinic, Inc. [38526]
Fredericksburg Dialysis Center • Fresenius Medical Care [27490]
Free at Last
      Intensive Outpatient Unit [39790]
      Malaika House [39791]
      Walker House [39792]
Free Library of Philadelphia • Library for the Blind and Physically Handicapped [3833]
The Free Medical Clinic of Greater Cleveland [51205]
Free Medical Clinic of • Greater Cleveland [47686]
Freedom Dialysis Center • Fresenius Medical Care [26711]
Freedom Healthcare Services [48304]
Freedom Home Health, Inc. [14295]
Freedom Hospice-Arlington [21383]
Freedom House [39288], [44808], [46003], [47345]
Freedom House Lake Area [47436]
Freedom House--Princeton [9243]
Freedom House Recovery Center
      Chapel Hill Outpatient Clinic [47245]
      Crisis Center [47246]
      Durham Access Center [47291]
      Francis Street Womens Halfway House [47292]
      Transitional Living [47293]
Freedom House--Weatherford [10518]
Freedom Institute Inc • Alcoholism Outpatient Clinic [46860]
Freedom Lake Dialysis Center • Fresenius Medical Care [25855]
Freedom Nursing Services [13659]
Freedom Recovery Center [49906]
Freedom to Speak [1672]
Freedom Village Psychosocial Club [31319]
Freeman Center
      Mens Residential [49573]
      Outpatient Unit [49574]
      Womens Residential [49575]
      Youth Outpatient Services [49576]
Freeman Health System
      Cancer Program [5444]
      Sleep Disorders Center [37275]
Freeman Nephrology and Dialysis Center [25218]
Freeman Sports Medicine Center [38658]
Freeport Clinic [6465]
Freeport Dialysis Satellite • Dialysis [23995]
Freeport Kidney Center • DaVita [25667]
Freeport Pride Inc [46643]
Freeport West, Inc. • Project Solo • Runaway and Homeless Youth Program [36035]
Fremont Alliance [10761]
Fremont Area Medical Center [20381]
      Cancer Program [5472]
Fremont Community Health Services, Inc. [6868]
Fremont Counseling Service [50587], [50595]
Fremont Counseling Service--Lander [33051]
Fremont Counseling Service--Riverton [33062]
Fremont County Group Homes • Runaway and Homeless Youth Program [36279]
Fremont County Public Health Department [7454]
Fremont Dialysis Center • Innovative Dialysis Centers [26124]
Fremont Family Medical Center [6390]
Fremont Hospital [33144], [39836]
Fremont RE--1 School District [320]
Fremont Regional Hospice [19089]
Fremont - Rideout Health Group [13458]
Fremont-Rideout Hospice [19082]
Fresenius Dialysis Services--Kaukauna [27727]
Fresenius Dialysis Services--Neenah [27762]
Fresenius Dialysis Services of Oshkosh [27769]
Fresenius Medical Care--Abbeville • Dialysis Facility [24452]
Fresenius Medical Care--Abilene [26931]

Fresenius Medical Care--Abington Inc., Willow Grove • Dialysis Facility [26612]
Fresenius Medical Care--Adrian [24824]
Fresenius Medical Care--Aguadilla • Dialysis Facility [26621]
Fresenius Medical Care--Airline • Dialysis Services [24462]
Fresenius Medical Care--Akron East • Dialysis Facility [26004]
Fresenius Medical Care--Akron West [26005]
Fresenius Medical Care--Albemarle • Dialysis Facility [25814]
Fresenius Medical Care - Alexander City [22305]
Fresenius Medical Care--Alexandria • Dialysis Services [24453]
Fresenius Medical Care--Alice [26934]
Fresenius Medical Care--Allegan • Dialysis Facility [24825]
Fresenius Medical Care--Allen [26935]
Fresenius Medical Care--Allentown • Dialysis Services [26364]
Fresenius Medical Care--Aloha Dialysis Center [23847]
Fresenius Medical Care--Alpharetta [23778]
Fresenius Medical Care--Altoona • Dialysis Facility [26370]
Fresenius Medical Care--Amarillo [26939]
Fresenius Medical Care--Amite • Dialysis Services [24455]
Fresenius Medical Care--Anchorage [22417]
Fresenius Medical Care--Andalusia [22306]
Fresenius Medical Care--Anderson [24112]
Fresenius Medical Care--Anderson Dialysis Clinic Inc. [26676]
Fresenius Medical Care--Ann Arbor [24995]
Fresenius Medical Care--Ann Arbor West [24829]
Fresenius Medical Care--Anne Arundel [24622]
Fresenius Medical Care--Anson County [25966]
Fresenius Medical Care--Antelope Valley [22749]
Fresenius Medical Care--Apache Junction • Dialysis Center [22423]
Fresenius Medical Care--Apex [25815]
Fresenius Medical Care--Appleton • Dialysis Care [27697]
Fresenius Medical Care--Aransas Pass [26942]
Fresenius Medical Care • Arcadia Dialysis Center [22473]
Fresenius Medical Care--Ardenwood • Dialysis Facility [22837]
Fresenius Medical Care--Ardmore • Dialysis Facility [26248]
Fresenius Medical Care--Arecibo • Dialysis Facility [26623]
Fresenius Medical Care--Arrowhead Dialysis [22440]
Fresenius Medical Care--Ascension [24570]
Fresenius Medical Care of Asheboro Inc • Dialysis Facility [25816]
Fresenius Medical Care--Ashland County [26012]
Fresenius Medical Care--Ashland • Dialysis Facility [24360]
Fresenius Medical Care--Astoria [26312]
Fresenius Medical Care--Atlanta [23645]
Fresenius Medical Care--Atlanta Downtown [23596]
Fresenius Medical Care--Atlantic City • Dialysis Center [25401]
Fresenius Medical Care--Atlantis [23235]
Fresenius Medical Care of Auburn [22309]
Fresenius Medical Care of Augusta Inc. [23611]
Fresenius Medical Care--Austintown [26015]
Fresenius Medical Care--Auxilio Mutuo Dialysis Center [26652]
Fresenius Medical Care - Avondale Dialysis [22425]
Fresenius Medical Care--Avondale • Dialysis Services [24456]
Fresenius Medical Care--Awhatukee [22474]
Fresenius Medical Care of Ayden [25818]
Fresenius Medical Care--Bainbridge [23623]
Fresenius Medical Care--Bakersfield [22595]
Fresenius Medical Care--Balboa--Marina Bay [22632]
Fresenius Medical Care--Baldwin [24834]
Fresenius Medical Care--Barataria [24531]
Fresenius Medical Care--Bardstown [24363]
Fresenius Medical Care--Bartlett [26805]
Fresenius Medical Care--Bastrop [26960]
Fresenius Medical Care--Batesburg Leesville [26738]
Fresenius Medical Care--Baton Rouge • Dialysis

Services [24463]
Fresenius Medical Care--Battle Creek North [24836]
Fresenius Medical Care--Battle Creek South [24837]
Fresenius Medical Care--Baxter Street, Charlotte [25834]
Fresenius Medical Care--Bay Minette [22310]
Fresenius Medical Care--Beatties Ford • Dialysis Facility [25835]
Fresenius Medical Care--Beaumont [26966]
Fresenius Medical Care--Beaverton [26313]
Fresenius Medical Care--Beckley [27662]
Fresenius Medical Care - Bellflower [22605]
Fresenius Medical Care--Belton Honea Path [26731]
Fresenius Medical Care--Belzoni [25102]
Fresenius Medical Care--Benton • Dialysis Facility [22527]
Fresenius Medical Care - Berkeley [22608]
Fresenius Medical Care--Berwick [26379]
Fresenius Medical Care--Berwyn [23899]
Fresenius Medical Care of Bethlehem • Dialysis Services [26381]
Fresenius Medical Care--Bewick [24871]
Fresenius Medical Care--Bexar County [27325]
Fresenius Medical Care--Big Rapids [24841]
Fresenius Medical Care--Birmingham [22317]
Fresenius Medical Care--Blackstone Valley [24781]
Fresenius Medical Care--Bloomfield [25406]
Fresenius Medical Care----Blue Ridge • Dialysis Facility [27463]
Fresenius Medical Care • Blue Springs Dialysis Center [25173]
Fresenius Medical Care--Blythe Desert • Dialysis Facility [22611]
Fresenius Medical Care--Blytheville • Dialysis Facility [22531]
Fresenius Medical Care • BMA--Northeast Washington [23220]
Fresenius Medical Care--Boardman [26022]
Fresenius Medical Care--Bolivar [25174]
Fresenius Medical Care--Bon Carre [24464]
Fresenius Medical Care--Boone County [24378]
Fresenius Medical Care--Boston Carney [24764]
Fresenius Medical Care--Botsford Park [24935]
Fresenius Medical Care--Bowling Green • Dialysis Facility [27466]
Fresenius Medical Care--Boynton Beach Gulf Stream [23249]
Fresenius Medical Care--Brandywine • Dialysis Facility [23203]
Fresenius Medical Care--Brawley [22612]
Fresenius Medical Care--Breaux Bridge [24473]
Fresenius Medical Care--Breman [23627]
Fresenius Medical Care of Brentwood [22614]
Fresenius Medical Care--Brevard [23382]
Fresenius Medical Care--Bridgeport [23923]
Fresenius Medical Care--Bridgeton [25177]
Fresenius Medical Care--Brighton [24843]
Fresenius Medical Care--Bristol • Dialysis Facility [26807]
Fresenius Medical Care--Brookhaven • Dialysis Facility [25106]
Fresenius Medical Care--Bruceton Mills [27666]
Fresenius Medical Care--Bryan [26025]
Fresenius Medical Care--Buchanan Road, Antioch • Dialysis Facility [22588]
Fresenius Medical Care--Buena Creek [23062]
Fresenius Medical Care--Bullhead City • Dialysis Center [22426]
Fresenius Medical Care--Bulloch County [23794]
Fresenius Medical Care--Bunkie • Dialysis Services [24474]
Fresenius Medical Care • Burbank Dialysis [22616]
Fresenius Medical Care--Burke County • Dialysis Facility [25914]
Fresenius Medical Care--Burlington [25825]
Fresenius Medical Care--Cadillac [24844]
Fresenius Medical Care--Cahaba Valley [22387]
Fresenius Medical Care--Calallen [27007]
Fresenius Medical Care--Caldwell Parish • Dialysis Services [24476]
Fresenius Medical Care--Calexico Desert • Dialysis Facility [22618]
Fresenius Medical Care--Camarillo • Dialysis Center [22620]
Fresenius Medical Care--Cambria [26516]
Fresenius Medical Care--Camden • Dialysis Facility [26684]

Fresenius Medical Care--Camellia • Dialysis Facility [22347]
Fresenius Medical Care--Camp Hill [26392]
Fresenius Medical Care--Camp Springs • Dialysis Facility [24732]
Fresenius Medical Care--Campbellsville [24366]
Fresenius Medical Care--Canovanas [26628]
Fresenius Medical Care--Canton [23908]
Fresenius Medical Care of Canton • Dialysis Facility [25108]
Fresenius Medical Care - Capitol City [22375]
Fresenius Medical Care of Carbon County • Dialysis Facility [26468]
Fresenius Medical Care--Carbondale [23909]
Fresenius Medical Care--Care Cheraw [26693]
Fresenius Medical Care • Carlsbad Dialysis [25541]
Fresenius Medical Care--Carmel [24121]
Fresenius Medical Care--Carolina • Dialysis Facility [26630]
Fresenius Medical Care--Carrollwood [23532]
Fresenius Medical Care - Carson [22624]
Fresenius Medical Care--Cartersville • Dialysis Facility [23639]
Fresenius Medical Care--Casa Grande • Dialysis Facility [22427]
Fresenius Medical Care--Caswell [25984]
Fresenius Medical Care--Cedar Park [26992]
Fresenius Medical Care--Centerpoint [25214]
Fresenius Medical Care--Centerville [26810]
Fresenius Medical Care--Central Delaware [23188]
Fresenius Medical Care • Central Fort Worth Dialysis Center [27085]
Fresenius Medical Care--Central Illinois Bloomington Home [23900]
Fresenius Medical Care--Central Illinois Pekin [24063]
Fresenius Medical Care--Central Ohio • Dialysis Center [26078]
Fresenius Medical Care--Central Ohio East • Dialysis Center [26079]
Fresenius Medical Care • Central Phoenix Dialysis [22475]
Fresenius Medical Care--Central Richmond • Dialysis Facility [24442]
Fresenius Medical Care--Centre Point • Dialysis Facility [27804]
Fresenius Medical Care--Centreville • Dialysis Facility [25110]
Fresenius Medical Care--Century [23262]
Fresenius Medical Care--Chabersburg [26399]
Fresenius Medical Care - Chambers [22362]
Fresenius Medical Care--Champlin [25012]
Fresenius Medical Care - Chandler [22429]
Fresenius Medical Care--Channel Islands • Dialysis Center [22865]
Fresenius Medical Care--Chanute • Dialysis Facility [24312]
Fresenius Medical Care--Charleston [27668]
Fresenius Medical Care--Charlestown [27677]
Fresenius Medical Care/Chase Dialysis Center [22353]
Fresenius Medical Care - Chatham Dialysis Center [23709]
Fresenius Medical Care--Chattahoochee Valley [23652]
Fresenius Medical Care--Chehalis [27599]
Fresenius Medical Care--Chester • Dialysis Facility [26694]
Fresenius Medical Care--Chesterfield [24850]
Fresenius Medical Care--Cheyenne • Dialysis Center [27811]
Fresenius Medical Care--Chicopee [24760]
Fresenius Medical Care--Chouteau [25270]
Fresenius Medical Care--Christiana • Dialysis Facility [23197]
Fresenius Medical Care/Chula Vista Dialysis Center, South [22936]
Fresenius Medical Care--Church Street [26712]
Fresenius Medical Care--Circle City [24176]
Fresenius Medical Care--Circleville [26057]
Fresenius Medical Care - Clairton [26403]
Fresenius Medical Care--Clanton [22322]
Fresenius Medical Care--Clarke County [23582]
Fresenius Medical Care--Clarksburg [27664]
Fresenius Medical Care--Clarksdale • Dialysis Facility [25111]
Fresenius Medical Care--Clayton [23644]
Fresenius Medical Care--Clayton County • Dialysis Facility [23726]
Fresenius Medical Care --Clermont [23269]
Fresenius Medical Care--Clermont [23416]
Fresenius Medical Care--Cleveland Clinic Eastside • Dialysis Facility [26066]
Fresenius Medical Care--Cleveland Clinic Westside • Dialysis Facility [26024]
Fresenius Medical Care--Cleveland • Dialysis Facility [25112]
Fresenius Medical Care--Clinton • Dialysis Facility [25845]
Fresenius Medical Care--Coldwater [24855]
Fresenius Medical Care--College Park [23646]
Fresenius Medical Care--Collierville [26823]
Fresenius Medical Care--Columbia [26825]
Fresenius Medical Care--Columbia Basin • Dialysis Facility [27608]
Fresenius Medical Care--Columbus Bartholomew • Dialysis Facility [24123]
Fresenius Medical Care--Columbus • Dialysis Facility [25114]
Fresenius Medical Care • Columbus Southside Dialysis Center [26080]
Fresenius Medical Care--Colville [27601]
Fresenius Medical Care--Concordia [24313]
Fresenius Medical Care--Conejo Valley Renal Center [23033]
Fresenius Medical Care--Conner [24872]
Fresenius Medical Care--Connersville [24124]
Fresenius Medical Care--Conway [22534]
Fresenius Medical Care--Conyers • Dialysis Facility [23658]
Fresenius Medical Care--Coon Rapids [25014]
Fresenius Medical Care--Coral Springs [23486]
Fresenius Medical Care--Corinth [25115]
Fresenius Medical Care--Corsicana • Dialysis Facility [27012]
Fresenius Medical Care--Corydon [24126]
Fresenius Medical Care--Coushatta [24477]
Fresenius Medical Care--Covington • Dialysis Facility [23662]
Fresenius Medical Care of Cranberry Township • Dialysis Facility [26410]
Fresenius Medical Care--Crestwood • Dialysis Facility [23968]
Fresenius Medical Care--Creve Coeur [25191]
Fresenius Medical Care--Crockett • Dialysis Facility [27013]
Fresenius Medical Care--Crowley • Dialysis Center [24481]
Fresenius Medical Care--Crown Point [24128]
Fresenius Medical Care--Crystal Coast • Dialysis Facility [25913]
Fresenius Medical Care - Culver City Dialysis [22652]
Fresenius Medical Care--Cumberland County • Dialysis Services [26396]
Fresenius Medical Care--Cumming [23665]
Fresenius Medical Care--Cynthiana [24373]
Fresenius Medical Care--Dallas Central [27024]
Fresenius Medical Care - Dallas County [22399]
Fresenius Medical Care--Dallas South • Dialysis Facility [27025]
Fresenius Medical Care Dalton [23668]
Fresenius Medical Care - Danville [24375]
Fresenius Medical Care--Danville • Dialysis Facility [27479]
Fresenius Medical Care • Dare County Dialysis [25906]
Fresenius Medical Care--Dauphin Island Parkway • Dialysis Facility [22365]
Fresenius Medical Care--De Funiak Springs [23285]
Fresenius Medical Care--Decatur [23677]
Fresenius Medical Care--Decatur East Home Dialysis [23972]
Fresenius Medical Care--Decatur Pike, Athens • Dialysis Facility [26804]
Fresenius Medical Care--Defiance [26100]
Fresenius Medical Care--Dekalb County [24113]
Fresenius Medical Care of Dekalb Gwinnett Inc. [23678]
Fresenius Medical Care--Del Rio [27046]
Fresenius Medical Care of Delco [26594]
Fresenius Medical Care--Delhi Dialysis Center [24484]
Fresenius Medical Care--Delta • Dialysis Facility [24485]
Fresenius Medical Care--Denham Springs [24487]

Fresenius Medical Care--Depot, Antioch [23893]
Fresenius Medical Care--Desert Valley Dialysis [22476]
Fresenius Medical Care--Detroit [24912]
Fresenius Medical Care
    Diablo Renal Services--Concord • Dialysis Facility [22883]
    Diablo Renal Services--Pittsburg [22881]
Fresenius Medical Care Dialysis--Buffalo • Buffalo Dialysis Center [25007]
Fresenius Medical Care • Dialysis Center [22740]
Fresenius Medical Care--Dialysis Center of Glendale [22441]
Fresenius Medical Care Dialysis Center--Snapfinger [23679]
Fresenius Medical Care Dialysis--Central Minnesota Regional Dialysis [25064]
Fresenius Medical Care Dialysis--Chequamegon Bay [27698]
Fresenius Medical Care Dialysis--Clinton [24853]
Fresenius Medical Care Dialysis of Craven County [25918]
Fresenius Medical Care Dialysis--Fergus Falls [25026]
Fresenius Medical Care Dialysis--Golden Valley [25029]
Fresenius Medical Care Dialysis--New Brighton [25056]
Fresenius Medical Care Dialysis--Roseville [25073]
Fresenius Medical Care Dialysis Services--Alachua [23230]
Fresenius Medical Care/Dialysis Services of Audubon [24411]
Fresenius Medical Care Dialysis Services of Burbank [23907]
Fresenius Medical Care Dialysis Services of the Capital Area [26439]
Fresenius Medical Care/Dialysis Services--Clewiston [23270]
Fresenius Medical Care/Dialysis Services of College [22937]
Fresenius Medical Care • Dialysis Services of Deer Valley [22477]
Fresenius Medical Care Dialysis Services Des Moines [24267]
Fresenius Medical Care Dialysis Services--First State, Inc. [23194]
Fresenius Medical Care - Dialysis Services of Forestville [23151]
Fresenius Medical Care Dialysis Services--Forsyth [23702]
Fresenius Medical Care Dialysis Services--Fort Lauderdale [23482]
Fresenius Medical Care Dialysis Services--Graduate [26517]
Fresenius Medical Care Dialysis Services of Hahnemann [26518]
Fresenius Medical Care Dialysis Services--Hawthorne [23316]
Fresenius Medical Care Dialysis Services of Kapolei [23857]
Fresenius Medical Care Dialysis Services--Live Oak [23373]
Fresenius Medical Care • Dialysis Services of Mount Oliver, Inc. [26552]
Fresenius Medical Care Dialysis Services of Nanticoke [26489]
Fresenius Medical Care Dialysis Services of Newton [23663]
Fresenius Medical Care Dialysis Services--North Myrtle Beach [26754]
Fresenius Medical Care Dialysis Services of Northwest Philadelphia [26519]
Fresenius Medical Care Dialysis Services--Ohio Valley [26553]
Fresenius Medical Care/Dialysis Services of Paradise [22938]
Fresenius Medical Care Dialysis Services of Parkview [26520]
Fresenius Medical Care Dialysis Services--Penn Hills [26554]
Fresenius Medical Care Dialysis Services of Philadelphia [26521]
Fresenius Medical Care Dialysis Services of Pittston [26567]
Fresenius Medical Care Dialysis Services--Pottsville [26570]
Fresenius Medical Care Dialysis Services--South

Ramsey [25865]
Fresenius Medical Care Dialysis Services--Terrell [27372]
Fresenius Medical Care Dialysis Services--Three Rivers [26555]
Fresenius Medical Care Dialysis Services--Vista Del Sol [27067]
Fresenius Medical Care Dialysis Services--West Palm Beach [23553]
Fresenius Medical Care Dialysis Services - Winter Park [23564]
Fresenius Medical Care Dialysis--South Minneapolis [25045]
Fresenius Medical Care--Diamondhead [25117]
Fresenius Medical Care--D'Iberville South • Mississippi Kidney Center [25116]
Fresenius Medical Care--Dickinson [27051]
Fresenius Medical Care--Dillon [26706]
Fresenius Medical Care/Discovery Dialysis [22354]
Fresenius Medical Care--Dodge City • Dialysis Facility [24315]
Fresenius Medical Care • Dominion Dialysis Center [27471]
Fresenius Medical Care--Donora • Dialysis Services [26413]
Fresenius Medical Care--Douglas County [23685]
Fresenius Medical Care--Downtown Houston [27136]
Fresenius Medical Care--Duluth [25018]
Fresenius Medical Care--Duluth/Lawrenceville [23730]
Fresenius Medical Care--Dundee [24887]
Fresenius Medical Care--Dunmore [26419]
Fresenius Medical Care of DuPage West [24105]
Fresenius Medical Care--DuQuoin [23978]
Fresenius Medical Care • Duval Kidney Center [23343]
Fresenius Medical Care--Dyer [24132]
Fresenius Medical Care--East Arkansas • Dialysis Facility [22579]
Fresenius Medical Care--East Carolina [25878]
Fresenius Medical Care--East Central Houston • Dialysis Center [27137]
Fresenius Medical Care--East Charlotte [25836]
Fresenius Medical Care--East County Dialysis Center [22667]
Fresenius Medical Care--East Detroit [24873]
Fresenius Medical Care--East Hills [26556]
Fresenius Medical Care--East Lafayette [24519]
Fresenius Medical Care--East Lansing [24888]
Fresenius Medical Care--East Los Angeles [22666]
Fresenius Medical Care--East Louisville • Dialysis Facility [24412]
Fresenius Medical Care--East Memphis [26885]
Fresenius Medical Care--East Minden [24537]
Fresenius Medical Care--East Mobile [22366]
Fresenius Medical Care--East Natchitoches • Dialysis Services [24545]
Fresenius Medical Care--East Orange Dialysis Center [25424]
Fresenius Medical Care--East Orlando • Dialysis Facility [23449]
Fresenius Medical Care--East Rocky Mount • Dialysis Facility [25937]
Fresenius Medical Care of East Stroudsburg • Dialysis Facility [26420]
Fresenius Medical Care--East Tulsa [26302]
Fresenius Medical Care--East Valley [22457]
Fresenius Medical Care--Eastern Shore • Dialysis Facility [22337]
Fresenius Medical Care--Eastern Tennessee [26842]
Fresenius Medical Care--Eastern Virginia [27472]
Fresenius Medical Care--Eastern Wake [25939]
Fresenius Medical Care of Eastman [23693]
Fresenius Medical Care of Easton • Dialysis Services [26422]
Fresenius Medical Care--El Centro Desert Valley Dialysis Center [22669]
Fresenius Medical Care--El Paso/Cliff View • Dialysis Facility [27068]
Fresenius Medical Care--El Paso/Gateway • Dialysis Facility [27069]
Fresenius Medical Care--El Reno • Dialysis Services [26257]
Fresenius Medical Care--Elizabeth [25428]
Fresenius Medical Care--Elizabethton [26834]
Fresenius Medical Care--Elk Grove • Dialysis Center [23986]

Fresenius Medical Care--Elk River Dialysis [26836]
Fresenius Medical Care--Elkins • Dialysis Facility [27671]
Fresenius Medical Care--Elkton • Elk River Kidney Center [24681]
Fresenius Medical Care - Ellijay [23696]
Fresenius Medical Care of Ellwood City • Dialysis Services [26429]
Fresenius Medical Care--Elwood [24136]
Fresenius Medical Care--Emporia • Dialysis Facility [24317]
Fresenius Medical Care--Ennis [27078]
Fresenius Medical Care--Escanaba • Dialysis Facility [24892]
Fresenius Medical Care--Espanola • Dialysis Services [25544]
Fresenius Medical Care--Estrella • Dialysis Center [22478]
Fresenius Medical Care--Eunice • Dialysis Facility [24490]
Fresenius Medical Care--Eupora [25118]
Fresenius Medical Care--Evans [23697]
Fresenius Medical Care--Eveleth [25023]
Fresenius Medical Care--Evergreen Park [23992]
Fresenius Medical Care--Ewing [25432]
Fresenius Medical Care--Fairbanks [22420]
Fresenius Medical Care--Fairfield [22336]
Fresenius Medical Care--Fairmont • Dialysis Center [27672]
Fresenius Medical Care--Fairmount [26522]
Fresenius Medical Care--Fairview [25434]
Fresenius Medical Care--Falfurrias [27079]
Fresenius Medical Care--Fall River [24766]
Fresenius Medical Care--Fallon [25252]
Fresenius Medical Care--Falls Drive, Abingdon [27450]
Fresenius Medical Care--Farmerville • Dialysis Services [24491]
Fresenius Medical Care--Farmville • Dialysis Facility [27487]
Fresenius Medical Care--Ferriday • Dialysis Facility [24493]
Fresenius Medical Care--Fifth Ward [27138]
Fresenius Medical Care--Florissant [25204]
Fresenius Medical Care--Floyd County • Dialysis Facility [24214]
Fresenius Medical Care--Foley [22342]
Fresenius Medical Care--Fondren [27139]
Fresenius Medical Care of Forest • Dialysis Center [25120]
Fresenius Medical Care--Forest Park [27026]
Fresenius Medical Care--Fort Belvoir • Dialysis Facility [27455]
Fresenius Medical Care--Fort Foote [24683]
Fresenius Medical Care--Fort Lawn [26713]
Fresenius Medical Care--Fort Mill [26715]
Fresenius Medical Care--Fort Payne [22343]
Fresenius Medical Care of Fort Valley [23705]
Fresenius Medical Care----Fort Vancouver • Dialysis Center [27657]
Fresenius Medical Care--Fort Washington • Dialysis Facility [24684]
Fresenius Medical Care--Fort Wayne Jefferson [24142]
Fresenius Medical Care--Fort Worth Parkway [27086]
Fresenius Medical Care--Framingham • West Suburban Artificial Kidney Center [24768]
Fresenius Medical Care--Frankfort [24381]
Fresenius Medical Care--Franklin County • Dialysis Facility [27561]
Fresenius Medical Care--Franklin, Indiana [24149]
Fresenius Medical Care--Franklin, Louisiana • Dialysis Services [24494]
Fresenius Medical Care--Franklin, Tennessee [26837]
Fresenius Medical Care--Franklinton [24495]
Fresenius Medical Care--Fremont • Dialysis Facility [22692]
Fresenius Medical Care--Gainesville [23706]
Fresenius Medical Care--Gallatin [26839]
Fresenius Medical Care--Gallipolis [26125]
Fresenius Medical Care--Gardendale [22345]
Fresenius Medical Care--Garrisonville • Dialysis Facility [27567]
Fresenius Medical Care--Gastonia [25870]
Fresenius Medical Care/Gateway Dialysis Center, East [22939]

Fresenius Medical Care--Georgetown • Dialysis Facility [26718]
Fresenius Medical Care--Giles • Dialysis Facility [27533]
Fresenius Medical Care--Gilmer [27106]
Fresenius Medical Care--Glendale [22442]
Fresenius Medical Care--Globe • Dialysis Facility [22460]
Fresenius Medical Care--Golden Isles [23628]
Fresenius Medical Care--Goochland [27497]
Fresenius Medical Care--Goodyear [22444]
Fresenius Medical Care--Graceland • Dialysis Facility [26886]
Fresenius Medical Care--Granbury • Dialysis Facility [27109]
Fresenius Medical Care--Grand Island [25322]
Fresenius Medical Care--Grand Prairie [27110]
Fresenius Medical Care--Grand Rapids [25030]
Fresenius Medical Care - Granite Valley [22505]
Fresenius Medical Care--Grant Park • Dialysis Facility [26081]
Fresenius Medical Care--Gray Court [26716]
Fresenius Medical Care--Grayson [24385]
Fresenius Medical Care--Great Bend • Dialysis Facility [24319]
Fresenius Medical Care--Greater Akron • Dialysis Facility [26006]
Fresenius Medical Care--Greater Baltimore • Dialysis Facility [24733]
Fresenius Medical Care--Greater Norfolk • Granby Dialysis Center [27524]
Fresenius Medical Care--Greenbriar County [27679]
Fresenius Medical Care--Greencastle [24154]
Fresenius Medical Care--Greene County • Dialysis Services [26397]
Fresenius Medical Care--Greenfield [24156]
Fresenius Medical Care of Greensburg Inc. • Dialysis Facility [26436]
Fresenius Medical Care--Greentree [23189]
Fresenius Medical Care--Greenup [24386]
Fresenius Medical Care--Greenville, Mississippi [25121]
Fresenius Medical Care--Greenville, South Carolina [26723]
Fresenius Medical Care--Greenwood • Dialysis Facility [25123]
Fresenius Medical Care--Greer [26726]
Fresenius Medical Care--Grenada • Dialysis Facility [25124]
Fresenius Medical Care--Guayama • Dialysis Facility [26632]
Fresenius Medical Care--Gulfport South Mississippi • Kidney Center [25125]
Fresenius Medical Care--Habersham [23681]
Fresenius Medical Care--Hagerstown [24692]
Fresenius Medical Care--Hamilton, Alabama [22351]
Fresenius Medical Care--Hamilton, Ohio [26131]
Fresenius Medical Care--Hamilton Square [25440]
Fresenius Medical Care--Hardin County [24377]
Fresenius Medical Care--Harlan [24388]
Fresenius Medical Care--Harlingen [27117]
Fresenius Medical Care--Harper Woods [24914]
Fresenius Medical Care of Harrisburg • Dialysis Services [26440]
Fresenius Medical Care--Harrison [25443]
Fresenius Medical Care--Harston Hall [26435]
Fresenius Medical Care--Hartford [23158]
Fresenius Medical Care--Hays • Dialysis Facility [24320]
Fresenius Medical Care--Hayward [27809]
Fresenius Medical Care--Hazard • Dialysis Facility [24389]
Fresenius Medical Care--Hazel Crest [24006]
Fresenius Medical Care of Hazlehurst [25132]
Fresenius Medical Care of Hazleton Inc. • Dialysis Facility [26443]
Fresenius Medical Care--Helena [22540]
Fresenius Medical Care--Hendricks County • Danville Dialysis Facility [24130]
Fresenius Medical Care--Henryetta [26260]
Fresenius Medical Care--Hereford [27122]
Fresenius Medical Care--Heritage Hunt [27493]
Fresenius Medical Care--Heritage Park • Dialysis Services [26268]
Fresenius Medical Care--Hermitage [26446]
Fresenius Medical Care of Hibbing • Dialysis Facility [25031]
Fresenius Medical Care--Hickory [25884]

Fresenius Medical Care--Highway 8 W, Aberdeen • Dialysis Services [25100]
Fresenius Medical Care--Highway 98, Destin [23293]
Fresenius Medical Care--Hillcrest • Dialysis Services [22940]
Fresenius Medical Care--Hillsboro [27123]
Fresenius Medical Care--Hiram [23721]
Fresenius Medical Care--Hobart [24164]
Fresenius Medical Care--Hoffman Estates [24008]
Fresenius Medical Care--Holly Springs [25133]
Fresenius Medical Care--Hollywood • Dialysis Center [26339]
Fresenius Medical Care--Homer [24505]
Fresenius Medical Care--Hoover [22352]
Fresenius Medical Care--Horizon Dialysis [27070]
Fresenius Medical Care--Houma • Dialysis Services [24507]
Fresenius Medical Care--Howell Place [24465]
Fresenius Medical Care--Huntington [24166]
Fresenius Medical Care - Huntsville [22355]
Fresenius Medical Care--Hurricane • Dialysis Services [27676]
Fresenius Medical Care--Hutchinson [25032]
Fresenius Medical Care--Imperial County [22670]
Fresenius Medical Care--Independence • Dialysis Center [25215]
Fresenius Medical Care--Indian Hills [26138]
Fresenius Medical Care • Indianapolis East Home [24177]
Fresenius Medical Care Indianapolis East Home Dialysis [24178]
Fresenius Medical Care--Indianapolis West • Dialysis Facility [24179]
Fresenius Medical Care--Indianola • Dialysis Facility [25134]
Fresenius Medical Care--Industrial Parkway, Aberdeen • Dialysis Center [27591]
Fresenius Medical Care--Inglewood • Dialysis Facility [22731]
Fresenius Medical Care--Irmo • Dialysis Services [26732]
Fresenius Medical Care--Iron Mountain [24919]
Fresenius Medical Care--Ironbound [25482]
Fresenius Medical Care--Irvington • Dialysis Facility [25447]
Fresenius Medical Care--Irwindale [22737]
Fresenius Medical Care of Jackson [24393] Dialysis Facility [25136]
Fresenius Medical Care--Jackson Oaks [24920]
Fresenius Medical Care--Jacksonville [23344]
Fresenius Medical Care--Jaguar [22367]
Fresenius Medical Care--Jefferson County • Dialysis Facility [22568]
Fresenius Medical Care--Jennings • Dialysis Services [24511]
Fresenius Medical Care--Jersey City [25448]
Fresenius Medical Care--Johnson City • Dialysis Facility [26852]
Fresenius Medical Care--Johnsonville [26733]
Fresenius Medical Care--Joplin East • Dialysis Facility [25219]
Fresenius Medical Care--Jourdanton [27197]
Fresenius Medical Care--Juneau [22421]
Fresenius Medical Care--Kalamazoo [24923]
Fresenius Medical Care--Kalamazoo East [24924]
Fresenius Medical Care--Kanawha County [27670]
Fresenius Medical Care • Kansas City Dialysis and Transplant Center [25223]
Fresenius Medical Care--Kaufman [27201]
Fresenius Medical Care--Kearney Mesa Dialysis Center [22941]
Fresenius Medical Care--Kenilworth [25451]
Fresenius Medical Care--Kenner Dialysis [24513]
Fresenius Medical Care----Kennett [25232]
Fresenius Medical Care--Kentwood [24515]
Fresenius Medical Care--Kenvil [25452]
Fresenius Medical Care--Kewanee [24017]
Fresenius Medical Care--Key West • Dialysis Facility [23354]
Fresenius Medical Care--Kiest Station [27027]
Fresenius Medical Care--Killeen • Dialysis Center [27205]
Fresenius Medical Care • Kingman Dialysis [22447]
Fresenius Medical Care--Kings Mills [26144]
Fresenius Medical Care--Kings Mountain • Dialysis Facility [25894]
Fresenius Medical Care--Kingsport [26855]

Fresenius Medical Care--Kingsville [27208]
Fresenius Medical Care--Kokomo [24186]
Fresenius Medical Care--Ko'Olau [23855]
Fresenius Medical Care of Kosciusko • Dialysis Facility [25140]
Fresenius Medical Care--Kuttawa [24394]
Fresenius Medical Care--Kutztown • Dialysis Services [26458]
Fresenius Medical Care--La Jolla [22942]
Fresenius Medical Care--La Plata • Dialysis Facility [24698]
Fresenius Medical Care--Lacey [27622]
Fresenius Medical Care--Lacombe [24518]
Fresenius Medical Care--Lafayette [24190]
Fresenius Medical Care--Lake Bluff [24018]
Fresenius Medical Care--Lake Havasu City • Dialysis Facility [22449]
Fresenius Medical Care--Lake Lanier [23707]
Fresenius Medical Care--Lake Marion [26774]
Fresenius Medical Care--Lakeview [22350]
Fresenius Medical Care--Lakeview/Thorek Hospital [23924]
Fresenius Medical Care--Lakewood Dialysis Center [25453]
Fresenius Medical Care--Lampasas [27216]
Fresenius Medical Care--Lancaster [25391]
Fresenius Medical Care--Landsdale [26465]
Fresenius Medical Care--Langdale • Dialysis Facility [22414]
Fresenius Medical Care--Lansing [24930]
Fresenius Medical Care--Lansing Road, Charlotte [24848]
Fresenius Medical Care--Laredo [27220]
Fresenius Medical Care--Las Cruces [25549]
Fresenius Medical Care of Latrobe • Dialysis Facility [26466]
Fresenius Medical Care--Lawrence County • Dialysis Unit [24116]
Fresenius Medical Care--Lawrenceburg [26867]
Fresenius Medical Care--Lawrenceville [23731]
Fresenius Medical Care--Lawton • Dialysis Facility [26261]
Fresenius Medical Care--Lawton East [26262]
Fresenius Medical Care of Lebanon [25393]
Fresenius Medical Care--Lebanon County • Dialysis Services [26499]
Fresenius Medical Care--Lebanon • Dialysis Facility [25236]
Fresenius Medical Care--Lebanon Marion County [24397]
Fresenius Medical Care of Lee County • Dialysis Center [26683]
Fresenius Medical Care--Lenoir • Dialysis Facility [25899]
Fresenius Medical Care--Leonardtown • Dialysis Facility [24704]
Fresenius Medical Care--Lewisburg [26870]
Fresenius Medical Care--Lexington [26739]
Fresenius Medical Care--Lexington East [24401]
Fresenius Medical Care--Lexington North [24402]
Fresenius Medical Care--Liberal [24336]
Fresenius Medical Care--Lillington [25901]
Fresenius Medical Care--Limerick [26470]
Fresenius Medical Care--Lincoln Kidney Center • Dialysis Facility [24573]
Fresenius Medical Care--Lincolnton [25902]
Fresenius Medical Care--Linton • Dialysis Center [24195]
Fresenius Medical Care--Lithonia [23735]
Fresenius Medical Care--Little Rock Dialysis [22554]
Fresenius Medical Care--Livingston ACC [25458]
Fresenius Medical Care--Livonia [24936]
Fresenius Medical Care--Logansport [24196]
Fresenius Medical Care--Loma Linda [22928]
Fresenius Medical Care--Londonderry [25394]
Fresenius Medical Care--Long Beach • Dialysis Center [22761]
Fresenius Medical Care--Longview [27615]
Fresenius Medical Care--Lorain County Elyria [26107]
Fresenius Medical Care--Lorton [27508]
Fresenius Medical Care--Los Gatos [22796]
Fresenius Medical Care--Louisville [25143]
Fresenius Medical Care--Low Country Dialysis [26760]
Fresenius Medical Care--Lower Richland • Dialysis Center [26699]
Fresenius Medical Care--Lubbock [27235]

Fresenius Medical Care--Lugoff Elgin [26742]
Fresenius Medical Care--MacClenny [23375]
Fresenius Medical Care--Macomb [24026]
Fresenius Medical Care--Macon [23743]
 Dialysis Facility [25145]
Fresenius Medical Care--Madison [24198], [26876]
Fresenius Medical Care of Magee • Dialysis Facility
 [25146]
Fresenius Medical Care--Magnolia Grove [22402]
Fresenius Medical Care--Mammoth [22451]
Fresenius Medical Care--Mamou [24528]
Fresenius Medical Care--Mancuso [24466]
Fresenius Medical Care--Mandarin [23345]
Fresenius Medical Care--Manistee [24942]
Fresenius Medical Care--Manning [26743]
Fresenius Medical Care--Many [24530]
Fresenius Medical Care--Maple Grove [25036]
Fresenius Medical Care--Maplewood Heights
 [25038]
Fresenius Medical Care--Marietta [23750]
Fresenius Medical Care--Marina Bay • Fresenius
 Medical Care [22633]
Fresenius Medical Care--Marlborough [24775]
Fresenius Medical Care--Marrero • Dialysis Services
 [24532]
Fresenius Medical Care--Martin [26878]
Fresenius Medical Care--Martinsburg • Dialysis
 Facility [27681]
Fresenius Medical Care--Martinsville [27512]
Fresenius Medical Care--Maryvale • Dialysis Facility
 [22479]
Fresenius Medical Care of Mashpee [24776]
Fresenius Medical Care--Mayaguez • Dialysis Facil-
 ity [26641]
Fresenius Medical Care--Mayaguez North [26642]
Fresenius Medical Care--Mayersville [25159]
Fresenius Medical Care--Mayfield [24424]
Fresenius Medical Care--McAllen [27250]
Fresenius Medical Care--McComb • Dialysis Facility
 [25147]
Fresenius Medical Care of McHenry [24038]
Fresenius Medical Care --McKinleyville [22804]
Fresenius Medical Care--McKinney [27255]
Fresenius Medical Care--McLean County [23901]
Fresenius Medical Care--McMinnville [26882]
 Dialysis Facility [26330]
Fresenius Medical Care--Memphis [26887]
Fresenius Medical Care--Memphis Germantown
 [26841]
Fresenius Medical Care--Mercer County • Dialysis
 Services [27688]
Fresenius Medical Care--Meridian [25148]
Fresenius Medical Care--Merrionette Park [24041]
Fresenius Medical Care Mesa [22458]
Fresenius Medical Care--Mesa • Dialysis Center
 [22437]
Fresenius Medical Care--Metairie • Dialysis Services
 [24535]
Fresenius Medical Care of Methuen [24779]
Fresenius Medical Care • Metro Dialysis Center--
 Normandy [25249]
Fresenius Medical Care of Metropolis [24042]
Fresenius Medical Care--Meyerland [27140]
Fresenius Medical Care--Miami Midwest • Dialysis
 Center [26265]
Fresenius Medical Care--Mid-America Evanston
 [23991]
Fresenius Medical Care--Mid Sussex County
 [23190]
Fresenius Medical Care--Mid-Wilshire [22781]
Fresenius Medical Care of Middletown [23192]
Fresenius Medical Care--Midfield Dialysis [22364]
Fresenius Medical Care--Midtown-South Carolina
 [26700]
Fresenius Medical Care--Midway Saint Paul [25081]
Fresenius Medical Care--Milford [23193]
Fresenius Medical Care--Millen • Dialysis Facility
 [23759]
Fresenius Medical Care--Millersburg [26480]
Fresenius Medical Care--Millington [26896]
Fresenius Medical Care--Mission Bend [27141]
Fresenius Medical Care--Mission Hills [22810]
Fresenius Medical Care--Mission Viejo [22812]
Fresenius Medical Care--Mobile [22368]
Fresenius Medical Care--Monroe [25909]
 Dialysis Facility [24539]
Fresenius Medical Care--Montgomery Baptist •
 Dialysis Facility [22376]

Fresenius Medical Care--Montgomery County •
 Dialysis Services [27464]
Fresenius Medical Care--Montgomery East [26495]
Fresenius Medical Care--Monticello • Dialysis Facil-
 ity [22562]
Fresenius Medical Care--Mora • Dialysis Center
 [25053]
Fresenius Medical Care--Morehead • Dialysis Facil-
 ity [24428]
Fresenius Medical Care--Morgan City [24542]
Fresenius Medical Care--Morgan County [24200]
Fresenius Medical Care--Morgantown • Dialysis
 Facility [27683]
Fresenius Medical Care--Morning Star [26274]
Fresenius Medical Care--Morris [24045]
Fresenius Medical Care--Morristown • Dialysis
 Services [26897]
Fresenius Medical Care--Moses Lake [27617]
Fresenius Medical Care--Mount Airy [26523]
Fresenius Medical Care--Mt. Carmel East [26082]
Fresenius Medical Care--Mount Carmel West
 [26083]
Fresenius Medical Care--Mount Sterling [24429]
Fresenius Medical Care--Mountain City • Dialysis
 Services [26898]
Fresenius Medical Care--Mountain Empire [27531]
Fresenius Medical Care--Mountain Grove [25247]
Fresenius Medical Care--Muncie [24209]
Fresenius Medical Care--Murfreesboro [26900]
Fresenius Medical Care--Murray Dialysis [23642]
Fresenius Medical Care--Murray • Dialysis Facility
 [24430]
Fresenius Medical Care--Muscogee County •
 Dialysis Center [23653]
Fresenius Medical Care--Museum District [27142]
Fresenius Medical Care--Myrtle Beach [26750]
Fresenius Medical Care NA--Thibodaux • Dialysis
 Services [24595]
Fresenius Medical Care--Nacogdoches [27269]
Fresenius Medical Care--Naranja [23330]
Fresenius Medical Care--Nassawadox • Dialysis
 Facility [27517]
Fresenius Medical Care--Natchez [25149]
Fresenius Medical Care--National City • Dialysis
 Center [22836]
Fresenius Medical Care--Nations Ford • Dialysis
 Facility [25837]
Fresenius Medical Care --Navarre [23425]
Fresenius Medical Care--Nazareth [26524]
Fresenius Medical Care--Nederland [27293]
Fresenius Medical Care--Neomedica--Gurnee
 [24002]
Fresenius Medical Care--Neomedica--Hoffman
 Estates [24009]
Fresenius Medical Care--Neomedica--Loop [23925]
Fresenius Medical Care--Neomedica--Marquette
 Park [23926]
Fresenius Medical Care--Neomedica--Melrose Park
 • Dialysis Center [24039]
Fresenius Medical Care--Neomedica--Munster •
 Dialysis Facility [24213]
Fresenius Medical Care--Neomedica--North Kil-
 patrick [23927]
Fresenius Medical Care--Neomedica--Rolling
 Meadows [24077]
Fresenius Medical Care--Neomedica--Round Lake
 [24078]
Fresenius Medical Care--Neomedica--South [23928]
Fresenius Medical Care--Neomedica--South Holland
 • Dialysis Center [24089]
Fresenius Medical Care--Neomedica--South Shore •
 Dialysis Center [23929]
Fresenius Medical Care Nephrology--Goshen
 [24153]
Fresenius Medical Care Nephrology--Marshall
 County [24222]
Fresenius Medical Care--Nephrology Mishawaka
 Home [24204]
Fresenius Medical Care--New Bailie [23612]
Fresenius Medical Care--New Bern • Dialysis Unit
 [25919]
Fresenius Medical Care of New Castle • Dialysis
 Facility [26491]
Fresenius Medical Care--New Iberia • Dialysis
 Services [24546]
Fresenius Medical Care--New Market [26913]
Fresenius Medical Care--New Orleans • Dialysis
 Center [24555]

Fresenius Medical Care--New Orleans--Ferncrest
 [24556]
Fresenius Medical Care--New River Valley • Dialysis
 Facility [27542]
Fresenius Medical Care--New Roads • Dialysis
 Services [24563]
Fresenius Medical Care--Newark • Dialysis Facility
 [25483]
Fresenius Medical Care of Newberry • Dialysis
 Facility [26752]
Fresenius Medical Care of Newburyport [24784]
Fresenius Medical Care--Newport [26915]
Fresenius Medical Care--Newport Pike [23204]
Fresenius Medical Care--Newton, Kansas • Dialysis
 Facility [24339]
Fresenius Medical Care--Newton, Mississippi
 [25150]
Fresenius Medical Care--Nicholasville [24431]
Fresenius Medical Care - Niles [24051]
Fresenius Medical Care--Niles • Dialysis Center
 [24052]
Fresenius Medical Care--Nixa [25248]
Fresenius Medical Care--Noblesville • Dialysis Facil-
 ity [24218]
Fresenius Medical Care--Norcross [23768]
Fresenius Medical Care--Norridge • Dialysis Center
 [24053]
Fresenius Medical Care--North Alabama [22356]
Fresenius Medical Care--North Bastrop [26961]
Fresenius Medical Care--North Baton Rouge--Airport
 • Dialysis Services [24467]
Fresenius Medical Care--North Boulevard • Dialysis
 Services [24468]
Fresenius Medical Care - North Boynton Beach
 Dialysis Services [23250]
Fresenius Medical Care--North Central Oklahoma
 City [26275]
Fresenius Medical Care--North Charlotte [25838]
Fresenius Medical Care--North Cobb [23751]
Fresenius Medical Care--North Fort Worth [27087]
Fresenius Medical Care--North Garland [27103]
Fresenius Medical Care--North Georgia [23636]
Fresenius Medical Care--North Houston Dialysis
 [27143]
Fresenius Medical Care--North Idaho • Dialysis
 Facility [23871]
Fresenius Medical Care--North Lafayette • Dialysis
 Services [24520]
Fresenius Medical Care--North Lima [26174]
Fresenius Medical Care--North Long Beach [22762]
Fresenius Medical Care--North Memphis • Dialysis
 Facility [26888]
Fresenius Medical Care--North Monroe • Dialysis
 Center [24540]
Fresenius Medical Care--North Orange County •
 Dialysis Facility [22586]
Fresenius Medical Care--North Phoenix Home
 [22480]
Fresenius Medical Care--North Pines [27649]
Fresenius Medical Care--North Platte [25335]
Fresenius Medical Care--North Rio Rancho [25556]
Fresenius Medical Care--North Roanoke • Dialysis
 Center [27559]
Fresenius Medical Care--North Salisbury [24724]
Fresenius Medical Care--North Scottsdale • Dialysis
 Facility [22496]
Fresenius Medical Care--North Suburban • Dialysis
 Facility [25015]
Fresenius Medical Care--North Tampa [23533]
Fresenius Medical Care--North Texas [27397]
Fresenius Medical Care--North Tulsa [26303]
Fresenius Medical Care--North Wilmington [23205]
Fresenius Medical Care • Northeast Louisiana
 Dialysis Center [24541]
Fresenius Medical Care--Northeast Louisville
 [24413]
Fresenius Medical Care of Northeast Philadelphia •
 Dialysis Facility [26525]
Fresenius Medical Care • Northwest Alabama
 Kidney Center [22416]
Fresenius Medical Care--Northwest Detroit [24874]
Fresenius Medical Care - Northwest Indiana Dialysis
 [24151]
Fresenius Medical Care--Northwest Oklahoma City
 [26276]
Fresenius Medical Care • Northwest Tucson Dialysis
 [22517]
Fresenius Medical Care--Northwestern [23930]

Fresenius Medical Care--Norwalk • Dialysis Facility [26177]
Fresenius Medical Care--Norwalk East [23000]
Fresenius Medical Care--Oak Grove • Dialysis Center [24564]
Fresenius Medical Care--Oak Hill [27673]
Fresenius Medical Care--Oak Park Dialysis Unit [24055]
Fresenius Medical Care--Oak Ridge • Dialysis Clinic [26916]
Fresenius Medical Care--Oceanside [23063]
Fresenius Medical Care--Oceanway [23346]
Fresenius Medical Care--Odyssey Dialysis [22363]
Fresenius Medical Care--Ohio Valley Dialysis Center [24138]
Fresenius Medical Care--Oklahoma City • Dialysis Services [26277]
Fresenius Medical Care--Oldham County [24395]
Fresenius Medical Care--Olney [26526]
Fresenius Medical Care--Oneonta [22382]
Fresenius Medical Care--Opelika • Dialysis Facility [22384]
Fresenius Medical Care--Opelousas • Dialysis Services [24566]
Fresenius Medical Care--Orange [25493]
Fresenius Medical Care--Orange County • Dialysis Center [27280]
Fresenius Medical Care--Orange Grove/South Mississippi Kidney Center [25126]
Fresenius Medical Care--Orland Park • Dialysis Facility [24060]
Fresenius Medical Care--Oshtemo • Dialysis Facility [24925]
Fresenius Medical Care--Oswego [24061]
Fresenius Medical Care--Ottumwa • Dialysis Facility [24294]
Fresenius Medical Care--Ouachita Dialysis [24598]
Fresenius Medical Care--Overland Trails [25325]
Fresenius Medical Care--Owosso [24955]
Fresenius Medical Care--Oxford, Mississippi [25152]
Fresenius Medical Care--Oxford, North Carolina [25921]
Fresenius Medical Care--Oxnard • Dialysis Facility [22866]
Fresenius Medical Care--Pacific Northwest • Dialysis Facility [26340]
Fresenius Medical Care----Paducah • Dialysis Center [24433]
Fresenius Medical Care--Paducah South [24434]
Fresenius Medical Care--Paintsville [24435]
Fresenius Medical Care--Palm Valley • Dialysis Services [22445]
Fresenius Medical Care--Palmetto • Dialysis Facility [26695]
Fresenius Medical Care--Palouse [23879]
Fresenius Medical Care--Pamlico • Dialysis Facility [25970]
Fresenius Medical Care--Pampa [27282]
Fresenius Medical Care--Paris [27283]
Fresenius Medical Care--Parker • Dialysis Center [22462]
Fresenius Medical Care--Parkway • Dialysis Center [22357]
Fresenius Medical Care--Patrick County [27572]
Fresenius Medical Care--Pauls Valley [26287]
Fresenius Medical Care--Pawtucket [26663]
Fresenius Medical Care--Pell City [22389]
Fresenius Medical Care--Peoria Downtown • Dialysis Facility [24065]
Fresenius Medical Care--Peoria North [24066]
Fresenius Medical Care--Perimeter • Dialysis Center [23597]
Fresenius Medical Care--Petaluma • Dialysis Facility [22879]
Fresenius Medical Care--Philadelphia [25155]
Fresenius Medical Care • Phoenix Artificial Kidney Center [22464]
Fresenius Medical Care--Picardy [24469]
Fresenius Medical Care--Pikeville [24438]
Fresenius Medical Care--Pinebrook [25484]
Fresenius Medical Care--Pinellas Park [23479]
Fresenius Medical Care--Pineville • Dialysis Services [24567]
Fresenius Medical Care--Pittsburg [24344]
Fresenius Medical Care--Pittsburgh [26557]
Fresenius Medical Care--Plainfield [24069]
Fresenius Medical Care--Plaquemine • Dialysis Services [24568]

Fresenius Medical Care--Plymouth Cordage [24794]
Fresenius Medical Care--Ponca City • Dialysis Facility [26288]
Fresenius Medical Care--Ponce Centro [26644]
Fresenius Medical Care--Ponce • Dialysis Facility [26645]
Fresenius Medical Care--Ponchartrain Kidney Center [24479]
Fresenius Medical Care--Pontiac [24070]
Fresenius Medical Care--Poplar Bluff [25256]
Fresenius Medical Care--Port City • Dialysis Center [22369]
Fresenius Medical Care--Port Gibson [25157]
Fresenius Medical Care--Port Huron [24959]
Fresenius Medical Care--Portage Dialysis Center [24223]
Fresenius Medical Care--Portland [26918]
Fresenius Medical Care--Portsmouth • Dialysis Facility [26187]
Fresenius Medical Care--Potomac Mills [27478]
Fresenius Medical Care--Powell [26859]
Fresenius Medical Care--Prairie [23931]
Fresenius Medical Care--Prattville [22392]
Fresenius Medical Care--Prestonsburg • Dialysis Facility [24439]
Fresenius Medical Care--Prichard • Dialysis Facility [22394]
Fresenius Medical Care--Princeton • Dialysis Facility [25501]
Fresenius Medical Care--Providence • Dialysis Center [26665]
Fresenius Medical Care--Rancho [22943]
Fresenius Medical Care--Rancho Cucamonga • Dialysis Services [22891]
Fresenius Medical Care--Randolph County • Dialysis Facility [23913]
Fresenius Medical Care - Rankin County [25105]
Fresenius Medical Care--Raytown [25258]
Fresenius Medical Care--Red Mountain • Dialysis Services [22459]
Fresenius Medical Care--Redmond [26350]
Fresenius Medical Care of Redstone [26387]
Fresenius Medical Care--Reedley [22900]
Fresenius Medical Care--Regency [26084]
Fresenius Medical Care of Rehoboth, Inc. • Dialysis Facility [23198]
Fresenius Medical Care--Reno County [24324]
Fresenius Medical Care--Richland County • Dialysis Services [26154]
Fresenius Medical Care--Richland Parish [24572]
Fresenius Medical Care--Richmond [24227]
Fresenius Medical Care--Rincon [23773]
Fresenius Medical Care - Rio Grande City [27296]
Fresenius Medical Care--Rio Piedras • Dialysis Facility [26653]
Fresenius Medical Care--Ripley [27689]
Fresenius Medical Care--Ripon South [27779]
Fresenius Medical Care--River City [23654]
Fresenius Medical Care--River Hills [27674]
Fresenius Medical Care--Riverside • Dialysis Services [22904]
Fresenius Medical Care--Riverside Park [23206]
Fresenius Medical Care--Roane County • Dialysis Facility [26843]
Fresenius Medical Care--Roanoke [27562]
Fresenius Medical Care--Roanoke Rapids • Dialysis Facility [25936]
Fresenius Medical Care--Robeson County [25862]
Fresenius Medical Care--Robstown [27298]
Fresenius Medical Care--Rockford Lane [24448]
Fresenius Medical Care--Rockport [27300]
Fresenius Medical Care--Rockville • Dialysis Facility [24721]
Fresenius Medical Care--Rocky Mount • Dialysis Facility [25938]
Fresenius Medical Care--Rogers Park • Dialysis Facility [23932]
Fresenius Medical Care--Romeo Plank [24940]
Fresenius Medical Care--Romulus [24963]
Fresenius Medical Care--Rose Quarter • Dialysis Center [26341]
Fresenius Medical Care--Roseland Dialysis [23933]
Fresenius Medical Care--Rowlett [27309]
Fresenius Medical Care--Royal Palm Beach [23554]
Fresenius Medical Care--Russell County • Dialysis Facility [27505]
Fresenius Medical Care--Ruston [24574]
Fresenius Medical Care--S Carroll Street, Athens •

Dialysis Facility [26947]
Fresenius Medical Care--Safford • Dialysis Facility [22492]
Fresenius Medical Care--Saint Augustine [23498]
Fresenius Medical Care--St. Barnabas S Orange Ave. [25459]
Fresenius Medical Care--Saint Charles Parish [24575]
Fresenius Medical Care--Saint Francis County • Dialysis Services [22539]
Fresenius Medical Care--St. Louis [25261]
Fresenius Medical Care--Saint Louis Park [25077]
Fresenius Medical Care--Saint Margaret Dialysis Center • Campus Dialysis Unit [24162]
Fresenius Medical Care--Saint Paul [25082]
Fresenius Medical Care--St. Pauls [25941]
Fresenius Medical Care--Salem South [26193]
Fresenius Medical Care--Saline County • Dialysis Facility [24003]
Fresenius Medical Care--Salisbury [24725]
Fresenius Medical Care--Salmon Creek • Dialysis Facility [27658]
Fresenius Medical Care--San Bernardino [22929]
Fresenius Medical Care--San Carlos [22465]
Fresenius Medical Care--San German • Dialysis Facility [26648]
Fresenius Medical Care--San Jose [22970]
Fresenius Medical Care--San Ysidro • Dialysis Center [22944]
Fresenius Medical Care--Sandusky [24971]
Fresenius Medical Care--Sandy Springs [23598]
Fresenius Medical Care--Sanford • Dialysis Facility [23508]
Fresenius Medical Care--Santa Barbara • Community Dialysis Center [22996]
Fresenius Medical Care--Santa Fe • Dialysis Facility [25561]
Fresenius Medical Care--Santa Juanita [26625]
Fresenius Medical Care--Santa Paula • Dialysis Facility [23005]
Fresenius Medical Care--Santa Rosa [26633]
Fresenius Medical Care Santa Rosa North [23008]
Fresenius Medical Care--Saratoga [27008]
Fresenius Medical Care--Sardis [25160]
Fresenius Medical Care--Scottsboro [22398]
Fresenius Medical Care - Scottsdale [22497]
Fresenius Medical Care--Seaford [23199]
Fresenius Medical Care - Selma [22400]
Fresenius Medical Care Services of Stoneham • Dialysis Facility [24805]
Fresenius Medical Care--Seymour [24234]
Fresenius Medical Care--Shadyside [26558]
Fresenius Medical Care--Shakopee [25088]
Fresenius Medical Care--Shaler [26559]
Fresenius Medical Care--Shawnee • Dialysis Services [26294]
Fresenius Medical Care--Shelby [22304], [24973]
Fresenius Medical Care--Shelbyville, Indiana • Dialysis Facility [24236]
Fresenius Medical Care--Shelbyville, Kentucky • Dialysis Facility [24443]
Fresenius Medical Care--Sheldon Corners [24845]
Fresenius Medical Care--Shelton [27646]
Fresenius Medical Care--Shepherdsville [24444]
Fresenius Medical Care--Shorewood [27785]
Fresenius Medical Care--Show Low • Dialysis Facility [22499]
Fresenius Medical Care--Shreveport Regional [24580]
Fresenius Medical Care--Sidney • Dialysis Facility [26199]
Fresenius Medical Care--Silver Spring [24729]
Fresenius Medical Care--Sinton [27362]
Fresenius Medical Care--Slidell [24591]
Fresenius Medical Care--Smyrna [23201], [23788]
Fresenius Medical Care--Snapfinger [23680]
Fresenius Medical Care of Snellville Inc. • Dialysis Facility [23790]
Fresenius Medical Care--Solon [26200]
Fresenius Medical Care--Somerset [24445]
Fresenius Medical Care--South Alexandria • Dialysis Services [24454]
Fresenius Medical Care--South Allentown [26365]
Fresenius Medical Care--South Annapolis • Dialysis Facility [24623]
Fresenius Medical Care - South Bay [22719]
Fresenius Medical Care--South Bossier [24472]
Fresenius Medical Care--South Boston • Dialysis

Facility **[27564]**
Fresenius Medical Care--South Central Louisville **[24414]**
Fresenius Medical Care--South Cobb **[23621]**
Fresenius Medical Care of South Dallas County • Dialysis Facility **[27028]**
Fresenius Medical Care--South Dekalb/Rockdale **[23736]**
Fresenius Medical Care--South Greensboro **[25875]**
Fresenius Medical Care--South Haven **[24974]**
Fresenius Medical Care of South Hills • Dialysis Facility **[26380]**
Fresenius Medical Care--South Laredo **[27221]**
Fresenius Medical Care--South Louisville • Dialysis Facility **[24415]**
Fresenius Medical Care - South Macon Dialysis **[23744]**
Fresenius Medical Care--South Mountain Dialysis Center **[22481]**
Fresenius Medical Care--South OKC **[26278]**
Fresenius Medical Care--South Orange County • Dialysis Facility **[22993]**
Fresenius Medical Care--South Phoenix Dialysis Services **[22482]**
Fresenius Medical Care--South Plainfield • Dialysis Facility **[25512]**
Fresenius Medical Care--South Saint Petersburg **[23503]**
Fresenius Medical Care--South Shreveport **[24581]**
Fresenius Medical Care--South Suburban **[24059]**
Fresenius Medical Care--South Tulsa **[26304]**
Fresenius Medical Care--Southaven • Dialysis Facility **[25162]**
Fresenius Medical Care--Southeast Missouri **[25182]**
Fresenius Medical Care • Southeast Valley Dialysis **[22490]**
Fresenius Medical Care - Southern Indiana **[24183]**
Fresenius Medical Care • Southern Maine Dialysis Facility **[24613]**
Fresenius Medical Care--Southern Ocean County • Dialysis Center **[25463]**
Fresenius Medical Care of Southington **[23179]**
Fresenius Medical Care--Southside **[27009]**
Fresenius Medical Care--Southside Dialysis Center **[23934]**
Fresenius Medical Care--Southtown **[25005]**
Fresenius Medical Care--Southwest Greensboro • Dialysis Facility **[25890]**
Fresenius Medical Care--Southwest Illinois **[23979]**
Fresenius Medical Care of Southwest Jackson • Dialysis Facility **[25137]**
Fresenius Medical Care--Southwest Oklahoma City **[26279]**
Fresenius Medical Care--Southwest Shreveport **[24582]**
Fresenius Medical Care--Southwest Virginia • Dialysis Facility **[27499]**
Fresenius Medical Care--Spencer • Dialysis Center **[24238]**
Fresenius Medical Care--Spirit Valley • Dialysis Center **[25019]**
Fresenius Medical Care--Spotsylvania **[27491]**
Fresenius Medical Care of Spring Hope **[25955]**
Fresenius Medical Care--Spring Valley **[24090]**
Fresenius Medical Care--Springfield, Missouri **[25291]**
Fresenius Medical Care--Springfield, Tennessee **[26926]**
Fresenius Medical Care--Starke **[23519]**
Fresenius Medical Care--Starkville • Dialysis Facility **[25163]**
Fresenius Medical Care--Stillwater • Dialysis Center **[17161]**, **[26296]**
Fresenius Medical Care--Stone Mountain **[23799]**
Fresenius Medical Care--Streator **[24096]**
Fresenius Medical Care--Streetsboro Kidney Center • Dialysis Facility **[26205]**
Fresenius Medical Care--Sturgis **[24981]**
Fresenius Medical Care--Stuttgart • Dialysis Center **[22576]**
Fresenius Medical Care--Suburban Louisville • Dialysis Facility **[24416]**
Fresenius Medical Care--Sullivan **[25294]**
Fresenius Medical Care--Sulphur Springs **[27368]**
Fresenius Medical Care--Sumter • Dialysis Center **[26777]**
Fresenius Medical Care--Sun City • Dialysis Facility **[22503]**

Fresenius Medical Care--Sun City West Dialysis **[22508]**
Fresenius Medical Care--Sun Lakes • Dialysis Facility **[22506]**
Fresenius Medical Care--Sunnyside **[27144]**
Fresenius Medical Care • Sunrise County Dialysis **[24609]**
Fresenius Medical Care--Sunset **[24594]**
Fresenius Medical Care--Swarthmore • Dialysis Services **[26587]**
Fresenius Medical Care--Sylacauga **[22405]**
Fresenius Medical Care--Talawanda **[26181]**
Fresenius Medical Care--Tamaqua • Dialysis Services **[26588]**
Fresenius Medical Care--Tawas Bay **[24890]**
Fresenius Medical Care--Taylor **[24982]**
Fresenius Medical Care--Tempe • Dialysis Facility **[22511]**
Fresenius Medical Care--Temple Episcopal **[26527]**
Fresenius Medical Care--Temple Germantown **[26528]**
Fresenius Medical Care--Terre Haute **[24240]**
Fresenius Medical Care--Terre Haute North **[24241]**
Fresenius Medical Care--Tesson Ferry Dialysis **[25271]**
Fresenius Medical Care--The Glades **[23396]**
Fresenius Medical Care--The Marshlands **[26762]**
Fresenius Medical Care--Thomasville, Alabama **[22409]**
Fresenius Medical Care--Thomasville, Georgia **[23807]**
Fresenius Medical Care - Thomson Dialysis **[23809]**
Fresenius Medical Care--Three Rivers **[24984]**
Fresenius Medical Care--Tipton County • Dialysis Facility **[26827]**
Fresenius Medical Care--Toccoa **[23812]**
Fresenius Medical Care - Tombigbee **[22358]**
Fresenius Medical Care--Topeka **[24348]**
Fresenius Medical Care--Toulminville • Dialysis Facility **[22370]**
Fresenius Medical Care--Tradition **[23491]**
Fresenius Medical Care--Trenton **[25518]**
Fresenius Medical Care--Tri-City **[26932]**
Fresenius Medical Care--Tri-Counties Dialysis Center **[24131]**
Fresenius Medical Care--Trigg County **[24365]**
Fresenius Medical Care--Trinity **[24592]**
Fresenius Medical Care - Troy **[22410]**
Fresenius Medical Care--Tualatin **[26359]**
Fresenius Medical Care Tucker • Dialysis Center **[23813]**
Fresenius Medical Care--Tullahoma **[26927]**
Fresenius Medical Care--Tunica **[25164]**
Fresenius Medical Care--Tupelo **[25165]**
Fresenius Medical Care--Tuskegee • Dialysis Facility **[22413]**
Fresenius Medical Care--Twin Oaks • Dialysis Facility **[26314]**
Fresenius Medical Care--Two Virginias • Dialysis Services **[27663]**
Fresenius Medical Care--Union **[25296]**
Fresenius Medical Care--Union City • Dialysis Center **[26928]**
Fresenius Medical Care--Union Parish • Dialysis Center **[24492]**
Fresenius Medical Care--Uniontown • Dialysis Facility **[26592]**
Fresenius Medical Care--University **[24875]**
Fresenius Medical Care--University City **[25297]**
Fresenius Medical Care--University of South Alabama • Dialysis Facility **[22371]**
Fresenius Medical Care--Valley Creek **[22401]**
Fresenius Medical Care--Vega Baja **[26657]**
Fresenius Medical Care--Ventura **[23056]**
Fresenius Medical Care--Vernon Dialysis Unit **[25895]**
Fresenius Medical Care--Vicksburg **[25167]**
Fresenius Medical Care--Vieques **[26647]**
Fresenius Medical Care--Villa Park **[24101]**
Fresenius Medical Care--Villa Rica **[23828]**
Fresenius Medical Care--Ville Platte • Dialysis Services **[24597]**
Fresenius Medical Care--Virginia Beach **[27581]**
Fresenius Medical Care--Wabash Valley **[24242]**
Fresenius Medical Care--Waldorf • Dialysis Services **[24735]**
Fresenius Medical Care--Walker **[22361]**
Fresenius Medical Care--Walnut Creek **[23064]**

Fresenius Medical Care--Walton **[23760]**
Fresenius Medical Care--Walton Way, New Bailie **[23613]**
Fresenius Medical Care--Warner Robins • Dialysis Facility **[23831]**
Fresenius Medical Care--Warren, Michigan **[24987]**
Fresenius Medical Care--Warren, Ohio **[26091]**
Fresenius Medical Care--Warrenton • Dialysis Facility **[27583]**
Fresenius Medical Care--Warsaw **[24245]**
Fresenius Medical Care--Warwick • Dialysis Facility **[26671]**
Fresenius Medical Care--Washington • Dialysis Facility **[24661]**
Fresenius Medical Care--Wasilla **[22422]**
Fresenius Medical Care--Watauga County **[25821]**
Fresenius Medical Care--Waupaca **[27797]**
Fresenius Medical Care--Waynesboro **[26602]**
Fresenius Medical Care--Welch • Dialysis Facility **[27692]**
Fresenius Medical Care--Wells County **[24119]**
Fresenius Medical Care--Wentzville **[25300]**
Fresenius Medical Care--West Belmont • Dialysis Center **[23935]**
Fresenius Medical Care--West Charlotte **[25839]**
Fresenius Medical Care--West Columbia • Dialysis Facility **[26781]**
Fresenius Medical Care--West Conway **[26704]**
Fresenius Medical Care--West Covina Kidney Center • Dialysis Facility **[23069]**
Fresenius Medical Care--West End • Dialysis Facility **[27549]**
Fresenius Medical Care--West Kingsport • Dialysis Facility **[26856]**
Fresenius Medical Care--West Knoxville • Dialysis Facility **[26860]**
Fresenius Medical Care--West Lafayette **[24521]**
Fresenius Medical Care - West Los Angeles **[22732]**
Fresenius Medical Care--West Louisville • Dialysis Facility **[24417]**
Fresenius Medical Care--West Metro • Dialysis Center **[23936]**
Fresenius Medical Care--West Mobile • Dialysis Facility **[22372]**
Fresenius Medical Care--West Nashville **[26907]**
Fresenius Medical Care--West Palm **[23555]**
Fresenius Medical Care--West Pennsylvania **[26560]**
Fresenius Medical Care--West Pensacola **[23471]**
Fresenius Medical Care--West Plano **[27291]**
Fresenius Medical Care--West Salem **[26353]**
Fresenius Medical Care--West Seguin **[27357]**
Fresenius Medical Care--West Shreveport **[24583]**
Fresenius Medical Care--West Suburban Dialysis Center **[24056]**
Fresenius Medical Care • West Texas Dialysis **[26973]**
Fresenius Medical Care--West Tucson **[22518]**
Fresenius Medical Care--Westbank **[24533]**
Fresenius Medical Care--Westchester • Dialysis Center **[24107]**
Fresenius Medical Care--Westchester Home **[24108]**
Fresenius Medical Care--Westerville Dialysis **[26233]**
Fresenius Medical Care--Weston **[27693]**
Fresenius Medical Care--Westport • Dialysis Facility **[24569]**
Fresenius Medical Care--Wheaton • Dialysis Facility **[24737]**
Fresenius Medical Care--Whetstone • Dialysis Facility **[22373]**
Fresenius Medical Care--Whitehall **[26609]**
Fresenius Medical Care--Whiteriver • Dialysis Facility **[22523]**
Fresenius Medical Care--Wichita • Dialysis Facility **[24352]**
Fresenius Medical Care--Wichita East **[24353]**
Fresenius Medical Care--Wichita West **[24354]**
Fresenius Medical Care--Wilcox County • Dialysis Services **[22320]**
Fresenius Medical Care of Wilkes-Barre **[26610]**
Fresenius Medical Care--Williamson County **[24029]**
Fresenius Medical Care--Willoughby **[26236]**
Fresenius Medical Care--Willowbrook **[24109]**
Fresenius Medical Care of Wilmington, Inc. • Dialysis Services **[23207]**
Fresenius Medical Care--Winchester, Kentucky **[24451]**
Fresenius Medical Care--Winchester, Tennessee **[26929]**

Fresenius Medical Care--Windsor • Dialysis Facility [25976]
Fresenius Medical Care--Winnfield • Dialysis Services [24599]
Fresenius Medical Care--Winnsboro • Dialysis Services [24600]
Fresenius Medical Care--Winona [25170]
Fresenius Medical Care--Winslow Dialysis Center Ltd. [22524]
Fresenius Medical Care--Winslow Twp. [25509]
Fresenius Medical Care--Winyah [26719]
Fresenius Medical Care--Woodland Hills • Dialysis Center [23080]
Fresenius Medical Care--Woodstock [23838]
Fresenius Medical Care--Woodward • Dialysis Center [26310]
Fresenius Medical Care--Wynnewood • Dialysis Unit [26615]
Fresenius Medical Care--Wytheville • Dialysis Facility [27590]
Fresenius Medical Care • Yankee Family Dialysis Center [24770]
Fresenius Medical Care of Yazoo City • Dialysis Facility [25171]
Fresenius Medical Care--York [26783]
Fresenius Medical Care--York County [26764]
Fresenius Medical Care--Youngstown [26241]
Fresenius Medical Care--Zachary Crossroad • Dialysis Facility [24601]
Fresenius Medical Care--Zebulon • Dialysis Facility [25985]
Fresenius Medical Center - Dadeville [22324]
Fresenius Medical Center--San Fernando • Dialysis Center [22952]
Fresenius Medical Services of Catawba Valley [25849]
Fresenius Medical Services Dialysis--Flint [24897]
Fresenius Medical Services Dialysis--Madison Heights [24941]
Fresenius Medical Services Dialysis--Milwaukee [27749]
Fresenius Medical Services Dialysis--Superior [27790]
Fresenius Medical Services of Mount Pleasant • Dialysis Facility [26488]
Fresenius Medical Services of Pendleton [26758]
Fresenius Medical Services of West Fayetteville [25866]
Fresenius Temple Dialysis Services--Germantown [26529]
Fresh Beginning Inc [40859]
Fresh Pond Physical Therapy [38815]
Fresh Start [8716], [46033]
Fresh Start Counseling Services [43154], [43218]
Fresh Start LLC [50045]
Fresh Start Ministries of Central FL [41859]
Fresno County Behavioral Health
    Adult System of Care [28505]
    Apollo Residential Treatment [33145]
    Reedley Regional Health Clinic [28716]
Fresno County Behavioral Health--Sanger [28506]
Fresno County Behavioral Health
    Southeast Asian Program [33146]
    West County Regional Clinic [28545]
Fresno County Board of Supervisors • Pathways to Recovery [39856]
Fresno County Department of Children and Family Services • Elkhorn Facility--Mental Health [33131]
Fresno County Economic Opportunities Commission • Runaway and Homeless Youth Program [35821]
Fresno County Hispanic Commission on Alcohol/Drug Abuse Services • DATE Prog [40710]
Fresno County Hispanic Commission on Alcohol/Drug Abuse Services Inc [39857]
Fresno County Human Services System
    East County Regional Clinic [28793]
    Orange Cove Community Clinic [28688]
Fresno County Mental Health • Intensive Services [33147]
Fresno County • Pinedale Clinic [33148]
Fresno County Public Library • Talking Book Library for the Blind [3753]
Fresno Dialysis Center • DaVita [22697]
Fresno New Connections [39858]
Fresno Veterans Affairs Medical Center • South Valley Outpatient Clinic [28830]
Friary • Lakeview Center Inc [41681]
Friberg Medical Associates • Chicago Women's

Wellness Center [22036]
Fridley Dialysis • DaVita [25028]
Friend Family Health Center [6658]
Friend to Friend [10022]
Friendly House [40110]
Friends of Abused Families [10744]
Friends of Alcoholics [45390]
Friends of Bridge Inc • Outpt Drug Abuse Treatment Program [47154]
Friends of Caroline Hospice [21270]
Friends Home Care [16348]
Friends Hospice [21128]
Friends Hospital [33817]
    Eating Disorder Program [11252]
Friends of Youth - Outreach [36252]
Friendship Center of Helena, Inc. [9750]
Friendship Home [9775]
Friendship Home Inc [47419]
Friendship House [34427], [45738]
    American Indian Lodge [40296]
Friendship House Assoc of Amer Indians [40607]
Friendship House Cloud Home [34424]
Friendship House--Hackensack [31134]
Friendship House--Johnson City [32321]
Friendship House--Knoxville [32335]
Friendship House at Woodsville • Tri County Community Action Prog Inc [45922]
Friendship Manor Dialysis Unit • Fresenius Medical Care [27560]
Friendship of Women, Inc. [10447]
Friendswood Dialysis • US Renal Care [27097]
Friman Home Health Service, PLC [15605]
Friona Intermediate School District/Parmer County SSA [789]
Friona Outpatient Clinic [32466]
Froedtert Memorial Hospital--Transplant • Froedtert & Medical College of Wisconsin [27750]
Froedtert Memorial Lutheran Hospital
    Cancer Center [6166]
    Froedtert Center for Sleep [37967]
    Inpatient Rehabilitation Programs [4492]
    Medical College of Wisconsin Clinics • MDA Clinic [34910]
Froedtert Sports Medicine Center • Froedtert Memorial Lutheran Hospital [39185]
Frog Box Inc. [2815]
From the Ashes Inc • DBA Kenneth Peters Center for Recovery [46682]
Front Range Community College • Office of Special Services [327]
Front Range Hospice [19104]
Front Range Therapists [1417]
Front Royal Dialysis Center • DaVita [27492]
Frontier Community Support Program [29849]
Frontier Health--Bristol • Tennessee Community Support [32274]
Frontier Health • Crisis Helpline [51356]
Frontier Health - Crossing Point [32270]
Frontier Health--Erwin [32308]
Frontier Health--Gray [32313]
Frontier Health--Greenville • Continuous Treatment Team [32315]
Frontier Health Inc
    Bristol Regional Counseling Center [49043]
    Lee County Behavioral Health Center [49803]
    Magnolia Ridge [49096]
    Nolachuckey Holston Mental Health Center [49079]
    Scott County Behavioral Health Service [49863]
    Watauga Mental Health Center [49097]
    Wise County Mental Health Center [49768]
Frontier Health--Johnson City [32322]
Frontier Health • Safeplace Program • Runaway and Homeless Youth Program [36205]
Frontier Health - Supported Living [32326]
Frontier Home Health and Hospice [20361]
Frontier Hospice--Bethany [20924]
Frontier Hospice--Pueblo [19123]
Frontline Foundations Inc [43006]
Frost Counseling Center [30308]
FRS Counseling [47778]
Frye Regional Medical Center • Cancer Center [5646]
F.S. DuBois Center [29044]
Fueling with Food [11188]
Full-Care Home Health, LLC [16910]
Full Care, Inc.--Rockville Centre [16619]
Full Care Inc.--West Nyack [16659]

Full Circle Healing [48136]
Full Circle Health Services [16281]
Full Circle Treatment Center [40474]
Full Circle Wellness Center Inc [43927], [44006]
Full Life Hospice, LLC • Centerpointe Resources, Inc. [20957]
Full Potential Behavioral Healthcare [47294]
Fuller Psychological & Family Services [28696]
Fullerton Dialysis • Davita [22702]
Fullerton Neurology and Headache Center • Multiple Sclerosis Center [34524]
Fulton County Addiction Services [46664]
Fulton County Health Center • Cancer Program [5759]
Fulton Friendship House Inc • Victorian Manor [46665]
Fulton--Mason Crisis Service [9197]
Fulton State Hospital [33630]
Function Junction [1839]
Functional Pain Center [35695]
Fundacion UPENS Inc
    Centro de Bayamon [48730]
    Centro El Camino [48836]
Fuquay Varina Kidney Center • Fresenius Medical Care [25869]
Fusion Home Health Care Agency [15681]
Future Surgical Supplies, Inc. [16529]
Future Visions Program Inc [49883]
Futures HealthCore [2525]
Futures Without Violence [8887]

G

G. A. Carmichael Family Health Center [6879]
G and A Home Health Services Corporation [13995]
G B Medical Services Inc [40029]
G & G Home Health Care Services [16153]
G. V. Montgomery Veterans Affairs Medical Center • Cancer Program [5427]
G. Werber Bryan Psychiatric Hospital [33833]
GAAMHA Inc • Pathway House [44476]
Gables [45276]
Gables Home Health, Inc. [13996]
Gablink, Inc. [18165]
Gadsden Independent School District [555]
Gadsden Regional Hospice [18676]
Gadsden Regional Medical Center [12668]
    Cancer Program [4733]
    Sleep Disorders Center [36583]
Gadsden Treatment Center [39250]
GaDuGi Safe Center [9366]
Gaines County Mental Health Center [32551]
Gainesville Dialysis & At Home • DaVita [23708]
Gainesville Hearing Services Inc. [1864]
Galax Treatment Center Inc • Life Center of Galax [49792]
Gale Houses Inc
    Gale House [44269]
    Olson House [44270]
Galesburg Veterans Affairs Clinic [29625]
Galilee Mission Inc [48857]
Galion Community Hospital • Sleep Center [37518]
Gallahue Behavioral Care Services • Community Hospitals of Indiana Inc [43198]
Gallahue Mental Health Center • Community Hospitals of Indiana Inc [43096], [43097]
Gallahue Mental Health Center/Hancock County • Community Hospital of Indiana Inc [43071]
Gallahue Mental Health Services--Hancock County [29735]
Gallahue Mental Health Services--Indianapolis [29744]
Gallatin Community Health [6926]
Galleria Home Training Dialysis and Training At Home • DaVita [26865]
Galleria Kidney Clinic • Dialysis Facility • DaVita [26866]
Gallipolis Developmental Center [8412]
Galloway Home Health Care [13997]
Gallup--McKinley County Schools [558]
Galter Life Center/Cardiac Rehabilitation • Swedish Covenant Hospital • Sports Medicine Therapy [38362]
Galveston--Brazoria Cooperative [803]
Galveston Recovery Program [49348]
Gambro Healthcare--Rock Prairie Rd. [27000]
Gandara Center Inc • Gandara Addiction Recovery Program [44579]

Gandara Mental Health Center **[30466]**, **[44580]**
Gandara Residential Services for Women **[44483]**
Ganix Home Health Care Services, Inc. **[17803]**
Gannon Counseling **[46196]**
GAO Therapy LLC • Gerald A Opthof **[46217]**
Garden City Dialysis Center • DaVita **[25669]**
Garden City Hospital **[2587]**
Garden State Sleep Center **[37345]**
Garden Terrace Nursing and Rehab Center **[1859]**
Gardenside Dialysis • DaVita **[24390]**
Gardner Family Care Corporation • Calworks Dual
    Diagnosis Program **[40658]**
Gardner Health Center **[6358]**
Gardner VNA Hospice **[19965]**
Gardnerville Dialysis • Dialysis Clinic Inc. **[25353]**
Garey Dialysis Center • Renal Advantage Inc.
    [22885]
Garfield Counseling Center Inc **[42508]**
Garfield County Human Services Pomeroy • Branch
    of Quality Behavioral Health **[50053]**
Garfield Fertility Center **[21914]**
Garfield Kidney Center **[23937]**
The Garham Home and Transitional Living Com-
    munity **[29303]**
Garland Dialysis • DaVita **[27104]**
Garner-Webb University • Noel Program for
    Students with Disabilities **[611]**
Garrard Community Mental Health Center **[30040]**
Garrard County Comprehensive • Care Center
    [43642]
Garrett County Health Department • Subst Abuse
    Prog/Behav Health Unit **[44316]**
Garrett Rehabilitation Services **[2423]**
Garrett's Voice **[36466]**
Garrisonville Dialysis Center • DaVita **[27568]**
Garvey House **[31315]**
The Gary Center **[39954]**
Gary Commission for Women • The Rainbow
    Shelter **[9277]**
Gary Community Health Center **[6687]**
Gary D Wood **[44786]**
Gary E Miller Candian County • Childrens Justice
    Center **[47928]**
Garza County Mental Health Center **[32534]**
Gastineau Human Services **[39335]**
Gaston County Schools **[617]**
Gaston Hospice County Inc. **[20668]**
Gaston Hospice, Inc-Robin Johnson House **[20643]**
Gaston Memorial Hospital • Caromont Cancer
    Center **[5640]**
Gate City Dialysis Center • DaVita **[23883]**
Gate House for Women **[48478]**
Gates Circle Dialysis Center **[25636]**
Gateway--20th Street S, Birmingham **[27856]**
Gateway--Airport Highway, Birmingham **[27857]**
Gateway • Allegheny Valley **[48590]**
Gateway Battered Women's Shelter **[8934]**
Gateway Behavioral Health Services **[29373]**
    Crisis Stabilization Program **[42052]**
Gateway Care Facility **[29903]**
Gateway Center for Domestic Violence Services
    [10246]
Gateway Center for Human Services **[28106]**
    Substance Abuse Services Division **[39341]**
Gateway Center of Monterey County **[7801]**
Gateway Community Health Center **[7298]**
Gateway Community Industries, Inc.--Kingston
    [31372]
Gateway Community Industries, Inc.--New Paltz
    [31399]
Gateway Community Initiative Inc **[47457]**
Gateway Community Services **[45699]**, **[51014]**
Gateway Community Services Inc
    Adolescent Outpatient Program **[41699]**
    Adolescent Residential Treatment Prog **[41700]**
    New Beginnings **[41701]**
    Substance Abuse Treatment Programs **[41702]**
Gateway Community Services • Runaway and
    Homeless Youth Services **[36017]**
Gateway Community and Technical College • Dis-
    ability Services **[440]**
GateWay Counseling Center **[48917]**
Gateway Counseling Center **[44907]**
Gateway Counseling Service, Inc. **[28980]**
Gateway Counseling Services **[50169]**
Gateway Dialysis Center **[25613]**
Gateway Dialysis Facility • US Renal Care **[27326]**
Gateway Education Center **[8377]**

Gateway Facility **[47754]**
Gateway Family Counseling Services • Shelby
    County **[28016]**
Gateway Family Services, Inc. **[10509]**
Gateway Foundation **[29563]**
Gateway Foundation Alcohol and
    Drug Treatment/Belleville **[42409]**
    Drug Treatment/Carbondale **[42438]**
    Drug Treatment/Caseyville **[42449]**
    Drug Treatment/Chicago Northwest **[42509]**
    Drug Treatment/Chicago West **[42510]**
    Drug Treatment/Kedzie **[42511]**
    Drug Treatment/Lake Villa **[42738]**
    Drug Treatment/Springfield **[42916]**
Gateway Foundation
    Dallas **[49284]**
    Gateway Recovery House **[40488]**
Gateway Foundation Inc **[45620]**
    Alcohol and Drug Treatment/Aurora **[42397]**
    Outpatient Counseling **[42398]**
Gateway--Great Falls **[30941]**
Gateway • Greentree **[48591]**
Gateway Health Care, Hospice and Palliative Care
    Services **[21138]**
Gateway Healthcare--Adult Crisis Services **[51306]**,
    [51309]
Gateway High School Youth • Fresno County
    Department of Children and Family Services
    [33135]
Gateway Home Care **[18524]**
Gateway Home Dialysis **[23059]**
Gateway Hospice **[21317]**
Gateway House Inc **[39532]**
Gateway House, Inc. **[9110]**
Gateway--Huntsville **[27951]**
Gateway Manor **[31400]**
Gateway Medical Center
    Behavioral Health Unit • Crisis Walk-In Center
        [32293]
    Cancer Care Program **[5925]**
Gateway--Mobile **[27981]**
Gateway
    Moffett House **[48283]**
    Monroeville **[48473]**
    North Hills **[48335]**
Gateway Outreach Center **[47642]**
Gateway • Pleasant Hills **[48690]**
Gateway to Prevention and Recovery **[47917]**,
    [48018], **[48019]**
Gateway Recovery **[50445]**
Gateway Recovery Systems • Outpatient Treatment
    Substance Abuse **[43830]**
Gateway Regional Hospice-Granite City **[19525]**
Gateway Regional Medical Center **[14808]**
Gateway Rehabilitation Center **[48261]**
Gateway • Rehabilitation Center **[48281]**
Gateway Rehabilitation Center • Liberty Station
    [48305]
Gateway Resources • Community Healthlink, Inc.
    [30484]
Gateway
    South **[48316]**
    Squirrel Hill **[48592]**
Gateways Community Mental Health Center •
    Hoover Street Programs **[33153]**
Gateways Forensic Community Treatment Program
    [33154]
Gateways Homeless Services **[33155]**
Gateways Hospital and Mental Health Center
    Effie Street, Los Angeles **[33156]**
    N Mariposa Avenue, Los Angeles **[33157]**
    Percy Street, Los Angeles **[33158]**
    Percy Village Adult Residential Program **[33159]**
Gateways • Outpatient Alcohol and Drug Services
    [47660]
The Gathering Place **[31347]**
Gathering Place • UCCODAR **[49654]**
Gaudenzia Erie Inc **[48361]**
    Community House I **[48362]**
    Community House II **[48363]**
    Dr Daniel S Snow Halfway House for Men
        [48364]
    Outpatient **[48365]**
Gaudenzia Inc **[48624]**
    Broad Street **[48512]**
    Chambers Hill Adolescent Program **[48392]**
    Common Ground **[48393]**
    Diagnostic and Rehabilitation Center **[48513]**

Focus House Men with Co-occ Disorders
    [48514]
Fountain Springs Women/Children Prog **[48280]**
Harrisburg Outpatient Services **[48394]**
House West Chester **[48686]**
Intensive Outpatient **[44132]**
Kindred House **[48687]**
New Image Women and Children **[48515]**
Non Hospital Residential **[44133]**
Outpatient West Chester **[48688]**
Outreach I **[48516]**
Owens Mills/Outpatient **[44320]**
People With Hope **[48517]**
Re-Entry House **[48518]**
Sunbury **[48651]**
Together House **[48519]**
Washington House **[48520]**
Weinberg Center **[44134]**
West Shore Outpatient **[48463]**
Gaudenzia Inc/Winner Co-occurring • Women and
    Children Program **[48521]**
Gaudenzia • Montgomery County Outpatient **[48488]**
Gavin Foundation Inc **[44569]**
    Center for Recovery Services **[44570]**
    Cushing House/Male and Female Programs
        [44571]
Gayle Seely LLC **[44841]**
Gaylord Hospital
    Department of Communication Disorders **[1497]**
    Gaylord Sleep Medicine, North Haven **[36740]**
Gaylord House **[34114]**
Gaylord Specialty Healthcare • Sleep Medicine
    Center **[36741]**
Gaylord Veterans Affairs Clinic **[30554]**
GBC Care Continuum Inc. **[12921]**
GBS Home Health **[17897]**
Geary County Hospital Home Health **[15131]**
Geary Rehabilitation and Fitness Center • Speech--
    Language Therapy **[2223]**
Geauga Sleep Center--Chardon **[37519]**
Geauga Sleep Center--Madison **[37520]**
Geauga Sleep Center--Medina **[37521]**
Geauga Sleep Center--Solon **[37522]**
Geisinger Health System **[26411]**
Geisinger Healthsouth Rehabilitation Center of Dan-
    ville **[38937]**
Geisinger Healthsouth Rehabilitation Hospital--
    Berwick **[38930]**
Geisinger Healthsouth Rehabilitation Hospital--
    Danville **[38938]**
Geisinger Medical Center
    Cancer Center **[5819]**
    Cystic Fibrosis Center **[7653]**
Geisinger Medical Center, Danville • ALS Center
    [143]
Geisinger Medical Center
    MDA Clinic **[34863]**
    Multiple Sclerosis Clinic **[34689]**
    Sleep Disorders Center--Bloomsburg **[37647]**
    Sleep Disorders Center--Coal Township **[37648]**
    Sleep Disorders Center--Danville **[37649]**
Geisinger Wyoming Valley Medical Center
    Henry Cancer Center **[5879]**
    MDA Clinic **[34864]**
    Sports Medicine Department **[38990]**
Geller House **[31474]**
G.E.M. Health Care Agency **[16620]**
Gem State Sports Medicine and Wellness Center
    [38337]
Gene Taylor community Based Outpatient clinic
    [16029]
Gene Taylor Veterans Affairs Community Based
    Outpatient Clinic **[30880]**
Gene Trek Genetics • Gene Trek Medical Clinic
    [12154]
GeneCare Medical Genetics Center **[12309]**
GeneCell International--Clermont **[34988]**
GeneCell International--Miami **[34989]**
Generations Family Health Center, Inc. **[6429]**
Generations Health Services **[47403]**
Generations Healthcare, LLC **[19583]**
Generations Hospice Service Corp. **[19841]**
Genesee County Community Mental Health **[30552]**
Genesee County Community Mental Health Services
    • Mental Health Crisis Clinic **[51016]**
Genesee County Youth Corporation • Reach •
    Runaway and Homeless Youth Program **[36018]**
Genesee District Library for the Blind and Physically

Handicapped • Talking Book Center [3805]
Genesee/Orleans Council on Alcohol and •
  Substance Abuse [46347]
Genesee/Orleans Council on Alcohol/SA • Atwater
  Home Community Residence [46368]
Genesee Valley Rural Preservation Corporation
  [9945]
Geneseo Central School [581]
Genesis A New Beginning [47277]
Genesis - A Place--New Beginning [9735]
Genesis Bank LLC [35031]
Genesis Behavioral Health [31077]
  Children's Center [31078]
Genesis Behavioral Services--Burlington [32958]
Genesis Behavioral Services Inc [50524]
  Comprehensive Womans Recovery [50563]
  Milwaukee Outpatient Clinics [50472]
  Racine Outpatient [50510]
  Residential Treatment Center [50473]
  Spring Place [50511]
  West Bend Outpatient [50564]
  Womens Residential Program [50474]
Genesis Behavioral Services--Milwaukee [32996]
Genesis Behavioral Services--Racine [33010]
Genesis Comprehensive Home Health Care
  Services [13998]
Genesis Counseling [41074], [41254], [41341]
Genesis Counseling Center [45951]
  Drug/Alcohol/Mental Outpatient Services [45965]
Genesis Counseling Services Inc [44471]
Genesis Detoxification Center [50475]
Genesis Family Center [28507]
Genesis/Good Samaritan Medical Center • Genesis
  Recovery Center [47897]
Genesis Health Care [21102]
Genesis Healthcare System • Cancer Program
  [5770]
Genesis HealthCare System • Rehabilitation Center
  • Pain Management Program [35607]
Genesis Healthcare System • Sleep Disorders
  Center [37523]
Genesis Home Health, Inc. [14266]
Genesis Hospice [19666]
Genesis Hospice and Palliative Care [20916]
Genesis House [50549]
Genesis House--Green Valley [8690]
Genesis • House Harrisburg [48395]
Genesis House Inc [41732], [48701]
  Genesis House I [40878]
  Genesis House II [40879]
Genesis House, Inc.--Cookeville [10398]
Genesis House--Lorain [10157]
Genesis II Inc • Caton Village [48522]
Genesis Medical Center [8012]
  Department of Speech and Hearing [2200]
  East Campus • Cancer Center [5185]
Genesis Medical Center, East Rusholme St. [24261]
Genesis Medical Center
  Genesis Regional Rehabilitation Program [4049]
  Genesis Sleep Disorders Center [36975]
Genesis Medical Park--Maplecrest [4050]
Genesis Outpatient Programs [41058]
Genesis Program Thousand Oaks [40850]
Genesis Programs Inc • Ventura [40905]
Genesis Recovery Services Inc [39309]
Genesis Sleep Disorders Center [36907]
Genesis Substance Abuse Services [47374]
Genesis - The Counseling Group [51085]
Genesis Treatment Services [44386]
Genesis Women's Shelter [10454]
Genesys Home Health Care, Inc. [18341]
Genesys Home Health and Hospice, Inc. [15662]
Genesys Hospice-Goodrich [20060]
Genesys Hurley Cancer Institute [5374]
Genesys Medical Equipment Services [15659]
Genesys Regional Medical Center
  Cancer Program [5377]
  Genesys Sleep Disorders Center [37157]
Genetic Counseling Center of Rhode Island [12330]
Genetic Medicine of Central California [12155]
Genetics and IVF Institute [12361], [22088], [22283]
Geneva County Clinic [27935]
Geneva County Day Treatment [28033]
  Our House--Specialized Residential Care
  [33096]
Geneva General Hospital [3026]
  Finger Lakes Health • Dialysis Unit [25671]
Geneva Hearing Services [2043]

Geneva Preschool Therapy Center [1606]
Gengras Center [7860]
The Genieve Shelter [10596]
Genpsych Site [45947]
Genter Healthcare, Inc. [16179]
Gentiva--Athens [12626]
Gentiva--Bessemer [12627]
Gentiva--Carson City [16134]
Gentiva--Clanton [12638]
Gentiva--El Centro [12982]
Gentiva--Encino [12991]
Gentiva--Exton [17317]
Gentiva--Fort Smith [12847]
Gentiva--Gilbertown [12670]
Gentiva--Greenwood Village [13495]
Gentiva Health Services--Albertville [12619]
Gentiva Health Services--Andalusa [12620]
Gentiva Health Services--Anniston [12622]
Gentiva Health Services--Apopka [13581]
Gentiva Health Services--Austin [17813]
Gentiva Health Services--Bedford [17827]
Gentiva Health Services--Birmingham [12632]
Gentiva Health Services--Boynton Beach [13599]
Gentiva Health Services--Bradenton [13604]
Gentiva Health Services--Cedar City [18192]
Gentiva Health Services--Charleston [18504]
Gentiva Health Services--Chiefland [13612]
Gentiva Health Services--Clarks Summit [17285]
Gentiva Health Services--Clearwater [13616]
Gentiva Health Services--Coeur D Alene [14657]
Gentiva Health Services--Crestview [13629]
Gentiva Health Services--Cullman [12641]
Gentiva Health Services--Daphne [12642]
Gentiva Health Services--Daytona Beach [13642]
Gentiva Health Services--Deland [13645]
Gentiva Health Services--Dothan [12649]
Gentiva Health Services--Enterprise [12654]
Gentiva Health Services--Eufaula [12657]
Gentiva Health Services--Florence [12663]
Gentiva Health Services--Foley [12665]
Gentiva Health Services--Fort Myers [13700]
Gentiva Health Services--Fort Payne [12667]
Gentiva Health Services--Fort Walton Beach [13705]
Gentiva Health Services--Gainesville [13708]
Gentiva Health Services--Geneva [12669]
Gentiva Health Services--Greenville [12671]
Gentiva Health Services/Healthfield, Inc. [12633]
Gentiva Health Services--Houston [17986]
Gentiva Health Services--Huntsville [12682]
Gentiva Health Services--Jacksonville [13813]
Gentiva Health Services--Jasper [12687]
Gentiva Health Services--Kissimmee [13828]
Gentiva Health Services--Lake City [13832]
Gentiva Health Services--Lakeland [13841]
Gentiva Health Services--Lancaster [17364]
Gentiva Health Services--Layton [18200]
Gentiva Health Services--Lecanto [13860]
Gentiva Health Services--Leesburg [13863]
Gentiva Health Services--Live Oak [13866]
Gentiva Health Services--Marianna [13875]
Gentiva Health Services--Menifee [13169]
Gentiva Health Services--Mesa [12796]
Gentiva Health Services--Miami [13999]
Gentiva Health Services--Mobile [12693]
Gentiva Health Services--Montgomery [12703]
Gentiva Health Services--Moulton [12704]
Gentiva Health Services--Muscle Shoals [12705]
Gentiva Health Services--Naples [14252]
Gentiva Health Services--New Smyrna Beach
  [14261]
Gentiva Health Services--Ocala [14280]
Gentiva Health Services--Opp [12707]
Gentiva Health Services--Orem [18209]
Gentiva Health Services--Palatka [14306]
Gentiva Health Services--Palm Bay [13882]
Gentiva Health Services--Panama City [14313]
Gentiva Health Services--Pell City [12711]
Gentiva Health Services--Pensacola [14334]
Gentiva Health Services--Phoenix [12808]
Gentiva Health Services--Piedmont [12713]
Gentiva Health Services--Plantation [14344]
Gentiva Health Services--Port Charlotte [14346]
Gentiva Health Services--Port Saint Lucie [14351]
Gentiva Health Services--Prattville [12715]
Gentiva Health Services--Racine [18620]
Gentiva Health Services--Rainbow City [12716]
Gentiva Health Services--Riverview [14356]
Gentiva Health Services--Russellville [12717]

Gentiva Health Services--Sacramento [13281]
Gentiva Health Services--Saint George [18214]
Gentiva Health Services--Saint Petersburg [14367]
Gentiva Health Services--Salt Lake City [18222]
Gentiva Health Services--San Antonio [18142]
Gentiva Health Services--Sanford [14371]
Gentiva Health Services--Sarasota [14376]
Gentiva Health Services--Sebring [14387]
Gentiva Health Services--Selma [12723]
Gentiva Health Services--Spring Hill [14390]
Gentiva Health Services--State College [17489]
Gentiva Health Services--Stockton [13369]
Gentiva Health Services--Sylacauga [12725]
Gentiva Health Services--Tacoma [18470]
Gentiva Health Services--Tallahassee [14398]
Gentiva Health Services--Tampa [14416]
Gentiva Health Services--Troy [12728]
Gentiva Health Services--Tucson [12831]
Gentiva Health Services--Viera [13883]
Gentiva Health Services--Wauwatosa [18642]
Gentiva Health Services--Wilkes Barre [17505]
Gentiva Health Services--Winston Salem [16805]
Gentiva Health Services--Winter Park [14462]
Gentiva Healthcare-Marietta [19406]
Gentiva Home Health Care-Flowood [20233]
Gentiva Home Health Care-Starkville [20264]
Gentiva Home Health Care-Tupelo [20268]
Gentiva Home Health Services [17491]
Gentiva Hospice, Bainbridge [19362]
Gentiva Hospice--Columbia [21218]
Gentiva Hospice-Cookeville [21323]
Gentiva Hospice--Cullman [18694]
Gentiva Hospice-Dothan [18704]
Gentiva Hospice of the Emerald Coast-Marianna
  [19252]
Gentiva Hospice-Enterprise [18707]
Gentiva Hospice - Eufaula [18708]
Gentiva Hospice-Florence [18711]
Gentiva Hospice Greenville [21241]
Gentiva Hospice-Huntsville [18726]
Gentiva Hospice - Jasper [18732]
Gentiva Hospice-Mobile [18738]
Gentiva Hospice, Montgomery [18744]
Gentiva Hospice--Oxford [18750]
Gentiva Hospice--Panama City [19294]
Gentiva Hospice--Stockbridge [19422]
Gentiva--Hot Springs Village [12858]
Gentiva--Houston [17987]
Gentiva--Little Rock [12871]
Gentiva--Marietta [14550]
Gentiva--Modesto [13176]
Gentiva--Orlando [14296]
Gentiva--Peoria [12799]
Gentiva--Pike Road [12714]
Gentiva--Port Saint Lucie [14352]
Gentiva--Pueblo [13507]
Gentiva Rehab Without Walls--Anchorage South
  Central Region [4480]
Gentiva Rehab Without Walls--Dallsa/Fort Worth
  [4444]
Gentiva Rehab Without Walls--Las Vegas and
  Southern Nevada [4263]
Gentiva Rehab Without Walls--Michigan [4162]
Gentiva Rehab Without Walls--Northern California/
  Bay Area [3899]
Gentiva Rehab Without Walls--Northern California/
  Greater Sacramento and Fresno Area [3900]
Gentiva Rehab Without Walls--Northern Nevada
  [4264]
Gentiva Rehab Without Walls • Pediatric Outpatient
  Center [4481]
Gentiva Rehab Without Walls--Phoenix and Tucson
  [3864]
Gentiva Rehab Without Walls--South Central Texas
  [4445]
Gentiva Rehab Without Walls--Southern California
  Los Angeles/San Diego [3901]
Gentiva Rehab Without Walls--Southwestern Utah
  [4467]
Gentiva Rehab Without Walls--Western Washington
  [4482]
Gentiva Respiratory Services & HME [17595]
Gentiva--Roseville [13276]
Gentiva--San Diego [13295]
Gentiva--San Jose [13315]
Gentiva--San Luis Obispo [13324]
Gentiva--Santa Ana [13328]
Gentiva--Santa Rosa [13340]

Pediatric Therapy Center [7780]
Glendale Adventist Medical Center--Psychiatric Institute [28518]
Glendale Adventist Medical Center • Sleep Disorders Center [36666]
Glendale Area Medical Assoc., inc. • Glendale Area Medical and Dental Center [7159]
Glendale Dialysis • DaVita [22708]
Glendale Family Health Care [6231]
Glendale Family Health Center [22443]
Glendale Guidance Center [31338]
Glendale Heights Dialysis Center • Fresenius Medical Care [23999]
Glendale Home Health Care, Glendale, CA [13035]
Glendale Home Healthcare Inc.--E Broadway, Glendale, CA [13036]
Glendale Kidney Center • Dialysis Facility [22709]
Glendive Clinical Office [30939]
Glendive VA Community Based Outpatient Clinic • VA Montana Health Care Center [4248]
Glendive Veterans Affairs Clinic [30940]
Glenmore Recovery Center [45139], [45329], [45330]
    Chemical Dependency Program [45118]
    Outpatient Clinic [45286]
Glenn County Health Services • Substance Abuse Department [40329]
Glenn County Perinatal Program • Discovery House [40330]
Glenn Leroy W Jr [47539]
Glenns Ferry Health Center [6637]
Glens Falls Hospital
    The Charles R. Wood Foundation • Cancer Center [5580]
    Dialysis Unit [25674]
    Rehabilitation Centers [3027]
Glens Falls Veterans Affairs Clinic [31339]
Glenview Dialysis Center • Fresenius Medical Care [24000]
Glenwood Home Health Agency [15380]
Glenwood, Inc. • Adult Day Habilitation [27858]
Glenwood Inc. • Adult Day Treatment [27859]
Glenwood Life Counseling Center [44140]
Glenwood Mental Health Services, Inc. [27860]
Glenwood Regional Medical Center
    Cancer Program [5267]
    Sleep Center [37064]
Glenwood Resource Center [8016]
Global Behavioral Health Inc [42924]
Global Healthcare Systems Inc [44372]
Global Home Care, Inc. [15861]
Global Home Health Inc. [13199]
Global Nursing Home Health, Inc. [14003]
Global Services Home Care Corporation [13745]
Global Speech Services [3585]
Globe-Miami VA Health Care Clinic • Division of Phoenix VA Health Care System [3865]
Globus Medical Inc. [35187]
Glorious Manor Inc II [40031]
Glory House of Sioux Falls [49021]
Glossa Speech--Language Services [2091]
Gloucester County Schools [851]
Gloucester Public Schools [474]
Glow Healthcare Solutions, Inc. [18042]
Glynn Academy High School [364]
GMC 4 West [48525]
GMC Outpatient Dialysis Unit--Justin Drive [26412]
GMO Urban Ministries Inc [47981]
GMS Counseling LLC [49606]
GMS Nursing Association [14004]
Go-Getters, Inc. [30300]
Go-Getters, Inc.--Day Program [30307]
Go-Getters, Inc.--Lower Shore Clinic [30310]
Go-Getters, Inc.--Peer Connection [30311]
Goddard Brockton Kidney Center [24806]
Gogebic County Community Mental Health Services [30649]
Gold Therapy Services Inc. [3250]
Golden Age Home Care of Broward, LLC [14243]
Golden Age Home Care, Inc. [13746]
Golden Age Home Health Care [15811]
Golden Age Home Health Inc. [13200]
Golden Bear Physical Therapy and Sports Injury Center [38106]
Golden Care of Northeastern Pennsylvania, Inc. [17451]
Golden Circle Behavioral Health [29854]
Golden Gate for Seniors [40608]

Golden Health Services [17252]
Golden Health Services, Inc. [17410]
Golden Heart Home Health Care Inc. [13037]
Golden Hills Healthcare Services Inc. [12922]
Golden Home Health Care, Inc.--Livonia [15718]
Golden Home Health Care, Inc.--Miami [14005]
Golden Rule Home Health Care, LLC [16911]
Golden Spread Domestic Violence Services [9864]
Golden State Donor Services [34947]
Golden Triangle Dialysis Center • Fresenius Medical Care [26967]
Golden Triangle Recovery Center Inc [45420]
Golden Valley Health Centers [6326]
Golden Valley Memorial Hospital Home Health Agency [15999]
Golden West College • Accessibility Center for Education [277]
Goldencare Home Health Agency, Inc.--Miami [14006]
Goldencare Home Health Agency--Lauderdale Lakes [13851]
Goldie B. Floberg Center [7970]
Goldsboro South Dialysis • Davita [25872]
Goldtree Kidney Center LLC • American Renal Associates [23492]
Gompers Center Inc. [7741]
Gonzales Mental Health Center [8065], [30138]
Gonzalez Counseling LLC [41195]
Goochland/Powhatan Community Services [49795]
Goochland Powhatan Community Services Board [32741]
Good Care by CPCI--Lancaster [16959]
Good Care by CPCI--Logan [16967]
Good Communications Etc. [1044]
Good Friends Inc [48476]
Good Friends Services [13783]
Good Home Care, Inc. [14007]
Good Hope Institute [41534]
Good Neighbor Community Health Center [6939]
Good Neighbor Healthcare Center [7295]
Good Neighbor Hospice [20943]
Good News Home for Women [45989]
Good Night Sleep Wellness Center • Sleep Disorders Center [36629]
Good Quality Home Health Care [13747]
Good Samaratin Shelter • Acute Care Detox [40759]
Good Samaritan Colony • Substance Abuse Center [48973]
Good Samaritan Community Healthcare • Cancer Care and Research Center [6109]
Good Samaritan Community Services [32847]
Good Samaritan Counseling PA • Donnie D Harrison [47458]
Good Samaritan Fit For Life Therapy and Wellness [1016]
Good Samaritan Healthcare Services [15053]
Good Samaritan Home Care Inc.--Vincennes [15059]
Good Samaritan Home Health • Nursing Sisters Home Care [16347]
Good Samaritan Hospice Inc-Christiansburg [21682]
Good Samaritan Hospice--Kearney [20386]
Good Samaritan Hospice--Roanoke [21729]
Good Samaritan Hospital [20615]
Good Samaritan Hospital--Baltimore [2370]
    Lorien Frankford Dialysis Unit [24640]
    Renal Dialysis Unit [24641]
Good Samaritan Hospital
    Bon Secours Sleep Disorder Institute [37392]
    Burn Program [4590]
Good Samaritan Hospital--Cincinnati
    Cancer Care Program [5694]
    Dialysis Unit [26046]
Good Samaritan Hospital - Corvallis [17185]
Good Samaritan Hospital--Cromwell Center [24642]
Good Samaritan Hospital--Harriman • Regional Kidney Center • Dialysis Facility [25677]
Good Samaritan Hospital and Health Center--Dayton • Cancer Program [5713]
Good Samaritan Hospital Home care [16660]
Good Samaritan Hospital Home Health [17201]
Good Samaritan Hospital • Inpatient [43223]
Good Samaritan Hospital--Kearney [16106]
    Cancer Center [5475]
Good Samaritan Hospital--Lindenhurst • Dialysis Unit [25696]
Good Samaritan Hospital--Los Angeles • Cancer Program [4797]

Good Samaritan Hospital of Maryland • Cancer Program [5283]
Good Samaritan Hospital Medical Center [16657]
Good Samaritan Hospital Medical Center--West Islip • Cancer Program [5624]
Good Samaritan Hospital/North Pavilion [42631]
Good Samaritan Hospital • Pediatric Cystic Fibrosis Center [7614]
Good Samaritan Hospital--Puyallup [18446]
Good Samaritan Hospital • Samaritan Sleep Center [37524]
Good Samaritan Hospital--San Jose • Regional Cancer Center [4846]
Good Samaritan Hospital
    SIDS [36516]
    Sleep Apnea Center [37393]
    Sleep Center [37525]
Good Samaritan Hospital Sleep Disorders Center [37101]
Good Samaritan Hospital Southwest [39634]
Good Samaritan Hospital--Suffern [16644]
    Cancer Program [5620]
Good Samaritan Hospital of Suffern
    Chemical Dependency Unit/Rehab [47108]
    Drug Abuse Treatment Unit/Detox [47109]
Good Samaritan Hospital--Vincennes [2194]
    Cancer Program [5178]
Good Samaritan Hospital--West Islip • Dialysis Unit [25802]
Good Samaritan Medical Center • Audiology-Speech Pathology Rehabilitation Services [2467]
Good Samaritan Medical Center--West Palm Beach • Helen & Harry Gray Cancer Institute [5002]
Good Samaritan Regional Health Center [14873]
Good Samaritan Regional Health Center-Mount Vernon • Cancer Program [5112]
Good Samaritan Regional Medical Center--Corvallis • Regional Cancer Center [5789]
Good Samaritan Regional Medical Center--Phoenix • Samaritan Rehabilitation Institute [967]
Good Samaritan Regional Medical Center--Pottsville • Department of Speech Therapy [3374]
Good Samaritan Services
    Another Road Detox [40008]
    Recovery Point [40760]
    Turning Point [40009]
Good Samaritan Society Home Care and Hospice [20184]
Good Samaritan Society Home Health and Hospice [19723]
Good Samaritan Society-Luther Manor [21303]
Good Samaritan Village [16102]
Good Shepherd Center [7953], [34172]
Good Shepherd Foundation Inc • Henry County [42683]
Good Shepherd Gracenter [40609]
Good Shepherd Health Care System [17195]
Good Shepherd Home Care--Linden [18044]
Good Shepherd Home Care--Longview [18050]
Good Shepherd Home Health and Hospice [21645]
Good Shepherd Home Health and Hospice Agency [16687]
Good Shepherd Home Health and Hospice Services [16736]
Good Shepherd Home Health Services [17989]
Good Shepherd Homecare [18066]
Good Shepherd Hospice--Bartow [19194]
Good Shepherd Hospice--Grove [20935]
Good Shepherd Hospice--Haines City [19231]
Good Shepherd Hospice--Hendricks [20169]
Good Shepherd Hospice Inc-Sebring [19312]
Good Shepherd Hospice--Kansas City [20308]
Good Shepherd Hospice--Lakeland [19246]
Good Shepherd Hospice--Melville [20577]
Good Shepherd Hospice of Mid-Florida [19192]
Good Shepherd Hospice--Oklahoma City [20958]
Good Shepherd Hospice--Tulsa [20980]
Good Shepherd Hospice-Wichita [19785]
Good Shepherd Rehabilitation Hospital
    Brain Injury Program [4388]
    MDA Clinic [34865]
    Multiple Sclerosis Center [34690]
Good Shepherd School for Children [8210]
Good Shepherd Shelter [8840]
Good Spirit Home Health Services Inc. [13128]
Good Talking People LLC [2949]
Good Will Home Association • Runaway and Homeless Youth Program [35980]

Gooden Center [40368]
Goodheart Healthcare Services, Inc. [18388]
Goodland Regional Medical Center [2218]
Goodman Addiction Services [47591]
Goodrich Center for the Deaf [3494]
Goodwill Industries [7838]
Goodwill Industries of the Coastal Empire [7917]
Goodwill Industries of Northern New England [4075]
Goodwill Industries of Santa Clara County • Institute for Career Development [1290]
Goodwill Industries of South Central Wisconsin Inc [3674]
Goodwill Industries Suncoast Inc [41917]
Goodwill Industries • Workforce Solutions • Lewiston/WestSide Neurorehabilitation Services [4076]
Goodwill Outpatient Services [41964]
Goodwin Center [28054]
Goodwin House Hospice [21691]
Gordon Hospice House [20742]
Gordon Hospital [14496]
Gordon Hospital Rehabilitation [1842]
Goretti Health Services Inc [39994]
Goshen County Task Force on Family Violence and Sexual Assault [10767]
Goshen Family Practice [7093]
Goshen General Hospital [2149]
   Cancer Center [5150]
   Center for Sleep Studies [36948]
Goshen Medical Center, Inc. [7051]
Goshen Veterans Affairs Outpatient Clinic [29731]
Gosnell Memorial Hospice House [19902]
Gosnold Inc
   Emerson House [44596]
   Gosnold at Cataumet [44438]
   Gosnold Thorne Counseling Center [44439]
   Gosnold/Thorne Counseling Outpatient Substance AbuseServices [44464]
   Miller House [44465]
Gosnold, Inc. [30375]
Gosnold Thorne Counseling Center [44430]
Gosnold-Thorne Counseling Center [44543]
Gosnold Treatment Center [30357]
Gospel Rescue Ministries [41535]
Gotham City Orthopedics [38718]
Gottfred--Lybolt Speech Associates [2085]
Gottlieb Home Health Services/Hospice [19543]
Gottlieb Memorial Hospital [2069], [14859]
Gottlieb Vision Group [7918]
Gould's Discount Medical [15220]
Goveia/Zeller Center [28774]
Governor Morehead School [3727]
GPA Treatment Inc [42084]
GPA Treatment of Macon Inc [42125]
GPASS Safe [48526]
Grace Center [8866], [44828]
Grace Counseling Services [45169]
Grace Court • Transitions Housing Facility [47414]
Grace G Johnston MSW LCSW LCAS [47359]
Grace Hill Neighborhood Health Centers, Inc. • Grace Hill Neighborhood Health Center [6917]
Grace Home Health Care, LLC [12789]
Grace Hospice--Kansas City [20309]
Grace Hospice of Oklahoma, LLC [20981]
Grace Hospice--Tempe [18823]
Grace Hospital • Cancer Center [5652]
Grace House [43871]
   Center for Human Development [44529]
Grace House Inc [49135]
   Extended [49136]
Grace Smith House [9979]
Gracemoor Inc. [10434]
Graceway Recovery Residence Inc [42018]
Gracewood State School and Hospital [7913]
Gracie Square Hospital Inc • Inpatient Dual Focus [46861]
Gracious Helpers [17876]
Graduate Hospital Human Performance & Sports Medicine Center [38988]
Grady Central Fulton Mental Health Center • Florida Hall [29350]
Grady County Dialysis Facility [23632]
Grady County Health Department/Sooner Start • Speech and Hearing Clinic [3264]
Grady County Hospital • Department of Speech and Language Pathology [3265]
Grady County Mental Health Center [29376]
Grady County Mental Health Older Persons Day

   Treatment [29377]
Grady Health System, Atlanta • Georgia Comprehensive Sickle Cell Center [36334]
Grady Memorial Hospital • Cancer Program [5717]
Grady Memorial Hospital--Chickasha [17110]
Grady Memorial Hospital--Delaware [16930]
Grady Memorial Hospital
   Georgia Cancer Center of Excellence [4668]
   Sleep Disorders Center [37526]
Graf Rheeneenhaanjii • Substance Abuse Services [39326]
Grafton VA Outpatient Clinic • ND State Developmental Center • Health Service Bldg. [4352]
Graham Dialysis Center • DaVita [27607]
Graham Hospital Home Health [14705]
Graham Hospital • Hospice Unit [19494]
Gramercy Park Medical Group PC • MMTP Clinic [46862]
Grammercy House [28453]
Grammy's House [9860]
Gran Recovery Center [42069]
Granada House Inc [44396]
Grand Blanc Dialysis • DaVita [24905]
Grand Care Home Health LLC [17923]
Grand Erie District School Board • Deaf/Hard of Hearing Program [676]
Grand Island Dialysis • DaVita [25323]
Grand Itasca Clinic & Hospital [15905]
Grand Junction Dialysis Center & At Home • DaVita [23122]
Grand Junction Regional Center for Developmental Disabilities [7842]
Grand Junction Vet Center [51906]
Grand Junction Veterans Affairs Medical Center [13493]
   Montrose Clinic [28938]
Grand Lake Home Health [17028]
Grand Lake Hospice [20889]
Grand Lake Mental Health Center [31874]
Grand Lake Mental Health Center, Inc. • Administrative Office [31898]
Grand Lake Mental Health Center, Inc.--Afton [31869]
Grand Lake Mental Health Center, Inc.
   Delaware County Office [31886]
   Nowata County Office [31899]
   Ottawa County Office [31892]
   Rogers County Office [31880]
Grand Lake Mental Health Center, Inc.--Vinita [31924]
Grand Prairie Dialysis Center Inc. [27111]
Grand Prairie Services
   Administrative Center [29681]
   Gloria McAfee Center [29630]
Grand Strand Regional Medical Center • Cancer Program [5911]
Grand Traverse Area Library for the Blind and Physically Handicapped [3806]
Grand Traverse Band of Ottawa and Chippewa Indians [9576], [44954]
Grand View Hospital [17473]
   Community Cancer Center [5872]
Grand View Hospital Community Nurse Home Care Department [17401]
Grand View Hospital Hospice [21156]
Grand View Hospital
   Speech Pathology/Physical Medicine and Rehab Department [3379]
   Sports Medicine Center [38982]
Grand Wood Area Education Agency, Number 10 [2198]
Grandcare Home Health Services [13038]
Grande Ronde Hospital Home Care Services [17199], [21011]
Grande Ronde Recovery [48141]
GrandView Behavioral Health Center--Anniston [27831]
Grandview Behavioral Health Center--Montgomery [27995]
Grandview Foundation Inc [40369]
   Marengo House [40370]
Grandview Hospital and Medical Center • Pain Management Center [35608]
Grandview Medical Center • Cancer Care Program [5714]
Grandview Regional Medical Center--Fort Payne [27930]

Granite Bay Speech--Roseville [1243]
Granite City Dialysis Center • DaVita [24001]
Granny's Home Health Care [14008]
Grant Addictive Disorders Clinic [43820]
Grant Blackford Mental Health Inc [43146]
   Cornerstone Behavioral Health [43147]
Grant Blackford Mental Health, Inc. • Hester Hollis Concern Center [29738]
Grant County Dialysis • Fresenius Medical Care [24199]
Grant County Hospice [21848]
Grant County Prevention and • Recovery Center [50023]
Grant Medical Center
   Cancer Care Program [5707]
   Sleep Diagnostic Center [37527]
Grant Memorial Home Care [18534]
Grant Memorial Hospital Hospice [21811]
Grant Mental Health and Family Service • Crisis Line [51450]
Grant Mental Healthcare [32840]
Grant Park Dialysis • daVita [23223]
Grant Street Partnership [41442]
Grants Dialysis • Dialysis Clinic, Inc. [25547]
Granville County Schools [628]
Grapevine--Colleyville Intermediate School District [790]
Grapevine Dialysis & At Home • DaVita [27113]
Grapevine Valley Hope [49351]
Grass Valley Dialysis Center • DaVita [22714]
Grassroots Crisis Intervention Center, Inc. [50972]
Gratiot Community Hospital • Ithaca Rehabilitation [2608]
Gratiot--Isabella Deaf/Hard of Hearing Program [493]
Gratitude House Inc [41995]
Gray Wolf Ranch • Port Townsend [50066]
Graybill Medical Group [38087]
Graydon Manor • Intermediate Residential Facility [49805]
Grays Harbor County Crisis Clinic [32830]
Great Bridge Dialysis Center • DaVita [27473]
Great Circle--St. James Campus [36054]
Great Falls Orthopedic Associates [38682]
Great Falls VA Community Based Outpatient Clinic • VA Montana Health Care Center [4249]
Great Falls Vet Center [52010]
Great Falls Veterans Affairs Clinic [30942]
Great Heights Family Medicine Ltd [42431]
Great Lakes Dialysis, LLC [24876]
Great Lakes Dialysis--Monroe • Fresenius Medical Care [24947]
Great Lakes Genetics [12374]
Great Lakes Hemophilia Foundation [12615]
Great Lakes Home Healthcare and Hospice [21083]
Great Lakes Home Healthcare Services--Bradford [17263]
Great Lakes Home Healthcare Services--Erie [17312]
Great Lakes Home Healthcare Services--Meadville [17383]
Great Lakes Home Patient Care--Dearborn Heights [15629]
Great Lakes Home Patient Care, LLC--Livonia [15719]
Great Lakes Hospice [20075]
Great Lakes Pain Consultants [35499]
Great Lakes Recovery Centers Inc
   Adult Residential Services [44913]
   Iron Mountain Outpatient Services [44855]
   Ironwood Outpatient Services [44859]
   Marquette Outpatient Services [44914]
   New Hope House for Men [45011]
   New Hope House for Women [45012]
Great Lakes Regional Rehabilitation Hospital [2648]
Great Lakes Renal Network--Alma • Dialysis Center [24827]
Great Lakes Renal Network--Greenville • Dialysis Facility [24911]
Great Lakes Renal Network--Mount Pleasant [24949]
Great Plains Hearing and Speech Associates [2243]
Great Plains Lions Eye Bank, Inc. [35228]
Great Plains Regional Medical Center [17117], [20394]
   Callahan Cancer Center [5478]
Great Plains Sports Medicine and Rehabilitation Center [38405]

Great River Hospice [19737]
Great River Hospice House [15114]
Great River Medical Center
    Addiction Services [43315]
    Sleep Disorders Center [36976]
Great River Recovery Resources Inc [42873]
Greatcare Home Health Inc. [13129]
Greater Ann Arbor Sleep Disorders Center [37158]
Greater Atlanta Speech and Language Clinics, Inc.
    [1884]
Greater Baden Medical Services [6792]
Greater Baltimore Medical Center [2371]
    Berman Cancer Institute [5284]
    Cochlear Implant Center [2372]
    Harvey Institute for Human Genetics • Prenatal
        Diagnostic Center [12227]
Greater Binghamton Health Center [33678]
Greater Boone Dialysis LLC [27669]
Greater Bridgeport Community Mental Health Center
    • Co-Occurring Treatment Unit [41364]
Greater Bristol Visiting Nurse Association [13516]
Greater Charleston Dialysis LLC [27690]
Greater Chesapeake Orthopaedic Associates •
    Baltimore [38515]
Greater Chesapeake Orthopedic Associates • Sports
    Medicine Center at Bel Air [38521]
Greater Cincinnati Behavioral Health Services--
    Madison Road [31693]
Greater Cincinnati Behavioral Health Services--
    Reading Road [31694]
Greater Columbia Behavioral Health RSN [51446]
Greater Columbus Regional Dialysis LLC • Fres-
    enius Medical Care [26085]
Greater Elgin Family Care Center [6671]
Greater Essex Counseling Services • Drug and
    Alcohol OP & IOP Treatment [46093]
Greater Health Home Health Care Inc. [13389]
Greater Hill Country Hospice • Hill Country Memorial
    Hospice [21467]
Greater Hudson Valley Family Health Center, Inc.
    [7033]
Greater Hudson Valley Family Hlth Center
    Center for Recovery/Outpt Chem Dep [46939]
    Center for Recovery/Rehab Services [46940]
    Methadone Maintenance Treatment Prog
        [46941]
Greater Lafayette Area Special Services [425]
Greater Lakes Mental Health Care--Lakewood
    [32832]
Greater Lakes Mental Health Center
    Independence Inn [32864]
    Sunset Inn [32873]
Greater Lakes Mental Healthcare [51447]
Greater Lawrence Family Health Center, Inc. [6818]
Greater Los Angeles Agency on Deafness Inc. •
    Employment Development Department [1161]
Greater Los Angeles Agency on Deafness Inc.
    (GLAD)--Los Angeles [1162]
Greater Los Angeles Agency on Deafness Inc.--West
    Covina • Employment Development Department
    [1360]
Greater Los Angeles Council on Deafness Inc.
    (GLAD)--Crenshaw • EDD/GLAD Job Service for
    Deaf and Hard of Hearing [1163]
Greater Los Angeles Dialysis Inc. [23018]
Greater Los Angeles Veterans Affairs Medical Center
    Bakersfield Community Based Outpatient Clinic
        [28390]
    East Los Angeles Community Based Outpatient
        Center [28443]
    Gardena Clinic [28512]
    PTSD Clinical Team [51689]
Greater Meridian Health Clinic, Inc. [6890]
Greater Miami Dialysis • DaVita • Dialysis Facility
    [23397]
Greater Minneapolis Council of Churches •
    Runaway and Homeless Youth Program [36036]
Greater Mount Calvary Holy Church • Cataada
    House/Outpatient Treatment Program [41536]
Greater Nashua Council on Alcoholism
    Cynthia Day Family Center [45912]
    Keystone Hall [45913]
Greater New Bedford Community Health Center Inc.
    [6821]
Greater New Bedford Women's Center [9493]
Greater Puyallup Dialysis Center [27630]
Greater Regional Hospice [19680]

Greater Rochester Physical Therapy and SportsCare
    [38826]
Greater Rumford AMI [50961]
Greater Saskatoon Catholic Schools • Deaf/Hard of
    Hearing Program [725]
Greater Southeast Community Dialysis Center • Fre-
    senius Medical Care [23224]
Greater Southern Tier BOCES [570]
Greater Tampa Home at Home • DaVita [23534]
Greater Trenton Adult Day Treatment [46189]
Greater Trenton C.M.H.C Inc. [31168]
Greater Waterbury Dialysis • DaVita [23185]
Greece Central Schools [595]
Greeley Medical Clinic • Audiology Department
    [1418]
Green Bay Northwood Dialysis • DaVita [27782]
Green Bay Program for Deaf and Hard of Hearing
    [885]
Green Brook Regional Center [8250]
Green Center of Growth and Development [47505]
Green Chimneys Children's Services, Inc. [34327]
Green Chimneys Children's Services • Runaway
    and Homeless Youth Program [36109]
Green Country Behavioral Health Services, Inc.
    [31893]
Green Country Behavioral Health Services •
    Integrated Services [47963]
Green County Human Services • Alcohol and Other
    Drug Abuse [50489]
Green County Mental Health Center [30022]
Green Door [29088]
Green Gables Haven [9540]
Green Haven Family Advocates, Inc. [10725]
Green Hills Women's Shelter [9731]
Green Lake County • Department of Health and Hu-
    man Srvs [50405]
Green Mountain at Fox Run [11293]
Green Mountain Speech and Hearing Services Inc.
    [3565]
Green Oaks Behavioral Healthcare of Plano [33879]
Green Oaks Hospital [33863]
Green Oaks at Medical City Dallas [49285]
Green Pine Home Health Care Services Inc. [13313]
Green Program for Hearing Handicapped [657]
Green River Hospice [19816]
Green River Medical Center [7323]
Green Tree School [32078]
Green Valley Community Based Outpatient Clinic
    [3866]
Green Valley Dialysis
    Diversified Specialty Insitutes [25356]
    Fresenius Medical Care [25364]
Greenbriar Children's Center • Runaway and Home-
    less Youth Program [35907]
Greenbriar Treatment Center [48674]
    Lighthouse for Men [48675]
    Lighthouse for Women [48676]
    Monroeville [48593]
    New Kensington [48483]
    North Strabane [48677]
    Robinson Township [48594]
    South Hills [48303]
    Squirrel Hill [48595]
    Wexford [48693]
Greene Area Medical Extenders, Inc. • Leakesville
    Medical Center [6886]
Greene County Dialysis Center • DaVita [25952]
Greene County General Hospital Home Healthcare
    Agency [15022]
Greene County Health Care [7058]
Greene County Health Care, Inc. • Snow Hill Medi-
    cal Center [7059]
Greene County Mental Health Center [31295]
Greene County Outreach [29769]
Greene Hall • Outpatient Services [47621]
Greene Memorial Hospital, Inc. [17085]
Greene Memorial Hospital • Ruth G. McMillan
    Cancer Center [5766]
Greene Regional Home Care [16781]
Greene Respiratory Services [17000]
Greene Valley Developmental Center [8517]
Greenfield Center [41703]
Greenfield Counseling Inc [48461]
Greenfield Health Systems--Dearborn • Dialysis
    Facility [24864]
Greenfield Health Systems--Detroit West Pavilion •
    Dialysis Facility [24877]
Greenfield Health Systems--Eastpointe • Dialysis

Facility [24891]
Greenfield Health Systems--Livonia • Dialysis Facil-
    ity [24937]
Greenfield Health Systems--Northwest Detroit
    [24878]
Greenfield Health Systems--Pontiac • Dialysis Facil-
    ity [24957]
Greenfield Health Systems--Taylor • Dialysis Facility
    [24983]
Greenfield Health Systems--Troy • Dialysis Facility
    [24986]
Greenfields Health Services Inc [39690]
Greenhill Wellness Center [2941]
Greenhope Services for Women Inc [46863]
Greenhouse Runaway Shelter • Runaway and
    Homeless Youth Program [36194]
Greenleaf Center • A Division of South GA Medical
    Center [42174]
Greenleaf Counseling Center • A Division of South
    GA Medical Center [42175]
Greenleaf Family Center • Community Services for
    the Deaf [3208]
GreenLight Home Health Care Services, Inc.
    [17936]
Greensboro Dialysis Facility LLC [23711]
Greensboro Kidney Center • Fresenius Medical
    Care [25876]
Greensboro Metro Treatment Center [47346]
Greensburg Dialysis and At Home • DaVita [24157]
Greenspring Dialysis Center • DaVita [24643]
Greenspring Village Hospice [21736]
Greenstein Neurology and Multiple Sclerosis Institute
    [34691]
Greensville Emporia Counseling Services [32729]
Greenview Regional Hospital • Cancer Care
    Program [5211]
Greenville Community Health Center [7292]
Greenville County Deaf and Hard of Hearing
    Program [730]
Greenville Dialysis [27114]
Greenville Dialysis Center • Fresenius Medical Care
    • Dialysis Facility [25879]
Greenville Genetic Center • Down Syndrome Clinic
    [10861]
Greenville Hospital System
    Cancer Treatment Center [5908]
    Center for Women's Medicine • Reproductive
        Endocrinology and Infertility [22243]
    University Medical Group • MDA Clinic [34872]
Greenville Intermediate School District [791]
Greenville Medical Center • Sickle Cell Disease
    Center [36424]
Greenville Mental Health Center • Crisis Intervention
    [51330]
Greenville Metro Treatment Center [48942]
Greenville Orthopedic Association [38946]
Greenville Outpatient Clinic [17596]
Greenville Psychiatric Associates • Winston E Lane
    III [47360]
Greenville Rape Crisis and Child Abuse Center
    [10351]
Greenville Recovery Center [47361]
Greenville Veterans Affairs Clinic--Moyle Boulevard
    [31540]
Greenville Veterans Affairs Clinic--S Colorado Street
    [30762]
Greenway Orchard [33201]
Greenwell Springs Hospital [33536]
Greenwich Hospital • Bendheim Cancer Center
    [4894]
Greenwich Hospital Hearing, Speech, & Language
    Center [1460]
Greenwich Hospital Home Hospice [19145]
Greenwich Hospital • Sleep Laboratory [36742]
Greenwich House Inc [46864]
    Greenwich House Chem Dependency Prog
        [46865]
Greenwich Otolaryngology [1461]
Greenwich Sports Medicine [38193]
Greenwich YWCA • Domestic Abuse Services
    [8994]
Greenwood Dialysis Center • Fresenius Medical
    Care [23938]
Greenwood Dialysis • DaVita [26305]
Greenwood Genetic Center • Genetics/Prenatal
    Diagnosis Clinic [12332]
Greenwood Holly Renal Center • Diversified
    Specialty Institutes [27010]

Greenwood House Hospice [20472]
Greenwood Leflore Hospital • Sleep Disorders Center [37247]
Greenwood Mental Health Clinic [32202]
Greer Kidney Center Inc. • DaVita [26727]
Greg Dumas LCSW [44052]
Gregory M Ortega LCSW LAC [41059]
Greil Memorial Psychiatric Hospital [33091]
Grenada Lake Medical Center [15962]
Gresham Dialysis Center • Innovative Dialysis Systems [26323]
GREY Physical Therapy & Sports Medicine Center [38191]
Greystone Park Psychiatric Hospital [33659]
Griffin Hospital [28989]
　　Center for Cancer Care [4892]
　　Chemical Dependency Service [41378]
　　Psychiatric Crisis Team [50725]
　　Sleep Wellness Center [36743]
Griffin Memorial Hospital [33779]
Griffin Mill Residential Care Home [28032]
Grinnell Regional Hospice [19696]
The GRIP Project, Justice Research Institute: Growing Responsibility and Independence in People • Runaway and Homeless Youth Program [36001]
Griswold Special Care [2499]
Gritman Medical Center [14665]
　　Gritman Sleep Laboratory [36876]
GRN Community Service Board [29456]
　　Beacon Place [29457]
　　Newton Mental Health Center [42070]
　　The Oaks Adaptive Group Residence [29458]
GRN CSB Lawrenceville • Alcohol and Drug Program [42120]
The Groden Center [8497]
Groden Center Inc. [33826]
　　Branch Pike House [33830]
　　Cove Center [33827]
　　Cowesett House [33831]
　　Livingston Center for Early Childhood [33828]
Grosse Pointe Audiology [2600]
Grosse Pointe Dialysis and At Home • DaVita [24879]
Grossman Burn Center - Santa Ana [4516]
Group Health • Behavioral Health Services [50170]
Group Health/Home & Community Services [21747]
Group Health/Home Health & Hospice [21773]
Group Home [31177]
Group Home for Girls [34008]
Group Home Number 2 [30923]
Group Home Number 3 [30924]
Group Home Support Services Inc • New Beginnings Addiction and Recovery [40420]
Group Homes for Children, Inc. • Runaway and Homeless Youth Program [35780]
Grove City Dialysis • DaVita [26130]
Grove Counseling Center Inc
　　The Grove Academy [42011]
　　Outpatient Services [41751]
Grove Counseling Center, Inc.--Longwood [29209]
Grove Counseling Center, Inc.
　　Outpatient in Altamonte [29103]
　　Outpatient in Lake Mary [29197]
Grove Counseling Center, Inc.--Winter Springs [29324]
Grove Hill Satellite Office [27941]
Grove School, Inc. • Therapeutic School For Emotionally Fragile Teenagers [34054]
Groves Community Hospice [20300]
Growing Minds Therapeutics [3059]
Growing Strong Sexual Assault Center [9220]
Growing Together Inc [47592]
　　STEP Program [47582]
Growth and Recovery Services [46048]
Growth Works Inc [44688], [44960]
Grundy Community Hospice [19546]
Grundy County Health Department [42786]
　　Mental Health Division [29650]
Grunewald-Blitz Clinic [7751]
Gryphon Place [51021]
Gryphon Place XI Inc [40381]
GSH Dialysis, Inc. • Dialysis Facility [26467]
Guadalupe County Domestic Violence Responders [9885]
Guadalupe Family Health Center [6234]
Guadalupe Kidney Disease Clinic • Fresenius Medical Care [27327]
Guadalupe Regional Hospice • Guadalupe Regional

Medical Center [21565]
Guadalupe Regional Medical Center [18156]
　　Teddy Buerger Center [49536]
Guadalupe Valley Family Violence Shelter [10507]
Guam Comprehensive Hemophilia Care Program [12512]
Guam Department of Health [36469]
Guam Dialysis Center--Tamuning [23842]
Guam Memorial Hospital • Dialysis Center [23843]
Guam Public School Systems • Division of Special Education [1931]
Guam Renal Care • Dialysis Facility [23841]
Guam Sleep Center [36867]
Guam Vet Center [51938]
Guaranteed Medical Services, Inc. [14732]
Guardian Angel Home [34111]
Guardian Angel Home Health [13469]
Guardian Angel Home Health Agency Inc. [13354]
Guardian Angel Home health, Inc. [16316]
Guardian Angel Home of Joliet, Inc. • Groundwork [9236]
Guardian Angel Hospice Care [20108]
Guardian Angel Hospice-Kokomo [19621]
Guardian Angel Hospice-Lafayette [19622]
Guardian Angel Hospice-Logansport [19626]
Guardian Angel Hospice-Marion [19627]
Guardian Angels HomeCare LLC [13517]
Guardian Care Services [14207]
Guardian Care Services of Broward [14244]
Guardian Health services, LLC [16740]
Guardian Health System [17149]
Guardian Healthcare, LLC [15503]
Guardian Hospice of Atlanta [19350]
Guardian Hospice Care, LLC-Alexandria [19832]
Guardian Hospice--Franklin [21332]
Guardian Hospice, Inc.--Metairie [19859]
Guardian Hospice of MA [19994]
Guardian Recovery Program [50112]
Guardian Shelter for Battered Families • Catholic Charities [9655]
Guernsey Counseling Center [31673]
Guernsey County Dialysis • DaVita • Dialysis Facility [26027]
Guest House Inc [45277]
Guidance Associates of Pennsylvania [48315], [48404]
Guidance Care Center Inc [41755]
Guidance/ Care Center Inc [41716]
Guidance Center [7786], [29939], [45023], [49075], [49150], [49190]
　　Adult and Family Services [45024]
The Guidance Center - Atchison County [29908]
The Guidance Center- Avalon [28386]
The Guidance Center--Bradford [31998]
Guidance Center of Brooklyn Inc [46503]
The Guidance Center--Flagstaff [28146]
Guidance Center Inc [39382]
　　Chemical Dependency Treatment Center [46800]
The Guidance Center - Jefferson County [29948]
The Guidance Center--Kane [32031]
Guidance Center of Lea County Inc [46277]
　　Lovington [46291]
Guidance Center of Lea County Inc. [31198]
The Guidance Center--Long Beach [28569]
The Guidance Center--New Rochelle [31401]
Guidance Center Recovery Services [43390], [43427]
Guidance Center Recovery Services of Atchison [43318]
The Guidance Center--Southgate [30639]
The Guidance Center--Williams [28227]
Guidance Clinic of the Middle Keys, Inc. [29210]
Guidance for Growing LLC [48647]
Guidance and Prevention Services Inc [45032]
Guidance Prevention Services Inc [44831]
Guided Life Structures [46169]
Guiding Light Counseling Inc [42420]
Guiding Light/Drug and Alcohol • Treatment Services [46076]
Guiding Light Mission [44809]
Guild for Infant Survival Orange County [36453]
Guildhaus Halfway House [42419]
Guilford Center [31546]
The Guilford Center [31536]
The Guilford Center/Bellemeade Center [31537]
Guilford County Area Mental Health/Mental Retardation/Substance Abuse Services [31538]

Gulf Bend Center [51395]
Gulf Bend Mental Health and Mental Retardation Center [8568]
Gulf Bend Mental Health/Mental Retardation Center [32565]
Gulf Breeze Dialysis Center & At Home • DaVita [23294]
Gulf Coast Assisting Hands [14253]
Gulf Coast Center [32468]
　　Adolescents in Recovery [49558]
The Gulf Coast Center--Alvin • Centralized Intake & Assessment [32399]
The Gulf Coast Center--Angleton [32403]
Gulf Coast Center • Angleton Recovery Program [49209]
The Gulf Coast Center--Texas City [32560]
Gulf Coast Dialysis Center Inc. [23295]
Gulf Coast Dialysis Inc. • DaVita [23487]
Gulf Coast Health Center, Inc. [7305]
Gulf Coast Hospice--D'Iberville [20232]
Gulf Coast Hospice of Houston [21483]
Gulf Coast Hospital [1580]
Gulf Coast Jewish Family Services
　　66th Street Group Home [29278]
　　Icot Boulevard [29127]
Gulf Coast Jewish Family Services Inc • 66th Street Group Home [41918]
Gulf Coast Jewish Family Services, Inc. • Chatlin [29180]
Gulf Coast Jewish Family Services • N Florida Avenue [29304]
Gulf Coast Kidney Center--Hudson [23333]
Gulf Coast Kidney Center--New Port Richey • Physicians Dialysis [23427]
Gulf Coast Medical Center [2754]
　　Cancer Program [4979]
Gulf Coast Recovery Inc [41982]
Gulf Coast Teaching Family Service • Runaway and Homeless Youth Program [35973]
Gulf Coast Treatment Center [39254]
Gulf Coast Veterans Healthcare System • Biloxi [45361]
Gulf Coast Women's Center for Non-Violence [9648]
Gulf Coast Youth Services [34071]
Gulf Medical Services [14399]
Gulf Medical Services--Daphne [12643]
Gulf Medical Services--Dothan [12650]
Gulf Medical Services--Milton [14229]
Gulf Medical Services--Panama City [14314]
Gulf Medical Services--Pensacola [14335]
Gulf Oaks Hospital • Behavioral Health Services [30744]
Gulf Shore Sleep Disorders Center [37248]
Gulf States Hemophilia and Thrombophilia Center [12599]
Gulfside Center for Hospice Care at Trinity [19328]
Gulfside Regional Hospice House at Edwinola [19213]
Gulfside Regional Hospice. Inc.--New Port Richey [19267]
Gulfside Regional Hospice Inc.--Zephyrhills [19338]
Gundersen Clinic • Pediatric Specialties [12616]
Gundersen Lutheran
　　Behav Health Unity House for Men [50431]
　　Behav Health Unity House for Women [50432]
　　Behavioral Health [50433], [50498], [50508], [50529], [50542], [50566]
Gundersen Lutheran Dialysis--Black River Falls [27703]
Gundersen Lutheran Dialysis Satellite--Prairie du Chien [27773]
Gundersen Lutheran Dialysis Satellite--Whitehall [27806]
Gundersen Lutheran Medical Center [18579]
Gundersen Lutheran Medical Center Behavioral Health [32983]
Gundersen Lutheran Medical Center • Cancer Program [6157]
Gundersen Lutheran Medical Center--La Crosse • Dialysis Center [27730]
Gundersen-Lutheran Medical Center • Speech-Language Pathology Department [3670]
Gundersen Lutheran Medical Center • Wisconsin Sleep Disorders Center [37968]
Gundersen--Lutheran Memorial Center [51508]
Gundersen-Lutheran SAT--Onalaska [27766]
Gundersen Lutheran Satellite--Tomah [27791]
Gundersen Lutheran Satellite--Viroqua • Dialysis

Facility [27792]
Gunderson Lutheran [8616]
Gunderson Lutheran At Home Hospice [21846]
Gunderson Lutheran Clinic • Developmental and Behavioral Pediatrics [10879]
Gunderson Lutheran Medical Center • Cystic Fibrosis Center [7699]
Gunderson Sports Medicine Center [39178]
Gunnison Valley Hospital [21606]
Gunter Speech and Hearing Services [1872]
Gurabo Community Health Center, Inc. [7199]
Guthrie Home Care DBA Guthrie Hospice [21163]
Guthrie Scottish Rite Center • Language Disorders Clinic [3269]
Gutierrez and Associates [42512]
Gutierrez and Associates Inc [42432]
G.V. Montgomery Veterans Affairs Medical Center [30777]
G.V. (Sonny) Montgomery Veterans Affairs Medical Center [4228]
GV Sonny Montgomery Veterans Affairs Medical Center [51594]
G.V. Sonny Montgomery Veterans Affairs Medical Center
    Multiple Sclerosis Center [34615]
    PTSD Residential Rehabilitation Program [51760]
    Substance Use PTSD Team [51761]
GW and Associates • A Wellness Organization [42513]
Gwinnett Children's Shelter • Runaway and Homeless Youth Program [35908]
Gwinnett County Public Schools [380]
Gwinnett Dialysis Facility [23732]
Gwinnett Hospital System • Cancer Program [5029]
Gwinnett Medical Center [1875]
    Center for Sleep Disorders [36840]
Gwinnett Pulmonary Group • Sleep Disorders Center [36841]
Gyft Clinic • In Vitro Fertilization Program [22295]
Gyst House Inc [39547]

H

H-Care Nursing Service [15663]
H Chandler and Associates LLC [47970]
H. Douglas Singer Mental Health Center [33438]
H and E Home Care [14009]
H Group BBT Inc
    Halfway House [42760]
    Illinois Centre Healthcare [42761]
    Matrix of Hope [42762]
    Outpatient and Intensive Outpatient [42763]
    West Frankfort Office [42957]
    Womens Halfway House [42764]
The H Group • Runaway and Homeless Youth Program [35927]
H and H Drug Stores, Inc. [13039]
H. Lee Moffitt Cancer Center [1777]
    Comprehensive Cancer Center [4666]
H & M Health Services, Inc. [13795]
HAART [40297]
    Hayward [39912]
Habersham County Medical Center [1857], [14517]
Habersham County Mental Health Center [50803]
Habersham Mental Health Center • Avita Community Partners [42083]
Habilitat Inc [42244]
Habilitative Systems Inc [42514]
Habit OPCO [44416], [44431], [44454], [44456], [44466], [44496], [44504], [44574], [44581], [44591], [45908], [45921]
Habit Opco • Allentown [48264]
Habit Opco Brattleboro [49728]
Habit OPCO • DBA New Street Treatment Associates [46018]
Habit Opco Inc • DBA Suburban Treatment Facility [46197]
Habit Opco
    Pottstown [48621]
    Satellite [44547]
HACC Inc • Harbor Area Substance Abuse Treatment [40695]
Hacienda Dialysis Center [22716]
Hackensack High School Program for the Deaf [545]
Hackensack Medical Center [25437]
    Renal Unit [25438]
Hackensack University Medical Center

Active Orthopedic and Sports Medicine [38727]
Burn Care Unit [4586]
Department of Audiology [2915]
Institute for Sleep/Wake Disorders [37346]
Judy Center for Down Syndrome [8252]
Hackensack University Medical Center--North • Active Orthopedic and Sports Mediicng [38769]
Hackensack University Medical Center
    North New Jersey Community Clinical Oncology Program [5515]
    Speech Pathology Department [2916]
    Tomorrow's Children Institute • Sickle Cell Disease Center [36378]
    University of Medicine and Dentistry of New Jersey • New Jersey Medical School Division of Reproductive Endocrinology and Infertility [22161]
Hackettstown Regional Medical Center
    The Counseling and Addiction Center [46010]
    Speech and Audiology Therapy Center [2917]
Hackley Community Care Center [6853]
Hackley Life Counseling [44937]
Hackley Visiting Nurse and Hospice Services, Inc. [20098]
Hadley School for the Blind [3706]
Hagedorn Little Village School • Jack Joel Center for Special Children [8354]
Hager Preschool [30090]
Hagerstown Veterans Affairs Clinic [30293]
Hahnemann Neurodiagnostic Sleep Center • Hahnemann University Hospital [37650]
Hahnemann University Hospital • Cancer Program [5852]
Haight Ashbury Free Clinics Inc [40610]
Haire Speech, Language and Learning Center [3451]
Hairston House [44530]
Hal Nichols Associates [43437]
Halcyon Center [28480]
The Halcyon Center [30432]
Halcyon Home [9125]
Halcyon Hospice & Palliative Care [19121]
Hale Ho'okupa'a [42255]
Hale Ho'okupa'a • Molokai High School/Molokai Middle Sch [42256]
Hale Ho'omalu Shelter and Alternatives to Violence [9152]
Hale House Center, Inc. [31415]
Hale Kipa, Inc. [29519]
Haley Center for Community Living [32759]
Haley House [45936]
Halfway Houses of Westchester Inc • Hawthorne House [47184]
Halifax Behavioral Health Services [29143]
Halifax County Dialysis Center • Fresenius Medical Care [25945]
Halifax County Mental Health • Roanoke Rapids Crisis Line [51174]
Halifax County Special Education [852]
Halifax Health-Hospice of Volusia Flagler [19216]
Halifax Health Hospice of Volusia/Flagler West Volusia Care Center [19279]
Halifax Health Medical Center • H.D. Kerman Regional Oncology Center [4938]
Halifax Medical Center [29144]
    Rehabilitation Department • Speech-Language Pathology [1569]
Halifax Regional Health System [18385]
Halifax Regional Hospice [21734]
Hall-Brooke Behavioral Health Services [33268]
Hall-Moore Medical Supplies, Inc. [13814]
The Hallmark Companies [17021]
Hallmark Health
    Cancer Care Center [5343]
    SleepHealth Centers [37116]
Hallmark Health System [30419]
Hallmark Health System, Inc. [15515]
Hallmark Health Visiting Nurse Association and Hospices, Inc. [19976]
Hallmark Health Visiting Nurse Association, Inc. [15513]
Hallmark Home Care, Inc. - West Union Branch [17069]
Hallmark Home Health Care [18286]
Hallmark Hospice, LLC [21203]
Hallwood Dialysis • DaVita [24898]
Halo Hospice [20917]
Halsey House [31264]

Haltom City Treatment Services LLC [49354]
Halton Hills Speech Centre [3298]
Hamakua Health Center [6616]
Hamburg Center [8464]
Hamburg Counseling Service, Inc. [31344]
Hamburg Dialysis • DaVita [24403]
Hamden Sleep Disorders Center [36744]
Hamilton--Boone--Madison Cooperative [416]
Hamilton Center [27877]
    Child and Adolescent Services [8008]
Hamilton Center Inc [42992], [43001], [43007], [43070], [43098], [43178], [43192], [43207], [43208], [43212], [43213]
    Child and Adolescent Services [43214]
    Eagle Street House [43215]
Hamilton Center, Inc.--Hendricks County Center [29800]
Hamilton Center, Inc.--Indianapolis [29745]
Hamilton Center, Inc.--Spencer [29818]
Hamilton Center, Inc.--Terre Haute [29820]
Hamilton Center, Inc. • Vermillion County Center [29704]
Hamilton Community Health Network, Inc. [6844]
Hamilton County Clinic [29190]
Hamilton County School Exceptional Education [748]
Hamilton Health Center, Inc. [7166]
Hamilton Health Sciences • Hamilton Firefighters Burn Unit [4614]
Hamilton--Madison House [31416]
Hamilton Madison House • Asian American Recovery Services [46866]
Hamilton Medical Center [14515]
    Cancer Program [5021]
Hamilton Medical Center Hospice [19378]
Hamilton Medical Equipment [15087]
Hamilton Memorial Home Health Agency [14858]
Hamilton Multiple Sclerosis Center [34680]
Hamilton Park Dialysis Center [25449]
Hamm Memorial Clinic [30722]
Hammond Addictive Disorders Clinic [43829]
Hammond Clinic, LLC [38443]
Hammond Developmental Center [8066]
Hammond Henry Hospital [14799]
Hammond Veterans Affairs Clinic [30139]
Hamot Medical Center
    Cancer Program [5827]
    Sleep Disorders Center [37651]
Hampden Health Solutions • at the Rail Inc [44141]
Hampden Hearing Center East [2475]
Hampshire County Dialysis Center • Fresenius Medical Care [24788]
Hampshire Hearing Services [2508]
Hampstead Hospital [33652]
Hampton Avenue Dialysis • DaVita [25272]
Hampton Dilaysis Clinic • Renal Advantage Inc. • Dialysis Center [26779]
Hampton Homecare [16622]
Hampton Hospital [33665]
Hampton Roads Clinic • Opioid Treatment Program [49814]
Hampton School District One [731]
Hampton VA Medical Center [4472]
Hampton Veterans Affairs Medical Center [32745]
Hampton Veterans • Medical Center/Mental Health SATP [49798]
Hana Community Health Center, Inc. [6613]
HANAC Inc • HANAC 822 Chemical Dependency Program [46362]
Hanbleceya Treatment Center [28548]
Hancock County Home Health and Hospice Agency [21364]
Hancock County Mental Health Clinic [32378]
Hancock County Office [30029]
Hancock County Schools [878]
Hancock Regional Home Health Care and Hospice [14988]
Hancock Regional Hospital [2151]
Hancock Regional Sleep Disorders Center [36949]
Hand County Memorial Hospital • Avera [21294]
Hand in Hand Homecare and Hospice [19752]
Hand of Hope [43522]
Hand In Hand [1104]
HAND Support Groups • Helping After Neonatal Death [36454]
Handelman Inc. [1520]
Handi Medical Supply, Inc. [15941]
The Handicapped Children's Association of Southern New York [8325]

Hands of Hope [9665]
    Division of Family Service Society Inc. [9297]
Hands of Hope Hospice [20332]
Hands of Hope Hospice, Inc. [19463]
Hands of Hope Resource Center--Little Falls [9605]
Hands of Hope Resource Center--Long Prairie [9606]
Hands of Life Against AIDS Program [29589]
Hands of Wellness [14704]
Hanford At Home Dialysis • DaVita [22717]
Hanford Community Medical Center [13070]
    Adventist Health Home Care [18937]
Hanford Dialysis • DaVita [22718]
Hanley Center Treatment Programs [41996]
Hanna Boys Center [34030]
Hannah Home Health Inc. [13130]
Hannah More School [8096]
Hannahs Aftercare and Rehab Center [44356]
Hannah's Place [10074]
Hannahville Behavioral Health Services [45064]
Hannahville Indian Community [9579]
Hannas House • Hannahs First Step Treatment Center [40112]
Hannibal Council on Alcohol/Drug Abuse Inc [45486]
    Canton [45449]
    Moberly [45569]
Hannibal Dialysis • Fresenius Medical Care [25210]
Hannibal Regional Hospital Home Health Services--Hannibal [16012]
Hannibal Regional Hospital Home Health Services--Hull [14825]
Hannibal Regional Hospital • James E. Cary Cancer Center [5442]
Hanniford House [30948]
Hanover County Community Service Board [49767], [49813]
Hanover County Community Services [32708]
Hanover Safe Place [10555]
Hansen House • For Men and Women [45978]
Hansen Orthopedics • Brent P. Hansen, DO [38033]
Hansen Speech and Language Services Inc. [2816]
Hanson and Hanson Addiction Specialist [45174]
Hanson Veterans Affairs Community Based Outpatient Clinic [30024]
Happy Heart Home Health Care [14208]
Happy Home Health [12710]
Happy Talkers [1097]
Haralson County Center for MH/MR/SA [29372]
Harambee Ombudsman Project Inc • Imani II Program [50476]
Harbel Prevention and Recovery Center
    Adolescent Clinic [44142]
    Adult Clinic [44143]
Harbin Clinic Cedartown Dialysis [23641]
Harbin Clinic Dialysis Center [23776]
Harbin Clinic Hearing Center [1846], [1897]
Harbin Clinic Summerville Dialysis Center [23802]
Harbinger Hospice [20908]
Harbinger House • Wayside Youth and Family Support Network [30382]
Harbor Apartment and Respite Program [28973]
Harbor Behavioral Health Care Institute [29232]
    Assertive Resource Management Service [33331]
    Children's Crisis Stabilization Unit [33332]
    Community Recovery Center [33333]
    Doris Cook Smith Counseling Center [33299]
Harbor Behavioral Healthcare Institute • Doris Cook Counseling Center [41609]
Harbor Care, LLC [16391]
Harbor City Counseling Center [41759]
Harbor City Unlimited [30261]
Harbor Counseling [48682]
Harbor COV [9475]
Harbor Crest Behavioral Health • Grays Harbor Community Hospital [49873]
Harbor Family Services [44049]
Harbor Grace Hospice [19384]
Harbor Hall Cheboygan Oupatient • Substance Abuse Program [44697]
Harbor Hall
    Outpatient Substance Abuse Program [44955]
    Residential [44956]
Harbor Health Services [28974]
    Substance Abuse Clinic [41360]
Harbor Homes Inc [45914]
Harbor Hospital Center • Harbor View Cancer Center [5285]

Harbor Hospital • SLP Services [2373]
Harbor House [28975]
Harbor House of Central Florida [9071]
Harbor House Collaborative • Harbor House Clinic [41060]
Harbor House Domestic Abuse Programs [10688]
Harbor House Inc [39533], [49137]
Harbor House, Inc.--New Philadelphia [10162]
Harbor House Program [40611]
Harbor House--Vincennes [9312]
Harbor Houses of Jackson Inc • Mens Transitional Program [45391]
Harbor, Inc. [10084]
Harbor Light [4163]
Harbor Light Hospice-Galesburg [19521]
Harbor Light Hospice Glen Ellyn [19523]
Harbor Light Hospice-Highland Heights [20846]
Harbor Light Hospice-Indianapolis [19610]
Harbor Light Hospice--Merrillville [19631]
Harbor Light Hospice--Munroe Falls [20874]
Harbor Light Hospice--Peoria [19559]
Harbor Light Hospice--South Bend [19652]
Harbor Light Hospice--Westerville [20907]
Harbor Light
    Outpatient Program/Unit 2 [47687]
    Substance Abuse Division Detox/Unit 1 [47688]
Harbor Lights Chem Dependency Services • Chemical Dependency Outpatient Clinic [46777]
Harbor Lights Shelter • Christian Associates at Table Rock Lake [9693]
Harbor Oaks Hospital [33599]
Harbor Schools--Amesbury [34180]
Harbor Schools • Newburyport Youth Home [34203]
Harbor Shelter and Counseling Center--Hastings [34250]
Harbor Shelter and Counseling Center--Stillwater [34258]
Harbor UCLA Medical Center • Division of Medical Genetics [12156]
Harbor/University of California, Los Angeles Medical Center [36297]
Harbor View Dialysis • DaVita [27574]
Harbors Home Health & Hospice [21755]
Harbortown Treatment Center PLLC [44665]
Harborview Center for Sexual Assault and Traumatic Stress [10645]
Harborview Medical Center Addictions Prog [50113]
Harborview Medical Center
    Northwest Regional Spinal Cord Injury System [4483]
    Sports Medicine Clinic [39147]
    University of Washington Medicine Sleep Institute [37911]
Harborview Sports Medicine & Physical Therapy [4095]
Harbour Haus [8638]
Harbour Hospice of Bexar County, LLC [21552]
The Harbour Inc. • Runaway and Homeless Youth Program [35928]
Hardeman County Community Health Center [7253]
Hardin County Hospice [20850]
Hardin County Regional Health Center, Inc. [7271]
Hardin Medical Center Home Health and Home Supply [17771]
Hardin Memorial Hospital • Cancer Program [5215]
Hardin Memorial Hospital Home Health Care [16951]
Hardin Memorial Hospital • Sleep Center [37026]
Hardin Mental Health Center [30946]
Hardwick Area Health Center [7335]
Harford Counseling LLC [44194]
Harford County Health Department • Division of Addiction Services [44195]
Harford County • Juvenile Drug Court [44196]
Harford Hearing Center Inc. [2387]
Harford Memorial Hospital • Cancer Care Program [5306]
Harford Road Dialysis Center • DaVita [24644]
Harford Road Dialysis • DaVita [24645]
Harlan Appalachian Regional [15186]
Harlan Dialysis • DaVita [24275]
Harlem Dialysis Center [25720]
Harlem East Life Plan
    Alcoholism Outpatient Clinic [46867]
    Outpatient Methadone Clinic/Chem Dep [46868]
    Outpatient Methadone Clinic/KEEP [46869]
Harlem Hospital Center

    Chem Depend Med Supervised Detox Unit [46870]
    Chemical Dependency Outpatient Service [46871]
    Harlem AIDS Treatment Group • Community Program for Clinical Research on AIDS [61]
Harlem Hospital • Dialysis Unit [25721]
Harlem Vet Center [52040]
Harlingen Dialysis • US Renal Care [27118]
Harlowton Mental Health Center [30953]
Harm Reduction Therapy Center [40612]
Harmony Care Hospice [21219]
Harmony Counseling and Consulting [49980]
Harmony Foundation Inc [41170]
Harmony Grove Counseling [50171]
Harmony Hearing and Speech Center [2976], [3029]
Harmony Hill School [34432]
Harmony Home Health [16301]
Harmony Home Health Care [14010]
Harmony Home Health Care Group, Corporation [14011]
Harmony Home Health Services, Inc. [14012]
Harmony Hospice LLC-Carnegie [21070]
Harmony House [8707], [44516]
    Park Center Inc [43049]
Harmony Place [40966]
Harnett County Home Health Agency [16747]
Harney Behavioral Health [31934]
Harney County Home Health/Hospice [20993]
Harney Helping Organization for Personal Emergencies [10224]
Harold W. Jordan Habilitation Center [8524]
Harper College • Access and Disability Services [408]
Harper Hospital Audiology Service [2572]
Harper House [8798]
Harper House/Hay - Madeira House Hospice [19313]
Harper University Hospital • Sleep Disorders Center [37159]
Harper's Hospice Care, Inc. [20251]
Harrell Home • JBS Mental Health Authority [27861]
Harrell's Hearing Services Inc. [1881]
Harriet Tubman Women and Children • Treatment Facility Residential Program [42515]
Harriet's House [8639]
Harrington Health Center [6775]
Harrington Memorial [2524]
Harrington Memorial Hospital • Recovery Services George B Wells Center [44575]
Harris County Children's Protective Services • Chimney Rock Center • Runaway and Homeless Youth Program [36223]
Harris County Hospital District • Cancer Program [5992]
Harris County Psychiatric Center • University of Texas [32480]
Harris County Vet Center [52109]
Harris Home Health [12877]
Harris Hospital Behavioral Health [28278]
Harris House Foundation [45621]
Harris Methodist Ft. Worth Transplant [27088]
Harris Methodist Hospital • Cancer Center [4709]
Harris Methodist Springwood [49245]
Harris YWCA [9206]
Harrisburg Dialysis Center • DaVita [25848]
Harrisburg Medical Center, Inc. Home Health Care [14811]
Harrison Clinic [28137]
Harrison Community Hospital [16859]
Harrison County Comprehensive Care [30000]
Harrison County Hospice [20279]
Harrison County Hospital [14972]
    Center for Sleep Disorders [36950]
Harrison County School District [520]
Harrison Home Health [18420]
Harrison House of Virginia [49757]
Harrison Medical Center
    Cancer Program [6095]
    Sleep Disorders Center [37912]
Harrison Memorial Hospital [18421]
Harrisonburg Rockingham Community Services Board [8588], [32747]
Harrisonburg/Rockingham • Community Services Board [49801]
Harrison's Hope...A Caring Place [19469]
Harrisonville Dialysis Center • Diversified Specialty Institutes [25211]

Harrold's Pharmacy, Inc. [17506]
Harry Hynes Memorial Hospice--Coffeyville [19748]
Harry Hynes Memorial Hospice-Newton [19764]
Harry Hynes Memorial Hospice-Parsons [19771]
Harry Hynes Memorial Hospice--Wichita [19786]
The Harry and Jeanette Weinberg Mental Health
  Center [31246]
Harry S Truman Memorial [51595]
Harry S. Truman Memorial Veterans Affairs Medical
  Center [30843]
Harry S Truman Memorial Veterans Hosp [45464]
Harry S. Truman Memorial Veterans' Hospital
  [16002]
Harry S. Truman Memorial Veterans Hospital
    Multiple Sclerosis Center [34617]
    PTSD Clinical Team [51762]
Harry's Nurses Registry, Inc. [16499]
Hart County Mental Health Center [29438]
Hart Foundation Inc. [11072]
Hart Group [44144]
Hartford Behavioral Health [29002]
    SATEP [41404]
Hartford Dialysis • DaVita [23159]
Hartford Dispensary [41405]
    Bristol Clinic [41372]
    Henderson/Johnson Clinic MMTP [41406]
    Manchester Clinic [41414]
    New Britain Clinic [41428]
    New London Clinic [41446]
    Norwich Clinic [41457]
    Willimantic Clinic [41496]
Hartford Health Services [13864]
Hartford Health Services or Orlando, Inc. [13870]
Hartford Home Health Care [14013]
Hartford Hospital
    Dialysis Unit [23160]
    Gray Cancer Center [4895]
    Sleep Disorders Center [36745]
Hartford Hospital Transplant Services [23161]
Hartford Interval House [8995]
Hartford Vet Center [51910]
Hartgrove Hospital [7940], [33413]
Hartselle Medical Center • New Day Unit [27947]
Hartung Place [29693]
Hartwell Chiropractic and Wellness Center [38916]
Harvard Medical School • Spaulding Rehabilitation
  Hospital • Pain Management [35491]
Harvard Park Hearing Centers [1396]
Harvard Street Neighborhood Health Center [6811]
Harvard University • Institute for Global Health •
  Centers for AIDS Research [53]
Harvard Vanguard Medical Associates
    Down Syndrome Program [10811]
    Genetics Department [12244]
Harvest House [47281]
Harvest of Wilmington [47520]
Harvey County Special Education Cooperative [435]
Harwichport Clubhouse [30393]
Hasting Dialysis Center • DaVita [25324]
Hastings Hemodialysis Center [25698]
Hastings Home Health Center [16883]
Hastings House [4265]
Hastings Orthopaedics and Sports Medicine Special-
  ists [38687]
Hastings Regional Center [33643]
Hatfield House [32007]
Hathaway Children's and Family Services [33992]
Hathaway Children's Services [33991]
Hathaway--Sycamores Child and Family Services
  [34033]
Hathaway-Sycamores Child and Family Services
  [28593]
    Family Resource Center [28594]
Hattie Larlham Foundation [8420]
Hattiesburg Clinic Dialysis [25129]
Hattiesburg Veterans Affairs Clinic [30769]
Hauula Clinic [6614]
Havasu Arthritis and Sports Medicine Institute
  [38036]
Havasu Regional Home Health [12795]
Havasu Regional Medical Center [946]
The Haven [33083]
HAVEN Against Violent Environments Now, Inc.
  [9679]
The Haven • Battered Women's Shelter [9127]
HAVEN--Bozeman [9740]
Haven Children's Center [28258]
Haven in Cloquet [45113]

HAVEN from Domestic Abuse [10259]
Haven • The Haven [39500]
Haven Hills, Inc. [8800]
Haven of Hope--Cambridge [10128]
Haven of Hope--Manchester [10417]
Haven Hospice-Chiefland [19205]
Haven Hospice--Gainesville [19230]
Haven Hospice-Jacksonville [19241]
Haven Hospice JFK Medical Center [20468]
Haven Hospice Lake City - Suwannee Valley
  Hospice Care Center [19245]
Haven Hospice--Murray [21621]
Haven House [34366]
Haven House--Allentown [31986]
Haven House for Boys [34367]
Haven House--Buffalo • Domestic Violence Program
  [9910]
Haven House--Everett [32827]
Haven House Family Shelter, Inc. [9660]
Haven House for Girls [34368]
Haven House--Hammond [9281]
Haven House Hospice-St. Augustine [19308]
Haven House Inc
    Inpatient [44253]
    Outpatient [44254]
Haven House, Inc.--Alcoa [10390]
Haven House, Inc.--Pasadena [8867]
Haven House, Inc.--Poplar Bluff [9711]
Haven House--McDonough [9119]
Haven House--Rio Rancho [9880]
Haven House • Runaway and Homeless Youth
  Program [36134]
Haven House--Wayne • Family Services Center
  [9785]
HAVEN, Inc. [10719]
The Haven, Inc. [9408]
Haven of Lake and Sumter Counties, Inc. [9062]
Haven in Lee County [10081]
Haven of Northeast Arkansas [8752]
Haven of Peace, Inc. • Women's Shelter [8814]
HAVEN--Pontiac [9569]
The Haven of RCS [9043]
Haven Recovery Center [41613]
    Serenity West Residential II [41624]
Haven Road Recovery Center LLC [45185]
Haven in Shakopee [45321]
Haven Shelter and Services, Inc. [10598]
Haven for Stuttering [3123]
Haven of Tioga County [10324]
Haven in Waconia [45337]
Haven Women's Center of Stanislaus [8849]
Haven in Woodbury Outpatient Program [45355]
Haven4Change Inc [43537]
Havenwyck Hospital [33588]
    Substance Abuse Services [44649]
Haverhill Clinic [30394]
Haviland Kidney Center • Northwest Kidney Center
  [27636]
Havre VA Community Based Outreach Clinic • VA
  Montana Health Care System [4250]
Hawaii Center for the Deaf and the Blind BKN 2205
  [3704]
Hawaii Center for Reproductive Medicine and
  Surgery [22027]
Hawaii Center for Sleep Medicine • Sleep Disorders
  Center [36868]
Hawaii Community Mental Health Center [29511]
Hawaii Cord Blood Bank [35016]
Hawaii Counseling and Educ Center Inc • Chemical
  Dependency Outpatient Treatment [42230]
Hawaii Department of Health • Child Wellness
  Program/Maternal Child Health • Hawaii SIDS
  Program [36470]
Hawaii Healthcare Professionals, Inc. [14618]
Hawaii Healthcare Professionals--Kahului [14629]
Hawaii Healthcare Professionals--Lihue [14640]
Hawaii Home Infusion Associates, Ltd. [14641]
Hawaii Island Recovery [42238]
Hawaii Lions Eye Bank & Makana Foundation
  [35017]
Hawaii Medical Center--East [23848]
Hawaii Medical Center - East • Institute of Cancer
  [5045]
Hawaii School for the Deaf and the Blind [382]
Hawaii Speech Pathology [1933]
Hawaii State Hospital [33396]
Hawaii State Library for the Blind and Physically
  Handicapped [3783]

Hawaii Youth Services Network • Runaway and
  Homeless Youth Program [35917]
Hawaiian Gardens Medical and Mental Health
  Services [39906]
Hawaiian Islands Medical Corp. [14619]
Hawkinsville Dialysis Center [23718]
Hawthorn Center [33600]
Hawthorn Medical Associates Sleep Center [37117]
Hawthorne Cedar Knolls School [34340]
Hawthorne Children's Psychiatric Hospital [33635]
Hawthorne Country Day School [8322]
Hawthorne Family Medical Center [6469]
Hawthorne Group Home [34341]
Haydel Memorial Hospice [19847]
Hayes Green Beach Memorial Hospital Home Health
  [15609]
Haymarket Dialysis • DaVita [27494]
Haypath House [31242]
Hays Caldwell Council on Alcohol and Drug Abuse
  [49535]
Hays--Caldwell Women's Center [10506]
Hays Medical Center
    Cancer Center [5198]
    Center for Health Improvement • Sleep
      Disorders Center [36990]
Hays Shelter Home [9160]
    Runaway and Homeless Youth Program [35920]
Hays Veterans Affairs Clinic [29928]
Haysville Mental Health and Substance AbuseSer-
  vices [43360]
Hayward Dialysis Center • DaVita [22721]
Hayward Group Home • Sheriffs Youth Programs of
  Minnesota [30658]
Haywood County Center [31606]
Haywood Regional Medical Center [16715]
Haywood Regional Medical Center Hospice [20641]
Hazard ARH Regional Medical Center • Cancer
  Program [5217]
Hazard Veterans Affairs Community Based
  Outpatient Clinic [30030]
Hazel Hawkins Memorial Hospital • San Benito
  Home Health Care [13078]
Hazel Pittman Center/Chester County • Commission
  on Alcohol and Drug Abuse [48914]
Hazel Street Recovery Center [49556]
Hazelden Foundation
    Center City [45110]
    Center for Youth and Families [45263]
    Chicago [42516]
    New York Outpatient Services [46872]
    Saint Paul [45305]
Hazelden Springbrook [48155]
Hazelwood ICF/MR [8054]
HBMC Hospice and Home Health Services [18184]
HCA Dominion Hospital [33902]
HCADA/Macon [45561]
HCADA/Mexico [45566]
HCCH Dental Clinic [6525]
HCS Hospice Specialists [21646]
HDC [50539]
Head Injury Rehabilitation and Referral Services
  [2428]
Head Injury Rehabilitation Services [3902]
Head Injury Therapy Services Inc. [2624]
Head--Neck Associates of Orange County [1181]
Head and Neck Group [2792]
Head and Neck Pain Center [35429]
Headache Associates [12458]
Headache Care Center [12438], [35528]
Headache Center of Atlanta [12417]
Headache Center of North Texas [12468]
The Headache Institute • Saint Luke's-Roosevelt
  Hospital Center [12450]
Headache Neurology of Central New Jersey
  Headache Clinic [12443]
Headache and Pain Center [35453]
Headache and Pain Center of Florida [12400]
Headache and Pain Center--Gray, Louisiana [12425]
Headache and Pain Center--New Iberia, Louisiana
  [12426]
Headache and Pain Center of Palm Beach [12401],
  [12402]
Headache and Pain Management Center of
  Southwest Florida [12403]
Headache Wellness Center [12456]
Headquarters Counseling Center [50921]
Headrest Inc [45903]
Headrest, Inc. [51086]

Headway Program • St. Vincent Healthcare [4251]
Headway Therapy PA [1696]
Healing with CAARE Inc [47295]
Healing Care [14014]
Healing Circle--Portland [10247]
Healing Club--Denver [8952]
Healing Hands Home Healthcare [13660]
Healing to Heal Another Home Healthcare, Inc. [14894]
Healing Hearts [9753]
Healing Hearts Therapeutic Services Inc [47394]
Healing House [9866]
Healing Lifes Pains [41129]
Healing Lives Therapeutic Services LLC [42007]
Healing Lodge • Butterfly PelPalWichiya Girls CD [50191]
Healing Place Church • Runaway and Homeless Youth Program [35974]
Healing Place • Womens Community [43687]
Healing Touch Healthcare, LLC [16927]
Healing Touch Home Care [15572]
Healing Touch Home Health Corporation [14015]
Healing Touch Homehealth Services [14689]
Healing Touch Pain Management Center [38778]
Healing Wings Home Healthcare, LLC [13627]
HealingTtouch Home Care, Inc. [15812]
Health 1st Home Health Services [17300]
Health Access Network [6779]
Health Access Washoe County [6955]
Health Alcohol and Drug Services • The Center [40216]
Health Alliance Hospitals--Leominster • Simonds-Simon Regional Cancer Center [5340]
Health Association of Niagara County, Inc. [16576]
Health Care for the Homeless [7446]
Health Care Options--Gonzales [15295]
Health Care Options--Greenwell Springs [15296]
Health Care Options, Inc-Greenwell Springs [19844]
Health Care Options--Plaquemine [15353]
Health Care Partners Inc. [7230]
Health Care Professional Inc. [13355]
Health and Care Professional Network [16154]
Health Care and Rehabilitation Service of Southeastern Vermont Programs--Union Street, Springfield [32682]
Health Care and Rehabilitation Service of Southeastern Vermont--River Street, Springfield [32683]
Health Care and Rehabilitation Service of Southeastern Vermont--White River Junction [32685]
Health Care and Rehabilitation Service of Southeastern Vermont--Woodstock [32690]
Health Care and Rehabilitation Services
    Community Rehabilitation Treatment [32643]
    Hartford Region Office [32656]
Health Care and Rehabilitation Services of Southeastern Vermont--Bellows Falls [32634]
Health Care and Rehabilitation Services of Southeastern Vermont--Brattleboro [32644]
Health Care and Rehabilitation Services of Southeastern Vermont • Mount Ascutney Hospital and Health Center [32686]
Health Care Solutions at Home, Inc.--Altoona [17240]
Health Care Solutions at Home, Inc.--Ambridge [17245]
Health Care Solutions at Home, Inc.--Broomall [17267]
Health Care Solutions at Home, Inc.--Butler [17271]
Health Care Solutions at Home, Inc.--Cheswick [17283]
Health Care Solutions at Home, Inc.--Erie [17313]
Health Care Solutions at Home, Inc.--Grove City [17330]
Health Care Solutions at Home, Inc.--Morgantown [18527]
Health Care Solutions at Home, Inc.--Mount Clare [18528]
Health Care Solutions at Home, Inc.--New Castle [17396]
Health Care Solutions at Home, Inc.--Orion [15766]
Health Care Solutions at Home, Inc.--Seneca [17474]
Health Care Solutions at Home, Inc.--Sharon [17477]
Health Care Solutions at Home, Inc.--Toledo [17054]

Health Care Solutions at Home, Inc.--Weirton [18544]
Health Care Solutions at Home, Inc.--Wheeling [18550]
Health Care Solutions at Home, Inc.Meadville [17384]
Health Care Unlimited, Inc.--Corpus Christi [17852]
Health Care Unlimited, Inc.--Harlingen [17944]
Health Care Unlimited, Inc.--Laredo [18035]
Health Care Unlimited, Inc.--McAllen [18072]
Health Center of Lake City [1623]
Health Center of the Piedmont--Chatham [7352]
Health Center of the Piedmont--Danville [7353]
Health Center for Plant City [1724]
Health Center Presentation Hospice of Carrington [20776]
Health Center Town & Country • Trinity Hospitals [16820]
Health Challenge [41061]
Health Delivery, Inc. [6857]
Health Dimensions Rehabilitation Inc. [2680]
Health-E-Quip [15127]
Health Education and Addictions • Recovery Training [45772]
Health and Education Services, Inc. [30332]
    Adolescent Crisis Center for Evaluation [30333]
    Bridgeview Residential Home [30334]
    Cape Ann Adult Treatment Center [30335]
    The Center for Family Development [30336]
Health & Education Services, Inc. • Gloucester Clinic [30389]
Health and Education Services, Inc. • Harmony House [30337]
Health & Education Services, Inc. • Ipswich Clinic [30401]
Health and Education Services, Inc.
    Rantoul Garden [30338]
    Salem Clinic [30461]
Health First Family Health Center [6959]
Health First Home Care, Inc.--Elk Grove Village [14779]
Health First Home Care--Melbourne [13884]
Health First Home Care--Merritt Island [13888]
Health First Home Health [14380]
Health Help, Inc. • White House Clinic [6737]
Health & Home Care Resources [13538]
Health Link [13307]
Health Management, Inc. - Home Health Agency [13571]
Health Management Institute • Canopy Cove Eating Disorder Treatment Center [11021]
Health Max Group LLC [12809]
Health Medical Equipment, Inc. [14016]
Health, Opportunity, Protection, Encouragement Center [10391]
Health Path Consulting Services LLC [46199]
Health Point Family Care [6726]
Health and Recovery Center at • Jackson Memorial Hospital [41782]
Health Recovery Center Inc [45214]
Health Recovery Clinic--Mississauga [35627]
Health Recovery Clinic--Toronto [35628]
Health and Recovery Institute of • Central FL [41860]
Health Recovery Services Inc
    Bassett House [47617]
    Vinton County Outpatient Clinic [47809]
Health Resources of Arkansas [28279], [39557], [39582]
Health Resources of Arkansas, Inc.
    Ash Flat Behavioral Health Care [28233]
    Augusta Behavioral Health Care [28234]
Health Resources of Arkansas Inc. • Batesville Behavioral Health Clinic [33113]
Health Resources of Arkansas, Inc.
    Clinton Behavioral Health Clinic [28255]
    Heber Springs Behavioral Health Center [28283]
    Melbourne Behavioral Health Clinic [28320]
    Mountain View Behavioral Health Clinic [28328]
    Newport Behavioral Health Care [28331]
Health Sciences Centre • Burn Unit [4556]
Health Services One • Central Pain Solutions [35539]
Health Signals Home Care, Inc. [13690]
Health South Deaconess Rehabilitation Hospital [2141]
Health South Emerald Coast Rehabilitation Hospital [3973]

Health South Rehabilitation Hospital [1008]
Health South Rehabilitation Hospital--Largo [3974]
Health South Rehabilitation Hospital of Miami [3975]
Health South Rehabilitation Hospital of Sarasota [3976]
Health South Rehabilitation Hospital of Spring Hill [3977]
Health South Rehabilitation Hospital of Tallahassee [3978]
Health South RidgeLake Hospital [3979]
Health South Sea Pines Rehabilitation Hospital [3980], [13885]
Health South Sunrise Rehabilitation Hospital [3981]
Health South Treasure Coast Rehabilitation Hospital [3982]
Health South/Tustin Rehabilitation Hospital [3903]
Health Star Physical Therapy [38985]
Health Systems 2000 [15314]
Health Touch, Inc. [17554]
Health and Wellness Center • Montrose Sleep Center [37528]
Health and Wellness Group [11046]
Health and Wellness Resource Center [38931]
Health West, Inc. [6642]
HealthAlliance Home Health and Hospice [19971]
HealthBridge Sleep Medicine [37394], [37395]
Healthcare Alternative Systems Inc [42517], [42518], [42519], [42686], [42775]
    Residential [42520]
    Transitional Housing Program [42521]
    Womens Program [42522]
Healthcare Alternatives of West FL Inc [41742]
Healthcare Commons Inc. [31115]
Healthcare Connection of Tampa Inc [41965]
Healthcare Corporation of America [18106]
Healthcare Etc. [17411]
Healthcare for the Homeless [6526], [6757]
Healthcare for the Homeless Inc [44145]
Healthcare and Rehabilitation Service of Southeast Vermont • HELPLINE [51408]
Healthcare and Rehabilitation Services of Southeastern Vermont [49736]
Healthcare and Rehabilitation Services • Southeastern Vermont [49718], [49746]
Healthcare Solutions & Medical Suppply, LLC [18347]
Healthcare STAT Home Care Services [17412]
Healthcare Unlimited of Florida [14017]
HealthEast Care System • Cancer Center [5417]
HealthEast Eagan Sleep Care Center [37219]
HealthEast Maplewood Clinic • Down Syndrome Clinic [10817]
Healthfirst Family Care Center [6814]
Healthkeepers Hospice, Inc. [21186]
HealthLinc--Michigan City [6696]
HealthLinc--Valpariso/Hilltop [6700]
Healthmark Counseling [45960]
Healthmax Home Care Services [13748]
Healthnet Home Care Services Inc. [12923]
Healthone Broncos Sports Medicine [38172]
HealthPartners-Hospice and Palliative Care [20148]
Healthplex Sports Medicine Institute [38986]
HealthPro Home Health Corporation [14018]
HealthQwest [42088], [42180]
Healthqwest [42179]
HealthReach HomeCare and Hospice [19906]
HealthReach Network [30181]
HealthReach Network--HomeCare and Hospice [30213]
HealthSouth [38575]
Healthsouth Bakersfield Rehabilitation Hospital [38074]
Healthsouth Bedford Rehabilitation Hospital [38928]
Healthsouth Bee Ridge Outpatient Therapy Center [38286]
Healthsouth Cane Creek Rehabilitation Hospital [39035]
Healthsouth Central Georgia Rehabilitation Hospital [1882]
Healthsouth--Chattanooga Center [35672]
HealthSouth Chesapeake Rehabilitation Hospital [15464]
Healthsouth City View Rehabilitation Hospital [17924], [39064]
HealthSouth Emerald Coast [1714]
HealthSouth of Erie [4389]
Healthsouth Harmarville Rehabilitation Hospital [38971]

HealthSouth Harmaville Rehabilitation Hospital [17440]
Healthsouth Hospital of Houston [39071]
Healthsouth Hospital of Pittsburgh [38961]
Healthsouth Lakeview Rehabilitation Hospital of Central Kentucky [38475]
Healthsouth Mountain View Regional Rehabilitation Hospital [3659], [39162]
HEALTHSOUTH Mountainview Regional Rehabilitation Hospital, Fairmont [35769]
Healthsouth Nittany Valley Rehabilitation Hospital [4390], [38976]
Healthsouth North Louisiana Rehabilitation Hospital Homer [38495]
HealthSouth Northern Kentucky Rehabilitation Hospital [2264]
HealthSouth Outpatient Rehabilitation [1753]
Healthsouth Plano Rehabilitation Hospital [39089]
HealthSouth of Reading, LLC--Reading [17461]
HealthSouth of Reading, LLC--York [17516]
Healthsouth Reading Rehabilitation Hospital [38979]
HealthSOUTH Rehabilitation Center [8533]
Healthsouth Rehabilitation Center--Beaumont [39052]
Healthsouth Rehabilitation Center--Ebensburg [38939]
Healthsouth Rehabilitation Center of Lewistown [38932]
Healthsouth Rehabilitation Center--Memphis [39036]
Healthsouth Rehabilitation Center of Mifflintown [38958]
Healthsouth Rehabilitation Center--New Cumberland [38956]
Healthsouth Rehabilitation Center--Shrewsbury [38984]
HealthSouth Rehabilitation Hospital--Albuquerque [16302]
Healthsouth Rehabilitation Hospital of Altoona [4391], [38926]
HealthSouth Rehabilitation Hospital of Austin [17814], [39045]
Healthsouth Rehabilitation Hospital--Chester Square [38954]
HealthSouth Rehabilitation Hospital of Colorado Springs [13466], [38168]
Healthsouth Rehabilitation Hospital--Columbia [39007]
Healthsouth Rehabilitation Hospital of Erie [38940]
Healthsouth Rehabilitation Hospital--Florence [39009]
Healthsouth Rehabilitation Hospital of Fort Smith [1014]
HealthSOUTH Rehabilitation Hospital of Fort Smith • Child and Adolescent Rehabilitation Program [7757]
Healthsouth Rehabilitation Hospital of Gasden [38006]
HealthSouth Rehabilitation Hospital of Henderson [16138]
Healthsouth Rehabilitation Hospital Holyoke [38553]
Healthsouth Rehabilitation Hospital--Humble [39079]
Healthsouth Rehabilitation Hospital of Huntington [35770], [39160]
Healthsouth Rehabilitation Hospital--Kingsport [39032]
Healthsouth Rehabilitation Hospital--Largo [1630]
HealthSouth Rehabilitation Hospital--Miami [1654]
Healthsouth Rehabilitation Hospital of Midland/Odessa [18088], [39085]
Healthsouth Rehabilitation Hospital--Milton [38959]
Healthsouth Rehabilitation Hospital of New Jersey [38762]
Healthsouth Rehabilitation Hospital of North Alabama [38007]
HealthSouth Rehabilitation Hospital of North Houston [17846]
HealthSouth Rehabilitation Hospital of Plano [18107]
Healthsouth Rehabilitation Hospital--Red Lion [38980]
HealthSouth Rehabilitation Hospital of San Antonio [18144]
Healthsouth Rehabilitation Hospital of Sarasota [38287]
Healthsouth Rehabilitation Hospital--Selinsgrove [38981]
Healthsouth Rehabilitation Hospital of Southern Arizona [38055]
Healthsouth Rehabilitation Hospital of Texarkana

[18173], [39099]
Healthsouth Rehabilitation Hospital--Tyrone [38987]
HealthSouth Rehabilitation Hospital of Utah [18227]
HealthSouth Rehabilitation Hospital of Virginia [35751], [39132]
Healthsouth Rehabilitation Hospital of Western Massachusetts [2492], [38555]
Healthsouth Rehabilitation Hospital of Wichita Falls [18190], [39103]
Healthsouth Rehabilitation Institute of Tucson [12832], [38056]
HEALTHSOUTH Rehabilitation of Mechanicsburg [35642]
Healthsouth Rehabilitation Specialists--Plano [39090]
Healthsouth Rock Hill [39015]
Healthsouth Sea Pines Rehabilitation Hospital [38251]
HealthSouth Sea Pines Rehabilitation Hospital • Pediatric/Adolescent Program [7893]
HealthSouth • Sleep Disorders Center [36646]
Healthsouth Southern Hills Rehabilitation Hospital [35771], [39168]
HealthSouth Sports Lakeshore Oupatient Center [37994]
Healthsouth Sports Medicine and Rehabilitation Center [39166]
HealthSouth Sunrise Rehabilitation Hospital [1767] Comprehensive Pain Care Center [35382]
HealthSouth--Tallahassee [1772]
Healthsouth Treasure Coast Rehabilitation Hospital [1788], [38294]
Healthsouth Tustin Rehabilitation Hospital [38155]
HealthSouth Valley of the Sun Rehabilitation Hospital [12791]
Healthsouth--Woburn • New England Rehabilitation • Keleher Ambulatory Care [2539]
Healthtrends, Ltd. [14767]
HealthWays Inc
    Adolescent Program [50349]
    Miracles Happen [50353]
    Passages for Growth [50350]
    Substance Abuse Program [50351]
HealthWest Spine and Joint Care [38140]
Healthwise Home Care Solutions Inc. [13229]
Healthworks Rehab and Fitness [39163]
Healthworks • Sports Nutrition Services [11089]
Healthworks of Staten Island [35576]
Healthy Babies Project
    Harriet Tubman Recovery Center [40298]
    Maudell Shirek Recovery Village [40299]
Healthy Choice Homecare, LLC [18108]
Healthy Connections Homecare Services, Inc. [17990]
Healthy Connections Inc [40824]
Healthy Families of Clallam County [10636]
Healthy Futures [10898]
Healthy Hearing and Balance Clinic [1628]
Healthy Heart Nurse, Inc. [14758]
Healthy Home • Blue Ridge Home Health Care [16789]
Healthy at Home - CMC [16712]
Healthy Life Home Care Inc. [13201]
Healthy Moms Program [39820]
Healthy Partnerships [39785], [40452], [40873]
Healthy Responses in a • Dysfunctional Society [48626]
Healthy Risk Counseling Center [50021]
Healthy Start [16115]
Healthy Steps Program • Nashua Area Health Center [45915]
Healthy Within [10955]
HealthyLife Home Care [14019]
Healy Counseling Associates [46184]
Hear Again Audiology Center [1581]
HEAR Center [1221]
Hear Inc • Gate House for Men [48453]
Hear Me Now! [2360]
Hear To Learn in Georgia [1901]
Hear USA [2513]
HearCare Audiology [1927]
Hearing Aid and Audiology Associates Inc. [1486]
Hearing Associates [1377]
Hearing and Balance Associates of Northwest Florida [1773]
Hearing and Balance Center [1260]
Hearing Balance and Speech Center [1464]
Hearing Care Associates--Encino [1105]

Hearing Care Associates--Northridge [1199]
Hearing Care Center [2522]
Hearing Center--Downers Grove [2020]
Hearing Center--Fort Wayne [2145]
Hearing Center of Glastonbury [1459]
The Hearing Center, Inc. [2009]
Hearing Center of San Clemente [1252]
Hearing Centers of Northern California [1279]
Hearing Clinic [2179]
The Hearing Clinic [905]
Hearing Consultants of California--Lompoc [1151]
Hearing Consultants of California--Santa Barbara [1306]
Hearing Diagnostics Center--South Bend [2184]
Hearing Diagnostics Center--Syracuse [2187]
Hearing Dynamics [1082], [1203]
Hearing Education Services [574]
Hearing Enhancement Center [1087]
Hearing Health Care Associates [1455]
Hearing Health Care Associates, Inc. [1472]
Hearing Health Care Center [1823]
Hearing Health Center--Chicago [1988]
Hearing Health Center--Naperville [2077]
Hearing Healthcare Associates--Augusta [2345]
Hearing Healthcare Associates--Baytown [3468]
Hearing Healthcare Associates--Beverly [2450]
Hearing Impaired Program of Bay County [353]
Hearing Improvement Center LLC [1503]
Hearing Institute [1232]
Hearing and Neurodiagnostic Centers--Murrieta [1191]
Hearing and Neurodiagnostics Centers--Encinitas [1101]
Hearing Pathways Dispensing Audiology [1365]
Hearing Plus Audiology [1928]
Hearing Resource Center of San Mateo [1300]
Hearing Science of the Foothills [1189]
Hearing Science of Walnut Creek [1358]
Hearing Sense Audiology [1249]
Hearing Services Associates--Centerbrook [1451]
Hearing Services Associates--Middletown [1469]
Hearing Services of Bad Axe and Sandusky [2557]
Hearing Services Center Inc. [1147]
Hearing Services of Pleasanton [1229]
Hearing Services of Vallejo [1353]
Hearing Solutions [1434]
Hearing and Speech Agency [2374]
Hearing and Speech Center [3650]
Hearing and Speech Center of Florida [1655]
Hearing and Speech Center of Northern California [1280]
Hearing and Speech Center of Rochester [3111]
Hearing and Speech Center of Saint Joseph County Inc. [2150]
Hearing, Speech and Deaf Center of Greater Cincinnati • Community Services for the Deaf [3220]
Hearing, Speech, & Deafness Center • Speech/Language Pathology and Audiology [3638]
Hearing and Speech Services [1291]
Hearing Zone [1944]
HearingCare Inc.--Arvada [1374]
HearingCare Inc.--Northglenn [1439]
HearingCare--North Glenn [1438]
HearingDocs, LLC [2244]
Hearne Dialysis Center • DaVita [27120]
Heart 2 Heart Home Healthcare Agency, Inc.--N State Rd., Miami [13856]
Heart 2 Heart Home Healthcare Agency--Miami [14020]
Heart of America Hospice--Kansas [19780]
Heart of America Hospice--Rugby [20792]
Heart City Health Center [6683]
Heart Connections PLLC [50250]
Heart of Florida Health Center [6519]
Heart of Georgia Hospice [19433]
Heart to Heart Home Care--Bronx [16363]
Heart to Heart Home Care--Brooklyn [16392]
Heart to Heart Home Care--East Orange [16198]
Heart to Heart Hospice of Austin [21387]
Heart to Heart Hospice of Fort Worth, LLC [21460]
Heart to Heart Hospice of Greater Houston [21484]
Heart to Heart Hospice-Lewisville [21510]
Heart to Heart Hospice-Lufkin [21526]
Heart to Heart Hospice of San Antonio, LLC [21553]
Heart of Hospice, LLC--Hood River [21006]
Heart of Hospice LLC--Lafayette [19848]
Heart and Lung Clinic • Cystic Fibrosis Center [7635]

Heart of the Mountains Hospice, Inc. [19113]
Heart 'n Home Hospice-Meridian [19470]
Heart 'n Home Hospice & Palliative Care-Baker City [20986]
Heart 'n Home Hospice & Palliative Care-Emmett [19457]
Heart 'n Home Hospice and Palliative Care--Fruitland [19460]
Heart of Ohio Dialysis Center • Fresenius Medical Care [26158]
Heart River Alcohol and • Drug Abuse Services [47566]
Heart Steps Counseling Services Inc [48142]
Heart of Texas Region Mental Health/Mental Retardation Center
    Bosque County Center [32512]
    Falls County Center [32507]
    Hill County Center [32478]
    Waco [32566]
Heartbeat Home Health Agency [14021]
Hearth 'n Home Hospice & Palliative Care-Caldwell [19453]
Hearthstone Fellowship Foundation Inc [41614]
Hearthstone of Minnesota [34257]
Heartland Alternative Service Program [45588]
Heartland Behavioral Health Services Inc. [33632]
Heartland Behavioral Healthcare [33756]
Heartland Center • Dual Recovery Program [28481]
Heartland Center for Reproductive Medicine [22149]
Heartland Community Health Clinic [6674]
Heartland Counseling and Consulting Clinic [51076]
Heartland Counseling and Consulting • Clinic/Region II Human Services [45778]
Heartland Counseling Services • Ainsworth Satellite [45723]
Heartland Counseling Services Inc [45815]
Heartland Dialysis • Davita • Dialysis Facility & At Home [26280]
Heartland Family Service [43252], [45793], [45794], [45808]
Heartland Family Service Domestic Abuse Program [9782]
Heartland Health [37313]
Heartland Health Center--Lincoln Square [6659]
Heartland Health Outreach, Inc. [6660]
Heartland Health Outreach • Pathways Home Outpatient [42523]
Heartland Home Care and Hospice--Portage [20107]
Heartland Home Health Care
    and Hospice--Allentown [21043]
    and Hospice--Grand Rapids [20062]
Heartland Home Health Care and Hospice--Bay City [20034]
Heartland Home Health Care and Hospice--Blue Bell [21055]
Heartland Home Health Care and Hospice--Caro [20043]
Heartland Home Health Care and Hospice-Chadds Ford [21071]
Heartland Home Health Care and Hospice-Columbus [20827]
Heartland Home Health Care and Hospice--Dallas [21431]
Heartland Home Health Care and Hospice--Dayton [20833]
Heartland Home Health Care and Hospice-De Pere [21829]
Heartland Home Health Care and Hospice--Fairfax [21689]
Heartland Home Health Care and Hospice--Fairview Heights [19519]
Heartland Home Health Care and Hospice--Flint [20056]
Heartland Home Health Care and Hospice--Fort Wayne [19598]
Heartland Home Health Care and Hospice Inc.--Indianapolis [19611]
Heartland Home Health Care and Hospice, Inc.--Richmond [21723]
Heartland Home Health Care and Hospice--Independence [20847]
Heartland Home Health Care and Hospice--Mason [20093]
Heartland Home Health Care and Hospice--Milwaukee [21856]
Heartland Home Health Care and Hospice--Newark [19180]

Heartland Home Health Care and Hospice--Orange [18983]
Heartland Home Health Care and Hospice--Pittsburgh [21139]
Heartland Home Health Care and Hospice--Portsmouth [20885]
Heartland Home Health Care and Hospice--Raleigh [20719]
Heartland Home Health Care and Hospice--Roseville [20200]
Heartland Home Health Care and Hospice--Saint Louis [20334]
Heartland Home Health Care and Hospice--San Antonio [21554]
Heartland Home Health Care and Hospice--Shawnee [20975]
Heartland Home Health Care and Hospice--Virginia Beach [21743]
Heartland Home Health Care and Hospice-West Branch [20133]
Heartland Home Health Care and Hospice--West Covina [19077]
Heartland Home Health Care and Hospice--Westminster [19131]
Heartland Home Health Care and Hospice--Wichita [19787]
Heartland Home Health Care and Hospice--Wyomissing [21178]
Heartland Home Health Care and Hospice-York [21180]
Heartland Home Health and Hospice-Fond Du Lac [21833]
Heartland Home Health and Hospice--Lancaster [21106]
Heartland Home Healthcare and Hospice--Ann Arbor [20029]
Heartland Home Healthcare and Hospice--Riverside [19002]
Heartland Home Healthcare and Hospice--Santa Clara [19038]
Heartland Home Healthcare and Hospice--Santa Rosa [19044]
Heartland Home Healthcare and Hospice--Southfield [20118]
Heartland Home HealthCare and Hospice--Toledo [20899]
Heartland Home Infusions, Inc. [14820]
Heartland Homecare and Hospice--Pittston [21144]
Heartland Hospice Care-Cartersville [19371]
Heartland Hospice Care-Dubuque [19689]
Heartland Hospice Care-Philadelphia [21056]
Heartland Hospice Care-Tucson [18829]
Heartland Hospice--Dickinson [20779]
Heartland Hospice--Fayetteville [19385]
Heartland Hospice House of Delaware [19185]
Heartland Hospice Service Inc-Fremont [20842]
Heartland Hospice Services--Albuquerque [20516]
Heartland Hospice Services--Augusta [19357]
Heartland Hospice Services--Baltimore [19912]
Heartland Hospice Services--Beltsville [19917]
Heartland Hospice Services--Brunswick [19366]
Heartland Hospice Services--Butler [20285]
Heartland Hospice Services--Catonsville [19918]
Heartland Hospice Services--Charleston [21211]
Heartland Hospice Services--Cincinnati [20811]
Heartland Hospice Services--Columbus [20828]
Heartland Hospice Services--Conway [21225]
Heartland Hospice Services--Davenport [19682]
Heartland Hospice Services--Erie [21084]
Heartland Hospice Services--Hillside [19529]
Heartland Hospice Services--Hurst [21497]
Heartland Hospice Services--Jacksonville [19242]
Heartland Hospice Services--Kansas City [20310]
Heartland Hospice Services--Macon [19403]
Heartland Hospice Services--McAlester [20939]
Heartland Hospice Services--Monterey [18971]
Heartland Hospice Services--Newport News [21707]
Heartland Hospice Services--Norman [20950]
Heartland Hospice Services--Palatine [19554]
Heartland Hospice Services--Rochester [20196]
Heartland Hospice Services--Rockford [19567]
Heartland Hospice Services--Saint Cloud [20202]
Heartland Hospice Services--Simpsonville [21278]
Heartland Hospice Services--Thorofare [20501]
Heartland Hospice Services--Topeka [19781]
Heartland Human Care Services Inc • Wellness and Prevention [42524]
Heartland Human Services [29615], [42652]

Heartland Kids [1690]
Heartland Lions Eye Bank--Hays, KS [35044]
Heartland Lions Eye Bank--Joplin, MO [35091]
Heartland Lions Eye Bank--Kansas City, MO [35092]
Heartland Lions Eye Bank--Saint Louis, MO [35093]
Heartland Lions Eye Bank--Springfield, IL [35024]
Heartland Lions Eye Bank--Springfield, MO [35094]
Heartland Lions Eye Bank--Wichita, KS [35045]
Heartland Recovery Services Inc [45081]
Heartland Regional Medical Center • Cancer Center [5458]
Heartland Regional Medical Center Home Services [16049]
Heartland Rehabilitation and Pilates - The Avenues [38234]
Heartland Rehabilitation Service--West Bloomfield [38610]
Heartland Rehabilitation Services [3594]
Heartland Rehabilitation Services - Alchua [38213]
Heartland Rehabilitation Services - Amelia Island [38224]
Heartland Rehabilitation Services - Arlington [38235]
Heartland Rehabilitation Services - Boca Raton [38218]
Heartland Rehabilitation Services, Chiefland [38221]
Heartland Rehabilitation Services - Emerson [38236]
Heartland Rehabilitation Services - Fleming Island [38259]
Heartland Rehabilitation Services - Gainesville [38229]
Heartland Rehabilitation Services - Homestead [38215]
Heartland Rehabilitation Services - Kennerly [38237]
Heartland Rehabilitation Services - Lake City [38247]
Heartland Rehabilitation Services - Live Oak [38249]
Heartland Rehabilitation Services - Middleburg [38255]
Heartland Rehabilitation Services - New Smyrna [38257]
Heartland Rehabilitation Services - North Mandarin [38238]
Heartland Rehabilitation Services - Northside [38239]
Heartland Rehabilitation Services - Onsite [38260]
Heartland Rehabilitation Services--Orange Park [38261]
Heartland Rehabilitation Services - Ortega [38240]
Heartland Rehabilitation Services--Palatka [38271]
Heartland Rehabilitation Services - Riverside [38241]
Heartland Rehabilitation Services - Saint John's [38280]
Heartland Rehabilitation Services - South Miami [38252]
Heartland Rehabilitation Services - Southside [38242]
Heartland Rehabilitation Services - The Beaches [38245]
Heartland Rehabilitation Services - Westside [38243]
Heartland Speech and Language Services [2849]
Heartline Inc • Lutheran Social Services of Michigan [44740]
Heartlite Hospice Care [18725]
Heartlite Hospice Care-Dalton [19379]
Heartly House, Inc. [9454]
Hearts & Hands Hospice • Pioneer Medical Center [20349]
Heart's Haven [10044]
Hearts & Homes for Youth • Runaway and Homeless Youth Program [35993]
Hearts for Hospice--American Fork [21596]
Hearts for Hospice--Meridian [19471]
Hearts for Hospice--Ogden [21627]
Hearts for Hospice--Phoenix [18807]
Hearts for Hospice--Salt Lake City [21647]
Hearts That Care, LLC Home Health Agency [16249]
Heart's Way Hospice of Northeast Texas [21517]
Heartspring [2248], [8037]
Heartstrings Hospice, Inc. [21220]
Heartsway Hospice of Northeast Texas [21417]
Heartview Foundation [47555]
Heathfield Hospice-Lawrenceville [19400]
Heathrow Psychology [11022]
Heaven and Earth Hospice • Christian Health Care [20941]
Heaven Home Health Care, Inc. [14269]

Heaven Home Health Inc. [13202]
Heavenly Health Care, LLC [18092]
Heavenly Home Health Agency Corporation [13784]
Heavenly Home Health Care Inc. [13131]
Heber Valley Counseling [49613]
Hebrew Academy for Special Children [8304]
Hebrew Health Care [19174]
Hebrew Rehabilitation Center [2519]
Hector Reyes House [44613]
Hedco Creative Living Center [28528]
Hedrick Medical Center Home Health Agency [15997]
Hegira House [30653]
Hegira Programs Inc
 Northville Counseling Center [44944]
 Oakdale Recovery Center [44689]
 Westland Counseling Center [45060]
Hegira Westland Counseling Center [30654]
Heidi Brockman Astrue LPC MAC • Astrue and Associates [48191]
Heights Hill Community Mental Health Center [31265]
Hein Speech-Language Pathology, Inc. [1261]
Helen B. Bentley Family Health Center, Inc. [6503]
Helen Devos Children's Hospital • Dialysis Unit [24909]
Helen DeVos Women and Children's Center
 Adult Cystic Fibrosis Center [7574]
 Pediatric Cystic Fibrosis Center [7575]
Helen Farabee Mental Health/Mental Retardation Center--Graham [32470]
Helen Farabee Mental Health/Mental Retardation Center--Quanah [32535]
Helen Farabee Mental Health/Mental Retardation Center--Wichita Falls [32571]
Helen Farabee Regional MH/MR Centers [49585], [49586]
 Wichita County Adult Probation [49587]
Helen Farabee Regional MHMR Center [51379], [51398]
Helen Hayes Hospital [4308]
Helen Herrmann Counseling Center [31166]
Helen Keller Center for Deaf--Blind Youth and Adults
 East Central Region--Region 3 [461]
 Great Plains Region--Region 7 [439]
 Mid--Atlantic Region--Region 2 [601]
 National Headquarters [602]
 New England Region--Region 1 [478]
 North Central Region--Region 5 [399]
 Northwestern Region--Region 10 [861]
 Rocky Mountain Region--Region 8 [325]
 South Central Region--Region 6 [768]
 Southeastern Region--Region 4 [370]
 Southwestern Region--Region 9 [298]
Helen Keller School of Alabama [213], [7727]
Helen Ross McNabb Center
 Adult Services [51359]
 Child and Youth Center [32336]
Helen Ross McNabb Center Inc
 CenterPointe Adult Services [49110]
 CenterPointe Detoxification Unit [49111]
 Sisters of the Rainbow [49112]
Helen Ross McNabb Center, Inc. • Blount County Mental Health Clinic [32265]
Helen Ross McNabb Center, Inc.--Maryville [32351]
Helen Ross McNabb Center--Knoxville [32337]
Helena Center for Mental Health [30949]
Helena Clinic [6384]
Helena Regional Medical Center [12851]
Helena Sleep Diagnostics [37298]
Helene Fuld Capital Health • Dialysis Unit [25519]
Helix Charter High School [280]
Helm DUI Services [42940]
Help for Abused Partners [8985]
Help for Abused Women and Their Children [9502]
Help for Brain Injured Children [7783]
Help on Call Crisis Line [50655]
HELP of Door County, Inc. • Helpline [51517]
Help and Emergency Response [10586]
Help End Abuse for Life Inc. [9882]
The Help Group [7828], [34029]
Help Hotline Crisis Center, Inc. [51237]
Help-in-Crisis, Inc. [10216]
HELP, Inc. [10097]
Help, Inc. [50687]
 Center Against Violence [10098]
Help Life Home Care [13661]
Help Line/Adapt [51223]

Help Ministry Fellowship YET • Help Center Inc [40113]
Help Now of Osceola County [9058]
HELP/PSI Inc [46419]
HELP of Southern Nevada • Youth Center [45841]
Helpful Hands Home Health, LLC [17877]
Helping Abused Victims In Need • HAVIN [10288]
Helping Associates Inc [39369]
Helping Hand Association • DBA The Haven [49685]
Helping Hand Home Health Services, Inc. [17349]
A Helping Hand LLC [44289]
A Helping Hand of Wilmington [47521]
Helping Hands [10093], [16479]
Helping Hands Against Violence, Inc. [10235]
Helping Hands Hawaii [29512]
Helping Hands Hawaii Bilingual Access Line [50814]
Helping Hands Hawaii IOP/OP [42207]
Helping Hands & Hearts Hospice [21506]
Helping Hands Home Health Care Services [13662]
Helping Hands Hospice--Hoover [18724]
Helping Hands Hospice, Inc.--Walnut Grove • Hospice in His Hands [20276]
Helping Hands Hospice--Tucumcari [20548]
Helping Hands Inc [46292]
Helping Hands Rehab & Home Health Services, Inc. [14022]
Helping Hearts Hospice [19659]
Helping Minnesota's Kids LLC [2711]
Helping Open Peoples Eyes Inc [49275]
 Outpatient [49264]
Helping Up Mission [44146]
Helpline Brevard 211 [50785]
Helpline of Carteret County, Inc. [51172]
HelpLine of Delaware and Morrow Counties, Inc.--Delaware [51214]
HelpLine of Delaware and Morrow Counties, Inc.--Mount Gilead [51227]
Helpline/Family Resources, Inc. [50786]
Helpline--Gaffney [51329]
Helpline Georgia [50812]
HelpLine--Hilton Head [51334]
HELPline--Huntsville [50617]
Helpline, Inc. [50767]
Helpline of the Midlands, Inc. [51323]
Helpline--Milwaukee [51512]
Helpline--Pittsburgh [51294]
Helpline/Ponca City [51244]
Helpline Referral Services [51253]
Helpline--Wilkes Barre [51301]
Helpline Youth Counseling Inc [40282]
Helpmate Crisis Center [10757]
Helpmate, Inc. [10014]
Hema-Quebec--Sainte-Foy [35198]
Hema-Quebec, Tissue Services--Saint-Laurent [35199]
HemaStem Therapeutics--Mississauga [35175]
HemaStem Therapeutics--Paramus • USA Lab [35115]
HemaStem Therapeutics--Toronto • Canadian Lab [35176]
Hemet Valley Medical Center [28532]
Heminger House [9303]
Hemophilia Center of Central Pennsylvania • Milton S. Hershey Medical Center [12586]
Hemophilia Center of Western New York--Adult [12562]
Hemophilia Center of Western Pennsylvania [12587]
 Sickle Cell Disease Center [36420]
Hemophilia Clinic of West Michigan Cancer Center [12537]
Hemophilia Foundation of Michigan [12538]
Hemophilia of Georgia [12511]
Hemophilia Outreach Centre [12617]
Hemophilia Treatment Center of Nevada • Children's Center for Cancer and Blood Diseases [12553]
Hemphill County Hospice [21416]
Hempstead County Clinic [28285]
Hempstead County Dialysis Unit [22541], [27374]
Henderson County Hospital Corporation • Sleep Center of Pardee [37471]
Henderson Dialysis Center • DaVita [27121]
Henderson Dual Diagnosis Treatment Center [29298]
Henderson House [10238]
Henderson Kidney Disease Center [27240]
Henderson Mental Health Center [7882], [29156]
Henderson Mental Health Center Inc • Central Henderson Mental Hlth Center Inc [41654]

Henderson Mental Health Center New Vista [29299]
Henderson Mental Health Center Rainbow [29203]
Henderson Mental Health Center South [29181]
Henderson Mental Health Office [31027]
Henderson Speech, Hearing and Language Center [2865]
Henderson Veterans Affairs Clinic [31028]
Henderson Village [29204]
Henderson Walk-In- Crisis Center [29157]
Hendersonville Speech and Hearing Services [3183]
Hendrick Hospice Care [21374]
Hendrick Housecalls [17783]
Hendricks House Inc [46203]
Hendricks Regional Health [2139]
 Cancer Program [5141]
Hendrix Health Care [33956]
Hendry-Glades Mental Health Clinic [29128]
Hendry/Glades Mental Health Clinic Inc
 Clewiston Unit [41601]
 LaBelle Unit [41723]
Hennepin County Medical Center
 Burn Center [4571]
 Cancer Program [5411]
 Crisis Intervention Center [51041]
 Department of Speech--Language Pathology [2712]
 Minnesota Regional Sleep Disorders Center [37220]
Hennepin County Medical Center Transplant [25046]
Hennepin Faculty Associates • Addiction Medicine Program [45215], [45216]
Hennepin House--People Incorporated [30698]
Henrico Area Mental Health/Mental Retardation Services--Glen Allen [32740]
Henrico Area Mental Health/Mental Retardation Services--Richmond [32778]
Henrico Doctors' Hospital--Forest • Cancer Program [6081]
Henrico Doctors Hospital--Transplant • HCA Virginia Health System [27550]
Henrietta D. Goodall Hospital • Cancer Care Center of York County [5277]
Henrietta Johnson Medical Center [6430]
Henrietta Weill Memorial • Child Guidance Clinic [28391]
Henry Booth House [42525]
Henry County Center [30008]
Henry County Counseling Center [29470]
Henry County Hospital • Help Center [47823]
Henry County Medical Center [17768]
Henry County Mental Retardation Day Training [33078]
Henry County Services [29793]
Henry Dialysis Center • Fresenius Medical Care [23796]
Henry Ford Behavioral Health--Clinton Township [33591]
Henry Ford Behavioral Health--Dearborn [33592]
Henry Ford Behavioral Health--Detroit [33593]
Henry Ford Behavioral Health Services
 Clinton Township [44709]
 Dearborn Office [44719]
Henry Ford Behavioral Health--Troy [33601]
Henry Ford Behavioral Health--West Bloomfield [33602]
Henry Ford Bi--County Hospital • Outpatient Rehabilitation Center [2662]
Henry Ford Cottage Hospital • Athletic Medicine and Physical Therapy Center [38591]
Henry Ford Health System
 Cancer Program [5371]
 Sleep Disorders and Research Center [37160]
Henry Ford Health Systems • Maplegrove Center for Chem Dependency [45056]
Henry Ford Hospice-Detroit Campus [20051]
Henry Ford Hospice-Kaleidoscope Kids & Henry Ford Hospice Wayne Team [20024]
Henry Ford Hospice Residence-Oakland [20119]
Henry Ford Hospice-Warren [20132]
Henry Ford Hospital
 Adult Hemophilia and Thrombosis Treatment Center [12539]
 Anesthesiology Pain Fellowship Program [35500]
 Department of Medical Genetics [12248]
 Department of Neurology • Multiple Sclerosis Clinic [34605]

Division of Infectious Diseases • Community Program for Clinical Research on AIDS [55]
Speech--Language Science and Disorders [2573]
Henry Ford Hospital--Transplant [24880]
Henry Ford Kingswood Hospital [33594]
Henry Ford Macomb Hospital • Josephine Ford Cancer Center [5369]
Henry Ford MaComb Hospital, Warren Campus • Sleep Medicine Center [37161]
Henry Ford Macomb Sleep Medicine Center [37162]
Henry Ford McComb • Behavioral Medicine Service OPD [44710]
Henry Ford Wyandotte Hospital
    Behavorial Services [45065]
    Speech Pathology/Audiology Department [2667]
Henry G Bannett Jr. Fertility Center • Integris Baptist Medical Canter [22220]
Henry J. Austin Health Center Inc. [6986]
Henry Lee Willis Community Center
    Channing House [44614]
    Linda Fay Griffin House [44615]
    Outpatient Substance Abuse Services [44616]
Henry Mayo Newhall Memorial Hospital • Cancer Program [4861]
Henry Medical Center • Cancer Program [5041]
Henry Occupational Therapy Services [7736]
Henry Ohlhoff North [40284]
Henry Street Shelter [9950]
Henry Viscardi School [8293]
Henrys Sober Living House [42526]
Herbert G. Birch School for Exceptional Children [8315]
Herbert Goodfriend LCSW LCADC [46069]
Hereford Physical Therapy and Sports Medicine [38531]
Heres Help Inc
    North Campus Residential/Outpatient [41843]
    South Campus/Outpatient [41783]
Heres Hope Counseling Center [49071], [49087]
Heritage Behavioral Health Center [29608], [42618]
Heritage Behavioral Health Center Inc. [50839]
Heritage Behavioral Health • Child and Adolescent Services [29609]
Heritage Dialysis Center LLC [24740]
Heritage Dialysis • Fresenius Medical Care [26108]
Heritage Health and Housing, Inc. [7030]
Heritage Home Care, Inc.--Ypsilanti [15886]
Heritage Home Care--Toronto, OH [17058]
Heritage Home Health Inc.--Reseda [13261]
Heritage Home Healthcare and Hospice [20517]
Heritage Hospice--Danville [19796]
Heritage Hospice, Inc.--Amory [20218]
Heritage Hospice, Inc.--Evansville [19594]
Heritage Hospice, Inc.--Marietta [19407]
Heritage Hospice LLC--Henryetta [20937]
Heritage Hospice of Texas [21401]
Heritage Hospital • Cancer Program [5661]
Heritage House--Eatontown [31124]
Heritage House--South Portland [30246]
Heritage Oaks Hospital [33179]
Heritage Outpatient Treatment Services [41130]
Herkimer Clinic and Club [33695]
Herkimer County Mental Health Services [31349]
Herman and Associates, Pediatrics [1697]
Hermanas Unidas [9027]
Hermiston Community Dialysis Center & At Home • DaVita [26324]
Hermitage Sleep Center [37765]
Hernando Home Health Care, Inc. [14391]
Hernando Kidney Center • DaVita [23518]
Herndon Clinic • Fort Hays State University [2220]
Heron Ridge Associates PLC [44642], [44674], [44700], [44961]
Herrick Memorial Hospital • D.B. Guild Rehabilitation Unit [2654]
Herrick Orthopaedic Clinic [38011]
Herring Houses of Dothan • Southeast Intervention Group Inc [39241]
Herrington Recovery Center [50495]
Hershey Physical Therapy Service--Lancaster [38951]
Hershey Physical Therapy Service--Lititz [38953]
Hertford--Gates Home Health Agency, Ahoskie [16686]
Hertford--Gates Home Health Agency, Gatesville [16728]
Hesperia Dialysis Center • DaVita [22725]

Hess Memorial Hospital • Dialysis Facility [27739]
Hess Memorial Hospital, Inc. [18589]
Hester Hollis Concern Center • Grant Blackford Mental Health Inc [43078]
Heuser Hearing and Language Academy [441]
Hexagram Home Health Care [14733]
HGA Home Care--Decatur [12646]
HGA Home Care--Huntsville [12683]
HHC/Bellevue Hospital
    CDOP Clinic [46873]
    Methadone Treatment Program [46874]
HHC/Metropolitan Hospital Center • Medically Managed Detoxification Unit [46875]
Hi-Desert Dialysis • DaVita [23086]
Hi Desert Medical Center [13087]
Hi-Line Recovery [45692]
Hi-Lines Help for Abused Spouses [9743]
Hi-Tech Healthcare, Inc. [14565]
Hi-Tech Medical Equipment, Inc [16586]
Hialeah Artificial Kidney Center • DaVita [23320]
Hialeah Medical Center--Flamingo Plaza [6473]
Hialeah Skills Center [6474]
Hiawatha Valley Mental Health--Caledonia [30669]
Hiawatha Valley Mental Health Center [45336], [45350]
Hiawatha Valley Mental Health Center--La Crescent [30691]
Hiawatha Valley Mental Health Center--Winona [30736]
Hibbing Veterans Affairs Clinic [30685]
Hickory Orthopedic Center [38835]
Hickory Street Center [32398]
Hickory Veterans Affairs Clinic [31545]
Hidden Brook Counseling Services PLLC [44957]
Hidden Garden Keepers Club • at Park West Health System Inc [44147]
Hidden Pines Rehabilitation [2344]
Higginsville Habilitation Center [8195]
High Ashbury Free Clinics Inc • Center for Recovery [40613]
High Country Counseling and Resource Center--Kemmerer [33050]
High Country Counseling and Resource Center--Pinedale [33058]
High Country Counseling abd Resource Centers--Afton [33030]
High Country Health Care System-Alleghany County [20739]
High Country Health Care System--Boone [16697]
High Country Health Care System Hospice--Boone [20624]
High Country Health Care System-Hospice--Jefferson [20685]
High Country Health Care System--Sparta [16783]
High Street Child Adolescent and • Family Services Center Inc [40914]
High Desert Domestic Violence Program, Inc. [8921]
High Desert Education Service District, Deaf/Hard of Hearing [681]
High Desert Family Medicine [38924]
High Desert Hemodialysis Inc. [22870]
High Desert Hospice LLC [21009]
High Desert Sleep Center [37613]
High Desert Sleep Disorders Center [36667]
High Desert Speech and Language Center Inc. [1356]
High Focus Centers [46116]
High Frontier, Inc. [34451]
High Hopes [3904], [8513]
High Peaks Hospice [20604]
High Peaks Hospice & Palliative Care, Inc. [20597]
High Plains Community Health Center, Inc. [6414]
High Plains Community Health Center Migrant Clinic [6408]
High Plains Counseling [41187], [41317]
High Plains Mental Health Center [8026]
    Colby Branch Office [29915]
High Plains Mental Health Center--Goodland [29926]
High Plains Mental Health Center--Hays [29929]
High Plains Mental Health Center--Norton [29946]
High Plains Mental Health Center
    Osborne Branch Office [29947]
    Phillipsburg Branch Office [29951]
High Point Kidney Center Inc. • Wake Forest University [25885]
High Point Regional Health System
    Hayworth Cancer Center [5647]
    Sleep Disorders Center [37472]

High Point Treatment Center Inc [44517]
    Dual Diagnosis Program [44540]
    Outpatient Program [44541]
    Section 35 WATC Program [44518]
High Point Youth [44432]
High Road Program [40456], [40894]
High Standard Health Services [14023]
Higher Goals [40114]
Higher Ground Services [43948]
Higher Ground • Tiyospaye [43490]
Higher Standards Senior Home Health Care [17878]
Highland Avenue Group Home [34106]
Highland County Dialysis • DaVita [26133]
Highland County Domestic Violence Task Force [10152]
Highland District Hospital Home Health [16945]
Highland Group Home [33422]
Highland Home Healthcare, Inc. [12911]
Highland Hospital [16614], [33916]
    Sickle Cell Disease Center [36298]
Highland House [48481]
Highland Lakes Family Crisis Center [10487]
Highland Park Dialysis • DaVita [25083]
Highland Park Hospital • Northshore University HealthSystem [24007]
Highland Park IVF Center [22037]
Highland Ridge Hospital [32590], [49630]
Highland Rim Orthopedics and Sports Medicine [39042]
Highland Rivers Center • Fannin/Gilmer Counties [29421]
Highland Rivers Community Service Board
    Adult Outpatient Services [29489]
    Bartow County Office [29384]
Highland Rivers Community Service Board--Blue Ridge [29371]
Highland Rivers Community Service Board--Calhoun [29378]
Highland Rivers Community Service Board--Dalton [29402]
Highland Rivers Community Service Board--Jasper [29444]
Highland Rivers Community Service Board
    Paulding County Office [29441]
    Polk County Office [29385]
Highland Rivers Community Services Board [42146]
    Drug Abuse Treatment and Education Prg [42075]
Highland Speech Services Inc. [3240]
Highlander Home Health Care, LLC [18596]
Highlands-Cashiers Hospice [20680]
Highlands Community Services Board
    Behavior Intervention Services [32715]
    Bristol Community Support Services [32716]
    Child and Adolescent Services [32717]
    Counseling Center [32693]
Highlands Community Services/ • Substance Abuse Intensive Treatment Program [49753]
Highlands Dialysis Center • American Renal Associates [23514]
Highlands Group Home [27913]
Highlands Home Health [12721]
Highland's Home Health Care [17251]
Highlands Medical Center [12722]
Highlands Regional Medical Center • Cancer Program [5236]
Highlands Regional Rehabilitation Hospital [4446]
Highlands Sleep Disorders Center [36584]
Highline Addiction Recovery Center • Highline Medical Center [50229]
Highline Hospice [21775]
Highline Medical Center [18452]
    Cancer Program [6096]
Highline Medical Center Specialty Campus [18474]
Highline Medical Pavilion • Highline Sleep Disorder Center [37913]
Highline Mental Health [33914]
Highline Physical Therapy & Sports Clinic--Burien [39141]
Highline Physical Therapy & Sports Clinic--Federal Way [39143]
Highline School District [862]
Highline-West Seattle Mental Health Center [32857]
HighPoint Rehabilitation Institute [35696]
Highway Christian Hospice Inc. [18808]
Hill Alcohol and Drug Treatment Center [40845]
Hill Alcohol and Substance Abuse Prog [42604]
Hill Country Community Clinic [6346]

Hill Country Community MH/MR
  Outpatient Treatment Services [49430]
  Villa Del Sol [49262]
Hill Country Community Needs Council [10463]
Hill Country Crisis Council, Inc. [10479]
Hill Country Dialysis Center of San Marcos • DaVita
  • Dialysis Facility [27354]
Hill Country Youth Ranch • Runaway and Homeless
  Youth Program [36224]
Hill County Council on AD Abuse Inc [49431]
Hill Crest Hospital • Hill Crest Behavioral Health
  Services [33079]
Hill Health Corporation [29024]
Hill Park Clinic • Pain Center [35313]
Hillandale Road Veterans Affairs Clinic [31528]
Hillcrest Baptist Medical Center • Cancer Center
  [4710]
Hillcrest Children and Family Center [41537]
Hillcrest Children's Center [29089]
Hillcrest Community Hospice [21586]
Hillcrest Educational Centers [34210]
Hillcrest Family Services [29862], [29876]
  Cedar Rapids Office [34138]
Hillcrest Family Services Clinic [29863]
Hillcrest Family Services
  Hillcrest Mental Health Center [29864]
  Marywood Home [29865]
  Vizaleea Home [29866]
Hillcrest Group Home [32728]
Hillcrest Home Care [20377]
Hillcrest Hospital
  Hirsch Cancer Center [5738]
  Sleep Disorders Center [37529]
Hillcrest Medical Center • Alexander Burn Center
  [4611]
Hillcrest of Ohio Valley Medical Center [51225]
Hillcroft Dialysis Center [27146]
Hillhaven Rehabilitation Center [3174]
Hilliard Dialysis Center LLC • American Renal As-
  sociates [23321]
Hills Medical Group [39046]
Hillsboro Area Hospital [14818]
Hillsboro Dialysis Center & At Home • DaVita
  [26325]
Hillsborough County Crisis Center [50790]
Hillsborough County Deaf/Hard of Hearing Program
  [357]
Hillside Center [15899], [32442]
Hillside Children's Center • Runaway and Homeless
  Youth Services [36110]
Hillside Dialysis Center
  Fresenius Medical Care [25521]
  KRU Medical Ventures [25444]
Hillside Home for Children [34009]
Hillside Homecare/Hospice • Beaver Dam Com-
  munity Hospitals, Inc. [21823]
Hillside, Inc. [29343]
Hillside Mental Health Center [28065]
Hillside Rehabilitation Hospital [4367]
Hillsides Family Center [28397]
Hilltop Counseling Services [43538]
Hilltop/Latimer House [8967]
Hilltop Recovery Services [40220]
  Residential Treatment [40221]
Hilltop Special Services • Runaway and Homeless
  Youth Program [35856]
Hilltop Speech and Language Services [1153]
Hilltop's Domestic Violence Program [8968]
Hillview Acres Children's Home [28437]
Hillview Terrace [27996]
Hillwood Home [28047]
Hilo Dialysis • Liberty Dialysis Hawaii [23846]
Hilo Family Health Center • Hilo Bay Clinic [6615]
Hilo Medical Center Home Care [14613]
Hilo Veterans Center [29513]
Hilo YMCA • Family Visitation Centers [9135]
Hilton Head Dialysis Center • Fresenius Medical
  Care [26729]
Hilton Head Health Institute [11268]
Hilton Head Sports Medicine [39010]
Hina Mauka/Teen Care
  Aliamanu Intermediate School [42208]
  Castle High School [42245]
  Kahuku High and Intermediate School [42229]
  Kailua Intermediate School [42231]
  Kalaheo High School [42232]
  Kalani High School [42209]
  Kamakehelei Middle School [42265]

Kapaa High School [42247]
Kapaa Middle School [42248]
Kauai High school [42266]
King Intermediate School [42246]
Mililani High School [42272]
Mililani Middle School [42273]
Olomana High School [42233]
Pearl City High School [42282]
Radford High School [42210]
Waimea Canyon Elem/Intermed School [42295]
Waimea High School [42296]
Hinchman House Outpatient Clinic [28570]
Hinds Behavioral Health Services [45392]
Hinds Feet Adventure • Hinds Feet Counseling
  [41062]
Hinds Hospice--Fresno [18929]
Hinds Hospice Home • Inpatient Services [18930]
Hinds Hospice--Merced [18967]
Hindsdale Orthopaedic Therapy Center--Naperville
  [38393]
Hindsdale Orthopaedic Therapy Center--New Lenox
  [38396]
Hines VA Hospital
  Aurora Clinic [4017]
  Elgin Clinic [4018]
  Joliet Clinic [4019]
  Kankakee Clinic [4020]
  LaSalle Clinic [4021]
  Oak Lawn Clinic [4022]
Hinesville Dialysis • DaVita [23719]
Hinsdale Center for Reproduction [22038]
Hinsdale Hospital • Adventist Health System,
  Midwest Region • Cancer Program [5098]
Hinsdale Orthopaedic Associates • Sports
  Performance Institute [38417]
Hinsdale Orthopaedic Therapy Center--Hinsdale
  [38380]
Hinsdale Othopaedic Therapy Center--Joliet [38384]
Hioaks Dialysis, PD & At Home • Dialysis Center •
  DaVita [27551]
Hiram G. Andrews Center • Deaf and Hard of Hear-
  ing Services Unit [3341]
HIRE/ProWork [4368], [35609]
Hirschfield Center for Children [34499]
HIS Acquisition XXX, Inc • US Bioservices [17258]
His Sheltering Arms Inc
  Family Service Center [40115]
  Outpatient [40116]
  Residential Long Term [40117]
Hispanic Battered Women's Program [9623]
Hispanic Clinic [33258]
Hispanic Counseling Center • Medically Supervised
  Outpatient Clinic [46692]
Hispanic Family Center [31111]
Hispanic Family Center of Southern • New Jersey
  Substance Abuse Services [45952]
Hispanic Partial Hospitalization Program • JFK
  Center for Mental Health & Retardation [32079]
Hispanic Urban Minority Alcoholism and Drug Abuse
  Outreach [10136]
Hitchcock Center for Women Inc [47689]
Hiwassee Mental Health [49125]
Hiwassee Mental Health Center [32267], [32294],
  [49059]
  Athens [49038]
HM Home Care & HM Home Pharmacy [16944]
HMS--Lordsburg HSHC [7000]
HMS School for Children with Cerebral Palsy [8474]
HMS--Silver City School Wellness Center [7005]
HMSD, LLC • Sleep Disorders Center [37816]
Ho Chunk Nation Behavioral Health [50434]
Ho Chunk Nation Dept of Hlth/Soc Services •
  Alcohol and Drug Program Services [50543]
Ho Ho Kus Speech and Language Practice [2911]
HO Program Office--Little House [6462]
Hoag Memorial Hospital
  Cancer Institute [4811]
  Chemical Dependency Recovery Center [40261]
  Judy & Richard Voltmer Sleep Center [36668]
Hobbs Dialysis • Fresenius Medical Care • Dialysis
  Services [25548]
Hobbs Municipal Schools [559]
Hobbs Orthopaedic and Sports Therapy [38771]
Hoboken Dialysis Center • Fresenius Medical Care
  [25445]
Hoboken University Medical Center
  Community Mental Health Center [51103]
  Giant Steps Program [46016]

Hocking Hills Dialysis Center • Fresenius Medical
  Care [26146]
Hoffler and Associates • Counseling Inc [41063]
Hoffman Homes [34413]
Hoffmann Hospice--Bakersfield [18888]
Hoffmann Hospice--Palmdale [18988]
Hogan Regional Center [8128]
Hogansville Dialysis Clinic • Renal Advantage Inc.
  [23722]
Hogar de Ayuda El Refugio Inc [48761]
Hogar Camino A La Salvacion II [48731]
Hogar Clara Lair [10331]
Hogar Compromiso de Vida Uno [48802]
Hogar Crea de Adultos • Barrio Real Anon [48797]
Hogar Crea Aguadilla [48719]
Hogar Crea Aibonito Adolescentes [48720]
Hogar Crea Arecibo Adolescentes [48723]
Hogar Crea Arecibo Adultos [48724]
Hogar Crea Barranquitas [48726]
Hogar Crea Cabo Rojo [48740]
Hogar Crea de Caguas [48742]
Hogar Crea Cayey [48749]
Hogar Crea Central Modelo Damas • Callejon los
  Marques Parcela D [48809]
Hogar Crea Ciudad Modelo [48813]
Hogar Crea Coamo Damas [48751]
Hogar Crea Coamo Varones [48752]
Hogar Crea Comerio [48753]
Hogar Crea Corozal [48754]
Hogar Crea Country Club [48814]
Hogar Crea El Conquistador [48831]
Hogar Crea Fajardo [48755]
Hogar Crea Guanica [48756]
Hogar Crea Guayama [48757]
Hogar Crea Guaynabo Adolescentes [48762]
Hogar Crea Guaynabo Adultos [48763]
Hogar Crea Gurabo [48767]
Hogar Crea Humacao [48771]
Hogar Crea Inc Posada de la Esperanza • Centro
  de Madres Con Ninos [48832]
Hogar Crea International of CT Inc [41407]
Hogar CREA International Inc of DE • Mens Center
  [41519]
Hogar Crea Isabela Adolescentes [48774]
Hogar CREA Juana Diaz Adolescentes • De Juana
  Diaz [48775]
Hogar Crea Juana Diaz Adultos [48776]
Hogar Crea Juncos [48777]
Hogar Crea La Quinta • Carlos Quevedo Estrada
  [48833]
Hogar Crea Las Americas [48803]
Hogar Crea Las Marias [48779]
Hogar Crea Loiza [48780]
Hogar Crea Luquillo [48781]
Hogar Crea Manati Damas [48782]
Hogar Crea Manati Varones [48783]
Hogar Crea Morovis [48788]
Hogar Crea Naguabo [48789]
Hogar Crea Naranjito [48790]
Hogar Crea Orocovis [48791]
Hogar Crea Parcelas Falu • Proyecto Especial
  [48815]
Hogar Crea Ponce Mercedita [48798]
Hogar Crea Ponce Playa • Posada Fe Y Esperanza
  [48799]
Hogar Crea Ponce Pueblo [48800]
Hogar Crea Rio Plantation [48732]
Hogar Crea Sabana Catano [48764]
Hogar Crea Sabana Grande [48807]
Hogar Crea Sabana Llana [48804]
Hogar Crea San German [48810]
Hogar Crea San Isidro [48745]
Hogar Crea San Jose [48816]
Hogar Crea San Lorenzo [48822]
Hogar Crea San Sebastian [48823]
Hogar CREA Santa Isabel [48824]
Hogar Crea Toa Alta [48827]
Hogar Crea Trujillo Pueblo [48834]
Hogar Crea Vega Alta [48835]
Hogar Crea Vega Baja [48837]
Hogar CREA Venezuela [48817]
Hogar Crea Villa Palmeras [48825]
Hogar Crea Vista Alegre [48733]
Hogar Crea Womens Center [41408], [48292]
Hogar Crea Yabucoa [48839]
Hogar Crea Yauco [48842]
Hogar Del Buen Pastor Inc [48818]
Hogar Dios Es Nuestro Refugio [48765]

Hogar Divino Nino Jesus Inc [48758], [48830]
Hogar JESUS Inc [48721]
Hogar Nueva Mujer Santa Maria de la Merced [10330]
Hogar Nueva Vida [48768]
Hogar Nueva Vida Humacao [48772]
Hogar Nueva Vida OCELI [48840]
Hogar Nuevo Pacto • Juncos [48778]
Hogar Posada la Victoria Inc [48828]
Hogar Resurreccion Inc [48743]
Hogar Ruth [10334]
Hogar Santisima Trinidad [48829]
Hogar Un Nuevo Camino [48759]
Hogares Casa--Casa Antigua [34307]
Hogares, Inc. [34308]
Hogares Outpatient [46234]
Hoke County Domestic Violence and Sexual Assault Center [10072]
Holbrook Counseling Center [29590]
Holbrook Counseling Center--Chciago [29591]
Holbrook Counseling Center--Cicero [29602]
Holbrook Counseling Center--Des Plaines [29610]
Holbrook Counseling Center--Highland Park [29632]
Holbrook Counseling Center--Mundelein [29652]
Holbrook Counseling Center--Worth [29687]
Holbrook Speech and Hearing Clinic [3038]
Holcomb Behavioral Health Systems [48665]
Holdaway Medical Services, LLC [15221]
Holden House [44883]
Holdrege Veterans Affairs Clinic [30991]
Holiness Home Healthcare Corporation [18104]
Holistic Health Care [18682]
Holistic Home Health Care [15357]
Holistic Home Health Care Corporation [14024]
Holistic Therapy Services • Linda Sue Gengelbach [43210]
Holistic Therapy Solutions [1727]
Holland Community Hospital • Behavioral Health Services [44843]
Holland Hospital Home Health [15683]
Holland Hospital
   Michigan Pain Consultants [35501]
   Sleep Disorders Center [37163]
Holland Public Schools [490]
Hollar Speech and Language Services [1135]
Hollins Communication Research Institute [3609]
The Holliswood Hospital [33696]
Holly Center [8101]
Holly Hill Children's Services [34150]
Holly Hill Clinic [32205]
Holly Hill Dialysis Center • Renal Advantage Inc. [26730]
Holly Hill Hospital [47459]
Holly Ridge Center • Infant-Toddler Program [8598]
Hollywood Artificial Kidney Center • Regional--KRU Medical Ventures [23323]
Hollywood Dialysis Center • DaVita [22782]
Hollywood Health Services Inc. [13132]
Hollywood Health System, Inc. [13133]
Hollywood Medical Supply Co. [13796]
Hollywood Mental Health Services [28595]
Hollywood Pavilion Hospital [33306]
Hollywood-Presbyterian Medical Center • Oncology Services [4798]
Hollywood Recovery Treatment Center [40831]
Hollywood and Vine Recovery Center [40278]
Holmdel Dialysis Center • DaVita [25446]
Holmes County Hospice [20869]
Holmes Regional Medical Center, Inc. • Regional Cancer Center [4961]
Holmes Street Foundation Inc
   Holmes Street Adolescent Residential [49286]
   Holmes Street Outpatient Program [49287]
Holmesview Center [48943]
Holston Children & Youth Services [32327]
Holston Counseling Center [32328]
Holston River Clinic • Dialysis Clinic Inc. [26861]
Holt House [31228]
Holton Community Hospital Home Health and Hospice [19756]
Holton Veterans Affairs Community Hospital [29931]
Holy Angel Home Health, Inc. [13134]
Holy Angels Residential Facility [8076]
Holy Comforter Saint Cyprian • Community Action Group Outpatient Prg [41538]
Holy Cross Childrens Services [44704]
Holy Cross Dialysis Center--Woodmore [24706]
Holy Cross Home Care and Hospice [15465]

Holy Cross Hospital [14734]
   Bienes Comprehensive Cancer Center [4941]
   Cancer Program [5314]
Holy Cross Hospital Home Health Services [13691]
Holy Cross Hospital Hospice Unit • Seasons Hospice Inc. [19501]
Holy Cross Hospital • Renal Dialysis Unit [24730]
Holy Cross Renal Center • Hemodialysis Inc. [22811]
Holy Family Hospice [20881]
Holy Family Hospice Care [18913]
Holy Family Hospital • Cancer Program [6121]
Holy Family Hospital and Medical Center • William L. Lance Cancer Management Center [5344]
Holy Family Hospital
   Sleep Disorders Center [37914]
   Speech and Hearing Center [3644]
Holy Family Institute [32107]
Holy Family Medical Center • Keys to Recovery [42625]
Holy Family Memorial Dialysis Center [27735]
Holy Family Memorial Hospice [21851]
Holy Family Memorial Inc. [18583]
Holy Family Memorial Medical Center • Cancer Center [6159]
Holy Family Social Services/Shores [48596]
Holy Name Home Care/Hospice [20500]
Holy Name Home Dialysis • Fresenius Medical Care [25515]
Holy Name Hospital • Dialysis Unit [25516]
Holy Name Hospital Home Care [16273]
Holy Name Hospital
   Multiple Sclerosis Center [34633]
   Northern New Jersey Center for Sleep Medicine [37347]
   Regional Cancer Center [5543]
Holy Redeemer Health System [17382]
Holy Redeemer Home Care and Hospice [21129]
Holy Redeemer Home Care NJ Shore-Hospice--Egg Harbor Township [20469]
Holy Redeemer Home Care NJ Shore-Hospice-- Toms River [20503]
Holy Redeemer Home Care--Runnemede [16261]
Holy Redeemer Home Care--Vineland [16284]
Holy Redeemer Home Health & Hospice Services-- Langhorne [17369]
Holy Redeemer Home Health & Hospice Services-- Philadelphia [17413]
Holy Redeemer Hospice [20493]
Holy Redeemer Hospice-Cape May Branch [20499]
Holy Redeemer Hospital and Medical Center
   Cancer Care Cancer [5841]
   Sleep Disorders Lab [37652]
Holy Redeemer Sports Medicine Center [38955]
Holy Redeemer Visiting Nurse Agency [16276]
Holy Redeemer Visiting Nurse Agency and Hospice-- Cape May Court House [16190]
Holy Redeemer Visiting Nurse Agency and Hospice- Egg Harbor Township [16207]
Holy Rosary Health Care [16091]
Holy Rosary Healthcare [20366]
Holy Rosary Home Care [17210]
Holy Spirit Hospital • Crisis Intervention/Teenline [51277]
Holy Trinity Hospice [20014]
Holy Trinity Program for Deaf and Hard of Hearing [394]
Holyoke Health Center, Inc. [6816]
Holyoke Medical Center [2487]
Holyoke Medical Center Inc • Partial Hosp and Intensive Outpatient Prog [44484]
Holyoke Medical Center • Massachusetts Oncology Services [5337]
Holzer Clinic, Gallipolis • Sleep Disorders Center [37530]
Holzer Clinic, Inc. • Holzer Sleep Center of Athens [37531]
Holzer Home Care - Jackson Branch [16950]
Holzer Home Care - Pomeroy Branch [17020]
Holzer Medical Center • Cancer Program [5724]
Holzer Sleep Center Jackson, LLC [37532]
Home Aides of Central New York, Inc. [16647]
Home Aides of Rockland, Inc. [16536]
Home Alive [10646]
Home Avenue Clinic [40555]
Home Bound Care, Inc. [14025]
Home Bound Healthcare [14944], [14949]
Home Call [15446]

Home Care Advantage, Inc. [17031]
Home Care of America / San Marino [13325]
Home Care Clinicians [17138]
Home Care Connection Hospice [20528]
Home Care Equipment, Inc. [16042]
Home Care of Fidelity [17991]
Home Care and Hospice, Inc [19763]
Home Care of Kittitas Valley [21752]
Home Care Medical Solutions [14026]
Home Care Options Houston, Inc. [17992]
Home Care Partners--Arlington [18246]
Home Care Partners--Washington DC [13572]
Home Care Plus, Inc.--Lewsville [18521]
Home Care Plus, Inc.--Milford [13532]
Home Care Professionals, LLC--Coral Springs [13628]
Home Care Professionals--Warren [15874]
Home Care Services, Inc. [16239]
Home Care Services Provider [14027]
Home Care Solutions [17659]
Home Care Specialists, Inc. [15498]
Home Care Supply [15315]
Home Care Supply, Inc. [17824]
Home Care Supply, LLC [17819]
Home Care Unlimited [14028]
Home Care USA [14029]
Home Choice Partners, Inc.--Chesterfield [15994]
Home Choice Partners, Inc.--Horsham [17345]
Home Companion Specialists [14336]
Home Counselors, Inc. • Runaway and Homeless Youth Program [35981]
Home for Creative Living [8186]
Home Detox Inc [41985]
Home Dialysis Network • Fresenius Medical Care [24012]
Home Dialysis of North Alabama [22327]
Home Dialysis of North Atlanta, Inc. [23599]
Home Dialysis Options of Baldwin County • Baldwin County At Home [22325]
Home Dialysis Services of Sandusky, Inc. [26195]
Home Dialysis Therapies of San Diego--North [22945]
Home Dialysis Therapies of San Diego - South [22634]
Home Free Shelter [9630]
Home of Grace • Addiction Recovery Program [45423]
Home of Guiding Hands [7775]
Home Health Advantage, Inc. [14735]
Home Health Agency of Alamogordo [20514]
Home Health of America [15813]
Home Health Care 2000--Alexandria [15263]
Home Health Care 2000--Baton Rouge [15270]
Home Health Care 2000--Crowley [15284]
Home Health Care 2000--Deridder [15289]
Home Health Care 2000--Jennings [15303]
Home Health Care 2000--Lafayette [15310]
Home Health Care 2000--Lake Charles [15316]
Home Health Care 2000--Laplace [15320]
Home Health Care 2000--New Iberia [15339]
Home Health Care 2000--Oakdale [15346]
Home Health Care 2000--Opelousas [15348]
Home Health Care 2000--Ville Platte [15378]
Home Health Care Associates [15720]
Home Health Care Center [16343]
Home Health Care of East Tennessee Inc. [21319]
Home Health Care Plus [17840]
Home Health Care Professionals & Hospice Inc. [21067]
Home Health Care of South Florida [14030]
Home Health Care of Sparrow, Inc.--Ionia [15692]
Home Health Care of Sparrow, Inc.--Lansing [15711]
Home Health Center of Thibodaux Regional Medical Center [15374]
Home Health of Coachella Valley Inc. [13231]
Home Health Connect--Bloomingdale [14690]
Home Health Connection--Chevy Chase [15429]
Home Health Connection, Inc.--Reston [18355]
Home Health Connections, Inc. [14928]
Home Health Corp. of America [14417]
Home Health Corporation of America [14434]
Home Health & Hospice Care [20447]
Home Health and Hospice Care [20446], [20677]
Home Health and Hospice Care-Clinton [20639]
Home Health and Hospice Care-Fayetteville [20661]
Home Health and Hospice Care-Maysville [20703]
Home Health and Hospice Care - Smithfield [20736]
Home Health and Hospice Care-Wilson [20768]

Home Health and Hospice of Person County [20727]
Home Health and Hospice of Sullivan County [19653]
Home Health Mates [14418]
Home Health Nursing Services, Inc. [14031]
Home Health One Ltd. [14821]
Home Health Partners Inc. [12963]
Home Health Pavilion, Inc. [16573]
Home Health--People Incorporated [30723]
Home Health Plus [17879]
Home Health Professional Services Corporation [14032]
Home Health Professionals [17993]
Home Health Quality Care, Inc. [14209]
Home Health 'R Us--Miami [14033]
Home Health R Us--Orlando [14297]
Home Health Resource [17241]
Home Health Resources, Inc. [17994]
Home Health Service of Self Regional Healthcare [17600]
Home Health Services of Florida AC, Inc. [14324]
Home Health Services--Jefferson City • University of Tennessee Medical Center [17688]
Home Health Services--Knoxville • University of Tennessee Medical Center [17705]
Home Health Services--La Follette • University of Tennessee Medical Center [17715]
Home Health Services--Loudon • University of Tennessee Medical Center [17722]
Home Health Services--Maryville • University of Tennessee Medical Center [17727]
Home Health Services--Morristown • University of Tennessee Medical Center [17741]
Home Health Services--Newport • University of Tennessee Medical Center [17764]
Home Health Services--Oak Ridge • University of Tennessee Medical Center [17766]
Home Health Services--Rogersville • University of Tennessee Medical Center [17770]
Home Health Services--Sevierville • University of Tennessee Medical Center [17772]
Home Health Services Unlimited, Inc. [15738]
Home Health Services of Venice [14438]
Home Health Specialists, Inc. [17385]
Home Health United Hospice [21822]
Home Health VNA--Chelmsford [15485]
Home Health VNA--Lawrence [15505]
Home Health VNA--Lowell [15511]
Home Health VNA--Newburyport [15524]
Home Healthcare Authority, Inc. [13592]
Home Healthcare, Hospice and Community Services [20437]
Home Healthcare Resources, Inc. [17253]
Home Healthcare Services--Knox [15011]
Home Healthcare Services--Plymouth [15041]
Home & Heart Health, Inc. [18299]
Home from Home Inc • Home from Home Counseling/Treatment Program [39980]
Home Hospice-Andrews [21382]
Home Hospice--Big Spring [21404]
Home and Hospice Care of RI • Philip Hulitar Inpatient Center [21196]
Home Hospice of Cooke County [21468]
Home Hospice of Grayson County [21567]
Home Hospice--Midland [21530]
Home Hospice--Odessa [21538]
Home and Hospital Medical Personnel, Inc. [16282]
Home Infusion Solutions--Canton [15483]
Home Infusion Solutions--Horsham [17346]
Home Infusion Solutions, Inc.--Somers Point [16268]
Home Infusion Solutions--York [17517]
Home I.V. Care, Inc. [15739]
Home IV Care and Nutritional Service [18406]
Home IV Services and Medical Supply [14674]
Home I.V. Specialists, Inc. [12841]
Home Kidney Care • Real Ventures Management, LLC [27029]
Home Life Healthcare [14923]
Home for Little Wanderers
    DBA Child and Family Counseling Center [44550]
    Longview Farm and Clifford School [34218]
Home-Med Equipment Co. [12954]
Home Med Solutions [14189]
Home Medical Specialties, Inc. [16516]
Home Medical Supply of Poplar Bluff, Inc. [16043]
Home Medix, Inc. [13112]
Home of New Vision [44643]

Home Nursing Agency Community Services • Alternatives [48274]
Home Nursing Agency Hospice [21047]
Home Nursing Co., Inc. [18315]
Home Nursing Company, Inc.--Chilhowie [18271]
Home Nursing Company, Inc.--Clintwood [18276]
Home Nursing Company, Inc.--Richlands [18356]
Home Nursing Service and Hospice • Marietta Memorial Hospital [20860]
Home Nursing Service of Southwest Virginia, Inc. [18241]
Home Options Hospice [20363]
Home Patient Services [14929]
Home Preferred Solution Corporation [14034]
Home Reach Hospice [20829]
Home Rehabilitation Healthcare Agency, Inc. [13135]
Home Respiratory Care and Hospital Equipment, Inc. [15636]
Home Respiratory Therapy and Equipment, Inc. [16539]
Home Safe in Wilson County [10415]
Home Solutions Infusion Network of the Cape and Islands [15494]
Home Solutions--Livingston [16235]
Home Stewards Health Services, LLC [14304]
Home Stretch Residential [40556]
Home Sweet Home Care [15123]
Home Touch Healthcare [12854]
Home Touch Healthcare, Inc. [14896]
Home Town Health Care [18279]
A Home for Us Foundation [40118]
Home Wellness, Inc. [16193]
Home With a Heart [48959]
Home for Women and Children [9886]
Homebound Health Care Services [13065]
Homebound Medical Supply Co., Inc. [16792]
HomeCall--Annapolis [15408]
HomeCall Baltimore [15416]
HomeCall--Easton [15434]
HomeCall--Hagerstown [15447]
HomeCall, Inc.--Frederick [15439]
HomeCall--Largo [15450]
HomeCall--Rockville [15460]
HomeCall--Waldorf [15468]
HomeCall--Westminster [15471]
HomeCare Advantage, Inc.--Cranston [17535]
Homecare Advantage, Inc.--Torrance [13390]
Homecare Alliance, Inc.--Dearborn [15620]
HomeCare Clinicians, LLC [17100]
Homecare with Heart, LLC [17088]
HomeCare and Hospice [20592]
HomeCare IV of Bend, Inc. [17180]
HomeCare Matters Home Health & Hospice [20843]
Homecare Medical, Inc. [18611]
HomeCare of Memorial Hospital [18393]
HomeCare of Metroplex [17847]
HomeCare of Michigan, Inc./Oakwood Home Medical Equipment [15573]
HomeCare of Mid-Missouri [20322]
Homecare Pharmacy LLC [18559]
HomeCare Providers Continuous Care • Alamance Regional Medical Center, Inc. [16703]
HomeCare Solutions [14736]
HomeCare Southwest [18476]
HomeChoice Partners--Augusta [14487]
HomeChoice Partners, Inc.--Ashland [18247]
HomeChoice Partners Inc.--Fayetteville [16724]
HomeChoice Partners, Inc.--Norfolk [18342]
HomeChoice Partners, Inc.--Roanoke [18376]
HomeChoice Partners, Inc.--Sterling [18392]
HomeChoice Partners--Norcross [14566]
Homecoming Project Inc [44197]
Homed Care Inc. [13749]
Homefront Health Care--East Providence [17540]
Homefront Health Care--Harmony [17541]
Homefront Health Care--Providence [17550]
Homefront Health Care--Warwick [17556]
Homefront Health Care--Westerly [17558]
Homefront Health Care--Woonsocket [17560]
HomeHealth Partnership [20153]
HomeHealth Solution Inc. [12992]
Homeland Hospice [21093]
Homeless Emergency Runaway Effort [35823]
Homeless Healthcare Los Angeles [40119]
Homeless Open Hands [6272]
Homeless Outreach and Advocacy Project [31974]
Homelink Health Services, Inc. [14835]
Homeliving Health Providers Inc. [12978]

Homemaker Service of the Metropolitan Area, Inc.--Philadelphia [17414]
Homemaker Services of the Metropolitan Area, Inc.--Chester [17282]
HomeReach Homecare and Hospice - Delaware [16931]
HomeReach Inc. [17083]
HomeSafe in Robertson County [10435]
HomeSafe in Sumner County [10403]
HomeSafeWemdAshtabula [10123]
Homeside Hospice LLC [20464]
Homestead Artificial Kidney Center • Fresenius Medical Care [23331]
Homestead Dialysis • DaVita • Dialysis Facility [26606]
Homestead Youth and Family Services [48171]
Hometown Hospice-Broken Arrow [20927]
Hometown Hospice--Collinsville [20227]
Hometown Hospice--Muskogee [20944]
Homeward Bound Inc • Trinity Recovery Center [49288]
Homeward Hospice [19664]
Homewatch Caregivers [13815]
Homewood/Brushton YMCA • Counseling Services [48597]
Honesdale Dialysis Center • DaVita [26448]
Honolulu Dialysis Center • Fresenius Medical Care • Dialysis Center [23849]
Honolulu Sports Medical Clinic [38334]
Honolulu Veterans Center [29520]
HONORehg • Middletown Addiction Crisis Center [46779]
Hood Home Health Service, LLC [15266]
Hook Rehabilitation Semi Independent Living • Program House [4037]
Ho'ola Lahui Hawaii [6626]
Hoomau Ke Ola • Residential and Outpatient Program [42289]
Hoonah Indian Association [39334]
Hoopa Valley Tribal Council • Division of Human Services [39930]
Hooper Detox • Stabilization Center [48192]
Hoosier Hearing Solutions [2129]
Hoosier Hills Dialysis • DaVita [24118]
Hoosier Hills PACT • Domestic Violence Shelter [9306]
Hoosier Orthopaedics and Sports Medicine [38433]
Hoosier Physical Therapy, PC [38428]
Hoosier Uplands Home Health and Hospice [19634]
Hop, Skip and Jump Inc. [1025]
Hope Action Care [49524]
Hope Again Dialysis Center • DaVita [25233]
HOPE Agency [10766]
Hope Alliance [10502]
HOPE Center [9596]
Hope Center [7895]
Hope Center ATS Step Down [44582]
Hope Center Children's Program [7839]
Hope Center
    Recovery Program [43660]
    Recovery Program for Women [43661]
Hope Center for Teens, Inc. • Runaway and Homeless Youth Program [35894]
Hope Community Resource, Inc. [33959]
Hope Community Resources [7732]
Hope Community Services [31901]
Hope Counseling Center [39327]
HOPE Crisis Center [9768]
Hope Dialysis Center [22542]
Hope of East Central Illinois [9200]
Hope of East Tennessee Inc [49172], [49173]
Hope Enterprises [8492]
Hope for Families [10075]
Hope Family Services, Inc. [9041]
Hope Found [44492]
Hope Foundation [8772]
Hope and Grace Recovery Services [39761]
Hope Harbor Home [10088]
Hope Haven of Cass County--Harrisonville [9683]
Hope Haven of Cass County--Pleasant Hill [9710]
Hope Haven Children's Clinic and Family Center • Down Syndrome Center [7886]
Hope Haven Clinic • Down Syndrome Center [10786]
Hope Haven Inc [47258]
Hope Haven of the Lowcountry [10344]
Hope Haven ME [1607]
Hope for Healing [10406]

Hope Healthcare Services [19223]
Hope Help and Healing Inc • Outpatient [39618]
Hope Help Health of Holton [43363]
Hope in Home Care, LLC [18335], [18402]
Hope Home Care Services [13750]
Hope Home Health Providers, LLC [14823]
Hope Home Health Services [14708]
Hope Horizon Center [41784]
Hope Hospice and Community Services, Inc. [19224]
Hope Hospice--Dublin [18918]
Hope Hospice and Healthcare, Inc. [19057]
Hope Hospice, Inc.--Anniston [18673]
Hope Hospice, Inc.--Birmingham [18683]
Hope Hospice Inc.--Pittsburgh [21140]
Hope Hospice Inc.--Rochester [19647]
Hope Hospice--New Braunfels [21536]
Hope Hospice--Owasso [20968]
Hope Hospice and Palliative Care-Medford [21854]
Hope House [30929]
Hope House--Baraboo [10690]
Hope House--Columbia [10397]
Hope House I [43050]
Hope House II [31366]
    Marthas Place [43051]
Hope House Inc [39592], [42043], [44501]
    Adolescent Residential Program [46331]
    Adult Residential Program [46332]
    CD Outpatient Clinic [46333]
    Recovery Home [44417]
    Women and Childrens Program [46334]
Hope House, Inc.--Independence [9685]
Hope House of Itasca County [45162]
Hope House • Outpatient Services [45967]
HOPE House of Scott County, Inc. [10570]
Hope House Treatment Center • Residential Medical
    Facility [44233]
HOPE, Inc.--Fairmont • Task Force on Domestic
    Violence [10674]
Hope Institute Center for Recovery and • Family
    Education Inc [39748]
Hope and Justice Project [9436]
Hope Kidney Clinic • Liberty Dialysis [27222]
Hope Medical Supply--Corpus Christi [17853]
Hope Medical Supply--San Antonio [18145]
HOPE--Mineral Wells [10491]
Hope Network Behavioral Health Services [30558]
Hope Network • Big Rapids Rehabilitation Services
    [4164]
Hope Network Insight [44884], [44945], [44998],
    [45061]
    Flint East [44787]
Hope Network • Lansing Rehabilitation Services
    [4165]
Hope Network Leadership Center [30559]
Hope Network • Mount Pleasant Rehabilitation
    Services [4166]
Hope Network Neurobehavior Program [4167]
Hope Network Rehabilitation Services [2595]
Hope Network Rehabilitation Services--Kalamazoo
    [4168]
Hope Network--South Michigan [4169]
Hope Network • VA Connecticut Healthcare System
    [3943]
Hope Neurology Clinic PLLC [34713]
Hope Nework Insight [44741]
Hope Psychological Services [11090]
Hope Recovery Center [43913], [44029]
Hope of Rochelle [9245]
The Hope School [7971]
Hope of South Texas [51396]
Hope Street Group Home LLC [47347]
HOPE for Tennessee • Frontier Health [32329]
Hope for Tomorrow Inc [42399]
Hope Unlimited [9361]
Hope Valley Inc [47279]
    Womens Division Treatment Center [47442]
Hope for Youth [34325]
Hopeline [51173]
Hope's Door--Caldwell [9166]
Hope's Door--Plano [10500]
Hopevale Inc. [34339]
Hopewell Center [30897]
Hopewell Center, Saint Louis [30898]
Hopewell Clinical [42874]
Hopewell/Prince George Counseling Services
    [32775]
Hopi Domestic Violence Program [8729]

Hopkins Children's Pediatric Burn Center • Burn
    Care Unit [4558]
Hopkinsville Clinic [30034]
Hopkinsville Dialysis & At Home • DaVita • Dialysis
    Center [24392]
Horace Mann School for the Deaf [466]
HoriSun Hospice, Inc. [20389]
Horizon Adolescent Treatment Center [39534]
Horizon Center [32845]
Horizon Counseling [41238]
Horizon Health Center [6974]
Horizon Health Services [31287]
Horizon Health Services Inc
    Addictions Outpatient Clinic/Bailey LaSalle
        [46560]
    Addictions Outpatient Clinic/Black Rock [46561]
    Addictions Outpatient Clinic/Central Park
        [46562]
    Addictions Outpatient Clinic/Niagara Falls
        [46949], [47129]
    Addictions Outpatient Treatment [46757]
    City Market Addictions CD [46950]
    Horizon Recovery Center CD OP [46369]
Horizon Healthcare Management, Inc. [18412]
Horizon Healthcare Services [17365]
Horizon Home Care & Hospice - Hartford [18573]
Horizon Home Care and Hospice, Inc.--Brown Deer
    [18562]
Horizon Home Health Care [13803]
Horizon Home Health and Hospice Inc. [19472]
Horizon Hospice--Elko [20407]
Horizon Hospice Inc-Silver City [20546]
Horizon Hospice Inc.--Chicago [19502]
Horizon Hospice & Palliative Care-Olympia Fields
    [19551]
Horizon Hospice--Poway [18995]
Horizon Hospice--Spokane [21770]
Horizon House--Centralia [29533]
Horizon House of Delaware, Inc. [29078]
Horizon House/First Step Shelter [32080]
Horizon House Inc • Behavioral Health Outpatient
    Center [48527]
Horizon House, Inc. • Old Baltimore Pike Group
    Home [29079]
Horizon House, Inc.--Stokley Street, Philadelphia
    [32081]
Horizon House--Ketchikan • Gateway Center for Hu-
    man Services [28107]
Horizon House--New Castle [32053]
Horizon House--Norristown [32060]
Horizon House--Phoenixville [32105]
Horizon House--S 30th Street, Philadelphia [32082]
Horizon House Therapeutic • Susquehanna Park
    Residential Community [48528]
Horizon Human Services [39370]
Horizon Human Services--Casa Grande [8680]
Horizon Human Services
    Casa Grande Office, E Cottonwood Lane
        [28135]
    Casa Grande Office, W Main Street [28136]
Horizon Human Services--Gila County Safehome
    [8688]
Horizon Human Services
    Globe Office [28156]
    Nogales Office [28167]
Horizon Medical Center • Cancer Care Program
    [5928]
Horizon Recovery and Counseling Center [45744]
Horizon Services
    Chrysalis [40300]
    Cronin House [39913]
    Horizon South [40659]
Horizon Treatment Center [45019]
Horizon Village • Drug Free Residential Treatment
    Prog [47064]
Horizons Community Development • Substance
    Abuse Services [46110]
Horizons Counseling Center [45897]
Horizons Day Treatment--Patrick Springs [32771]
Horizons Day Treatment Programs--Martinsville
    [32766]
Horizons • Daybreak [47243]
Horizons Developmental Remediation Center [2564]
Horizons Mental Health Center [50911]
    Harper County Area Office [29907]
Horizons • Outpatient Services [47259]
Horizons Rehabilitation Services, Inc. [1964]
Horizons School [7707]

Horizons Speech Language and Voice [1424]
Horizons Unlimited of • San Francisco Inc [40614]
Horn Hospice • Horn Memorial Hospital [19698]
Karen Horney Clinic [31417]
Horse Play Productions Healing Center [49008]
Horsham Clinic [48277]
The Horsham Clinic [33795]
Hortense & Louis Rubin Dialysis Center [25791]
Hortense & Louis Rubin Dialysis Center II [25774]
Hortense & Louise Rubin Dialysis Center [25642]
Horton Dialysis • DaVita [24321]
Hosparus Grief Counseling Center [19812]
Hospicare and Palliative Care Services of Tompkins
    County [20572]
Hospice of Acadiana, Inc. [19849]
Hospice Advantage-Athens [19343]
Hospice Advantage--Cass City [20044]
Hospice Advantage-Fayetteville [19386]
Hospice Advantage-Fond Du Lac [21834]
Hospice Advantage, Inc-Bay City [20035]
Hospice Advantage, Inc-Blue Springs [20280]
Hospice Advantage, Inc-East Ellijay [19383]
Hospice Advantage, Inc-Fond Du Lac [21835]
Hospice Advantage, Inc-Lansing [20083]
Hospice Advantage, Inc-Overland Park [19769]
Hospice Advantage, Inc-Southfield [20120]
Hospice Advantage, Inc.--Kennesaw [19396]
Hospice Advantage, Inc.--Liberty [20318]
Hospice Advantage--Troy [18766]
Hospice Advantage-Wetumpka [18773]
Hospice Alliance [21863]
Hospice of Amador [18945]
Hospice of Anchorage [18776]
Hospice Angels [18874]
Hospice of Arizona--Avondale [18781]
Hospice of Arizona--Phoenix [18809]
Hospice of Ashtabula County [20801]
Hospice Associates-Baton Rouge [19836]
Hospice Associates of Greater New Orleans Area
    [19860]
Hospice Associates-Mandeville [19853]
Hospice At Cherry Meadows [21819]
Hospice of Athens Limestone County [18675]
Hospice Atlanta-Visiting Nurse Health System
    [19351]
Hospice Austin [21388]
Hospice Austin-Williamson City [21469]
Hospice Austin's at Christopher House [21389]
Hospice of Baton Rouge [19837]
Hospice of Benewah County [19477]
Hospice of the Big Country Inc. [21375]
Hospice of the Big Horns [21882]
Hospice of the Bluegrass-Corbin [19794]
Hospice of the Bluegrass--Cynthiana [19795]
Hospice of the Bluegrass--Frankfort [19801]
Hospice of the Bluegrass--Hazard [19805]
Hospice of the Bluegrass - Jessamine County
    [19823]
Hospice of the Bluegrass--Lexington [19809]
Hospice of the Bluegrass-Pikeville [19827]
Hospice of the Bluegrass-St Joseph In-Patient Unit
    [19810]
Hospice of Boston Inc./Hospice of Greater Brockton
    [19950]
Hospice of Boulder and Broomfield Counties • Care
    Center [19119]
Hospice Brazos Valley-Brenham [21408]
Hospice Brazos Valley Inc-Bryan [21412]
Hospice Brazos Valley Inc-La Grange [21505]
Hospice of Bristol Hospital [19137]
Hospice By the Bay-Larkspur [18956]
Hospice By the Bay-San Francisco [19023]
Hospice By the Bay-Sonoma [19051]
Hospice By Loving Care [20947]
Hospice By Loving Care-Purcell [20974]
Hospice By the Sea
    Boca Care Center [19198]
    Hollywood Inpatient Unit [19232]
Hospice of the Calumet Area [19637]
Hospice of the Calumet Area Inc. [19534]
Hospice Care of America [19568]
Hospice Care of America-Pecatonica [19558]
Hospice Care of Avoyelles Parish [19857]
Hospice Care of Avoyelles Parish-Opelousas
    [19870]
Hospice Care of Boulder/Broomfield Counties
    [19115]
Hospice Care of California [18951], [19041]

Hospice Care Center of the Renaissance [20878]
Hospice Care Corporation--Arthurdale [21783]
Hospice Care Corporation-Burnsville [21791]
Hospice Care Corporation-Carmichaels [21069]
Hospice Care Corporation--Fairmont [21798]
Hospice Care Corporation-Grafton [21800]
Hospice Care Corporation--Morgantown [21806]
Hospice Care Corporation-Parsons [21810]
Hospice Care Corporation--Philippi [21812]
Hospice Care in Douglas County [19761]
Hospice Care of Greater Taunton [19998]
Hospice Care Inc.--Park Hills [20328]
Hospice Care Inpatient Unit-Elkins [21796]
Hospice Care of the Lowcountry, Inc. [21207]
Hospice Care of Middletown Inc. [20868]
Hospice Care of Nantucket [19979]
Hospice Care Network-Hospice Inn [20578]
Hospice Care of Northern Utah, LLC [21628]
Hospice Care of the NOrthwest [21031]
Hospice Care of the Northwest [21020]
Hospice Care Options, Inc. [19404]
Hospice Care Plus, Inc. [19792]
Hospice Care of St. Elizabeth Healthcare [19798]
Hospice Care of Sangamon [19576]
Hospice Care of South Carolina [21215]
Hospice Care of South Carolina-Abbeville [21198]
Hospice Care of South Carolina-Aiken [21199]
Hospice Care of South Carolina-Barnwell [21205]
Hospice Care of South Carolina-Bishopville [21206]
Hospice Care of South Carolina-Cherokee [21236]
Hospice Care of South Carolina-Colleton [21285]
Hospice Care of South Carolina-Edgefield [21230]
Hospice Care of South Carolina-Georgetown [21238]
Hospice Care of South Carolina-Greenville [21242]
Hospice Care of South Carolina-Greenwood [21247]
Hospice Care of South Carolina-Hampton-Allendale [21232]
Hospice Care of South Carolina-Horry [21226]
Hospice Care of South Carolina-Lancaster [21254]
Hospice Care of South Carolina-McCormick [21258]
Hospice Care of South Carolina-Newberry [21271]
Hospice Care of South Carolina-Pickens [21231]
Hospice Care of South Carolina-Spartanburg [21280]
Hospice Care of South Carolina-Williamsburg [21253]
Hospice Care of South Carolina-York [21272]
Hospice Care of Southeast Florida, Inc. [19219]
Hospice Care of the Southwest [21379], [21514]
Hospice Care of Southwest Michigan [20077], [20103]
Hospice Care Team, Inc.--Lake Jackson [21507]
Hospice Care Team, Inc.--Texas City [21578]
Hospice Care of Tri-County--Columbia [21221]
Hospice Care of Tri-County--Sumter [21284]
Hospice Care of the Washington Hospital [21168]
Hospice Care of the West [18884]
Hospice of Caring Hearts [19842]
Hospice of the Carolina Foothills Inc. [20642]
Hospice of Carroll County [20810]
Hospice of Carteret County [20709]
Hospice of Cedar Lake--Vital Signs [21426]
Hospice Center • Hospice of Charleston-Gentiva [21263]
Hospice of the Central Coast [18972]
Hospice of Central Georgia [19405]
Hospice of Central Iowa-Boone [19668]
Hospice of Central Iowa • The Bright Center [19743]
Hospice of Central Iowa, Centerville [19674]
Hospice of Central Iowa
    Knoxville [19705]
    Mount Ayr [19715]
Hospice of Central Iowa-Mount Pleasant [19716]
Hospice of Central Iowa--Osceola [19721]
Hospice of Central Iowa - Perry [19726]
Hospice of Central Kentucky-Campbellsville [19793]
Hospice of Central Kentucky-Elizabethtown [19799]
Hospice of Central New York [20574]
Hospice of Central Ohio [20882]
Hospice of Central PA--Carlisle [21068]
Hospice of Central PA--Harrisburg [21094]
Hospice of Central Virginia--Farmville [21693]
Hospice of Central Virginia--Richmond [21724]
Hospice of Central Virginia--Tappahannock [21739]
Hospice of the Champlain Valley [21662]
Hospice of Charles County [19930]
Hospice of Charleston [21261]

Hospice at Charlotte [20634]
Hospice of Chattanooga [21315]
Hospice Chautauqua County [20573]
Hospice of Chenango County [20591]
Hospice of the Cherokee [20978]
Hospice of the Chesapeake--Annapolis [19909]
Hospice of the Chesapeake--Landover [19931]
Hospice of Chesterfield County, Inc. [21214]
Hospice of Chippewa County • Chippewa County
    Health Department [20115]
Hospice of Cincinnati [20812]
Hospice of Cincinnati - Western Hills Unit [20813]
Hospice Circle of Love [20934]
Hospice of Citrus County-Care Unit [19235]
Hospice of Citrus County Inc.--Beverly Hills [19196]
Hospice of Citrus County, Inc.--Inverness [19236]
Hospice of Citrus County, Inc.--Lecanto [19249]
Hospice of Cleveland [21320]
Hospice of Cleveland Clinic [20848]
Hospice of Cleveland County-Wendover • The Kath-
    leen Dover Hamrick Hospice House [20732]
Hospice of Comfort • Regional Medical Center
    [19708]
Hospice of the Comforter Horizons Bereavement
    Center [19190]
Hospice and Community Care [21273]
Hospice Community Care-Glen Allen [21699]
Hospice Community Care-Newport News [21708]
Hospice of Community VNA [19946]
Hospice Compassus-Albuquerque [20518]
Hospice Compassus-Alexandria [19833]
Hospice Compassus-Baton Rouge [19838]
Hospice Compassus-Baytown [21397]
Hospice Compassus-Branson [20284]
Hospice Compassus--Casa Grande [18784]
Hospice Compassus--Cedar Rapids [19672]
Hospice Compassus-Columbia [21322]
Hospice Compassus-Dallas [21432]
Hospice Compassus-Davenport [19683]
Hospice Compassus-Financial Support Center [18684]
Hospice Compassus-Flagstaff [18789]
Hospice Compassus-Houston [21485]
Hospice Compassus-Jefferson City [20303]
Hospice Compassus-Joplin [20305]
Hospice Compassus-Lakeside [18796]
Hospice Compassus-League City [21509]
Hospice Compassus-Macon [20319]
Hospice Compassus-McComb [20250]
Hospice Compassus-Meridian [20252]
Hospice Compassus-Monett [20323]
Hospice Compassus-Monroe [19863]
Hospice Compassus-Mountain Grove [20324]
Hospice Compassus-Natchez [20253]
Hospice Compassus-New Orleans [19867]
Hospice Compassus-North Richland Hills [21537]
Hospice Compassus-Osage Beach [20326]
Hospice Compassus-Osceola [20327]
Hospice Compassus-Peoria [19560]
Hospice Compassus-Pittsburg [19773]
Hospice Compassus-Princeton [21813]
Hospice Compassus--San Antonio [21555]
Hospice Compassus--Sedona [18820]
Hospice Compassus-Shreveport [19876]
Hospice Compassus-Southfield [20121]
Hospice Compassus-Spartanburg [21281]
Hospice Compassus-Springfield [20341]
Hospice Compassus-Tullahoma [21371]
Hospice Compassus-Waveland [20277]
Hospice Compassus-Welch [21815]
Hospice Compassus-Willow Grove [21174]
Hospice Compassus-Yuma [18836]
Hospice of the Conejo [19059]
Hospice of Crawford County [21113], [21162]
Hospice of Cullman County [18695]
Hospice of Cumberland County, Inc. [21327]
Hospice of Davidson County [20694]
Hospice of Dayton Inc. [20834]
Hospice De La Luz [20519]
Hospice of Dickinson County [19745]
Hospice Direct, Inc. [20274]
Hospice Division of South MS Home HLT-
    Hattiesburg [20244]
Hospice of Douglas County [20140]
Hospice of Dubuque [19690]
Hospice East [19831]
Hospice of East Alabama Medical Center [18678]
Hospice of the East Bay--Pleasant Hill [18993]

Hospice of East Texas [21581]
Hospice of Eastern Connecticut [19148]
Hospice of Eastern Idaho, Inc. [19464]
Hospice of El Paso Inc. [21450]
Hospice of Emanuel [19066]
Hospice of the Emerald Coast-Ft. Walton [19228]
Hospice of Englewood Hospital [20471]
Hospice of the Estes Valley [19105]
Hospice Family Alliance, LLC [19864]
Hospice Family Care [18727]
Hospice Family Care, Inc-Mesa [18798]
Hospice Family Care Inc-Prescott [18819]
Hospice Family Care-Peoria [18801]
Hospice Family Care-Tucson [18830]
Hospice of Fayette Medical Center [18710]
Hospice of the Finger Lakes [20553]
Hospice of the Florida Keys [19243]
Hospice of the Foothills [18936]
Hospice of Foothills Visiting Nurse/Home Care •
    Foothills Hospice [19176]
Hospice of Franklin County [19966]
Hospice of Frederick County • Division of Frederick
    Memorial Hospital [19926]
Hospice of Garrett County [19935]
Hospice at Geary Community Hospital [19759]
Hospice of Gladwin Area [20058]
Hospice of the Golden Isles [19367]
Hospice of the Good Shepherd [19982]
Hospice of the Gorge [21007]
Hospice of Green Country Inc. [20982]
Hospice of Guernsey, Inc. [20806]
Hospice of Hamilton [20845]
Hospice of Harnett County, Inc. [20645]
Hospice of Havasu [18795]
Hospice Hawaii Inc. [19438]
Hospice Hawaii, Inc. Molokal [19444]
Hospice Hawaii, Inc. • Palolo House [19439]
Hospice Hawaii Kailua House [19441]
Hospice of Health First, Inc. [19332]
Hospice of the Heart Inc. [21591]
Hospice with Heart, Inc. [19678]
Hospice of the Heartland--Algona [19662]
Hospice of Helping Hands [20134]
Hospice of Henry County [20875]
Hospice of Henry Ford - Downriver [20136]
Hospice of Henry Ford Health System [20088]
    Saint Joseph's Team [20048]
Hospice of the Hills--Harrison [18854]
Hospice of the Hills--Rapid City [21298]
Hospice of Hillsdale County [20067]
Hospice of Hilo [19436]
Hospice in His Care, LLC [19839]
Hospice in His Hands--Carthage [20223]
Hospice of Hocking County [20854]
Hospice of Holland [20068]
Hospice at Home - A Program Visiting Nurse
    Services of Connecticut [19169]
Hospice at Home-A Program of VNS of CT [19170]
Hospice and Home Care of Alexander County Inc.
    [20751]
Hospice and Home Care of Juneau [18779]
Hospice at Home • Program of VNS of Connecticut
    [19158]
Hospice at Home-St. Joseph [20114]
Hospice at Home-South Haven [20116]
Hospice Hope [21839]
Hospice of Hope [19817], [20872]
Hospice of Hope-Ohio Valley Inpatient Center
    [20891]
Hospice House-Bend [20990]
Hospice House--Charlottesville [21678]
Hospice House of Holland [20069]
Hospice House of Home Hospice [21539]
Hospice House--Mountain Home [18869]
Hospice House--Sun City Center [19317]
Hospice House West [21461]
Hospice House-Woodside [19300]
Hospice of Humboldt [18923]
Hospice of Huntington [21802]
Hospice In His Hands-Magee [20249]
Hospice, Inc. [20599]
Hospice Inpatient Unit [19109]
Hospice Inspiris [18810]
Hospice Inspiris-King of Prussia [21103]
Hospice Inspiris, LLC [21556]
Hospice of Iredell County [20743]
Hospice of Jackson County, Inc. [19710]
Hospice of Jasper County [19718]

Hospice of Jefferson County [19766], [20612]
Hospice of Jennings County [19641]
Hospice Journey of California [18933]
Hospice of Kankakee Valley, Inc. [19492]
Hospice of Kitsap County [21748], [21769]
Hospice of Knox County [20873]
Hospice of Kona [19442]
Hospice of Lake Cumberland [19830]
Hospice of Lake Cumberland-Monticello [19818]
Hospice of Lancaster [21255]
Hospice of Lancaster County [21107]
The Hospice of Lansing [20084]
Hospice of Lansing-Residence [20085]
Hospice of Laramie [21879]
Hospice of Las Vegas [20417]
Hospice of Laurens County [19382]
Hospice of Laurens County Inc. [21216]
Hospice of Lenawee [20022]
Hospice of Licking County, Inc./Hospice of Central Ohio [20876]
Hospice Life Care [19968]
Hospice of Light [20235]
Hospice of Lincoln County [20696]
Hospice of Little Traverse Bay [20104]
Hospice of Louisville--Main Street [19829]
Hospice of Louisville • Norton Healthcare Pavilion Inpatient [19813]
Hospice of Lubbock [21521]
Hospice of the Madlyn & Leonard Abramson Center for Jewish Life [21123]
Hospice of Marion County [19273]
Hospice of Marshall County [18670]
Hospice of Martha's Vineyard [19992]
Hospice Maui [19446]
Hospice of McAlester [20940]
Hospice of McDowell County Inc. [20702]
Hospice of Medina County [20866]
Hospice of Memorial Hospital [20825]
Hospice of Metropolitan Erie [21085]
Hospice of Miami County, Inc. [20902]
Hospice of the Miami Valley [20913]
Hospice of Michigan Alpena [20026]
Hospice of Michigan Big Rapids [20038]
Hospice of Michigan Detroit [20052]
Hospice of Michigan-Grand Rapids [20021]
Hospice of Michigan-Saginaw [20110]
Hospice of Michigan-Southfield [20122]
Hospice of Midland Inc. [21531]
Hospice of Missoula [20367]
Hospice of Monroe County-Albia [19661]
Hospice of Montezuma [19096]
Hospice of Montgomery [18745]
The Hospice of Moorestown VNA [20481]
Hospice of Morongo Basin [18946]
Hospice of Morrow County, Inc. [20871]
Hospice of Muskegon-Oceana/dba Harbor Hospice • The Leila and Cyrus Poppen Hospice Residence [20099]
Hospice of Napa Valley and Adult Day Services [18978]
Hospice of Nashoba Nursing Service [19999]
Hospice of Nelson County • Flaget Memorial Hospital [19791]
Hospice of New Jersey--Bloomfield [20459]
Hospice of New Jersey--Toms River [20504]
Hospice of North Alabama, LLC [18728]
Hospice of North Central Ohio, Inc.--Ashland [20800]
Hospice of North Central Ohio, Inc.--Mansfield [20858]
Hospice of North Central Oklahoma, Inc. [20969]
Hospice of the North Coast [18899]
Hospice of the North Country [20596]
Hospice of North Idaho [19462]
Hospice of North Iowa [19712]
Hospice of North Ottawa Community [20127]
Hospice of the North Shore [19954]
Hospice of Northeast Georgia Medical Center [19389]
Hospice of Northeast Kansas-Multi-County [19755]
Hospice of Northeast Missouri [20315]
Hospice of Northeastern Connecticut • Day Kimball Home Care and Hospital [19160]
Hospice of Northeastern Illinois [19485]
Hospice of the Northern Hills • Spearfish Regional Hospital [21305]
Hospice of Northern Kentucky [19800]
Hospice of the Northwest [21761]

Hospice of Northwest Alabama Inc. [18774]
Hospice of Northwest Connecticut--Hospital Hill Road • Sharon Healthcare Center [19162]
Hospice of Northwest Connecticut--Law Road • Sharon Health Care Center [19163]
Hospice of Northwest Iowa [19734]
Hospice of Northwest Michigan [20045]
Hospice of Northwest Ohio-Lambertville [20081]
Hospice of Northwest Ohio--Perrysburg [20883]
Hospice of Northwest Ohio--Toledo [20900]
Hospice of Nursing Placement, Inc. [21194]
Hospice of Ochiltree General Hospital [21545]
Hospice of Ohio County [19804]
Hospice of Okeechobee [19277]
Hospice of Oklahoma County [20959]
Hospice of Olathe Medical Center [19765]
Hospice of Orange & Sullivan Counties, Inc.--Middletown [20579]
Hospice of Orange & Sullivan Counties, Inc.--Newburgh [20589]
Hospice of Orleans, Inc. [20551]
Hospice Outreach [19961]
Hospice of the Owens Valley [18895]
Hospice of the Ozarks [18870]
Hospice & Palliative Care of Cabarrus County [20686]
Hospice & Palliative Care of Cape Cod, Inc. [19969]
Hospice and Palliative Care Center [20770]
Hospice & Palliative Care Center of Alamance Caswell [20629]
Hospice and Palliative Care Center of Mitchell County [20740]
Hospice and Palliative Care - Cleveland County [20733]
Hospice and Palliative Care of the Eastern Shore [21713]
Hospice and Palliative Care of Greater Wayne County [20912]
Hospice & Palliative Care of Greensboro [20673]
Hospice and Palliative Care Group, Inc. • Niagara Hospice [20575]
Hospice and Palliative Care of the Gunnison Valley [19112]
Hospice and Palliative Care, Inc.--New Hartford [20583]
Hospice and Palliative Care of Iredell County [20707]
Hospice and Palliative Care of Northern Colorado. Inc. [19110]
Hospice and Palliative Care Program of VNA of Central Connecticut, Inc. [19159]
Hospice and Palliative Care of Saint Lawrence Valley, Inc. [20598]
Hospice & Palliative Care of Visiting Nurse Service [20796]
Hospice and Palliative Care of Westchester [20617]
Hospice and Palliative Care of Western Colorado [19091], [19097], [19108], [19122]
Hospice & Palliative CareCenter of Davie County [20704]
Hospice & Palliative CareCenter of Rowan County [20728]
Hospice & Palliative CareCenter of Stokes County [20759]
Hospice of Palm Beach County--Boynton Beach • Bethesda Memorial Hospice and Palliative Care Center [19199]
Hospice of Palm Beach County, Inc-Palm Beach Gardens Medical Center [19286]
Hospice of Palm Beach County, Inc.--West Palm Beach [19333]
Hospice of the Palm Coast [19215]
Hospice of Palo Alto County [19691]
Hospice of Pamlico County [20623]
Hospice of the Panhandle [21805]
Hospice of the Panhandle-Morgan County [21787]
Hospice Partners of the Central Coast [19032]
Hospice Partners of Southern California [19043]
Hospice Peachtree/dba Peachtree Hospice, LLC - Arkansas [18881]
Hospice Peachtree/dba Peachtree Hospice LLC--Rogers Ave., Fort Smith [18850]
Hospice Peachtree/dba Peachtree Hospice LLC--Towson Ave., Fort Smith • Palliative Care Unit [18851]
Hospice of Pella-Comfort House [19725]
Hospice of Petaluma [18992]
Hospice of the Piedmont--Charlottesville [21679]

Hospice of the Piedmont--High Point [20679]
Hospice in the Pines [21527]
Hospice of the Pines [18788]
Hospice of the Plains Inc. - Sterling Office [19129]
Hospice of the Plains, Inc. - Wray Office [19136]
Hospice Plus [21433]
Hospice of the Prairie Inc. [19749]
Hospice of Presbyterian [18950]
Hospice Program of VNA Health at Home Inc. [19173]
Hospice of Queen Anne's, Inc. [19919]
Hospice of Randolph County [20620]
Hospice of the Rapidan [21686]
Hospice of the Red River • Valley/Detroit Lakes [20155]
Hospice of the Red River Valley--Fargo [20780]
Hospice of the Red River Valley - Grand Forks [20783]
Hospice of the Red River Valley/Lisbon [20786]
Hospice of the Red/River Valley/Mayville Ofc. [20788]
Hospice of the Red River Valley/Valley City [20793]
Hospice of Redmond, Sisters, and Grant County [21028]
Hospice of Reno County, Inc. [19757]
Hospice/Respite Care of Hamilton County [19741]
Hospice of the Rock River Valley [19513]
Hospice of Rockingham County, Inc. [20761]
Hospice of Rutherford County [20664]
Hospice of Sacred Heart [20998]
Hospice of the Sacred Heart [21172]
Hospice of Saddleback Valley [18952]
Hospice of Saint Francis, Inc. [19327]
Hospice of Saint John Foundation, Inc. [19116]
Hospice of Saint John-Inverness Drive [19103]
Hospice of Saint Peter's Hospital [20362]
Hospice of Saint Tammany [19854]
Hospice of Salina, Inc. [19776]
Hospice of Salmon Valley [19478]
Hospice of San Angelo, Inc. [21548]
Hospice of San Joaquin [19056]
Hospice of the Sandias, LLC [20520]
Hospice of the Sandias, LLC-Clovis [20532]
Hospice of Sanford Hospital Luverne [20177]
Hospice of Santa Barbara Inc. [19035]
Hospice of Santa Cruz County [19046]
Hospice Savannah, Inc. [19415]
Hospice of Scotland County [20690]
Hospice by the Sea--Solona Beach [19050]
Hospice Services of Alabama [18685]
Hospice Services, Inc. [19772]
Hospice Services of Lake County [18954]
Hospice Services of Massachusetts [19957], [20008]
Hospice Services of Southwest General [20895]
Hospice of the Shoals [18712]
Hospice of Shreveport/Bossier [19877]
Hospice of Siouxland [19733]
Hospice of Siouxland Nebraska [20402]
Hospice of Siouxland North [19707]
Hospice SMDC & Palliative • Care-East Range Team [20212]
Hospice of South Carolina-Saluda [21276]
Hospice of South Central Indiana-Decatur [19603]
Hospice of South Central Indiana, Inc.--Columbus [19589]
Hospice of South Central Indiana-Shelby County [19650]
Hospice of South Georgia, Inc.--Baxley [19364]
Hospice of South Georgia, Inc.--Jesup [19394]
Hospice of South Georgia--Valdosta [19428]
Hospice of the South Plains [21522]
Hospice of South Texas, Hallettsville [21478]
Hospice of South Texas--Victoria [21585]
Hospice of Southeastern Connecticut [19156]
Hospice of Southeastern Illinois [19550]
Hospice of Southern Illinois Inc.--Belleville [19487]
Hospice of Southern Illinois Inc.--Marion [19541]
Hospice of Southern Indiana [19638]
Hospice of Southern Maine [19903]
Hospice of Southern Ohio [20886]
Hospice of Southwest [21778]
Hospice of the Southwest [18799]
Hospice of Southwest Georgia--Bainbridge [19363]
Hospice of Southwest Georgia--Thomasville [19425]
Hospice of Southwest Montana [20353]
Hospice of Southwest Ohio [20814]
Hospice of Southwest Oklahoma [20938]
Hospice of Southwest Virginia--Abingdon • Wythe

County Community Hospital [21670]
Hospice of Southwest Virginia--Wytheville [21746]
Hospice of Spokane [21771]
Hospice of Stanly County [20619]
Hospice of Stark County [20809]
Hospice of the Straits [20046]
Hospice of Sturgis [20128]
Hospice of Summa [20797]
Hospice of the Sunrise Shore [20027]
Hospice Support Services of Washington County [21671]
Hospice of Sweetwater County [21881]
Hospice of Tabitha [20390]
Hospice of the Tanana Valley [18778]
Hospice of Texarkana, Inc. [21575]
Hospice of Texas [21398]
Hospice of The Gorge-The Dalles Office [21035]
Hospice of Tift Area [19426]
Hospice Touch Tomah Memorial Hospital [21836]
The Hospice Touch Tomah Memorial Hospital [21869]
Hospice Touch Tomah Memorial Hospital-Mauston [21853]
Hospice of Tuscarawas County, Inc. [20838]
Hospice of Twin Cities [20192]
Hospice of Union County--Monroe [20706]
Hospice of Union County--Wadesboro [20756]
Hospice of the Upstate [21204]
Hospice del Valle [19084]
Hospice of the Valley-Basalt [19087]
Hospice of the Valley--Decatur [18701]
Hospice of the Valley Hospice House--Poland [20884]
Hospice of the Valley--San Jose [19029]
Hospice of the Valley--Youngstown [20914]
Hospice of the Valleys--Murrieta [18976]
Hospice Visions [19480]
Hospice Visions Hospice Home [19466]
Hospice of the Visiting Nurse • Association of Southeast • Michigan [20101]
Hospice at Visiting Nurse Service of Newport Bristol County [21192], [21195]
Hospice of the VNA of Greater Philadelphia [21130]
Hospice Volunteers of Waldo County [19887]
Hospice Volunteers of Waterville Area [19907]
Hospice of Volusia/Flager [19287]
Hospice of Volusia/Flagler [19283], [19303]
Hospice of the Wabash Valley [19654]
Hospice of Wake County [20720]
Hospice of Wapello [19724]
Hospice of Warren County [21167]
Hospice of Washington County--Hillsboro [21005]
Hospice of Washington County Inc.--Hagerstown [19927]
Hospice of Washington County--Washington [19738]
Hospice of West Alabama [18770]
Hospice of the West LLC [18811]
Hospice of West Tennessee [21339]
Hospice of Western Kentucky [19824]
Hospice of the Western Reserve-Cleveland Office [20821]
Hospice of the Western Reserve, Inc-Lorain [20856]
Hospice of the Western Reserve Inc. Hospice House--Cleveland [20822]
Hospice of the Western Reserve, Inc.--Mentor [20867]
Hospice of the Western Reserve, Inc. - University Circle Office [20823]
Hospice of the Western Reserve, Inc.--Warrensville Heights [20904]
Hospice of the Western Reserve Inc.--Westlake [20909]
Hospice of the Western Reserve-Lakewood [20851]
Hospice of Westmoreland [21099]
Hospice of Wichita Falls Inc. [21592]
Hospice of the Wood River Valley [19467]
Hospice for Wright County [19676]
Hospice of Wyandot County [20903]
Hospice of Yancey County [20631]
Hospice of Yuma [18837]
HospiceCare in the Berkshires, Inc. [19995]
HospiceCare of Boulder and Broomfield Counties-Longmont [19118]
HospiceCare Inc. [21842], [21849]
HospiceCare of the Piedmont, Inc. [21248]
HospiceCare of Southeast Florida, Inc. [19324]
Hospicio La Guadalupe Inc. [21188]
Hospicio La Paz Inc. [21185]

Hospicio San Judas [21189]
Hospital Center at Orange [2939]
Hospital of Central Connecticut at New Britain [1474]
Hospital of Central Connecticut-New Britain Campus • George Bray Cancer Center [4900]
Hospital of Central Connecticut • Sleep Disorders Center [23166], [36746]
Hospital for Children • University of Maryland • Department of Medical Genetics [10807]
Hospital Damas, Inc. [17528]
Hospital Doctor Pila [17529]
Hospital Home Health and Hospice [21331]
Hospital for Joint Diseases Orthopedics Institute • Language Pathology Division [3060]
Hospital of Saint Raphael
    Down Syndrome Adult Assessment Clinic [10784]
    Father McGivney Cancer Center [4901]
Hospital for Sick Children [7873]
    Burn Unit [4615]
    Eating Disorders Program [11221]
    Sickle Cell Disease Center [36416]
    Tissue and Stem Cell Laboratory [35177]
Hospital for Special Care [3944]
    MDA/ALS Clinic [106]
    MDA Clinic [34773]
Hospital for Special Surgery
    Department of Biomechanics & Biomaterials • Musculoskeletal Disorders Core Center [171]
    Sports Rehabilitation and Performance Center [38794]
Hospital of the University of Pennsylvania
    Division of Medical Genetics [12325]
    MDA Clinic [34866]
    Reproductive Endocrinology and Infertility • In Vitro Fertilization Program [22231]
    Speech and Hearing Center [3360]
Hospital of the University of Pennsylvania Transplant Unit [26531]
Hospitality House • Therapeutic Community Inc [46335]
Hospitality House for Women, Inc. [9121]
Hot Springs County Counseling Center [33071]
    Common Ground [33072]
Hot Springs County Counseling Service [50605]
Hot Springs Diagnostic Associates • Arkansas Nephrology Services, Ltd. [22545]
Hot Springs Rehabilitation Center [7758]
Hot Springs Sports Medicine [38060]
Hotel Dieu Hospital • Eating Disorder Program for Adults [11222]
Hotline/Family Centers [50727]
Hotline--Fargo [51188]
Hotline Help Center [50666]
Hotline and Referral/Project Help, Inc. [50777]
HOTLINE--Salina • Crisis, Information, and Referral Program [50923]
Hotline of San Luis Obispo [50696]
Hotline of Southern California [50676]
Houma Veterans Affairs Community Based Outpatient Clinic [30141]
House of Acts
    Substance Abuse Prog/House of Acts II [40880]
    Substance Abuse Program [40881]
House Call Providers [21021]
House of Charity • Day By Day Program [45217]
House Ear Clinic • CARE Center [1164]
House of Freedom Inc [41719]
House of Good Shepherd [9207]
House of Hope for Alcoholics Inc [47718]
    Outpatient [47719]
House of Hope--Douglas [8685]
House of Hope Foundation [40696]
House of Hope Inc [45193], [45194], [47938]
    Residential/1st Street [41655]
    Stepping Stones Residential [41656]
House of Hope, Inc.--Lexington [9696]
House of Hope--Jacksboro [10404]
House of Hope of Madison County Inc [42980]
House of Hope Provo [49662], [49677]
House of Imagene [9028]
House of Mercy [9906], [43264]
House of Metamorphosis Inc • Residential [40557]
House of Refuge for Abused and Battered Women [9728]
House of Ruth [29090]
House of Ruth--Dothan [8640]

House of Ruth, Inc.--Baltimore [9444]
House of Ruth, Inc.--Claremont [8804]
House of Ruth Madison Program [29091]
House of Ruth • Madison Program [33280]
House of Ruth Mothers' Program [29092]
House of Ruth • Mother's Program [33281]
House of Ruth Transitional/Unity [29093]
House of Ruth • Transitional/Unity [33282]
House of Ruth--Washington [9029]
House of Ruth • Washington DC [33283]
The House of The Good Shepherd--New Hartford [34343]
The House of The Good Shepherd--Utica [34360]
HouseCall Home Healthcare--Bartlett [17644]
Housecall Home Healthcare--Elizabethton [17666]
Housecall Home Healthcare--Jackson [17683]
Housecall Home Healthcare--Knoxville [17706]
Housecall Home Healthcare--Morristown [17742]
Housecall Home Healthcare--Salem [18382]
Housecalls Home Health--Hartsville [18515]
Housecalls Home Health--Parkersburg [18533]
Housecalls for the Homebound [18597]
Houser Street Care Facility [29887]
Houses of Hope of Nebraska Inc [45756]
Housing Works Inc • Chemical Dependence Outpatient Service [46504]
Houston Area Women's Center [10474]
Houston County Board of Education [377]
Houston County Clinic and Daycare Treatment [27898]
Houston Dialysis • DaVita [27147]
Houston Fertility Institute [22260]
Houston Group Home [28346]
Houston Headache Clinic [12469]
Houston Home Dialysis [27148]
Houston Independent School District • Deaf and Vision Program [793]
Houston Infertility Clinic [22261]
Houston IVF [22262]
Houston Kidney Center--Cypress • Dialysis Facility • DaVita [27149]
Houston Kidney Center Southwest • DaVita [27150]
Houston Launch Pad [49375]
Houston--Love Memorial Library • Department for the Blind and Physically Handicapped [3747]
Houston Maintenance Clinic Inc [49376]
Houston Northwest Medical Center • Cancer Program [5993]
Houston Recovery Campus • Adolescent Program [49377]
Houston Sleep Center • Sleep Disorders Center [37817]
Houston Sleep Disorders Center, Katy [37818]
Houston Solari Hospice Care [21402]
Houston Street Dialysis and PD • US Renal Care [27328]
Houston Substance Abuse Clinic [49378], [49478]
Houston Treatment Center [39282]
Houston Treatment Center Inc [49379]
HOUT of Saint Lawrence County [9977]
Howard A. Rusk Rehabilitation Center [4234]
Howard Center [32681]
    Act One/Bridge Program [49731]
    Chittenden Clinic [49732]
Howard Center for Human Services--Burlington [32648]
Howard Center for Human Services
    Group Home [32654]
    Howard Community Services [32649]
    Pine Street Counseling Center [32650]
    Westview House [32651]
Howard Center
    Pine Street Counseling Services [49733]
    Substance Abuse Treatment Services [49743]
Howard Community Health Center [7246]
Howard Community Hospital [2168]
Howard County Community Hospice [19679]
Howard County General Hospital [2408]
    Cancer Program [5298]
Howard County Halfway House [44256]
Howard County Health Department • Bureau of Substance Abuse Services [44227]
Howard County Home Health and Hospice [20296]
Howard County Mental Health Center [32413]
Howard County Physical Therapy and Sports Rehabilitation [38525]
Howard Regional Health System [15015]
Howard Regional Hospital • Cancer Program [5161]

Howard University
College of Medicine • Department of Pediatrics and Child Health [12179]
Comprehensive Sickle Cell Center [36316]
Department of Communicative Sciences & Disorders [1527]
Howard University Hospital
Cancer Center [4921]
Drug Abuse Institute [41539]
Renal Dialysis Unit [23225]
Howard Young Medical Center • Dialysis Center [27808]
Howell Center Bear Creek [8384]
Hoy Recovery Program Inc [46245], [46261]
Hoyleton Youth and Family Services/Children First • Runaway and Homeless Youth Program [35929]
Hoyos Home Health Care [14035]
HPH Hospice Care Center • North Pasco Office [19233]
HPH Hospice - Central West Pasco [19268]
HPH Hospice - Citrus Office [19197]
HPH Hospice
East Pasco Office [19214]
West Hernando Office [19203]
HRC Mental Health Center [33015]
HRDC District 7 • Runaway and Homeless Youth Program [36061]
HSA Behavioral Health [32260]
Sisseton Outpatient Mental Health [32256]
HSA Counseling Inc [48356], [48427]
HSA Greenbrier Hospital [33535]
HSC Medical Center • Behavioral Health Services [28314]
Hualapai Health Department • Alcoholism and Drug Abuse Program [39415]
Hub City Services LLC [43581]
Hubbard Hospice House [21793]
Hubbard House [9057]
Huber and Associates Counseling Center [44148]
Hubs Home Oxygen & Medical Supplies [17510]
Huckleberry House, Inc. [31730]
Huckleberry House • Runaway and Homeless Youth Program [36145]
Huckleberry Youth Programs • Huckleberry House and Nine Grove • Runaway and Homeless Youth Program [35824]
Hudson Hospice House [19234]
Hudson Hospice Volunteers, Inc. [20475]
Hudson Hospital and Clinics • Programs For Change [50414]
Hudson House [32760]
Hudson Mohawk Recovery Center • Elizabeth House-Womens Comm Resident [47133]
Hudson Mohawk Recovery Center Inc
Chemical Dependency Outpatient Clinic [47134]
Intensive Outpatient Alcohol Rehab Program [47135]
Outpatient Alcoholism Clinic [46611]
Hudson Mohawk Supportive Living [47136]
Hudson River Healthcare, Inc. • Peekskill Community Health Center [7035]
Hudson River Housing, Inc. • Runaway and Homeless Youth Program [36111]
Hudson River Psychiatric Center [33716]
Hudson Valley Developmental Disabilities Service Office [8359]
Hudson Valley Home Care [16601]
Hudson Valley Hospital Center • Methadone Maintenance Treatment Prog [46605]
Hudson Valley Orthopedics and Sports Medicine, PC [38813]
Hudson Valley Rehabilitative and Extended Care Center [16489]
Hudspeth Mental Retardation Center [8193]
Hueytown Elementary [912]
Hugh E. Sandefur Training Center [8046]
The Hughen Center [8562]
Hughston Clinic [38332]
Hughston Clinic, PC [38314]
HUGS Recovery Center • Humanity United with God for Society [42092]
Huguley Home Health Agency [17836]
Huguley Memorial Medical Center [17925]
Huguley Psychotherapy Clinic • Addiction Center [49265]
Hui Ho ola O Na Nahulu O Hawaii [42260]
Huiras Center [50465]
Hull Institute [11195]

Humacao Dialysis Center • Fresenius Medical Care [26635]
Human Development Center [7755]
Human Development Center--Cloquet [30671]
Human Development Center--Duluth [30674]
Human Development Center--Grand Marais [30680]
Human Development Center Jonesboro [7759]
Human Development Center--Two Harbors [30730]
Human Development and Research Services [39567]
Pine Bluff Outpatient Office [39568]
Human Dynamics and Diagnostics LLC [42337]
Human Energy Research Laboratory • University of Pittsburgh [38972]
Human Options, Inc. [8822]
Human Performance Center
Saint Alexius Medical Center [38840]
Santa Barbara [38138]
Human Resources Administration • Office of Domestic Violence [9951]
Human Resources Center [50864]
Human Resources Center of • Edgar and Clark Counties [42765], [42849]
Human Resources Development Council, District IX • Runaway and Homeless Youth Program [36062]
Human Resources Development Institute
BRAS II/ [42527]
Brass I/Outpatient Opioid Treatment [42528]
SW Opioid Treatment Program [42529]
Womens Program [42530]
Human Resources Inc
Outpatient Methadone Program [49826]
Willow Oaks [49769]
Human Response Network [10612], [51431]
Human Response Network/Family Crisis Line [8926]
Human Service Agency [49031]
Human Service Agency--Milbank [32233]
Human Service Center [42856]
Human Service Center on Hamilton Blvd [42857]
Human Service Center--Peoria [29661]
Day Treatment Program [29662]
Outpatient Services [29663]
Women at the Crossroads [29664]
Human Service Center on Richard Pryor Place [42858]
Human Service Center/Rochelle [42859]
Human Service Center of South Metro East [29670]
Human Service Center on Willow Knolls Road [42860]
Human Services and • Resources and Associates Inc [41586], [41868]
Human Services Associates Inc
Addictions Receiving Facility [41861]
Adult and Youth Outpatient [41862]
Human Services Center--New Castle [32054]
Human Services Center--Waukesha [33019]
Human Services Inc [45724]
Detoxification Center [45811]
Human Services, Inc.--Downington [32011]
Human Services, Inc.--Stillwater [30729]
Human Services, Inc.--West Chester [32129]
Human Services, Inc. • West Chester Office and Crisis Services [32130]
Human Skills and Resources Inc [47920], [48015], [48039]
Human Support Services [29684]
Substance Abuse Alternatives [42943]
Human Touch Home Health Care Agency--Allentown [17232]
Human Touch Home Health Care Agency, Inc.--Christiansburg [18273]
Human Touch Home Health Care Agency, Inc.--Washington DC [13573]
Human Touch Home Health Care--Falls Church [18292]
Humana Hospital Southwest • Speech-Language Pathology [2281]
Humana Hospital Suburban [2282]
HUMANIM Inc. [4096]
Humanity Home Care Services [14036]
Humanity Home Health Care, Inc. [14037]
Humanly Home Health Care Agency [14038]
Humble RDSPD [800]
Humboldt Addictions Services Progs [39768]
Humboldt County Alcohol and Other Drug • Children Youth and Family Services [39821]
Humboldt County Mental Health • Alcohol and Other Drug Programs [39822]

Humboldt County Mental Health Services [28491]
Children, Youth and Family Services [28492]
Outpatient Clinic [28510]
Humboldt Dialysis • DaVita • Dialysis Facility [26847]
Humboldt Family Service Center [28380]
Humboldt Recovery Center Inc [39823]
Mens Counseling Center [39824]
Humboldt Volunteer Hospice [20430]
Humboldt Women for Shelter [8811]
Hume-Lee Transplant Center • VCU Medical Center [27552]
Humility of Mary Health Partners • Cancer Program [5767]
Hunt Regional Home Care [17938]
Hunt Street House [32141]
Hunter Health Center [43491]
Hunter Health Clinic, Inc. [6723]
Hunter Holmes Maguire Veterans Affairs Medical Center • PTSD Clinical Team [51837]
Hunter Holmes McGuire Richmond VA Medical Center • Spinal Care Center [4473]
Hunter Holmes McGuire • Veterans Affairs Hospice Unit [21725]
Hunter Holmes McGuire Veterans Affairs Medical Center [32779]
Cancer Program [6082]
Hunter Medical Services, Inc. [17899]
Hunterdon Developmental Center [8245]
Hunterdon Drug Awareness Program [45990]
Hunterdon Helpline [51090]
Hunterdon Hospice [20473]
Hunterdon Med Center/Addictions Treatment Services • Hunterdon Behavioral Health [45991]
Hunterdon Medical Center • Child Development Center • Special Child Health Services Case Management [8249]
Hunterdon Medical Center Home Health Services [16216]
Hunterdon Medical Center
Regional Cancer Program [5513]
Speech and Hearing Department [2913]
Hunterdon Medical Sleep Disorders Center [37348]
Hunterdon Prevention Resources [45992]
Huntingdon Family Practice [7167]
Huntingdon Valley Dialysis • DaVita [26450]
Huntington Artificial Kidney Center • DaVita [25685]
Huntington Beach Dialysis • DaVita [22726]
Huntington Beach Partial Hospitalization Program [28535]
Huntington Beach Youth Shelter [28536]
Huntington Dialysis Center • Hemodialysis Inc. [22877]
Huntington Hearing and Speech Center [3032]
Huntington Hospital
Cancer Program [5582]
Dialysis Unit [25684]
Huntington Memorial Hospital
Cancer Program [4820]
Pediatrics Unit [7805]
Huntington Reproductive Center--Fullerton [21915]
Huntington Reproductive Center--Laguna Hills [21916]
Huntington Reproductive Center--Pasadena [21917]
Huntington Reproductive Center--Tarzana [21918]
Huntington Reproductive Center--West Los Angeles [21919]
Huntington Reproductive Center--Westlake Village [21920]
Huntington Treatment Center [50307]
Huntington Youth Bureau • Huntington Drug and Alcohol Project [46706]
Huntington Youth Bureau Sanctuary • Runaway and Homeless Youth Program [36112]
Hunts Point Multi Service Center Inc • Chemical Dependency Program [46420]
Hunts Point Multi Service Prog Center Inc • Methadone Maintenance Program [46421]
Huntsville Achievement School [7716]
Huntsville Adult and Adolescent • Bradford Health Services [27973]
Huntsville City Schools H.I. Program [197]
Huntsville Clinic Inc [49424]
Huntsville Dialysis • DaVita [27190]
Huntsville Hospital • Comprehensive Cancer Institute [4734]
Huntsville Hospital East • Tennessee Valley Pain Consultants • Center for Pain Management and

Rehabilitation [35273]
Huntsville Hospital
 Huntsville Sleep Center [36585]
 Madison Sleep Center [36586]
 MDA Clinic [34749]
Huntsville Madison County Mental Health Center •
 New Horizons Recovery Center [39261]
Huntsville Memorial Hospital [18016]
Huntsville Metro Treatment Center [39262]
Huntsville Primary Care Center [7258]
Huntsville Recovery Inc [39263]
Huntsville Reproductive Medicine, PC [21886]
Huntsville Subregional Library for the Blind and
 Physically Handicapped [3748]
Hurley Drug Home Health [18552]
Hurley House • Recovery Home [44594]
Hurley Medical Center
 Burn Unit [4567]
 Center for Reproductive Medicine [22119]
 Max E. Dodds Cancer Center [5375]
 Pediatric Sickle Cell Clinic [36363]
 Physical Medicine and Rehabilitation Services
  [4170]
 Sleep Diagnostics Center [37164]
Hurlock Medical Center [6797]
Huron Behavioral Health [30507]
Huron Behavioral Health Services [44650]
Huron County Victim Assistance Program [10164]
Huron Hospital • Cancer Program [5718]
Huron Regional Medical Center [3412]
 Dialysis Facility [26789]
 Home Care Agency [21292]
Hurricane Dialysis Center • University Health Care
 [27404]
Huss Recovery--People Incorporated [30699]
Hutcheson Hospice [19388]
Hutcheson Medical Center, Inc. [14530]
Hutchings Psychiatric Center [31477]
 Children and Youth Services [33726]
 Outpatient Services [33727]
Hutchinson Area Healthcare [45178]
Hutchinson Clinic Renal Dialysis Center [24322]
Hutchinson County Crisis Center [10446]
Hutchinson Medical, Inc. [15538]
Hutchinson Speech and Language Services [2221]
Hutchinson Veterans Affairs Community Based
 Outpatient Clinic [29932]
Huther Doyle [47038]
 Esperanza Latina [47039]
 Memorial Institute Inc [47040]
Hutzel Hospital • Department of Obstetrics and
 Gynecology • Division of Reproductive Genetics
 [12249]
Hyattsville Speech and Language Center [2399]
Hyde Park Counseling Center [11023], [41966]
Hyde Park Dialysis Center • Fresenius Medical Care
 [24771]
Hyde Park Headache Center [12404]
Hye Quality Home Health [13349]
Hygieia Home Health, Inc. [12896]
Hyndman Area Health Center [7168]

I

I-ADARP [40895]
I Am New Life Ministries [39920]
I Believe In Me Ranch Inc. [34284]
I Care Home Health Providers, LLC [14930]
I and Y Senior Care [16393]
IA Lutheran Hospital • Powell Chemical Dependency
 Center [43265]
IAA Project Special Delivery [39328]
Iberia Comprehensive Community Health Center,
 Inc. [6755]
Iberia Medical Center Home Health Agancy [15340]
IC Quality Health Corp. [14039]
ICAN Community Services Inc NFP [42912]
ICAN of Washington Inc. [2392]
ICD/International Center for the Disabled • Addiction
 Recovery Services [46876]
Icon Home Health Services [14040]
ICP, Inc. [17051]
ICS Speech--Language Services LLC [2092]
Idaho Center for Reproductive Medicine [22030]
Idaho Division of Health • Bureau of Clinical and
 Preventive Services [36471]
Idaho Elks Rehabilitation Hospital [4013]
 MDA Clinic [34789]

Idaho Falls School District Number Ninety-One [390]
Idaho Falls Sleep Institute [36877]
Idaho Home Health and Hospice, Inc.--Buhl [14652]
Idaho Home Health and Hospice, Inc.--Gooding
 [14658]
Idaho Home Health and Hospice, Inc.--Hailey
 [14659]
Idaho Home Health and Hospice, Inc.--Idaho Falls
 [14661]
Idaho Home Health and Hospice, Inc.--Meridian
 [14664]
Idaho Home Health and Hospice, Inc.--Pocatello
 [14668]
Idaho Home Health and Hospice, Inc.--Rigby
 [14670]
Idaho Home Health and Hospice, Inc.--Rupert
 [14671]
Idaho Home Health and Hospice, Inc.--Twin Falls
 [14675]
Idaho Kidney Center--Blackfoot • Liberty Dialysis
 [23867]
Idaho Kidney Center - Pocatello • Liberty Dialysis
 [23884]
Idaho Lions Eye Bank [35019]
Idaho Panhandle Dialysis • Fresenius Medical Care
 [23885]
Idaho Physical Therapy--Caldwell [38339]
Idaho Physical Therapy--Nampa [38343]
Idaho Regional Hemophilia Center • Saint Luke's
 Regional Medical Center • Mountain States Tumor
 Institute • Pediatric/Hematology Department
 [12514]
Idaho School for the Blind [3705]
Idaho School for the Deaf and the Blind [389]
Idaho Sleep Health • Sleep Disorders Center
 [36878], [36879]
Idaho Sports Medicine Institute [38338]
Idaho State Hospital South [29538]
Idaho State School and Hospital [7924]
Idaho State University • Speech and Hearing Center
 [1951]
Idaho Suicide Prevention Hotline Service [50818]
Idaho Youth Ranch [33403]
 Anchor House [42330]
Idaho Youth Ranch Emancipation Home [33397]
Idaho Youth Ranch--Main Campus [34094]
Idaho Youth Ranch • Runaway and Homeless Youth
 Program [35921]
Idant Laboratories [35132]
Idarola and Associates [1800]
Idea Home Health Care, Inc. [14444]
Ideal Care and Health Services Inc [40403]
Ideal Care Home Health, Inc.--Aurora [14684]
Ideal Care Home Health Inc.--Chatsworth [12940]
Ideal Health Care, LLC [16237]
Ideal Home Health [14041]
Ideas Directed at Eliminating Abuse [8953], [41000],
 [41024], [41131]
 Sago Center [41328]
IDS Group Inc [42400], [42894]
IDS Group Inc/Chicago [42531]
IFA Universal Health Care [14325]
IGO Medical Group of San Diego • In Vitro Fertiliza-
 tion Program [21921]
IHC Home Care [18224]
IHC Home Care of Cedar City [18193]
IHC Home Care of Delta [18196]
IHC Home Care of Fillmore [18197]
IHC Home Care of Heber City [18198]
IHC Home Care of Logan [18203]
IHC Home Care of Mount Pleasant [18206]
IHC Home Care of Ogden [18207]
IHC Home Care of Orem [18210]
IHC Home Care of Richfield [18213]
IHC Home Medical Equipment, Home Health &
 Hospice [18215]
IHC Hospice [21632]
IHC Hospice and Home Care [14654]
IHC Hospice--Richfield [21634]
IHC Hospice--Salt Lake City [21648]
IHS Acquisitions XXX, Inc. [17480]
IJEGBA Community Inc [42532]
IKRON Corporation [47661]
IL Alcohol and Drug Evaluation Services [42861]
IL Institute for Addiction Recovery [42917]
 at Advocate BroMenn Medical Center [42811]
 at Ingalls Memorial Hospital [42698]
 at Proctor Hospital [42862]

Illini Renal Dialysis & At Home • Davita [23912]
Illinois Bone and Joint Institute • Sports Medicine
 [38363]
Illinois Department of Public Health
 Family Health [36473]
 Illinois Statewide SIDS/Infant Mortality Program
  [36474]
Illinois Drug and Alcohol Services • IDDACS Inc
 [42863]
Illinois Eye-Bank, Chicago [35025]
Illinois Eye-Bank, Watson Gailey [35026]
Illinois/Iowa Center for Independent Living [2102]
Illinois Neurological Institute • Sleep Center [36908]
Illinois Planned Parenthood Council • Springfield
 Health Center--Family Planning and Abortion
 Services [11524]
Illinois School for the Deaf [402]
Illinois School for the Visually Impaired [3707]
Illinois Service Resource Center [2086]
 Centerview Therapeutic School [2087]
Illinois Sportsmedicine and Orthopaedic Centers
 [38378]
Illinois State Library • Talking Book and Braille
 Service [3786]
Illinois State University--Student Counseling Services
 [50861]
Illinois Valley Hospice [19563]
Illinois Valley Safe House Alliance [10225]
Illiuliuk Family and Health Service [6218]
Image Hospice • Faith Hospice Services [20925]
Imagine Programs LLC [49489]
Imani House - Substance Abuse [30860]
Immaculate Care Center Inc [40243]
Immanuel Home Care Services [14737]
Immanuel Saint Joseph's Hospital [2703]
Immanuel-Saint Joseph's Hospital • Dialysis Unit
 [25035]
Immanuel-Saint Joseph's Hospital--New Ulm •
 Dialysis Center [25058]
Immanuel Saint Joseph's - Mayo Health System
 [15911]
Immanuel Saint Josephs/Mayo Health System •
 Sleep Disorders Center [37221]
Immediate Homecare and Hospice [21051]
Immediate HomeCare, Inc. [17254]
Impac Rehabilitation Inc. [2327]
IMPACT [44564]
Impact [40371], [51324]
IMPACT Center for Independent Living [1953]
IMPACT Counseling Services • Medically
 Supervised Outpatient [46744]
IMPACT • National Sudden & Unexpected Infant/
 Child Death • Tomorrow's Child • Michigan SIDS
 [36492]
Impact Rehabilitation and Wellness [38296]
Imperial Beach Health Center [6307]
Imperial County Behavioral Hlth Services
 Adolescent Programs [39800]
 Adult Outpatient Alcohol and Drug [39801]
Imperial County Mental Health [28483]
Imperial Dialysis • DaVita [22733]
Imperial Point Medical Center • Fitness and
 Rehabilitation Services [38226]
Imperial Professional Healthcare Services, Inc.
 [17880]
Imperial Valley Drug and Rehab Clinic [39802]
Imperial Valley Home Therapies • Fresenius Medical
 Care [22671]
Imperial Valley Methadone Clinic [39672]
Imperial Valley Methadone Clinic Inc • Medical
 Treatment Center [39803]
Imperial Valley Sleep Center [36669]
Improving Life Home Care [14042]
In Care of Families First [33149]
In--Home Care Nursing [15834]
In Home Health Services [17387]
In Home Health Services--Sparta [16271]
In Home Healthcare, LLC [17995]
In Home Program/Preferred Home Care [17415]
In-House Hospice Services-Kalamazoo [20078]
In-House Hospice Solutions [20039], [20049]
In-House Hospice Solutions-Akron [20798]
In-House Hospice Solutions-Grand Rapids [20063]
In-House Hospice Solutions-Howell [20070]
In Touch Home Health, LLC [14282]
In Touch Hospice Program • Somerset Hospital
 [21158]
InCare At Home Health and Hospice [20905]

InCare Home Health--Conway [17581]
InCare Home Health--Georgetown [17591]
InCare Home Health--Myrtle Beach [17608]
InCare Home Health--North Myrtle Beach [17616]
Incare Home Health Services--San Francisco [13308]
InCare Homemakers, Inc. [17609]
Incentives Inc [47389]
Incredible Kids Program [28642]
Independence Dialysis Center • DaVita [24325]
Independence Family Health Center [6260]
Independence Hall Industries [4392]
Independence Health Services, LLC [17551]
Independence House [9482], [32710]
Independence House South Side [41132]
Independence Park Medical Services • Sports Injury Rehabilitation [38018]
Independence Place [31945]
Independence Project LLC [43928]
Independence Rehab Services [4279]
Independence Renal Center • DaVita [24508]
IndependenceFirst [3682]
Independent Dialysis Foundation--Allegany Center [24672]
Independent Dialysis Foundation--Arundel Center [24691]
Independent Dialysis Foundation--Calvert Center [24714]
Independent Dialysis Foundation--Deaton • Dialysis Center [24646]
Independent Dialysis Foundation • Garrett Dialysis Center [24707]
Independent Dialysis Foundation--Parkview Center [24647]
Independent Dialysis FoundationF--Lions Manor [24673]
Independent Home Health Care, Inc.--Coeburn [18278]
Independent Home Health Care, Inc.--Jonesville [18313]
Independent Home Health Care, Inc.--Rosedale [18381]
Independent Home Health Care, Inc.--Weber City [18407]
Independent Living Facility • Mobile Community Mental Health Center [27982]
Independent Living--Pediatrics [1778]
Independent Living Resource Center [303]
Communications Department [1307]
Independent Nephrology Services--Charlotte [25840]
Independent Nephrology Services--Franklin County [25887]
Independent Nephrology Services--Huntersville [25888]
Independent Nephrology Services--Iredell County [25911]
Independent Rehabilitation Associates [38426]
Indian Bay Services • Mouskegon County [30606]
Indian Health Board of Billings • Substance Abuse Program [45680]
Indian Health Board of Minneapolis • Indian Health Board [6869]
Indian Health Center of Santa Clara Valley, Inc. [6359]
Indian Health Services [8739]
Indian Healthcare Resource Center of • Tulsa Inc [48040]
Indian Mountain Clinic [7260]
Indian Path Pavilion [33844]
Indian Pueblo Legal Services, Inc. [9862]
Indian River Dialysis • DaVita [23549]
Indian River Memorial Hospital • Regional Cancer Center [5001]
Indian River Mental Health Center [27881], [50623]
Indian Rivers Community Mental Health/Mental Retardation Administration [28055]
Indian Rivers Mental Health [39284]
Indian Rivers Mental Health Center
Bibb County Satellite [27873]
Substance Abuse Intensive Outpatient [39232], [39233]
Substance Abuse Services [39296]
Indian Township Health Center • Passamaquoddy Tribe [44044]
Indian Wells Valley Dialysis Center • DaVita [22902]
Indiana Avenue DUI Service [42533]
Indiana Deaf and Hard of Hearing Services • FSSA

Division of Disability and Rehabilitation Services [2160]
Indiana Health Center at South Bend [6699]
Indiana Health Centers [6690]
Indiana Hemophilia and Thrombosis Center [12521]
Indiana Hemophilia and Thrombosis Center Inc. • Sickle Cell Clinic [36343]
Indiana Juvenile Justice Task Force • Runaway and Homeless Youth Services [35950]
Indiana Lions Eye and Tissue Transplant Bank [35032]
Indiana Organ Procurement Organization--Indianapolis • Eye and Tissue Bank [35033]
Indiana Organ Procurement Organization--Northeast • Eye and Tissue Bank [35034]
Indiana Organ Procurement Organization--Northwest Indiana • Eye and Tissue Bank [35035]
Indiana Organ Procurement Organization--Southern Indiana • Eye and Tissue Bank [35036]
Indiana Orthopedic Hospital [38434]
Indiana Perinatal Network [36477]
Indiana Regional Medical Center • Cancer Center [5833]
Indiana School for the Blind and Visually Impaired [3708]
Indiana School for the Deaf [421]
Indiana Sleep Center [36951]
Indiana State Department of Health • Maternal and Child Health Services • Sudden Infant Death Syndrome of Indiana [36478]
Indiana State Library • Indiana Talking Book & Braille Library [3792]
Indiana State University • Indiana Deafblind Services Project • Blumberg Center [2189]
Indiana United Methodist Children's Home • Centenary Hall [34132]
Indiana United Methodist Children's Home, Inc [34133]
Indiana University • Department of Speech and Hearing [2130]
Indiana University Health
Arnett Health Clinic • Sleep Disorders Center [36952]
Bedford Hospital • Center for Sleep Disorders Medicine [36953]
Indiana University Health West Hospital • Cancer Center [4672]
Indiana University Medical Center [2161]
Riley Hospital for Children • Adult Cystic Fibrosis Center [7539]
Riley University Hospital and Outpatient Center • Pediatric Cystic Fibrosis and Chronic Pulmonary Disease Center [7540]
Wishard Health Services • Burn Center [4543]
Indiana University Multiple Sclerosis Center [34578]
Indiana University • Riley Children's Hospital • Riley Burn Unit [4544]
Indiana University School of Medicine • Department of Medical and Molecular Genetics • Medical Genetics Clinic [12211]
Indiana University School of Medicine, Northwest • Genetics Center [12212]
Indiana University
School of Medicine • Pain Management [35442]
West Hospital • Sleep Disorders Center [36954]
Indianapolis Community Hospital, Inc. • Access Services [50892]
Indianapolis Counseling Center LLC [43099]
Indianapolis Neurosurgical Group • Pain Clinic [35443]
Indianapolis Treatment Center LLC [43100]
Indianhead Medical Center, Inc. [18629]
Indiantown Community Health Center [6478]
Individual Care Center Inc [47662]
Indus Home Health Care [16982]
Indy Cottage Counseling LLC [43101]
Indy Interventions [43073]
Infant Toddler Program [7923]
Infanzon and Twins Home Health [14043]
Infertility Center of Saint Louis at Saint Luke's Hospital [22144]
Infertility & Invitro Fertilization Medical Associates of WNY, PLLC [22182]
Infertility Solutions [22232]
Infinite Care, Inc. [17416]
Infinite Home Health, Inc.--Westlake Village [13447]
Infinite Home Health Inc.--Woodland Hills [13455]
Infinity Care of Tulsa [20983]

Infinity Home Care Providers [12984]
Infinity Hospice Care--Las Vegas [20418]
Infinity Hospice Care--Phoenix [18812]
Infirmary Health Systems Inc. • Infirmary West Sleep Disorders Center [36587]
Infirmary Home Care--Grove Hill [12673]
Infirmary Home Care--Mobile [12694]
Infirmary Home Care--Saraland [12720]
Infirmary Hospice Care [18739]
Information and Crisis Service [51222]
Infusal Partners [14210]
InfuScience--Egan [15902]
InfuScience, Inc.--Chantilly [18256]
InfuScience--Omaha [16124]
Infusion Network of Louisiana [15271]
Infusion Options, Inc. [16394]
Infusion Partners [17707]
Infusion Plus, Inc. [15548]
Infusion Services, LLC [12651]
Ingalls Center for Outpatient Rehabilitation [1972]
Ingalls Home Care--Flossmoor [14793]
Ingalls Home Care--Harvey [14812]
Ingalls Hospice & Palliative Care [19528]
Ingalls Hospital • Cancer Program [5095]
Ingham Intermediate School District [496]
Ingham Regional Medical Center
Cancer Program [5382]
Ingham Regional Center for Sleep and Alertness [37165]
Inglewood Dialysis • DaVita [22734]
Ingraham [50960]
InHome Care, Inc.--Midland [18089]
InHome Care, Inc.--San Antonio [18146]
Initiative for Violence Free Families [9616]
Injury 1 Treatment Center [35697]
Inland Behavioral and Health Services Inc [40523]
Inland Counseling Network [32819]
Day Treatment Center [32820]
Inland Empire Community Health Center and Dental Clinic [6291]
Inland Hospice Association [18906]
Inland Medical and Rehab, Inc. [18463]
Inland Valley Drug and Alcohol • Recovery Services/Men/Women/Children [40871]
Inland Valley Hospice [18965]
Inland Valley Recovery Services
San Bernardino Recovery Center [40524]
Upland Recovery Center [40872]
inMotion [15192]
Inn Transition [44536]
Inner Access Therapy Center [44852]
Inner Change Counseling [41133]
Inner City Counseling Services [46125]
Inner Harbour Hospitals • The Shoals [33378]
Inner Harbour Outpatient Services [33379]
Inner Journey Community Counseling [41208]
inner Journey Healing Arts [48238]
Inner Journey Healing Arts Center [48130]
Inner Peace Counseling Inc [49925]
inner Voice Inc [42534]
InnerBalance Health Center [41267]
Innerchange [32906]
InnerSolutions [10956]
Innersport Chiropractic [38075]
Innis Community Health Center [6748]
Innovation Home Health--Doral [13663]
Innovations Club [31460]
Innovative Dialysis of Toledo [26211]
Innovative Health Systems Inc • Chemical Dependency Outpatient Clinic [47185]
Innovative Home Health--Lawton [17126]
Innovative Nursing Management, Inc./Innovated Nursing, Inc. [13579]
Innovative Pain Treatment Solutions [35314]
Innovative Recovery Solutions Inc [48632]
Innovative Renal Care--Webster Inc. [27151]
Innovative Senior Care Home Health--Denver [13474]
Innovative Senior Care Home Health--Jacksonville [13816]
Innovative Senior Care Home Health at Park Regency [12785]
Innovative Senior Care Home Health, Summit at Westlake Hills [17815]
Innovative Senior Care Home Health--Tucson [12833]
Innovative Sleep Solution [37733]

Innovative Solutions Addiction Treatment Center [43454]
Innovative Speech and Communication Services [2617]
Innovative Therapy 4-Kids [1076]
Innovative Therapy Associates Inc. [1318]
Innovative Therapy Solutions LLC [2677]
Innovative Treatment Services [41840]
Innovis Health/Dakota Clinic • Cancer Program [5670]
InnVision [28775]
    Julian Street Inn [28776]
Inova Alexandria Hospital • Northern Virginia Cancer Center [6051]
Inova Comprehensive Addiction • Treatment Services [49782]
Inova Fair Oaks Hospital • Cancer Program [6058]
Inova Fairfax Hospital [18293]
    Life With Cancer [6059]
    Pediatric Lung Center • Cystic Fibrosis Center [7686]
INOVA Hospital for Children • Northern Virginia Sickle Cell Center [36439]
Inova Kellar Center Behavioral [49780]
Inova Mount Vernon Hospital
    Cancer Program [6052]
    Rehabilitation Department [3568]
Inova VNA Home Health [18389]
Inpatient Hospice Program of Hackensack University Medical Center [20474]
Inpatient Rehabilitation Unit • Addiction Institute of New York [46877]
Inpatient Unit at Community Medical Center [21154]
Inroads Counseling and DUI Center [42446]
INS Statesville [25957]
Inside Out Counseling Services [48137]
Insight Counseling/Eating Disorder Foundation of Orange County [10957]
Insight Counseling of Tecumseh LLC [45033]
Insight House Chem Depend Services Inc
    Day Rehabilitation Program [47148]
    Drug Abuse Inpatient Treatment Program [47149]
    Substance Abuse Outpatient Clinic [47150]
Insight Human Services [47540]
    Womens Recovery Center [47210]
The Insight Program [42149]
Insight Psychological Center [11047]
Insight Services PLLC [41064]
Insight Therapy LLC [39310]
Insights [48956]
Insights Counseling Center [41845]
Insights in Recovery [47321]
Inspiration Hospice-Salt Lake City [21649]
Inspirations Outpatient Counseling Center [28342]
Inspirations for Youth and Families [41657]
Inspire [3028]
Institute for Alcohol Awareness of • Greeley [41215]
Institute for Arthroscopy & Sports Medicine [38128]
Institute of Athletic Medicine - Eagan Clinic [38615]
Institute for Athletic Medicine - Eden Prairie Clinic [38616]
Institute for Athletic Medicine--Edina [38618]
Institute for Athletic Medicine--Elk River [38619]
Institute for Athletic Medicine--Maple Grove [38622]
Institute for Athletic Medicine--Maplewood [38624]
Institute for Athletic Medicine--Minneapolis [38625]
Institute for Athletic Medicine - Minnetonka Clinic [38634]
Institute for Athletic Medicine - Oxboro Clinic [38613]
Institute for Athletic Medicine--Plymouth [38632]
Institute for Athletic Medicine - Uptown Minneapolis [38626]
Institute for Basic Research in Developmental Disabilities • Down Syndrome Clinic [10831]
Institute for Child & Family Health • Sunset Clinic [29216], [50774]
Institute for Cognitive Therapy Inc [49655]
Institute for Communicative Disorders [2078]
Institute for Community Living • Continuing Day Treatment Program [31266]
Institute for Community Living, Inc. [31418]
Institute for Family • Adolescent Services [46147]
Institute for Family Health [9952]
Institute for the Hispanic Family • Hispanic Alcohol/Substance Abuse Prog [41409]
Institute Home Care Services, Inc. • Innovative Health Care Systems [16553]

Institute for Human Resources [42870]
Institute for Learning and Development [8133]
Institute for Life Enrichment [29094]
Institute of Life and Health Alcohol • Drug Assessment and Therapy Program [44375]
Institute of Living • Grace S. Webb School [7849]
Institute of Living Hartford Hospital • Addiction Recovery Program [41410]
Institute for Personal Development [42787]
Institute of Physical Medicine and Rehabilitation [2098]
The Institute for Rehabilitation and Research [8552]
Institute for Rehabilitation and Research
    Texas Model Spinal Cord Injury System [4447]
    UPMC Passavant [4393]
Institute for Reproductive Health [22214]
Institute for Reproductive Health and Infertility [22183]
Institute for Reproductive Medicine and Science at Saint Barnabas Medical Center • Department of Obstetrics and Gynecology • In Vitro Fertilization Program [22162]
Institute of Sleep Medicine • DuPage Medical Group [36909]
Institute for Stress Management and Psychotherapy [50850]
Institute for the Study of Disadvantage and Disability • Adult Down Syndrome Program • Down Syndrome Clinic [10789]
Institute for Stuttering Treatment and Research [936]
Institutes for the Achievement of Human Potential [8494]
Institutes for Behavior Resources Inc • REACH Mobile Health Services /Outpt Services [44149]
Instituto Psicoterapeutico de PR [48769]
Instituto de Reeducacion de PR [48746]
Integracare Hospice--Decatur [21442]
Integracare Hospice-Grapevine [21475]
Integracare Hospice-Lubbock [21523]
Integracare Hospice--Mineral Wells [21532]
Integral Home Health Agency, Inc. [14225]
Integral Home Health Services, Inc. [14044]
Integral Youth Services • Runaway and Homeless Youth Program [36168]
Integrated Behavioral Healthcare • Clinics [39743]
Integrated Care Systems [13428]
Integrated Healing Associates [10958]
Integrated Health Clinics [48153]
Integrated Health Clinics of Eugene [48103]
Integrated Health Professionals, Inc. [18464]
Integrated Health Resources [50795]
Integrated Home Care [15660]
Integrated HomeCare Services--East Dundee [14770]
Integrated HomeCare Services--Rockford [14914]
Integrated Life Center Inc [42161]
Integrated Medical, Inc. [16884]
Integrated Neurology Services • Multiple Sclerosis Center [34729]
Integrated Speech and Language Services [1640]
Integrated Spine Care • Pain Clinic [35632]
Integrated Treatment Unit [44559]
Integrative Counseling LLC
    Congruent Counseling Services [44228]
    Outpatient Services [44229]
Integrative Counseling Services [43079]
Integrative Medicine and Psychotherapy of Greenwich [11004]
Integrative Recovery & Wellness Clinic [45987]
Integrative Treatment Centers [35352], [38184]
Integris Baptist Medical Center--Transplant [26281]
Integris Baptist Medical Center • Troy and Dollie Smith Cancer Center [5777]
Integris Baptist • Paul Silverstein Burn Center [4612]
Integris Bass Baptist Health Center Home Health [17119]
Integris Blackwell Regional Hospital Home Health [17105]
Integris Hospice of Mayes County [20973]
INTEGRIS Marshall County Medical Center [17127]
INTEGRIS Mayes County Medical Center [17157]
Integris Mental Health Center [33781]
Integris Mental Health
    Oklahoma City Campus [33782]
    Spencer Campus [33783]
INTEGRIS Regency Home Care [17130]
Integris Regency Hospice [20942]

Integris Sleep Disorders Center of Oklahoma Yukon [37600]
Integris Southwest Medical Center
    Central Oklahoma Cancer Center [5778]
    MDA/ALS Center [139], [34856]
Integris Western Oklahoma Hospice [20930]
Integrity Counseling Inc [41593], [41743]
    Outpatient Services [41744]
Integrity Hospice LLC-Brigham City [21600]
Integrity House Inc
    Intensive Outpatient [46094]
    Mens Facility [46095]
Integrity Inc [46160]
Integrity Physical Therapy [38381]
Integrity Wellness Group [42340]
Inteli Home Healthcare, Inc. [17996]
Intensive Fluency Clinic • Department of Neurology [3508]
Intensive Home HealthCare, Inc [15375]
Intensive Outpatient Care Inc [42649]
Intensive Renal Care [22653]
Intensive Residential Support [28982]
Intensive Residential Treatment Center • Center for Developmental Disabilities [33322]
Intensive Training Residence [29329]
Intensive Treatment Systems LLC [39432], [39433], [39434]
Intensive Treatment Unit [34195]
Inter Act of Michigan Inc • Substance Abuse Services [44868]
Inter-Active Health Care, Inc. [17997]
Inter Care Ltd • Chemical Dependency Outpatient [46878]
Inter-Coastal Home Health Care, Inc. [13593]
Inter-Community Mental Health Group [29052]
Inter-Community Mental Hlth Group Inc • Co-Occurring Disorder Program [41379]
Inter County Council on Drug/Alc Abuse Administration • Drug Free Counseling [46026]
Inter County Council on Drug/Alc Abuse • Opiate Treatment Clinic [46027]
Inter Tribal Substance Abuse • Prevention and Treatment Center [47957]
Interact [10073]
Interactiv Children's Therapy Services [1889]
Interactive Speech Associates [2123]
Interactive Speech Services Inc. [3322]
InterActive Therapy Group--East Syracuse [3013]
Interactive Therapy Group--New York [3061]
Interactive Therapy Inc. [2783]
Interamerican Dialysis Center & At Home • DaVita [23398]
InterCare Community Health Network--Bangor • InterCare [6834]
Intercare Community Health Network--Holland [6847]
Intercare North Hospital [33871]
Intercept Associates [49960]
Intercept Programs Inc [42829]
Intercommunity Action Inc • Alcohol and Drug Education Family [48529]
Intercommunity Action, Inc. [32083]
    Group Home 2 [32084]
    Group Home 3 [32085]
    Group Home 4 [32086]
    Group Home 5 [32087]
    Outpatient Services [32088]
Intercommunity Dialysis Center [23076]
Intercommunity Mental Health Group [28990]
Interconnections SC [50424]
Intercultural Family Services Inc [48530]
Interdynamics Inc [44303]
Interface Children/Family Services [8799]
Interface Children and Family Services • Runaway and Homeless Youth Program [35825]
Interface Environments dba • Winways [3905]
Interfaith Community Health Center [7374]
Interfaith Medical Center [16395]
    Chemical Dependency Outpatient Services [46505]
    Detoxification [46506]
    MMTP [46507]
    Sickle Cell Program [36394]
    Substance Abuse Detoxification [46508]
    Substance Abuse Rehabilitation [46509]
Intergrative Counseling Services [50114]
Interim Healthcare [20960]
Interim Healthcare--Escondido [12993]

Interim HealthCare Hospice of Western PA, Inc. [21141]
Interim Healthcare Inc.--San Jose [13316]
Interim Healthcare--Modesto [13177]
Interim Healthcare--Pasadena [13241]
Interim Healthcare--Riverside [13269]
Interim HealthCare--Sacramento [13282]
Interim Healthcare--San Diego [13296]
Interim Healthcare Specialty Services [1388]
Interim Healthcare Staffing of Northern California Inc. [13283]
Interim House Inc [48531]
    Recovery Home [44448]
    West [48532]
Interior Alaska Center for Non-Violent Living [8661]
Interior Alaska Orthopedic and Sports Medicine [38021]
Interior Neighborhood Health Corp. • Interior Community Health Clinic [6210]
Interline Employee Assistance Prog Inc • Alcoholism Substance Abuse Clinic [46723]
Interlink Counseling Services Inc [43688]
Interlude [28983]
Intermed Home Care Services [12985]
Intermediate School District Number 287 [515]
Intermediate School District Number 709 • Deaf and Hard of Hearing Services [509]
Intermediate School District Number 917 [516]
Intermediate Unit Number 29, Schuylkill [704]
Intermediate Unit One [695]
Intermountain American Fork Hospital Sleep Center [37871]
Intermountain American Fork Hospital • Sleep Center [37870]
Intermountain • Center for Cognitive Therapy [49638]
Intermountain Children's Home & Services [34281]
InterMountain Education Service District • Speech--Language Program [3316]
Intermountain Healthcare Cancer Program Network • Jon and Karen Huntsman Cancer Center [6038]
Intermountain Healthcare Hospice [19452]
Intermountain Homecare-Cedar City [21601]
Intermountain Homecare-Delta [21603]
Intermountain Homecare-Fillmore [21604]
Intermountain Homecare-Heber City [21609]
Intermountain Homecare--Logan [21616]
Intermountain Homecare-Mt. Pleasant [21618]
Intermountain Hospice--Ogden [21629]
Intermountain Hospital [33398]
Intermountain Hospital of Boise [42313]
Intermountain
    Specialized Abuse Treatment Center [49661], [49672], [49686]
    Substance Abuse [49639]
Intermountain Transplant Center [27422]
International Biologics LLC [34924]
International Center for the Disabled • Speech and Hearing Department [3062]
International Community Health Services [7386]
International Cornea Project [34948]
International Eating Disorders Institute [11303]
International Home Health Care, Inc. [13136]
International Sight Restoration Inc. [34991]
International Speech and Language [2990]
International Women's House [9105]
Internet Behavioral Care PC [48615]
Interpore Cross International [34949]
Interval Brotherhood Homes Inc • Alcohol and Drug Rehabilitation Center [47606]
Interval House Crisis Shelters [8910]
Intervenemd • Pain Care Center [35663]
Intervention Institute [40851]
Intervention and Rehab Associates Inc [44796]
Intervention Specialist LLC [45982]
Interventional Pain Center [12405]
Interventional Pain Services of Western North Carolina--Clyde [35590]
Interventional Pain Services of Western North Carolina--Franklin [35591]
InterWorld Health Care, Inc. [17911]
Intracare Hospital [51382]
Intracare Medical Center Hospital [49380]
Intravene [18323]
Intuitive Eating Counseling [10959]
Inverness Dialysis Center • Fresenius Medical Care [23334]
InVia Fertility [22039]

Inwood Community Services Inc • Comp Outpatient Addiction Program [46879]
Inyo County Mental Health [28415]
    South County Office [28566]
The Ionia Area Hospice [20071]
Ionia Cnty Substance Abuse Initiative [44853]
Ionia County Community Mental Health, Belding [30512]
Ionia County Community Mental Health, Ionia [30573]
Ionia County Memorial Hospital Corp. [15693]
Ionia Dialysis • DaVita [24918]
Iowa Braille School [3709]
Iowa City Hospice [19700]
Iowa City VA Medical Center [19701]
Iowa City Veterans Affairs Medical Center [4051] Multiple Sclerosis Center [34580]
Iowa Department of Education • Iowa's Deafblind Services Project [2202]
Iowa Department of Human Services, Des Moines • Runaway and Homeless Youth Program [35956]
Iowa Department of Public Health • Family Services Bureau • Iowa SIDS Program [36480]
Iowa Donor Network--Johnston [35039]
Iowa Donor Network--North Liberty [35040]
Iowa Donor Network--Sioux City [35041]
Iowa Health Des Moines • Des Moines University Clinic • Medicine and Rehabilitation [4052]
Iowa Health Home Care-Intrust [19736]
Iowa Lions Eye Bank--Iowa City [35042]
Iowa Medical Center • Des Moines Sleep Disorders Center [36977]
Iowa Methodist Medical Center • John Stoddard Cancer Center [5186]
Iowa Methodist Orthopaedic and Sports Medicine Centre--West Des Moines [38459]
Iowa Methodist Orthopaedic and Sports Medicine Centres--Des Moines [38451]
Iowa Methodist Sports Medicine Centre [38452]
Iowa River Hospice [19711]
Iowa School for the Deaf [429]
Iowa Sleep Disorders Center [36978]
Iowa Sudden Infant Death Syndrome Alliance [36481]
Iowa Western Community College • Disability Services [430]
IPR Healthcare System, Inc.--Baytown [17820]
IPR Healthcare System, Inc.--Houston [17998]
IPR Healthcare System, Inc.--Kingwood [18030]
Iredell Memorial Hospital • Cancer Center [5660]
Iredell Memorial Hospital, Inc. [16785]
Irene Stacy CMHC • Drug and Alcohol Unit [48312]
Irene Stacy Community Mental Health Center [51276]
Iris Center Womens Counseling and • Recovery Services [40615]
Iris City Dialysis • DaVita [23713]
Irlen Institute for Perceptual and Learning Development [7787]
Iron County Human Services • Department and Associates [50415]
Iron Mission Dialysis Center [27403]
Ironton Family Medical Center [7087]
Ironton/Lawrence County Community • Action Org Family Guidance Center [47780]
Iroquois Center for Human Development [8025] Crisis Line [50917]
Iroquois Community Health Center [6679]
Iroquois Memorial Hospice [19581]
Iroquois Memorial Hospital and Iroquois Resident Home [14953]
Iroquois Mental Health Center [42944], [50879]
Iroquois Special Education Association [396]
Irvine Head Injury Home [4171]
Irving Dialysis Center • Fresenius Medical Care [27192]
Irving Place Dialysis • Beth Israel Medical Center [25722]
Irving Regional Day School for the Deaf [796]
Irwin Army Community Hospital • Cancer Program [5197]
A Is for Apple--Saratoga [1313]
A Is For Apple Inc.--Los Gatos [1173]
A Is For Apple--San Jose [1292]
Isa Marrs Speech Language Feeding [2980]
Isaac Coggs Heritage Health Center [7433]
Isabel Community Clinic [7247]
Isabella Geriatric Center Home Care [16554]

Isabella House [50172]
Iselborn Chiropractic & Sports Medicine [38244]
Isis Center [28752]
Island Assessment and Counseling Center [50033] Seattle Branch [50115]
Island Assessment and Counseling • Freeland Branch [49966]
Island Dialysis Center • DaVita [27100]
Island Health Care--Beaufort [17564]
Island Health Care, Inc.--Savannah [14581]
Island Health Northwest • Cancer Program [6091]
Island Healthcare--Pooler [14572]
Island Hospice--Hardeeville [21250]
Island Hospice - Savannah [19416]
Island Hospital [18414]
Island Mental Health Center [32818]
Island Rehabilitation Center [1642]
Island Rehabilitative Service Inc. • Dialysis Unit [25780]
Island Rehabilitative Services, Bronx [25588]
Island Rehabilitative Services • Clove Lakes Extension [25781]
Island Rehabilitative Services--Queens • Dialysis Facility [25694]
Island Rehabilitative Servicescommitteemack [25643]
Island Reproductive Services [22184]
Island Speech Language and Rehabilitation--Oak Harbor [3631]
Islands Community Medical Services [6786]
Islands Counseling [11114]
IsoTis OrthoBiologics [34950]
iSPORT [39114]
ISTO Technologies Inc. [35095]
Italian Home for Children [34197]
Ithaca Dialysis Clinic • DaVita [25686]
Ithaca Veterans Affairs Clinic [31360]
Its About Change/Sober Living [42433]
Its About Change/Sober Living Inc [42656]
ITxM Clinical Services • Cord Blood Services [35027]
Iuka Sleep Disorders Lab • Iuka Hospital [37249]
IV Care Options--Eastman [14525]
IV Care Options--Macon [14544]
IV League [12969]
IV Solutions of Amarillo [17793]
IV Specialist, Inc. [17565]
IVF Florida Reproductive Associates [21997]
IVF Michigan, PC--Ann Arbor [22120]
IVF Michigan, PC--Brighton [22121]
IVF Michigan, PC--Dearborn [22122]
IVF Michigan, PC--Flint [22123]
IVF Michigan, PC--Rochester Hills [22124]
IVF Michigan, PC--Saginaw [22125]
IVF Michigan, PC--Toledo [22215]
IVF New Jersey [22163]
IVF Phoenix [21898]
IVF Plano [22263]
IVF1 [22040]
Ivinson Memorial Hospital • Dialysis Center [27816]
Ivor Medical Center [7355]
Ivy House Center for Self Sufficiency [47541]
The Ivymount School [8098]
IWK Health Centre [11189]
    Burn Unit [4601]
Iyana House [31419]

J

J. Arthur Trudeau Memorial Center [8499]
J Bar J Ranch • Runaway and Homeless Youth Program [36169]
J Cole Recovery Homes Inc • Cole House [39607]
A J Counseling and Associates Inc [41001]
J. D. McCarty Center for Children with Developmental Disabilities [8437]
J & D Ultracare Corp. [16645]
J. David Collins and Associates LLC [44347]
J-Jireh Healthcare Services, LLC [17881]
J and L Medical Services [13530]
J Luis Hospital Saint Croix • Dialysis Center [27448]
J. Martin Carnell Residence [31452]
J Michael Horsley MI Residential Home [27878]
J. Oliver Speech Pathology Services Inc. [1789]
J. R. Medical, Inc. [13083]
J Robert Pritchard Dialysis Center • Cabell Huntington Hospital [27675]
J-Shalom Home Health Services, Inc. [18109]

J. U. Kevil Memorial Foundation [8055]
Jabberjaws Pediatric Speech Pathology [2866]
Jacinto Dialysis Center • DaVita [27193]
Jacinto Sleep Evaluation Center [37819]
Jack Barth Family Health Center [6788]
Jack Brown Regional Treatment Center [48023]
Jack C Montgomery VAMC [47964]
Jack C. Montgomery Veterans Affairs Medical Center
    [17134], [31894], [51630]
Jack C. Montgomery Veterans Hospital • PTSD
    Clinical Team [51801]
Jack Clarks Family • Recovering Community Inc
    [42535], [42536], [42887]
Jackie Myland and Associates--Boulder [1382]
Jackie Myland and Associates--Denver [1397]
Jackie Nitschke Center Inc [50400], [50401]
Jackson Area Council on Alcoholism and Drug
    Dependency [49090]
Jackson Counseling Agency [44644]
Jackson County Health and Human Services
    [31952]
Jackson County Memorial Hospital Home Care and
    Hospice [17096]
Jackson County Mental Health Center--Jefferson
    [29445]
Jackson County Mental Health Center--Scottsboro
    [28034]
Jackson County Regional Health Center [15093]
Jackson County Schneck Memorial Hospital [15050]
Jackson County Schools [631], [880]
Jackson Dialysis • DaVita [24921]
Jackson Dialysis & Kidney Center [26139]
Jackson Hearing Clinic [2610]
Jackson Hole Community Counseling Center
    [33046]
Jackson Home Health [18538]
Jackson Hospital
    Jackson Sleep Disorders Center [36588]
    Sports Medicine Unit [38010]
Jackson Jade and Associates, A Speech Pathology
    Corporation [1238]
Jackson-Madison County General Hospital [17684]
Jackson-Madison County General Hospital • Sleep
    Disorders Center [37766]
Jackson-Madison County General Hospital • West
    Tennessee Cancer Center [5933]
Jackson Medical Clinic • Premier Sleep Disorders
    Center [37250]
Jackson Memorial Hospital
    Cancer Program [4964]
    Pain Management [35383]
    Pediatric Dialysis Unit [23399]
Jackson Memorial Hospital Rehabilitation Center
    [3983]
Jackson Memorial Hospital Transplant Center
    [23400]
Jackson North Community Mental Health Center
    [29249]
    South Florida Provider Coalition [41844]
Jackson Park Dialysis Center • Fresenius Medical
    Care [23939]
Jackson Professional Associates [49091]
Jackson Recovery Centers Inc
    Grandview House/Men [43302]
    Mapleton Satellite Office [43287]
    Marienne Manor [43303]
    Outpatient [43304]
    Plymouth County Satellite [43285]
    Women and Childrens Center [43305]
Jackson Speech and Rehabilitation [1644]
Jackson State University • Central Mississippi
    Speech/Language/Hearing Clinic [2763]
Jackson Veterans Affairs Clinic [30601]
Jacksonville Beach Dialysis • Fresenius Medical
    Care [23347]
Jacksonville Center for Reproductive Medicine
    [21998]
Jacksonville Developmental Center [7957]
Jacksonville Dialysis Center • Fresenius Medical
    Care [27194]
Jacksonville Mental Health [27955]
Jacksonville Metro Treatment Center [41704]
Jacksonville Public Library • Talking Books/Special
    Needs Library [3762]
Jacksonville South Dialysis Center and At Home •
    DaVita [23348]
Jacksonville Speech and Hearing Center Inc.--N
    Laura Street [1608]

Jacksonville Speech and Language Center--N 5th
    Street [3311]
Jacksonville State University • Disability Support
    Services [198]
Jacksonville Treatment Center [47395]
Jacksonville VA Outpatient Clinic [13817]
Jacksonville Veterans Affairs Clinic [31551]
Jacob Center [41175]
The Jacob Crouch Foundation [50945]
Jacob Perlow Hospice [20585]
Jacobi Medical Center
    Burn Unit [4591]
    Chemical Dependence Inpatient [46422]
    Comprehensive Addiction Treatment Center/
        Outpatient [46423]
Jacobs Family Chiropractic • Pain Clinic [35315]
Jacobs Neurological Institute and William C. Baird
    Multiple Sclerosis Research Center [34646]
Jacqueline Brill [45904]
Jade Wellness Center [48474]
JAEL Health Services Inc [44257]
Jalopy Shoppe, Inc.--Longview [18051]
Jalopy Shoppe, Inc.--Sherman [18157]
Jalopy Shoppe, Inc.--Victoria [18182]
Jamaica Community Services [33697]
Jamaica Continuing Day Treatment [31367]
Jamaica Continuing Support System [31368]
Jamaica Hospital Medical Center [16500]
Jameco Home Health Agency, Inc. [13182]
James A. Haley Veterans Affairs Hospital, Tampa •
    Multiple Sclerosis Center [34555]
James A. Haley Veterans Affairs Medical Center
    New Port Richey Clinic [29233]
    Zephyrhills Clinic [29325]
James A. Haley Veteran's Hospital • Physical
    Medicine and Rehabilitation Service [35384]
James A. Haley Veterans Hospital
    PTSD Clinical Team [51713]
    Spinal Cord Injury Service [3984]
James A. Simon, MD, PC • In Vitro Fertilization
    Clinic [21984]
James B. Haggin Memorial Hospital [15187]
The James Cancer Hospital and Solove Research
    Institute [5708]
James E. Cartwright Care Center [20111]
James E. Scott Satellite [6504]
James E Van Zandt VA Medical Center [17242]
James E. Van Zandt Veterans Affairs Medical Center
    [17243], [31989]
James E. van Zandt Veterans Affairs Medical Center
    - Altoona [51634]
James Graham Brown Cancer Center • Adult Sickle
    Cell Disease Center [36346]
James H Quillen VAMC [49149]
James H. Quillen Veterans Affairs Medical Center
    [32364]
    Cancer Program [5942]
    PTSD Clinical Team [51820]
The James Harrigan Center Dialysis [23140]
James House [10574]
James J. Howard, Brick NJ • VA NJ Health Care
    System [4280]
James J. Peters Bronx VA Medical Center [16364]
James J. Peters Veterans Affairs Medical Center
    [4309], [31247], [51610]
James L. Dennis Developmental Center [1026]
James Lawrence Kernan Hospital • William Donald
    Schaefer Rehabilitation Center [4097]
James Madison University • Communication Sci-
    ences and Disorders Applied Laboratory • Speech
    and Hearing Center [3586]
James Oldham Treatment Center [49917]
James Quarles 1 [27997]
James Quarles 2 [27998]
James R Gage and Associates [42733], [42836]
James River Special Education Cooperative [641]
James Wortham Counseling Services Inc [43143]
Jameson Hospice of Lawrence County • Jameson
    Hospital North Campus [21120]
Jamestown Hospital [16815]
Jamestown Hospital Hospice [20785]
Jamestown VA Outpatient Clinic [4353]
Jamestown Veterans Affairs Clinic--5th Street NE
    [31633]
Jamestown Veterans Affairs Clinic--W 3rd Street
    [31370]
Jamieson Total Health Care Center [38594]
Jan Kaminis Platt Regional Library • Hillsborough

County Talking Book Library [3763]
Jane Addams Place [10304]
Jane Brooks School for the Deaf [665]
Jane H. Booker Outpatient Dialysis Center • Jersey
    Shore University Medical Center [25478]
Jane Phillips Dialysis Facility [26249]
Jane Phillips Home Care [17103]
Jane Phillips Regional Home Care [15115]
Janesville Community Health Center [7426]
Janesville Psychiatric Clinic [50418]
Janesville Veterans Affairs Clinic [32979]
Janet Wattles Center [29672]
Janey Tolliver Speech Pathology Services [3432]
Jansen Hospice and Palliative Care [20610]
Janus Community Clinic [40744]
Janus Perinatal • Mondanaro Baskin Center [40745]
Janus of Santa Cruz [40746]
Janus Youth Programs Inc. • Runaway and Home-
    less Youth Program [36170]
Jarrett Fertility Group LLC [22058]
Jary Barreto Crisis Center [28753]
Jason Foundation Inc. [51354]
Jasper County Health Department [42810]
Jasper County Hospital • Home Health Care/
    Hospice [19644]
Jasper County Outreach [10445]
Jasper Dialysis • DaVita [24182]
Jasper Mountain Center [31948]
Jasper Mountain SAFE Center [31981]
Jawonio [8329]
Jawonio Inc. [3052]
Jayne Shover Easter Seal Rehabilitation Center
    [2024]
Jayron Home Care, Inc. [14879]
Jaywalker Lodge [41034]
Jaywalker Lodge LLC [41035]
J.B. Summers Center [32380]
JBL Behavioral Health Systems [29161]
JBS Mental Health Authority [27862]
    Beverly Health Care Center - West [27911]
    Crestline Home [28003]
    Day Treatment Program [27863]
    Greenwood Homes [28019]
JC Audiology [1639]
JCC on the Palisades • Therapeutic Nursery [8272]
JCH Dialysis LLC [24011]
JCS Home Health/dba Home Instead Senior Care
    [13609]
Jean Massieu Academy [767]
Jean Weingarten Peninsula Oral School for the Deaf
    [294]
Jeanes Hospital [37653]
Jeanes Hospital Home Health [17417]
Jeanette Egan [48352]
Jeanine Schultz Memorial School [34117]
Jeanne Barth Speech/Language Pathology Services
    [1779]
Jedburg Dialysis and At Home • DaVita [26775]
Jeff Anderson Regional Medical Center • Regional
    Cancer Center [5431]
Jeff Davis ADC Inc [43833]
Jefferson Avenue Dialysis • DaVita [27519]
Jefferson Behavioral Health System [31842]
    Addiction Services [47862]
Jefferson Center for Mental Health [28900], [50709]
    Carr Street Center and Older Adults [28921]
    Clear Creek Community Service Center [28916]
    Fenton Place [28922]
    Gilpin Mental Health Services [28857]
    HAF House [28923]
    Hilltop Residential Facility [28924]
    Jefferson Hills I [28925]
    North Outpatient Office [28962]
    The ROAD [28963]
    Sobesky Academy Day Treatment [28926]
    Summit Center [28964]
    Teller Residential Facility [28927]
    Transitions in Community Living [28928]
    Transitions Meadowlark Day Treatment [28929]
    Wellness on Wadsworth [28965]
    West Colfax Outpatient/Emergency Services
        [28930]
    Westminster Counseling Service [28960]
    Westminster Office [28961]
Jefferson City Veterans Affairs Clinic [30854]
Jefferson Cnty Committee for Economic Opportunity
    • Community Substance Abuse Program [39223]

Jefferson Community Health Care Centers, Inc. [6741]
Jefferson Community Technical College • Deaf and Hard of Hearing Student Services [442]
Jefferson Comprehensive Health Center, Inc. [6881]
Jefferson County Board of Education [188]
Jefferson County Clubhouse [30758]
Jefferson County Comp Services Inc • Vantage Point [42795]
Jefferson County Dialysis Center • Fresenius Medical Care [25202]
Jefferson County Human Services Dept [50422]
Jefferson County Public Schools ECE [443]
Jefferson County Service Center [29461]
Jefferson County Women's Center [10001]
Jefferson Dialysis • DaVita [26427]
Jefferson/DuPont Children's Health Program • Pediatric Headache Program [12462]
Jefferson Health Care Hospice [21765]
Jefferson Healthcare--Port Townsend • Sleep Medicine [37915]
Jefferson Healthcare--Silverdale • Sleep Medicine Center [37916]
Jefferson Hills II [28855]
Jefferson Home Health Care [17501]
Jefferson House [44742]
Jefferson Intensive Outpatient Program [48533]
Jefferson Medical College • Women's Medical Specialties • In Vitro Fertilization Program [22233]
Jefferson Memorial Hospital [18537]
Jefferson Mental Health Services • Community Counseling Service [51458]
Jefferson Pain and Rehabilitation Center [35643]
Jefferson Parish Human Services Authority • Westbank Center [43857]
Jefferson Regional Medical Center [12880]
Behavioral Health [28341]
Jefferson Sleep Disorders Center [37654]
Jefferson Sports Medicine Center [38966]
Jefferson Trail Treatment • Center for Children [49773]
Jefferson University Hospitals
Headache Center [12463]
Magee Rehabilitation • Regional Spinal Cord Injury System of Delaware Valley [4394]
Jelani Inc [40616]
The Family Program [40617]
JEM Treatment Inc [42948]
Jenesse Center, Inc. [8841]
Jenkins Memorial Children's Center [7762]
Jennersville Dialysis Center • DaVita [26605]
Jennersville Regional Hospital • Cancer Center [5878]
Jennie Edmundson Memorial Hospital • Cancer Program [5184]
Jennie Stuart Medical Center • Cancer Program [5218]
Jennie Stuart Medical Center Home Health [15193]
Jennie Stuart Medical Center • Sleep Disorders Center [37027]
Jennifer Beach Foundation [10615]
Jennings Behavioral Health [30144]
Jennings County • Centerstone of IN Inc [43144]
Jennings Outreach [30152]
Jennings Place [32462]
Jennings Veterans Affairs Clinic [30145]
Jeremiahs Hospice Inc • Jeremiahs Inn [44617]
Jericho Project [39775]
Jerry L. Pettis Memorial Veterans Affairs Medical Center [28563]
Multiple Sclerosis Center [34525]
Jerry's Drug and Surgical Supply [16184]
Jersey Battered Women's Service [9837]
Jersey City Artificial Kidney Center--North Bergen • KRU Medical Ventures [25490]
Jersey City Medical Center
Addiction Services Outpatient [46023]
Liberty Health [25450]
Sickle Cell Disease Center [36379]
Jersey City Vet Center [52024]
Jersey Hospital--Cumberland County Guidance Center [51093]
Jersey Shore Medical Center
Addiction Recovery Services [46077]
Dialysis Unit [25476]
Sickle Cell Disease Center [36380]
Jersey Shore Sports Medicine Center [38746]
Jersey Shore University Medical Center

Cancer Center [4687]
Child Development Division • Down Syndrome Clinic [10828]
Jessamine Counseling & Education Center [30089]
Jesse Brown Addiction Programs • Drug Dependency Treatment Program [42537]
Jesse Brown VA Medical Center [14738]
Addiction Treatment Program [42538]
SARRTP [42539]
Jesse Brown Veterans Affairs Medical Center [29592]
PTSD Clinical Team [51722]
Jessie Trice Center for Community Health [6505]
Jessie Trice Community Health Center Inc [41785]
Jessie's Hope Society • North Fraser Eating Disorders Program [10915]
Jesup Dialysis • DaVita [23724]
Jewett Orthopaedic Clinic of Central Florida--Stirling Center [38248]
Jewett Orthopaedic Clinic of Central Florida--University [38266]
Jewett Orthopaedic Clinic of Central Florida--Winter Park [38298]
Jewish Board of Family and Children's Services--Bronx [31248]
Jewish Board of Family and Children's Services, Inc. • Child Development Center [31420]
Jewish Board of Family and Children's Services • Kingsbrook ICF [31267]
Jewish Board of Family and Children's Services--New York [31421]
Jewish Board of Family and Children's Services • Older Adult Services [31463]
Jewish Board of Family and Children's ServicesManhattan North • Madeline Borg Counseling Service [31422]
Jewish Child Care Association [8344]
Jewish Child and Family Services [29561]
Jewish Community Services [44150]
Jewish Community Services of South FL [41786], [41787], [41805]
Jewish Deaf and Hearing Impaired Council [2925]
Jewish Family and Children Services • Eleanor Haas Koshland Center [28788]
Jewish Family and Children Services--Glendale [28151]
Jewish Family and Children Services--San Rafael [28790]
Jewish Family and Childrens Service [39407], [39435]
Jewish Family and Children's Service of Sarasota-Manatee, Inc. [29289]
Jewish Family and Children's Services • Administrative Headquarters [28174]
Jewish Family and Children's Services--Long Beach [28571]
Jewish Family and Children's Services of Southern Arizona [8740]
Jewish Family and Community Services [29186]
Jewish Family Service [44946], [45057]
Jewish Family Service Association of Cleveland • Drost Family Center [31660]
Jewish Family Service Association • Project Chai • Family Violence Project [10126]
Jewish Family Service of Los Angeles [28596]
Alcohol Drug Action Program [40120]
Jewish Family Service of Los Angeles--North Hollywood [28656]
Jewish Family Service of Metrowest [31143]
Jewish Family Service of Seattle [10647]
Jewish Family Service of Tidewater, Inc. [18343]
Jewish Family Services • Copeline Crisis Line [50948]
Jewish Family Services--Home Care [18366]
Jewish Healthcare Center [15565]
Jewish HealthCare Center/dba Jewish Home Hosice [20015]
Jewish Home and Hospital [16365]
The Jewish Home and Hospital Life Care [16555]
The Jewish Home Lifecare [16556]
Jewish Hospital • Cancer Program [5695]
Jewish Hospital Renal Dialysis--Acute Dialysis [24418]
Jewish Hospital and Saint Mary HealthCare • Saints Mary and Elizabeth Sleep Disorders Center [37028]
Jewish Hospital and Saint Mary's Healthcare--Bardstown [15161]

Jewish Hospital and Saint Mary's Healthcare • Cancer Program [5223]
Jewish Hospital and Saint Mary's Healthcare--Churchman, Louisville [15222]
Jewish Hospital and Saint Mary's Healthcare--Clarksville [14969]
Jewish Hospital and Saint Mary's Healthcare--Elizabethtown [15175]
Jewish Hospital and Saint Mary's Healthcare • Frazier Rehab Institute [38484]
Jewish Hospital and Saint Mary's Healthcare--S 4th-Street, Louisville [15223]
Jewish Hospital and Saint Mary's Healthcare--US Hwy. 42, Louisville [15224]
Jewish Renaissance Medical Center [6983]
Jewish Social Service Agency [8099]
Jewish Social Service Agency Hospice [19940]
JFK Alcohol and Drug Abuse Treatment Center [47222]
JFK Center for Behavioral Health [45977]
JFK Hartwyck at Edison Estates [4281]
JFK Johnson Rehabilitation Institute
Brain Trauma Unit [4282]
Health and Fitness Center [4283]
Outpatient Center at Old Bridge [4284]
Pediatric Rehabilitation Department [8246]
Speech Pathology and Audiology Department [2908]
JFK Johnson Rehabilitation Institution
Center for Head Injuries [4285]
Outpatient Center [4286], [4287]
Shore Rehabilitation Institute [4288]
JFK Medical Center [16204]
JFK Medical Center--Edison • Comprehensive Cancer Program [5509]
JFK Medical Center at Home [16257]
JFK Medical Center--Lake Worth • Cancer Care Program [4956]
JFK Pediatric Rehabilitation Department [2909]
JHHLCS [3063]
JHU/Cornerstone [44151]
Jim 'Catfish' Hunter ALS Clinic [135]
Jim Gilmore Jr. Community Healing Center [30580]
Jim Taliaferro CMHC [47946]
Jim Taliaferro Community Mental Health Center--Altus [31870]
Jim Taliaferro Community Mental Health Center--Anadarko [31871]
Jim Taliaferro Community Mental Health Center--Duncan [31882]
Jim Taliaferro Community Mental Health Center--Lawton [31888]
Jim Taliaferro Community Mental Health Center • Psychosocial Clubhouse [31889]
Jims Alcohol and Drug Services [47391]
Jireh Counseling Center [41002]
Jireh Home Health Agency [14045]
JMB Nursing Service [16342]
JNS Counseling Services Inc • CD Outpatient Clinic [46510]
Jo Wells Education Center [374]
Joab Home Health Agency, LLC [18110]
Joan Chomark and Associates [1214]
Joan and Howard Woltz Hospice Home [20644]
The Job Site [31016]
Joe DiMaggio Children's Hospital • Cystic Fibrosis Center [7502]
Joe Healy Medical Detoxification • Project [40618]
Joel Nevers - Private Practice [43991]
John and Arloine Mandrin Chesapeake Hospice House [19928]
John Brooks Recovery Center [45926]
John C. Fremont Healthcare District Hospice [18963]
John C. Lincoln Hospital [968]
John Cunio Dialysis Center • Fresenius Medical Care [23401]
John D. Archbold Memorial Hospital
Lewis Hall Singletary Oncology Center [5042]
Sleep Disorders Center [36842]
John D Dingel Veteran Affairs Med Center • Chemical Dependence Treatment Services [44743]
John D. Dingell VA Medical Center [4172], [15637], [20053]
John D. Dingell Veterans Administration Medical Center • Sleep/Wake Disorders Center [37166]
John D. Dingell Veterans Affairs Medical Center [30542]

Cancer Program [5372]
PTSD Clinical Team [51755]
John Darby Assisted Living Facility [6556]
John Dempsey Hospital • University of Connecticut
Health Center • Neag Comprehensive Cancer
Center [4893]
John E Davis MA • 2Xtreme PC [41255]
John F. Keever Solace Center [20622]
John F. Kennedy Community Mental Health/Mental
Retardation Center [32089]
Life Acceptance Clinic--Partial Hospital [32090]
John F Kennedy Drug Treatment Clinic [48534]
John G. Leach School [7866]
John Glen and Associates [45824]
John H. Kinzie Elementary School [395]
John H. Stroger Jr. Hospital of Cook County
Cancer Care Program [5069]
Division of Nephrology [23940]
John Heinz Institute of Rehabilitation Medicine
[4395]
The John Henry Foundation [28796]
John Hopkins Children's Center [19913]
John Hopkins Hospital Sleep Disorders Center
[37102]
John Hopkins Pediatric Sleep Center • John Hop-
kins Hospital [37103]
John J. Doherty [38444]
John J. Pershing VA Medical Center [16044]
John J. Pershing Veterans Affairs Medical Center
[51597]
PTSD Clinical Team [51764]
John L. Gildner Regional Institute for Children and
Adolescents Rockville [34178]
John L. McClellan Memorial VA Medical Center •
Multiple Sclerosis Center [34518]
John L. McClellan Memorial VAMC • Mental Hygiene
Unit [28299]
John L Norris • Addiction Treatment Center [47041]
John Lewis Coffee Shop • Runaway and Homeless
Youth Program [35957]
John Muir Behavioral Health • Center for Recovery
[39738]
John Muir Medical Center [13436]
John Muir Medical Center-Concord • Cancer Center
[4767]
John Muir Medical Center-Walnut Creek •
Comprehensive Cancer Center [4865]
John P. Murtha Neuroscience and Pain Institute •
ALS Center [144]
John Randolph Medical Center • Cancer Care
Program [6064]
John S. Charlton School [7863]
John S. Dunn, Sr. Burn Center [4636]
John T. Mather Hospital • Sleep Disorders Center
[37396]
John T. Mather Memorial Hospital
Cancer Program [5608]
Eating Disorder Partial Hospitalization and
Intensive Outpatient Program [11159]
Eating Disorder Program [11160]
John T Mather Memorial Hospital • Mather
Outpatient Alcoholism Clinic [46986]
John Umstead Hospital • Children's Psychiatric
Institute [33734]
Johns Community Hospital [18169]
Johns Creek Sleep Disorders Center [36843]
Johns Creek Technology Park • Fusion Center for
Sleep Disorders [36844]
Johns Hopkins Bayview Medical Center [37104]
Audiology Department [2375]
Center for Addiction and Pregnancy [44152]
Comm Psychiatry Prog/Adult Outpatient/MISA
[44153]
Sports Medicine [38516]
Johns Hopkins Eating Disorders Program [11081]
Johns Hopkins Fertility Center & IVF Program • Div.
Of Reproductive Endocrinology & Infertility • Fertil-
ity Center [22090]
Johns Hopkins Health Care and Surgery Center--
White Marsh • Sports Medicine [38537]
Johns Hopkins Home Care Group [15417]
Johns Hopkins Hospital Broadway Center [44154]
Johns Hopkins Hospital
Department of Neurosurgery [35478]
kimmel Comprehensive Cancer Center [5286]
Mount Washington Pediatric Sleep Center
[37105]
Pediatric Cystic Fibrosis Center [7561]

School of Medicine • Johns Hopkins Outpatient
Center Multiple Sclerosis Center [34593]
Johns Hopkins Medical Institutions • Johns Hopkins
Outpatient Center [2376]
Johns Hopkins Outpatient Care • Dialysis Unit
[24648]
Johns Hopkins Regional • Burn and Wound Unit
[4559]
Johns Hopkins Sports Medicine • Division of Sports
Medicine & Shoulder Surgery [38527]
Johns Hopkins University
Adult Cystic Fibrosis Center [7562]
Center for Immunization Research • HIV Vac-
cine Trials Unit [82]
Johns Hopkins University Hospital • Pain Manage-
ment [35479]
Johns Hopkins University • Institute of Genetic
Medicine [12228]
Johns Hopkins University at JHBMC • Behavioral
Pharmacology Research Unit [44155]
Johns Hopkins University Medical Center •
Hemophilia Program [12528]
Johns Hopkins University
School of Medicine
Adult AIDS Clinical Trials Unit [12]
MDA/ALS Center [34809]
Sickle Cell Center for Adults [36355]
Johnson and Associates • Counseling and Consulta-
tion Group PC [45974]
Johnson City Medical Center
Cancer Program [5934]
Center for Sleep Disorders [37767]
Johnson County Community College • Access
Services [437]
Johnson County Counseling Center [32363]
Johnson County Crisis Center [50905]
Johnson County Dialysis • DaVita [24334]
Johnson County Family Crisis Center--Buffalo
[10747]
Johnson County Family Crisis Center--Cleburne
[10450]
Johnson County Healthcare Center [18645]
Johnson County Hospice Care [20345]
Johnson County Mental Health Center [33509]
ACT Olathe [43424]
Adolescent Center for Treatment [34147]
ADU Shawnee [43459]
FACT [43438]
Outpatient Mission [43408]
Outpatient Substance Abuse Services [43425]
Johnson County Safe Haven, Inc. [10422]
Johnson County SSA [813]
Johnson Dialysis Center [23469]
Johnson/Ellis/Navarro Mental Health Mental
Retardation • Ellis County Clinic [32568]
Johnson/Ellis/Navarro Mental Health/Mental Retarda-
tion Services [32426]
Johnson Memorial Hospital [41469]
Audiology Department [2147]
Cancer Center [4714], [5148]
Johnson Mental Health Center [49052]
Main Center [32280]
Johnson Mental Retardation Group Home [33954]
Johnson Physical Therapy, Inc. [38903]
Johnson Regional Medical Center [1000]
Sleep Laboratory [36647]
Johnson Street Home [32986]
Johnston Counseling Services [47497]
Johnston County Mental Health Center [31592]
Johnston Dialysis Center • Fresenius Medical Care
[25951]
Johnston Memorial Home Care & Hospice [20737]
Johnston Memorial Hospital [16780]
Johnston Memorial Hospital Home Care [18242]
Johnston Recovery Services [47271]
Joint Ambulatory Care Clinic [14337]
Joint Military Family Abuse Shelter [9141]
Joint Rehabilitation & Sports Medical Center, Inc.
[38097]
Joint Township District Memorial Hospital [17029]
Joliet Area Community Hospice [19531]
Joliet Orthopedic & Sportsmedicine Center [38397]
Jonahs Place [49381]
Jonathan M. Wainwright Memorial VA Medical
Center [21779]
Jonathan M. Wainwright Memorial Veterans Affairs
Medical Center [18480], [32881], [51671]
Jonathan M Wainwright VA Medical Center • SAR-

RTP/Res and Outpatient Treatment [50251]
Jonathan Wade Center • Growth and Development
[41594]
Jones Behavioral Health Inc [42044]
Jones County Medical Supplies, Inc. [15969]
Jones Institute for Reproductive Medicine [22285]
Jones Memorial Health Center • Adult Mental Health
Unit • Jamestown Crisis Line [51142]
Jones Regional Medical Center [29839]
Jonesboro Mental Health Clinic [30146]
Jonesville Addictive Disorders Clinic [43834]
Joni Fair Hospice House [19124]
Joplin Health Care Center [2794]
JOPPA Health Serices Inc [44302]
Jordan Hospital Rehabilitation [2515]
Jordan Recovery Center [39769], [39770]
Jordans Crossing Inc [47982]
Jos--El Care Agency [16652]
Josdan Home Health Care [14836]
Joseph D. Brandenburg Center [8090]
Joseph H. Tyler Jr. Mental Health Center [33539]
Joseph M. Smith Community Health Center, Inc.
[6801], [6828]
Joseph P. Addabbo Family Health Center [7008]
Joseph R Briscoe Treatment Center [43844]
Joseph Richey Hospice, Inc. [19914]
Josephine Chen Center for Speech and Language
Pathology--Greenwich [1462]
Josephine Chen Center for Speech and Language
Pathology--Norwalk [1483]
Josephine County Community Corrections •
Substance Abuse Treatment Program [48121]
Josephine County Humane Services Department
[31942]
Josephine County Mental Health [51254]
Joshua Center of Brooklyn [33240]
Joshua Center Mansfield [33250]
Joshua Center of Montville [33264]
Joshua House [49633]
Joshua Intermediate School District [797]
Josie's Place [28628]
Josselyn Center for Mental Health [29655]
Journey Center Inc [48944]
Journey Counseling Services [45149]
Journey Home [45318]
The Journey Home [43824]
Journey Hospice [20350]
Journey House [29005]
Journey LLC [49663]
Journey Malibu [40195]
Journey to Self Understanding
Outpatient Substance Abuse [44334]
Outpatient Substance Abuse Program [44357]
Journey to Wellness Inc [46131]
Journey at Willowcreek • Family Tree Center LLC
[49687]
Journeys Counseling Center Inc [41355]
Journeys End Counseling • Consulting and Training
LLC [42008]
Journeys Hospice, Inc. [19474]
Journeys Program [45728]
Journeys for Women Adult Program [44335]
Joyce C Williams Center for Battered Women and
Children [9363]
Joyce Fails Home • JBS Mental Health Authority
[27864]
Joyce Goldenberg Hospice Inpatient Residence
[19298]
Joyce Marty K Frazho • Independent Contractor
[44673]
Joyful Noise Speech and Language Therapy
Services [1861]
Joyner Sportsmedicine Institute [39011]
Joyner Therapy [1559]
JP Sleep Diagnostic Services [37601]
JPK Home Care, LLS • DBA/ Care Minders Home
Care [15880]
JPS Health Network • Center for Cancer Care
[4711]
JSAS Healthcare [46078]
The Juanita Center [50029]
Jubilee House of Gunnison County, Inc. [8970]
Jude House Inc [44201]
Judge Blair Reeves Rehabilitation Center [4448]
Judith Karman Hospice Inc. [20976]
Judson Center [30626]
Judson Washtenaw Regional Center [30504]
Judy Center for Down Syndrome • Hackensack

University Medical Center [10829]
Judy Haymon 3 • Wigley Home [27931]
Judy Haymon - Holiday Home [28036]
Julia M. Davis Speech-Language-Hearing Center
[2713]
Julian Center, Inc. [9286]
Julian F. Keith Alcohol and Drug Abuse Center
[31506]
Julien Care Facility [29867]
Jump Street [28597]
Junction City Veterans Affairs Clinic [29934]
June Jenkins Women's Shelter [9405]
Juneau County Human Service Center [50460]
Juneau School District [221]
Juneau Urgent Care and Family Medical Clinic •
Pain Clinic [35277]
Juneau Youth Services • Chemical Dependency
Program [39336]
Juneau Youth Services, inc. [33961]
Juneau Youth Services, Inc. • Wallington House
[33962]
Juneau Youth Services • Runaway and Homeless
Youth Program [35788]
Junta Centro de Salud [7212]
Jupiter Kidney Center LLC • American Renal Associ-
ates [23353]
Jupiter Medical Center [34778]
   Foshay Cancer Center [4955]
   Sleep Disorders Center [36788]
Jupiter Vet Center [51923]
Just Kids Learning Center [1281]
Justice Resource Institute, Inc. [34183]
Justice Services [39393], [39467]
Justine Sherman and Associates Inc. [1320]
Juvenile Justice • Stanislaus County Behavioral
Health [28629]
J.V. Home Health Services [13751]
JWCH/Clinic Institute • Safe Harbor Women's Clinic
[6318]
Jzanus Home Care, Inc.--Floral Park [16457]
Jzanus Home Care, Inc.--New York [16557]
Jzanus Home Care--Patchogue [16590]

K

K and S Health Care [14046]
Ka Hale Pomaikai [42257]
Kachemak Bay Sports Medicine [38023]
Kadlec Medical Center • Cancer Program [6111]
Kaerbear's Healthcare [13797], [14047]
Kahala Elementary School [383]
Kahana Dialysis • Liberty Dialysis Hawaii [23859]
Kahi Mohala Behavioral Health [29510]
Kailua-Kona Veterans Center [29527]
Kaimuki Dialysis • Liberty Dialysis [23850]
Kairos Healthcare Inc
   Family Care Center [44675], [44999]
   Outpatient Clinic [44676]
Kaiser Department of Mental Health and Chemical
Depend Services [40395]
Kaiser Foundation Hospital - Anaheim [12891]
Kaiser Foundation Hospital - Bellflower [12907]
Kaiser Foundation Hospital • Cancer Program
[5787]
Kaiser Foundation Hospital - Fontana [12999]
Kaiser Foundation Hospital - Fremont/Hayward
Medical Center [13075]
Kaiser Foundation Hospital • Genetic Services
[12157]
Kaiser Foundation Hospital Home Health [13284]
Kaiser Foundation Hospital
   Home Health [13365]
   Home Health Agency, Redwood City [13259]
   Home Health Agency, Santa Clara [12971]
   Home Health Department [13245]
   Home Health--San Francisco [13309]
   Hospice and Home Health [13403]
   Kaiser Valley MSA--Lancaster • Home Health/
   Hospice/Continuing Care [13100]
Kaiser Foundation Hospital - Los Angeles Medical
Center [13137]
Kaiser Foundation Hospital Medical Center--
Anaheim • Kaiser Permanente • PD Unit [23082]
Kaiser Foundation Hospital Medical Center--Downey
• Kaiser Permanente [22663]
Kaiser Foundation Hospital Medical Center--Fontana
• Kaiser Permanente [22687]
Kaiser Foundation Hospital Medical Center--

Riverside • Kaiser Permanente [22905]
Kaiser Foundation Hospital Medical Center--Sunset
• Kaiser Permanente [22783]
Kaiser Foundation Hospital Medical Center--West
Los Angeles • Kaiser Permanente • Acute Dialysis
Center [22784]
Kaiser Foundation Hospital--Metro Los Angeles •
Home Health and Hospice [13138]
Kaiser Foundation Hospital • Oakland Genetics
Department [12158]
Kaiser Foundation Hospital - Oakland/Richmond
[13220]
Kaiser Foundation Hospital - Riverside [13270]
Kaiser Foundation Hospital Roseville [13277]
Kaiser Foundation Hospital - San Diego/El Cajon
[13297]
Kaiser Foundation Hospital - San Francisco [13310]
Kaiser Foundation Hospital, San Rafael [13327]
Kaiser Foundation Hospital--San Rafael • Home
Health [13219]
Kaiser Foundation Hospital - Santa Clara [13331]
Kaiser Foundation Hospital - Santa Rosa [13341]
Kaiser Foundation Hospital
   Santa Teresa Home Health and Hospice [13317]
   Tri--Central Home Health and Hospice [12975]
Kaiser Foundation Hospital--Vallejo [13408]
Kaiser Foundation Hospital - Valley Service Area
[13235]
Kaiser Foundation Hospital - Walnut Creek [13437]
Kaiser Foundation Rehabilitation Center [3906]
Kaiser Hayward Hospice Program [19067]
Kaiser Hospital ESRD PD Unit [22722]
Kaiser Hospital Hemodialysis [22955]
Kaiser Milpitas Chem Dependency Services •
Department of Psychiatry [40224]
Kaiser Permanente [40943], [50007]
   Addiction Medicine [40121]
Kaiser Permanente--Atlanta [1824]
Kaiser Permanente--Aurora [19086]
Kaiser Permanente • Behavioral Health Services
[42211], [42294], [42298]
Kaiser Permanente Behavioral Healthcare Helpline
[50685]
Kaiser Permanente--Bellflow • Pain Block Center
[35316]
Kaiser Permanente/Bellflower Med Center •
Orchard/Imperial Outpatient Clinic [39786]
Kaiser Permanente
   Chemical Dependency Recovery Program
   [39859], [40301], [40882]
   Chemical Dependency Services [40870],
   [40933]
Kaiser Permanente Continuing Care [21022]
Kaiser Permanente Continuing Care Service [17216]
Kaiser Permanente • Department of Addiction
Medicine [48193]
Kaiser Permanente Fontana • Home Health and
Hospice Agency [13000]
Kaiser Permanente--Hayward • Department of
Genetics [12159]
Kaiser Permanente--Honolulu • Hawaii Speech
Language Services Department [1934]
Kaiser Permanente Hospice [18915]
Kaiser Permanente Hospital • Chemical
Dependency Recovery Program [39830]
Kaiser Permanente--Martinez [18964], [22802]
Kaiser Permanente Medical Care Program
   Adult Cystic Fibrosis Center [7470]
   Pediatric Cystic Fibrosis Center [7471]
Kaiser Permanente Medical Center [47835]
   Chemical Dependency Services [40490],
   [40539]
Kaiser Permanente Medical Center--San Francisco •
Genetic Services Department [12160]
Kaiser Permanente Medical Center--San Jose •
Department of Genetics Services [12161]
Kaiser Permanente Medical Group • Chemical
Dependency Recovery Program [39773], [40558]
Kaiser Permanente Mental Health [28377]
Kaiser Permanente • Mental Health and Chemical
Dependency [39608]
Kaiser Permanente Merrifield Mental Health Center
[32731]
Kaiser Permanente Northwest Region • Cystic
Fibrosis Center [7646]
Kaiser Permanente Oahu Home Health Agency
[14620]
Kaiser Permanente--Sacramento • Department of

Genetics [12162]
Kaiser Permanente--Santa Clara [22998]
Kaiser Permanente • Sickle Cell Disease Center for
Children [36299]
Kaiser-Permanente Southern California • Cystic
Fibrosis Center [7472]
Kaiser Permanente--Walnut Creek • Department of
Genetics [12163]
Kaiser Permanente--Woodland Hills • Dialysis
Center [23081]
Kaiser San Jose • Alcohol and Drug Abuse
Programs [40660]
Kalamazoo Central Dialysis • DaVita [24926]
Kalamazoo Mental Health & Substance Abuse
Services [30581]
Kalamazoo PD Unit • Fresenius Medical Care
[24927]
Kalamazoo Psychiatric Hospital [33597]
Kalamazoo Psychology LLC [44869]
Kalamazoo West Dialysis and At Home • DaVita
[24928]
Kaleida Health • Buffalo Therapy Services--
Williamsville [3000]
Kali Brewer LLC • DBA Asheville Institute [47211]
Kalihi-Palama Health Center [6617]
Kalispel Tribe • Social Services Alcohol Program
[49932]
Kalispell VA Community Based Outpatient Clinic •
VA Montana Health Care System [4252]
Kalispell Vet Center [52011]
Kalispell Veterans Affairs Clinic [30950]
Kalkaska Dialysis Center [24929]
Kaltag Counseling Center [28103]
Kamara Center for Learning and Communication
Disorders [2429]
Kamp Talk-a-Lot [980]
Kanasas Rehabilitation Hospital [38468]
Kanawha Hospice Care--Charleston [21794]
Kanawha Hospice Care-Lewisburg [21803]
Kanawha Hospice Care-Madison [21804]
Kanawha Hospice Care-Summersville [21814]
Kandiyohi County Boys Group Home [34259]
Kane School District [837]
Kankakee County Coalition Against Domestic
Violence--Kankakee • Harbor House [9237]
Kankakee County Coalition Against Domestic
Violence--Watseka • Watseka Office • Harbor
House [9256]
Kankakee County Dialysis and At Home • DaVita
[23904]
Kanmar Place [18831]
Kannapolis City Schools [621]
Kansas Children's Service League • Runaway and
Homeless Youth Program • Oasis I [35961]
Kansas City Anti--Violence Project [9688]
Kansas City Community Center [45596]
   Community Supervision Center [45438], [45640]
   Independence Site [45501]
   R-2 [45518]
Kansas City Hospice House [20311]
Kansas City Hospice & Palliative Care--
Independence [20301]
Kansas City Hospice & Palliative Care--Kansas City
[20312]
Kansas City Hospice & Palliative Care--Overland
Park [19770]
Kansas City Indian Center • Morningstar Outpatient
Program [45519]
Kansas City Metro Methadone Program [43376]
Kansas City Missouri School District [527]
Kansas City Psychiatric and • Psychological
Services LLC [45502]
Kansas City Regional Hemophilia Center • The
Children's Mercy Hospital [12549]
Kansas City VA Medical Center [4235]
Kansas City Vet Center [52005]
Kansas City Veterans Affairs Medical Center
[16022], [30861]
Kansas Department of Health and Environment •
Bureau for Children, Youth and Families [36482]
Kansas Department of Human Services • Kansas
City Metro Region [2237]
Kansas Dialysis Services--Lawrence [24331]
Kansas Dialysis Services--Manhattan [24338]
Kansas Dialysis Services--Ottawa [24342]
Kansas Dialysis Services--Sabetha [24346]
Kansas Dialysis Services--Topeka [24349]

Kansas Elks Training Center for the Handicapped [8038]
Kansas Eye Bank and Cornea Research Center [35046]
Kansas Neurological Institute [2245], [8036]
Kansas Orthopedics and Sports Medicine [38469]
Kansas Rehabilitation Hospital [15154]
Kansas School for the Deaf [436]
Kansas State Library • Kansas Talking Books Regional Library [3794]
Kansas State School for the Blind [3710]
Kansas Statewide Farmworker Health Program [6721]
Kansas Treatment Services LLC [43377]
Kansas University Department of Neurology • Sleep Medicine Clinic [36991]
Kanza Mental Health & Guidance Center [29930]
Kapahulu Dialysis Center • Fresenius Medical Care [23851]
Kapi Olani Medical Center for Women and Children • Cancer Program [4671]
Kapiolani Community College/Gallaudet University Regional Center • Program for Deaf and Hard of Hearing Students [384]
Kapiolani Medical Center for Women and Children
    Fetal Diagnostic Center and Genetic Counseling [12193]
    Hemophilia and Thrombosis Center of Hawaii [12513]
Kaplan Family Hospice [20590]
Kaplan Family Hospice House [19955]
Kappa Home Health Services, Inc. [18166]
KAR House • Residential Substance Abuse Program [39342]
Kara Lee and Associates [44962]
Karen Ann Quinlan Hospice - Northwest New Jersey [20486]
Karen Glick Ed S [46153]
Karmanos Cancer Institute • Cancer Center [5373]
Kartini Clinic for Disordered Eating [11249]
Karuk Tribe • Health and Human Services Program [39904]
Kassy Home Health Care [13871]
Katahdin Valley Health CenterPatten [6781]
Kate B. Reynolds Hospice Home [20771]
Kathadin Valley Health Center--Houlton [6776]
Katherine and Duncan Phillips LifeCare & Counseling Center [20765]
Katherine Vickery MI Residential Home [27889]
Kathi Cullop • DBA ACCENT Counseling [42452]
Kathleen Mary House [9901]
Kathryn Benson Clinical Consulting [49156]
Kathryn Klein LCSW [44014]
Kathy J. Weinman Shelter for Battered Women and Their Children [9717]
Katy Cinco Ranch Dialysis • DaVita [27198]
Katy Dialysis Center • DaVita [27199]
Katz Head and Neck [2240]
Katz Orthopaedic Surgery & Sports Medicine [38336]
Kauai Dialysis Facility • Liberty Dialysis [23861]
Kauai Hospice [19445]
Kauai Vet Center [51941]
Kauai YWCA • Alternatives to Violence [9154]
Kaufman Children's Center for Speech and Language Disorders [2665]
Kaufman Dialysis • DaVita [27202]
Kavannagh House on 56th St. [19686]
Kaw Valley Center • Runaway and Homeless Youth Services [35962]
Kaw Valley Psychiatric Hospital [33505]
Kaweah Delta Dialysis Facility [23060]
Kaweah Delta District Hospital • Sleep Disorders Center [36670]
Kaweah Delta Health Care District [13429]
    Cancer Care Program [4864]
    Hospice of Tulare County, Inc. [19071]
Kaweah Delta Mental Health Hosptial • Kaweah Delta Family Recovery Center [40920]
Kay Freeman Health Center [6554]
Kayenta Outpatient Treatment Center [39398]
Kayne--Eras Center [7772]
KBICSAP • Outpatient Counseling Services [44653]
KBTCAP • New Day [44877]
KC Services [39874]
KCCS LLC [43731]
KCI--USA Anchorage [12739]
Ke Ala Pono/Hawaii Counseling and Education

Center, Inc. [9150]
Keaau Elementary School [387]
Kearney Public Schools [537]
Kedish House • Domestic Violence Program [10111]
Kedren Community Mental Health Center [33152]
Keeler Center for the Study of Headache [12387]
Keeler's Medical Supply, Inc. [18488]
Keep the Faith Foundation [42540]
Keeping the Faith [8784]
Keesler Air Force Base • ADAPT Program [45398]
Keesler Air Force Base Medical Center • Cancer Program [5423]
Keetoowah Cherokee Treatment Services [48041]
Keller Chiropractic and Sports Rehabilitation [38112]
Kelley Drive Home [30239]
Kelley's Rainbow--Albertville [8635]
Kelly Center FHSU Drug and Alcohol • Wellness Network Hays [43358]
Kelly Home Healthcare, Inc. [14794]
Kelly Street Supervised Community Residence [31249]
Kelowna General Hospital • Multiple Sclerosis Clinic [34520]
Kelsey--Seybold Clinic • Crump Cancer Center [5994]
Kempsville Dialysis Center • Fresenius Medical Care [27525]
Ken-O-Sha Preschool and Diagnostic Center [2596]
Kenai Peninsula Community Care Center [33963]
Kenai Peninsula Orthopaedics [38025]
Kenaitze Indian Tribe • Nakenu Family [39340]
Kendall Comprehensive Inc. [14048]
Kendall County Health Department [42975]
Kendall Home Care [14049]
Kendall Home Health Agency, LLC [14050]
Kendall Manor [31731]
Kendall Speech and Language Center Inc. [1656]
Kendallville Dialysis Center • Diversified Specialty Institutes [24184]
Kendallwood Hospice-Riverside [20330]
Kene Me-Wu Family Healing Center, Inc. [8911]
Kennebec Behavioral Health [44059], [44077]
Kennebec Behavioral Health--Augusta [50954]
Kennebec Behavioral Health--Skowhegan [30242], [50964]
Kennebec Behavioral Health--Stone Street, Augusta [30182]
Kennebec Behavioral Health • Substance Abuse Services [43915]
Kennebec Behavioral Health--Waterville [30249], [50965]
Kennebec Behavioral Health--Western Avenue, Augusta [30183]
Kennebec Behavioral Health--Winthrop [50966]
Kennebec Kidney Center • Fresenius Medical Care [24603]
Kennebec Valley Mental Health Center [8085]
Kennebunk Community Residence • Sweetser [34163]
Kennedy Brothers Physical Therapy [38544]
Kennedy Child Study Center [8332]
Kennedy Home Dialysis • DaVita [23941]
Kennedy Hospital Dialysis Center--Stratford [25525]
Kennedy Hospital--Washington • Dialysis Unit [25507]
Kennedy Krieger Children's Hospital--Fairmount [4098]
Kennedy Krieger Institute
    Down Syndrome Clinic [10808]
    Genetics Laboratory [12229]
    Speech and Language Department [2377]
Kennedy Learning Center [637]
Kennedy Mem Hosp/Cherry Hill Division • Substance Abuse Services /Detox and Outpatient [45957]
Kennedy Memorial Hospital • Behavioral Health Services [46162]
Kennedy Memorial Hospital--University Medical Center [31116]
Kennedy Memorial Hospitals - University Medical Center Home Healthcare [16285]
Kennedy-Willis Center on Down Syndrome [10832]
Kenner Orthopedic & Sports Therapy, Inc. [38496]
Kenner Regional Dialysis • DaVita [24514]
Kennestone Dialysis and At Home • DaVita [23752]
Kenneth Peters Center for Recovery • Outpatient Alcoholism Clinic [47111]

Kennewick General Hospital [18433]
    Cancer Program [6101]
    Columbia Sleep Center [37917]
Kenosha Community Health Center [7427]
Kenosha Hospital and Medical Center Rehabilitation West [39177]
Kenosha Human Development Services Inc. • Runaway and Homeless Youth Program [36266]
Kenosha Kidney Dialysis [27728]
Kensington Hospital
    Addiction Services [48535]
    Methadone Maintenance Program [48536]
Kent Center [48888]
The Kent Center - Cedar House [32145]
The Kent Center - Hillsgrove House [32182]
The Kent Center for Human and Organizational Development [32183]
Kent County Behavioral Health [44218]
Kent Dialysis Center • DaVita [27609]
Kent District Library for the Blind and Physically Handicapped • Wyoming Branch Library [3807]
Kent General Sports Medicine Center [38202]
Kent Hospital • Cancer Program [5896]
Kent Kidney Center • Northwest Kidney Center [27610]
Kent Sussex Counseling Services [41502], [41507], [41509]
Kent/Sussex Mobile Crisis Unit [50742]
Kent Youth and Family Services [49985]
Kentuckiana Pain Specialists Inc. [35459]
Kentucky Children's Hospital [44404]
Kentucky Correctional Psychiatric Center [33523]
Kentucky Department of Public Health • Child Fatality/Injury Prevention [36484]
Kentucky Nephrology [24405]
Kentucky Organ Donor Affiliates--Bowling Green [35048]
Kentucky Organ Donor Affiliates--Huntington, WV [35262]
Kentucky Organ Donor Affiliates--Lexington [35049]
Kentucky Organ Donor Affiliates--Louisville [35050]
Kentucky Organ Donor Affiliates--Paducah [35051]
Kentucky River Community Care [50933]
Kentucky River Community Care Inc
    Breathitt Outpatient [43638]
    Knott County Outpatient Office [43585]
    Lee Outpatient [43530]
    Leslie County Outpatient [43635]
    Letcher County Outpatient Office [43711]
    Perry County [43621]
    Project Advance [43622]
    Sewell Family and Childrens Center [43639]
    Wolfe County Outpatient [43551]
Kentucky River Community Care, Inc.--Beattyville • Riverbend Treatment Center [29972]
Kentucky River Community Care, Inc.--Hazard [30031]
Kentucky River Community Care, Inc.--Isom [30036]
Kentucky River Community Care, Inc.--Jackson • Breathitt County Outpatient Services [30037]
Kentucky School for the Blind [3711]
Kentucky School for the Deaf [2262]
Kentucky Talking Book Library [3798]
Kentucky United Methodist Homes for Children and Youth [34158]
Keokuk Area Hospital Home Health Care [15092]
Keokuk Area Hospital • Sleep Disorders Center [36979]
Kerlan-Jobe Beverly Hills [38076]
Kerlan--Jobe Orthopaedic Clinic [38098]
Kerlan-Jobe Orthopaedic Clinic [38072], [38114]
Kerman Recovery Center [39952]
Kern County Mental Health Department • Wasco Clinic [40935]
Kern County Mental Health Services • Adult Outpatient Service-Rehab 3 [28392]
Kern County Superintendent of Schools [263]
Kern High School District [264]
Kern Medical Center • Regional Oncology Center [4760]
Kernan Outpatient Neuro Services [2378]
Kerr Youth and Family Center [34401]
Kerrs Counseling Concordia [43328]
Kerrville Dialysis • DaVita • Dialysis Center & At Home [27203]
Kerrville Division - South Texas Veterans Health Care System [18025]
Kerrville Intermediate School District [798]

Kerrville State Hospital [33875]
Kerrville Veterans Affairs Hospital [32491]
Kershaw County Medical Center [17566]
Kershaw Health Hospice [21209]
Kershaw Health • Sleep Diagnostics Center [37734]
Kesling Home Health Care Center [15023]
Kessler Foundation Research Center • Multiple Sclerosis Center [34634]
Kessler Institute for Rehabilitation [2945], [8280]
Kessler Institute for Rehabilitation--East Orange Facility • Speech Services [2955]
Kessler Institute for Rehabilitation, Inc.
    Saddle Brook Facility [4289]
    Welkind Facility [4290]
Kessler Institute for Rehabilitation
    Northern New Jersey Spinal Cord Injury System [4291]
    West Orange Facility [4292]
Kessler Physical Therapy and Fitness [38742]
Kessler Physical Therapy and Rehabilitation--Chester [38717]
Kessler Physical Therapy and Rehabilitation--Saddle Brook [38758]
Kessler Physical Therapy and Rehabilitation--West Orange [38767]
Ketchikan General Hospital [12755]
Ketchikan General Hospital--Washington Street [12756]
Ketchikan Indian Community • Tribal Clinic Behavioral Health Dept [39343]
Kettering Dialysis & At Home • DaVita [26143]
Kettering Home Health Service [16992]
Kettering Medical Center Home Health Service [16954]
Kettering Medical Center Network • Cancer Program [5728]
Kettering Medical Center • Sleep Disorders Center [37533]
Kettering Sports Medicine Center [38882]
Kevin and Associates Inc [42660]
Kewaunee County Dept of Human Services • Alcohol and Drug Abuse Treatment Prog [50428]
Keweenaw Bay Indian Community • VOCA [9515]
Key Development Center [44680]
Key to Life Counseling [41003]
Key Point Health Services--Aberdeen [30254]
Key Point Health Services--Baltimore [30262]
Key Point Health Services, Inc.--Catonsville • Outpatient Clinic [30273]
Key Point Health Services, Inc.--Dundalk • Outpatient Clinic [30281]
Key Program, Inc.--Framingham [30383]
Key Program, Inc.--Pittsfield [30447]
Key Program, Inc. - Western Key [30467]
Keys to Communication [2771]
Keys Health Care [13664]
Keyserling Cancer Center [4704]
Keystone [45870]
Keystone Care, LLC [21176]
Keystone Community Resources [8453]
Keystone Family Medicine [7155]
Keystone Hall [45916]
Keystone House, Inc. [29031]
    Group Home [29032]
    Halfway House and DBT [29033]
Keystone Outpatient Program [49022]
Keystone Rural Health Center • Keystone Family Medical Center [7156]
Keystone Substance Abuse Services [48972]
Keystone Treatment Center • Bowling Green Inn of SD [48994]
Khaleidoscope Health Care Inc [46024]
Khepera House [40906], [40907], [40908], [40909], [40910]
KI BOIS Community Action Foundation • DBA The Oaks RSC [48009]
Kiamichi Council on Alcoholism and Other Drug Abuse Inc [47925], [47943], [47944]
Kiamichi Family Medical Center [7102]
Kibler Hall [31647]
KiBois Community Action Foundation, Inc. [10214]
Kickapoo Emergency Shelter [9359]
Kid Partners Inc. [2787]
Kid Talk [1609]
Kid Talk Inc. [2748]
Kid Talk and Play [969]
Kid Talk Speech Therapy Services [1913]
Kidability Speech Therapy [932]

Kidcare Nursing Services [13692]
Kidney Care of Acadiana--Lafayette [24522]
Kidney Care of Acadiana--New Iberia • Dialysis Facility [24547]
Kidney Care Center of the North Valley [22713]
Kidney Care Centers of Zanesville • American Renal Associates [26243]
Kidney Care of Largo • DaVita [24702]
Kidney Care of Laurel • DaVita [24703]
Kidney Care Services of Brookville [26386]
Kidney Care Services of DuBois [26417]
Kidney Care Services of Philipsburg [26541]
Kidney Center of Arvada • American Renal Associates [23089]
Kidney Center of Columbus East • American Renal Associates [26086]
Kidney Center of Columbus North • American Renal Associates [26087]
Kidney Center of Columbus South • American Renal Associates [26088]
Kidney Center of Greater Hazelton • American Renal Associates [26444]
Kidney Center Inc. • Kidney Dialysis Center of Ventura LLC [23057]
Kidney Center of Jasper • American Renal Associates [27195]
Kidney Center of Lafayette • American Renal Associates [23126]
Kidney Center of Lakewood • American Renal Associates [23128]
Kidney Center of Longmont • American Renal Associates [23131]
Kidney Center of Los Angeles [22785]
Kidney Center of Lubbock [27236]
Kidney Center at Millville • South Jersey Healthcare [25468]
Kidney Center of Panorama City • Dialysis Facility [22874]
Kidney Center of Van Nuys [23055]
Kidney Center of Westminster • American Renal Associates [23144]
Kidney Dialysis Center LLC • DaVita [23745]
Kidney Dialysis Center of Northridge, LLC [22842]
Kidney Dialysis Center of Pismo Beach [22880]
Kidney Dialysis Center of San Luis Obispo [22984]
Kidney Dialysis Center of Templeton LLC • Kidney Center Inc. [23032]
Kidney Disease Clinic--Central San Antonio • Dialysis Facility • Fresenius Medical Care [27329]
Kidney Disease Clinic of San Antonio • Fresenius Medical Care [27330]
Kidney Disease Clinic--Seguin • Fresenius Medical Care [27358]
Kidney Disease Clinic--Uvalde • Fresenius Medical Care [27384]
Kidney Home Center • DaVita [24649]
Kidney Home Center, Dialysis and At Home • DaVita [24650]
Kidney Institute of the Desert [22727]
The Kidney Institute--Eisenhower Medical Center • Dialysis Facility [22892]
Kidney Institute of Naples • Naples Nephrology [23420]
Kidney Institute of North Dakota • Aurora Medical Park [25995]
Kidney Services of West Central Ohio--Mercer County [26033]
Kidney Spa LLC [23402]
Kidney Treatment Center--East • Dialysis Facility [27331]
Kidney Treatment Center--Miami [23403]
Kidney Treatment Center--Northwest PA [27332]
Kidney Treatment Center--San Antonio [27333]
Kidney Treatment Center of Slatebelt • Dialysis Facility • Fresenius Medical Care [26613]
Kids Are People, Inc. • Runaway and Homeless Youth Program [35789]
KIDS Behavioral Health of Montana [34279]
Kids Can Do Inc. [2071]
Kids Communication Center [1528]
Kids in Crisis • Runaway and Homeless Youth Program [35864]
Kids in Distress--Hollywood [29182]
Kids in Distress • Palm Beach County [29149]
Kids in Distress--Wilton Manors [29323]
Kids Hope United • Lake/Cook Behavioral Health Center [33406]
Kids Kampus [7993]

Kid's Link Rhode Island [51310]
Kids Only Inc. [2162]
Kids Path • Hospice and Palliative Care of Greensboro [20674]
Kids Peace--Aberdeen [31499]
Kids Talk [1196]
Kids Therapy--Lake Barrington [2055]
Kids Therapy Ltd.--Libertyville [2060]
Kids Under Twenty One [51062]
Kidship [1149]
KidsPeace [34404]
KidsPeace Broadway Campus [34409]
KidsPeace Cumberland County [34419]
KidsPeace Lackawanna County [34428]
KidsPeace--Lewiston [30217]
KidsPeace Luzerne County [34417]
KidsPeace Lycoming County [34431]
KidsPeace Montour County [34411]
KidsPeace Orchard Hills Campus [34420]
KidsPeace Schuylkill County [34426]
KidsPeace Wayne County [34416]
KidSpeak--Grapevine [3498]
KidSpeak LLC [3453]
Kidspeak--Oneida [3089]
KidSpeak Speech Therapy [1610]
Kidspeech--Crystal Lake [2011]
Kidspeech Inc.--Lawrenceville [1876]
Kidsplay Therapy Center [1879]
KidsTLC [43426]
KidTalk Inc.--New Lenox [2080]
KidTalk, PA [1760]
Kidtalk--Thomasville [3196]
Kidz Kare at Home, Inc. [18367]
Kidz Therapy Services LLC [3024]
Kilgo Headache Clinic [12377]
Kilgore Community Crisis Center [10480]
Kilgore Dialysis Center • DaVita [27204]
Killeen Diversified Family Counseling [10482]
Killeen Heights Vet Center [52108]
Killeen Intermediate School District [799]
Kim Logan Communication Clinic Inc [44744]
Kimball Medical Center • Cancer Program [5518]
KinderMourn, Inc. [36526]
Kindness-Care Home Health [12959]
Kindred Hospital [2514]
King Drive Counseling Assessment and • Referral Services Inc [42541]
King Group Home [34277]
King Home Medical Equipment, Inc. [15580]
King of Kings Community Center • Mens Recovery Home [39860]
King of Kings Community Centers • Pregnant and Postpartum Womens Program [39861]
King Medical Supply, Inc. [13391]
King of Prussia West Specialty Care Center [17354]
King State Veterans Home [18578]
Kingdom Living Outreach Services Inc [42830]
Kingman Aid to Abused People, Inc. [8692]
Kingman CBOC • Division of Prescott VAMC [3867]
Kingman Kidney Clinic Inc. • Dialysis Facility [22448]
Kingman Regional Medical Center [12793]
Kingman Regional Medical Center Hospice [18794]
Kings Alcohol and Drug Treatment Center
    Brad G Recovery [43492]
    Community Based Outpatient [43493]
    The Light House [43494]
    Winfield [43518]
    Winfield Outpatient [43519]
Kings Care • A Safe Place [40353]
Kings Community Action Organization • Domestic Violence Program [8820]
Kings County Hospital Center
    Cancer Program [5565]
    Chemical Dependency Inpatient Detox [46511]
    Chemical Dependency/TOPS [46512]
    Dialysis Unit [25614]
    HHC MMTP C12 Clinic II [46513]
    HHC MTA C13 Clinic III [46514]
    Polydrug Unit [46515]
Kings Court Dialysis--Flemington • Fresenius Medical Care [25435]
Kings Daughter Hospital • Mississippi Sports Medicine and Orthopaedic Center [38647]
King's Daughter Medical Center [2254]
King's Daughters' Home Health--Ashland [15160]
King's Daughters Home Health--Louisa [15214]
King's Daughters' Hospital and Health Services •

Cancer Program [5164]
King's Daughters' Medical Center • Cancer
  Resource Center [5209]
The King's Daughters' School and Center for Autism
  [8515]
Kings Daughters Spine and Pain Center [35460]
Kings Harbor Health Services LLC [25589]
Kings Health Care, LLC [17787]
Kings View Counseling Services for King County
  [28387]
Kings View Rural Services [40711]
Kings View • Substance Abuse Program Tulare
  County [40863]
Kingsboro Psychiatric Center [31268]
    Brooklyn Manor/CSS [33682]
    Canarsie Service [33683]
Kingsbrook Jewish Medical Center [8305]
    Dialysis Unit [25615]
    Kingsbrook Rehabilitation Institute [4310]
Kingsbury Center [7874]
The Kingsbury Day School [1529]
Kingston City School District [586]
Kingston Hospital
    Dialysis Center Satellite [25695]
    Pain Management Service [35577]
Kingston House [6803]
Kingston Veterans Affairs Clinic [31373]
Kingstree Dialysis • Fresenius Medical Care [26734]
Kingsway Learning Center [8254]
Kingwood Dialysis Center • DaVita [27209]
Kingwood Health Center [33876]
Kingwood Pines Hospital [49432]
Kingwood Sleep Disorders Center [37820]
Kingwood Speech Pathology Services [3520]
Kinnic Falls • Alcohol and Drug Abuse Services
  [50521]
Kinston Community Health Center, Inc. [7053]
Kinston Dialysis Unit • Fresenius Medical Care •
  Dialysis Unit [25896]
Kipnuk Traditional Council • Community Suicide
  Prevention Program [50637]
Kirby Forensic Psychiatric Center • Ward Island
  [33704]
Kirby Kidney Disease Center • Fresenius Medical
  Care [27211]
Kirchner Headache Clinic [12442]
Kirkbride Center [48537]
Kirksville Regional Center [8203]
Kirkwood House [31017]
Kishwaukee Community Hospital
    Cancer Program [5084]
    Pain Management Program [35430]
Kissimmee Dialysis • DaVita • Dialysis Facility
  [23356]
The Kitchen, Inc. • Runaway and Homeless Youth
  Program [36055]
Kitsap Children's Speech Therapy [3642]
KITSAP Mental Health Services [49914]
Kitsap Mental Health Services [32810]
Kittson County Hospice [20168]
Kitty Askins Hospice Center [20671]
Kivalliq School Operations • Deaf/Hard of Hearing
  Program [642]
Kiwanis Center for Child Development [8518]
Klallam Counseling Services [50055]
Klamath Falls Dialysis • DaVita [26327]
Klamath Hospice, Inc. [21010]
Klamath Open Door Family Practice [7134]
Klamath Pain Clinic, PC [35633]
Klamath Sleep Medicine Center [37614]
KLH Therapy Services [1154]
Klickitat Valley Health, Home Health & Hospice
  [21754]
Kline Galland Hospice Services • Kline Galland
  Home [21767]
Kline Hospice House [19934]
Kline Welsh Behavioral Hlth Foundation • Sand
  Island Treatment Center [42212]
Klingberg Family Centers--Hartford [33244]
Klingberg Family Centers--New Britain [33254]
Klingensmith HealthCare, Inc. [17325]
Kluge Children's Rehabilitation Center [34898]
KM Pediatric Therapy, Inc. [3163]
Knapp Medical Center [18189]
Kno-Wal-Lin Home Care, • Hospice Program
  [19900]
Kno-Wal-Lin Home Care
    [19899]

Visiting Nurse Associations of America [19888]
Knowledge Counseling Services [50049]
Knox Center Inc Wichita [43495]
Knox Community Hospital • Cancer Center [4694]
Knox County Kidney Center • Fresenius Medical
  Care • Dialysis Facility [26169]
Knox County Schools Hearing Services [754]
Knoxville Central Dialysis and At Home • DaVita
  [26862]
Knoxville Orthopedic Clinic [39034]
Kobeissi Speech Language Services [2569]
Kodiak Women's Resource and Crisis Center [8667]
Kohler Child Development Center [8282]
Koinonia Foster Homes Inc
    Koinonia Group Homes [40050]
    Koinonia Treatment Clinic [40051]
Koinonia Residential Treatment Center [50517]
Koke Mill Medical Center/Lohman Family Center for
  Rehabilitation [4023]
Kokomo Area Special Education Cooperative [424]
Kokua Kalihi Valley Main Clinic [6618]
Kokua Nurses--Hilo [14614]
Kokua Nurses--Honolulu [14621]
Kolburne School, Inc. • The Brigham Center [34198]
Koller Behavioral Health Services [32964]
Kolmac Clinic [41540], [44230], [44277], [44358],
  [44373]
Kolob Oxygen & Medical Equipment--Cedar City
  [18194]
Kolob Oxygen & Medical Equipment--Saint George
  [18216]
KOLPIA Counseling Services Inc [48064]
Komed/Holman Health Center [42542]
Komfort and Kare [16291]
Kona Community Hospital • Behavioral Health
  [29530]
Konza Prarie Commuity Health Center [6718]
Koochiching Counseling Center [30688]
Kootenai Medical Center
    North Idaho Cancer Center [5052]
    Sleep Disorders Center [36880]
Kootenay Hearing Aid and Audiology Clinic [1047]
Korean American Family Service Center [9922]
Korean American Women in Need [9208]
Korean Community Services Inc [40122]
Korean Family Enrichment Program • Korean
  Service Center [9617]
Korean Women's Association • We Are Family
  Home [10662]
Kornegay Foster Home [33084]
Kosair Children's Hospital
    Alliant Health System • Cancer Program [5224]
    Burn Unit [4550]
Kosair Children's Hospital, Hearts & Hands Palliative
  Care Program [19814]
Kosciuske Home Care & Hospice [19658]
Kosciusko Community Hospital • Cancer Center
  [5180]
Kosciusko Veterans Affairs Clinic [30778]
Kossuth Regional Health Center [29837]
Kotlik City Council • Suicide Prevention Program
  [50638]
KP Counseling Inc [42888]
KPHC Downtown [6619]
Krause Speech and Language Services [1989]
Kreg Therapeutics, Inc. [14739]
KRU Medical Ventures
    Saint Augustine Kidney Center [23499]
    Silver Spring Artificial Kidney Center • Dialysis
      Facility [24731]
Kruse Group Home [34283]
Krystal's Wish Foundation for SIDS [36517]
KSB Hospice [19514]
KSB Hospital Audiology Services [2018]
KSTAR, Inc. • Runaway and Homeless Youth
  Program [36225]
Ku Aloha Ola Mau Inc • East Hawaii Treatment
  Clinic [42198]
Ku Aloha Ola Mau • Methadone Maintenance
  [42213]
Kuakini Medical Center • Cancer Program [5046]
Kuruk Tribal Health Program of • River of Health
  and Wellness [40968]
Kuumba Community Health and Wellness Center
  [7367]
KV Consultants and Associates [47309]
KVC Behavioral Health Care [33511]
Kwenyan Professional Health Services [45975]

L

L E Phillips Libertas Center [50376]
L. Medical Center [14051]
L and N Counseling [43800]
L and P Services Inc [47801]
L and S Medical Group [13665]
LA Best Health Care, Inc. [13139]
La Buena Vida Inc [46250]
L.A. Care Provider [13262]
La Caridad Home Health Services Corporation
  [14052]
La Casa de Buena Salud--Clovis [6993]
La Casa de Buena Salud--Hondo [6997]
La Casa de Esperanza • Outpatient Clinic [50550]
La Casa, Inc. [9875]
La Casa de las Madres [8888]
La Casa de Nuestra Gente [7213]
La Casa Psychiatric Health Facility [28567]
La Casa Quigg Newton Family Health and Counsel-
  ing Center [6398]
La Casa Ramona Counseling [28740]
La Clinica de los Campesinos • Family Health Medi-
  cal and Dental Center [7443]
La Clinica del Carino Family Health Care Center
  [7133]
La Clinica del Carino--The Dalles [7150]
La Clinica Del Valle [7137]
La Clinica de Familia, Inc. [6998]
La Clinica Noroeste de Comportamientos Modifica-
  dos [50271]
La Clinica Noroeste de Comportamientos • Modifica-
  dos [50050]
La Clinica del Pueblo [9030]
La Clinica del Pueblo de Rio Arriba [7006]
La Clinica de la Raza-Fruitvale Health Project, Inc.
  [6335]
La Clinica--Saint Louis [6918]
LA County Department Public Health • Acton
  Rehabilitation Center [39584]
La Crosse County Human Services • Chemical
  Health and Justice Sanctions [50435]
La Crosse Cryobank [35264]
La Crosse Vet Center [52148]
La Esperanza Clinic [7309]
La Esperanza HCS • Renton Branch [50082]
La Esperanza Health Counseling Services [50014]
La Familia Home Health, Inc. [17912]
La Familia Medical [7004]
La Fe Family Health Center • La Fe Clinic [7289]
La Follette Dialysis Center • Fresenius Medical Care
  [26864]
La Follette Outpatient Clinic • Ridgeview Psychiatric
  Hospital and Center [33846]
La Frontera Casa Alegre [28210]
La Frontera Casa de Vida [28211]
La Frontera Center
    Casa de Vida [39501]
    East Clinic [39502]
    Hope Center [39503]
La Frontera Center, Inc. [28212]
La Frontera Center • Substance Abuse Outpatient
  Services [39504]
La Frontera East Clinic [28213]
La Frontera Hope Center [28214]
La Frontera La Pagosa [28215]
La Frontera Main Clinic • Child and Family Center
  [28216]
La Frontera Pima House [28217]
La Frontera Psychiatric Health Facility [28218]
La Frontera Rapp Programs [28219]
La Grange Dialysis Center • DaVita [24396]
La Hacienda College Station [49268]
La Hacienda Treatment Center [49423]
La Haciendas Solutions [49230]
La Isla Pacifica/South County Alternatives, Inc.
  [8817]
La Luna Center [10999]
La Mariposa Hospice at Providence Hospital [21451]
La Palma Dialysis Center, LLC [22741]
La Paloma Family Services • Runaway and Home-
  less Youth Program [35794]
La Paloma Treatment Center [49138]
La Perla de Gran Precio [48734]
La Porte Dialysis Facility • Fresenius Medical Care
  [27213]
La Porte Regional Health System • Cancer Program
  [5162]
La Posta Substance Abuse Center • Outpatient

Substance Abuse Services [39665]
La Pryor Intermediate School District [801]
La Puente Dialysis Center • California Kidney Specialists [22742]
La Trenza Counseling Inc [41075]
La Ventana Eating Disorder Programs--San Francisco [10960]
La Ventana Eating Disorders Programs--San Jose [10961]
La Ventana San Jose [10962]
La Ventana Thousand Oaks [10963]
La Vida [9529]
LAAM and Methadone Program • VA North Texas Healthcare System [49335]
LaAmistad Behavioral Health Services • LaAmistad Residential Treatment Center [34074]
The Lab School of Washington [1530]
Labelle Home Health care Services, LLC [16912]
Labelle House [32160]
Labette Center for Mental Health Services [43443]
Labette Health • Sleep Laboratory [36992]
Laboratory for Elite Athlete Performance [38311]
Laboratory Services • WuXi AppTec Inc. [35084]
Laboratory of Speech and Language Disorders [2856]
Lac Courte Oreilles • Alcohol Drug and Mental Health Program [50411]
Lac Courte Oreilles Oakwood Haven Program and Shelter [10705]
Lac du Flambeau Domestic Abuse Program [10711]
LAC Harbor--UCLA Medical Center [23036]
LAC/USC Women's and Children's Hospital
    Adult Sickle Cell Disease Center [36300]
    Children's Sickle Cell Disease Center [36301]
Lac Vieux Desert Band [45053]
Lac Vieux Desert • Behavioral Health Services [45054]
Lackawanna Veterans Affairs Clinic [31376]
Lackland AFB Alcohol and Drug Abuse • Prevention and Treatment Program [49435]
Lad Lake [34482]
Ladacin Network [8279]
Lady Lake Outpatient Center [33312]
Lady of the Sea Dialysis Center • Lady of the Sea General Hospital [24482]
Lady of the Sea General Hospital [15285]
Lafayette Addictive Disorders Clinic [43843]
Lafayette County • Department of Human Services /AODA Prog [50377]
Lafayette Crisis Center [50894]
Lafayette General Medical Center [15311]
    Cancer Program [5248]
Lafayette House [9687]
LaFayette Outpatient Clinic [42116]
Lafayette Pediatric Center [7110]
Lafayette Veterans Affairs Clinic [30149]
LaForges Addiction Therapy [43338]
    Winds of Change [43496]
Lafourche Mental Health Center [30170]
LaGrande Community Based Outpatient Clinic [17200]
LaGrange Area Department of Special Education [2053]
LaGrange Dialysis Clinic [22743]
LaGuardia Community College • Program for Deaf Adults [588]
Laguna Family Shelter Program [9874]
Laguna Honda Hospital and • Rehabilitation Center SATS [40619]
Laguna Psych • Eating Disorders Therapy [10964]
Lahey Clinic • Department of Orthopaedic Surgery • Sports Medicine Center [38548]
Lahey Clinic Hospital • Cancer Program [5327]
Lahey Clinic, Inc. • Multiple Sclerosis Clinical Center [34596]
Lahey Clinic Medical Center • Sleep Disorders Center [37118]
LAJ Home Health [13622]
LaJunta Dialysis • Fresenius Medical Care [23125]
Lake Area Citizens Advisory Board • LACAB [45447]
Lake Area Recovery Center
    Outpatient Drug Free Program [47615]
    Turning Point [47616]
Lake Arrowhead Treatment Center [39974]
Lake Avenue Dialysis Center [24143]
    Diversified Specialty Institutes [24144]
Lake Charles Behavioral Health Center [43845]
Lake Charles Dialysis Center [24524]

Lake Charles Memorial Hospital
    Cancer Program [5252]
    Kid's Team [8068]
Lake Charles Mental Health Center [30153]
Lake Charles Subst Abuse Clinic Inc [43846]
Lake City Kidney Center • Northwest Kidney Centers [27612]
Lake City Medical Center • Department of Rehabilitation Services [1624]
Lake City VA Medical Center [13833]
Lake City VAMC • PRRTP Unit [41725]
Lake Cliff Dialysis Center • DaVita [27030]
Lake Country Physical Therapy and Sportscare, PC [38779]
Lake County Alcohol and Other Drug Services [39978]
    Clearlake Clinic [39717]
Lake County Counseling Services [50502]
Lake County Crisis Intervention Center [10237]
Lake County Dialysis • DaVita [26153]
Lake County Dialysis Services Inc. • DaVita [24020]
Lake County Health Dept Behav Health • Addictions Treatment Program [42949]
Lake County Health Dept /CHC • Behav Health/Womens Resid Services [42941]
Lake County Home Health and Hospice [20372]
Lake County Mental Health [48085]
Lake County Mental Health Emergency Service [50675]
Lake County Public Library • Northwest Indiana Subregional Library for the Blind and Physically Handicapped [3793]
Lake County Substance Abuse Program [42950]
Lake Cumberland Regional Hospital
    Cancer Center [5237]
    Sleep Disorders Center [37029]
Lake Dialysis • DaVita [23369]
Lake Ellenor Dental Center [6527]
Lake Forest Hospital [14830]
    Center for Rehabilitation [35431]
Lake Forrest Hospital • Outpatient and Acute Care • Center for Sleep Medicine [36910]
Lake Griffin East Dialysis • DaVita [23370]
Lake Havasu City Clinic [3868]
Lake Havasu City Salvation Army Safehouse [8694]
Lake Havasu Interagency Council [8695]
Lake Hearn Dialysis • DaVita [23600]
Lake Hospital System [17015]
    Cancer Program [5762]
    Sleep Center [37534]
Lake Jackson Dialysis and Kidney Center [27215]
Lake Martin Hospice [18698]
Lake Norman Dialysis Center • Wake Forest University [25912]
Lake Norman Regional Medical Center • Cancer Center [4693]
Lake Norman Regional Medical Center Home Health [16755]
Lake Owasso Residence [8184]
Lake of the Ozarks Veterans Affairs Clinic [30835]
Lake Park Chronic Hemodialysis Unit • University of Chicago Medical Center [23942]
Lake Place Retreat Center [45089]
Lake Placid Sports Medicine [38790]
Lake Plains Dialysis at Batavia [25574]
Lake Plains Dialysis Center [25702]
Lake Powell Medical Center [6237]
Lake Preston Community Health Center [7248]
Lake Region Halfway Homes Inc [45152]
Lake Region Human Service Center [51186]
    Chemical Dependency Program [47564]
Lake Region Outreach Office [47597]
Lake Regional Health System Home Health [16036]
Lake St. Louis Dialysis • DaVita [25235]
Lake Shore Behavioral Health [31288]
Lake Shore Behavioral Health Inc
    Drug and Alcohol Abuse Services Prog [46563]
    Drug Free Resid Prog for Women [46564]
Lake Shore Bone & Joint Institute • Northwestern Memorial Hospital [23943]
Lake Shore Center for Psychological Services • Better Way Chem Dep Treatment Program [49577]
Lake Sunapee Region VNA Hospice and Palliative Care [20449]
Lake Superior Community Health Center [7441]
Lake Superior Health Center [6864]
Lake Superior Hospice Association [20091]
Lake Superior Medical Equipment, Inc. [15900]

Lake Superior Treatment Center [45132]
Lake Underhill Family Health Center [6528]
Lake View Memorial Hospital • Chemical Dependency Unit [45332]
Lake Villa Dialysis & At Home • DaVita [24019]
Lake Wales Dialysis • DaVita • Dialysis Facility [23360]
Lake Washington Kidney Center • Northwest Kidney Center [27595]
Lake West Hospital [17072]
Lake of the Woods District Hospital • Saint Joseph's Health Centre • Eating Disorders Treatment [11223]
Lake Worth Dialysis • DaVita [23556]
Lakeland Area Hospice [21086]
Lakeland Centers Atlanta [42141]
Lakeland Centres [41737]
Lakeland Community Hospital [12676]
Lakeland Dialysis • DaVita [23363]
Lakeland Health and Healing [2646]
Lakeland Home Care [15584]
Lakeland Homecare Niles [15758]
Lakeland Hospice [20036]
Lakeland Hospice and Home Care [20162]
Lakeland Mental Health Center [30678]
Lakeland Primary Care [6485]
Lakeland Regional Health System • Cancer Care Center [5397]
Lakeland Regional Hospital [33638]
Lakeland Regional Medical Center [19247]
    Cancer Program [4957]
Lakeland South Dialysis & At Home • DaVita • Dialysis Facility [23364]
Lakeland Village School [8601]
Lakemary Center • Children's Residential Program [8031]
Lakeport Dialysis Center • DaVita [22746]
Lakeridge Outpatient Treatment • Transitional Housing [44745]
Lakes Area Hospice [21501]
Lakes Counseling Center [45124]
Lakes Crisis and Resource Center [9593]
Lakes Homehealth Corporation [14211]
Lakes Region • Chemical Dependency LLC [45084]
Lakes Region General Hospital • Nathan Brody Chemical Dependency Prog [45886]
Lakes Regional Hospice [19713]
Lakes Regional Mental Health/Mental Retardation Center--Paris [32524]
Lakes Regional Mental Health/Mental Retardation Center--Sulphur Springs [32555]
Lakes Regional MH/MR Center [49353], [49468], • [49538], [49554]
    Lakes Behavioral Health [49249]
Lakeshore ENT [2605]
Lakeshore Healthcare Services, Inc. [17882]
Lakeshore Hearing Centers [2606]
Lakeshore Home Health Care [15732]
Lakeshore Hospice [19855]
Lakeshore Mental Health Institute [33845]
Lakeshore Pediatrics Annex [6521]
Lakeshore Sleep Disorder Center [36589]
Lakeside Behavioral Health System [32353]
Lakeside Behavioral System [51363]
Lakeside Center [34274]
Lakeside Counseling Center [29739]
Lakeside Dialysis Center [27402]
Lakeside Hospice, Inc. [18753]
Lakeside Milam Recovery Centers Inc [49961], [50116]
    Auburn [49884]
    Edmonds [49941]
    Everett Branch [49954]
    Issaquah [49973]
    Kirkland [49990]
    Kirkland Inpatient [49991]
    Puyallup [50072]
    Renton [50083]
    Seattle/Eastlake [50117]
    Tacoma [50210]
Lakeside Recovery Centers • Spokane [50173]
Lakeside Residential Care [27957]
Lakeside Treatment and Learning [34232]
Lakeview Center [29261]
Lakeview Center Inc
    Adult Outpatient [41587]
    Adult Residential [41890]
    Avalon [41808]

Child Outpatient Substance Abuse Services [41891]
DAART [41892]
Outpatient Counseling [41893]
Pathway [41894]
Pathway/Shalimar [41935]
Lakeview Center, Inc. • Pensacola Help Line [50780]
Lakeview Center • Southeast Vocational Services [33342]
Lakeview Christian Hospice Care [20529]
Lakeview Health Systems LLC [41705], [41706]
Lakeview Healthcare Systems--Blackburg • Blue Ridge [4474]
Lakeview Healthcare Systems--Sebago Place • Mentor ABI [4077]
Lakeview Healthcare Systems--Waterford • Reach House [4493]
Lakeview Healthcare Systems--Weyers Cave [4475]
LakeView Home [18948]
LakeView Home Health [15769]
Lakeview Home Health and Hospice [21013]
Lakeview Hospice [20210]
Lakeview Hospital
New Vision [49599]
Outpatient Substance Abuse Program [49600]
Lakeview Lodges [33343]
Lakeview Medical Center [18624]
Dialysis Center [27778]
Lakeview Medical Center Home Health Care & Hospice [21864]
Lakeview Medical Center
Satellite Dialysis [27786]
Speech Pathology Department [3686]
Lakeview Memorial Hospital [15944]
Lakeview Mental Health Services Community Residence [31298]
Lakeview NeuroRehabilitation Center [4268]
Lakeview Place [33344]
Lakeview Public Schools • Hearing Impaired Center Program [501]
Lakeview School [8247]
Lakeview Villas [33345]
Lakeview Virginia NeuroCare [4476]
Lakeview Virginia NeuroCare LLC [4477]
Lakewood Community Dialysis Center & At Home • DaVita [27613]
Lakewood Counseling Service TMC • Drug Addiction Recovery Center [45551]
Lakewood Day Treatment [27865]
Lakewood Hospice [20144]
Lakewood Hospital • Cancer Program [5729]
Lakewood Ranch OB/GYN [6486]
Lakewood University Dialysis Center • Diversified Specialty Institutes [23546]
Lakewoods Center [7439]
Lamar Area Hospice Association [19117]
Lamar Community Reintegration • Hope [28062]
Lamar Dialysis • Fresenius Medical Care [23129]
Lamar University • Speech and Language Clinic [3470]
Lamb of God Recovery Centers [41841]
Lambda Gay and Lesbian Anti-Violence Project [10460]
Lambs Farm [7961]
Lamm Institute for Child Neurology [2991]
Lamoille County Mental Health Service [32670]
Day Treatment Program [32671]
Intensive Family-Based Service [32672]
Lamoille Home Health and Hospice [21664]
LAMP Community • Frank Rice SafeHaven [28598]
LAMP Day Center/Shelter [28599]
LAMP Lodge [28600]
LAMP Village [28601]
Lamplighter Plaza Dialysis • DaVita [25273]
Lamprey Health Care [6964]
Lanai Community Dialysis • Fresenius Medical Care [23860]
Lancaster Audiology Services [1145]
Lancaster Child Guidance Residential Treatment • Lincoln [30995]
Lancaster Clinical Counseling Assoc [48428]
Lancaster County Community Mental Health Center [30996]
The Heather [30997]
Transitional Living Facility [30998]
Lancaster County Helpline • Family Services [51287]

Lancaster County School District [732]
Lancaster Dialysis • DaVita [26736], [27217]
Lancaster Family Center [7146]
Lancaster Freedom Center [48429]
Lancaster General Hospital
Cancer Program [5836]
Department of Physical Medicine and Rehabilitation [3346]
Sleep Disorders Center of Lancaster [37655]
Lancaster Regional Medical Center [17366]
Behavioral Health Unit [32033]
Lancaster Shelter for Abused Women [10289]
Lancaster Vet Center [52076]
Lancaster Veterans Affairs Outpatient Clinic [17367]
Land Manor Inc • Franklin House North Women/ Children [49238]
Landauer Metropolitan [16530]
Lander County Committee Against Domestic Violence [9786]
Lander Regional Hospital [33052]
Lander Valley Medical Center L.L.C. [18654]
Landmark Medical Center • Cancer Program [5898]
Landsun Hospice [20530]
Lane County Behavioral Health • Methadone Treatment Program [48104]
Lane Physical Therapy Center [38069]
Lane Purcell House [19316]
Lane Regional Medical Center Home Health [15381]
Lane Regional Program, Deaf and Hard of Hearing [683]
Lane Speech-Language Pathology Services [3393]
Lane Treatment Center [44156]
Lane's Learning Center [7796]
Lang Home Medical Equipment, Inc. [14702]
Langdale Hospice House [19429]
Langel House [30943]
Langhorne Dialysis Center • American Renal Associates [26464]
Langlade Health Care Center [32945]
Emergency Mental Health [51500]
North Central Health Care [50357]
Langlade Memorial Dialysis [27696]
Langlade Memorial Hospital [18555]
Langley Porter Psychiatric Hospital & Clinics [33189]
Langley School District Number 35 • Deaf/Hard of Hearing Program [254]
Language and Cognitive Development Center [8136]
Language Experience [2400]
The Language Experience [2430]
The Language Group [1825]
Language Interaction Pathology Service LLC [3410]
Language Learning Associates [3209]
Language and Learning Center [1974]
Language and Learning Concepts [3536]
Language and Learning Disability Solutions [2474]
Language and Speech Associates [1368]
Language, Speech and Hearing Center [1200]
Language and Speech Services for the Hard of Hearing [227]
Language and Speech Therapy [1122]
Lanham Counseling and Therapy [43644]
Lanier Health Services Home Health [12733]
Lanier Treatment Center [42103]
The Lankenau Hospital
Cancer Program [5883]
Sleep Medicine Services [37656]
Lansdale Hospital • Cancer Program [5838]
Lansing Central Dialysis • Fresenius Medical Care [24931]
Lansing Chiropractic Clinic [38386]
Lansing Community College • Physical Fitness and Wellness Department [38595]
Lansing Home Hemodialysis • DaVita [24889]
Lansing Psychological Associates PC [44771]
Lantana Chiropractic/Delaware Health and Fitness [38203]
Lantana/Lake Worth Health Center [6488]
Lanterman Developmental Center [7808]
Program 4, Sensory and Positive Behavior Development [1230]
Lanza, Inc. [17441]
Lanza Pediatrics [6537]
Lapeer Area Citizens Against Domestic Assault [9553]
Lapeer County Community Mental Health Center [44897], [51022]
Lapeer Regional Medical Center • Great Lakes Cancer Institute [4678]

LaPlace Dialysis Center [24516]
LaPorte Cty Comprehensive Mental Health Council • Swanson Center [43158]
LaRabida Children's Hospital • Down Syndrome Clinic [10794]
Laradon [7840]
Laramie Youth Crisis Center • Runaway and Homeless Youth Program [36280]
Laraway Youth and Family Services [34462]
Larchmont--Mamaroneck Branch Clinic [31386]
Laredo Dialysis Ltd. • US Renal Care [27223]
Laredo Family Violence Center/Casa De Misericordia [10484]
Laredo Hospice [21508]
Laredo Regional Day School for the Deaf [802]
Laredo South Dialysis Center • US Renal Care [27224]
Laredo Veterans Affairs Outpatient Clinic [32498]
Laredo Visiting Nurses, Inc. [18036]
Lares Health Center, Inc. • Centro de Salud de Lares Inc. [7202]
Largo Medical Center • Cancer Program [4959]
Larimer Center for Mental Health [28899], [41176], [41268]
Adult Services [28901]
Children and Family Services [28902]
Loveland Branch [28936]
The Larkin Center [34107]
The Larkin Centers • Transitional Skills Center [34108]
Larkin Home Health Services, Inc. [14388]
Larkin Street Youth Center • Runaway and Homeless Youth Program [35826]
Larned State Hospital [33507]
Larry E. Hoyle BS CADC • Action Consultants [42642]
Larry Savage, DC • Pain Clinic [35287]
Larry Simmering Recovery Center [45442]
Larson East PAU
Downey [272]
Selaco High School [273]
Larson West PAU • Redondo Beach [293]
Larue D. Carter Memorial Hospital [33474]
Las Clinicas del Norte [6994]
Las Colinas Spine and Sports Medicine [39081]
Las Cruces Mobile Vet Center [52028]
Las Cruces Public Schools [560]
Las Cruces Renal Center • Diversified Specialty Institutes [25550]
Las Cruces South Dialysis • Fresenius Medical Care [25551]
Las Cumbres Learning Services [8290]
Las Encinas Hospital [33171], [40372]
Las Palmas Del Sol Medical Center • Cancer Program [5982]
Las Palmas Dialysis Center • DaVita [27334]
Las Trampas [7784]
Las Vegas Dialysis Center & At Home • DaVita [25365]
Las Vegas Dialysis • Diversified Specialty Institutes [25366]
Las Vegas Home Health Care [16155]
Las Vegas Indian Center [45842]
Las Vegas Kidney Clinic [25378]
Las Vegas Medical Center [33671]
Community Mental Health Program [31203]
Las Vegas Medical Clinic [6999]
Las Vegas NM Dialysis Center • Fresenius Medical Care [25552]
Las Vegas Pain Institute [35547]
Las Vegas Pediatrics Dialysis Center • DaVita [25367]
Las Vegas Recovery Center [45843]
Las Vegas VA Outpatient Clinic [45844]
Las Vegas Veterans Affairs Medical Center [31031]
LaSalle Addictive Disorders Clinic [43832]
LaSalle Outpatient [42734]
Lashley & Associates, Inc. [3509]
Laskin Therapy Group [2764]
Lassen County Alcohol and Drug Program [40835]
Lassen Family Services, Inc. [8916]
Lassen Indian Health Center • Substance Abuse Services [40836]
Lasting Recovery Outpatient • Substance Abuse Treatment Center [40559]
Lasting Solutions • Legal Services of Eastern Missouri [9718]
Latham Centers [8114]

Latimer Counseling Services [41134]
Latin American Community Center [9012], [41520]
Latin American Health Institute • Oasis Substance Abuse Clinic [44418]
Latin American Youth Center
    Runaway and Homeless Youth Program [35872]
    Substance Abuse Program [41541]
Latinas United for a New Dawn • Latinas Unidas Nuevo Amanecer [9329]
Latino Commission on Alcohol and • Drug Abuse Services BASN [40817]
Latino Commission on Alcohol/DA Services
    Casa Los Hermanos [40540]
    Casa Quetzal [40620]
    Latina Perinatal Women [40621]
Latino Commission on Alcohol/Drug Abuse Services • Casa Adelita [40541]
Latino Family Services Inc [44746]
Latino Treatment Center • Chicago Outpatient [42543]
Latrobe Area Hospital
    Cacer Care Center [5839]
    Department of Speech Pathology [3349]
Lattimore Physical Therapy and Sports Rehabilitation [38816]
Laughlin Home Health Agency [17673]
Laughlin Memorial Hospital • Cancer Program [5931]
Laughlin Mental Health Center [31037]
Laura Baker Services Association [8182]
Laura T Fetters LPC CAC III [41065]
Laural Manor Dialysis Center • DaVita [23542]
Laura's House [8826]
Laureate Psychiatric Clinic and Hospital [33786]
Laureate Psychiatric Clinic & Hospital • Eating Disorders Program [11202]
Laurel Behavioral Health [48683]
Laurel Center Intervention for Domestic and Sexual Violence [10600]
Laurel Dialysis Center [25141]
Laurel Fertility Care [21922]
Laurel Fork Health Commission • Tri-Area Health Clinic [7356]
Laurel Heights Hospital [34090]
Laurel Hill Center [31941]
Laurel Hill Inn [11091]
Laurel Home Health / Hospice [21169]
Laurel House [10301]
Laurel Learning Intervention Center [2767]
Laurel Manor Dialysis Center at the Villages • DaVita [23357]
Laurel Mountain Medical [18547]
Laurel Oaks Behavioral Health Center [27899]
Laurel Ridge Psychiatric Hospital • Treatment Center [33882]
Laurel Ridge Treatment Center [49525]
Laurel Shelter, Inc. [10571]
Laurelwood Hospital [33761], [42104]
Laurelwood • Transitional Living [50308]
Laurence Learning Center [2403]
Laurens County Deaf/Hard of Hearing Program [372]
Laurens County--Dublin • DaVita [23686]
Laurens County Safe Homes [10346]
Laurens Mental Health Center [32192]
Laurie LaViolette LCSW CCS [43969]
Laurie Silverman and Associates [1262]
Laurinburg Dialysis Center • Fresenius Medical Care [25897]
Lavelle School for the Blind [3724]
Lavelle Youth Homes • The Lavelle Center [39892]
Laverna Lodge • Fairbanks Hospital [43004]
Lawley Premier Hospice Care [18761]
Lawndale Christian Health Center [6661]
Lawndale Medical and Mental Health Services [39995]
Lawrence County Domestic Violence Task Force [10153]
Lawrence County Health Department/ • Behavioral Health [42743]
Lawrence Court Halfway House [44336]
Lawrence General Hospital • Cancer Program [5339]
Lawrence Hall Youth Services [34103]
Lawrence Hospital Center • Cancer Program [5563]
Lawrence and Memorial [1488]
Lawrence Memorial Hospital [2495]
Lawrence and Memorial Hospital • Community

Cancer Center [4903]
Lawrence Memorial Hospital/Kreider Rehabilitation Services [2224]
Lawrence Memorial Hospital • Sleep Disorders Center [36993]
Lawrence and Memorial Hospital Speech/Audiology Services [1480]
Lawrence Otolaryngology Associates [2225]
Lawrence Schmidt Center • Vera Lloyd Presbyterian Home [28300]
Lawrence Veterans Affairs Clinic [29937]
Lawrenceburg Dialysis Center • DaVita [24155]
Lawrenceburg Veterans Affairs Clinic [29734]
Laws Support Center [40123]
Lawton Chiles Children and Family HCC [6439]
Lawton/Fort Sill Veterans Affairs Clinic [31885]
LDS & Associates [1347]
LDS Hospital
    Cancer Program [6042]
    Intermountain Sleep Disorders Center [37872]
L.D.S. Hospital • Speech-Language Pathology Department [3556]
Le Bonheur Children's Hospital • Transplant/Dialysis Center [26889]
Le Penseur Youth and Family Services • Runaway and Homeless Youth Program [35930]
Le Penseur Youth and Family Srvs Inc [42544]
LEAD Institute • Leadership through Education and Advocacy for the Deaf [9672]
Leading Edge Recovery Center [46058]
A Leaf DME [18101]
League for the Deaf and Hard of Hearing--Nashville [3446]
League for the Hard of Hearing--Florida [1678]
League School of Greater Boston [8122]
League Treatment Center [2992]
Leah Layne Dialysis Center • Fresenius Medical Care [27625]
Leake and Watts Services [31250]
Leake & Watts Services, Inc. [31498]
Leanne Young Professional Counseling Services [11128]
LEAP Inc [43689]
Lear Communication • Speech Language Voice Cognitive Therapy [3296]
Learn2Balance [11000]
Learning Center [7823]
The Learning Center for Deaf Children [473] Audiology Unit [2480]
Learning Center for the Deaf, Randolph Campus [2517]
Learning Clinic [7954]
Learning and Developmental Disabilities Evaluation and Rehabilitation Services [8156]
Learning Edge [2274]
Learning Resource Center [2309]
Learning Services Corp.--California [3907]
Learning Services Corporation--Georgia [4004]
Learning Services Corporation--Michigan [4173]
Learning Services-Gilroy [3908]
Learning Services Neurobehavioral Institute [4330]
Learning Services Neurobehavioral Institute-West [3939]
Learning Services--Northern California [3909]
Learning Services Residential Rehabilitation--Draper [4468]
Learning Services Residential Rehabilitation--Riverton [4469]
Learning Web • Runaway and Homeless Youth Program [36113]
Leary Educational Foundation [34465]
Leavenworth Dialysis • DaVita [24332]
Lebanon Dialysis, At Home and Home Training Center • DaVita [26147]
Lebanon Dialysis • Liberty Dialysis [24194]
Lebanon Therapeutic Rehabilitation Programs [30043]
Lebanon Treatment Center [48442]
Lebanon VA Medical Center • Cancer Center [4702]
Lebanon Veterans Affairs Medical Center [32037]
LeBonheur Children's Medical Center • Pediatric and Adolescent Sleep Disorders Center [37768]
Lecanto VA Community Based Outpatient Clinic [13861]
The Ledges [8129]
Ledyard Regional Visiting Nurse Agency [13528]
Lee Ballard RN LCSW CAP [41875]
Lee Center [48906]

Lee College • Hearing Impaired Program [3469]
Lee Conlee House [9072]
Lee County Cooperative Clinic [6274]
Lee County Counseling Center [32751]
Lee County Health Department Hospice [19694]
Lee County Mental Health Center [29459]
Lee County Mental Health Crisis Line [51177]
Lee County Talking Books Library [3764]
Lee County Youth and Family Services • Runaway and Homeless Youth Program [36135]
Lee Davis Health Center [6557]
Lee-Harnett Emergency Crisis and Suicide Intervention Service [51158]
Lee Memorial Health System • ALS Clinic [107]
Lee Memorial Health System, Cape Coral • Pain Management Center [35385]
Lee Memorial Health System, HealthPark • Pain Management Center [35386]
Lee Memorial Health System • Regional Cancer Center [4942]
Lee Memorial Hospital • MDA Clinic [34779]
Lee Mental Health Center • Crisis Stabilization Unit [50757]
Lee Shore Center [8665]
Lee Woodward Counseling Center for Women • AARS [40622]
Leeanne S Taylor MS LADC [43929]
Leech Lake
    Opioid Program [45108]
    Outpatient Program [45109]
Lee's Summit Dialysis • Fresenius Medical Care [25239]
Leesburg Community Health Center [6492]
Leesburg Dialysis Center • DaVita [23371]
Leesburg Dialysis • DaVita [27506]
Leesburg Regional Medical Center [1634]
    Cancer Program [4960]
Leesville Developmental Center [8070]
Leesville Dialysis • Fresenius Medical Care [24525]
Leesville Mental Health Center [30154]
Leeward Dialysis Facility • Liberty Dialysis [23845]
Leflore County Health Department • Speech and Hearing Clinic [3282]
Legacy Community Health Services, Inc. [7296]
Legacy Emanuel Hospital and Health Center • Department of Medical Genetics • Center for Maternal Fetal Medicine [12322]
Legacy Emmanuel Hospital • Oregon Burn Center [4619]
Legacy Good Samaritan Hospital and Medical Center • Legacy Sleep Disorders Center [37615]
Legacy Health System • Cancer Services [5799]
Legacy Home Care Services, Inc. [18093]
Legacy Home Health Care--Euless [17918]
Legacy Home Health Care--Mesquite [18083]
Legacy Home Health Care--Norwalk [13217]
Legacy Home Health Care--Plano [18111]
Legacy Hopewell House Hospice [21023]
Legacy Hospice-Gilmer [21472]
Legacy Hospice, Inc. Livingston [18735]
Legacy Hospice Longview [21518]
Legacy Hospice McMinnville [21015]
Legacy Hospice Meridian [19473]
Legacy Hospice-Paris [21544]
Legacy Hospice • Preferred Hospice [21719]
Legacy Hospice Services [21024]
Legacy Hospice-Sulphur Springs [21572]
Legacy House [9287], [19274]
Legacy of Life Tissue Foundation [35229]
Legacy of Love Hospice [21513]
Legacy Meridian Park Hospital • Cancer Program [5808]
Legacy Meridian Park Sleep Center [37616]
Legacy Mount Hood Medical Center • Cancer Program [5790]
Legacy Portland Hospitals • Good Samaritan Hospital Campus • Cancer Program [5800]
Legacy Salmon Creek Hospital • Cancer Program [6127]
Legacy Salmon Creek Medical Center • Genetics Clinic [12366]
Legacy Strategy [11037]
Legacy Transplant Services • Legacy Health [26342]
Legal Advocates for Abused Women [9719]
Legal Aid Society of Hawaii • Hawaii Immigrant Justice Center [9142]
Legal Aid Society of Hawaii--Waianae Branch [9143]
Legal Aid Society of Mid--New York Inc. [9996]

Legal Aid Society of Middle Tennessee and the Cumberlands [10424]
Legal Aid Society--Washington [9031]
Legal FACS [9855]
Legal Momentum [9032]
Legend Home Care [15588]
Lehigh Acres Dialysis • DaVita [23372]
Lehigh Acres Medical and Dental Office [6493]
Lehigh Valley Hospice [21044]
Lehigh Valley Hospital
    ALS Center [145]
    Burn Center [4621]
    Dialysis Center [26366]
Lehigh Valley Hospital and Health Network • Cystic Fibrosis Center [7654]
Lehigh Valley Hospital • Hemophilia Treatment Center [12588]
Lehigh Valley Hospital Home Health & Hospice Services [17234]
Lehigh Valley Hospital • John and Dorothy Morgan Cancer Center [5810]
Lehigh Valley Hospital--Muhlenberg • Cancer Program [5813]
Lehigh Valley Hospital
    Multiple Sclerosis Center of the Lehigh Valley [34692]
    Sleep Disorders Center [37657]
Lehigh Valley Hospital Transplant Center • Lehigh Valley Health Network [26367]
Lehman College • Program for Deaf and Hard of Hearing Students [571]
Lehua Elementary School [388]
Leigh Dialysis Center • DaVita [27526]
Leister and Associates Inc. [3169]
Leitchfield Dialysis • DaVita [24398]
Leitchfield Therapeutic Rehabilitation Program [30046]
Lela L Lyons LADC • Hope Recovery Services [43961]
Lemak Sports Medicine [37995]
Lemhi County Crisis Intervention • Mahoney Family Safety Center [9187]
LeMoyne Center [27983]
Lemuel Shattuck Hospital • Dialysis Unit [24773]
Lena Pope Home Inc • Family Matters Counseling [49336]
Lena Pope Home, Inc. [32405]
Lena Street Group Home [33085]
Lenawee County Community Mental Health [30495]
Lenawee Intermediate School District [480]
Lenexa Dialysis & At Home • DaVita [24335]
Lennard Clinic Inc [45983]
The Lennard Clinic Inc [46096]
Lenoir Memorial Hoapital [37473]
Lenoir Memorial Hospital, Inc. • Cancer Program [5648]
Lenoir-Rhyne College • Support Services for Deaf/Hard of Hearing Students [620]
Lenox Baker Children's Hospital [8374]
Lenox Hill Hospital [16558]
    Dialysis Unit [25723]
    Nicholas Institute of Sports Medicine and Athletic Trauma [38795]
Leo A. Hoffmann Center [34256]
Leon County Treatment Center [41948]
Leonard J. Chabert Medical Center [30142]
Leone Home Health Care Agency, Inc.--Rowlett [18130]
Leone HomeHealth Care Agency, Inc.--Mesquite [18084]
LeRoyer Hospice [21818]
Lesbian and Gay Community Services Center
    CD Outpatient [46880]
    Mental Health and Social Services [46881]
Leslie R. Peterson Rehabilitation Center [35297]
Leslie S Berkley and Associates [42424]
Lesly Home Health Care, Inc. [14053]
Lester A Drenk Behavioral Health Center [46074]
Lester A. Drenk Behavioral Health Center [31137]
Lester Dierksen Memorial Hospice [21576]
Lester E. Cox Medical Centers • Hulston Cancer Center [5465]
Letholt Dialysis Center • Fresenius Medical Care [25259]
Let's Communicate Inc. [1142]
Let's Grow Well Together Inc [41634]
Let's Talk--Chicago [1990]
Let's Talk LLC--Saint Clair Shores [2644]

Let's Talk Solutions, Speech Pathology Inc. [1053]
Levi Hospice [18856]
Levine Children's Hospital
    Down Syndrome Center [10840]
    Pediatric Rehabilitation Pavilion [4331]
Levine & Dickson Hospice House • Hospice & Palliative Care [20682]
Levittown Union Free School District [587]
Levy County Clinic [29121]
Lewin Services, Inc. [16611]
Lewis & Clark Behavioral Health Services, Inc.--Lake Andes • CARE Program & Crisis Intervention [51342]
Lewis & Clark Behavioral Health Services, Inc.--Vermillion [32259]
    CARE Program & Crisis Intervention [51349]
Lewis & Clark Behavioral Health Services, Inc.--Yankton [32264]
    CARE Program & Crisis Intervention [51350]
Lewis and Clark Behavioral Hlth Services • Alcohol and Drug Program [49035]
Lewis & Clark Behavioral Services, Inc.--Lake Andes [32231]
Lewis & Clark City-County Health Department • Cooperative Health Center, Inc. [6932]
Lewis County Community Recovery • Treatment Center [46766]
Lewis County Hospice [20576]
Lewis County Opportunities, Inc.--Lowville [9942]
Lewis County Opportunities Inc.--Watertown [10002]
Lewis County Primary Care Center, Inc. [6739]
Lewis Gale Center for Behavioral Health [49839]
Lewis-Gale Medical Center • Regional Cancer Center [6085]
Lewis-Gale Physicians Sleep Center [37888]
Lewis School and Diagnostic Clinic [8269]
Lewiston Auburn Kidney Center • Fresenius Medical Care [24611]
Lewiston Hospital • Sleep Center [37658]
Lewiston Idaho Veterans Affairs Clinic [29547]
Lewiston Independent School District Number One [391]
Lewiston VA Community Based Outpatient Clinic • VA Montana Health Care System [4253]
Lewistown Dialysis Center • DaVita [26469]
Lewistown Hospital • Cancer Services [5840]
Lewistown Mental Health Center [30954]
Lewisville Dialysis Clinic • Renal Ventures Management [27226]
Lexington Center for Mental Health Services [3034]
Lexington Center for Recovery [46994]
    CD Outpatient/Airmont Clinic [46320]
    Outpatient Clinic [46795]
    Outpatient Rehabilitation [46321]
Lexington Clinic • Sleep Center [37030]
Lexington Clinic Sports Medicine Center [38479]
Lexington Community Counseling Center [44899]
Lexington Dialysis Center Inc. • Wake Forest University [25900]
Lexington Dialysis • Dialysis Facility • DaVita [27507]
Lexington-Fayette County Health Department [6732]
Lexington-Fayette Urban County Government • Division of Youth Services • Runaway and Homeless Youth Program [35968]
Lexington Hearing and Speech Center [2275]
Lexington Kidney Clinic • Dialysis Facility • DaVita [26872]
Lexington Medical Center
    Cancer Center [5915]
    Sleep Solutions [37735]
Lexington Medical Services • PLLC Sleep Disorders Center [37397]
Lexington Memorial Hospital [3184]
    Pain Center [35592]
Lexington Professional Associates [43662]
Lexington School for the Deaf [584]
Lexington Treatment Associates [47408]
Lexington VA Medical Center [4061]
Lexington Veterans Affairs Medical Center--Leestown Division [30055]
Lexington Veterans Affairs Medical Center • Leestown Division [51574]
Lexington Vocational Services Inc. [585]
Leyden Family Service and Mental Health Center [29622]
Leyden Family Service
    Mental Health Center [42677]

Share Program [42710]
LGA Home Health Inc. [13040]
LGE Sports Medicine Institute [38267]
LH Transitional Center Inc [49382]
LHC Home Care--Andalusa [12621]
LHC Home Care--Opp [12708]
LHRC • Reality House [43812]
Liberal Area Rape Crisis and Domestic Violence Services [9369]
    Satanta Outreach Office [9377]
Liberal Veterans Affairs Clinic [29940]
Liberation Programs Inc
    Darien Family and Youth Options [41377]
    Families in Recovery Program [41471]
    Greenwich Family and Youth Options [41387]
    Liberation House [41472]
    Methadone Program [41365]
    Stamford Outpatient Services [41473]
Libertae Inc
    Family House [48288]
    Halfway House [48289]
Libertas of Sheboygan [50525]
Libertas Treatment Center [50402]
Liberty Centre Services Inc. [31003]
Liberty Community Health Care [6448]
Liberty Counseling Center [42712], [42933]
Liberty County Mental Health Center [29440]
Liberty Dayton Dialysis FAC • Fresenius Medical Care [27227]
Liberty Dialysis--Anchorage [22418]
Liberty Dialysis--Anchorage Home Program [22419]
Liberty Dialysis--Baden [26372]
Liberty Dialysis--Banksville [26561]
Liberty Dialysis--Berlin [25405]
Liberty Dialysis--Brenham [26978]
Liberty Dialysis--Bryan [26984]
Liberty Dialysis--Carson City [25350]
Liberty Dialysis--Castle Rock [23098]
Liberty Dialysis--Charring Cross [24651]
Liberty Dialysis--Chippewa [26375]
Liberty Dialysis--College Station [27001]
Liberty Dialysis--Colorado Springs Central [23099]
Liberty Dialysis--Crawfordsville [24127]
Liberty Dialysis • DaVita • Dialysis Center [25240]
Liberty Dialysis--Doylestown [26598]
Liberty Dialysis--Duncanville [27053]
Liberty Dialysis--Duneland-Coffee Creek [24122]
Liberty Dialysis--Fairfield [23156]
Liberty Dialysis--Frankfort [24147]
Liberty Dialysis--Friendship Ridge [26373]
Liberty Dialysis--Hammond [24163]
Liberty Dialysis--Hammonton [25442]
Liberty Dialysis--Hayden [23872]
Liberty Dialysis--Hopewell [26363]
Liberty Dialysis--Idaho Falls [23873]
Liberty Dialysis--Kenwood [26142]
Liberty Dialysis--Kokomo [24187]
Liberty Dialysis--Kona [23853]
Liberty Dialysis--Lafayette II [24191]
Liberty Dialysis at Lakeland [24952]
Liberty Dialysis at Lakeland--Royalton [24970]
Liberty Dialysis Lancaster [27218]
Liberty Dialysis--Las Vegas [25368]
Liberty Dialysis--Layton [27406]
Liberty Dialysis--Linwood [25457]
Liberty Dialysis--Meridian [23876]
Liberty Dialysis--Mesquite [27256]
Liberty Dialysis--Monticello [24206]
Liberty Dialysis--Nampa [23881]
Liberty Dialysis--North Colorado Springs [23100]
Liberty Dialysis--North Haven [23173]
Liberty Dialysis--Northwest Reno [25381]
Liberty Dialysis--Norwood [26178]
Liberty Dialysis--Ogden [27410]
Liberty Dialysis--Oquirrh [27430]
Liberty Dialysis--Orange [23178]
Liberty Dialysis--Petersburg [27535]
Liberty Dialysis--Pueblo [23136]
Liberty Dialysis--Reno Home [25382]
Liberty Dialysis--Rockwall [27302]
Liberty Dialysis--Runnemede [25505]
Liberty Dialysis--Saint George [27420]
Liberty Dialysis
    Saint Joseph's Hospital--Camillus • Dialysis Unit [25639]
    Saint Joseph's Hospital ESRD--Seneca Campus • Dialysis Facility [25697]
Liberty Dialysis--Sandpoint [23888]

Liberty Dialysis--Seaford [23200]
Liberty Dialysis--South Colorado Springs [23101]
Liberty Dialysis--Southpointe [26394]
Liberty Dialysis--Vestal [25798]
Liberty Dialysis--Washington [26600]
Liberty Dialysis--West Jordan [27436]
Liberty Dialysis--Wilmington [23208]
Liberty Dialysis--Woods Cross [27437]
Liberty Healthcare Services, LLC [16913]
Liberty Home Care & Hospice [21200], [21687]
Liberty Home Care and Hospice-Burgaw [20626]
Liberty Home Care and Hospice-Burlington [20630]
Liberty Home Care and Hospice-Clinton [20640]
Liberty Home Care and Hospice-Dunn [20646]
Liberty Home Care and Hospice-Jacksonville [20684]
Liberty Home Care and Hospice-Lumberton [20699]
Liberty Home Care and Hospice-Raleigh [20721]
Liberty Home Care and Hospice Services-Durham [20651]
Liberty Home Care, Inc.--Jersey City [16228]
Liberty Home Care--Taylor [15847]
Liberty Home Health Care Inc. [13041]
Liberty HomeCare & Hospice-Raeford [20717]
Liberty HomeCare and Hospice-Sanford [20730]
Liberty HomeCare & Hospice Services-Supply [20744]
Liberty HomeCare and Hospice-Silery /City [20735]
Liberty HomeCare & Hospice-Thomasville [20752]
Liberty HomeCare & Hospice-Wadesboro [20757]
Liberty HomeCare & Hospice-Whiteville [20763]
Liberty Hospital • Cancer Center [5453]
Liberty Hospital Home Health [16027]
Liberty House of Albany [9085]
Liberty Pain Relief [35560]
Liberty Place Recovery Center • For Women [43771]
Liberty Resources, Inc.--Canastota [31299]
Liberty Resources, Inc.--Fulton [31330]
Liberty Resources, Inc.--Oneida • Venture House [31443]
Liberty Resources, Inc.--Syracuse [31478]
Libra Substance Abuse Counseling Services [43947]
Library for the Blind and Physically Handicapped [3751]
Library Park Rehabilitation Center [2152]
Library Services for the Deaf and Hard of Hearing [3447]
LICA Program for Students Who Are Deaf/Hard of Hearing [405]
Licking County Alcoholism Prev Program • Outpatient Services [47827]
Licking Memorial Hospital [17010]
    Cancer Program [5742]
Life Alaska Donor Services, Inc. [34918]
Life--Alysis Kidney Center [24881]
Life By Design PA [43979], [43987], [44043]
Life Care Center of Fort Wayne [2146]
Life Care Center of Orlando [1698]
Life Care Center of Punta Gorda [1741]
Life Care Center of Sierra Vista [986]
Life Care Hospice, Inc. [18696]
Life Care Sleep and Health Center, Allegan [37167]
Life Care Sleep and Health Center, Carson City [37168]
Life Care Sleep and Health Center, Cheboygan [37169]
Life Care Sleep and Health Center, Eaton Rapids [37170]
Life Care Sleep and Health Center, Jackson [37171]
Life Care Sleep and Health Center, Kalamazoo [37172]
Life Care Sleep and Health Center, Lansing [37173]
Life Care Sleep and Health Center, Marshall [37174]
Life Care Sleep and Health Center, Sheridan [37175]
Life Care Sleep and Health Center, Traverse City [37176]
LIFE Center--Bloomington [1967]
LIFE Center--Pontiac [2101]
Life Change Center [45881]
Life Changes Counseling [47334], [47481]
    Life Changes DWI Center [47301]
Life Changing Behavioral Health Srvs [47513]
Life Choice Hospice--Dresher [21078]
Life Choice Hospice--Waltham [20006]
Life Choices Treatment Services Inc [40661]
Life Crisis Center [50980]

Life Crisis Center, Inc. [9462]
Life Currents Counseling [11073]
Life Development Institute [7735]
Life Dimensions [11068]
Life Enhancement Center [49664]
Life Happens [10916]
Life Healing Center of Santa Fe [11151]
Life Health Services Inc [40124]
Life Help
    Attala County Office [45399]
    Denton House [45379]
Life Help Mental Health Center - Region 6 • Grenada County Office [30765]
Life Help Mental Health Center-Region 6 • Indianola Office-Sunflower County [30774]
Life Help Mental Heath Center-Region 6 • Winona Office-Montgomery County [30825]
Life Help • Montgomery County Office [45430]
Life Help Region VI Mental Health [30743]
Life Help • Sunflower County Office [45384]
Life Home Health Services [14054]
Life Home Healthcare Corporation [14055]
Life & Hope Healthcare [13666]
Life House [45323]
Life Improvement Counseling Center LLC [43122]
Life Journeys [44885]
Life Line Counseling Center [49781]
Life-Line Home Health, Inc.--Dearborn [15621]
Life Link [46303]
Life Management Center
    Adult Day Program [29255]
    Calhoun County Facility [29111]
    Gulf County Facility [29268]
    Holmes County [29115]
    Jackson County Facility [29211]
Life Management Center of Northwest Florida, Inc. [29256]
Life Management Center of Northwest Florida Inc.--Bonifay [50750]
Life Management Center of Northwest Florida Inc.--Marianna [50773]
Life Management Center of NW Florida [41885]
Life Management Counseling and Consulting Inc [47947]
Life Management Inc [43690]
Life Management Resources [49490]
Life Medical Home Care Services, Inc. [12976]
Life Medical Supplies, Inc. [16234]
Life Options Health Services, Inc. [14740]
Life Path Hospice [19321]
Life Path Hospice Care Services, LLC [19878]
Life Path Systems [32510], [32531]
Life Point Solutions [43565]
Life Recovery Center [43102], [43103]
A Life Recovery Center Inc [41949]
Life Skills • Children's Crisis Stabilization Unit [29980]
Life Skills Helpline--E Main Street, Bowling Green [50929]
Life Skills Helpline--Suwannee Trail, Bowling Green [50930]
Life Skills Learning Center [46256]
Life Skills Service Center, Morgantown [30084]
Life Skills Service Center, Scottsville [30111]
Life Source Consultants [9720]
Life Source Services, LLC [19856]
Life Span Inc. [9222]
Life Stride Inc [41542]
Life Supply Corp. [15486]
Life Support Behavioral Institute • IOP for Adolescent and Adult Drug/Alc [41040]
Life Touch Hospice [18845]
Life Treatment Centers [43025]
Life Treatment Centers Inc [43203]
Life and Work Solutions Inc [41863]
Life and Work Soulutions [41720]
LifeBanc [35163]
Lifebank Cryogenics Corporation [34930]
LifeBank USA [35116]
LifeBridge Health Network • Lapidus Cancer Institute [5287]
LifeCare Home Health Services Inc. [13435]
LifeCare Hospice of South Carolina, LLC [21251]
LifeCare Medical Center [15932], [20199]
Lifecare Options Home Health Services, Inc. [18124]
Lifecare Psychiatric Services--Lafayette [30150]
Lifecare Psychiatric Services--Opelousas [30168]
Lifecare Resources, Inc. [17999]

LifeCell Corp. [35117]
LifeCenter Northwest [35257]
LifeCenter Organ Donor Network [35164]
Lifeforce Cryobanks [34992]
LifeGift Organ Donation Center [35230]
LifeLegacy Foundation [34925]
Lifeline Center for Sleep Disorders, Forest Hills [37659]
Lifeline Center for Sleep Disorders, Greensburg [37660]
Lifeline Center for Sleep Disorders, Johnstown [37661]
Lifeline Center for Sleep Disorders, Latrobe [37662]
Lifeline Center for Sleep Disorders, McMurray [37663]
Lifeline Center for Sleep Disorders, Monaca [37664]
Lifeline Center for Sleep Disorders, Monroeville [37665]
Lifeline Center for Sleep Disorders, Mount Pleasant • Frick Hospital [37666]
Lifeline Center for Sleep Disorders, New Castle [37667]
Lifeline Center for Sleep Disorders, North Hunting-don [37668]
Lifeline Center for Sleep Disorders, Pennsylvania [37669]
Lifeline Center for Sleep Disorders, Washington [37670]
Lifeline Center for Sleep Disorders, Waynesburg [37671]
Lifeline Connections [50240]
Lifeline Counseling Center Inc [42687]
Lifeline Cryogenics, LLC [34978]
Lifeline Health Services, Inc./Lifetech [14786]
Lifeline Home Care, LLC [14833]
Lifeline Home Health Care--Lakeland [13842]
Lifeline Home Health Care--Marathon [13872]
Lifeline Home Health Care--Port Charlotte [14347]
Lifeline Home Health Care--Springfield, TN [17773]
Lifeline Home Health, Inc.--Springfield, PA [17486]
Lifeline Hospice, Inc. [20928]
Lifeline of Laredo, Inc. [51385]
Lifeline of Miami Inc [41690], [41822]
Lifeline of Ohio [35165]
Lifeline Sleep Disorders Center--Warrendale Labora-tory [37672]
Lifeline Treatment Services Inc [40302]
Lifelink Health Providers Inc. [13060]
LifeLink Home Health Services, Inc. [15875]
LifeLink Tissue Bank [34993]
LifeLinks, Inc. [29641]
    Psychosocial Rehabilitation Center [29642]
    Supervised Group Homes [29643]
Lifelong Care Over 60 Health Center [6290]
LifeMark Health Center--Calgary [35279]
LifeMark Health Center--Dartmouth [35603]
LifeMark Health Center--Vancouver [35298]
LifeMark Health Institute [35280]
LifeMatters Counseling and • Health Center Inc [49688]
LifeNet Health of Florida [34994]
LifeNet Health--Virginia Beach [35253]
LifePath Hospice and Palliative Care, inc. [14419]
LifePath Hospice and Palliative Care--Ruskin • Sun City Center Community Resource Center [19307]
LifePath Hospice and Palliative Care--Temple Ter-race [19326]
LifePath Systems
    ECI Frisco [32467]
    ECI Rockwell [32539]
Lifepoint Inc.--Charleston • Vision Share [35201]
Lifepoint Inc.--Greenville • Vision Share [35202]
Lifepoint Inc.--West Columbia • Vision Share [35203]
Life's Doors Hospice [19449]
Lifes Journey Center [40349]
Life's Resources Inc. [2549]
Life's Work of Western Pennsylvania [8480]
Lifesavers [13843]
LifeScape Medical Associates [38048]
Lifeshare Eye Facility--Asheville [35146]
Lifeshare Eye Facility--Charlotte [35147]
LifeShare Transplant Services of Oklahoma [35170]
Lifesharing Tissue Services [34951]
LIFESIGNS Inc. • Interpreter Services [1165]
LifeSkills Adult Crisis Stabilization [29981]
LifeSkills Inc [43774]
    Barren County Service Center [43606]

Butler County Office [43722]
Edmonson County Office [43545]
Hart County Office [43727]
Scottsville Counseling Center [43778]
Simpson County Office [43596]
LifeSkills Service Center [29982], [30119]
Lifeskills South Florida [41620]
LifeSource [35085]
LifeSource Cryobank LLC [35057]
LifeSouth Community Blood Center Headquarters • Civitan Regional Blood Center--Donor Testing Laboratory [34995]
LifeSouth Community Blood Centers, Inc. • Civitan Region [34996]
LifeSouth • LifeCord [34997]
LifeSpan--Albermarle [31500]
LifeSpan--Burlington [31510]
LifeSpan--Charlotte [31519]
LifeSpan--Concord [31520]
LifeSpan--Dobson [31522]
Lifespan Good Samaritan Hospice [20032]
LifeSpan--Greensboro [31539]
LifeSpan--High Point [31547]
Lifespan, Inc. [15581], [20033]
LifeSpan of Minnesota, Inc. [30666]
LifeSpan--Monroe [31561]
LifeSpan--Mount Airy [31567]
LifeSpan--Troutman [31601]
LifeSpan--Waynesville [31607]
Lifespeak [3623]
Lifespire [8333]
LifeSport Medicine & Wellness Center [38079]
Lifespring [43123]
Center Place I [29748]
Center Place II [29749]
LifeSpring • Floyd County Office [29790]
LifeSpring Inc [43013]
Turning Point Center [43124]
Lifespring Inc • Washington County Office [43195]
LifeSpring, Inc. [29750]
LifeSpring • Jefferson County office [29778]
Lifespring Mental Health Services [43196]
LifeSpring Mental Health Services • Harrison County Office [29709]
LifeSpring • Scott County Office [29815]
Lifespring • Substance Abuse Residential Services [29751]
LifeSpring Turning Point Center [29752]
LifeSpring • Washington County Office [29814]
LifeStream Academy--Altoona [33286]
LifeStream Behavioral Center • Crossroads [33313]
Lifestream Behavioral Center • Crossroads II [41583], [41749]
LifeStream Behavioral Center
Crossroads II - Safer Communities [33300]
Full Circle/Geriatric Residential Treatment [33314]
Phoenix House [33356]
Lifestream Behavioral Center • Southlake Counseling [41600]
LifeStream- Bushnell Outpatient [33294]
LifeStream--Lake Region Homes [33315]
LifeStream - Southlake Outpatient Center [33298]
Lifestrength Physical Therapy [38536]
Lifestyle Counseling of • Richfield Bloomington [45088]
Lifestyle Counseling Services [45267]
Lifestyles Changes Counseling [42379]
LifeTek OrthoBiologics, LLC [34998]
Lifetime Care Hospice [20602]
LifeTime Center at Timber Ridge [1682]
Lifetime Recovery Residential Services [49526]
Lifetrack Resources [2742]
Lifeways Inc [48162]
Lifeways, Inc. [31953]
Lifeways--Jackson [51020]
Lifeways--Ontario [51262]
Lifeworks Alliance of Youth and Family Services • Runaway and Homeless Youth Services [36226]
Lifeworks Northwest Albina [31960]
LifeWorks Northwest--Hillsboro [31944]
Lifeworks Northwest Seaside [31979]
LifeWorks Northwest--Tigard [31984]
LifeWorks NW • Albina Site [48194]
Lifeworks NW • Cedar Mill Site [48195]
LifeWorks NW
Gresham Site [48123]
Hillsboro Site [48131]

Millikan Site [48074]
Project Network [48196]
Rockwood Site [48197]
Lifeworks NW
Southwest Site [48198]
Tigard Site [48199]
Light Home Care [14056]
Light for Life Foundation of America [50723]
LightBridge Hospice [13298], [19016]
Lighted Pathways Health Services, Inc. [21566]
Lighted Way Association • Children's Developmental Center [7960]
The Lighthouse [8651]
Lighthouse Addiction Services [41902]
Lighthouse Care Center of Augusta [33372]
Lighthouse Care Center of Conway [48924]
Lighthouse Care Center of Oconee [32216]
Lighthouse Convalescent Care, Inc. [28042]
Lighthouse Counseling [49787]
Lighthouse Counseling Center [47310]
Lighthouse Counseling Center Inc [41256]
Intensive Outpatient Unit [39280]
Lighthouse Counseling Inc [46235]
Lighthouse Counseling Service Inc. [51242]
Lighthouse Counseling Services Inc [43625], [43735], [47983]
Lighthouse Eastland [21448]
Lighthouse Hospice-Austin [21390]
Lighthouse Hospice-Brownwood [21410]
Lighthouse Hospice--Cherry Hill [20463]
Lighthouse Hospice-Conroe [21420]
Lighthouse Hospice-Georgetown [21470]
Lighthouse Hospice-Salt Lake City [21650]
Lighthouse Hospice-Tomball [21579]
Lighthouse Inc [39236]
The Lighthouse, Inc. [4174]
Lighthouse--Juneau • Juneau Youth Services, Inc. [28099]
Lighthouse--Lancaster [10154], [31786]
Lighthouse at Manahawkin [46042]
Lighthouse for Recovery [42327], [42361]
Lighthouse Recovery Center [49631]
Lighthouse--Russellville [28347]
Lighthouse School [8139]
Lighthouse Shelter--Annapolis [9439]
Lighthouse Shelter--Marshall [9699]
Lighthouse Substance Abuse Services of • Northwest Center Behavioral Health [48057]
Lighthouse of Tallapoosa County Inc • Substance Abuse Rehab Program/Resid [39204]
Lighthouse--Weirton [10681]
Lighthouse Youth Services • Runaway and Home-less Youth Program [36146]
Like Family Home Nursing Services [13338]
Lillian Smith Home [27964]
Lilly's Home Care [13667]
Lima Memorial Health System • Cancer Institute [5731]
Lima Memorial Hospital • Dialysis Center [26148]
Lima Memorial Hospital Home Health [16964]
Lima Memorial Hospital • Speech and Hearing Center [3243]
Lima Veterans Affairs Community Based Outpatient Clinic [31789]
Limed Home Health Care [13752]
Limestone District School Board • Deaf/Hard of Hearing Program [677]
Limited Home Health Care [14212]
Lincoln Avenue Branch Clinic [31402]
Lincoln Behavioral Health Clinic Inc. [11130]
Lincoln Child Center [28665]
Kinship Support Services [28529]
Lincoln Community Health Center [7050]
Lincoln County Board of Education [873]
Lincoln County Community Health Center Inc. [6934]
Lincoln County Council on Alcohol and • Drug Abuse Inc/DBA KenTrueman Recovery [48157]
Lincoln County Counseling Center [51435]
Lincoln County Health and Human Services • Addictions Recovery Program [48158]
Lincoln County Memorial Hospital Home Health Agency [16080]
Lincoln Developmental Center [7951]
Lincoln Dialysis • DaVita [24021]
Lincoln Health Care Center [33934], [33948], [51510], [51518]
Lincoln Health Center [7126]
Lincoln Healthcare Center

Merrill Office [50467]
Tomahawk Office/Substance Abuse Services [50545]
Lincoln Home Health Care, Inc. [14837]
Lincoln Hospital • Hemodialysis Unit [25590]
Lincoln House [32152]
Lincoln Lakes Regional Dialysis [24612]
Lincoln/Lancaster County • Child Guidance Center [45757]
Lincoln Medical Center - Hospital Home Health & Hospice [17670]
Lincoln Medical Education Partnership [45758]
Lincoln Medical & Mental Health Center • Cancer Center [5560]
Lincoln Medical/Mental Health Center • Lincoln Recovery Center [46424]
Lincoln Park Dialysis • DaVita [23944]
Lincoln Park Home Health Care [14741]
Lincoln Regional Center [33645]
Lincoln School [8171]
Lincoln Trail Behavioral Health System • United Healthcare of Hardin Inc [43770]
Lincoln Trail Hospital • Lincoln Trail Behavioral Health System [33533]
Lincoln Treatment Center [45759]
Lincoln Veterans Affairs Clinic [30225]
Lincolnland Hospice of Sarah Bush Lincoln--Casey [19498]
Lincolnland Hospice of Sarah Bush Lincoln--Effingham [19516]
Lincolnland Hospice of Sarah Bush Lincoln--Mattoon [19542]
Lincolnview [30118]
Linda J. Roos, MD [39072]
Linda Page LMHC CAP [41834]
Lindbergh Dialysis Center [23601]
Linden Dialysis • DaVita [23602]
Linden Oaks Hospital [33432]
Linden Oaks Hospital at Edward [42805]
Linden Oaks Hospital--Edwards [33433]
Lindencroft Program • Community Care Services, Inc. [30331]
Lindner Center of HOPE • Sibcy House [11196]
Linguistic Alternatives [1207]
Linguistic Solutions [981]
The Link of Behavioral Connections [51197]
Link Crisis Intervention Center [51008]
Link House [32330]
Link House Inc [44523]
Link Inc [45775]
Linn County • Alcohol and Drug Treatment Program [48061]
Linn County Crisis Services [51246]
Linn County Health Services [48143], [48252]
Linn County Health Services--Lebanon [31949]
Linn County Health Services--Sweet Home [31982]
Linn County Mental Health Division [31927]
Linn County Mental Health Services--Crisis Services, Lebanon [51258]
Linn County Mental Health Services--Crisis Services, Sweet Home [51267]
Linwood Center [8091]
Lion Hospice, Inc. [21434]
Lionel R John Health Center • Behavioral Health Unit [47063]
Lions Eye Bank at Albany • Sight Society of Northeastern New York [35133]
Lions Eye Bank, Alberta Society [34920]
Lions Eye Bank of Delaware Valley [35188]
Lions Eye Bank for Long Island • North Shore University Hospital [35134]
Lions Eye Bank of Manitoba and Northwest Ontario Inc. [35061]
Lions Eye Bank of New Jersey • Midwest Eye Banks [35118]
Lions Eye Bank of North Dakota [35151]
Lions Eye Bank of Northwest Pennsylvania, Inc. [35189]
Lions Eye Bank of Oregon [35182]
Lions Eye Bank of Oregon, Medford • Southern Oregon Laboratory [35183]
Lions Eye Bank of Puerto Rico [35195]
Lions Eye Bank of Saskatchewan [35200]
Lions Eye Bank of Texas • Baylor College of Medicine • Department of Ophthalmology [35231]
Lions Eye Bank of West Central Ohio [35166]
Lions Eye Bank of Wisconsin [35265]

Lions Eye Institute for Transplant and Research [34999]
Lions Medical Eye Bank and Research Center of Eastern Virginia [35254]
Lions Organ and Eye Bank of District 2-E2 [35232]
Lions Sight and Tissue Foundation--District 2-X1 [35233]
Lions Tissue and Eye Bank Inc.--District 2-El [35234]
Lipton Center [8131]
Lisa Harmon Mollicone LLC • MA LCADC ICADC CJC CPS [45999]
List Psychological Services PLC [44660], [44661], [44690], [44691], [44898], [45000]
List Psychological Services, PLC [30588]
Listen to Kids [10248]
Listening Ear Crisis Center--Alexandria [51035]
Listening Ear Crisis Center, Inc.--Mount Pleasant [51024]
Listening Ear Crisis Center • Runaway and Homeless Youth Program [36019]
Listening Ear Crisis Intervention Center [9532]
The Listening Ear, Inc. [51015]
Listening Ears LLC [943]
Listening Ears NYC [3064]
Listening and Language Connections LLC [2553]
Lister Hill Health Center [6195]
Litchfield Area Hospice [20174]
Litchfield Dialysis • DaVita [24023]
Lithia Springs Programs [34391]
Little Angels Center [2979]
Little City Foundation [7963]
Little Colorado Behavioral Health Centers [28196]
Little Colorado • Behavioral Health Centers [39463], [39478]
Little Colorado Behavioral Health Centers, Saint Johns [50650]
Little Colorado Behavioral Health Centers, Springerville [50652]
Little Company of Mary Home Based Care Services [14889]
Little Co. of Mary Home Based Services [19549]
Little Company of Mary Hospital [13392]
Behavioral Health [42666]
Little Company of Mary Hospital and Health Care Centers [36911]
Little Company of Mary Hospital and Healthcare Centers • Regional Cancer Center [5093]
Little Hill • Alina Lodge [45937]
Little House Inc [39652]
Little River Medical Center, Inc. [7237]
Little Rock Community Health Center [6273]
Little Rock Community Mental Health Center [28301]
Mid-Arkansas Substance Abuse Center [28302]
Pinnacle House [28303]
Up and Out Rehabilitative Day Treatment [28304]
Little Rock School District [247]
Little Rock Vet Center [51871]
Little Sister's Place [10370]
Little Steps Preschool [28075]
Little Talkers Inc. [2678]
Little Traverse Bay Bands of Odawa • Anishnaabe Life Srvs Substance Abuseand Mental Health Prog [44958]
Little Treasures--Petits Tresors [3003]
Little Village Dialysis • DaVita [23945]
Little Works In Progress [2338]
Littlestown Dialysis Center • Wellspan Dialysis [26471]
Littleton Dialysis • Davita [23130]
Live Again Recovery Homes • Live Again Ministries [40791]
Live Oak Center for Communication Disorders [3461]
Live Oak Dialysis • DaVita [27228]
Live Oak Inc. [11048]
Live Oak Public Libraries • Subregional Library for the Blind and Physically Handicapped [3776]
Live True Therapy [10965]
Livengrin Counseling Center [48341], [48449]
Hanover Office Plaza [48265]
Highland Office Center [48374]
Livengrin Foundation Inc [48290]
Livermore Dialysis Center • DaVita [22751]
Livermore VAMC [40003]
Liverpool Dialysis Center, LLC [25787]
Living Center [40865]

Living Center Modesto
Inpatient [40227]
Outpatient [40228]
Living Free Health Services [49758]
Living Free Recovery Services [45095]
Living Hope International Ministry • New Beginning Transitional Program [41864]
Living Hope Texarkana [33118]
Living Legacy Foundation [35062]
Living New Inc • Real Families Inc [46097]
Living Proof Recovery Center [39612]
Living Solutions [47506]
Living Trees Center Inc [42545]
Living Water [8771]
Living Waters Program [44300]
Livingsprings Home Health Care, Inc. [14824]
Livingston Area Council Against Spouse Abuse [9544]
Livingston County Council on Alcohol and Substance Abuse Inc [46606]
Livingston County Hospice [20581]
Livingston Family Center • Runaway and Homeless Youth Program [36020]
Livingston Hospice Care [20365]
Livingston Infusion Care [16270]
Livingston Medical Group [6311]
Livingston Memorial Visiting Nurse Association [13423]
Livingston Memorial Visiting Nurse Association and Hospice [13384]
Livingston Memorial VNA [19069]
Livingston Tennessee Dialysis • DaVita [26873]
Livingston Wyoming Association for Retarded Citizens Children's Services [8318]
Living Care Home Health, Inc. [13668]
Livi's Home Health Care Inc. [13042]
Livonia Counseling Center [30592], [44903]
LKLP Safe House [9388]
LLC Counseling Services • Outpatient Treatment Clinic [39436]
Llerena Home Health Care [14057]
Lloyd C Elam Mental Health Center • Meharry Medical College [49157]
Lloyd Wolfe Juvenile Justice Network • Wolfe Center [40253]
LMAS Home Health & Hospice of Mackinac County [20113]
LMH Satellite at Saint Mary's • Dialysis Center [26191]
LNHSatellite at St. Marys [26192]
Loch Raven Veterans Affairs Outpatient Clinic [30263]
Loch RavenVeterans Affairs Rehabilitation and Extended Care Center [51580]
Lochland School [8319]
Lock Raven VA Community Living & Rehab Ctr. [4099]
Locke Speech/Language Services [2922]
Lockehill Kidney Disease Clinic • Dialysis Facility • Fresenius Medical Care [27335]
Lockport Center for Behavioral Health [33424]
Lockport Home Dialysis and At Home • DaVita [24024]
Lockport Veterans Affairs Clinic [31380]
The Lodge [9065], [30862]
Lodi Dialysis Center • DaVita [22752]
Lodi Memorial Hospital [13106]
Lofink [1211]
Logan [8006]
Logan Community Services Inc [47941]
Logan County Board of Mental Retardation and Developmental Disabilities [8400]
Logan Dialysis • DaVita [26151]
Logan Heights Family Health Centers of San Diego [6351]
Logan-Mason Mental Health Center • Lincoln Crisis Clinic [50855]
Logan/Mingo Area Mental Health • Futures [50322]
Logan/Mingo Area Mental Health Inc [50323]
Mingo County Office [50292]
Logan Square Dialysis Services Inc. • DaVita [23946]
Logan Vet Center Outstation [52139]
Logansport State Hospital [33481]
Loganville Dialysis Center [23737]
Logic Homehealth Services, Inc. [18120]
Logical Behaviors Counseling [11001]
Logistics Home Services, Inc.--Miami [14058]

Logopaedics LLC [3221]
Logopedica LLC [2973]
Logos Healthcare Services [18118]
Lokahi Treatment Centers [42202]
Kona Office/Hillside Plaza [42239]
Lohala Town Center [42251]
Waiakea Villas [42199]
Loma Linda Home Health Care [13077]
Loma Linda Sleep Disorders Center [36671]
Loma Linda University
Behavioral Medicine Center [40436]
Behavioral Medicine Eating Disorder Program [10966]
Center for Fertility and In Vitro Fertilization [21923]
Loma Linda University Health Care - ALS Center [101]
Loma Linda University Kidney Center [22755]
Loma Linda University • MDA Clinic [34760]
Loma Linda University Medical Center [22756]
Loma Linda University Medical Center - Cancer Program [4790]
Loma Linda University Medical Center and Children's Hospital [13107]
Loma Linda University Medical Center - Cystic Fibrosis Center [7473]
Loma Linda University Medical Center - Pain Management [35317]
Loma Linda University • Medical Center • Rehabilitation Clinic [1150]
Loma Linda University Medical Center - Sickle Cell Disease Center for Children [36302]
Loma Linda Veterans Affairs Medical Center
Corona Community Based Outpatient Clinic [28458]
Sun City Outpatient Clinic [28825]
Upland Clinic [28834]
Loma Vista Dialysis • DaVita [27071]
Lombard Home Therapies • Fresenius Medical Care [24025]
Lompoc Artificial Kidney Center • Dialysis Facility [22758]
Lompoc Mental Health Services [28564]
Londin Place--People Incorporated [30724]
London Dialysis Clinic • Renal Advantage Inc. [24407]
London Health Sciences Centre • Speech Language Pathology [3299]
London Health Sciences Complex • Thompson Regional Burn Unit [4616]
London Speech and Language Centre [3300]
Lone Peak Dialysis • DaVita [27400]
Lone Star Community Health Center [7280]
Lone Star Dialysis Center • DaVita [27152]
Lone Star Lions Eye Bank [35235]
Lonetree Dialysis • DaVita [23118]
Long Beach Adult Services [28572]
Long Beach Asian Mental Health Services [28573]
Long Beach Community Medical Center • Comprehensive Cancer Center [4792]
Long Beach Dialysis Center [22763]
Long Beach Harbor (UCLA) Dialysis Center • DaVita [22764]
Long Beach Medical Center • FACTS CD Outpatient Clinic [46759]
Long Beach Medical Center Home Care [16512]
Long Beach Medical Center
Methadone Maintenance Clinic [46760]
Speech Language-Pathology Department [3046]
Long Beach Memorial Medical Center
Adult Cystic Fibrosis Center [7474]
Memorial Care Sleep Disorders Center [36672]
Miller Children's Hospital • Pediatric Cystic Fibrosis Center [7475]
Long Beach Mental Health Services • Child and Adolescent [28574]
Long Beach Reach Inc • Medically Supervised Drug Abuse Clinic [46761]
Long Beach Sleep Disorder Center [36673]
Long Beach Unified School District [281]
Long Beach Veterans Affairs Medical Center • Villages at Cabrillo [28575]
Long Creek Youth Development Center [30243]
Long Island Care at Home [16662]
Long Island Center for Recovery Inc
Alcohol Primary Care Program [46675]
Drug Abuse Inpatient Rehabilitation [46676]
Outpatient Drug Abuse Clinic [46677]

Long Island College Hospital [2993]
   Cystic Fibrosis Center [7615]
   Dialysis Center [25616]
   Neuromuscular Disease Clinic [12288]
   Othmer Cancer Center [5566]
   Stanley S. Lamm Institute for Child Neurology and Developmental Medicine [8306]
Long Island Consultation Center Inc • Chemical Dependency Clinic [47006]
Long Island Counseling Center [47174]
Long Island Crisis Center [51135]
   Runaway and Homeless Youth Program [36114]
Long Island Developmental Disabilities Service Office [8311]
Long Island Health Care [16458]
Long Island Home
   DBA South Oaks Hosp Acute Care Program [46351]
   DBA South Oaks Hosp CD Outpatient Clinic [46352]
   DBA South Oaks Hosp SWI/SWIIA CH Rehab [46353]
Long Island In Vitro Fertilization [22185]
Long Island Jewish Certified Home Health Agency [16540]
Long Island Jewish Medical Center
   Cancer Program [5591]
   Chem Dependence Outpatient Rehab [46636]
   Daehrs Outpatient Drug Free [46656]
   Dialysis Unit [25709]
   Hemophilia Treatment Center [12563]
   MDA Clinic [34836]
   Methadone Maintenance Treatment Program [46657]
   Project Outreach/Outpatient Drug Free [47175]
Long Island Renal Care, Inc. [25708]
Long Island Sleep Center [37398]
Long Island Talking Book Library • Suffolk Cooperative Library System • Outreach Services [3824]
Long Island University • J.M. Ladge Speech and Hearing Center [2997]
Long Island Women's Coalition [9931]
Long-Term Group Home Program • Naperville Group Home [29653]
Long Valley Families in Crisis [9168]
Long Valley Health Center [6310]
Longcare Home Health Corporation [14059]
Longevity home Health Care, Inc. [14060]
Longevity Home Health Services [13857]
Longmont Clinic PC [1430]
Longmont Dialysis • DaVita [23132]
Longmont Hearing Center [1431]
Longmont United Hospital • Cancer Program [4884]
Longs Dialysis • DaVita [26740]
Longview Dialysis Center • DaVita • Dialysis Center & At Home [27232]
Longview Home Medical Equipment [18052]
Longview Regional Speech and Hearing Center [3521]
Longview Wellness Center Inc [49446]
Longwood Rehabilitative Services [38250]
Lonoke County Safe Haven [8753]
Look Who's Talking LLC [2192]
Looking Glass • Adolescent Recovery Program [48105]
Looking Glass Counseling Center [39680]
Looking Glass Youth Family Services, Inc. • Runaway and Homeless Youth Program [36171]
Looking for My Sister [9565]
Lookout Mountain Community Services [29449], [42162]
   ANCOR- Chickamauga [29388]
   ANCOR - La Fayette [29450]
   Cornerstone Psychosocial Rehabilitation Services [29451]
Lookout Mountain Community Services- Horizons [29428]
Loomis Road Dialysis and At Home • DaVita [27724]
Loop Dialysis Center • Diversified Specialty Institutes [23947]
Loop Pharmacy and Home Medical [18539]
Looper Speech & Hearing Center [1851]
Lorain County Alcohol and • Drug Abuse Services Inc [47755], [47793]
Lorain County Alcohol and DA Services Inc • Adolescent Treatment Center [47794]
Lorain County Elyria Home • Fresenius Medical

Care [26109]
Lorain County Health and Dentistry [7092]
Lorain Veterans Affairs Clinic [31793]
Lord Elementary School [8227]
Loretta Adams Ashby Health Center [44652]
Loretto Hospital • Addiction Center [42546]
Loring Family Hospice [19728]
Loris Dialysis Center • Fresenius Medical Care [26741]
Los Alamitos Hemodialysis Center [22767]
Los Alamitos Medical Center • Cancer Program [4795]
Los Alamos Family Council [31206]
Los Alamos Family Council Inc [46288]
Los Alamos VNS Hospice [20540]
Los Angeles Centers for Alcohol and Drug Abuse
   Allen House [40751]
   Downtown [40125]
   Santa Fe Springs [40752]
Los Angeles Child Guidance Clinic [28602]
Los Angeles Community Dialysis South [22786]
Los Angeles Conservation Corps [35827]
Los Angeles County DPH AVRCs • High Desert Recovery Services [39988]
Los Angeles County-Harbor-UCLA Medical Center • Cancer Program [4857]
Los Angeles County Mental Health [28603]
Los Angeles County University of Southern CA Medical Center [13140]
Los Angeles County-University of Southern California Medical Center • Cancer Program [4799]
Los Angeles Drug Treatment Center [39944]
Los Angeles Ear, Nose and Throat Associates [1166]
Los Angeles Gay & Lesbian Center • Mental Health Services [28604]
Los Angeles Gay and Lesbian Youth Services • Runaway and Homeless Youth Program [35828]
Los Angeles Hospice [18959]
Los Angeles Hospice Care Inc. [18943]
Los Angeles Hospice North Branch [18990]
Los Angeles New Life Center Inc [40126]
Los Angeles Pierce College • Special Services [316]
Los Angeles Scottish Rite Childhood [1167]
Los Angeles Speech and Language Therapy Center [1089]
Los Angeles Trade Tech College • Disabled Students Programs and Services [282]
Los Angeles Unified School District • Program for Adults with Disabilities [283]
Los Angeles Vet Center [51886]
Los Angeles Youth Network • Runaway and Homeless Youth Program [35829]
Los Banos Dialysis Center • DaVita [22795]
Los Barrios Unidos Community Clinic [7283]
Los Gatos Orthopedic Sports Therapy [38100]
Los Jazmines Home Care Corporation [14061]
Los Lunas Hospital and Training School [8291]
Los Lunas Schools • Special Services [561]
Los Ninos Pediatrics [7003]
Los Padrinos Juvenile Hall Mental Health Unit [28476]
Los Robles Regional Medical Center [1336]
   Cancer Program [4856]
   Outpatient Services [1362]
Lott Physical Therapy and Sports Medicine [39062]
Lotus Group • Intensive Outpatient Program for Eating Disorders [11062]
Lotus Path Center for Eating Recovery [10967]
Loudon County Mental Health Center [32753]
Loudon Dialysis • Fresenius Medical Care [26869]
Loudoun Abused Women's Shelter [10575]
Loudoun County Mental Health Center
   Eastern Loudon Office [49847]
   Substance Abuse Program [49806]
Loudoun County Public Schools [848]
Loudoun Hospital Center • Mary Elizabeth Miller Radiation Oncology Center [6065]
Louis A. Johnson Veterans Affairs Medical Center [32894]
   PTSD Residential Rehabilitation Program [51845]
Louis A. Weiss Memorial Hospital • Cancer Program [5070]
Louis B. Stokes Cleveland VA Medical Center [20824]
Louis Landau Health Center • Near North Health Service Inc [42547]

Louis Stokes Cleveland Department of VA Medical Center • Spinal Care Center [4369]
Louis Stokes, Cleveland Department of Veterans Affairs Medical Center [16885]
Louis Stokes Cleveland • VA Medical Center [47627]
Louis Stokes Cleveland Veterans Affairs Medical Center--Brecksville Campus [51624]
Louis Stokes Cleveland Veterans Affairs Medical Center--Wade Park Campus [51627]
Louis Stokes Veterans Affairs Medical Center
   Cancer Care Program [5702]
   Multiple Sclerosis Center [34671]
   PTSD Clinical Team [51793]
Louisa--Fort Gay Regional Dialysis [24408]
Louisburg-Paola Veterans Affairs Clinic [29949]
Louisiana Center for Bleeding Disorders and Clotting Disorders • Tulane University Health Science Center • Hematology/Medical Oncology TB-31 [12526]
Louisiana Center for Disordered Eating [11069]
Louisiana Coalition Against Domestic Violence [9404]
Louisiana Department of Education • Louisiana Services to Children and Youth with Deafblindness [2303]
Louisiana Headache Center [12427]
Louisiana Home Care or Alexandria [15264]
Louisiana Home Care--Lafayette [15312]
Louisiana Home Care--Mamore [15322]
Louisiana Home Care--Shreveport [15360]
Louisiana Home Care--Slidell [15368]
Louisiana Home Health of Houma [15301]
Louisiana HomeCare--Jonesville [15304]
Louisiana HomeCare/Minden [15332]
Louisiana HomeCare Mississippi--Louisiana [15291]
Louisiana HomeCare of Monroe [15335]
Louisiana HomeCare of Northwest Louisiana [15324]
Louisiana HomeCare--Ruston [15355]
Louisiana HomeCare--Springhill [15370]
Louisiana Homecare--Vidalia [15376]
Louisiana Homecare of Zwolle [15382]
Louisiana Hospice of Mamou [19852]
Louisiana Office of Public Health • Department of Health and Hospitals • SIDS Information and Counseling Program [36486]
Louisiana Organ Procurement Agency [35058]
Louisiana School for the Deaf [447]
Louisiana School for the Visually Impaired [3712]
Louisiana Sleep Diagnostics, LLC • Sleep Disorders Center [37065]
Louisiana Sleep Foundation [37066]
Louisiana State University Health Science Center, Shreveport • MDA Clinic [34803]
Louisiana State University • Health Sciences Center [2339]
Louisiana State University Health Sciences Center
   LSU Sleep Disorders Center [37067]
   Regional Burn Center - Shreveport [4554]
   School of Medicine in New Orleans • Department of Pediatrics Genetics Clinic [12222]
Louisiana State University Health Sciences Center, Shreveport • Pain Management [35467]
Louisiana State University Health Sciences Center University Hospital
   Cystic Fibrosis and Pediatric Pulmonary Center [7555]
   Gene Therapy Program [12223]
Louisiana State University • Heath Sciences Center • Headache Center [12428]
Louisiana State University Interim Hospital • Cancer Care Program [5257]
Louisiana State University Medical Center • Feist-Weiller Cancer Center [5263]
Louisiana State University • Medical Center of Louisiana • New Orleans Sickle Cell Clinic [36350]
Louisiana State University Medical School • Sickle Cell Center [36351]
Louisiana State University
   Speech and Hearing Clinic [2304]
   Touro Infirmary • Pain Management [35468]
Louisiana University, Monroe • Speech and Hearing Clinic [2331]
Louisville-Jefferson County Board of Health • Family Heath Centers, Inc. [6735]
Louisville Veterans Affairs Medical Center [4062], [30068]
Lourdes Chemical Dependency Program [50051]

Lourdes Counseling Center [51462]
Lourdes Dialysis at Innova, Inc. • Lourdes Health System [25472]
Lourdes Health Support [16349]
Lourdes Home Care--Illinois [14862]
Lourdes Home Care--Mayfield [15231]
Lourdes Homecare and Hospice Wickliffe [15258]
Lourdes Hospice--Metropolis [19544]
Lourdes Hospice--Paducah [19825]
Lourdes Hospice-Vestal [20611]
Lourdes Hospital • Diller Regional Sleep Disorders Center [37031]
Lourdes Hospital, Inc. [15243]
Lourdes Hospital • Speech Pathology Department [2977]
Lourdes Medical Center of Burlington County • Community Cancer Program [5548]
Lourdes Medical Center • Cancer Program [6107]
Lourdesmont Good Shepherd Youth and Family Services [34410]
Love Lines Crisis Center [51042]
Lovejoy Hospice [21002]
Lovejoy Medical--Grundy [18308]
Lovejoy Medical--Lexington [15207]
Lovelace Medical Center • Cancer Center [5549]
Lovelace Rehabilitation Hospital [2963], [4303]
Loveland Dialysis • Fresenius Medical Care [23133]
Lovelock Mental Health Center [31038]
Loving Angles Health Care, Inc. [14062]
Loving Care Hospice [20855]
Loving Care Hospice-Marysville [20862]
Loving Hands Adult and Senior Care Services [15664]
Loving Home Care [16396]
Loving Nursing Home Health Care [14063]
Loving Touch Home Health Care [14064]
Low Country Health Care System [7231]
Lowell Community Health Center Inc • Behavioral Health Services Outpatient [44505]
Lowell General Hospital • Cancer Center [5341]
Lowell House Inc
    Outpatient Substance Abuse Services [44506]
    Residential Services [44507]
Lower Bucks Hospital • Sleep Disorders Center [17265], [37673]
Lower Cape Fear Hospice and Life Care Center
    Bladen County Office [20654]
    Columbus County Angel House Hospice Care Center [20764]
Lower Cape Fear Hospice and Life Care Center--Supply [20745]
Lower Cape Fear Hospice and LifeCare Center=Burgaw [20627]
Lower Columbia Hospice [20985]
Lower Columbia Hospice Adult Foster Care Home • Lower Columbia Hospice [21038]
Lower Columbia Mental Health [51449]
Lower East Side Drop-In Center • Runaway and Homeless Youth Program [36115]
Lower Eastside Service Center DRS • Drug Abuse Outpatient Clinic [46882]
Lower Eastside Service Center
    Methadone Treatment Program [46883]
    Pregnant Women and Infants Program [46884]
    Short Stay Methadone Residence [46885]
    Su Casa Methadone To Abstinence Res. [46886]
    Unit I [46887]
Lower Elwha Health Clinic [50056]
Lower Keys Medical Center • Psych and Chemical Dependency Unit [41717]
Lower Kuskokwim School District [219]
Lower Manhattan Dialysis Center [25724]
Lower Manhattan Dialysis Center II [25725]
Lower Merion Counseling Services [48307]
Lower Sioux Community Center • Runaway and Homeless Youth Program [36037]
Lower Valley Crisis and Support Services [10660]
Lower Valley Home Care Services [18492]
Lower Valley Hospice [21772]
Lowry Dialysis Center • DaVita [23112]
Lowry Speech Therapy [1398]
Loxley Family Dental Center [6191]
Loyal Home Health [14065]
Loyola Center for Health at Hickory Hills [14817]
Loyola Clinical Centers [2379]
Loyola College Alcohol and • Drug Education and Support Services [44157]

Loyola Primary Care [2014]
Loyola Primary Care Center--Wheaton [2119]
Loyola University Medical Center [2093]
    Burn Center [4540]
    Cancer Program [5109]
    Center for Sleep Disorders [36912]
    Cystic Fibrosis Center [7528]
    Multiple Sclerosis Clinic [34569]
Loyola University • Pain Center [35432]
LPG Health Care Inc. [13043]
LRADAC/Behavioral Health Center of the Midlandsx [48919]
LRADAC/The Behavioral Health Center of
    The Midlands [48957]
    The Midlands/WCR [48986]
LRC Substance Abuse and • Behavioral Programs [48958]
LRG Healthcare Sleep Evaluation Center [37331]
LRMC Home Health [13829], [13865]
LSSI BHS in the Northwest Suburbs [42903]
lst Choice Rehabilitation and Sports Medicine [1506]
LSU Center, Department of Communication Disorders • Mollie Webb Speech/Hearing Center [2340]
LT Health Care Corporation [14066]
Lt. Joseph P. Kennedy Institute [7875]
Lt. Joseph P.Kennedy School for Exceptional Children [7973]
Lubbock Dialysis Center--Redbud • Fresenius Medical Care [27237]
Lubbock Faith Center Inc [49449]
Lubbock Intermediate School District--RDSPD [806]
Lubbock Lighthouse [49450]
Lubbock Regional Mental Health/Mental Retardation Center [32502]
Lubbock Regional MH/MR Center • Methadone Clinic [49451]
Lubbock Regional MHMR Center [51387]
Lubbock State School [8556]
Lucas County Health Center [43245]
Lucedale Dialysis • DaVita [25144]
Lucent Home Health, LLC [18119]
Lucid Speech and Language [1192]
Lucila Camacho Craft [40761]
Lucile Packard Children's Hospital at Stanford, Mountain View • Comprehensive Eating Disorders Program [10968]
Lucile Packard Children's Hospital at Stanford, Palo Alto • Comprehensive Eating Disorders Program [10969]
Lucile Packard Stanford Pediatric Transplant • Lucile Packard Children's Hospital at Stanford [22872]
Lucile Salter Packard Children's Hospital at Stanford [12490], [13233]
Lucille Greene Home • JBS Mental Health Authority [27866]
Lucille Packard Stanford Ped Transplant [22873]
Ludlow Street • Community Healthlink, Inc. [30485]
Lufkin Dialysis • DaVita • Dialysis Facility [27241]
Lufkin State School [8557]
Luis E. Martinez House [30425]
LUK Crisis Center Inc • LUK Behavioral Health Clinic [44467]
L.U.K. Crisis Center, Inc. • Runaway and Homeless Youth Program [36002]
LUK, Inc. [30378]
Luke Dorf Inc [48254]
Lumberton Dialysis Center • DaVita [25461]
Lumberton Dialysis Unit • Fresenius Medical Care [25904]
Lumina of Elizabethtown [2267]
Lummi Counseling Services [49901]
Lummi Indian Nation • Runaway and Homeless Youth Program [36253]
Lummi Victims of Crime [10607]
Lumpkin House • Transitional Housing [40127]
Luna Counseling LLP [41203]
Lund Family Center [49734]
Lund and Sleep Center PC [37177]
Lung Associates of Sarasota • Sleep Center of Sarasota [36789]
Lung Clinic • Center for Sleep Medicine [37617]
LUNNS Home Corporation [39945]
Lupe Quintero Wellness Center • Corazon [39437]
Ann and Robert H. Lurie Children's Hospital of Chicago [1991], [14742]
Lurline Smith Mental Health Center [30155]
Luther Hospital--Mayo Clinic Dialysis [27710]

Luther Midelfort • Dunlap Cancer Center [4718]
Luther Midelfort/Mayo Health System • Luther Midelfort Sleep Disorders Center [37969]
Lutheran Association for Special Education [8211]
Lutheran Child and Family Services [44947]
Lutheran Community Service Northwest [32831]
Lutheran Community Services [31961]
Lutheran Community Services Northwest [32811], [51264], [51474]
Lutheran Community Services NW [48138], [48200]
    Crook County Alcohol and Drug [48223]
Lutheran Family Health Centers [7018]
Lutheran Family Services [30975], [45795], [45810]
    Bellevue [45729]
    McCook [45769]
    Papillion Clinic [45809]
    Substance Abuse Program [45760]
Lutheran General Children's Hospital • Cystic Fibrosis Center [7529]
Lutheran General Hospital
    Adult Cystic Fibrosis Center [7530]
    Genetics Services [12198]
Lutheran General Sports Medicine Center [38404]
Lutheran Home Care Hospice of Hope [20057]
Lutheran Home Care Services [21090]
Lutheran Home Care Services Inc. [21072]
Lutheran Hospice-Low Country [21262]
Lutheran Hospice-Upstate [21249]
Lutheran Hospice--White Rock [21288]
Lutheran Hospital
    Cleveland Clinic Sports Health [38867]
    Cystic Fibrosis and Pediatric Pulmonary Clinic [7541]
Lutheran Hospital of Indiana
    Cancer Center [5146]
    MDA Clinic [34797]
    Sleep Disorders Center of Indiana [36955]
Lutheran Hospital of Indiana Transplant • Lutheran Health Network [24145]
Lutheran Medical Center
    Acute Care Addiction Program [46516]
    Pain Management Center [35610]
Lutheran Metro Ministry • Runaway and Homeless Youth Program [36147]
Lutheran Services Florida--Pensacola • Runaway and Homeless Youth Program [35895]
Lutheran Services Florida--Tampa • Runaway and Homeless Youth Program [35896]
Lutheran Services in Iowa, Inc.--Ames [34135]
Lutheran Services in Iowa, Inc.--Waverly [34143]
Lutheran Settlement House • Bilingual Domestic Violence Project [10305]
Lutheran Social Services [50565]
Lutheran Social Services--Aberdeen [34435]
Lutheran Social Services • Alcohol and Drug Treatment Unit [50419]
Lutheran Social Services--Beloiot [32953]
Lutheran Social Services
    Bethany Crisis Shelter • Runaway and Homeless Youth Program [36038]
    Branch Office [30576]
    Cephas Halfway House [33020]
    Eastern Region Office [47764]
Lutheran Social Services--Eau Claire [32970]
Lutheran Social Services--Germantown [32974]
Lutheran Social Services • Homme Youth and Family Programs [33029]
Lutheran Social Services--Hudson [32978]
Lutheran Social Services of Illinois [42628], [42925]
    Behavioral Health Services [42548]
    Behavioral Health Services/Edgewater [42549]
    Elgin [42657]
    Mens Residence North [42550]
    Mens Residence South [42551]
    Nachusa Lutheran Home [42799]
    Womens Residence/North Kenmore [42552]
Lutheran Social Services--Janesville [32980]
Lutheran Social Services--Madison [32987]
Lutheran Social Services--Menominee [30598]
Lutheran Social Services of the National Capital Area [29095]
Lutheran Social Services
    Northeast Regional Office [32947]
    Northern Region Office [47866]
Lutheran Social Services--Rapid City [34438]
Lutheran Social Services • Runaway and Homeless Youth Program [36039]
Lutheran Social Services of South Dakota [34442]

Residential and Outpatient Services [34440]
Runaway and Homeless Youth Program [36198]
Lutheran Social Services--Superior [33016]
Lutheran Social Services--Waukesha [33021]
Lutheran Social Services • Wazee House [32955]
Lutheran Social Services of Wisconsin and Upper
Michigan [32997]
Lutheran Social Services of Wisconsin and Upper
Michigan--Appleton, WI • Runaway and Homeless
Youth Program [36267]
Lutheran Social Services • Wisconsin and Upper
Michigan Inc [50360], [50361], [50446]
Lutheran Social Services of Wisconsin and Upper
Michigan--Marquette, MI • Runaway and Homeless
Youth Program [36021]
Lutherbrook Children's Center • Lutheran Child &
Family Services [34097]
Lutherwood Residential Treatment Center for
Troubled Youth [34128]
Luverne Nursing Facility [27970]
Luz Health Care Corporation [13753]
Luz Home Care, Inc. [14067]
Luzerne Intermediate Unit [703]
L.V. Stabler Memorial Hospital [12672]
Neuropsychiatric Care [28068]
LXR Home Health Services [13754]
Lydia's House [9721]
Lynchburg Counseling Center [32761]
Lynchburg Speech Therapy Inc. [3592]
Lynn Agency, Inc. [16503]
Lynn Canal Counseling Services [39333]
Lynn Canal Counseling Services--Haines [28093]
Lynn Canal Counseling Services--Skagway [28121]
Lynn Community Health Center [30410]
Lynn Community Health, Inc. • Lynn Community
Health Center [6819]
Lynn Laucik [46198]
Lynnfield Drugs, Inc./Hemophilia of the Sunshine
State [14283]
Lynnwood Behavioral Health Clinic [32835]
Lyon Council on Alcohol and Other Drugs [45825],
[45828], [45879], [45882], [45884]
Lyon County Health Department • Flint Hills Com-
munity Health Center [6716]
Lyons Campus of the Veterans Affairs • New Jersey
Healthcare System [51605]
Lyons Home health Care, LLC [16914]

M

M & D Home Health Care [13755]
M D Respiratory Services, Inc. [16185]
M & G Home Health Care Group, Inc. [14068]
M & K Home Health Care [14069]
M-R Medical, Inc.--Arlington [17804]
M-R Medical, Inc.--Waco [18185]
M & S Home Health Group, Inc. [13669]
MA Home Health Agency [14070]
Ma-Lowe Home Care Agency, Inc.--Alexandria
[18245]
Ma-Lowe Home Care Agency, Inc.--Manassas
[18325]
MAAC Project
Nosotros [39708]
Recovery Home/Casa de Milagros [40560]
MAB Addiction Counseling Services [47578]
Mabank Intermediate School District [807]
Mabee Physical Medicine and Rehabilitation Center
• Harris Methodist Fort Worth [4449]
Mableton Dialysis [23740]
MacDonald Training Center [7906]
MacDonell United Methodist Children's Services, Inc.
[34159]
Mackay Center • Deaf Education Program [719]
Mackey Speech and Language Services [3347]
Maclay Rehabilitation Center [40838]
MacNeal Family Practice Sports Medicine Center
[38346]
MacNeal Hospital [14687]
Cancer Program [5063]
Macomb Audiology Services [2652]
Macomb County Community Mental Health Access
Center • Survivors of Suicide [51011]
Macomb County Vet Center [51991]
Macomb Family Services Inc [44711], [44985],
[44990]
Macomb Family Services, Inc. [30625]
Macomb Heart and Rehabilitation Institute [38606]

Macomb Infant Preschool Program [485]
Macomb Kidney Center • DaVita • Dialysis Facility
[24988]
Macomb Library for the Blind and Physically
Handicapped [3808]
Macomb Regional Dialysis Center • Greenfield
Health Systems [24854]
Macomb Rehabilitation Center • Children's Hospital
of Michigan [4175]
Macon Behavioral Health System [33385]
Macon County Dialysis • DaVita [23973]
Macon County Satellite [28057]
Macon County Schools [217]
Macon Health Care Center [2805]
Macon--Piatt Special Education [2016]
Mad River Dialysis Center • Fresenius Medical Care
[26018]
Madawaska Group Home [30228]
Madden Mental Health Center [33431]
Made Free Community Church Inc • Countryside
Christian Center - ATR [41595]
Madear's Kinship Village [31732]
Madeleine Borg Counseling Service--Boro Park
[31269]
Madelia Community Hospital [15909]
Madeline Borg Counseling Service--Manhattan West
[31423]
Madeline's House • Southside Center for Violence
Prevention [10566]
Madera County Behavioral Health Services [28618]
Madera County Behavioral Hlth Services
Oakhurst Counseling Center [40286]
Perinatal Alcohol and Drug Services [40190]
Supervision and Treatment Program [40191]
Madera County Community Action Partnership
[8844]
Madigan Army Medical Center
Cystic Fibrosis Center [7693]
Tumor Registry [6124]
Madison Center for Children [33489]
Madison Center Elkhart [33451]
Madison Center Harris House [33490]
Madison Center and Hospital [33491]
Madison Center Inc • Quiet Care [43204]
Madison Center Metcalfe House [33492]
Madison Center New Passages and Community
Support Program [33493]
Madison Center Plymouth [33484]
Madison Center Portage Manor [33494]
Madison Center Providence House [33495]
Madison Cnty Mental Health Prog/ADAPT/Medically
• Supervised Chemical Dependence Outpatient
Serv [47159]
Madison Community Hospice • Avera McKennan
Branch [21293]
Madison County Afterschool [30107]
Madison County Community Health Center [6680]
Madison County Schools [523]
Madison Dialysis Center • DaVita [25905]
Madison Dialysis of Sioux Valley Hospital [26790]
Madison Health Services • A CRC Hlth Group Facil-
ity/Suboxone Treatment [50447]
Madison House [51416]
Madison Kidney Center [23748]
Madison Pediatrics and Dental [7430]
Madison State Hospital [8000]
Madisonville Clinic [30073]
Madisonville Dialysis Center • DaVita [24423]
Madisonville Dialysis • Fresenius Medical Care
[24427]
Madonna Manor Pain Program [35492]
Madonna Rehabilitation Hospital [4260]
Madonna School for Exceptional Children [8228]
Madonna University • Office of Disability Resources
[495]
Madrone Hospice Inc./Adult Day Healthcare
Services [19081]
Mady and Mules Physical Therapy and Sports
Rehabilitation [38528]
Maehnowesekiyah Wellness Center [50407]
Magaziner Center for Wellness • Pain Clinic [35561]
Magee General Hospital • Mississippi Sports
Medicine and Orthopaedic Center [38646]
Magee General Hospital Sleep Lab [37251]
Magee Rehabilitation Hospital [4396]
Magee Riverfront [4397]
Magee-Women's Hospital
Cancer Program [5858]

Department of Center for Medical Genetics
[12326]
Magee-Women's Hospital of UPMC • Pediatric
Genetics [12327]
Magers Associates [2219]
Maggie Carroll Smith Group Home [31746]
Maghakian Place--People Incorporated [30725]
Magna Healthcare Services [14377]
Magnifique Home Health Care, Inc.--Miami [14071]
Magnifique Home Healthcare--Hialeah [13756]
Magnolia Creek Treatment Center for Eating
Disorders [10882]
Magnolia Dialysis Center and At Home • DaVita
[27243]
Magnolia Hospital Home Health Agency [12873]
Magnolia House Counseling Center [42553]
Magnolia House/Waycross Area Shelter [9130]
Magnolia Oaks Dialysis • DaVita [23720]
Magnolia Regional Health Center Home • Health
and Hospice Agency [20231]
Magnolia Regional Health Center • Home Health
and Hospice Agency [15957]
Magnolia Speech School, Inc. [521]
Magnolia West Dialysis & At Home • DaVita [22906]
Mahaska County Community Health [15098]
Mahaska Health Partnership • New Directions
[43294]
Mahaska Hospice [19722]
Mailman Center for Child Development [7896]
Maimonides Developmental Center [8307]
Maimonides Medical Center
Cancer Center [4688]
Linda Morgante Multiple Sclerosis Care Center
[34647]
Medical Genetics [12289]
Main Gate Counseling Services [49033]
Main Line Health • Lawrence Park Sleep Center
[37674]
Main Line Hospital Lankenau Transplant Center
[26616]
Main Line Rehabilitation Associates, Inc. [4398]
Main Line Speech Consultants [3337]
Main Street Center [30468]
Main Street Clinic [32463]
Main Street Human Resources • The Brien Center
[30390]
Main Street Opportunities Day Support [32724]
Main Street Physicians [7371]
Main Street Transitional Living Program • Runaway
and Homeless Youth Program [35830]
Maine Center [42852]
Maine Center for Integrated Rehabilitation--Brewer
[4078]
Maine Center for Integrated Rehabilitation--Rockland
[4079]
Maine Center for Integrated Rehabilitation--Winslow
[4080]
Maine Coast Memorial Hospital • Rehabilitation
Services [2356]
Maine Educational Center for the Deaf and Hard of
Hearing [457]
Maine General Counseling • Family Medicine
Institute [43916]
Maine General Health [43983]
Maine General Medical Center • Thayer Campus •
Dialysis Center [24617]
Maine General Medical Center - Waterville Campus
• Harold Alfond Center for Cancer Care [5268]
Maine General Sports Medicine [38513]
Maine Health and Human Services • Public Health
Nursing Division • Maine SIDS Program [36487]
Maine Medical Center
Cancer Program [5274]
Maine Hemophilia and Thrombosis Center
[12527]
Maine Pediatric Specialty Group
Adult Cystic Fibrosis Center [7559]
Pediatric Cystic Fibrosis Center [7560]
MDA Clinic [34808]
Special Care Unit [4555]
Sports Medicine Services [38511]
Maine Medical Center--Transplant [24614]
Maine Medical Partners • Division of Reproductive
Endocrinology and Infertility [22084]
Maine Medical Partners Neurology • Multiple
Sclerosis Clinic [34591]
Maine Migrant Health Program [6765]
Maine Sleep Institute [37091]

Maine State Library • Library Services for the Blind and Physically Handicapped **[3800]**
Maine Veterans Affairs Medical Center **[4081]**
MaineGeneral Counseling **[44088]**
MaineGeneral
  Counseling **[43917]**, **[44078]**
  Intensive Outpatient Program **[44079]**
  Residential Services for Men **[44057]**
  Residential Services for Women **[43918]**
Mainland Dialysis Facility • DaVita **[27212]**
Mainline **[50949]**
Mainline Clinic • Adult Sickle Cell Clinic **[36291]**
Mainline Health Systems, Inc. • Portland Health Care Center **[6277]**
Mainstay **[10045]**
Mainstream Counseling **[48410]**
Maintenance and Recovery Services Inc (MARS) **[49231]**
  South **[49232]**
Maitland Audiology, PA **[1641]**
Maiu's Home Health Care, Inc. **[14213]**
Maize Dialysis Center • DaVita **[24337]**
Majesty Home Health, Inc. **[13209]**
Major Hospital **[2182]**
MAK Medical **[14498]**
Makah Chemical Dependency Program **[50030]**
Malama Na Makua A Keiki • DBA Malama Family Recovery Center **[42270]**
Malcolm Grow Medical Center Addiction • Services Program **[44094]**
Malcolm Grow Medical Center • Cancer Program **[5280]**
Malcolm Randall VA Medical Center **[13709]**
Malcolm Randall Veterans Affairs Medical Center • North Florida--South Georgia Healthcare System • PTSD Clinical Team **[51709]**
Malcom Randall Veterans Affairs Medical Center
  Lecanto Clinic **[29205]**
  Ocala Clinic **[29243]**
  Saint Augustine Clinic **[29275]**
  Tallahassee Clinic **[29297]**
  Valdosta Clinic **[29499]**
  The Villages Clinic **[29312]**
Malibu Horizon • Residential Treatment **[40196]**
Mallard Lane Center **[31586]**
Malone Veterans Affairs Clinic **[31384]**
Malvern Institute **[48454]**, **[48622]**
  Trevose **[48659]**
MAM Unique Health Services, Inc. **[17788]**
Man Alive Inc **[44158]**
Managed Care Center Inc
  Adult Outpatient General Population **[49452]**
  Mens Residential Program **[49453]**
  Specialized Female Outpatient **[49454]**
  Womens Residential Programs **[49455]**
Managed Care at Home LLC **[13004]**
Management Consulting Services **[41556]**
Manatee Children's Services • The Flamiglio Center **[34064]**
Manatee County Drug Court **[41570]**
Manatee County Rural Health Services, Inc. • Parrish Clinic **[6535]**
Manatee County School District • Deaf/Hard of Hearing Program **[345]**
Manatee General Surgery **[6440]**
Manatee Glens • Adult Outpatient Substance Abuse Program **[41571]**
Manatee Glens Corporation **[29116]**
Manatee Glens Corp. HELPline **[50752]**
Manatee Glens Corporation • Substance Abuse Treatment Services **[41572]**
Manatee Glens Counseling Services • Youth Addiction Outpatient Services **[29118]**
Manatee Glens Hospital and Crisis Center **[29119]**
Manatee Glens West Counseling Services **[29120]**
Manatee Hearing & Speech Center **[1550]**
Manatee Memorial Hospital • Cancer Program **[4933]**
Manatee Palms Youth Services **[33292]**
Manatee Pediatrics and Westgate OB/GYN **[6441]**
Manavi, Inc. **[9839]**
Manchester Community Health Center **[6961]**
Manchester Dialysis Center • Dialysis Clinic Inc. **[23162]**
Manchester House • Residential Treatment Center **[31622]**
Manchester Kidney Center • Fresenius Medical Care **[25396]**

Manchester Memorial Hospital **[1468]**
  Eastern Connecticut Cancer Institute **[4897]**
  ECHN Sleep Disorders Center **[36747]**
Manchester Public Schools **[330]**
Manchester Sports and Physical Therapy **[38706]**
Manchester VA Medical Ctr. • VA New England Healthcare System **[4269]**
Manchester Veterans Affairs Medical Center **[31081]**
Mandarin Hearing and Balance Center **[1611]**
Mandel Center **[10899]**
Mandell Center for Comprehensive Multiple Sclerosis Care and Neuroscience Research **[34547]**
Mandy • Turning Point Community Programs, Inc. **[28732]**
Mandy's Special Farm **[8286]**
Manet Community Health Center, Inc. • Manet Community Health Center at North Quincy **[6822]**
Manhattan Cougar House **[33430]**
Manhattan Eye, Ear and Throat Hospital **[3065]**
Manhattan Psychiatric Center--125th Street Clinic **[33705]**
Manhattan Psychiatric Center--Ward's Island **[33706]**
Manhattan Vet Center **[52041]**
Maniilaq Counseling and Recovery Center **[39345]**
Maniilaq Counseling Services **[28109]**
Maniilaq's Family Crisis Center **[8668]**
Manistee-Benzie CMH • DBA - Centra Wellness Network **[44667]**
Manistee-Benzie Community Mental Health Services **[30595]**
Manitoba School for the Deaf **[458]**
Manitowoc County Community Hospice • HomeCare Health Services & Hospice **[21850]**
Manitowoc County Domestic Violence Center **[10714]**
Mann House Inc **[44198]**
Manna House • Faith Based Treatment **[49578]**
Manna Inc
  Derek House **[43930]**
  Northern Region Outpatient **[44015]**
Mannboro Medical Center **[7345]**
Manning Regional Healthcare Center • Manning Family Recovery Center **[43286]**
Manny Esh Respiratory Care, Inc. **[17481]**
The Manor **[8175]**, **[34231]**
Manor Care Dialysis Center **[24652]**
Manor Clinic • Capital Nephrology Associates **[26952]**
Manor Healthcare Center **[6442]**
Manor House I • Life Spring **[29791]**
Manor House II **[29753]**
Mansfield Dialysis Center • DaVita **[27244]**
Mansfield Kidney Center • Fresenius Medical Care **[26155]**
Mansfield Mental Health Center **[30156]**
Mansfield Veterans Affairs Clinic **[31799]**
Mantachie Rural Health Care, Inc. **[6889]**
Manteca Dialysis Center • DaVita **[22800]**
Manteno Dialysis Center • Kankakee Valley Dialysis **[24027]**
Manus Academy **[8373]**
Manzanita Dialysis Center • DaVita **[22622]**
MAP Behavioral Health Services Inc **[48874]**
Maple Avenue Kidney Center **[24057]**
Maple Grove Dialysis Unit and At Home • DaVita **[25037]**
Maple Lake Recovery Center **[45196]**
Maple Leaf Family & Sports Medicine, LLC **[38854]**
Maple Leaf Farm Associates Inc **[49747]**
Maple Shade Youth & Family Services, Inc. **[30299]**
Maple Valley Plaza Dialysis • DaVita **[25199]**
Mapleton Community Mental Health Center **[31270]**
Maplewood Dialysis Center • Fresenius Medical Care **[25465]**
Maplewood Dialysis • DaVita **[25039]**
Maplewood Veterans Affairs Clinic **[30694]**
MAPS/Stepping Stones • Runaway and Homeless Youth Program **[35982]**
Maquoketa Kidney Center LLC **[24284]**
Marana Health Center **[6236]**
Marathon Health Care Center • North Central Health Care-Crisis Intervention **[51520]**
Marathon Health Center **[6494]**
Marathon Physical Therapy, PC **[38949]**
Marbridge Foundation **[8558]**
Marc Center **[29978]**
  Marc Graphics **[30108]**

MARC Physical Therapy/Sports Medicine--Dumont **[38719]**
MARC Physical Therapy/Sports Medicine--Fairview **[38723]**
Marcelo E Lopez Claros **[47460]**
Marcey Halfway House **[44310]**
Marcialed Healthcare Corporation **[14072]**
Marco Island Pediatrics **[6495]**
MARCO Services Inc **[50454]**
Marcus Daly Center for Hospice & Palliative Care **[20359]**
Marcus Daly Memorial Hospital **[2835]**
Marcus Institute • Down Syndrome Clinic **[10790]**
Marden Rehabilitation--Beckley **[39157]**
Marden Rehabilitation--Columbus **[38869]**
Marden Rehabilitation--Oceana **[39165]**
Marden Rehabilitation - Wesley Ridge **[38891]**
Marden Rehabilitation--Woodsfield **[38902]**
Mare Island Home Health Inc. **[13409]**
Marengo Memorial Hospital • Dialysis Unit **[24285]**
M.A.R.G. Home Health Care **[14073]**
Margaret Dumas Mental Health Center **[30129]**
Margaret J. Weston Health Center **[7226]**
Margaret Mary Community Hospital • Cancer Care Program **[5136]**
Margaret Mary Home Care & Hospice **[14962]**
Margaret R. Pardee Memorial Hospital **[16739]**
  Cancer Program **[5643]**
Margarets House **[45200]**
Margie's Haven House, Inc. **[8763]**
MARI Home Healthcare Services • comet Home Healthcare, Inc. **[14853]**
MARI Home Healthcare Services, LLC **[14854]**
Maria Parham Medical Center **[16737]**
Maria de los Santos Health Center **[7176]**
Maria Sardinas Center **[40561]**
Maria Sardinas Clinic **[28754]**
Marian Anderson Sickle Cell Anemia Care and Research Center **[36421]**
Marian Center • Services for Developmentally Handicapped and Mentally Retarded **[7901]**
Marian Educational Outreach **[7988]**
Marian Hall Emergency Shelter • Runaway and Homeless Youth Program **[36056]**
Marian Hill Chemical Dependency Center **[45424]**
Marian Hospice **[19042]**
Marian Manor Pain Management Program **[35493]**
Marian Medical Center
  Cancer Program **[4851]**
  Hospital Home Care/Hospice/Infusion **[13337]**
  Hospital Home Care--Lompoc Branch **[13109]**
  Hospital Home Care--Templeton Branch **[13382]**
Marianas Psychiatric Services LLC **[42187]**
Marianjoy **[2094]**
Marianjoy, Oakbrook Terrace • Pain Management Program **[35433]**
Marianjoy Rehabilitation Hospital and Clinics **[2120]**, **[4024]**, **[38418]**
Marianna Dialysis Center • DaVita **[23380]**
Maria's Home Health Services **[14298]**
Maricopa County Department of Public Health Services **[6243]**
Maricopa Medical Center
  Dialysis Center **[22483]**
  Pain Clinic **[35288]**
Maricopa Special Healthcare District **[12810]**
  Attendant Care **[12811]**
Marie Detty Youth and Family Service Center • Runaway and Homeless Youth Program **[36155]**
Marie H. Katzenbach School for the Deaf **[551]**
Marie Lorenz Dialysis Center • Olean General Hospital • Hemodialysis Unit **[25748]**
Marie Steiner Kelting Hospice Home **[20152]**
Marietta City Schools **[376]**
Marietta Dialysis • Dialysis Facility • DaVita **[26157]**
Marietta Memorial Hospital • Stecker Cancer Center **[5735]**
Marietta Neurology and Headache Center **[12418]**
Marillac **[8030]**
Marillac Center **[33513]**, **[34267]**
Marillac/IMPACT • Overland Park **[43439]**
Marilu Home Health Care **[13757]**
Marimor School **[8417]**
Marin Abused Women's Services **[8901]**
Marin Community Clinic--Greenbrae **[6304]**
Marin Community Clinic--Novato **[6332]**
Marin County Community Mental Health Services **[28791]**

West Marin Service Center [28708]
Marin General Hospital [13068]
Cancer Institute [4784]
Marin Outpatient and Recovery Services [40707]
Marin Reproductive Medical Associates [21924]
Marin Services for Men [40708]
Marin Services for Women • Residential Program [39993]
Marin Treatment Center • Outpatient Services [40709]
Marina Sports Medicine Clinic [38116]
Mariners Inn [44747]
Marinette County Hlth and Human Services • ADAPT Clinic [50457]
Marion Area Counseling Center [31803]
Alcohol and Drug Program [47803]
Marion Area Counseling Center, Inc. • CONTACT Care Line [51224]
Marion Area Health Center II • Sleep Disorders Center [37535]
Marion Area Health Center • Industrial Rehabilitation [35611]
Marion Citrus Mental Health Center [29244]
Citrus Outpatient Service [29206]
Marion-Citrus Mental Health Center--Lecanto Campus [50771]
Marion Citrus Mental Health Center • Northern Landing Transitional Program [29245]
Marion County Drug Court • Vision of Strength [41835]
Marion County Health Department • Alcohol and Drug Treatment Program [48241]
Marion County Industries [30044]
Marion County Schools [872]
Marion County Treatment Center [39257]
Marion Dialysis & At Home • DaVita [24030]
Marion Dialysis Center • Fresenius Medical Care [26744]
Marion General Hospital
Cancer Center [5165]
Cancer Program [5736]
Marion General Hospital Home Care & Hospice [16980]
Marion General Hospital • Quality of Life Hospice [20861]
Marion Medical Center Behavioral Health Annex [28175]
Marion Regional Medical Center, Inc. [12677]
Marion Stamm dba Abusive Partners/PB • Delray Beach - ATR [41635]
Marion Veterans Affairs Medical Center [29640]
Mariposa Community Health Center [6240]
Mariposa Counseling Center [50679]
Mariposa County Behavioral Health and Recovery Services [28462]
Mariposa County Behavioral Health • Recovery Services [40202]
Mariposa Rehabilitation Center [1441]
Mariposa Women and Family Center [40322]
Marjan Rafeii Speech Pathology Inc. [1067]
Marjorie Basser Dialysis Center • Saint John's Episcopal Hospital [25658]
Mark Bontreger Inc [49032]
Mark Lindsay Dialysis • University Health Care [27434]
Mark Twain Area Counseling Center [30850]
Mark Youth and Family Care • Campus Inc [39505]
Markham House [31362]
Marklund Children's Home [7929]
Marksville Home Care [15326]
Markus Mittermeyer [29279]
Marlborough Medical Center • Center for Sleep Disorders [37119]
Marlee C Poulin LCSW [43919]
Marlette Regional Hospital • Sleep Lab ww. marletteregionalhospital.org [37178]
Marliere Hospice Care Center [19269]
Marlon P. Rimando, MD, Inc. [38335]
Marlowe House [31695]
Marlton Dialysis Center • Diversified Specialty Institutes [25466]
Marlton School [284]
Marnie Millington Speech--Language Pathology [2535]
Marquette General Health System [2623]
Behavioral Health Service [44915]
Cancer Center [5385]
Marquette General Home Health and Hospice--

Escanaba [15648]
Marquette General Home Health and Hospice--Menominee [15749]
Marquette General Home Health Parent Organization [15745]
Marquette General Hospital • Dialysis Center [24944]
Marquette University • Speech and Hearing Clinic [3683]
MARR Inc
Mens Recovery Center [42085]
Womens Recovery Center [42121]
Marra's Homecare Equipment & Supplies, Inc. [16655]
Marrero Dialysis • DaVita [24504]
Marriage and Family Counseling Center [45932]
Marsh Creek Residence • Carelink Community Support Services [32012]
Marshall Center [7364]
Marshall County Association for Retarded Citizens [7714]
Marshall County Family Support Service [10201]
Marshall County Hospital Home Health Agency [15163]
Marshall County Schools [877]
Marshall Dialysis Center • Diversified Specialty Institutes [25243]
Marshall Habilitation Center [8204]
Marshall Hospital • Cancer Program [4821]
Marshall I Pickens Hospital • Addlife Addiction Services [48945]
Marshall Manor Nursing Home [27942]
Marshall Medical Center [13247]
Marshall Medical Center North [12674]
Marshall Medical Center
Pain Clinic [35673]
Sleep Disorders Center [36590]
Marshall-Starke Development Center [8003]
Marshall University • Speech and Hearing Center [3652], [3656]
Marshfield Clinic--Chippewa Center [7422]
Marshfield Clinic - Cystic Fibrosis Center [7700]
Marshfield Clinic Inc. [8621]
Marshfield Clinic
Marshfield Sleep Disorders Center [37970]
MDA Clinic [34911]
Medical Genetic Services 1A4 [12375]
Multiple Sclerosis Center [34743]
Psychiatry & Behavioral Health Department [32991]
Speech Pathology Section [3679]
Marshfield Sports Medicine • Marshfield Clinic • Saint Joseph's Hospital [39182]
Marshville Dialysis Center • DaVita [25908]
Martha Jefferson Hospital [18259]
Cancer Program [6054]
Sleep Medicine Center [37889]
Martha Lloyd Community Services [8489]
Martha Morehouse Medical Plaza • Outpatient Rehabilitation [4370]
Martha's House, Inc. [9069]
Marthas Place [44159]
Martha's Vineyard Community Services--CONNECT to End Violence [9505]
Marthas Vineyard Community Services • Island Counseling Center/Outpatient [44534]
Martha's Vineyard Hospital • Dialysis Unit [24790]
Martin Audiology Associates [3547]
Martin Bowen Hefley Knee and Sports [38066]
Martin County Home Health [15194]
Martin County Office/Samaritan Center • Knox County Hospital [43142]
Martin County Schools Exceptional Children Program [634]
Martin and Edith Stein Hospice [20496]
Martin Lott Group Home [29280]
Martin Luther King Health Center [6953]
Martin Luther King Jr. Clinica Campesina [6475]
Martin Luther King, Jr. Family Clinic, Inc. [7284]
Martin Luther King • Multipurpose Center [47087]
Martin Memorial Health Systems • Weissman Cancer Center [4994]
Martin Memorial Medical Center • Sleep and Audiology Department [1762]
Martin Sleep Clinic [37602]
Martindale/Brightwood Community Health Center [6691]
Martin's Florida Elder Care [14074]

Martinsburg Institute [50328]
Martinsburg Veterans Affairs Medical Center [32919]
Marvels Home Health, Inc. [13758]
Marvina Home Health and Hospice--Cheriton [18264]
Marvina Home Health and Hospice--Chesapeake [18268]
Marvina Home Health and Hospice--Newport News [18336]
Marvina Home Health and Hospice--Virginia Beach [18403]
Marworth [48680]
Mary Ann Barr PhD [40222]
Mary Anne Ruane LCSW CADC [46149]
Mary Benson House • ARP Phoenix [47212]
Mary Bird Perkins Cancer Center--Baton Rouge [5242]
Mary Bird Perkins Cancer Center--Covington • Cancer Center [5245]
Mary Bridge Children's Health Center
Cystic Fibrosis Center [7694]
Genetics Clinic [12367]
Mary Bridge Children's Hospital & Health Center [18471]
The Mary Campbell Center [7869]
Mary E Watts Recovery Center • Inpatient [49168]
Mary Eliza Mahoney Dialysis Center • Fresenius Medical Care [24796]
Mary Free Bed Hospital • MDA/ALS Clinic [125]
Mary Free Bed Hospital and Rehabilitation Center [2597], [35502]
Mary Free Bed Professional Building [4176]
Mary Free Bed Rehabilitation Hospital [4177]
MDA/ALS Clinic [34815]
MDA Clinic [34816]
Mary Greeley Hospital • McFarland Clinic • Cystic Fibrosis Center [7544]
Mary Greeley Medical Center--Ames [24249]
Mary Greeley Medical Center--Homeward [15063]
Mary Greeley Medical Center--Iowa Falls • Iowa Falls Dialysis Center [24281]
Mary Greeley Medical Center--Marshalltown • Marshalltown Dialysis [24286]
Mary Greeley Medical Center
Sleep Disorders Center [36980]
William R. Bliss Cancer Center [5181]
Mary Hall Freedom House Inc [42028]
Mary Imogene Bassett Hospital • Dialysis Center [25644]
Mary Koening Center • Day Activity Center [29281]
Mary L Bonsant LCPC [43941]
Mary Lanning Hospice [20384]
Mary Lanning Hospital--Clay County Branch • Home Health Services [16097]
Mary Lanning Hospital--Webster County • Home Health Services [16096]
Mary Lanning Memorial Healthcare • Pain Clinic [35540]
Mary Lanning Memorial Hospital--Hastings [16103]
Mary Lanning Memorial Hospital • Morrison Cancer Center [5474]
Mary Lee Foundation [8530]
Mary Lee Foundation Rehabilitation Center [4450]
Mary Lind Recovery Centers
Rena B Recovery Center [40128]
Royal Palms Recovery Home [40129]
Mary M. Gooley Hemophilia Center [12564]
Mary Mavec Euclid Opportunity School [8411]
Mary Parrish Center [10425]
Mary Rutan Hospital • Sleep Disorders Center [37536]
Mary Shaw Butler Shelter • Victim Center [9684]
Mary Starke Harper Geriatric Psychiatry Center [28056]
Mary Washington Home Health [18300]
Mary Washington Home Health and Hospice [21696]
Mary Washington Hospital [18301]
Cancer Center of Virginia [6061]
Sleep Wake Disorders Center of Fredericksburg [37890]
Maryhaven Adult Outpatient Services--Columbus [31733]
Maryhaven Center for Hope Inc [47021]
Maryhaven--Delaware [31757]
Maryhaven Inc
Inpatient/Outpatient for Youths/Adults [47720]
Womens Extended Care Program [47721]
Maryhaven--Main Campus [31734]

Mays and Schnapp Pain Clinic and Rehabilitation Center [35674]
Maysville At Home--Kentucky • DaVita [24426]
Maysville Medical Center [6194]
Mayview State Hospital [33796]
MAZE Cord Blood Laboratories [35135]
Mazzitti and Sullivan Inc [48396]
MB Home Health Care [15721]
MBA Southeast Baltimore County [44262]
MBA Wellness Centers LLC [42160]
MBL Associates [15441]
McAlester Regional Dialysis Center LLC [26264]
McAlester Regional Health Center [3301]
McAlester Regional Health Center - Home Health Services [17128]
McAlester Regional Home health [17129]
McAlester Scottish Rite Center • Language Disorders Clinic [3271]
McAlister Institute for Treatment and Educ
    East Region North Teen Recovery Center [39796]
    North Rural Teen Recovery Center [40418]
    South Bay Womens Recovery [40255]
McAlister Institute for Treatment and Education
    East County Adolescent Detox [39997]
    East County Regional [39797]
    East Region South Teen Rec Center [39958]
    McAlister Institute Group Home [40819]
    North Central Teen Recovery Center [40562]
    North Coastal Regional [40313]
    North County Adolescent Detox [40314]
    Options Residential/Kiva [39998]
    South Bay East TRC [39709]
    South Bay Regional Recovery Center [39710]
McAllen Dialysis Center • Diversified Specialty Institutes [27251]
McAllen Dialysis Ltd. • US Renal Care [27252]
McAllen Intermediate School District [808]
McAllen Regional School for the Deaf [809]
McAndrews House--People Incorporated [30667]
McBride Clinic, Inc. [38908]
MCC Healthcare Services [14790]
MCCA [41465]
    Trinity Glen [41468]
McCabe Speech and Language Services [2031]
McCafferty Vet Center Outstation [52057]
McCafferty Veterans Affairs Clinic [31716]
McCain LLC • DOT - SAP [44748], [44780]
McCall Foundation Inc • Carnes Weeks Center/ Intensive Residential [41478]
McCall Foundation
    McCall House [41479]
    Outpatient Program [41480]
    Winsted Satellite Office [41498]
McCallum Place [11121]
McClain County Health Department [31875]
McClanahan and Associates [44099]
McClellan Outpatient Clinic [13168]
McCook Dialysis Center • DaVita [25333]
McCormack Place Apartments [28259]
McCormick Mental Health Clinic [32208]
Mccormick Speech & Language [1348]
McCready Hospital and Outpatient Clinic [2409]
McCreary County DUI Services [43798]
McCullough-Hyde Memorial Hospital • Sleep Disorders Center [37538]
McCullough Vargas and Associates [44627], [44864]
McDermott Center/Haymarket Center
    Adolescent Outpatient/Haymarket South [42554]
    IOP [42555], [42556]
    Mater Hall A [42557]
    Mens Detox [42558]
    MISA [42559]
    West [42904]
McDermott/Haymarket Center • Womens Treatment [42560]
McDonough Dialysis Facility • Davita [23754]
McDonough District Hospital [14849]
    Cancer Program [5107]
    The MDH Hospice [19540]
McDowell County Dialysis • DaVita [25907]
The McDowell Hospital • Home Care Agency [16752]
MCDS Home Health Group [13761]
McFarland Clinic [29877]
MCG Reproductive Medicine and Inferility Assocites [22016]

MCG Reproductive Medicine and Infertility Associates [22017]
McGaughey-Creswell-Mann, Inc. [17939]
McGowan House • Community Healthlink, Inc. [30486]
McGuire Memorial Home [8471]
McGuire Veterans Affairs Medical Center • Substance Abuse Treatment Program [49827]
MCH Home Health Department/Muhlenberg Surgical Association [15184]
McHenry County Crisis Program [50882]
McHenry County Youth Service • Runaway and Homeless Youth Program [35931]
McIntosh Trail Community Service Board [29436]
McIntosh Trail MH/MR/Substance Abuse Comm Serv Brd • DBA Pine Woods [42050]
McIntyre Center [47836]
McIntyre House [40132]
McKay-Dee Hospital Center • Cancer Program [6039]
McKean County Visiting Nurse Association Hospice [21060]
McKee Medical Center • Cancer Center [4885]
McKeesport Dialysis • Dialysis Center • DaVita [26607]
McKeesport West Dialysis • DaVita [26474]
McKenna Pain Management [35548]
Mckenna Recovery Center • Ke Ala Pono Kauai [42267]
McKenna Sports Fitness and Rehabilitation Center [39087]
McKennan Hospital [35670]
McKenzie--Willamette Sleep Solutions Center [37618]
McKinley Hall Inc [47857]
    Mens Residential Program [47858]
    Women and Children Program [47859]
McKinley Intervention Services [29593]
McKinney Community Health Center, Inc. [6609]
McKinnon Speech and Language Services Inc. [3387]
McLaren Regional Medical Center
    Great Lakes Cancer Institute [5376]
    Sleep Diagnostic Center [37179]
    Speech and Audiology Department [2585]
McLaren Visiting Nurse and Hospice--Bay City [15583]
McLaren Visiting Nurse and Hospice--Davison [15615]
McLaren Visiting Nurse and Hospice--Sterling Heights [15838]
McLean Ambulatory and Residential • Treatment Center [44397]
McLean Ambulatory Treatment Center, Naukeag [33569]
McLean Center at Fernside [44542]
McLean County Center for Human Services [29566]
    Emergency Crisis Intervention Team [50831]
Mclean Family Resource Center [10118]
McLean Homecare and Hospice [19165]
McLean Hospital [33571]
    Alcohol and Drug Abuse Treatment [44401]
    East House II Acute Rehabilitation [44402]
    Klarman Eating Disorder Center [11092]
McLean Hospital Southeast [33574]
McLean Residence at The Brook [44595]
McLeod Addictive Disease Center [47225], [47260], [47261], [47278], [47322], [47420]
    Hickory [47382]
    Marion [47415]
    Statesville [47503]
McLeod Behavioral Health Services [48926]
McLeod Hospice • McLeod Regional Medical Center [21234]
McLeod Regional Medical Center - Home Health [17587]
McLeod Regional Medical Center of the Pee Dee, Inc. [17588]
MCM Substance Abuse Center [42661]
The McMains Children's Developmental Center [8059]
McMaster Children's Hospital • Pediatric Eating Disorders Program [11224]
McMathis Counseling Services [44886], [45008]
McMinn/Meigs/Monroe CONTACT [51351]
McNair Academic High School • Total Communication Program [548]

McNeal Hospital • Behavioral Health Services [42412]
McNulty Center [32748]
McPherson Counseling Services Inc [42012]
McPherson County Council on Violence Against Persons [9372]
McPike Addiction Treatment Center • CD Inpatient Rehab Program [47151]
McRory Pediatric Services [1106]
MD Nursing Corporation [13670]
MDA/ALS Center of Memphis Mid-South [150], [34877]
MDA/ALS Clinic [97]
MDC Home Health Care [14075]
MDPA Sleep Disorders Center • Gowani Medical Associates [36791]
MDT Home Health Care Agency [14076]
Me Without Measure [10888]
Meade County Industries [29984]
Meadow Creek [45261]
Meadow Lane health Services • Meadowbrook [33564]
Meadow Wood Behavioral Health System [41511]
Meadow Wood Hospital [33274]
Meadowlake Dialysis • Fresenius Medical Care [26701]
Meadowlark Hospice [19747]
Meadowridge Behavioral Health Center [34215]
The Meadows [28224], [39514]
Meadows Behavioral Healthcare [33445]
The Meadows of Chambersburg [32002]
Meadows East Dialysis • DaVita [24419]
Meadows Edge • North Kingstown [48860]
Meadows Hospital [33446]
Meadows Psychiatric Center [33798]
The Meadows Psychiatric Center [31992], [32040], [32042], [32104], [32134], [33797]
Meadows Sleep Center at Vidalia [36845]
Meadowview Psychiatric Hospital [33661]
MeadowWood Behavioral Health System [29070]
Meadville Dialysis • DaVita • Dialysis Center & At Home [26475]
Meadville Medical Center • Cancer Program [5842]
Meadville Veterans Affairs Clinic [30789]
Mease Hospital • Cancer Center [4988]
MECCA Services [43266], [43279]
Mechanicsville Dialysis • American Renal Associates [27514]
Mecklenburg County Provided Srvs Org • Substance Abuse Services Center [47262]
Mecklenburg County Women's Commission [10024]
Mecosta County Medical Center [15587]
Med Assist Home Health Services Inc. [13346]
Med-Care Home--Fort Worth • Care South Home Care [17926]
Med-Care Home--Grapevine [17937]
Med Care Home Health Care [15814]
Med-Care Home--Waxahachie [18186]
Med Care Plus Inc. [13242]
Med-Center At Home • DaVita [27153]
Med Center Dialysis • DaVita [27154]
Med Central Health System • Sleep Disorders Center [37539]
Med-Equip, Inc. [17466]
Med Equip Services [18422]
Med-Fast Home Care [17231]
Med North Health Center [7063]
Med Pro Home Health Services [14077]
Med--Solutions Home Health Care [14078]
Med-South, Inc. [12688]
Med South Mental Health [30130]
MedCare at Home • Care South Home Health [17883]
Medcare Home Health, Inc [14744]
MedCare Home Health Services--Coral Gables [13623]
MedCare Home Health Services--Lauderdale Lakes [13852]
Medcare--Temecula Home Health Agency Inc. [13380]
Medcenter One
    Communication Disorders [3200]
    Dialysis Unit [25986]
Medcenter One Health Systems • Cancer Program [5668]
Medcenter One Home Health and Hospice [20787]
Medcenter One, Inc.--Bismarck [16806]
Medcenter One, Inc.--Mandan [16817]

Medcenter One Satellite--Fort Yates • Dialysis Facility [25993]
Medcenter One Satellite--Jamestown • Dialysis Unit [25996]
Medcenter One Sleep Center [37498]
MedCentral Health System • Cancer Program [5734]
MedCentral Health System Home Health--Mansfield [16972]
MedCentral Health System - Shelby Hospital [17038]
MedCentral Hospice [20859]
Medco Health Solutions Inc. [16218]
Mederi Caretender--Brooksville [13607]
Mederi Caretenders--Naples [14254]
Mederi Caretenders--Port Saint Lucie [14353]
Mederi Caretenders--Punta Gorda [14354]
Mederi Caretenders--Vero Beach [14439]
Mederi Caretenders Visiting Services of Broward [13693]
Mederi Caretenders Visiting Services of Gainesville [13710]
Mederi Caretenders Visiting Services of Southwest Florida [13701]
Medex Home Healthcare [14745]
Medford Dialysis Center • Fresenius Medical Care [24777]
Medford Kidney Center • DaVita [25701]
Medi-Cure Health Services Inc [40133]
Medi-Fair [16526]
Medi Home Care--Columbia [17574]
Medi Home Care--Mount Airy [16761]
Medi-Home Health Agency--Altoona [17244]
Medi Home Health Agency--Barboursville [18493]
Medi-Home Health Agency--Belpre [16851]
Medi-Home Health Agency--Butler [17272]
Medi Home Health Agency--Chesapeake [18269]
Medi Home Health Agency--Chirstiansburg [18274]
Medi-Home Health Agency--Clifton Forge [18275]
Medi-Home Health Agency--Coraopolis [17291]
Medi Home Health Agency--Daytona Beach [13643]
Medi Home Health Agency--Fort Myers [13702]
Medi Home Health Agency--Fredericksburg [18302]
Medi Home Health Agency--Gallipolis [16942]
Medi Home Health Agency--Lakeland [13844]
Medi-Home Health Agency--Largo [13849]
Medi-Home Health Agency--Ligonier [17379]
Medi Home Health Agency--Manassas [18326]
Medi-Home Health Agency--Monogahela [17389]
Medi Home Health Agency--New Port Richey [14260]
Medi-Home Health Agency--Pensacola [14338]
Medi-Home Health Agency--Pittsburgh [17442]
Medi Home Health Agency--Pulaski [18351]
Medi Home Health Agency--Raleigh [16769]
Medi Home Health Agency--Richmond [18368]
Medi Home Health Agency--Roanoke [18377]
Medi Home Health Agency--Saint Clairsville [17027]
Medi-Home Health Agency--State College [17490]
Medi Home Health Agency--Tampa [14420]
Medi Home Health Agency--Wintersville [17076]
Medi Home Health Agency--Woodsfield [17077]
Medi Home Health and Hospice-Chesapeake [21680]
Medi Home Health and Hospice--Richmond [21726]
Medi Home Health and Hospice--Roanoke [21730]
Medi Home Health and Hospice--Saint Clairsville [20887]
Medi Home Health--Jacksonville [13818]
Medi Home Private Care--Hixson [17679]
Medi Home Private Care--Johnson City [17693]
Medi Home Private Care--Knoxville [17708]
Medi Home Private Care--Lebanon [17718]
Medi Home Private Care--Rock Hill [17618]
Medi-Plex Health Professionals, LLC [16056]
Medi-Rents, Inc./Praxair Healthcare Services [15554]
Medi-Speech Service/Rehab Team [2583]
Mediassist Home Health Care Services Agency Corporation [14079]
Medic Help Home Health Care [14080]
Medic Home Health Care [16886]
Medical Advanced Pain Specialists [35520]
Medical Arts Chemists and Surgicals [16397]
Medical Care Products, Inc. [13819]
Medical Center of Arlington • Cancer Care Program [5959]

The Medical Center of Aurora • Cancer Program [4867]
The Medical Center at Bowling Green • Cancer Center [5212]
Medical Center at Bowling Green • Sleep Disorders Center [37032]
Medical Center of Central Georgia • Cancer Life Program [5031]
Medical Center Clinic • Sleep Diagnostic Center [36792]
Medical Center of Georgia • Central Georgia Fertility Institute [22018]
Medical Center Health Care Services, Inc. [16288]
The Medical Center Home Care Program [15166]
Medical Center Home Health--Bolivar [17645]
Medical Center Home Health--Jackson [17685]
Medical Center Home Health--Trenton [17779]
Medical Center Hospital--Odessa • Cancer Care Program [6015]
Medical Center Hospital of Vermont • Fletcher Allen Healthcare [27441]
The Medical Center • J. B. Amos Community Cancer Center [5019]
Medical Center Kidney Clinic • Fresenius Medical Care [27155]
Medical Center at Lancaster [32495]
Medical Center of Lewisville • Sleep Diagnostic Institute [37821]
Medical Center of McKinney Behavioral Health [32511]
Medical Center of McKinney
    Behavioral Medicine Services [49464]
    Sleep Specialties Center [37822]
Medical Center of Ocean County • Cancer Program [5503]
Medical Center of Plano • Cancer Program [6017]
Medical Center of South Arkansas [1004]
    Home Health [12842]
Medical Center of Southeastern Oklahoma [17116]
Medical Centers Home Care [12675]
Medical City Dallas Hospital
    Cancer Program [5974]
    Rehabilitation Services [35698]
Medical City Dallas Renal Transplant [27031]
Medical College of Georgia
    Adult Cystic Fibrosis Center [7520]
    Comprehensive Sickle Cell Center [36336]
    Department of Pediatrics • Down Syndrome Clinic [10791]
Medical College of Georgia - Department of Pediatrics • Section of Pulmonology • Pediatric Cystic Fibrosis Center [7521]
Medical College of Georgia Health Inc. • Sleep Disorders Center [36846]
Medical College of Georgia Health • MDA Clinic [34788]
Medical College of Georgia • Hospital and Clinics [42045]
Medical College of Georgia Hospital and Clinics
    Cancer Program [5012]
    Department of OB/GYN • Reproductive Endocrinology, Infertility and Genetics Section [12190]
Medical College of Georgia • Pain Management [35408]
Medical College Hospital • Transplant/Dialysis Center [26212]
Medical College of Virginia
    Chester Sports Medicine [39123]
    Children's Medical Center • Pediatric Comprehensive Sickle Cell Center [36440]
    Cystic Fibrosis Center [7687]
Medical College of Virginia Hospitals
    Cancer Program [6083]
    Evans-Haynes Burn Center [4644]
    House Calls Program [18369]
Medical College of Virginia
    MDA Clinic [34899]
    OBGYN [22286]
    Speech Pathology Department [3603]
    Sports Medicine Center [39133]
Medical College of Wisconsin/Children's Hospital of Wisconsin • Froedtert Hospital • Pediatric Cystic Fibrosis Center [7701]
Medical College of Wisconsin
    Department of Neurology • Multiple Sclerosis Clinic • Lutheran Hospital [34744]

Froedtert Hospital • Adult Cystic Fibrosis Center [7702]
    Pain Management [35775]
Medical Comfort Systems [17694]
Medical Decision Services, LLC [13694]
Medical Eye Bank of Florida [35000]
Medical Eye Bank of Maryland [35063]
Medical Eye Bank of West Virginia • Vision Share [35263]
Medical Kidney Services of Central Georgia [23758]
Medical Mall Dialysis [25138]
Medical One • Pain Clinic [35562]
Medical Pain Center [35541]
Medical Pain Relief Clinic [35542]
Medical Park Hospital • Cancer Program [5666]
Medical Plaza Dialysis • Fresenius Medical Care • Dialysis Services [26282]
Medical Rehabilitation Associates--Augusta [35474]
Medical Rehabilitation Associates--Brunswick [35475]
Medical Rehabilitation Associates--Lewiston [35476]
Medical Rehabilitation Center--East Campus [4229]
Medical Rehabilitation Program • Active Duty Rehabilitation Program • Veterans Affairs Medical Center--Augusta, Georgia [4005]
Medical Services of America [17602]
Medical Services of America Home Health and Hospice [20409]
Medical Services Group [15410]
Medical Services of Northwest Florida [14315]
Medical Services of Northwest Florida, Inc. [14257]
Medical Sigma Equipment [17460]
The Medical Store, Inc. [14452]
Medical Supply, Inc. [18459]
The Medical Team, Inc. [18147]
Medical Technical Rehab Services LLC [48382]
Medical Technology of Louisiana Inc. [15265]
Medical University of South Carolina
    Adult Cystic Fibrosis Center [7659]
    ALS Center [148]
    Children's Hospital • Burn Center [4632]
    College of Dental Medicine • Department of Pediatric Dentistry/Orthodontics • Division of Craniofacial Genetics [12333]
    Department of Medicine - Rheumatology • Multi-disciplinary Clinical Research Center [179]
    Department of Pediatrics • Genetics and Child Development Clinics [12334]
    Down Syndrome Center [10862]
    Evelyn Trammell Institute • Voice and Swallowing Center [3397]
    IOP CDAP [48911]
    MUSC Medical Center • MDA Clinic [34873]
    Pediatric Cystic Fibrosis Center [7660]
    Pediatric Sickle Cell Center [36425]
    Rehabilitation Unit [35664]
Medical University of South Carolina--Transplant [26690]
Medicine-in-Motion • San Marcos Ambulatory Care Center [38137]
Medicine Wheel Clinic [42039]
Medicor Healthcare [14421]
MediGroup Sleep Centers [37120]
Medilink Homecare, Inc. [16222]
Medina County Board of Mental Retardation and Developmental Disabilities [8422]
Medina County Kidney Center • Fresenius Medical Care [26161]
Medina Dialysis Facility • US Renal Care [27124]
Medina General Hospital
    Cancer Program [5739]
    Sleep Related Breathing Disorders Laboratory [37540]
Medina Memorial Health Care System Home Care Services [16520]
MediServe Medical Equipment, Inc.--Gray [17672]
Mediserve Medical Equipment--Knoxville [17709]
Mediserve Medical Equipment--Morristown [17743]
Medley and Mesaric Therapy Associates [3325]
Medlife Home Care--Farmington Hills [15655]
Medlife Home Care, Inc.--Nampa [15651]
MedLink Colbert [6587]
Medlink Gainesville [6593]
Medlock Bridge Dialysis • DaVita [23689]
MedMark Treatment Centers Inc [39862]
    MedMark Treatment Centers Fairfield [39827]
    Sacramento [40491]
MedMark Treatment Centers • Stockton [40825]

Men's Group Home [32663]
Mental Health 8 East • UMASS Memorial Medical Center [44618]
Mental Health America of Boone County [50896]
Mental Health America of Greenville County [51331]
Mental Health America of the Heartland - Kansas City, Kansas [50919]
Mental Health America of North Dakota [51183]
Mental Health America of Wisconsin [51513]
Mental Health Assoc of PB County • Peer Place - Support [41997]
Mental Health Associates and New Leaf • Recovery Services of North Central PA [48658]
Mental Health Associates of North Central Pennsylvania [48439]
Mental Health Association in Abilene [51369]
Mental Health Association of Columbia • Children and Families Division [31304]
Mental Health Association of Columbia-Greene Counties [31354]
Mental Health Association of Frederick County Hotline [50975]
Mental Health Association of Greater Lowell [30408]
Mental Health Association of Illinois Valley--Bartonville [50829]
Mental Health Association of Illinois Valley--Peoria [50867]
Mental Health Association • Indian Res./Saint Lucie Crisis Line [50793]
Mental Health Association of Marion County • Crisis and Suicide Intervention Service [50893]
Mental Health Association of the New River Valley [32713]
Mental Health Association in North Dakota [51184]
Mental Health Association in Orange County, Inc. • Help Line [51140]
Mental Health Association of Rockland County [31485]
Mental Health Association in Waukesha County, Inc. • First Call for Help [51519]
Mental Health Association of Westchester • Abused Spouse Assistance Services [10008]
Mental Health Association of Westchester County • Sterling Center [51139]
Mental Health Association of Westchester--Elmsford [31318]
Mental Health Association of Westchester--Mount Kisco [31395]
Mental Health Care [50791]
Mental Health Care, Inc.
    Baylife Adult Center [29264]
    East Panos Center [29265]
Mental Health Center [30925]
The Mental Health Center [30294]
Mental Health Center of Boulder County
    Boulder Office [28861]
    Broomfield Office [28865]
Mental Health Center of Boulder County, Inc.
    Halcyon Office [28862]
    Lafayette Office [28920]
    Saint Vrain ATP [28934]
Mental Health Center of Boulder County • Longmont Office [28935]
Mental Health Center of Boulder, Inc. • Emergency Psychiatric Services [50712]
Mental Health Center of Broomfield County [50713]
Mental Health Center of Central Louisiana [8058]
Mental Health Center of Champaign County [29574]
    Community Elements • Runaway and Homeless Youth Program [35932]
Mental Health Center of Dane County • Integrated Alcohol and Drug Services [50448]
Mental Health Center of Denver [41135]
    Adult Outpatient [28883]
Mental Health Center of East Central Kansas--Burlington [29911]
Mental Health Center of East Central Kansas • Children's Services [8023]
Mental Health Center of East Central Kansas--Emporia [29919]
Mental Health Center of East Central Kansas • Emporia Emergency Services [50915]
Mental Health Center of Greater Manchester [8239], [31082], [51087]
Mental Health Center • Helpline [51069]
Mental Health Center of Jacksonville [29187]
Mental Health Center of Madison County [27952]

Mental Health Center of Mid-Iowa • Center Associates [29881]
Mental Health Center of North Central AL • Quest Rec Center Subst Abuse Treatment [39238]
Mental Health Center of North Central Alabama, Inc. [27895]
Mental Health Center of North Iowa [8019]
Mental Health Center of North Iowa, Inc. [29884]
Mental Health Center of Saint Clair County [29612]
Mental Health Center--The Hub [30926]
Mental Health Centers of Central Illinois [50875]
Mental Health Centers of Illinois • Crisis Hotline [50876]
Mental Health Centers of Western IL
    Brown Site [42793]
    Hancock Site [42447]
    Pike Site [42867]
Mental Health and Deafness Resources Inc. [407]
Mental Health Group Home [32636]
    Children's Service Center [32050]
Mental Health Institute [33500]
Mental Health Institute Cherokee [33497]
Mental Health Institute • Iowa Residential Treatment Center [43291]
Mental Health Kokua--Duplex I [29533]
Mental Health Kokua--Duplex II [29534]
Mental Health Kokua--East Hawaii Office [29514]
Mental Health Kokua--Kauai County Office [29531]
Mental Health Kokua--Main Office [29521]
Mental Health Kokua • Maui County Services [29536]
Mental Health Kokua--West Hawaii Office [29528]
Mental Health/Mental Retardation Association of Harris County • NeuroPsychiatric Center [51383]
Mental Health/Mental Retardation Authority of Brazos Valley--Bryan [32422]
Mental Health/Mental Retardation Authority of Brazos Valley
    Grimes County Outpatient Program [32520]
    Robertson County [32475]
    Washington County [32416]
Mental Health/Mental Retardation Authority of Harris County [32481]
    Bayshore Mental Health/Mental Retardation Center [32410]
    Behavioral Training Program [32482]
    Branard Street [32483]
    Early Childhood Intervention South Team [32484]
    New Day Treatment Program [32485]
    Ripley Clinic [32486]
    Safe Haven [32487]
Mental Health/Mental Retardation and Drug Abuse of Clarion County [32003]
Mental Health/Mental Retardation Services for the Concho Valley [32542]
Mental Health/Mental Retardation of Tarrant County [51378]
Mental Health of North Central Alabama [50612]
Mental Health and Recovery Centers of
    Clinton County [47886]
    Warren County [47787], [47805], [47856]
Mental Health Recovery Services of Warren & Clinton Counties [31787]
Mental Health Resource Center [51110]
Mental Health Resources [51130]
Mental Health Resources Inc [46257], [46319]
Mental Health Resources, Inc. [31209]
Mental Health Resources PLLC [49141]
Mental Health Services of Catawba County [8380]
Mental Health Services for Clark County [31836]
    Bridge House [31837]
    Center for Community Support [31838]
    Child, Adolescent and Family Center [31839]
Mental Health Services Community Support Center [32149]
Mental Health Services--Helena [51072]
Mental Health Services for Homeless Persons, Inc. [31717]
Mental Health Services Inc [47692]
Mental Health Services--Johnston [32150]
Mental Health Services • Mount Vernon [32700]
Mental Health Services of the New River Valley [32772]
Mental Health Services of
    South Oklahoma/Pontotoc County [47901]
    Southern Oklahoma [47910]
    Southern Oklahoma/Bryan County [47926]

Mental Health Services of Southern Oklahoma--Ada [31867]
Mental Health Services of Southern Oklahoma • Ada Clinic [31868]
Mental Health Services of Southern Oklahoma--Ardmore [31872]
Mental Health Services of Southern Oklahoma--Durant [31883]
Mental Health Services of Southern Oklahoma
    Madill Clinic [31890]
    Pauls Valley Clinic [31908]
    Seminole Clinic [31917]
    Sulphur Clinic [31919]
Mental Health Substance Abuse Division
    Adult Day Treatment Program [49853]
    Child and Youth Services [49854]
Mental Health Substance Abuse Program • La Clinica del Pueblo Inc [41543]
Mental Health/Substance Abuse Services [29330]
Mental Health Systems Inc
    Central East Regional Recovery Center [40563]
    East County Center for Change [39798]
    Fresno Center for Change [39863]
    Harmony Womens Recovery Center [40564]
    Hemet Center for Change [39921]
    Indio Center for Change [39693]
    Mid Coast Counseling and Recovery Center [40565]
    North County Center for Change [40932]
    North Inland Regional Recovery Center [39811]
Mental Health Systems Inc/ • Probationers Rec Thru Interv/Drug Educ [40525]
Mental Health Systems Inc
    Providence Place [40566]
    Redlands Center for Change [40437]
    Riverside Center for Change [40457]
    San Bernardino Center for Change [40526]
    San Diego Center for Change [40567]
    Santa Maria Center for Change [40762]
    Teen Recovery Center/North Inland [40675]
Mental Health Systems PC [45356]
Mental Health of Umatilla County [51261]
Mental Healthcare of Cullman [27892]
Mental Morphosis Inc [45042]
Mental Retardation Group Home [32637]
Mental Retardation/ICF Group Home [32638]
Mental Wellness Center [42338]
Mental Wellness Centers [42303]
Mentor ABI [4380]
MEPCO Home Health Agency--Berea [15164]
MEPCO Home Health Agency--Irvine [15195]
MEPCO Home Health Agency--Richmond [15249]
MEPCO Home Health Agency--Stanton [15254]
MER Home Health Care Services [15815]
Meramec Recovery Center Inc [45663]
Merced County Alcohol and Drug Services
    Division of Mental Health [40004]
    Recovery Assistance for Teens [40217]
Merced County Mental Health--Administration Office [28623]
Merced County Mental Health Department • Division of Alcohol and Drug Services [40183]
Merced County Mental Health
    Livingston Clinic [28562]
    Recovery Assistance for Teens [28624]
    Westside Community Counseling Center [28616]
Merced County SACPA Drug Treatment Program [40218]
Mercer County Family Crisis Center [9191]
Mercer County Fellowship Home Inc [50286]
Mercer County Joint Township Community Hospital [16893]
Mercer Outpatient Services • Alcoholism Addictions Program [46190]
Merci [7793]
Mercury Medical [13618]
Mercy Behavioral Care • Chemical Dependency Services [43306]
Mercy Behavioral Health [48598], [48599], [48600]
    Center for Hearing and Deaf Services [48601]
Mercy Canton • Dialysis Center • DaVita [26032]
Mercy Capitol Hospital [15077]
Mercy Care-Loris [21257]
Mercy Care Mor [15081]
Mercy Care-Myrtle Beach [21264]
Mercy Care-Treasures of the Heart [21227]
Mercy Catholic Medical Center • Fitzgerald Mercy Hospital Campus • Cancer Program [5820]

Mercy Catholic Medical Center of Southwestern Pennsylvania [17418]
Mercy Center for Pain Management [35450]
Mercy Centre for Developmental Disabilities [8160]
Mercy Children's Hospital • Genetics Center NW Ohio [12316]
Mercy Clinic Downtown [6582]
Mercy Clinic North [6583]
Mercy College Speech and Hearing Center [3008]
Mercy Crystal Lake East Medical Center [2012]
Mercy Dialysis Center--Mason City [24287]
Mercy Dialysis--Vinton • Covenant--Mercycare, Inc. • Dialysis Unit [24303]
Mercy Fitzgerald Hospital • Sleep Disorders Center [37675]
Mercy Franciscan Hospital--Mount Airy • Cancer Program [5696]
Mercy Franciscan Hospital--Western Hills • Cancer Program [5697]
Mercy General Health Partners • Johnson Family Center for Cancer Care [5388]
Mercy General Hospital • Cancer Program [4828]
Mercy Harvard Sleep Disorders Center [36915]
Mercy Health Center • Cancer Program [5779]
Mercy Health Center at Home [17150]
Mercy Health Center Medical Plaza • Mercy Home-care [15121]
Mercy Health Clinic [6837]
Mercy Health Partners • Cancer Center [5752]
Mercy Health System • Cancer Program [6154]
Mercy Health System of Kansas, Inc. [15122]
Mercy Health System • Mercy Regional Sleep Disorders Center [37972]
Mercy Healthcare Bakersfield [12903]
Mercy Heath Center-North Iowa • Cancer Center [5192]
Mercy Home for Boys and Girls
    Boys Campus [34104]
    Girls Campus [33414]
Mercy Home Care Branch--Hawarden [15086]
Mercy Home Care--Cedar Rapids [15066]
Mercy Home Care, Grayling and Houghton Lake [20065]
Mercy Home Care and Hospice [14919]
Mercy Home Care--Independence [15088]
Mercy Home Care and Medical Supplies, Inc. [16398]
Mercy Home Care & Medical Supply, Inc. [16203]
Mercy Home Care--Pender [16129]
Mercy Home Health Care--Iowa City [15097]
Mercy Home Health Care, LLC--Highland [14989]
Mercy Home Health Care, LLC--Madison Heights [15740]
Mercy Home Health and Hospice--Durango [13482]
Mercy Home Health and Hospice--Pagosa Springs [13504]
Mercy Home Health and Mercy Hospice [13248]
Mercy Home Health--Norristown [17398]
Mercy Home Health--Philadelphia [17419]
Mercy Home Health--Rogers • Saint Mary's Hospital [12881]
Mercy Home Health Services [17487]
Mercy Home Healthcare [15095]
Mercy at Home-Hospice • Mercy Health System of Oklahoma [20961]
Mercy Homecare--Mason City [15129]
Mercy HomeCare--North Canton [17012]
Mercy Homecare--Southfield [15816]
Mercy Hospice--Bloomfield Hills [20040]
Mercy Hospice Cadillac [20042]
Mercy Hospice--Des Moines [19687]
Mercy Hospice--Devils Lake [20778]
Mercy Hospice--Folsom [18927]
Mercy Hospice Inpatient Unit--Fort Smith [18852]
Mercy Hospice-Johnston [19704]
Mercy Hospice-Lewisville [21511]
Mercy Hospice - Mount Shasta [18975]
Mercy Hospice--Redding [18998]
Mercy Hospice--Roseburg [21030]
Mercy Hospice-Scranton [21155]
Mercy Hospice--Williston [20794]
Mercy Hospital Anderson • Cancer Center [5698]
Mercy Hospital-Bakersfield • Florence R. Wheeler Cancer Center [4761]
Mercy Hospital Clermont • Cancer Center [5681]
Mercy Hospital--Coon Rapids [2684]
Mercy Hospital Council Bluffs • Alegent Health at Home [15070]

Mercy Hospital--Fairfield • Cancer Care Center [5721]
Mercy Hospital--Iowa City • Cancer Program [5190]
Mercy Hospital and Medical Center • Alcoholism and Drug Dependency Program [42561]
Mercy Hospital and Medical Center--Chicago • Cancer Program [5071]
Mercy Hospital Medical Center • Mercy Sleep Center [36981]
Mercy Hospital--Miami [14082]
    Community Comprehensive Cancer Center [4965]
    Kohly Center for Outpatient Therapy [1657]
Mercy Hospital of Philadelphia • Department of Psychiatry [48538]
Mercy Hospital of Pittsburgh • Burn Center [4622]
Mercy Hospital-Port Hurno • Regional Cancer Center [5392]
Mercy Hospital--Portland • Cancer Center [5275]
Mercy Hospital--Scranton [17471]
Mercy Hospital of Scranton • Cancer Center [5871]
Mercy Hospital • Sleep Disorders Center [36793]
Mercy Hospital of Tiffin, Ohio [17052]
Mercy Hospital of Tiffin • Sleep Improvement Center [37541]
Mercy Hospital of Willard [17071]
    Sleep Disorders Center [37542]
Mercy Hospital--Williston • Dialysis Unit [26000]
Mercy Hospitals of Bakersfield [18889]
Mercy House [9893]
Mercy McHenry Medical Center • Sports Medicine and Rehabilitation [38391]
Mercy Medical [12644]
Mercy Medical Center--Baltimore • Cancer Program [5288]
Mercy Medical Center • Behavioral Health [29868]
Mercy Medical Center--Canton [3211]
    Cancer Program [5687]
Mercy Medical Center--Cedar Rapids • Cancer Care Program [5182]
Mercy Medical Center Cedar Rapids • Dialysis Unit [24253]
Mercy Medical Center - Centerville [24255]
Mercy Medical Center--Clinton • Dialysis Facility [24257]
Mercy Medical Center--Des Moines • Cancer Center [5187]
Mercy Medical Center Dialysis--Mercy Plaza [24254]
Mercy Medical Center--Dubuque [15082]
Mercy Medical Center Home Health & Hospice [17220]
Mercy Medical Center Hospice [20877]
Mercy Medical Center--Merced Community Campus [13172]
Mercy Medical Center • Mercy Turning Point Treatment Center [43270]
Mercy Medical Center Mt. Shasta [13194]
Mercy Medical Center--Nampa [14667]
Mercy Medical Center North [15083]
Mercy Medical Center--Oshkosh • Cancer Program [6171]
Mercy Medical Center Outpatient BHS • Family Counseling CD Outpatient Clinic [46648]
Mercy Medical Center Redding [13255]
Mercy Medical Center--Redding
    Cancer Program [4825]
    Speech/Language Pathology Department [1233]
Mercy Medical Center--Rockville Centre • Long Island Cancer Institute [5615]
Mercy Medical Center--Roseburg • Cancer Program [5805]
Mercy Medical Center • Sedlacek Treatment Center [43244]
Mercy Medical Center - Sioux City [15104]
Mercy Medical Center--Sioux City • Cancer Program [5194]
Mercy Medical Center • Sleep Center [37543]
Mercy Medical Center South [15069]
Mercy Medical Center-Springfield • Cancer Program [5357]
Mercy Medical Center--Springfield • Weldon Hearing Center [2526]
Mercy Medical Center--Williston [16822]
Mercy Medical--Daphne • Calling All Angels [906]
Mercy Medical--Dyersville Homecare • Oakcrest Manor [15083]
Mercy Memorial Health Center [17101]
Mercy Memorial Hospice of Monroe [20095]

Mercy Memorial Hospital • Family Center [44924]
Mercy Memorial Hospital Home Health Care [15751]
Mercy Memorial Hospital
    Mercy REACH [47860], [47873]
    Speech and Language Department [2627]
Mercy Memorial Hospital System • Cancer Center [4679]
Mercy Multiple Sclerosis Center [34526]
Mercy Options [50420]
    Behavioral Health Clinic [50369]
Mercy Perinatal Recovery Network [40492]
Mercy Regional Dialysis Center [27726]
Mercy Regional Health Center • Sleep Disorders Services [36994]
Mercy Regional Medical Center [1406]
Mercy Regional Medical Center--Durango [13483]
    Durango Cancer Center [4876]
Mercy Regional Medical Center--Lorain [16968]
Mercy Residential Services • Runaway and Home-less Youth Program [36116]
Mercy Saint Anne Sleep Disorders Center [37544]
Mercy San Juan Medical Center [12932]
    Cancer Program [4763]
    Mercy Sleep Center [36674]
Mercy Sleep Center • Saint Mary's North [37771]
Mercy Sports Medicine Center [38887]
Mercy Sports Medicine Center and Rehab Center [39176]
Mercy Suburban Hospital • Cancer Program [5846]
Mercy Tiffin Hospital • Cancer Program [4695]
Mercy Walworth Sports Medicine and Rehabilitation Center [39179]
Mercy Whitewater Sports Medicine and Rehabilita-tion Center [39191]
Mercy Woodstock Medical Center • Sports Medicine and Rehabilitation [38421]
Meremark Inc • DBA Clarity at Seven Ponds [47915]
Meridell Achievement Center [34453]
Meriden--Wallingford Chrysalis, Inc. [8996]
Meridia Center for Rehabilitation and Pain Manage-ment [35612]
Meridia Sports Medicine Center [38892]
Meridian Behavior Health Care • Suwannee County Office [29208]
Meridian Behavioral Health • Cedar Ridge [45327]
Meridian Behavioral Health Services [47317], [47504], [47510]
Meridian Behavioral Healthcare [50762]
    Gateway Acute Care/Recovery Center [29196]
Meridian Behavioral Healthcare Inc [41577], [41750]
    Addictions Outpatient and Residential [41679]
    Bradford Guidance Clinic [41939]
    Columbia County [41726]
    Union Office [41724]
Meridian Behavioral Healthcare, Inc. [29171]
    Alachua County Campus [29172]
    Joyce House [29173]
Meridian Behavioral Healthcare Union County Office [29195]
Meridian Community Care [47893]
    Adolescent Center [47830]
    Co-occurring Treatment Program [47894]
Meridian Dialysis Center • DaVita [27214]
Meridian Health Group • Pain Care Center [35444]
Meridian Health System • Riverview Medical Center • Booker Cancer Center [5538]
Meridian Home Care [20485]
Meridian Home Care--Monmouth County [16247]
Meridian Home Care--Ocean County [16189]
Meridian Home Care--Whiting [16294]
Meridian House [30369]
Meridian Nursing and Rehabilitation at Brick • Merid-ian Health [20460]
Meridian Park Dialysis Center & At Home • DaVita [26360]
Meridian • Professional Psychological Consultants [44772]
Meridian Services [43163], [43167]
Meridian Services Corp • Jay Outpatient Services [43183]
Meridian Services - Delaware County Services [29786]
Meridian Veterans Affairs Clinic [30792]
Merit Care Sports Medicine [38841]
Merit Home Health Care, Inc. [15606]
Merit Hospice Services LLC [19537]
Merit Resource Services [50195], [50225], [50272]
    Wapato Branch [50254]

MERIT Sleep Technologies, Inc. [14845]
Sleep Disorders Center [36916]
MeritCare Bemidji • MeritCare Reproductive
Medicine [22136]
MeritCare Broadway Health Center [4354]
MeritCare Children's Hospital • Coordinated Treat-
ment Center • Down Syndrome Outpatient Service
[10841]
Meritcare Dialysis--Morris [25054]
Meritcare Dialysis--Red Lake • Red Lake Hospital
[25065]
MeritCare Health System • Roger Maris Cancer
Center [5671]
Meritcare Home Health services, Inc. [17884]
MeritCare Hospital
DBA Roger Maris Cancer Center • Hemophilia
and Thrombosis Treatment Center [12572]
MDA Clinic [34849]
MeritCare Hospital Rehabilitation Services [4355]
MeritCare Medical Center • Pediatric Cystic Fibrosis
Center [7636]
MeritCare Reproductive Medicine [22205]
MeritCare South University • Eating Disorder
Institute [11181]
MeritCare Southpointe [4356]
Meriter Home Health [18581]
Meriter Hospital Inc. • Speech Pathology Depart-
ment [3675]
Meriter Hospital • Physical Medicine and Rehabilita-
tion Program [8619]
Meritus Medical Center • Total Rehab Care [4101]
Merle Wallace Purvis Center [27872]
Meroke House [31388]
Merrill Kidney Center [27743]
Merrillville Dialysis Center • Fresenius Medical Care
• Dialysis Center [24202]
Merrimack River Medical Associates • Somersworth
Methadone Clinic [45919]
Merrimack River Medical Services [45900], [45918]
Merrimack Special Education Collaborative [2471]
Merrimack Valley Hospice [19970]
Merrimon W. Baker, MD [39053]
Merritt Speech and Learning [1613]
Merwin Home Medical--Robbinsdale [15928]
Merwin Home Medical--Saint Cloud [15935]
Mesa County Criminal Justice Services [41209]
Mesa County Dialysis • DaVita [23123]
Mesa Family Counseling [45845]
Mesa Family Health Center [6238]
Mesa Vista Dialysis Center • DaVita [27072]
Mescalero Care Center--Dialysis [25554]
Mesilla Valley Hospice Inc. [20539]
Mesilla Valley Hospital [33670]
Mesquite Mental Health Center [31039], [45857]
Mesquite Regional Day School for the Deaf [810]
Mesquite Specialty Hospital [3524]
Meta House Inc
Meta House Women and Childrens Prog
[50478]
Outpatient Program [50479]
Metairie Kidney Center [24536]
Metamorphosis Ogden Inc [49645]
Metamorphosis Salt Lake Inc [49689]
Methadone Clinic of East Texas [49564]
Methadone/Opiate Rehabilitation and • Education
Center [43691]
Methodist Alliance Hospice [21348]
Methodist Children's Home Society [34235]
Methodist Children's Hospital of South Texas •
Pediatric Cancer Care Program [6025]
Methodist Dallas Medical Center • Cancer Program
[5975]
Methodist Healthcare • Sleep Disorders Center
[37772]
Methodist Healthcare Sleep Disorders Center -
Desoto [37252]
Methodist Healthcare System--San Antonio • Cancer
Program [6026]
Methodist Healthcare-University Hospital--Memphis •
Cancer Center [5943]
Methodist Healthwest • Methodist Hospital • Sleep
Disorders Center [37314]
The Methodist Home Care Services [14987]
Methodist Home for Children • Bridges Program
[47461]
Methodist Home Health and Hospice [20399]
Methodist Hospital [21487]

Methodist Hospital Dallas Transplant Institute
[27032]
Methodist Hospital • Department of Speech Pathol-
ogy [2148]
Methodist Hospital ESRD Transplant Services
[27158]
Methodist Hospital--Henderson • Sleep Related
Breathing Disorders Laboratory [37033]
Methodist Hospital Home Care [15907]
Methodist Hospital Hospice [20204]
Methodist Hospital--Houston
Cancer Program [6000]
Sleep Disorders Center [37823]
Methodist Hospital of Indianapolis • Methodist Sleep
Disorders Center [36957]
Methodist Hospital • Neurological Institute • MDA/
ALS Center [34884]
Methodist Hospital/Park Nicollet [2736]
Methodist Hospital/Park Nicollet Health • HealthSys-
tem Minnesota Cancer Program [5412]
Methodist Hospital Rehabilitation Center • Speech
Pathology Department [2857]
Methodist Hospital--Saint Louis Park • Sleep
Disorders Center [37223]
Methodist Hospital of Southern California [1058]
Methodist Hospital Southern California • Cancer
Program [4757]
The Methodist Hospitals, Inc. • Cancer Care
Program [5149]
Methodist Lebonheur Health Care • MDA Clinic
[34878]
Methodist Medical Center • Hospice Services
[19561]
The Methodist Medical Center of Illinois [14904]
Methodist Medical Center of Illinois
C. Duane Morgan Sleep Disorders Center
[36917]
Cancer Program [5120]
The Wellness Center [38406]
Methodist Medical Center of Oak Ridge • Regional
Cancer Program [5954]
Methodist Medical Center • Sleep Disorders Center
[37773]
Methodist Mission Home/Southwest Center for
Higher Independence [3537]
Methodist Rehabilitation Center [4230]
Methodist Richardson Medical Center [49496]
Cancer Care Program [6019]
Methodist Specialty/Transplant Hosp • Inpatient Unit
Behavioral Medicine [49527]
Methodist Sports Medicine Center [38435]
Methodist Sugar Land Hospital [3542]
Metrio Healthcare Services, LLC [18161]
Metro Community Provider Network • MCPN/Engle-
wood Clinic [6401]
Metro Counseling Center Inc [45393]
Metro Counseling Services Inc [44337]
Metro Deaf School [517]
Metro Dialysis Center--North • Fresenius Medical
Care [25205]
Metro East Dialysis & At Home • DaVita [23897]
Metro East Dialysis Center • Fresenius Medical
Care [27257]
Metro East • Substance Abuse Treatment Corpora-
tion [44749]
Metro Family Support Counseling PC [45026]
Metro Health • AIDS Clinical Trials Unit [27]
Metro Hearing Services [944]
Metro Home Medical Supply [15638]
Metro-Med, Inc. [12924]
Metro New York Developmental Disabilities Service
Office [8334]
Metro Saint Louis Dialysis Center, LLC [25274]
Metro Treatment of Alabama LP • Sumter County
Treatment Center [39267]
Metro Treatment Center Inc • Wichita [43497]
Metro Treatment of Florida LP
DBA Pensacola Metro Treatment [41584]
DBA Pompano Treatment Center [41899]
DBA West Palm Beach Treatment Center
[41727]
Sunrise Treatment Center [41943]
Metro Treatment of Georgia LP • Northwest Georgia
Treatment Center [42099]
Metro Treatment of Maryland LP • DBA Hagerstown
Treatment Center [44293]
Metro Treatment of Minnesota LP
Rochester Metro Treatment Center [45279]

Saint Cloud Metro Treatment Center [45293]
Metro Treatment of Missouri LP • Cape Girardeau
Metro Treatment Center [45453]
Metro Treatment of New Hampshire LP
Keene Metro Treatment Center [45920]
Manchester Metro Treatment Center [45909]
Metro Treatment of New Mexico • Central New
Mexico Treatment Center [46236]
Metro Treatment of North Carolina LP [47383]
Charlotte Treatment Center [47263]
Fayetteville Treatment Center [47311]
Metro Treatment of Texas LP
Dallas County Treatment Center [49289]
DBA San Antonio Treatment Center [49528]
Metro Treatment of Virginia LP • DBA Richmond
Treatment Center [49828]
MetroCare Givers Inc. [16399]
Metrocare Services • Westside Family Center
[32443]
MetroHealth Medical Center
Burn Unit [4604]
Comprehensive Care Program for Children with
Disabilities [8407]
MetroHealth Medical Center • MDA Clinic [34852]
MetroHealth Medical Center
MetroHealth Center for Rehabilitation [4371]
Northeast Ohio Regional Spinal Cord Injury
System [4372]
Speech Pathology/Audiology [3230]
The MetroHealth System • Cancer Program [5703]
MetroHealth System • MetroHealth Center for Sleep
Medicine [37545]
Metrolina Orthopedic Sportsmedicine [38829]
Metron Health Care Products [15676]
Metron People Care [15677]
Metroplex Adventist Hospital, Inc. [18027]
Metroplex Home Health Services [17895]
Metroplex Pulmonary & Sleep Center [37824]
Metropolitan Arts Complex Inc • DBA Metro Arts
Therapy Services /Main Off [44750]
Metropolitan Center for Mental Health • CD
Outpatient Clinic/Families/Indiv in Recov [46889]
Metropolitan Center for Women and Children [9409]
Metropolitan Corporation for • Life Skills/Outpatient
[46890]
Metropolitan Developmental Center [8060]
Metropolitan Dialysis Center LLC • Innovative
Dialysis Systems [22910]
Metropolitan Family Health Center [6975]
Metropolitan Family Services [9209]
Metropolitan Hospital Center
AIDS Clinical Trials Unit [20]
Dialysis Unit [25726]
Methadone Treatment Program [46891]
Metropolitan Jewish Home Care--Bronx [16366]
Metropolitan Jewish Home Care--Brooklyn [16400]
Metropolitan Jewish Home Care--New York [16559]
Metropolitan Jewish Hospice and Palliative Care
Program [20558]
Metropolitan Organization to Counter Sexual Assault
[9689]
Metropolitan Orthopedics [38665]
Metropolitan Pain Management Consultants [35318]
Metropolitan Pulmonary Sleep Center [37276]
Metropolitan Rehabilitation Clinics [44948]
Metropolitan Saint Louis Psychiatric Center [33636]
Metropolitan Speech and Language Center--
Livingston [2926]
Metropolitan Speech and Language Center--Saint
Louis [2817]
Metropolitan Speech Pathology Group [1532]
Metropolitan State Hospital [33169]
MetroSouth Hospice [19491]
MetroSouth Medical Center • Speech Pathology
Department [1970]
MetroWest Hospice [19963]
MetroWest Hospice-Framingham [19964]
MetroWest Medical Center [38552]
Cancer Program [5335]
Metwork Health Services Inc [44250]
Mexia State School [8560]
Mexican American Alcoholism Program Inc [40493]
Mi Casa Recovery Home [40494]
Mexico Veterans Affairs Clinic [30875]
Meyer Medical Group • Mental Health Services
[50863]
Meyer Pediatric Therapy Services [1035]
Meyer Treatment Center of the Washington School

of Psychiatry [29097]
M.F. Home Care Services, Inc. [14083]
MFI Recovery Center [39641], [40250], [40458]
    A Womens Place [40459]
    Woodcrest Facility [40460]
MH/MR of Tarrant County
    Add Serv Div Tarrant Yth Recov Campus
        [49337]
    Addiction Recovery Center [49426]
    Pine Street Resid/Billy Gregory Detox [49338]
MH Providers of Western Queens Inc • Western
    Queens Recovery Services [47194]
MHCTI • DBA Step Two Recovery Center [39388]
MHMRSA of Alexandria [51411]
MHS Central Valley • Regional Recovery Center
    [39722]
MHS South County Center for Change • Treatment
    and Testing Program [40568]
MHT--Neopolitan LightHouse [6662]
Miami Artificial Kidney Center, LLC • KRU Medical
    Ventures • Dialysis Facility [23404]
Miami Beach Community Health Center, Inc. [6514]
Miami Beach Community Health Center--North
    [6506]
Miami Behavioral Health Center
    Casa Nueva Vida [41788]
    CRISIS [41789]
Miami Behavioral Health Center, Inc.
    Coconut Grove [29217]
    Opalocka [29250]
    S Dixie Highway, Coconut Grove [29129]
    W Flagler Street, Miami [29218]
    Westchester [29219]
Miami Behavioral Health Center • Substance Abuse
    Outpatient Unit [41790]
Miami Bridge • Runaway and Homeless Youth
    Program [35897]
Miami Campus Dialysis • DaVita [23405]
Miami Children's Hospital
    Cancer Care Program [4966]
    Dan Marino Center [1795]
Miami Children's Hospital Dialysis Unit [23406]
Miami Children's Hospital
    Division of Clinical Genetics [12181]
    Pediatric Cystic Fibrosis Center [7503]
    Sickle Cell Clinic [36322]
    Sleep Disorders Center [36794]
Miami Comprehensive Hemophilia Center-Pediatrics
    [12503]
Miami Counseling Services [41791]
Miami County Recovery Council [47871]
Miami-Dade Advocates for Victims [9066]
Miami Dade Bureau of Rehab Services
    Diversion and Treatment Prog/Northside [41792]
    New Direction Residential Treatment Program
        [41793]
    TASC Diversion and Treatment Pgm - MDCC
        [41794]
    TASC Diversion and Treatment Pgm South
        [41643]
Miami Dade Community Services Inc [41795]
Miami--Dade Home Health Care [13762]
Miami--Dade Public Library System • Talking Books
    Library [3765]
Miami East Dialysis • DaVita [23407]
Miami Fluency Clinic [1658]
Miami Gardens Dialysis • DaVita [23440]
Miami Home Care Services, Inc. [14445]
Miami Home Health Agency, Inc. [14084]
Miami Lakes Artificial Kidney Center • DaVita
    [23411]
Miami North Dialysis • DaVita [23430]
Miami Regional Dialysis Center Inc. • American
    Renal Associates [23431]
Miami Sleep Disorders Center [36795]
Miami United Home Health Care [13672]
Miami University • Speech and Hearing Clinic [3252]
Miami Valley Hospital
    Center for Sleep and Wake Disorders [37546]
    David L. Riker Cancer Center [5715]
    Dialysis Center [26096]
    Fertility Program [22216]
    Pain Center [35613]
    Regional Adult Burn Center [4605]
    Rehabilitation Institute of Ohio [4373]
Miami Valley Hospital Sports Medicine Center
    [38858]
Miami Valley Hospital • Turning Point [47741]

Miami Veterans Affairs Healthcare System
    Deerfield Beach Clinic [29147]
    Homestead Clinic [29184]
    Key Largo Clinic [29191]
    Key West Clinic [29192]
    Pembroke Pines/Hollywood Clinic [29183]
    PTSD Clinical Team [51711]
    Spinal Cord Injury Services [3985]
MICA Community Residence [31251]
Micah's Place [9048]
Michael Brubaker Counseling [39371]
Michael C. Bach Treatment Center [6443]
Michael Chenkin LCSW LCADC [46170]
Michael E. DeBakey VA Medical Center • Spinal
    Cord Injury Center--SCRSC [4451]
Michael E. DeBakey-Veterans Affairs Medical Center
    [18000]
Michael E. Debakey Veterans Affairs Medical Center
    • PTSD Clinical Team [51828]
Michael Home Health Providers [14190]
Michael J. Gill Rehabilitation Center [30403]
Michael Lane Behavioral Healthcare • Cornerstone
    [44080]
Michael R Gildea PC [48450]
Michael Reese Hospital • Department of Speech
    Language Pathology [1992]
Michael S Levy • Center for Addiction Medicine
    [45846]
Michael S. Melnick, DMD, MAGD [35644]
Michaels House [40350]
Michelle Stewart Therapies [1263]
Michiana Behavioral Health Center [33485]
Michiana Regional Sleep Disorders Center [37181]
Michigan Access Center Inc [44887]
Michigan Behavioral Health Institute [44775]
Michigan Behavioral Medicine [30647]
Michigan Center for Fertility and Women's Health
    [22126]
Michigan Commission for the Blind • Braille and
    Talking Book Library [3809]
Michigan Community Blood Centers [35078]
Michigan Department of Community Health [36493]
Michigan Ear, Nose and Throat [2634]
Michigan Head Pain and Neurological Institute
    [12432], [35503]
Michigan Headache TMJ Clinic • Michigan
    Neurological Craniofacial Pain Management
    [12433]
Michigan Hearing Aid Center [2613]
Michigan Heart Sleep Center [37182]
Michigan Institute for Neurological Disorders
    MDA/ALS Clinic [126]
    MDA Clinic [34817]
    Multiple Sclerosis Center [34606]
Michigan Interventional Pain Center [35504]
Michigan Multispecialty Physicians' Sleep Disorders
    Center [37183]
Michigan Neurological Craniofacial Pain Manage-
    ment • Michigan Headache TMJ Clinic [12434]
Michigan Neurology Associates • Multiple Sclerosis
    Center [34607]
Michigan Neurology Institute • Sleep Disorders
    Center [37184]
Michigan Pain Consultants [35505]
Michigan ResCare Premier [4178]
Michigan School for the Blind [3715]
Michigan School for the Deaf and Blind [488]
Michigan Spine and Pain [35506]
Michigan Sports Medicine and Orthopedic Center
    [38611]
Michigan State University
    Center for Bleeding Disorders and Clotting
        Disorders [12540]
    Clinical Center • MDA/ALS Clinic [34818]
    Cystic Fibrosis Center [7576]
    Department of Pediatrics and Human Develop-
        ment • Division of Human Genetics [12250]
    Kalamazoo Center for Medical Studies
        Cystic Fibrosis Center [7577]
        MDA Clinic [34819]
    Mary Free Bed Rehabilitation Hospital • ALS
        Center [127]
    Rehabilitation Medicine Clinic [35507]
    Safe Place [9533]
    Sexual Assault Program [9534]
    West Michigan Pediatric, Bronson • Kalamazoo
        Center for Medical Studies [12541]

Michigan Therapeutic Consultants PC [44888],
    [44929]
Michigan Therapy Center [38586]
Michigan Therapy Center Inc. [38604]
Michigan Therapy Centre [38600]
Michigan Visiting Nurses - Ann Arbor [15577]
Michigan Visiting Nurses--Bloomfield [15591]
Michigan Visiting Nurses - Brighton [15596]
Michigan Visiting Nurses - Dearborn [15622]
Michigan Visiting Nurses, Jackson [15701]
Michigan Visiting Nurses - Plymouth [15772]
Micks Alcohol and Drug Treatment [49673]
Mid--America Dialysis LLC • Liberty Dialysis [26089]
Mid America Home Health [16057]
Mid America Psychological Services [44980]
Mid America Rehabilitation Hospital [38464]
Mid-America Transplant Services [35096]
Mid Arkansas Substance Abuse Services [39548]
Mid-Atlantic Fertility Centers [22091]
Mid Atlantic Rehabilitation Services
    ATP Program [46011]
    (MARS ATP) [48293]
Mid-Bergen Center, Paramus [51118]
Mid--Carolina Homecare Specialists [16760]
Mid Cities Dialysis Center and At Home • DaVita
    [27191]
Mid Cities Speech and Hearing Clinic Inc. [3492]
Mid--Coast Family Services--San Antonio [10505]
Mid-Coast Family Services--Victoria [10516]
Mid Coast Hospital [2353]
    Addiction Resource Center [43950]
    Sleep Disorders Center [37092]
Mid-Coast Mental Health Center [30196], [30235]
Mid-Coast Speech and Hearing Center [2363]
Mid Columbia Center for Living [48253]
Mid-Columbia Center for Living [31983], [51256],
    [51268]
Mid Columbia Center for Living • Hood River Alcohol
    and Drug Program [48132]
Mid-Columbia Center for Living
    Hood River Care Center [31946]
    Woods Court, Hood River [31947]
Mid-Columbia Kidney Center • Dialysis Facility & At
    Home • DaVita [27626]
Mid-Columbia Medical Center
    Cancer Care Program [5807]
    Center for Sleep Medicine [37619]
    Visiting Health Services [17227]
Mid--County Health Center [7140]
Mid-County Mental Health Services [28701]
Mid--Del Clinic [7103]
Mid Del Youth and Family Center Inc [47961]
Mid-Delta Health Systems, Inc. • Mid-DeltaHealth
    Center [6262]
Mid-Delta Hospice--Batesville [20220]
Mid-Delta Hospice--Belzoni [20222]
Mid-Delta Hospice-Charleston [20224]
Mid-Delta Hospice--Clarksdale [20225]
Mid-Delta Hospice-Cleveland [20226]
Mid-Delta Hospice--Greenville [20236]
Mid-Delta Hospice-Greenwood [20237]
Mid-Delta Hospice-Indianola [20245]
Mid-Delta Hospice--Lexington [20248]
Mid-Delta Hospice-Yazoo City [20278]
Mid-Delta Kidney Center, Inc. [25122]
Mid-East Tennessee Speech and Hearing Center
    [3426]
Mid Eastern Council on Chemical Abuse [43280]
Mid Erie Counseling and Treatment Services
    [46590]
Mid-Erie Counseling and Treatment Services
    [31289]
Mid Erie Counseling and Treatment Services •
    Chemical Dependency Clinic [46565]
Mid Florida Metro Treatment Center [41721]
Mid-Florida Rehabilitation Services • Winter Haven
    Hospital [1796]
Mid Hudson Addiction Recov Centers Inc • Florence
    Manor Community Residence [46638]
Mid Hudson Addiction Recovery Center
    Bolger House Community Residence [46995]
    Dowling House [46996]
    Medically Monitored Withdrawal [46997]
Mid-Hudson Forensic Psychiatric Center [33703]
Mid Iowa Fertility Clinic [22064]
Mid-Island Medical Supply Co. [16654]
Mid--Kansas ENT Associates [2249]
Mid-Michigan Center for Sleep Disorders [37185]

Mid--Michigan Ear, Nose and Throat [2579]
Mid Michigan Home Health Care [15665]
Mid Missouri Counseling [45597]
Mid Ohio Psychological Services [47785]
Mid Ohio Sleep Center [37547]
Mid-Peninsula Speech and Language Clinic [1217]
Mid-Plains Center [30976]
Mid-Plains Center for Behavioral Healthcare
  Services [30985]
Mid Plains Center for • Behavioral Healthcare
  Services Inc [45739]
Mid-Shore Council on Family Violence, Inc. [9452]
Mid-South Arc [8520]
Mid-South Eye Bank for Sight Restoration, Inc.
  [35208]
Mid-South Health Systems, Inc.
  Craighead County [28294]
  Greene County [28337]
Mid-South Health Systems, Inc.--Lawrence County
  [28361]
Mid--South Home Health [12689], [12690]
Mid-South Speech Pathology Group [3441]
Mid-South Tissue Bank [35209]
Mid State Health Center [6965]
Mid State Orthopaedic and Sports Medicine Clinic
  [38488]
Mid-State Sports Medicine [39028]
Mid Texas Council on Alcohol/Drug Abuse [49256]
Mid Valley Recovery Services Inc
  Court Program [39808]
  Omni Center Casa de Paz [39809]
Mid-Valley Speech & Hearing Center [3302]
Mid Valley Weslaco Dialysis • US Renal Care
  [27393]
Mid-Valley Women's Crisis Service [10258]
MidAmerica Neuroscience Institute • Multiple
  Sclerosis Center [34583]
MidAmerican Neuroscience Institute • Sleep
  Disorders Center [36995]
Middle Country Schools [603]
Middle Flint Behavioral HealthCare [29333]
Middle Flint Behavioral Healthcare • Adult Mental
  Health Day Treatment [29397]
Middle Flint Behavioral HealthCare
  Alcohol/Drug Day Treatment [29334]
  Breezeway Adult Mental Health Day Services
  [29335]
  Group Homes and Residences [29336]
  Residential Services [29337]
Middle Peninsula Northern Neck Community
  Services Board [32788]
  Warsaw Counseling Center [32795]
Middle Peninsula Northern Neck • Counseling
  Center [49794]
Middle River Hospice [19744]
Middle Tennessee Medical Center • Cancer Center
  [5945]
Middle Tennessee Mental Health Institute [33850]
Middle Way House, Inc. [9266]
Middleburg Dialysis LLC • American Renal Associ-
  ates [23413]
Middleburg Early Education Center [8424]
Middleburg Heights Dialysis Center • DaVita [26164]
Middledorf Medical Group [38608]
Middlesboro Appalachian Regional Hospital Home
  Health [15233]
Middlesex Dialysis Center LLC • DaVita [23164]
Middlesex Home Care and Supplies Inc. [13521]
Middlesex Hospice and Palliative Care [19151]
Middlesex Hospital
  Cancer Center [4899]
  Center for Behavioral Health [29009]
  Crisis Assessment and Triage Service [50730]
Middlesex Hospital Homecare [13519]
Middlesex Human Service Agency Inc
  Answer House Recovery Home [44420]
  Middlesex DUIL/Tewksbury Hospital [44592]
Middlesex Rehabilitation Associates Inc. [38560]
Middleton Group Home [27900]
Middletown Community Health Center [7095]
Middletown Crossroads at • Croydon Hall [46035]
Middletown Dialysis Center [25703]
Middletown Medical LLC [46061]
Middletown Medical Sleep Center [37399]
Middletown Pediatric Community Health Center, Inc.
  [7023]
Middletown Psychiatric Center • Newburgh Mental
  Health Clinic [33709]

Middletown Residential Treatment Center [34060]
Middletown Veterans Affairs Clinic [32155]
Middletown Veterans Affairs Community Based
  Outpatient Clinic [31809]
Midland Dialysis Center [27258]
Midland Health Care Services, Inc. [18162]
Midland Hospice Care [19782]
Midland Memorial Hospital • Allison Cancer Center
  [6013]
Midlands Regional Center [8502]
Midlothian Dialysis • DaVita [27516]
MidMichigan Health Services • MidMichigan Health
  Park - Houghton Lake [6848]
MidMichigan Home Care--Alma [20025]
MidMichigan Home Care-Clare [20047]
MidMichigan Home Care-Gladwin [20059]
MidMichigan Medical Center, Clare [2566]
MidMichigan Medical Center--Midland • Speech--
  Language Pathology Program [2625]
MidMichigan Medical Center • Pardee Cancer
  Center [5386]
MidMichigan Visiting Nurse Hospice [20094]
Midsouth Neurology Clinic • Sleep Disorders Center
  [37774]
Midsouth Treatment Center [49072]
Midstate Behavioral Health System • Crisis Stabliza-
  tion Program [50729]
MidState Medical Center--Behavioral Health [29006]
MidState Medical Center • Cancer Program [4898]
Midtown Center [30999]
Midtown Community Health Center [7324]
Midtown Community Mental Health Center
  Health/Hospital Corp of Marion Cnty [43104]
  Health/Hospital Corp of Marion County [43105]
  Narcotics Treatment [43106]
Midtown Counseling Center [32355]
Midtown Dialysis Center [22555]
Midtown Habilitation Center [8212]
Midtown Kidney Center • Fresenius Medical Care
  [27159]
Midtown Mental Health Center [32356]
Midtowne Norfolk Dialysis • DaVita [27527]
Midvale Park Dialysis • Fresenius Medical Care
  [22519]
Midway Dialysis • Fresenius Medical Care [23948]
Midway Recovery Systems Inc [42107]
Midwest Addiction Psychiatric • Psychological
  Services [43052]
Midwest Brain Injury Clubhouse [1993]
Midwest Center for Eating Disorders [11122]
Midwest Center for Reproductive Health
  CentraCare Women's and Children's Clinic
  [22137]
  Denali OB/GYN [21889]
  Duluth Clinic [22138]
  Innovis Health [22206]
  Mankato Clinic [22139]
  Mid Dakota Clinic [22207]
Midwest Center for Sleep Disorders, Aurora [36918]
Midwest Center for Sleep Disorders, Brighton
  [37186]
Midwest Center for Sleep Disorders, Lansing
  [37187]
Midwest Center for Sleep Medicine, Bloomington •
  Sleep Disorders Center [36919]
Midwest Center for Youth and Families [34131]
Midwest Chiropractic and Sports Medicine [38649]
Midwest City--Del City School District [666]
Midwest City--Del City Schools [667]
Midwest Companies [15920]
Midwest Cord Blood Bank [35037]
Midwest Counseling Associates [43107]
Midwest Dialysis--27th Street Branch [27751]
Midwest Dialysis--Appleton Avenue Branch [27752]
Midwest Dialysis--Capitol Branch [27753]
Midwest Dialysis • Fresenius Medical Care [24298]
Midwest Dialysis--Glendale [27754]
Midwest Dialysis--Good Hope Branch • Dialysis
  Center [27755]
Midwest Dialysis--Lakeshore [27781]
Midwest Dialysis--Ryan Road [27763]
Midwest Dialysis--South Milwaukee [27756]
Midwest Dialysis--West Bend [27805]
Midwest Ear Institute [2797]
Midwest Ear, Nose, and Throat [2232]
Midwest Eye Banks • Michigan Eye Bank [35079]
Midwest Fairborn Dialysis • DaVita [26112]
Midwest Fertility Center • In Vitro Fertilization

  Program [22041]
Midwest Fertility Specialists [22059]
Midwest Kidney Care--Kenosha [27729]
Midwest Kidney Care--Racine [27774]
Midwest Kidney Care--Waukesha [27794]
Midwest Pain Management Centers [35445]
Midwest Pain Relief Center, P.A. [38467]
Midwest Palliative and Hospice Care Center--
  Glenview [19524]
Midwest Palliative and Hospice Care Center--
  Libertyville [19536]
Midwest Palliative and Hospice Care Center -
  Skokie, Illinois [19572]
Midwest Palliative and Hospice CareCenter [14805]
Midwest Regional Medical Center [17131]
Midwest Rehabilitation Associates • Pain Center
  [35454]
Midwest Reproductive Center [22068]
Midwest Sports Medicine [38874]
Midwest Springfield Dialysis • DaVita [26203]
Midwest Surgery Center • Pain Clinic [35455]
Midwest Therapy Associates Inc. [3242]
Midwest Transplant Network [35047]
Midwest Treatment Center [42742]
Midwest Urbana Dialysis • DaVita [26222]
Midwest Woman's Healthcare [22145]
Midwest Youth Services • Runaway and Homeless
  Youth Program [35933]
Midwestern Colorado Mental Health Center [41086],
  [41222], [41273], [41281], [41321]
  Center for Mental Health [28878], [28956]
Midwestern CT Council on Alcohol
  McDonough House/Intensive Residential
  [41375]
  Outpatient [41376]
Midwestern CT Council on Alcoholism • New Milford
  [41450]
Midwood Chaim Aruchim • Dialysis Facility [25617]
Midwood Chayim Auchim Dialysis Site II [25618]
MIGHTYSPEECHWORKS Inc. [2008]
Migrant Camps [7065]
Migrant Health Center Western Region [7204]
Migrant Health Program [7452]
Migrant Health Service [6871]
Migrant Health Services, Inc. • Battered Women's
  Program [9592]
Mike Conley Hospice House [19207]
Miland E. Knapp Rehabilitation Center [4222]
Milder Physical Therapy & Sports Medicine PC
  [38589]
Mildred Mitchell-Bateman Hospital [33917]
The Mile High Council [41004]
The Mile High Council On Substance Abuse and
  Mental Health [41136]
Mile High Counseling Inc [41279]
Miles City VA Community Based Outpatient Clinic
  and Community Living Ctr. • VA Montana Health
  Care Center [4254]
Miles City Veterans Affairs Clinic and Nursing Home
  [30956]
Miles Foundation [9002]
Miles Home Health and Hospice [19891]
Milestone Centers, Inc. [32108]
Milestone Centers Inc. • Day Treatment and Deaf
  Services [3367]
Milestone Counseling Services Inc [41005], [41041],
  [41239], [41280]
Milestone Foundation • Extended Care [44020]
Milestone Group LLC [45927]
Milestones Eating Disorders Program [11024]
Milestones Family Recovery Program • Womens
  Residential [48091]
Milestones in Language and Speech [3590]
Milestones Outpatient Program [48092]
Milestones Speech and Language Center [1363]
Milestones Therapeutic Services Inc. [1228]
Milford Audiology Center [2497]
Milford Dialysis • DaVita [23165]
Milford Memorial Hospital [13561]
Milford Regional Medical Center • Cancer Center
  [5345]
Milford Regional Medical Center, Inc. • VNA of
  Greater Milford [15518]
Milhous Center [34014]
Milhous Children's Services, Inc [28649]
Mill Creek Community Hospital • Substance Abuse
  Services [48368]
Mill Creek Dialysis Center • DaVita [27597]

Mill Creek Outpatient Services [43440]
Mill Neck Manor School for the Deaf [589]
Mill Swan Communication Skills Center [8161]
Millard Health [35281]
Millbrook Continuing Treatment Center [31391]
Millcreek of Arkansas [7756], [33117]
Millcreek Behavioral Health Services [34262]
Millcreek Home Health and Hospice [21651]
Mille Lacs Band
    Halfway House [45253]
    Outpatient Program [45177], [45254]
Mille Lacs Home Care Hospice [20188]
Millennium Healthcare [16293]
Miller Children's Hospital [18957]
    Sickle Cell Disease Center for Children [36303]
Miller County Dialysis Unit • Texarkana Regional
    Dialysis Center [27375]
Miller County Mental Health Center [29390]
Miller-Dwan Medical Center • Burn Center [4572]
Miller Dwan Rehabilitation Center [4223]
Miller Home Care [14085]
Miller House--Denver [28884]
Miller House--Juneau • Juneau Youth Services, Inc.
    [28100]
Miller St. Dialysis Center [25978]
Miller & Standel Speech Pathology [1319]
Miller & Standel Speech Pathology Services [1127]
Millhon Clinic • OhioHealth Sleep Center [37548]
Millroy • Turning Point Community Programs, Inc.
    [28733]
Mills Dialysis Center [22986]
Mills-Peninsula Health Center [1301]
Mills Peninsula Health Services • Behavioral Health
    Department [40679]
Mills-Peninsula Health Services • Schneider Cancer
    Center [4848]
Millstone Counseling Center [43746]
Millwood Hospital [32404], [49215]
Milne Detoxification Center [45740]
Milner House [29013]
Milner-Rushing Home Care [12664]
Milstein Pediatric Speech and Language Services
    [2666]
Milton & Ethyl Warner Dialysis Unit--Spencer •
    Spencer Municipal Hospital [24300]
Milton S. Hershey Medical Center • Sleep Research
    and Treatment Center [37676]
Milwaukee Community Mental Health Complex •
    Psychiatric Crisis Service [51521]
Milwaukee County Executive Office for Persons with
    Disabilities [3684]
Milwaukee County Mental Health [33936]
    Community Support Program [33937]
    Day Hospital [33938]
    Metro-North Community Clinic [33939]
    Southside Community Support Program [33940]
Milwaukee Dialysis Center • American Renal Associ-
    ates [27757]
Milwaukee Health Service Systems [50480]
Milwaukee Health Service Systems II • 10th Street
    Clinic [50481]
Milwaukee Health Services Inc. [7434]
Milwaukee Public Schools • Hearing Impaired
    Program [888]
Milwaukee Veterans Affairs Medical Center [32998]
Milwaukee Womens Center • Horizon House
    [50482]
Milwaukee Women's Center, Inc. [10723]
MIMA Sleep Disorders Center [36796]
Mimbres Valley Home Health and Hospice [16310]
Mimbres Valley Hospice [20534]
Mind Body Soul Wellness [10889]
Mind Body Wellness Center [11144]
Mindbody Medicine Clinic • Pain Center [35748]
Minden Dialysis • Fresenius Medical Care [24538]
Minden Medical Center Home Health Agency
    [15333]
Mindful Health [11025]
Mineola Dialysis • Fresenius Medical Care [27260]
Mineral County Advocates to End Domestic Violence
    [9791]
Mineral Wells Clinic [32516]
Mingo-Wayne Home Health [18553]
Mingus Center • Rio de Esperanza [39377]
Mini Twelve Step House Inc [40135]
    The Solution Family Resource Center [39727]
Ministerio Evangelistico • El Eterno Yo Soy [48843]
Ministerio Renovados En El Espiritu de • Vuestra

Mente Inc [48766]
Ministerio de Restauracion • Cristo Mi Fortaleza
    [48841]
Ministry Behavioral Health [50532]
    Residential Treatment Center [50533]
Ministry Behavioral Health--Rhinelander [33011]
Ministry Behavioral Health--Wisconsin Rapids
    [33028]
Ministry of Children and Family Development • North
    Fraser Eating Disorders Program [10917]
Ministry Dialysis--Marshfield [27738]
Ministry Door County Medical Center • Sleep
    Disorders Facility [37973]
Ministry of Health [39200]
Ministry Home Care • Hospice Services - Stevens
    Point [21868]
Ministry Home Care, Inc.--Marshfield [18586]
Ministry Home Care--Marshfield [18587]
Ministry Home Care--Rhinelander [18622]
Ministry Home Care--Stevens Point [18630]
Ministry Home Care--Wausau [18641]
Ministry Koller Behavioral Health [50518]
Ministry Saint Josephs Hospital • Alcohol and Drug
    Recovery Services [50458]
Minneapolis Clinic of Neurology
    Headache Clinic [12436]
    Shapiro Center for Multiple Sclerosis [34610]
Minneapolis Dialysis Unit • DaVita [25047]
Minneapolis Veterans Affairs Medical Center [4224]
Minnesota Alternative LLC [45114]
Minnesota Braille and Talking Book Library [3815]
Minnesota Community Hospice [20173]
Minnesota Deaf and Hard of Hearing Services
    Division--Central [2733]
Minnesota Deafblind Project [2732]
Minnesota Department of Health • Maternal and
    Child Health Section [36496]
Minnesota Department of Human Services • Deaf
    and Hard of Hearing Services [2688]
Minnesota Extended Treatment Options [8178]
Minnesota Foot & Ankle Clinics, PA [38638]
Minnesota Interventional Pain Associates [35521]
Minnesota Lions Eye Bank [35086]
Minnesota Orthopedic Sports Medicine Institute/Twin
    City Orthopedics [38627]
Minnesota Program Development • Domestic Abuse
    Intervention Project [9594]
Minnesota Speech Language [2743]
Minnesota Sport & Spine Rehabilitation, Inc. [38614]
Minnesota Sports Medicine Center--Eden Prairie
    [38617]
Minnesota Sports Medicine Center--Minneapolis
    [38628]
Minnesota State Academy for the Blind [3716]
Minnesota State Academy for the Deaf [510]
Minnesota State University, Moorhead • Speech/
    Language & Hearing Clinic [2720]
Minnesota Teen Challenge [45133], [45218]
Minnesota Voice and Speech Clinic [2691]
Minnetonka Dialysis • DaVita [25050]
Minnetonka Pediatric Therapy Center [2717]
MinnHealth SportsCare Consultants • MinnHealth
    PA [38639]
Minnie Jones Family Health Center [7046]
Minocqua Behavioral Health Center [32999]
Minot Infant Development Program [8395]
Minot State University • Department of Communica-
    tion Disorders [3207]
Minot VA Outpatient Clinic [4357]
Minot Veterans Affairs Clinic [31635]
Minsec at Erie Outpatient [48539]
MinSec Hazleton Treatment Center [48402]
Minto Village Council • Suicide Prevention Line
    [50639]
Miracle Hill Renewal Center [48946]
Miracle Home Health Care Inc. [13141]
Miracles Detox/Recovery Program • at Brotman
    Medical Center [39772]
Miracles Inc
    Miracles House [43498]
    Outpatient [43499]
Miracles Inc/Sanctuary House Program • Women
    With Co-occuring Mental Illness [43500]
Miramar Kidney Center • DaVita [23325]
Miramar Recovery [39969]
Miramar Top Health Care [14246]
Mirasol Eating Disorder Recovery Center [10900]
Mirasol Family Health Center [7131]

Mirasol Transitional Living Center [10901]
MiRehab PC [2565]
Miriam Hospital
    Cancer Program [5890]
    Dialysis Unit [26666]
    Sleep Disorders Center of Lifespan Hospitals
        [37725]
Mirian Worthy Women's Health Center [6578]
Mirmont Treatment Center [48466]
Mirror Inc [43319]
    Hiawatha [43361]
    Hutchinson [43365]
    Medicine Lodge [43406]
    Mens Program [43412]
    Newton [43413]
    Shawnee [43460]
    Topeka [43465]
    Wellington [43472]
    Womens Program [43414]
    Wyandotte [43378]
Misericordia Home-South [7941]
Mission Rescate Drug Abuse Treatment • de Sabana
    Grande [48808]
Mission Area Health Associates • Mission Neighbor-
    hood Health Center [6353]
Mission Children's Clinic • Pediatric Cystic Fibrosis
    Center [7631]
Mission Council on Alcohol Abuse for the Spanish
    Speaking [40623]
Mission Council Family Day Treatment [40624]
Mission Detox Center [45264]
Mission Dialysis • US Renal Care [27261]
Mission Health Care Providers Inc. [13236]
Mission Hills Dialysis • DaVita [27073]
Mission Hospice, LLC [20962]
Mission Hospice of San Mateo County [19033]
Mission Hospital • Mountain Area Cancer Center
    [5627]
Mission Hospital Regional Medical Center
    Acute Rehabilitation Unit [3911]
    Cancer Care Center [4806]
Mission Kidney Center • Fresenius Medical Care
    [27262]
Mission Road Developmental Center [8566]
Mission/Saint Joseph Health System • Ruth and
    Billy Graham Children's Health Center • Sickle Cell
    Program [36405]
Mission Sleep Disorders Clinic [36675]
Mission Treatment Center [39468]
Mission Treatment Centers [45831], [45847],
    [47985], [48042]
Mission Treatment Services Inc
    Escondido [39812]
    San Diego [40569]
Mission Unity Inc [41903]
Mission Valley Dialysis • DaVita [27263]
Mission Viejo Dialysis • DaVita [22813]
Mission Vista Behavioral Health [33883]
Mississippi Baptist Health Systems • Hederman
    Cancer Center [5428]
Mississippi Baptist Medical Center
    Mississippi Sports Medicine and Orthopaedic
        Center [38642]
    Sleep Disorders Center of Mississippi [37253]
Mississippi Children's Home Society • Runaway and
    Homeless Youth Program [36042]
Mississippi Children's Home/Warren County
    Children's Shelter • Runaway and Homeless Youth
    Program [36043]
Mississippi Department of Health • SIDS Information
    and Counseling Program [36497]
Mississippi Fertility Institute • Woman's Specialty
    Center [22142]
Mississippi HomeCare of Bay Saint Louis [15952]
Mississippi HomeCare of Gulfport [15963]
Mississippi HomeCare of Picayune [15974]
Mississippi HomeCare of Wiggins [15983]
Mississippi Library Commission • Blind and Physi-
    cally Handicapped Library Services [3816]
Mississippi Lions Eye Bank [35089]
Mississippi School for the Blind [3717]
Mississippi School for the Deaf [522]
Mississippi SIDS Alliance [36498]
Mississippi Sports Medicine and Orthopaedic
    Center--Brookhaven [38640]
Mississippi Sports Medicine and Orthopaedic
    Center--Jackson [38644]

Mississippi State Community Counseling Services [51048]
Mississippi State Hospital [33624], [33627]
    Chemical Dependency Unit [45429]
    Claiborne House [33617]
    Kitty Mitchell Group Home [33618]
    Opportunity House [33619]
    Villa Hope Group Home [33620]
Mississippi University for Women • Speech and Hearing Center [2757]
Mississippi Valley Sleep Disorder Center [36982]
Missoula City County Health Department [6937]
Missoula County Public Schools [535]
Missoula Indian Center [45713]
Missoula Veterans Affairs Clinic [30957]
Missouri Alcohol Drug Assessment and • Consultants Inc [45664]
Missouri Alcohol Drug Assessment • Consultants [45581]
Missouri Baptist Medical Center
    Cancer Program [5461]
    Multiple Sclerosis Center for Innovations in Care [34618]
    Orthopedic and Spine Center [38666]
Missouri Baptist Sullivan Hospital [45656]
Missouri City Dialysis • Fresenius Medical Care [27266]
Missouri Department of Health and Senior Services • Division of Maternal, Child and Family Health [36499]
Missouri Highlands Medical Clinic [6914]
Missouri Lions Eye Banks, Headquarters • Heartland Lions Eye Bank [35097]
Missouri Rehabilitation Center [2808], [4236]
Missouri School for the Blind [3718]
    Missouri Deafblind Technical Assistance Project [2818]
Missouri School for the Deaf [526]
Missouri Shores Domestic Violence Center [10379]
Missouri Southern Healthcare [2788]
Missouri Veterans Affairs Clinic [30899]
Mitchell Clinic [48353]
Mitchell Community Dialysis • DaVita [26791]
Mitchell Community Hospice at Avera Queen of Peace [21295]
Mitchell County Dialysis Center [23634]
Mitchell County Hosital • Somnograph Sleep Laboratory [36996]
Mitchell County Mental Health Center [32428]
Mitchell County Mental Health Children & Youth [29379]
Mitchell County SafePlace [10086]
Mize and Associates [2325]
Mizell Memorial Hospital • Sleep Disorders Center [36591]
MJ Leadenham Center [51003]
MJB Transitional Recovery [40136]
M.J.G. Nursing Home Co., Inc. [16401]
MK Place Adolescent Substance Abuse • Treatment Center [42362]
MLF Speech Therapy [3241]
MMH DCNWJ Succasunna Dialysis Center of Northwest Jersey [25513]
MMLD Inc • DBA New Beginnings Counseling Services [47986]
MNAP Diagnostics • MNAP Sleep Disorders Center [37677]
MNP Enterprises • Nextep [41300]
Moapa Mental Health Center [31041]
Moberly Regional Medical Center [2807]
Mobilcare Medical [17738]
Mobile Association for Retarded Citizens [7719]
Mobile Audiology--Gobles [2588]
Mobile Audiology--Holland [2607]
Mobile County Health Department [12695]
Mobile County Home Health Office [12696]
Mobile Crisis Intervention Service • New Castle CMHC [50745]
Mobile Crisis Team [51206]
Mobile Crisis Unit [51360]
Mobile Dialysis Services, Inc.--Compton [22644]
Mobile Infirmary Medical Center [12697]
    Cancer Program [4735]
Mobile Infirmary Sleep Disorders Center [36592]
Mobile Metro Treatment Center [39276]
Mobile Therapy Centers of America LLC [2061]
MobileCare Medical, Inc. [12727]
Mobility Designs [14480]

Mobility Home Health Services Inc. [13210]
Mobility Plus Home Health Care--Flint [15666]
Mobility Plus Home Health Care, Inc.--Warren [15876]
Moccasin Bend Mental Health Institute [33841]
Moccasin Bend Ranch [33776]
Mockingbird Peritoneal Dialysis • Fresenius Medical Care [27033]
Modesto Kidney Center, LLC • Innovative Dialysis Systems [22814]
MODOC County Alcohol and Drug Services [39589]
Modoc County Mental Health Services [28230]
Modus Vivendi LLC [48201]
H. Lee Moffitt Cancer Center & Research Institute [4996]
Mofrankel Healthcare Services [15419]
Mohan Dialysis Center of Covina [22650]
Mohan Dialysis Center of Glendora [22711]
Mohan Dialysis Center of Industry [22638]
Mohave Hospice [18782]
Mohave Mental Health Clinic [39368], [39399]
Mohave Mental Health Clinic--Bullhead City [28133]
Mohave Mental Health Clinic • Lake Havasu [39400]
Mohave Mental Health Clinic--Lake Havasu City [28161]
Mohave Mental Health Clinic--Sycamore Avenue, Kingman [28158]
Mohave Mental Health Clinic--Western Avenue, Kingman [28159]
Mohawk Valley Psychiatric Center [31481]
Mojave Mental Health
    Adult Services [31032]
    Children's Services [31033]
Mokena Dialysis • Fresenius Medical Care [24043]
Moline District 40 Deaf/Hard of Hearing Program [404]
Molokai Community Health Center [6623]
Molokai Dialysis Facility • Liberty Dialysis [23858]
MOMA's [8696]
Momentum for Health [28777]
Moms and Womens Recovery Center
    East/Puyallup Branch [50073]
    South Parkland Branch [50211]
    Tacoma Branch [50212]
Mon Yough Community Services, Inc. [32043]
Monadnock Community Hospital [31088]
Monadnock Dialysis Center • Fresenius Medical Care [25389]
Monadnock Family Services
    Administrative Office [31074]
    Community Support Programs [31075]
    Eastern Regional Office [31089]
    Jaffrey District Office [31073]
    Monadnock Region Substance Abuse [45901]
Monarch Hospice & Palliative Care [19483]
Monarch House [44519]
Monarch Inc [47965]
Monarch Pain Care and Rehabilitation Center, Inc. [35699]
Moncrief Dialysis Center • DaVita [26953]
Mondanock Family Services/Emerald House • Momndanock Family [31076]
Monfort Children's Clinic [6409]
Monfort Family Clinic [6402]
Monica House [31369]
Monmouth County • Division of Social Services [46107]
Monmouth Family Health Center [6976]
Monmouth Medical Center
    Adult Cystic Fibrosis Center [7602]
    Cystic Fibrosis and Pediatric Pulmonary Center [7603]
    Leon Hess Cancer Center [5520]
    Sleep Disorders Center [37349]
Monmouth Psychological Associates • Eating Disorders Program [11145]
Mono County Alcohol and Drug Program [40200]
Monocacy Counseling Center LLC [44271]
Monongahela Valley Assoc. of Health Centers, Inc. • Fairmont Clinic [7404]
Monongahela Valley Association of Health Centers, Inc. [18513]
Monongahela Valley Hospital • Regional Cancer Treatment Center [5844]
Monroe 2--Orleans BOCES [604]
Monroe Addictive Disorders Clinic [43860]
Monroe Behavioral Health Clinic [32837]
Monroe Clinic Dialysis • Liberty Dialysis [27760]

The Monroe Clinic Home Care [18604]
Monroe Clinic Hospice [21861]
Monroe Community Dialysis • Fresenius Medical Care [25764]
Monroe Counseling Center LLC [46118]
Monroe County BOCES Number One [579]
Monroe County Community Mental Health Authority [30605]
Monroe County Counseling Center [29427]
Monroe County Domestic Abuse Project--Sparta [10737]
Monroe County Domestic Abuse--Tomah [10740]
Monroe County Health Center • Monroe Health Center [7417]
Monroe County Health Department [6852]
Monroe County Hospital [12699]
Monroe County Medical Center [15255]
Monroe County Program for Children with Hearing Impaired [492]
Monroe County Public Schools [203]
Monroe Home Care Shoppe, Inc. [15752]
Monroe House [28885]
Monroe Nursing Facility [27989]
Monroe Veterans Affairs Clinic [30160]
Monroeville Dialysis • DaVita [26483]
Monsey Medical and Dental Care [7024]
Monsignor Carr Institute • Outpatient Clinic [46566]
Monsignor Patrick J. Frawley Mental Health Clinic [31476]
Monsignor Wall Social Services Center [46113]
Monson Developmental Center [8110]
Monsoon • United Asian Women of Iowa [9330]
Monta Vista High School/Fremont UHSD [271]
Montana Center on Disabilities • Montana State University/Billings [8222]
Montana Chemical Dependency Center [45691]
Montana Department of Public Health and Human Services • Family and Community Health Bureau [36503]
Montana Developmental Center [8223]
Montana Healthcare Services • Outpatient Program [45695]
Montana House • Juneau Youth Services, Inc. [28101]
Montana Legal Services Association • Domestic Violence Unit [9751]
Montana Migrant and Seasonal Farmworker Council • Migrant Health Project [6924]
Montana Office of Public Instruction • Montana Idea Services for Children and Youth with Deafblindness [2836]
Montana School for the Deaf and the Blind [534], [3719]
Montana State Hospital [33642]
Montana State University • Victim Options in the Campus Environment [9741]
Montana Talking Book Library [3818]
Montcalm Center for Behavioral Health [30641]
Montclare Dialysis • DaVita [23949]
Monte Nido [10970]
Montebello Artificial Kidney Center [22822]
Montebello Dialysis Center LLC [22823]
Montecatini [28425]
Montecatini Comprehensive Treatment Center for Women with Eating Disorders [10971]
Montefiore [16849]
Montefiore Dialysis Center--Unit III [25591]
Montefiore Dialysis Center--Unit IV [25592]
Montefiore Family Health Center [7010]
Montefiore Hospice [20803]
Montefiore Hospital and Medical Center [25593]
Montefiore Hospital Medical Center, Rosenthal Main • Comprehensive Sickle Cell Center [36395]
Montefiore Medical Center
    Cancer Care Program [5561]
    Chemical Dependence Outpatient Program [46425]
Montefiore Medical Center Detox [46426]
Montefiore Medical Center • Headache Unit [12451]
Montefiore Medical Center Home Health Agency [16367]
Montefiore Medical Center
    Institute for Human Communication [2981]
    MDA Clinic [34837]
Montefiore Medical Center--North Division • Hemodialysis Unit [25594]
Montefiore Medical Center
    Sleep Disorders Center [37400]

Subst Abuse Treatment Program Unit I [46427]
Subst Abuse Treatment Program Unit III [46428]
Montefiore North Division OP CD [46429]
Montefiore's Institute of Reproductive Medicine and Health [22186]
Monterey County Behavioral Health Services [28736]
Monterey County Mental Health [28546]
Monterey County Mental Health--Monterey [28641]
Monterey County Mental Health--Salinas [28737]
Monterey Peninsula Dialysis • Innovative Dialysis Systems [22825]
Montevideo Dialysis • DaVita [25051]
Montevideo Veterans Affairs Clinic [30701]
Montevista Hospital [33647]
Montezuma Dialysis • DaVita [23762]
Montgomery Academy High School [8263]
Montgomery Area Mental Health Authority • Autanga County Satellite Office [28026]
Montgomery Area Mental Health Authority, Inc. • Montgomery [27999]
Montgomery Area Mental Health Authority
Lowndes County Satellite Office [27948]
Lowndesboro [27966]
Wetumpka Nursing Facility [28066]
Montgomery County Abused Persons [9461]
Montgomery County Community Clinic [6276]
Montgomery County Dept Health/Human • Services/ Outpatient Addiction Services [44338]
Montgomery County Emergency Service Inc. [33812], [51290]
Montgomery County Exceptional Child Program [632]
Montgomery County Health Department [42706]
Division of Mental Health Helpline [50849]
Montgomery County Hotline • Mental Health As-sociation [50979]
Montgomery County Methadone Center [48489]
Montgomery County School District [444]
Montgomery County United Way [51375]
Montgomery County Women's Center [10512]
Montgomery County Youth Services • Runaway and Homeless Youth Services [36228]
Montgomery Crisis Residential Facility [28000]
Montgomery Developmental Center [8415]
Montgomery Dialysis Center • DaVita [25820]
Montgomery General Hospital [19936]
Addiction and Mental Health Center [44318]
Cancer Program [5309]
Sleep Center [37107]
Montgomery General Hospital,Inc. [15453]
Montgomery Home Care, LLC [16876]
Montgomery Hospice [19941]
Montgomery Hospital Hospice Program [21121]
Montgomery Hospital Medical Center • Cancer Program [5847]
Montgomery Hospital Medical Center Home Care [17399]
Montgomery Hospital Medical Center • Sleep Laboratory [37678]
Montgomery Metro Treatment Center [39281]
Montgomery Primary Achievement Center [8103]
Montgomery Recovery Services Inc [44339]
Montgomery Renal Center, LLC [24689]
Montgomery Surgery Center [35645]
Montgomery Transitional Services Inc • Alcoholism Halfway House [46357]
Monticello Dialysis Center • Renal Advantage Inc. [23763]
Montreal Children's Hospital • Burn Unit [4626]
Montreal General Hospital • Burn Unit [4627]
Montreal Neurological Hospital • Multiple Sclerosis Research Clinic [34702]
Montreal Oral School for the Deaf, Inc. [720]
Montrose Counseling Center [10475], [49385]
Montrose Dialysis • Dialysis Clinic, Inc. [23134]
Monument Counseling Center [41275]
Moody Health Systems Corporation [18001]
Moody Park Dialysis • Fresenius Medical Care [27160]
Moog Center for Deaf Education [530]
Moonlite Home Health Services, Inc. [15782]
Moore Center for Eating Disorders [11304]
Moore Counseling and Mediation Services Inc [47757]
Moore Counseling Services [48662]
Moore Norman Technology Center • Career and Technical Education for Students [668]

Moore Regional Hospital • Department Pyschiatry [47445]
Moore's Home Health and Medical Supply--Kokomo [15016]
Moore's Home Health and Medical Supply--Marion [15024]
Mooresville Center [29784]
Moorhead Health Care Center • Speech Therapy Department [2721]
Mooring Programs Inc [50362]
Moorpark Health Care Center [18973]
Mora Valley Community Health Services, Inc. [7001]
More Than Words [1184]
More Than Words Speech and Language Services [1155]
More Than Words Speech Pathology Services [910]
Morehead City Veterans Affairs Clinic [31562]
Morehead Hill Program • Learning Services Residential Rehabilitation • Durham, North Carolina [4332]
Morehead Memorial Hospital • Smith McMichael Cancer Center [5638]
Morehead VA Outpatient Clinic [15234]
Morehead Veterans Affairs Outpatient Clinic [30081]
Morehouse Community Medical Centers [6742]
Morehouse Parish Dialysis Center, LLC • Fresenius Medical Care [24457]
Morehouse Parish Dialysis • Fresenius Medical Care [24458]
Morgan Behavioral Health Choices [47810]
The Morgan Center [7819]
Morgan City Dialysis Center [24543]
Morgan County Health Council, Inc. • Morgan County Medical Center [7276]
Morgan County Schools [191]
Morgan County System of Services • Runaway and Homeless Youth Program [35781]
Morgan Hospital and Medical Center [2170]
Morgan Hospital & Medical Center • Cancer Center [5166]
Morgan Treatment Center [45219]
Morgantown Hospice [21807]
Morgantown Mobile Vet Center [52142]
Morgantown Physical Therapy Associates [39164]
Morning Star Sanctuary [10426]
Morningstar Home Health Agency, Inc. [14247]
Morningstar Treatment Services, Inc.--Reynolds [29486]
Morningstar Treatment Services, Inc.--Rome [29490]
Morningstar Treatment Services, Inc.--Waycross [29504]
Morningstar Treatment Services, Inc.--West Point [29507]
Morongo Basin Mental Health Services
Barstow Recovery Services [39644]
Joshua Tree Drug Court [39950]
Panorama Ranch [39951]
Panorama Ranch Outpatient [39645], [40974]
Morongo Basin Unity Home [8824]
Morovis Community Health Center, Inc. [7205]
Morris County Sexual Assault Center [9838]
Morris Foundation Inc
Outpatient Services [41488]
Therapeutic Shelter [41489]
Women and Childrens Program [41490]
Morris Heights Health Center [7011]
Morris Hospital • Cancer Program [5111]
Morris House [41491]
Morris L. Black Community Counseling Center [31475]
Morris Village [48920]
Morrison Center [31962]
Breakthrough [48202]
Morrison Child and Family Services • Rosemont Treatment Center and School [48203]
Morrison Manor • Hospice of Scotland County [20691]
Morristown Memorial Hospital
Atlantic Health Sleep Disorder Center [37350]
Center for Human Development [8258]
Department of Communication Disorders [2933]
Goryeb Children's Hospital • Child Development Center [10830]
Hemodialysis Unit • Dialysis Center [25471]
Psychiatric Emergency Service • Crisis Hotline [51112]
Simon Cancer Center [5524]
Morrow County Hospital [17004]

Morton Bakar Center [33150]
Morton Center Inc [43663], [43692]
Morton Comprehensive Health Services • Morton Health Center [7121]
Morton F. Plant Hospital • Barnett Rehabilitation Center [7881]
Morton Hospital and Medical Center [15551]
Cancer Program [5358]
Speech, Hearing, and Language Center • North Woods Medical Center [2528]
Morton Plant Hospital • Sleep Center [36797]
Morton Plant Mease Health Care • H. Lee Moffitt Cancer Center [4935]
Mosaic [8229]
Mosaic Community Services [33566]
Dual Diagnosis Program [44368]
Mosaic Medical [7143]
Mosaic Recovery [43108]
Moscow Dialysis Center • DaVita [23880]
Moses Cone Health System [20675]
Behavioral Health Center [33738], [33739], [33742]
Regional Cancer Center [5641]
Moses Dialysis Unit [24969]
Moses H. Cone Health System • Sleep Disorders Center [37474]
Moses H. Cone Memorial Hospital
Internal Medicine Division • AIDS Clinical Trials Unit [24]
Rehabilitation Center [4333]
Moses Lake Community Health Center [7379]
Moses Lake SLP Services [3598]
Moses Taylor Hospital [17472]
Renal Unit • DaVita [26577]
Moss Regional Hospital • Sickle Cell Center [36352]
Moss Speech & Language Center, Inc. [1746]
Mossglen • Turning Point Community Programs, Inc. [28734]
MossRehab--Elkins Park [4399]
MossRehab, Tabor Road [4400]
MossRehab at Woodbury [4293]
Mother Theresa Sister of Charity [6507]
Motivated Youth Recovery Program [44619]
Motivating Individuals for Learning and Living • Mill School [34122]
Motivational Frame Works LLC [41358]
Motivational One Counseling [41066]
Motivational Services, Inc. [30184]
Augusta Supported Living Center [30185]
Elm Street House [30186]
Sunrise House [30187]
Transitional Intensive Residential [30188]
Young Adult Housing and Support Services [30189]
Motivations Treatment Center [50262]
Motor City Dialysis • DaVita [24882]
Motor City Medical [15741]
Mott Children's Health Center • Hurley Children's Clinic • Outreach Program • Cystic Fibrosis Center [7578]
Moulton Center • Southwestern Behavioral Health-care Inc [43035]
Moulton-Lawrence Counseling Center [28002]
Moultree County Counseling Center • Sullivan Crisis Line [50877]
Moultrie County Counseling Center • Moultrie County DUI Referral [42930]
Moultrie Dialysis Center • DaVita [23765]
Moundbuilders Guidance Center [31815], [31821]
Mount Adams Kidney Center • DaVita [27653]
Mount Airy Dialysis Center • Wake Forest University [25915]
Mount Auburn Dialysis & Home • DaVita [26047]
Mount Auburn Health Center [7079]
Mount Auburn Hospital [2470]
Cancer Program [5329]
Mount Auburn Hospital I Home Health [15482]
Mount Auburn Hospital • Multiple Sclerosis Care Center [34598]
Mount Baker Kidney Center [27596]
Mount Baker Planned Parenthood
Bellingham Clinic [12051]
Friday Harbor Clinic [12052]
Mount Vernon Health Center [12053]
Mount Carmel Guild Behavioral Healthcare • PACT [31155]
Mount Carmel Health • Cancer Institute [5709]
Mount Carmel Health System

Network Cancer Program [5710]
 Saint Ann's Sports Medicine [38899]
Mount Carmel Home Health Services [15149]
Mount Carmel Hospital • Central Ohio Sleep
 Medicine [37549]
Mount Carmel Regional Medical Center
 Outpatient Rehabilitation Services [2239]
 Regional Cancer Center [5203]
Mount Carmel Saint Ann's Medical Center • Cancer
 Care Program [5760]
Mount Clemens Regional Medical Center • Ted B.
 Wahby Cancer Center [5387]
Mount Desert Island Hospital • Behavioral Health
 Center [43939]
Mount Dora Dialysis • DaVita [23417]
Mount Enterprise Community Health Center [7302]
Mount Evans Hospice, Inc. [19106]
Mount Graham Regional Medical Center [12814]
Mount Graham Safe House, Inc. [8726]
Mount Greenwood Dialysis • DaVita [23950]
Mount Hood Hospice [21034]
Mount Laurel Dialysis Center [25473]
Mount Nittany Medical Center • Cancer Center
 [5875], [26585]
Mount Olive Counseling and Clinic [46034]
Mount Olive Dialysis • DaVita [25916]
Mt. Pleasant Dialysis Center [26747]
Mount Pleasant Dialysis Center Inc. • Fresenius
 Medical Care [27267]
Mount Pleasant Medical Center [7177]
Mount Pleasant RDSPD [811]
Mount Pleasant Regional Center for Developmental
 Disabilities [8177]
Mount Pleasant Treatment Center • Mental Health
 Institute [33502]
Mount Pocono Dialysis • DaVita [26589]
Mount Rainier Kidney Center • Northwest Kidney
 Center [27632]
Mount Regis Center [49840]
Mount Rogers Community Service Board [32799]
 Friendship House [32764]
 Grayson County Mental Health Center [32750]
 Transitions [32765]
Mount Saint Mary's Hospital and Health Center
 Sleep Disorders Clinic [37401]
 Speech Rehabilitation Services [3085]
Mount Saint Ursula Speech Center [2982]
Mount Saint Vincent Home [34044]
Mount Saint Vincent University • Eating Disorders
 Program [11190]
Mount San Antonio College • DSPS--Services to
 Deaf/Hard of Hearing Students [313]
Mount Sinai Allograft Technologies [35178]
Mount Sinai Hospital Medical Center [14746]
Mount Sinai Hospital Medical Center of Chicago •
 Cancer Program [5072]
Mount Sinai Hospital Medical Center • Deaf and
 Hard of Hearing Services [1994]
Mount Sinai Hospital and Medical Center
 MDA Clinic [34838]
 Renal Unit [23951]
Mount Sinai Hospital/Miami Heart Institute [1665]
Mount Sinai Hospital • Pediatric and Adult
 Comprehensive Sickle Cell Program [36396]
Mount Sinai Kidney Center • Dialysis Center [25727]
Mount Sinai Medical Center
 Comprehensive Cancer Center [4971]
 Corrine Goldsmith Dickinson Center for Multiple
 Sclerosis [34648]
 Cystic Fibrosis and Pediatric Pulmonary Center
 [7616]
 Dialysis Center [25728]
 Genetics Center [12290]
 Headache Center [12452]
 Mount Sinai Rehabilitation Center [4311]
 Mount Sinai Spinal Cord Injury Model System
 [4312]
 RMA of NY [22187]
Mount Sinai Medical Rehabilitation Center • Center
 for Advanced Medicine [4313]
Mount Sinai Physical Therapy & Health Promotion at
 Asphalt Green [38796]
Mount Sinai School of Medicine
 Eating and Weight Disorders Program [11161]
 Pain Management [35579]
 Regional Comprehensive Hemophilia Treatment
 Center [12565]

Mount Sinai Sports Therapy • Mount Sinai Medical
 [38797]
Mount Tom Center for Mental Health and Recovery •
 Satellite [44583]
Mount Tom Mental Health Center [30397], [50992]
Mount Vernon Behavioral Health Clinic [32843]
Mount Vernon Community Service Center [31396]
Mount Vernon Developmental Center [8426]
Mount Vernon Dialysis & At Home • DaVita [24047]
Mount Vernon Dialysis, LLC [25707]
Mount Vernon Girls Residence [31397]
Mount Vernon Hospital • Methadone Maintenance
 Treatment Prog [46796]
Mount Vernon Neighborhood Health Center [7025]
Mount Vernon Veterans Affairs Clinic [29651]
Mount Washington Pediatric Hospital [8088]
Mountain Area Recovery Center Inc [47213]
Mountain Area Recovery Center West [47273]
Mountain Brook Schools [205]
Mountain Case Management [28220]
Mountain Comprehensive Care Center [43532]
 Community Support Program [30098]
Mountain Comprehensive Care Center--Inez [30035]
Mountain Comprehensive Care Center
 Johnson County Clinic [43750]
 Layne House [43763]
 Magoffin County Clinic [43776]
Mountain Comprehensive Care Center--Martin
 [30074]
Mountain Comprehensive Care Center
 Martin County Clinic [43636]
 Outpatient [43764]
Mountain Comprehensive Care Center--Paintsville
 [30097]
Mountain Comprehensive Care Center
 Pike County Outpatient Clinic [43757]
 Pikeville Clinic [30099]
Mountain Comprehensive Care Center--Prestonburg
 [30101]
Mountain Comprehensive Care Center • Preston-
 burg Helpline [50940]
Mountain Comprehensive Care Center--Salyersville
 [30109]
Mountain Comprehensive Care Center--South Will-
 iamson [30115]
Mountain Comprehensive Health Corp. • Whitesburg
 Medical/Dental Clinic [6740]
Mountain Crest Behavioral Healthcare System/PVHS
 [33219]
Mountain Crisis Services, Inc. [8847]
Mountain Empire Family Medicine [6296]
Mountain Family Health Center [6407]
Mountain Health Solutions [47214]
Mountain Heritage Hospice [19803]
Mountain Home Health Hospice [20547]
Mountain Home Veterans Affairs Medical Center
 [51651]
Mountain Hospice--Belington [21786]
Mountain Hospice-Davis [21795]
Mountain Hospice-Elkins [21797]
Mountain Hospice-Franklin [21799]
Mountain House [33047]
Mountain House Clubhouse [32784]
Mountain House Day Treatment [32892]
Mountain Lakes Behavioral Healthcare [27943]
 Geriatric Services [27944]
Mountain Land Ortho and Sports Physical Therapy
 [39109]
Mountain Land Sports and Ortho Physical Therapy
 [39104]
Mountain Manor Outpatient Services [44272]
Mountain Manor Safe Harbor Project • Potomac
 Health Services Pregnant Clients [44258]
Mountain Manor Treatment Center [44387]
 Emmitsburg Rehabilitation [44259]
 Outpatient/Baltimore/Frederick Avenue [44161]
 Outpatient Site [44162]
 Residential/Frederick Avenue [44163]
Mountain Park Dialysis • DaVita [23800]
Mountain Park Health Center--Goodyear [6232]
Mountain Park Health Center--Phoenix [6244]
Mountain Park Health Center--Tempe [6251]
Mountain Peace Shelter [8936]
Mountain Plains Network For Youth • Runaway and
 Homeless Youth Program [36139]
Mountain Region Speech and Hearing Center [3431]
Mountain Regional Hospice [21683]
Mountain Regional Services • DBA Cornerstone

Behavioral Health [50582]
Mountain Ridge Dialysis • Liberty Dialysis [27691]
Mountain States Chemical Dependency and
 Counseling Services Inc [42356]
Mountain States Regional Hemophilia Center-Utah •
 Primary Children's Medical Center [12604]
Mountain States Regional Hemophilia and Thrombo-
 sis Center • University of Colorado at Denver and
 Health Sciences Center [12496]
Mountain Treatment Center [47215]
Mountain Valley Hospice--Gloversville [20570]
Mountain Valley Hospice and Palliative Care-Elkin
 [20655]
Mountain Valley Hospice and Palliative Care-Galax
 [21697]
Mountain Valley Hospice and Palliative Care--Mount
 Airy [20710]
Mountain Valley Hospice and Palliative Care--Stuart
 [21737]
Mountain Valley Hospice and Palliative Care--
 Yadkinville [20773]
Mountain Valley Mental Health Center • Volunteer
 Behavioral Healthcare System [49094]
Mountain Valley Mental Health Programs, Inc. •
 Crisis Intervention [51248]
Mountain Valley Regional Rehabilitation Hospital
 [976]
Mountain View--Birch Tree R--III [528]
Mountain View Dialysis Center, Inc. [22819]
Mountain View Dialysis • DaVita • Dialysis Facility
 [25369]
Mountain View Hospital [32607], [33088]
Mountain View Hospital District Hospice [21014]
Mountain View Hospital
 Intensive Outpatient Program [39287]
 Outpatient Services [39251]
 Partial Hospitalization Program [39252]
Mountain Vista Dialysis Center • DaVita [22930]
Mountain Vista Farm [39887]
Mountain West Hospice • Mountain West Medical
 Center [21658]
Mountain West Medical Center • Speech Therapy
 Department [3560]
Mountain Women's Rescue Center [8912]
Mountain Youth Resources • Runaway and Home-
 less Youth Program [36136]
Mountaineer Community Health Center, Inc.--Paw
 Paw [7412]
Mountaineer Home Care [18505]
Mountainlands Community Health Center--Provo
 [7325]
Mountainside Hospital
 Atlantic Health System • Cancer Program [5523]
 Audiology and Speech Pathology Department
 [2930]
 Dialysis Unit [25470]
Mountainside Treatment Center [41373]
Mountaintop Area Medical Center [7188]
Moving to End Sexual Assault [28863]
Moving Forward Assessment Services [45322]
Mowhawk Valley Community Action Agency •
 Runaway and Homeless Youth Program [36117]
MPI Treatment Services [40303]
MPTS CASA ALMA/CASA MARIA [47693]
Mr. Jill's Body Firm [38156]
MRB Counseling Services Inc [44278], [44301]
MRPT Physical Therapy [38798]
MRS Homecare, Inc. [14597]
Mrs Wilsons Halfway House [46070]
MS/Hershey Medical Center • Transplant/Dialysis
 Center [26447]
MS Supply and Home Health Company [14422]
MSA Home Health [16139]
MST Speech and Language Center [1297]
Muasher Center for Fertility and IVF [22287]
Muckleshoot Behavioral Health Program [49885]
Mueller Speech and Hearing Associates, Inc. [1088]
Mujeres Latinas en Accion [9210]
Mujeres Unidas/Women Together [10488]
Mukilteo Evaluation and Treatment Program [32844]
Muleshoe Dialysis • AccessCare [27238]
Multi Addictions Processing Agency • (MAPA)
 [41137]
Multi Counseling Inc • Tahlequah [48024]
Multi Cultural Counseling Services • DBA Renew
 Counseling Services [50483]
Multi--Organ Transplant Program, QEII Health Sci-
 ences [35152]

Multi-Service Eating Disorders Association [11093]
Multi Systemic Therapy Unit [47694]
MultiCare - Good Samaritan Home Health & Hospice [18472]
MultiCare Home Health Agency, Inc. [17420]
Multicare Hospice of Tacoma [21774]
Multicare International Home Health Agency Inc. [12908]
MultiCare Regional Cancer Center • Cancer Program [6125]
MultiCare Sleep Disorders Center at Tacoma [37918]
Multicultural Counseling Services Ltd [50118]
Multilingual Development Agency [3051]
Multiple Sclerosis Care of Connecticut [34548]
The Multiple Sclerosis Center [34586]
Multiple Sclerosis Center of Atlanta [34565]
Multiple Sclerosis Center of Greater Orlando [34556]
Multiple Sclerosis Center for the Greater Quebec Area [34703]
Multiple Sclerosis Center of Northeastern New York [34649]
Multiple Sclerosis Center of South Texas [34718]
Multiple Sclerosis Comprehensive Care Center of Central Florida [34557]
Multiple Sclerosis Treatment and Research Center [34611]
Multipractice Clinic [6747]
Muncie/Anderson Veterans Affairs Clinic [29787]
Munroe Regional Home Care [13830]
Munroe Regional Medical Center
    Home Care [14281]
    Speech and Hearing Center [1683]
Munson Dialysis Center [24985]
Munson Hospice House [20129]
Munson Hospice and Palliative Care [20130]
Munson Medical Center
    Alcohol and Drug Treatment Center [45037]
    Cancer Program [5399]
    Hemophilia Center [12542]
    Memory and Attention Training Center [4179]
    Munson Sleep Disorders Center [37188]
Murdoch Center [8369]
Murfreesboro Dialysis • Dialysis Center • DaVita [26901]
Murphy Pain Center [35461]
Murray-Calloway County Hospital [19821]
Murray--Calloway County Hospital • Cancer Program [5232]
Murray Calloway County Hospital • Center for Sleep Studies [37034]
Murray-Calloway County Hospital Home Care Services [15237]
Murray-Calloway County Hospital Hospice [19822]
Murtis H. Taylor Multi-Service Center [31718]
MUSC Sports Medicine [39005]
Muscala Chemical Health Clinic [45220]
Muscle Shoals Dialysis • DaVita [22380]
Muscogee County Program for Exceptional Students [369]
Muscular Dystrophy Association [8444]
Musculoskeletal Transplant Foundation--Edison, NJ [35120]
Musculoskeletal Transplant Foundation (MTF)--Costa Mesa, CA [34952]
Musculoskeletal Transplant Foundation (MTF)--Jessup, PA [35190]
Musculoskeletal Transplant Foundation (MTF)--Redlands, CA [34953]
Muskegon Area District Library for the Blind and Physically Handicapped [3810]
Muskegon Area Intermediate School District [497]
Muskegon County CMHSP • John Halmond Center [30609]
Muskegon Hearing and Speech Center • Audiology Service [2630]
Muskingum Behavioral Health [47898]
Muskingum Valley Health Centers [7101]
Muskogee County • Council of Youth Services [47966]
Muskogee County Health Department [31895]
    Speech and Hearing Clinic [3273]
Muskogee Dialysis Center • Fresenius Medical Care [26270]
Muskogee Regional Medical Center [17135]
    Cancer Program [5774]
    Speech Therapy Department [3274]
Musomed Healthcare Corporation [14086]

Mutual Ground, Inc. [9193]
MVI HospiceCare Inc. [20915]
MVP Health Inc. [14087]
MVP Physical Therapy at Lakewood [39145]
mvpsportsmed.com [38529]
My Angels Home Health Agency, Inc. [14226]
My Family Inc [40461]
My Fathers House Inc [46004]
My Friend Home Care/Saint Kevin Home Health Agency [14088]
My Home Care, LP [17892]
My Home Inc [45306]
My Sister's House--Gallup [9871]
My Sister's House Inc.--North Charleston [10358]
My Sister's House--Rocky Mount [10078]
My Sister's House--Statesville [10087]
My Sister's Place--Athens [10124]
My Sister's Place--Chandler [8682]
My Sister's Place, Inc.--Tuckahoe [9995]
My Sisters' Place, Inc.--White Plains [10009]
My Sister's Place--Marshall [10060]
My Sister's Place--Newport [10241]
My Sisters Place • Thomas Jefferson University [48540]
My Sister's Place--Washington [9033]
MYG Home Care Agency, Inc. [14089]
Myofunctional Center of Connecticut [1493]
Myrtle Beach Dialysis • DaVita [26751]
Myrtle C. Robinson Home • JBS Mental Health Authority [27867]
Myrtle Hilliard Davis Comprehensive Health Center, Inc. • Comprehensive Health Center [6919]

N

9th Judicial Juvenile Drug Court Treatment [43881]
N and D Health Care Services Inc. [13278]
N. E. Washington Health Programs [18423]
N Street Village • Luther Place • Night Shelter/Safehouse [9034]
Na Nihzhoozhi Center Inc [46271]
Naaman Center [48351]
Nacogdoches Memorial Hospital [18098]
    Dialysis Facility [27270]
Nacogdoches Regional Day School for the Deaf [812]
Nadeene Brunini Comprehensive Hemophilia Care Center • Saint Michael's Medical Center [12556]
NAIC/Norman Addiction Information and • Counseling [47969]
Nalco, LLC • Dialysis Center [24406]
Namaqua Center [7843], [34050]
Namaste Child and Family Development Center [31207]
Namaste Child & Family Development Center--Las Vegas [34313]
Namaste Child & Family Development Center--Roswell [34316]
Namaste Child and Family Development Center--Santa Fe [34317]
Namaste Comfort Care [19100]
Namaste, Inc. [31195], [31204]
Nampa Dialysis Center • DaVita • Dialysis Center [23882]
Nampa Group Home [33401]
Nan Coley Murphy Counseling Center [27824], [50608]
Nancy C Craft Counseling Services [45956]
Nancy L. Foreman and Associates [3472]
Nannie Hogan Boyd Down Syndrome Resource Center and Clinic • Cook Children's Medical Center [10870]
Nanticoke Memorial Hospital • Cancer Care Center [4916]
Nantucket Cottage Hospital [15520]
    Dialysis Unit [24782]
Nanuet House Congregate Treatment Residence [31398]
Nany Home Health Care and Medical Supply [14090]
Naomis Nest [44839]
Napa County Health and Human Services • Alcohol/Drug Program Services Division [40254]
Napa Dialysis Center • DaVita [22834]
Napa Emergency Women's Services [8852]
Napa State Hospital [33167]
    Deaf and Hearing Impaired Adult Programs [1193]

Napa Valley Dialysis [22835]
Napa Valley Fertility Center--Greenbrae [21925]
Napa Valley Fertility Center--Napa [21926]
Napa Valley Fertility Center--Sonoma [21927]
Naperville Dialysis Center • Fresenius Medical Care • Dialysis Center [24048]
Naperville Foot Clinic [38394]
Naperville North Dialysis Center • Fresenius Medical Care [24049]
Naperville Psychiatric Ventures • DBA Linden Oaks Hospital [42806]
Naples AKC--North Collier Branch • Fresenius Medical Care [23246]
Naples Artificial Kidney Center • Fresenius Medical Care [23421]
Naples Center for Voice, Speech and Swallowing Disabilities [1673]
Naples Community Hospital Healthcare System • Cancer Program [4972]
Naples Community Hospital Inc • Dept of Psychiatric Medicine [41813]
Naples Dialysis Center • DSI Corp [23422]
Naples Dialysis • DaVita • Dialysis Facility [23423]
Naples Veterans Affairs Primary Care Clinic [29229]
Naptime Homecare [12914]
NARA of the Northwest Inc [48204]
Narco Freedom Inc
    Alternatives [46430]
    Alternatives II/CD Outpatient [46517]
    Bridge Plaza [46763]
    Independence CD Outpatient Tx Program [46431]
    Methadone Maintenance Treatment Prog [46432]
    Methadone Treatment Clinic [46433]
Narco Freedom Inc/Regeneration • Women and Children Residential Treatment Prg [46434]
Narconon Colorado • A Life Worth Saving [41177]
Narconon Florida Inc [41596]
Narconon • Freedom Center [44628]
Narconon Georgia/Atlanta [42142]
Narconon Gulf Coast Inc [41639]
Narconon Louisiana • New Life Retreat Inc [43825]
Narconon of Oklahoma Inc • Narconon Arrowhead [47916]
Narconon Vista Bay [40937]
Narcotic Addiction Treatment Agency Inc • (NATA) [40832]
Narcotic Drug Treatment Center Inc • Center for Drug Problems [39311]
Narcotics Prevention Project/Methadone • Maintenance Treatment Program [40137]
Nardin Park • Recovery Center [44751]
NARIKA: A Helpline for Abused South Asian Women [8794]
Narrows Kidney Center • Dialysis Clinic Inc. [25619]
Nash General Hospital • Coastal Plain Hospital [47477]
Nash Health Care Systems • Cancer Program [5657]
Nash Hospitals, Inc. [16775]
Nashoba Valley Medical Center [2446]
Nashua Dialysis • DaVita • Dialysis Center & At Home [25397]
Nashville Alternative Center [29481]
Nashville CARES [49158]
Nashville Clinic [28329]
Nashville General Hospital • Cancer Program [5948]
Nashville Home Training Dialysis PD and At Home Training • DaVita [26908]
Nashville Neuroscience Group [12465]
Nashville Pain Center [35675]
Nason Hospital Home Health Agency [17467]
Nason Hospital Hospice [21151]
Nassau Alternative Advocacy Program • Nassau Alternative Counseling Center [46784]
Nassau Community College • Center for Students with Disabilities [580]
Nassau County Coalition Against Domestic Violence [9928]
Nassau County Medical Center • Dialysis Center [25650]
Nassau County Mental Health Association [31348]
Nassau County MMTP • Division of Chemical Dependency Services [46614]
Nassau Cty Mental Health Alcohol/Drug Abuse Council • Sutton Place at Hilliard [41686]
Nassau University Medical Center

Burn Center [4592]
Department of Pediatrics • Division of Medical Genetics [12291]
Detox Unit [46615]
Hospital IP Rehab [46616]
Nassau Vet Center [52038]
Natchaug Hospital Inc
River East Day Hospital and Treatment Center [41481]
Sachem House [41416]
Natchaug Hospital, Inc. • Joshua Center/Sachem House [33251]
Natchaug Hospital • Joshua Center--Enfield [33241]
Natchez Veterans Affairs Clinic [30797]
Natchitoches Center for Addictive Disorders [43865]
Natchitoches Mental Health Center [30161]
Natchitoches Outpatient Medical Center [6754]
Nathan Adelson Hospice - North West [20419]
Nathan Adelson Hospice - Pahrump [20426]
Nathan Adelson Hospice--Swenson Street, Las Vegas [20420]
Natick VNA, Inc. [19980]
National Athletic Training & Fitness Institute [38546]
National Biblical Institute for the Deaf • Program for Deaf Students [189]
The National Birth Defects Center [8154]
National Birth Defects Center • Down Syndrome Clinic [10813]
The National Center for Children and Families [34175]
National Center for Speech and Language Inc. [1562]
National Center for Victims of Crime [9035]
National Children's Center [7876]
National Council on Alcohol and Drug Dep [40495], [40854]
Dependence of the San Fernando Valley [40743]
East San Gabriel and Pomona Valley [40404]
East San Gabriel and Pomona Valleys [39762]
San Fernando Valley [40896]
South Bay [40032], [40033]
Woman to Woman Recovery Program [40034]
Womens Residential Program [40035]
National Council on Alcohol/Drug Depend • Central Arizona [39438]
National Council on Alcoholism and Drug Depend GDA Vantage Point West [44752]
National Council on Alcoholism • Lansing Regional Area [44889]
National Deaf Academy [1669]
National Disease Research Interchange [35191]
National Eye Bank Center [35210]
National Health Services [6367]
National Healthcare Center of Fort Oglethorpe [1863]
National Home Care Services [2341]
National Hospice/dba Promises Kept Hospice [19788]
National Hospice and Palliative Care Organization [21673]
National Institute for Change [41006], [41199], [41240], [41258]
National Institutes of Health • VRC--Vaccine Evaluation Clinic • HIV Vaccine Trials Unit [83]
National Jewish Medical and Research Center [1399]
The Sleep Center [36727]
National Latina Lesbian, Gay, Bisexual, Transgender Organization [9036]
National Medicine Center [14299]
National Naval Medical Center--Bethesda • Cancer Program [5295]
National Naval Medical Center • Cystic Fibrosis Center [7563]
National Nephrology Associates--Central [26954]
National Nephrology Associates--Marble Falls [27246]
National Nephrology Associates--North • Dialysis Facility [26955]
National Nephrology Associates--Round Rock • Dialysis Facility [27306]
National Nephrology Associates--San Marcos [27355]
National Nephrology Associates--South • Dialysis Facility [26956]
National Pain Institute, Bradenton [35388]
National Pain Institute--Delray Beach [35389]

National Pain Institute, Holiday [35390]
National Pain Institute--Lady Lake [35391]
National Pain Institute--Lake Mary [35392]
National Pain Institute--New Port Richey [35393]
National Pain Institute--Port Saint Lucie [35394]
National Pain Institute--Sand Lake [35395]
National Pain Institute, Winter Park [35396]
National Pharmacy Acquisition, LLC [15272]
National Quality and Review Corporation--Baltimore [15420]
National Quality and Review Corporation--Frederick [15440]
National Quality and Review Corporation--Riverdale [15459]
National Rehabilitation Hospital [3946]
National Rehabilitation Hospital--Metro Center, Bethesda • Pain Clinic [35480]
National Rehabilitation Hospital • National Capital Spinal Cord Injury Model System/Brain Injury Program [3947]
National Rehabilitation Hospital--Rockledge Drive, Bethesda, MD • Pain Program [35481]
National Rehabilitation Hospital
Sleep Center [36763]
Suburban Regional Rehabilitation at Montrose [2431]
National Rehabilitation Hospital--Washington DC • Pain Program [35375]
National Renal Institutes--Tampa Central [23535]
National Sleep Centers, Inc. [37825]
National Speech-Language Therapy Center [2393]
National Stem Cell Bank [35266]
National Therapeutic Services Inc [39749]
Joshua House [39750]
The RAP Center [40262]
Nations Home Infusion [15456]
Nationwide Childrens Hospital • Behavioral Health [47722]
Nationwide Children's Hospital
Cystic Fibrosis Center [7640]
Down Syndrome Clinic [10847]
Hemophilia Treatment Center [12577]
Region IV Genetics Center [12317]
Sleep Disorders Center [37550]
Nationwide Home Health Care, Inc. [15817]
Native American Community Health • Center [39439]
Native American Connections Inc
Guiding Star [39440]
Indian Rehabilitation [39441]
Outpatient Clinic [39442]
Native American Health Center [40304]
Family and Child Guidance Clinic [40625]
Native American Rehabilitation • Association of The Northwest Inc [48205]
Native American Resource Center [47598]
Native American Women's Health Education Resource [10372]
Native Angels Hospice-Pembroke [20714]
Native Directions Inc • Three Rivers Lodge [40201]
Native Project [50174]
Natomas Dialysis • DaVita [22920]
Natrona County Health Department • Denver Genetics Clinic [12376]
Natural Balance Nutrition [10972]
Nature Coast Community Health Center--Brooksville [6449]
Nature Coast Community Health Center--Dental Office, Spring Hill [6549]
Nature Coast Community Health Center--Spring Hill Campus [6550]
Nature and Nurture Eating Disorder Intensive Outpatient Program [10973]
Nature's Place Therapy Services Inc. [1564]
Nava Counseling Services [46281]
Navajo Mountain Community Health Center [6239]
Navajo Nation • DBHS [46272], [46317]
Navajo Regional Behavorial Health Center • Outpatient/Adult Men Residential [46308]
Navajo United Methodist Center [9869]
Naval Ambulatory Care Center • Chronic Pain Management Center [35656]
Naval Branch Health Clinic • Substance Abuse Rehabilitation Program [43951]
Naval Health Clinic • Substance Abuse Rehabilitation Program [42283]
Naval Hospital [39676]
Naval Hospital Bremerton • Substance Abuse

Rehabilitation Program [50158]
Naval Medical Center • Naval Hospital Portsmouth • Pain Management [35753]
Naval Medical Center--Portsmouth • Cancer Program [6076]
Naval Medical Center, Portsmouth • Cystic Fibrosis Center [7688]
Naval Medical Center Portsmouth • Substance Abuse Rehabilitation Program [49816]
Naval Medical Center San Diego • Cancer Program [4834]
Naval Medical Center, San Diego • Cystic Fibrosis Center [7476]
Naves Foster Home • JBS Mental Health Authority [27868]
Navos Outpatient Services--Burien Campus [32812]
Navy Substance Abuse Rehab Department • Naval Base San Diego [40570]
Nazareth Home for Boys [34199]
Nazareth Home Care [17421]
Nazareth Hospital Hospice • Inpatient Unit - VITAS [21131]
Nazareth Hospital • Northeast Sleep Disorders Center [37679]
NC Development Services [14091]
N.C. Little Memorial Hospice [20159]
NCC Associates • North Central Mental Health/Satellite [47765]
NCC Reynoldsburg • North Central Mental Health/Satellite [47723]
NCED Mental Health Center [33866]
NCO Youth and Family Services • Runaway and Homeless Youth Program [35934]
NEA Hospice of Arkansas [18877]
Neale and Associates Inc. [1645]
Near North Health Service Corporation • Winfield Moody Health Center [42562]
Near West Family Health Center [6663]
Near West Woodworks [31719]
Neat Home Care Inc. [13142]
Nebo School District [841]
Nebraska Center for the Education of the Children Who are Blind or Visually Impaired [3720]
Nebraska Commission for the Deaf and Hard of Hearing [2850]
Nebraska Department of Education • Services for Children and Youth Who are Deafblind • Nebraska Deafblind Project [2858]
Nebraska Department of Health • Perinatal Child and Adolescent Health Program [36504]
Nebraska Health Center • Clarkson Hospital Burn Center [4582]
Nebraska Library Commission • Talking Book and Braille Service [3819]
Nebraska Medical Center
Clarkson Hospital • Storz Cancer Institute [5482]
Eppley Cancer Center [5483]
Sleep Disorders Center [37315]
Nebraska Methodist Hospital • Eastbrook Cancer Center [5484]
Nebraska Methodist Hospital Home Health [16125]
Nebraska Orthopaedic Hospital [38690]
Nebraska Orthopaedic and Sports Medicine [38689]
Nebraska SIDS Foundation [36505]
Nebraska Spine and Pain Center [35543]
Nebraska Urban Indian Health Coalition • Inter Tribal Treatment Center [45796]
Ned Behnke Speech and Deafness School • Hearing, Speech and Deafness Center • Early Childhood Program [863]
Needles Counseling Center • Child/Adolescent/Adult Outpatient Clinic [28648]
Needs, Inc. [51525]
NEFA [49656]
NeghborCare at Home--Pittsburgh [17443]
NeghborCare at Home--Reading [17462]
Nehemiah Family Services [45126]
NeighborCare--Boothwyn [17259]
NeighborCare HME [18390]
NeighborCare - San Bernardino [13289]
NeighborCare of Windsor [13555]
Neighborhood Coalition for Shelter Inc • NCS Outpatient Services [46892]
Neighborhood Counseling Center [45339]
Neighborhood Health Care, Inc. • Neighborhood Family Practice [7080]
Neighborhood Health Care Services, Inc. [17945]

Neighborhood Health Clinics, Inc. [6685]
Neighborhood Home Care, LLC [15512]
Neighborhood Hospice [21170]
Neighborhood House Inc • Alcohol and Drug
  Outpatient Treatment [47724]
Neighborhood House of North Richmond • West
  County Human Development Center [40449]
Neighborhood Justice Project [10003]
Neighborhood Service Organization [51013]
Neighborhood Union Health Center [29351]
Neighboring [47814]
Neighbors Consejo [41544]
Neil Dobbins Center [47216]
Neil Kennedy Recovery Clinic [47875], [47895]
Neil Kennedy Recovery Clinic/Dublin [47752]
Neili Home Health Care Agency [14092]
Nelo Health Care Services, Inc. [18024]
NELSA [43878]
Nelson Behavioral Center Inc [48631]
Nelson Counseling [39571]
Nelson County Industries [29970]
Nelson L Price Treatment Center [42131]
Nemaha County Home Health and Hospice [19775]
Nemaha Valley Veterans Affairs Community Hospital
  [29954]
Nemours/Alfred DuPont Hospital for Children •
  Down Syndrome Clinic [10785]
Nemours Children's Clinic [1699]
    Cystic Fibrosis Center [7504]
    Division of Pediatric Hematology/Oncology •
      Hemophilia Treatment Center [12504]
Nemours Children's Clinic, Jacksonville • Division of
  Genetics and Metabolism [12182]
Nemours Children's Clinic • MDA Program [34781]
Nemours Children's Clinic Orlando
    Central Florida Pulmonary Group
        Adult Cystic Fibrosis Center [7505]
        Pediatric Cystic Fibrosis Foundation [7506]
Nemour's Children's Clinic Pensacola • Cystic
  Fibrosis Center [7507]
Nemours Children's Clinic • Wolfson Children's
  Hospital • Cancer Program [4952]
Nemours Sickle Cell Clinic/Arnold Palmer Hospital
  [36323]
NeoCells [35001]
NeoFight [36479]
NeoHealth Pediatrics [7116]
Neomy Dialysis Center [25620]
Neopolitan Lighthouse [9211]
Neosho Memorial Veterans Affairs Medical Center
  [29912]
NeoStem • Adult Stem Cell Operations [35136]
NeoStem Family Stem Cell Banking [35121]
Nephro Care Inc.--West • Fresenius Medical Care
  [25621]
Nephrocare Inc. • Fresenius Medical Care [25622]
Nephrology Center of Crestview • Fresenius Medical
  Care [23274]
Nephrology Center of Milton • Fresenius Medical
  Care [23415]
Nephrology Center of Pensacola • Fresenius Medi-
  cal Care [23472]
Nephrology Center--South Augusta • DaVita •
  Dialysis Facility [23614]
Nephrology Center of Statesboro • DaVita [23795]
Nephrology Center of Vidalia • DaVita [23825]
Nephrology Center of Waynesboro [23835]
Nephrology Centers of America--Grovetown [23715]
Nephrology Centers of America--Louisville [23739]
Nephrology Foundation of Brooklyn East • Dialysis
  Facility [25623]
Nephrology Foundation of Brooklyn North [25624]
Nephrology Foundation of Brooklyn South [25625]
Nephrology Physicians LLC [24205]
Nephron Dialysis Center of Lakewood, LLC [22765]
Nephron Dialysis Center Ltd. [23952]
Neptune Dialysis Center • DaVita [25477]
Ness Counseling Center Inc [40138]
Nestor's Health Services--Hieleah [13790]
Nestor's Health Services, Inc.--Miami [14093]
Net Care Access [31735]
The Net Domestic Violence Program [9897]
Network Against Domestic Abuse [8993]
Neuro-Audiological Associates of Boca Raton [1543]
Neuro Care of Washington [39142]
Neuro Institute of Austin, LP dba • Texas NeuroRe-
  hab Center [4452]
The Neuro Medical Center • MDA Clinic [34804]

Neuro--Recovery [2655]
Neuro Rehab Program [4063]
Neuro--Rehabilitation Center at Middleboro [4137]
Neuro--Rehabilitation Center at Worcester [4138]
Neurobehavioral Health Institute [1728]
Neurobehavioral Resources Ltd./dba Touchstone
  Neurorecovery Center [4453]
NeuroCare Center • Sleep Center [37551]
Neurocare, Inc.--Brockton [37121]
Neurocare Inc.--Newton • Center for Sleep
  Diagnostics [37122]
Neurodevelopmental Therapy Services [3519]
Neurodiagnostic Center of Kansas • Comprehensive
  Sleep Disorders Center [36997]
Neurological Associates • Mid--Ohio Multiple
  Sclerosis Center [34672]
Neurological Associates of Northeastern New York
  [12453]
Neurological Clinic of Texas • MDA Clinic [34885]
Neurology Associates [12419], [12441], [34875]
Neurology Associates of Arlington • MDA Clinic
  [34886]
Neurology Associates • Great Plains Multiple
  Sclerosis Center [34709]
Neurology Center of Fairfax • Multiple Sclerosis
  Center [34730]
Neurology Center
    MDA Clinic [34887]
    Pain Clinic [35319]
Neurology & Headache Clinics of NWO [12459]
The Neurology & Headache Treatment Center
  [12474]
Neurology Neuro Pain Consulting [35621]
Neurology and Pain Management--Lafayette [35446]
Neurology and Pain Management--Rensselaer
  [35447]
Neurology & Sleep Clinic [37826]
The Neurology and Sleep Clinic [37068]
Neurology Specialists Inc. • Multiple Sclerosis
  Center [34673]
NeuroMedical Center Hospital [37069]
NeuroRestorative--Braintree [4139]
NeuroRestorative--Carbondale [4026]
NeuroRestorative Center [3884]
NeuroRestorative--Chichester • Mentor ABI [4270]
NeuroRestorative--Florida [3986]
NeuroRestorative--Georgetown [4064]
NeuroRestorative--Louisville [4065]
NeuroRestorative--Lutz • Clement House [3987]
NeuroRestorative Oklahoma [4377]
NeuroRestorative--Paducah • Barkley House [4066]
NeuroRestorative--Phoenix [3869]
NeuroRestorative--Raynham [4140]
NeuroRestorative Rhode Island [4425]
NeuroRestorative Specialty Services [4454]
NeuroRestorative Tennessee [4433]
Neuroscience Consultants • Comprehensive Multiple
  Sclerosis Center [34558]
NeuroTherapy Specialist Inc. [2305]
Neuse River Dialysis Center • Fresenius Medical
  Care [25922]
Nevada Center for Reproductive Medicine [22151]
Nevada Community Enrichment Program [4266]
Nevada County Behavioral Health [28522]
Nevada County Mental Health [28650]
Nevada Department of Human Resources • Division
  of Health • Special Children's Clinic [8233]
Nevada Dialysis Center • DaVita [25357]
Nevada Donor Network, Inc. [35107]
Nevada Fertility CARES [22152]
Nevada Habilitation Center [8206]
Nevada Home Health Providers [16156]
Nevada Lung Center • Desert Sleep Disorders
  Center [37319]
Nevada Medical Systems Inc • Center for Behavioral
  Health [45859]
Nevada Regional Medical Center [16031]
Nevada State Division of Health • Bureau of Family
  Health Services • SIDS Information Services
  [36506]
Nevada State Library and Archives • Nevada Talking
  Book Services [3820]
Nevada Treatment Center [45848]
Nevada Veterans Affairs Clinic [30882]
Never Alone Inc • Never Alone RCDFY [46711]
Never Lake Home Health [14094]
New Advances for People with • Disabilities (NAPD)/
  Genesis Program [39635]

New Age Home Care Inc. [16637]
New Age Services Corporation [42563]
New Albany Dialysis • DaVita [24215]
New Albany--Floyd County Schools [427]
New Alternatives Center LLC [47987]
New Alternatives Inc [44692]
New Beacon--Alabaster [18669]
New Beacon--Anniston [18674]
New Beacon--Gadsden [18718]
New Beacon, Inc.--Birmingham [18686]
New Beacon of Jasper [18733]
New Beacon of Oneonta [18749]
New Beacon of Scottsboro [18759]
New Bedford Dialysis & At Home • DaVita • Dialysis
  Center [24783]
New Beginning with Advantages
    Port Orchard [50062]
    Poulsbo [50068]
New Beginning Center [10465]
New Beginning Fellowship Center [39834]
New Beginning Home Health Care Inc. [13211]
A New Beginning PA [11026]
A New Beginning--Scottsdale [10902]
New Beginnings [31937], [47421], [48093]
New Beginnings Addiction Recovery Center [43879]
New Beginnings • Behavioral Health Services
  [49315]
New Beginnings CASA [39581]
New Beginnings Counseling [11197]
New Beginnings Counseling Centers [45849],
  [45860]
New Beginnings CSTAR Inc [45622]
New Beginnings Detox [41989]
New Beginnings--Laconia [9810]
New Beginnings at Litchfield [45182]
New Beginnings of
    Gaston County [47323]
    Southern Piedmont LLC [47264]
New Beginnings • Outpatient Services [49324]
New Beginnings Recovery Services [47799]
New Beginnings Res Transitional • Trt Program of
  Catholic Charities Inc [45394]
New Beginnings • Runaway and Homeless Youth
  Program [35983]
New Beginnings at Saint Peter • Outpatient Program
  [45317]
New Beginnings--Seattle [10648]
New Beginnings--Springfield [10550]
New Beginnings of Tampa Inc [41967]
New Beginnings Therapy Associates LLC [45779]
New Beginnings at Waverly [45341]
New Beginnings • Womens Program [45342]
New Braunfels Dialysis Center • DaVita [27271]
New Braunfels Kidney Disease Clinic • Dialysis
  Facility • Fresenius Medical Care [27272]
New Bridge Family Shelter [10503]
New Bridge Foundation [28368]
New Bridge Foundation Inc
    Bridge 1 [39655]
    Bridge 2 [39656]
New Bridge Services Inc [46065]
    Partial Care Program Visions [46210]
New Bridges • Outpatient Rehabilitation Center
  [49855]
New Brunswick Counseling Center [46081]
New Brunswick Eye and Tissue Bank [35112]
New Care Concepts, Inc. [18453]
New Care Home Health Agency [14095]
New Castle Dialysis Center • American Renal As-
  sociates [26492]
New Center Community Mental Health Services
  [30564]
New Center Community Mental Health Services--
  Detroit [30544]
New Center Community Mental Health Services--
  Highland Park [30545]
New Center Community Mental Health Services--
  North Park [30546]
New Center Dialysis • DaVita [24883]
New Century Dialysis Center of Jasper [27196]
New Century Home Care [16402]
New Century Home Health Inc. [13418]
New Chance Inc [43335]
New Choice Inc [48043]
New Choice Recovery Treatment Center [40139]
New Choices [10171], [45681]
New Choices for Recovery [45328]

New Choices Recovery Center • Purcell House [47074]
New Choices for Recovery
    Forest Lake HSI [45154]
    Human Services Inc [45117]
N.E.W. Community Clinic [7424]
New Community Corporation • Runaway and Home-less Youth Program [36080]
New Connection Programs • Coon Rapids Outpatient Programs [45115]
New Connections [39739]
    Runaway and Homeless Youth Program [36263]
N.E.W. Curative Rehabilitation, Inc. [4494]
New Dawn Eating Disorders Recovery Center [10974]
New Dawn Enterprises [49030]
New Dawn Recovery Centers
    Outpatient Services [39712]
    Residential Rehab [40328]
New Dawn Wellness and Recovery Center [43466]
A New Day [41826]
New Day of Avery County [10069]
A New Day, Inc. [31182]
New Day Recovery • Youth and Family Services Inc [47988]
New Day Treatment Center [42029]
New Day Treatment Services [48106]
New Destiny Treatment Center [47707]
New Dimension Homecare [15818]
New Dimension Inc [43501]
New Dimensions [32207]
New Dimensions Day Hospital LLC [49386]
New Dimensions Inc. [3212]
A New Direction [39302]
New Direction Treatment Services [47663]
New Directions [34497], [39961]
New Directions Alcohol and • Substance Abuse Treatment Program [46518]
New Directions Behavioral Health Center [46098]
New Directions • Blue Mountains Addictions [48070]
New Directions Center [30944]
New Directions Center, Inc.--Staunton [10595]
New Directions Counseling Center [42871]
New Directions at Cove Forge [48417]
New Directions of Cross County, Inc. [8788]
New Directions of Decatur County Inc. [9280]
New Directions Eating Disorders Center [10975]
New Directions • Hightower Place Womens Facility [43249]
New Directions Inc [40140], [40141], [47695]
New Directions Inc of North Central CT
    Day Treatment Program [41381]
    Outpatient [41382]
New Directions, Inc.--Crawfordsville [29710]
New Directions, Inc.--Enfield [28993]
New Directions--Lawton [10200]
New Directions--Mount Vernon [10161]
New Directions Northwest Inc • Recovery Village [48071]
New Directions
    A Service Area/SA Council/King House [43250]
    A Service of Area/Subst Abuse Council [43251]
New Directions Treatment Center [42612]
New Directions Treatment Services [48294], [48692]
New Directions--Yuma [8988]
New Dominion School of Maryland, Inc. [34177]
New England Aftercare Ministries Inc • The Bridge House/Recovery Home [44472]
The New England Center for Children [8146]
New England Center • Deafblind Project [2533]
New England Center for Headache, PC [12394]
New England Cord Blood Bank--Dallas [35236]
New England Cord Blood Bank--Houston [35237]
New England Cord Blood Bank Inc.--Newton, MA [35069]
New England Cord Blood Bank--Miami [35002]
New England Cryogenic Center, Inc. [35070]
New England Eye & Tissue Transplant Bank [35071]
New England Fertility Institute [21970]
New England Home Care--Cromwell [13522]
New England Home Care Inc.--Bridgeport [13541]
New England Home Care Inc.--New Haven [13534]
New England Home Care--Waterbury [13550]
New England Home Care--West Hartford [13556]
New England Learning Center for Women in Transition [9480]
New England Life Care--Concord [16171]
New England Life Care--Portland [15397]

New England Life Care--Woburn [15563]
New England Medical Center • Department of Speech Language Pathology and Audiology [2460]
New England Network • Runaway and Homeless Youth Program [36239]
New England Neurological Associates [8137]
New England Organ Bank • Tissue Banking Services [35072]
New England Orthopaedic Surgeons Sports Medical Center [38570]
New England Pediatric Care [8138]
New England Salem Children's Village [34295]
New England Sinai Hospital and Rehabilitation Center [8151]
New England Speech Services--Biddeford [2351]
New England Speech Services--Dover [2879]
New England Therapy Options [2886]
New England Village [8140]
New Era Health Center [41796]
New Era Home Care [14838]
New Era Rehabilitation Center Inc [41443]
    NERC [41366]
New Field High School [3118]
New Focus Program • Buddies of New Jersey [46009]
New Found Life [40036]
New Foundation [33970], [39469]
New Foundations Children and Family Services, Inc. [32187]
New Freedom Center [47556]
New Freedom Inc [43859]
New Generation Home Health Services [14270]
New Hampshire Department of Health and Human Services • Bureau of Maternal and Child Health • New Hampshire SIDS Program [36507]
New Hampshire Hospital [33651]
New Hampshire Kidney Center • Fresenius Medical Care [25387]
New Hampshire Orthopaedic Center [38707]
New Hampshire Palliative Care Services, LLC [20455]
New Hampshire SIDS Alliance [36508]
New Hampshire State Library • Talking Book Services [3821]
New Hanover Metro Treatment Center [47522]
New Hanover Regional Medical Center • Cancer Program [5663]
New Haven [49626]
New Haven Dialysis • DaVita [23167]
New Haven Home Dialysis • Fresenius Medical Care [23168]
New Haven Hospice Care, Inc. [18885]
New Haven Youth and Family Services [7831]
New Heritage Christian Worship Center • ATR Site [41968]
New Hope [40921]
New Hope/Attleboro [50983]
New Hope Behavioral Health Center [46019]
New Hope Behavioral Health Center Inc [39408], [39506]
A New Hope Center [9973]
New Hope Community Service Center [42564]
New Hope Cord Blood Bank [35003]
New Hope CORPS • Substance Abuse Treatment Program [41695]
New Hope Counseling Center [47274]
New Hope Dialysis • Fresenius Medical Care [25927]
New Hope Domestic Violence and Sexual Assault Services [10628]
New Hope Drug and Alcohol Treatment Prog Inc [40142]
New Hope Foundation Inc
    Open Door [46082]
    Outpatient [46000]
    Substance Abuse Services [46047]
New Hope Hospice--Eddington [19894]
New Hope Hospice-Laughlin • National Hospice Management, Inc. [20423]
New Hope Hospice--Marion [19628]
New Hope Hospice of Nevada [20410]
A New Hope, Inc. [18465]
New Hope, Inc. [9467]
New Hope of Mangum [47904]
    Chemical Dependency Unit [47951]
New Hope Manor Inc
    Residential [41415]
    Residential Drug Abuse Treatment Unit [46366]

New Hope Ranch [8727]
New Hope Recovery [40229]
New Hope Recovery Center [42565]
New Hope Recovery Center LLC [42684]
New Hope Services [7996]
New Hope--Taunton [51000]
New Hope Telephone Counseling Center [50673]
New Hope--Webster [51001]
New Hope for Women [9437]
New Horizon [29164]
New Horizon Advancement Center [40833]
New Horizon Counseling Center [31446]
New Horizon Counseling Services
    Outpatient [50175]
    Valley Branch of New Horizon Care Centers [50249]
New Horizon Family Center [10444]
New Horizon Family Health Services [7232]
New Horizon Home Health Care Inc. [13044]
New Horizon Recovery [45694]
New Horizon Treatment Services Inc [46191]
New Horizons [32201], [42165], [43736], [48126], [49625]
New Horizons--Alma [10686]
New Horizons • Child and Adolescent Substance AbuseProgram [42060]
New Horizons Community Mental Health Center, Inc. [29220]
New Horizons Community Mental Health Center
    NW 36th Street, Miami [29221]
    Substance Abuse Unit [41797]
New Horizons Community Service Board • Adaptive Group Residence [29391]
New Horizons Community Service Board--Columbus [29392]
New Horizons Community Service Board • Family Enrichment Services [29393]
New Horizons Community Service Board--Georgetown [29432]
New Horizons Community Service Board
    Harris County MH/SA Services [29437]
    Springlake Intensive Day Treatment [29394]
    Substance Abuse/ Adult Day Services [29401]
New Horizons Counseling [42274], [43630], [43705]
New Horizons Counseling Center • Eating Disorders Program [11135]
New Horizons Counseling Service Inc [39443]
New Horizons Crisis Center--Richfield [10531]
New Horizons Health Services Inc [44206]
New Horizons, Inc. [34445]
New Horizons--Middletown [8997]
New Horizons NCS [49646]
New Horizons North • Community Support Services [32948]
New Horizons Rehabilitation [7979]
New Horizons Residential Treatment Facility [34498]
New Horizons--Rockingham [10076]
New Horizons Substance Abuse • Counseling Agency [42847]
New Horizons of the Treasure Coast • Fact Florida Assertive Community Treatment [29165]
New Horizons of the Treasure Coast--Fort Pierce [29166]
New Horizons of the Treasure Coast Inc [41941]
    Detox [41674]
New Horizons of the Treasure Coast, Inc. [50759]
New Horizons of the Treasure Coast • Martin County Outpatient Program [29293]
New Horizons of the Treasure Coast--Okeechobee [29247]
New Horizons of the Treasure Coast • Saint Lucie County Outpatient Center [29167]
New Horizons of the Treasure Coast--Vero Beach [29315]
New Horizons Treatment Center [42147]
New Horizons Youth Service Bureau • Runaway and Homeless Youth Program [35975]
New House Inc • Residential Programs [40527]
New House Inc/Women With Children • Under 12 Years and Pregnant Women [40528]
New Hyde Park Dialysis Center [25710]
New Iberia • Behavioral Health Clinic [43866]
New Iberia Mental Health Center [30162]
New Insights DWI Services /Counseling Center [47396], [47471]
New Insights Inc
    Lemoyne [48448]
    York [48712]

New Insights Programs [39890]
New Jersey Center for Orthopaedics and Sports Medicine [38712]
New Jersey Center for Pain Management [35563]
New Jersey Cord Blood Bank • Ellie Katz Umbilical Cord Blood Program [35122]
New Jersey Department of Health and Senior Services • Primary and Preventive Health Services [36509]
New Jersey Medical School • Division of Infectious Diseases • AIDS Clinical Trials Unit [16]
New Jersey Neuroscience Institute at JFK Medical Center • Center for Sleep Disorders Treatment, Research, and Education [37351]
New Jersey Orthopedics & Sports Medicine, LLC [38754]
New Jersey Pediatric Feeding Associates LLC [2906]
New Jersey SIDS Alliance [36510]
New Jersey Speech Consultants [2918]
New Jersey Sports Medicine and Performance Center [38726]
New Jersey State Library Talking Book and Braille Center [3822]
A New Journey Eating Disorder Center [10976]
New Journeys in Recovery [48541]
New Leaders in Fertility and Endocrinology [21999]
New Leaf [42864]
New Leaf Autumn House [8698]
New Leaf Center Inc [42009]
New Leaf Counseling Services [39619], [39620] Residential [39621]
A New Leaf--E University Drive, Mesa [28163]
A New Leaf • Jag Center [28152]
New Leaf Residential [39622]
New Leaf Retreat for Women [29665]
A New Leaf Substance Abuse Service [45013]
New Leaf Treatment Center [39967]
A New Leaf--Wickenburg [28225]
New Life • Addiction Counseling Services Inc [44323]
New Life Center for Change/Teen University • Runaway and Homeless Youth Program [35782]
New Life Center Commission on Alcohol and Other Drug Abuse Services [48953]
New Life Center--Goodyear [8689]
New Life Centers [11291]
New Life Community Services Inc [40747]
New Life Connections Inc [41869], [41924]
New Life Generation Inc. [35038]
New Life Home Health Agency [14096]
New Life Home Health Care Agency [17348]
New Life Hospice Center of St. Joseph [20857]
New Life Hospice--Elyria [20839]
New Life Outpatient Center Inc [43258]
New Life Recovery Center [46214]
New Life Recovery Centers Inc [40662]
New Life Shelter--Litchfield Park [8697]
New Life Treatment Center [43063], [45358]
New Life for Women Inc [45395]
New Light Consultants Inc [44922]
New Light Recovery Center Inc [44753]
New Lisbon Developmental Center [8262]
New Lite Counseling Center Inc [49387]
New London Dialysis • DaVita [23171]
New Madrid Family Clinic [6912]
New Martinsville Dialysis Facility [27685]
A New Me, Speech Language Pathology [3019]
New Memories Inc [41210]
New Mexico Artificial Kidney Center • Fresenius Medical Care [25535]
New Mexico Library for the Blind and Physically Handicapped [3823]
New Mexico Lions Eye Bank/Lions Eyebank of District 2T1 [35124]
New Mexico Rehabilitation Center • Chemical Dependency Unit [46300]
New Mexico Rehabilitation La Residencia [2967]
New Mexico School for the Blind and Visually Impaired [3722], [3723]
New Mexico School for the Deaf [564]
New Mexico State University • Edgar R. Garrett Speech and Hearing Center [2966]
New Mexico Treatment Services LLC [46262], [46304]
New Mexico VA Health Care System [4304], [16303]
New Mexico Veterans Affairs Health Care System [51606]

Spinal Care Center [4305]
New Mexico Veterans Health Care System • Artesia Clinic [31186]
New Milford Hospital • Cancer Center [4904]
New Milford Supervised Apartment Program [29026]
New Milford Visiting Nurse Association Hospice [19154]
New Millennium Sports Medicine and Wellness [39159]
New Moon Lodge [46293]
New Morning Youth and Family Services [40393] Runaway and Homeless Youth Program [35832]
New Opportunities Inc • Substance Abuse/Prevention Services [43238], [43241], [43275], [43283], [43300]
New Options • Richard M Burns [43080]
New Options of Royal Palm Beach Inc [41990]
New Orleans Adolescent Hospital [33544]
New Orleans Family Justice Center [9420]
New Orleans Kidney Center [24558]
New Orleans Mental Health Center [30165]
New Orleans Speech and Hearing Center [2333]
New Orleans Veterans Resource Center [51969]
New Paradigm Counseling LLC [41037]
New Paths Inc [44788]
New Pathway Counseling [46114], [46134]
New Pathway Counseling Services Inc [45930]
New Pathways Halfway House [47948]
New Perspective at • White Deer Run [48443]
A New Perspective Counseling Centers [41178], [41269], [41352]
New Perspectives • Behavioral Health Systems LLC [45271]
New Philadelphia Veterans Affairs Clinic [31819]
New Port Richey Kidney Center • DaVita [23489]
New Realities Eating Disorders Recovery Centre-- Salt Lake City [11225]
New Realities Eating Disorders Recovery Centre-- Toronto, Ontario [11226]
New Resource Institute • DBA Clear Path Counseling Center [39728]
New River Behavioral Health Care • Sparta [31593]
New River Behavioral Health • Elkin Outpatient Office [31530]
New River Behavioral Healthcare [47406], [47429], [47433], [47501]
    Ashe County Outpatient Services [47399]
    Avery Cares Center [47434]
    Avery Outpatient Center [31572]
    Family Solutions [47226]
New River Behavioral Healthcare/Serenity Farms [31507]
New River Behavioral Healthcare
    Substance Abuse Services [47227]
    Wilkes County [47437]
    Willow Place [31609]
New River Community College • Center for the Deaf and Hard of Hearing [849]
New River Health Assoc., Inc. [7415]
New River Medical Center [37224]
New River Mental Health Program [31508]
New River Treatment Center [49793]
New River Valley Community Services • ACCESS Services [51414]
New River Valley Community Services--Blacksburg [32714]
New River Valley Community Services--Floyd [32734]
New River Valley Community Services
    New Life Recovery Center [49822]
    Pulaski Center [49821]
A New Safehaven [50008]
New Smyrna Beach Artificial Kidney Center • KRU Medical Ventures [23428]
New Smyrna Beach Dialysis • DaVita • Dialysis Facility [23429]
New Spirit II Inc • Outpatient Chemical Dep Program [46724]
A New Spirit Recovery Program Inc [49942]
A New Start [41257]
New Start Center [9423]
New Start Drug Treatment Center [42030]
New Start Home Health Care, Inc. [13212]
New Start Home Medical Equipment, Inc. [13213]
New Start Peer Support Center [32379]
New Start Program Meriter Hospital
    Addiction Med Consult and Eval Service [50449]
    New Start Outpatient Services [50450]

New Start Treatment LLC [42166]
New Traditions [50119]
New Ulm Medical Center [15922]
    Substance Abuse Services [45249]
New Vision at Jackson Hospital [41758]
NEW Visions [28886]
New Visions Center • Inpatient Program [45071]
New Visions Center of Morris [45243]
New Visions Center • Outpatient Program [45072]
New Visions Chemical Dependency Prog • Conemaugh Memorial Medical Center [48418]
New Visions Counseling Services Inc [42632]
New Visions Home Health Care [14815]
New Visions Home Health Care, Inc. [14816]
New Visions Program [47523]
New Visions Substance Abuse Counseling [43036]
New Visions Unlimited Inc [47777]
New Vistas [28755]
New Way Clinic Inc [44231]
New Way Counseling Center [44870]
New Way Foundation [39668]
    Aware Program [39669]
New Way of Life Counseling [43737]
New Way of Life Inc [42448]
New Wellness Associates [50403]
New West Sports Medicine [38688]
New York AKC, Inc. • Dialysis Center [25626]
New York Asian Women's Center [9953]
New York Blood Center • National Cord Blood Program [35137]
New York Catholic Deaf Center [3066]
New York Center for Learning and Child Development [2984]
New York Center for Living Inc • Outpatient Youth [46893]
New York City Gay and Lesbian Anti-Violence Project [9954]
New York Couseling for Change LCS PLLC [46719]
New York Cryo [35138]
New York Downtown Hospital • Hemodialysis Unit [25729]
New York Eye and Ear Infirmary [3067]
New York Firefighter's Skin Bank [35139]
New York Foundling Hospital • Pathways [46894]
New York Harbor Healthcare System • Brooklyn Campus SATP [46519]
New York Headache Center--New York [12454]
New York Headache Center--White Plains [12455]
New York Health Care--Hempstead [16480]
New York Health Care, Inc.--McDonald Ave., Brooklyn [16403]
New York Health Care--Jay St., Brooklyn [16404]
New York Health Care--Mount Vernon [16531]
New York Health Care--Newburgh [16574]
New York Health Care--Spring Valley [16631]
New York Home Health Care Equipment [16663]
New York Hospital Medical Center of Queens • The Cancer Center [5577]
The New York Hospital Medical Center of Queens • Hemodialysis Unit [25666]
New York Hospital • Weill Cornell Medical Center • William Randolph Hearst Burn Center [4593]
New York Institute for Special Education [3725] Readiness Program [8300]
New York Legal Assistance Group [9955]
New York Medical College
    Mental Retardation Institute • Down Syndrome Interdisciplinary Clinic [10833]
    Westchester Medical Center • Adult Cystic Fibrosis Center [7617]
New York Medical College/Westchester Medical Center • Children's Hospital • Pediatric Cystic Fibrosis Center [7618]
New York Methodist Hospital
    Cancer Program [5567]
    Center for Sleep Disorders Medicine and Research [37402]
    Fertility Institute [22188]
    Sickle Cell Center [36397]
New York Organ Donor Network [35140]
New York Presbyterian Hospital, Columbia Campus • Pain Management [35580]
New York-Presbyterian Hospital/Columbia University Medical Center • Herbert Irving Comprehensive Cancer Center [5597]
New York Presbyterian Hospital, Cornell Campus • Pain Management [35581]
New York Presbyterian Hospital-Cornell University

Weill Medical College • Department of Pediatrics • Division of Human Genetics [12292]
The New York Presbyterian Hospital • Division of Clinical Genetics [12293]
New York and Presbyterian Hospital Inc • Westchester Div/Alc Inpt Rehab Program [47186]
New York-Presbyterian Hospital • Sleep Disorders Center [37403]
New York Presbyterian Hospital • Weill-Cornell Medical Center [5598]
New York Presbyterian Medical Center [3068]
New York-Presbyterian Weill Cornell Medical Center • Hemodialysis Unit [25730]
New York Psychiatric Institute [33707]
New York Public Library • Andrew Heiskell Braille and Talking Book Library [3825]
New York Renal Associates • Dialysis Facility [25595]
New York School for the Deaf [608]
New York Service Network Inc • Outpatient Chemical Dependency Clinic [46520]
New York Sleep Disorder Center [37404]
New York Sleep Institute [37405]
New York Sleep Wake Institute [37406]
New York Speech Consultants [3091]
New York Speech and Hearing--Maspeth [3049]
New York Speech and Hearing--New York [3069]
New York Speech and Voice Connection [3070]
New York State Center for SIDS • Western Satellite Office [36518]
New York State Center for Sudden Infant Death • NYC--Satellite Office/MHRA [36519]
New York State Center for Sudden Infant Death Syndrome [36520]
    Central New York Satellite Office [36521]
    Western Satellite Office [36522]
New York State Department of Health • Division of Family Health [36523]
New York State Health Department • Division of Family Health • Child Morbidity and Mortality Prevention Program [36524]
New York State Institute for Basic Research in Developmental Disabilities • Department of Human Genetics [12294]
New York State Psychiatric Institute
    Eating Disorders Clinic [11162]
    Washington Heights Community Service [33708]
New York State School for the Blind [3726]
New York State School for the Deaf [600]
New York State Talking Book and Braille Library [3826]
New York Therapeutic Communities Inc • NYC DOP/CD Outpatient Clinic [46521]
New York University • Fertility Center [22189]
New York University Hospital for Joint Diseases • Multiple Sclerosis Comprehensive Care Center [34650]
New York University Hospital for Joint Diseases Orthopedic Institute [4314]
New York University Langone Medical Center • Dialysis Unit [25731]
New York University Medical Center
    Bellevue Hospital Center • Adult AIDS Clinical Trials Unit [21]
    Department of Pediatrics • Human Genetics Program [12295]
    Howard A. Rusk Institute of Rehabilitation Medicine • Speech-Language Pathology Department [3071]
    Institute of Rehabilitation Medicine • MDA Clinic [34839]
    School of Medicine
        Centers for AIDS Research [62]
        Pain Management [35582]
New York University • School of Medicine • Sleep Medicine Associates of NYC, LLC [37407]
The New You Center Inc [40143]
Newark Beth Israel Medical Center [31156]
Newark Beth Israel Medical Center/Children's Hospital of New Jersey • Valerie Fund Children's Center • Sickle Cell Disease Center [36381]
Newark Beth Israel Medical Center
    Comprehensive Hemophilia Treatment Center [12557]
    Dialysis Unit [25485]
    Flo Okin Oncology Center • Valerie Fund Children's Center [5528]
Newark Beth Israel Medical Center--Primary Screen-

ing Center • Essex County [51115]
Newark Beth Israel Medical Center • Sleep Disorders Center [37352]
Newark Community Health Centers, Inc. [6979]
Newark Dialysis Center • DaVita [25486]
Newark Renaissance House Inc [46099]
Newberg Dialysis Center • Fresenius Medical Care [26333]
Newberry Hospice [21012]
Newberry Mental Health Center [32209]
Newbridge Services [8267]
NewBridge Services, Inc.--Boonton [31105]
NewBridge Services, Inc.--Montville [31147]
    Adult and Family Services [31148]
NewBridge Services, Inc.--Pompton Lakes • Adult and Family Services [31163]
NewBridge Services, Inc.--Pompton Plains [31164]
NewBridge Services, Inc.--Wayne • Visions [31171]
NewBridge Services, Inc.--West Milford • Adult and Family Services [31173]
Newday Youth and Family Services • Safe Home • Runaway and Homeless Youth Program [36086]
Newfoundland Eating Disorder Treatment [11170]
Newfoundland School for the Deaf [610]
Newhouse [9690]
Newlife Family Services • Christian Counseling Center [49962]
Newman Counseling Alternatives PA • Outpatient Services [41615]
Newman Regional Health [2216]
    Sleep Disorders Center [36998]
Newnan Dialysis Services • Renal Advantage Inc [23767]
NewPoint Behavioral Healthcare [31178]
    Emergency Screening Services [31179]
Newport Audiology Centers [970]
Newport Bay Hospital [33168]
Newport Beach Dialysis • Renal Research Institute [22838]
Newport County • Community Mental Health Center [48856]
Newport County Community Mental Health Center
    Case Management [32156]
    Child and Adolescent Services [32157]
    Day Treatment [32158]
Newport County Community Mental Health Center Main Office [32159]
Newport Dialysis Center [22564]
Newport Hospital
    Cancer Program [5887]
    Sleep Disorders Center of Lifespan Hospitals [37726]
Newport Integrated Behavioral Healthcare [29408]
Newport Intergrated Behav Hlthcare Inc [42080]
Newport Language Speech Center--Fountain Valley [1111]
Newport Language Speech Center--Mission Viejo [1182]
Newport Language Speech Center--Yorba Linda [1370]
Newport Language Speech Centers--Cerritos [1080]
Newport Mesa Dialysis Services • Avantis Renal Therapy [22648]
Newport Richey Hospice House [19270]
Newton Center • GRN Community Services Board [29398]
Newton Dialysis Center • DaVita [24340]
Newton Dialysis • DaVita [24291]
Newton Medical [2231]
Newton Medical Center Home Health [14512]
Newton Memorial Hospital
    Cancer Program [5532]
    Center for Mental Health [46103]
Newton--Wellesley Eating Disorders and Behavioral Medicine [11094]
Newton Wellesley Hospital • Multiple Sclerosis Clinic [34599]
Newton-Wellesley Hospital • Vernon Cancer Center [5347]
Newton Youth and Family Services [29028]
NewTown Dialysis Center • DaVita [26494]
Newtown Dialysis Center Inc. [25572]
Next Door Inc [49159]
    Knoxville [49113]
Next Door, Solutions to Domestic Violence [8893]
Next Level HealthCare Outreach [14747]
Next Step • Adolescent Residential [45325]
The Next Step--Ellsworth • Domestic Violence

Project [9431]
Next Step Foundation [48457]
The Next Step Inc [46336]
The Next Step--Machias [9432]
Nextron, Inc. [16215]
Nexus Adolescent Chemical Health [42831]
Nexus Home Healthcare Holdings, LLC [15691]
Nexus Pain Care [35743]
Nexus Recovery Center Inc
    Nexus Outreach Center [49290]
    Nexus Residential Facility [49291]
Nez Perce County Court Services [42341], [42342]
Nez Perce Tribal Victims Advocate Project [9177]
NH Div Alcohol/Drug Abuse Prevention and Recovery Tirrell Halfway House [45910]
NHC HealthCare [2806]
NHC of Rossville [1898]
NHR Regional Rehab at 19th St. NW [3948]
NHR Regional Rehab at K St., NW [3949]
NHRB Regional Rehab • Good Samaritan Hospital Rehabilitation Services [4102]
NHS Human Services • Delaware County [48640]
NHS Montgomery County [48438]
Nia Children and Family Services [47531]
Niagara County Mental Health Hotline and Crisis Intervention [51147]
Niagara Falls Memorial Medical Center Renal Center [25742]
Niagara Falls Outpatient Clinic [31437]
Niagara Falls Veterans Affairs Clinic [31438]
Niagara Renal Center • Apollo Healthcare [25743]
Niagara Sleep Center [37408]
NICASA Bridgehouse [42951]
NICASA NFP [42703]
Nicasas Judy H Fried Center [42817]
Nicol Group Home [34005]
Nieves M. Flores Memorial Library • Guam Public Library for the Blind and Physically Handicapped [3782]
The Night Ministry • Runaway and Homeless Youth Program [35935]
Nightingale Home Care, Inc. [13299]
Nightingale Home Health Agency Inc. [13250]
Nightingale Home Health Care of Miami--Miami [14097]
Nightingale Home Health Care of Miami--Miami Springs [14227]
NIH/NIDA • Archway [44164]
Nikkari Elementary School [503]
Niles Home for Children [45520]
Niles Home for Children, Inc. [34268]
Nilsson House [44165]
Nirvana Drug and Alcohol Institute [40230]
    Outpatient [40231]
    Women of Hope [40232]
Nisqually Indian Tribe • Substance Abuse and Prevention Program [50039]
Niwot Center for Integrative Therapies [1432]
Nix Home Care [18148]
NJ Department of Veteran Affairs [46040]
NM Department of Health • Turquoise Lodge Hospital [46237]
NMFLAG [9856]
NMHU Wellness Program [38773]
NNA Kidney Dialysis Center--Sarasota • Fresenius Medical Care [23510]
No to Abuse--Pahrump [9797]
No Other Place Like Home [13649], [13873]
No To Abuse--Tonopah [9801]
No Turning Back [44166]
NOA--No-One Alone • Noa's Ark [9103]
Noah Project, Inc.--Abilene [10436]
Noah Project, Inc. - North [10470]
Noah's Anchorages YMCA • Runaway and Homeless Youth Program [35833]
Noble Behavioral Health Choices Inc [47631]
Noble Counseling Center [31672]
Noble County Office • Otis R Bowen Cntr for Human Services Inc [42977]
Noble Hospital • Cancer Program [5359]
Noble House, Inc. [9261]
Noble Visiting Nurse and Hospice Services [20011]
Noble Visiting Nurse and Hospice Services, Inc. [15560]
Noblesville Outpatient Office • Aspire IN Inc [43170]
Nocturna Sleep Center of Tulsa [37603]
Nolachuckey-Holston Area Mental Health Center [32316]

Nondalton Suicide Prevention [50640]
Nonviolent Alternatives Counseling [43074]
Noran Clinic Sleep Center [37225]
Noran Neurological Clinic • Minnesota Headache
  Center [12437]
Norbert Sander, Jr., MD [38777]
Norco Dialysis Center • DaVita [22839]
Norcon Family Counseling Services [45556]
Norcross Mental Health Clinic • GRN Community
  Services Board [29483]
Nord Center • Addiction Services [47795]
The Nord Center • Elyria Counseling Office [31762]
Nord Community Mental Health Center [31794]
  Group Home [31795]
Norfolk Community Health Care Clinic [6942]
Norfolk Community Services Board [32769]
  Substance Abuse Services [49817]
Norfolk County Speech Services [2511]
Norfolk Dialysis Center • DaVita [27528]
Norfolk Regional Center [33646]
Norfolk Speech and Language Services [3601]
Norfolk Veterans Affairs Clinic [31004]
Norland Medical Center [6508]
Norman Public Schools [669]
Norman Regional Hospital [17139]
  Oncology Services [5775]
Norman Westlund Child Guidance Clinic [30628]
Normandy Village Dialysis Center • American Renal
  Associates [23350]
Norris Adolescent Center [34490]
Norristown Sports Medicine Center [38963]
Norristown State Hospital [33813]
North Adams Regional Hospital
  Cancer Program [5348]
  Greylock Pavilion [44526]
North Alabama Audiology, Inc. • Decatur Hearing Aid
  Center [907]
North Alabama Regional Hospital [33081]
North Alabama Sleep Disorders Center, LLC [36593]
North Albuquerque Dialysis Center • Fresenius
  Medical Care [25536]
North American Family Institute, Inc.--Danvers
  Emergency Placement Intervention Center
  [34186]
  Massachusetts [34187]
North American Family Institute, Inc.--Peabody
  [34208]
North American Family Institute--Winooski [34463]
North Andover Renal Center • Diversified Specialty
  Institutes [24785]
North Arkansas Regional Medical Center [1015]
North Atlantic Vet Center [51934]
North Aurora Family Health Services [6385]
North Austin Medical Center • Cancer Care Program
  [5961]
North Austin Medical Center Transplant [26957]
North Avenue Dialysis Center • Fresenius Medical
  Care [24040]
The North Baltimore Center • Booker T. Middle
  School [30264]
The North Baltimore Center, Inc. [30265]
North Bay Hospice and Bereavement [18924]
North Bay Sleep Medicine Institute, Inc. • Sleep
  Disorders Center [36676]
North Beach Dialysis Center [23408]
North Benton County Health Care, Inc. • Benton
  Medical Center [6876]
North Boulder Physical Therapy Sports Rehabilita-
  tion, LLC [38165]
North Broward Medical Center • Cancer Center
  [4939]
North Buckner Dialysis Center • Fresenius Medical
  Care [27034]
North Care Adult Services [31902]
North Care Center [31903]
  Program of Assertive Community Treatment
  [47989]
North Carolina Baptist Hospital [4334]
North Carolina Behavioral Health [47462]
North Carolina Department of Health and Human
  Services • Division of Public Health and Human
  Services • North Carolina Sudden Infant Death
  Syndrome Program [36527]
North Carolina Department of Public Instruction •
  North Carolina Project for Children and Young
  Adults Who are Deafblind • Exceptional Children
  Division [3190]
North Carolina Division of Services for the Deaf and

Hard of Hearing • Wilson Regional Center for the
  Deaf and the Hard of Hearing [3198]
The North Carolina Eye Bank • Vision Share
  [35148]
North Carolina Eye and Human Tissue Bank, Inc.,
  Durham • Vision Share [35149]
North Carolina Farmworker Health Program [7056]
North Carolina Healthy Start Foundation • ITS-SIDS
  Project [36528]
North Carolina Pain Management Services [35593]
North Carolina School for the Deaf [626]
North Carolina Services for the Deaf and Hard of
  Hearing • Morgantown Regional Center [627]
North Carolina Solutions [47524]
North Central Alabama Early Childhood Services •
  Centers for the Developmentally Disabled [7710]
North Central Alcohol and • Drug Counseling Inc/
  Ord [45807]
North Central Behavioral Health System [42735],
  [42837], [42872], [42929]
    at Fulton and McDonough Counties [42435],
    [42756]
North Central Behavioral Health Systems
  La Salle Office [29636]
  Princeton Area Office [29668]
North Central Community Mental Health [51010]
  Grayling Office [30560]
  Houghton Lake Office [30570]
North Central Counseling Associates [31769]
North Central Counseling Services [50726]
North Central Health Care [33950]
North Central Health Center [44754]
North Central Healthcare Facilities [50556]
North Central Hospice/Visiting Nurse and Health
  Services of Connecticut Inc. [19171]
North Central Human Service Center • Chemical
  Dependency Program [47593]
North Central Human Service
  Newtown Outreach Center [31637]
  Rugby Outreach Center [31638]
  Stanley Outreach Center [31639]
North Central Human Services [44477]
North Central Human Services--Gardner [30388]
North Central Indiana Rural Crisis Center, Inc.
  [9304]
North Central Kidney Disease Center • Dialysis
  Facility • Fresenius Medical Care [27337]
North Central Mental Health Services--Columbus
  [31736]
North Central Mental Health Services
  Drug and Alcohol Treatment Program [47725]
  Family Focus [31737]
  Fowler House [31738]
  Norwich House [31739]
  Soaring Sober [31740]
North Central Missouri Mental Health Center--
  Brookfiled [30833]
North Central Missouri Mental Health Center--
  Chillicothe [30840]
North Central Missouri Mental Health Center--
  Hamilton [30849]
North Central Missouri Mental Health Center--Milan
  [30877]
North Central Missouri Mental Health Center--
  Trenton [30910]
North Central Missouri Mental Health Center--
  Unionville [30911]
North Central Pennsylvania Dialysis Clinics • Lock
  Haven Dialysis Clinic [26472]
North Central Quad County Task Force Against
  Domestic Violence [9784]
North Central Texas Community Health Care Center
  [7317]
North Central University • Carlstrom Deaf Studies
  [513]
North Central Washington Regional Support Network
  [51439]
North Central Washington Respiratory Care [18485]
North Charles Institute • For the Addictions [44565]
North Charleston Dialysis • DaVita [26691]
North Charlotte Dialysis Center • DaVita [25841]
North Chester Clinic • Adult Outpatient [28394]
North Chicago VA Medical Center [14882], [19548]
North Chicago Veterans Affairs Medical Center
  [4027], [29654]
North Coast Behavioral Healthcare System • West
  Campus [33759]
North Coast Kidney Center • Fresenius Medical

Care [22853]
North Coast Subst Abuse Council Inc • Crossroads
  [39825]
North Coastal Mental Health Center [28685]
North Collier Sleep Diagnostic Center [36798]
North Colorado Behavioral Health of • Fort Collins
  [41179]
North Colorado Medical Center [1419]
  Cancer Care Program [4882]
  Western States Burn Center [4528]
North Colorado Sportsmedicine [38174]
North Colorado Springs Dialysis • Davita [23102]
North Community Counseling Centers Inc • The
  Bridge [47726]
North Cottage Program Inc • Halfway House
  [44531]
North Country Center for Independence [8343]
North Country Community Health Center
  Ash Fork Clinic [6223]
  Flagstaff [6230]
  Kingman Clinic [6235]
  Round Valley Clinic [6249]
North Country Community Mental Health [30619]
  Petoskey Club [30620]
North Country Counseling Services PC [44949]
North Country Dialysis Unit • Fletcher Allen Health-
  care [27442]
North Country Freedom Homes
  The Canton House [46578]
  John E Murphy Community Residence [46768]
  Supportive Living Facility [46579]
North Country Home Health and Hospice Agency
  [20441]
North Country HomeCare & Hospice [20145]
North Country Orthopaedic Group Sports Medicine
  Center [38825]
North Country Sports Medicine [38814]
North County Audiology [1264]
North County Family Resource Center [32805]
North County Health Services [6360]
North County Healthcare Center [6548]
North County Hospice • St. Joseph Health System-
  Synoma County [18939]
North County Hospital • Northern Vermont Center
  for Pulmonary/Sleep Medicine [37878]
North County Learning [7777]
North County Mental Health Center [28467]
North County Pain Clinic [35555]
North County Serenity House Inc
  Alcohol and Drug Residential Service [39813]
  Serenity Too [39814]
North County Women's Resource Center/Shelter
  [8868]
North Crest Hospice [21367]
North Crown Heights Family Outreach • CD
  Outpatient [46522]
North Cypress Medical Center • Sleep Center
  [37827]
North Dakota Center for Sleep [37499]
North Dakota Department of Health • Maternal and
  Child Health Division • North Dakota SIDS
  Management Program [36529]
North Dakota School for the Deaf [640]
North Dakota Southeast Human Service Center
  [51189]
North Dakota State Hospital [33748]
  Chemical Dependency Services [47587]
North Dakota State Library • Talking Book Services
  [3828]
North Dakota Vision Services
  School for the Blind [3728]
  School for the Deaf • North Dakota Dual
  Sensory Project [3202]
North Dallas Drug Rehabilitation Center [49261]
North East Counseling Services LLC [45998]
North East Medical Services [6354]
North East Texas Dialysis Center • Diversified
  Specialty Institutes [27115]
North East Treatment Centers • Kirkwood Detoxifica-
  tion Center [41521]
North End Community Health Committee, Inc. •
  North End Community Health Center [6806]
North Essex Mental Health Center • Crisis Service
  and Central Intake [50990]
North Evansville Dialysis • DaVita [24139]
North Florida Center for Speech and Hearing [1587]
North Florida Regional Medical Center
  Cancer Center [4944]

Sleep Disorders Center [36799]
North Florida/South Georgia Veterans Health System [13711]
  Gainesville Division • Malcolm Randall VAMC [51552]
  Lake City Division [51553]
  Lake City Veterans Affairs Medical Center [3988]
  Malcolm Randall Veterans Affairs Medical Center [3989]
North Fork Valley Community Health Center [6730]
North Fresno Dialysis • Fresenius Medical Care [22698]
North Fulton Dialysis • DaVita [23779]
North Fulton Outpatient Rehabilitation [1902]
North Fulton Treatment Center • The Renaissance Recovery Group Inc [42150]
North Georgia Mountain Crisis Network, Inc. [9092]
North Glendale Dialysis • DaVita [22710]
North Granville Dialysis Clinic • Renal Advantage Inc. [24210]
North Gwinnett Dialysis • Fresenius Medical Care [23803]
North Haven Community Services [29029]
North Haven Dialysis Center • Hospital of St. Raphael [23174]
North Hawaii Community Hospital [14636]
  Sleep Disorders Center [36870]
North Hawaii Dialysis • Liberty Dialysis [23854]
North Hawaii Hospice, Inc. [19443]
North Henry Dialysis • DaVita [23797]
North Hills Dialysis [22538]
  DaVita [27273]
North Hills Medical Center • Sleep Disorders Center [37736]
North Hills Orthopedic and Sports Physical Therapy [38983]
North Hollywood Dialysis • DaVita [22841]
North Houston Center for Reproductive Medicine [22264]
North Houston Dialysis Center • DaVita [27161]
North Hudson Community Action Center • Mental Health and Addictive Services [46215]
North Hudson Community Action Corporation Health Center [6981]
North Hudson Community Action Corp. • North Hudson Community Action Corp. Health Center [6988]
North Idaho Physical Therapy and Medical Exercise--Coeur d'Alene [38340]
North Idaho Physical Therapy and Medical Exercise--Hayden [38342]
North Idaho Physical Therapy and Medical Exercise--Post Falls [38344]
North Iowa Crisis Center [50907]
North Iowa Mercy Dialysis Center--Algona [24248]
North Iowa Mercy Dialysis Center--Charles City [24256]
North Islands Counseling and Psychotherapy • Crisis Service [51442]
North Jersey Community Research Initiative • Community Program for Clinical Research on AIDS [57]
North Jersey Developmental Center [8274]
North Kansas City Hospital [16032]
  Cancer Center [5455]
  Sleep Disorders Center [37277]
North Kent Guidance Services LLC [44811], [44829]
North Key Community Care
  Campbell County Substance Abuse Srvs [43730]
  Carroll County Out Patient Center [43554]
  Employment Rehabilitation Program [29996]
  Gallatin County Substance Abuse Services [43794]
North Key Community Care of Owen County [43743]
North Key Community Care • Pendleton County Substance Abuse Services [43586]
North Knoxville Dialysis Center • Fresenius Medical Care [26863]
North Las Vegas Awareness School and • Treatment Center [45861]
North Las Vegas Dialysis Center • DaVita [25379]
North Las Vegas Family Health Center [6954]
North Manatee Health Center [6533]
North Melbourne Dialysis Inc. [23385]
North Memorial Health Care • Hubert H. Humphrey Cancer Center [5414]
North Memorial Healthcare [2727]
North Memorial Home Health & Hospice [15929]
North Memorial Sleep Health Center [37226]

North Memorial Speech Pathology [2705]
North Merced Dialysis Center • DaVita [22806]
North Metro Denver Dialysis • DaVita [23145]
North Metro Medical Center [12859]
  Rebsamen Medical Center [36648]
North Mississippi Hospice of Oxford [20256]
North Mississippi Hospice of Oxford/Southaven [20262]
North Mississippi Medical Center [30815]
  Behavioral Health Center [45421]
  Cancer Program [5434]
  Home Health Agency--Amory Branch [15950]
  Home Health Agency--Eupora Branch [15958]
  Home Health Agency--Fulton Branch [15960]
  Home Health Agency--Pontotoc Branch [15975]
  Home Health Agency--Ripley Branch [15979]
North Mississippi Medical Center Hospice [20269]
North Mississippi Medical Center, Inc. [15980]
North Mississippi Medical Center • Sleep Disorders Center [37254]
North Mississippi Regional Center [8191]
North Mississippi State Hospital [33626]
North Naples Dialysis LLC [23424]
North Oakland Counseling Associates [44701]
North Oakland Kidney Center • DaVita • Dialysis Facility [24958]
North Oakland Medical Center [2635]
North Oaks Medical Center [15298]
  Sleep Disorders Center [37070]
North Oaks Podiatry [38317]
North Oaks Sports Medicine/Rehabilitation Services • North Oaks Health System [38492]
North Okaloosa Dialysis Center • DaVita [23275]
North Okaloosa Medical Center [13630]
North Ottawa Community Hospital - In Home Care [15672]
North Palm Beach Dialysis Center • DaVita [23461]
North Penn Visiting Nurse Association [17372]
North Philadelphia Health System • Miracles in Progress [48542]
North Philadelphia Health Systems • Eleven Tower Dual Diagnosis [48543]
North Platte Veterans Affairs Clinic [31007]
North Port Health Center [6517]
North Port Health Center--Dental [6564]
North Providence Dialysis Center • Diversified Specialty Institutes [26661]
North Puget Sound Center for Sleep Disorders [37919]
North Ranch, Marshall [30870]
North Range Behavioral Health [28913], [41171], [41183], [41216], [41217], [41218], [41219], [41220]
  ACT Program [33226]
  Acute Treatment Unit [33227]
  Adult Recovery Program [33228]
  Adult Services [28914]
  Children's Residential Treatment Center [33229]
  Monfort Children's and Clinic [33230]
  Outpatient Child and Family Services [33231]
  South County Clinic [33220]
  Stanek Center [34048]
North Rio Rancho Dialysis • Fresenius Medical Care [25557]
North Rockland Mental Health Clinic [31345]
North Saint Louis County Dialysis • DaVita [25206]
North Seminole Family and Sports Medicine [38283]
North Shepherd Kidney Clinic • Fresenius Medical Care [27162]
A North Shore Center for Eating Disorders [11163]
North Shore Center for Weight Management [11049]
North Shore Child/Fam Guidance Center • Chemical Dependency Outpatient Clinic [47180]
North Shore Fertility [22042]
North Shore Headache Clinic [12421]
North Shore Health Care Foundation [20165]
North Shore Horizons [9641]
North Shore-LIJ Glen Cove Hospital • Adolescent Services Unit [46654]
North Shore LIJ Health System • Mineola Community Treatment Center [46785]
North Shore Long Isl Jewish Health Sys • Elmont Treatment Center/Chemical Dep [46632]
North Shore-Long Island Jewish home Care Network [16664]
North Shore Long Island Jewish Health System
  North Shore University Hospital • Sleep Disorders Center [37409]

Schneider Children's Hospital
  Adult Cystic Fibrosis Center [7619]
  Pediatric Cystic Fibrosis Center [7620]
North Shore-Long Island Jewish Hospital System
  Adults and Children with Learning and Developmental Disabilities, Inc.
    ACLD Career and Community Service [8328]
    ACLD Hauppage [8320]
    ACLD Kramer Learning Center [8295]
    ACLD Linder Center [8297]
    ACLD Oasis/Bridges [8314]
North Shore Medical Center • Griffith Community Cancer Center [4967]
North Shore Medical Center, Inc. • Cancer Program [5354]
North Shore Regional Dialysis Center • Fresenius Medical Care [24742]
North Shore/Regional Health Center [6695]
North Shore Speech--Language Associates [3048]
North Shore Sports Medical Center [38549]
North Shore Univ Hospital at Glen Cove • Subst Abuse Treatment/Womens/Childrens Prog [46655]
North Shore University Health System • Doreen E Chapman Center [42663]
North Shore University Hospital
  Drug Treatment and Education Center/ Outpatient [46771]
  Drug Treatment Education Center/Outpatient Detox [46772]
  Genetic Counseling Center [12296]
North Shore University Hospital at Glen Cove Hospital • Don Monti Cancer Center [5579]
North Shore University Hospital • In Vitro Fertilization Program • Center for Human Reproduction [22190]
North Shore University Hospital--Manhasset TC [25699]
North Shore University Hospital • Monter Cancer Center [5592]
North Shore University Hospital--Plainview • Cancer Program [5606]
North Shore University Hospital • Walbaum Dialysis Center [25675]
North Shreveport Dialysis • Fresenius Medical Care [24584]
North Side Christian Health Center at Northview [7182]
North Side Medical Center • Cancer Program [5768]
North Slope Borough Community Mental Health Center [50629]
North Slope Borough • Integrated Behavioral Health Services [28078]
North Sound Evaluation and Treatment Facility [32861]
North Star Behavioral Health--Anchorage [28076]
North Star Behavioral Health--Palmer Residential Treatment Center [28114]
North Star Behavioral Health Services--Malone [31385]
North Star Behavioral Health Services--Saranac Lake [31469]
North Star Behavioral Health System [50627]
North Star Centre [29114]
North Star Dialysis Center • DaVita [27163]
North Star Hospice [20170]
North Star Hospice-International Falls [20172]
North Star Hospital [33106]
North Star Substance Abuse Services [31470]
North Suburban Dialysis Center • Fresenius Medical Care [24798]
North Suffolk Mental Health Association
  Boston Emergency Service Team [30344]
  Harbor Area Early Childhood Services [30345]
North Suffolk Mental Health Association, Inc.-- Chelsea [30360]
North Suffolk Mental Health Association--PACT [30356]
North Suffolk Mental Hlth Association • Meridian House [44452]
North Summit Clinic [31747]
North Texas Addiction
  Counseling and Education Inc [49339]
  Counseling Inc/Outpatient [49216]
North Texas Comprehensive Hemophilia Center • Pediatric Program [12600]
North Texas Healthcare System [49292]

North Texas Lung and Sleep Clinic--Fort Worth [37828]

North Texas Lung and Sleep Clinic--Southlake [37829]

North Texas Pain Recovery Clinic [35700]

North Texas Rehabilitation Center--Dallas [35701]

North Texas Rehabilitation Center--Fort Worth [35702]

North Texas Sleep Lab [37830]

North Texas State Hospital--Vernon Campus [33886]

North Texas State Hospital
　Vernon Campus/Adolescent Forensic Prog [49568]
　Wichita Falls Campus [33889]

North Texas Veterans Affairs Health Care System [17885]

North Texas Youth Connection • Runaway and Homeless Youth Services [36229]

North Valley Health Center [6990]

North Vernon Dialysis • DaVita [24219]

North West Essex Community • Healthcare Network [45933]

North West Physical Therapy and Spine Rehabilitation [39149]

North Woods Medical Cooperative • North Woods Community Health Center [7437]

Northampton County Crisis Intervention [51279]

Northampton VA Medical Center [15506]

Northampton Veterans Affair Medical Center [51585]

Northampton Veterans Affairs Med Center • Substance Abuse Treatment Program [44500]

Northampton Veterans Affairs Medical Center [30405]
　PTSD Clinical Team [51751]

NorthBay Center for Primary Care [38071]

NorthBay Healthcare Group [12998]

NorthBay Medical Center • Cancer Center [4773]

NorthCare Hospice & Palliative Care [20325]

Northcenter Dialysis • Fresenius Medical Care [23953]

Northcoast Behavioral Healthcare • Cleveland Campus [33753]

Northcoast Behavioral Healthcare System • Northfield Campus [33757]

Northeast Alabama Health Services [6188]

Northeast Alabama Health Services--North Sand Mountain [6182]

Northeast Alabama Health Services--Paint Rock Valley [6200]

Northeast Alabama Health Services--Scottsboro [6198]

Northeast Alabama Regional Medical Center
　Behavioral Health [27832]
　Cancer Program [4722]
　Sleep Disorders Center [36594]

Northeast Arkansas Council on Family Violence • Women's Crisis Center [8767]

Northeast Bakersfield Dialysis • DaVita [22596]

Northeast Cambridge Dialysis • DaVita • Dialysis Center [24758]

Northeast Career Planning [3050]

Northeast Communication Specialists [3339]

Northeast Community Center for Mental Health and Mental Retardation [32091]
　Adult Adjustment Center [32092]
　The Gathering Place [32093]

Northeast Community Center for MH/MR • Outpatient Addiction Recovery Program [48544]

Northeast Counseling Services [51288]

Northeast Counseling Services--E Broad Street, Nanticoke [32051]

Northeast Counseling Services--Hazleton [32026]

Northeast Counseling Services--W Washington Street, Nanticoke [32052]

Northeast Family Mental Health Services [28605]

Northeast Florida Dialysis Center • American Renal Associates [23442]

Northeast Florida State Hospital [33316]

Northeast Fort Worth Dialysis Center • Fresenius Medical Care [27116]

Northeast Georgia Council on Domestic Violence [9112]

Northeast Georgia Medical Center [14532]
　Cancer Program [5026]
　Sleep Disorders Center [36848]

Northeast Georgia RESA [381]

Northeast Georgia Sleep Medicine • Sleep Disorders Center [36849]

Northeast Georgia Speech Center Inc. [1865]

Northeast Guidance Center [8169]
　Adult Triage/Outpatient Services [44755]

Northeast Health Service [7039]

Northeast Health Systems • Beverly Hospital [34182]

Northeast Hearing Center [1747]

Northeast Hearing and Speech Center [2362]

Northeast Human Service Center [51190]
　Chemical Dependency Program [47583]

Northeast Human Service Center--Grafton [31629]

Northeast Human Service Center--Grand Forks [31631]

Northeast Independent School District [818]

Northeast Insomnia and Sleep Medicine [37410]

Northeast Iowa Mental Health Center • DBA Northeast Iowa Behavioral Health [43259]

Northeast Kingdom Human Services [32655]

Northeast Kingdom Mental Health Service--Newport [32673]

Northeast Kingdom Mental Health Service--Saint Johnsbury [32680]

Northeast LA Substance Abuse Inc [43909]

Northeast Life Skills Associates Inc [46119]

Northeast Med-Equip [17344]

Northeast Medical Canter--NorthEast • George A. Batte Jr. Center for Cancer and Blood Disorders [5636]

Northeast Medical Center • Sleep Medicine Services [37475]

Northeast Metro 916 • EARS [2699]

Northeast Michigan Community Mental Health Authority--Harrisville [30562]

Northeast Michigan Community Mental Health Authority--Hillman [30565]

Northeast Michigan Community Mental Health Authority • Light of Hope Clubhouse [30501]

Northeast Michigan Community Mental Health Authority--Rogers City [30624]

Northeast Michigan Community Mental Health Services Board--Alpena [30502]

Northeast Mississippi Health Care, Inc. • Byhalia Family Health Center [6878]

Northeast Missouri Family Health Clinic--Edina [6902]

Northeast Missouri Family Health Clinic--Milan [6911]

Northeast Missouri Health Council, Inc. • Northeast Missouri Family Health Clinic [6910]

Northeast Nebraska Dialysis Center [25334]

Northeast Occupational Exchange [30205], [43931], [43965], [44018], [44030]

Northeast Ohio Neighborhood Health Services, Inc. • Hough Health Center [7081]

Northeast Ohio Sports Medicine & Physical Therapy [38849]

Northeast Oregon Renal Center • Diversified Specialty Institutes • Dialysis Services [26343]

Northeast Otolaryngology [2175]

Northeast Panhandle Substance Abuse Center [45731]

Northeast Panhandle • Substance Abuse Center [45737]

Northeast Pennsylvania Lions Eye Bank, Inc [35192]

Northeast Physical Therapy [38582]

Northeast Psychiatric Services--Albemarle [31501]

Northeast Psychiatric Services--Concord [31521]

Northeast Regional Program for Deaf/Hard of Hearing Children [538]

Northeast Rehabilitation Hospital [16182]

Northeast Speech and Language Center [3517]

Northeast Spine and Pain Center [35544]

Northeast Spine and Sports Medicine [38731]

Northeast Texas Dialysis Center [26948]

Northeast Treatment Centers
　Frankford [48545]
　NET STEPS [48546]
　Spring Garden Counseling Center [48547]

Northeast Valley Health Corporation • Van Nuys Contract [40592]

Northeast WA Alliance Counseling Services • Colville Branch [49931]

NorthEast Washington Alliance Counseling Services--Chewelah [32815]

Northeast Washington Alliance • Counseling Services Chewelah [49928]

NorthEast Washington Alliance Counseling

Services--Colville [32817], [51434]

Northeast Washington Alliance • Counseling Services--Republic [50088]

Northeast Washington Health Program [7376]

Northeast Washington • Treatment Alternatives [50176]

Northeast Wichita Dialysis Center • DaVita [24355]

Northeastern Center [33477]

Northeastern Center Inc [42985], [43133]
　Dekalb County [42986]
　Noble County Office [43126]

Northeastern Center, Inc. [29755]
　La Grange County Office--OP [29760]
　Ligonier Outpatient [29768]
　Noble County office/Administration [29756]
　Steuben County Satellite/Community Support [29694]
　Vision Quest Auburn [29695]

Northeastern Center • Kendallville Outpatient [29757]

Northeastern Counseling Center [49670], [49713]

Northeastern Counseling Center--Duchesne [32581]

Northeastern Counseling Center--Roosevelt [32614]

Northeastern Counseling Center--Vernal [32629]

Northeastern Family Institute, Inc.
　Keystone [34204]
　Wakefield Lodging House [34217]
　Washington Manor [34209]

Northeastern Family Institute • North Crossing [34205]

Northeastern Health Center [6370]

Northeastern Mental Health Center [32238]
　Dakota House [32218]
　Main Center [32219]
　Podoll Center [32220]
　Redfield [32246]
　Webster Clinic [32261]

Northeastern Oklahoma Community Health Center [7106]

Northeastern Oklahoma Council on Alcoholism Inc [47958]

Northeastern University
　Disability Resource Center [469]
　Speech-Language and Hearing Center [2461]

Northern Arizona Orthopaedics [38031]

Northern Arizona Regional Behavioral Health Authority [28147]

Northern Arizona Rehabilitation and Fitness, PC [38029]

Northern Arizona • Substance Abuse Services [39383]

Northern Arizona VA Health Care System [3870], [12812]
　Anthem CBOC [3871]
　Bellemont CBOC [3872]

Northern Arizona Veterans Affairs Health Care System [51533]
　PTSD Clinical Team [51686]

Northern Arizona Veterans Affairs Healthcare System [28192]

Northern Berkshire Counseling Center • The Brien Center [30431]

Northern California Family Center • Runaway and Homeless Youth Program [35834]

Northern California Fertility Medical Center [21928]

Northern California Institute of Sports Medicine [38083]

Northern California Spine and Rehabilitation Association [3912]

Northern California Treatment Services [40334]

Northern California VAHCS [40211]

Northern California Veterans Affairs Healthcare System • Mather Mental Health Outpatient Clinic • PTSD Clinical Team [51694]

Northern Chesapeake Hospice • Seasons VNA Hospice and Palliative Care [19925]

Northern Cheyenne Recovery Center [45707]

Northern Colorado Kidney Center • Fresenius Medical Care [23119]

Northern Counties Health Care, Inc. • Saint Johnsbury Family Health Center [7337]

Northern Country Community Mental Health--Bellaire [30513]

Northern Country Community Mental Health--Charlevoix [30526]

Northern Country Community Mental Health--Gaylord [30555]

Northern Country Community Mental Health--

Kalkaska [30582]
Northern Educational Services Inc [44584]
Northern Greenbrier--Southern [7418]
Northern Health Centers [7428]
Northern Health • Porch Multiple Sclerosis Clinic [34521]
Northern Hearing Services [2552]
Northern Hearing Services, Inc. [933]
Northern Hills Alcohol/Drug Services
    Spearfish [49028]
    Sturgis [49029]
Northern Hills Training Center [8510]
Northern Hospital District of Surry County [16762]
Northern Human Services [45891]
Northern Human Services--Berlin [31050]
Northern Human Services--Conway [31065]
Northern Human Services Mental Health Center [31051]
Northern Illinois Council on Alcohol and • Substance Abuse [42425], [42895], [42952]
Northern Illinois Hospice and Grief Center [19569]
Northern Illinois Medical Center • Centegra Hospital [2068]
Northern Illinois University
    Center for Access-Ability Resources [398]
    Department of Communicative Disorders [2015]
Northern Indiana Neurological Institute/dba Certified Sleep Centers of Northern Indiana [36958]
Northern Kentucky Mental Health/Mental Retardation Regional Center
    Boone County Adult Unit • NorthKey Community Care [30011]
    Boone County Children's Unit [30012]
Northern Lakes Community Mental Health • Missaukee/Wexford County [30518]
Northern Lakes Community Mental Health Service Program [30646]
Northern Louisiana Medical Center • Sleep Center [37071]
Northern Michigan Hospital • Sleep Center [37189]
Northern Michigan Regional Health System • Cancer Center [5390]
Northern Michigan Regional Hospital • Dialysis Center [24956]
Northern Michigan SLPs [2632]
Northern Michigan Sports Medicine Center--Harbor Springs [38592]
Northern Michigan Sports Medicine Center--Petoskey [38599]
Northern Michigan Sports Medicine Center--Rogers City [38601]
Northern Michigan University • HPER Department • Exercise Science Laboratory [38596]
Northern Montana Hospital • Dialysis Unit [25309]
Northern Nevada Child and Adolescent Services [31044]
Northern Nevada Medical Center • Northern Nevada Sports Medicine [38702]
Northern New Jersey Maternal/Child Health Consortium • Black Infant Mortality Reduction Resource Center [36511]
Northern Ohio Recovery Association [47696]
Northern Oswego County Health Services, Inc. [7037]
Northern Physical Therapy Services [38609]
Northern Region Community Health Center [6611]
Northern Rockies Brain and Spine Center • Pain Clinic [35536]
Northern Rockies Regional Spinal Injury Center • Saint Vincent Healthcare [4255]
Northern State University [48990]
Northern Tier Counseling--Mansfield [32041]
Northern Tier Counseling--Monroe Township [32047]
Northern Tier Counseling--South Waverly [32122]
Northern Tier Counseling--Towanda [32124]
Northern Virginia Diagnostic and Evaluation Clinic [8578]
Northern Virginia Hotline [51412]
Northern Virginia Mental Health Institute [33903]
Northern Virginia Sleep Diagnostic Center [37891]
Northern Virginia Training Center [8583]
Northern Westchester Hospital • Cancer Program [5590]
Northern Westchester Shelter [9976]
Northern Westchester Shelter, Inc. [9993]
Northern Winds Treatment Center [45269]
Northern Wisconsin Center for the Developmentally Disabled [8611]

Northern Wyoming Mental Health Center [50592]
    Hulett Medical Clinic [33069]
    Johnson County Outpatient Office [33032]
    Kaycee Family Clinic [33049]
Northern Wyoming Mental Health Center--Newcastle [33057]
Northern Wyoming Mental Health Center • Substance Abuse Services [50569], [50600]
Northern Wyoming Mental Health Center--Sundance [33070]
Northern Wyoming Mental Health Center--W 5th Street, Sheridan [33066]
Northern Wyoming Mental Health Center--W Brundage, Sheridan [33067]
Northfield Group Home [28994]
Northfield Hospice [20185]
Northfield Hospital [15923]
Northgate Dialysis Center • DaVita [22989]
NorthKey Community Care
    Children's Intensive Services [29997]
    Dixie Pike Family Health Center [29998]
    Grant County Substance Abuse Services [43801]
    Greenup Haus, Inc. [29999]
    Kenton County Substance Abuse Services [43566]
    Owen County Office [30093]
NorthKey Community Care--Williamstown [30122]
Northlake Addictive Disorders Clinic [43854]
Northlake Dialysis • DaVita [23814]
Northlake Medical Supply, Inc. [15280]
Northland [47819]
Northland Community Center [45557]
Northland Community Health Center--McCluskey [7071]
Northland Community Health Center--Rolla [7073]
Northland Community Services, Inc.--Adams [32944]
Northland Counseling Center [30681]
Northland Dependency Services LLC [45521] [45558]
Northland Dialysis • DaVita [25250]
Northland Family Help Center [8686]
    Runaway and Homeless Youth Program [35795]
Northland Health Partners • Community Health Center [7074]
Northland Hospice and Palliative Care [18790]
Northland Recovery Center [51040]
    Adolescent Center [45163]
    Substance Abuse Services [45164]
Northland Recovery Womens Center [45165]
Northpoint Consulting and Behavioral • Health Services [47849]
NorthPoint Health and Wellness Inc • NorthPoint Inc Renaissance [45221]
Northpoint Pioneer Inc • DBA Pioneer Counseling Center Clinton [44712]
Northpointe Behavioral Healthcare System [30584]
Northpointe Behavioral Healthcare System--Iron River [30575]
Northpointe Behavioral Healthcare System--Menominee [30599]
Northpointe Council Inc
    Methadone Maintenance Treatment Prg [46951]
    Outpatient [46758]
    Outpatient Treatment Program [46952]
Northpointe Counseling Services [44981]
Northpointe Dialysis Unit • Fresenius Medical Care--Northpointe [27650]
Northport Veterans Affairs Medical Center [31440]
    PTSD Clinical Team Outpatient [51785]
    PTSD Clinical Team Residential Rehabilitation Program Intensive/Inpatient [51786]
Northridge Hospital Medical Center [40279]
    Center for Rehabilitation Medicine [3913]
Northridge Hospital Medical Center--Roscoe Blvd. Campus • Thomas & Dorothy Leavey Cancer Center [4812]
Northridge Hospital Medical Center • Sleep Evaluation Center [36677]
Northridge Reproductive Medicine and Surgery • Fertility Clinic [22288]
Northshore Neurosciences • MDA Clinic [34867]
NorthShore Regional Medical Center • Sleep Disorders Center [37072]
Northshore Sleep Medicine [36920]
Northshore STARS Program • Center for Human Services [49909]
Northshore Treatment Center [49388]

NorthShore University Health System
    Evanston Hospital
        Center for Medical Genetics [12199]
        Eating Disorders Unit [11050]
    Glenbrook Hospital • Eating Disorders Unit [11051]
    Highland Park Hospital • Evanston Northwestern Healthcare [11052]
    Skokie Hospital • Eating Disorders Unit [11053]
    Sleep and Behavior Medicine Institute [36921]
    Sleep Center [36922]
NorthShore University HealthSystem Home and Hospice Services [19573]
Northshore Youth and Family Services [49910]
Northside Behavioral Health and Specialty Services [6267]
Northside Center for Child Development [8335]
Northside Center for Child Development, Inc. [31424]
Northside Community Outpatient Services [6425], [41444]
Northside Dialysis Center • Wake Forest University [25979]
Northside Dialysis • DaVita [26562]
Northside Home Infusion [17093]
Northside Hospital Behav Health Services [42031]
Northside Hospital
    Cherokee Sleep Disorders Center [36850]
    Institute for Cancer Control [5009]
    Sleep Medicine Institute [36851]
    Speech Pathology and Audiology Department [1826]
Northside Intermediate School District--RDSPD [819]
Northside Medical Center [7365]
Northside Mental Health Center
    Access House [29305]
    Access Manor [29306]
Northside Mental Health Center--Atlanta [29352]
Northside Mental Health Center--Fasst [29311]
Northside Mental Health Center • Satellite II Apartments [29307]
Northside Mental Health Center--Tampa [29308]
Northstar DUI Counsulting LLC [42918]
Northstar Health System--Dialysis [24857]
Northstar Health System Home Care [15698]
Northstar Health Systems--Crystal Falls • Dialysis Center [24858]
Northstar Home Care & Hospice-Iron River [20072]
NorthStar Medical Specialists • Sleep Center [37920]
Northumberland Dialysis • DaVita [26486]
Northville Counseling Center [30615]
Northwest Alabama Easter Seal Rehabilitation Center [7723]
Northwest Alabama Mental Health Center [39265]
    Adam Bishop (Wee Care) Day Treatment [27958]
    Fayette County Office [27914]
    Group Home [27959]
    Jasper Apartments [27960]
    Lamar County Office [28063]
    Marion County Office [27946]
    Walker County Office [27961]
    Winston County Office [27945]
Northwest Alabama Treatment Center [39214]
Northwest Arkansas Crisis Intervention Center [50665]
Northwest Arkansas Psychological Group [39529]
Northwest Arkansas Rape Crisis, Inc. [8785]
Northwest Arkansas Regional Health Center • Fayetteville Health Center [11335]
Northwest Arkansas Women's Shelter [8751]
Northwest Audiology [1885]
Northwest Baltimore Youth Services Inc [44167]
Northwest Behavioral Health Services [41707]
Northwest Behavioral • Healthcare Services [48115]
Northwest Buffalo Community Health Care Center [7020]
Northwest Cardiac Rehabilitation Center • William Rainey Harper College [38402]
Northwest Center for Behavioral Health--Alva [33763]
Northwest Center for Behavioral Health--Enid [33764]
Northwest Center for Behavioral Health--Fairview [33765]
Northwest Center for Behavioral Health--Fort Supply [33766]

Northwest Center for Behavioral Health--Guthrie [33767]

Northwest Center for Behavioral Health--Guymon [33768]

Northwest Center for Behavioral Health--Kingfisher [33773]

Northwest Center for Behavioral Health--Woodward [33790]

Northwest Center for Change [49992]

Northwest Center for Integrative Medicine, Inc. [35756]

Northwest Change Program • Tri County Community Corrections [45119]

Northwest Children's Home
    Residential Treatment--Main Campus [34095]
    Syringa House [34096]

Northwest Clinic [32464]

Northwest Colorado Visiting Nurse Association [19128]

Northwest Community Counseling Service [42974]

Northwest Community Counseling Services [42607]

Northwest Community Health Care [7220]

Northwest Community Health Center [6929]

Northwest Community Hospital [5059], [14680]
    Mental Health Network [42390]
    Sleep Disorders Center [36923]

Northwest Community Mental Health Center • Kenmore Center [31371]

Northwest Counseling Services [47727]

Northwest Counseling and Wellness Center [49233]

Northwest Dade Community Mental Health Center • Children/Adolescent Crisis Service [50764]

Northwest Detroit Dialysis--Lahser Satellite • Greenfield Health Systems [24977]

Northwest Domestic Crisis Services, Inc. [10219]

Northwest Family Center • DC Department of Mental Health [29098]

Northwest Family Services • Family Resource Centers [31790]

Northwest Family Services, Inc. • Runaway and Homeless Youth Program [36156]

Northwest Florida Community Hospital Home Health [13613]

Northwest Georgia Family Crisis Center, Inc. [9104]

Northwest Georgia Regional Hospital [33387]
    Developmental Services Unit [7916]

Northwest Greensboro Kidney Center • Fresenius Medical Care [25877]

Northwest Habilitation Center [8213]

Northwest Harris County Cooperative • Deaf Education Program [794]

Northwest Home Health--Russellville [12718]

Northwest Home Health Services [15656]

Northwest Home Health--Winfield [12734]

Northwest Home Medical [18467]

Northwest Hospital • Cancer Program [6114]

Northwest Hospital Center • Cancer Program [5311]

Northwest Hospital Speech Language Services [3639]

Northwest Houston Dialysis Center • Fresenius Medical Care [27164]

Northwest Human Service [31640]

Northwest Human Service Center [51194]

Northwest Human Services • Administration and Connections Program [31975]

Northwest Human Services Center • Developmental Disabilities Office [8396]

Northwest Human Services--Crisis & Information Hotline [51266]

Northwest Human Services, Inc. • Host Youth & Family Center • Runaway and Homeless Youth Program [36172]

Northwest Indiana Dialysis • Fresenius Medical Care [24152]

Northwest Indiana Special Education Cooperative [417]

Northwest Indiana Treatment Center [43155]

Northwest Infant Survival and SIDS Alliance [36555]

Northwest Intermediate School District [788]

Northwest Iowa Dialysis Center [24276]

Northwest Kansas Family Shelter, Inc. [9358]

Northwest Kansas Library System • Western Kansas Talking Books [3795]

Northwest Kidney Center
    Dialysis Facility • DaVita [27165]
    Diversified Specialty Institutes [23894]

Northwest Las Vegas Dialysis • Fresenius Medical Care [25370]

Northwest Louisiana Developmental Center [8062]

Northwest Louisiana Lions Eye Bank [35059]

Northwest Medical Center Behavioral Health [28067]

Northwest Medical Center Oro Valley [959]

Northwest Michigan Health Services, Inc. • Traverse City Clinic [6861]

Northwest Missouri Psychiatric Rehabilitation Center [33634]

Northwest Neurology • Multiple Sclerosis Clinic [34570]

Northwest Occupational Medicine Center, LLP [35634]

Northwest Ohio Developmental Center [8431]

Northwest Ohio Hemophilia Treatment Center • Toledo Hospital--Children's Medical Center [12578]

Northwest Orthopedics and Sports Medicine [38683]

Northwest Pediatric Therapy [1009]

Northwest Physical Therapy Sports Rehabilitation [39146]

Northwest Primary Care Group • Northwest Sleep Health [37620]

Northwest Recovery Centers LLC [50084]

Northwest Regional Center for Addictive Disorders [43898]

Northwest Regional Consultant Services • Deaf and Hard of Hearing Program [845]

Northwest Rehabilitation Associates, Inc. [39139]

Northwest Resources II Inc [50040], [50149]

Northwest Resources One LLC [49936]

Northwest Respiratory Services [13497], [15942]

Northwest Safeline [10400]

Northwest San Antonio Dialysis Center • DaVita [27338]

Northwest School for Hearing Impaired Children [864]

Northwest Sleep Center [36924]

Northwest Speech Center [3315]

Northwest Speech and Hearing Center Ltd. [1957]

Northwest Speech and Hearing Clinic--Corvallis [3307]

Northwest Speech and Hearing Clinic--Eugene [3309]

Northwest Substance Abuse Treatment • Women and Children [48056]

Northwest Suburban Physical Therapy • Sports Medicine Center, Ltd. [38382]

Northwest Texas Healthcare System
    Cancer Program [5958]
    The Pavillion [49207]

Northwest Tissue Services--Missoula [35101]

Northwest Tissue Services--Renton [35258]

Northwest Tissue Services--Spokane [35259]

Northwest Treatment [48167]

Northwest VA Health Care Clinic-Sun City, AZ [3873]

Northwest Veterans Affairs Healthcare Clinic [28203]

Northwest Youth Services • Runaway and Homeless Youth Program [36254], [36255]

Northwestern Bone and Tissue [35108]

Northwestern Community Service Center [32736]

Northwestern Community Service--Luray [32755]

Northwestern Community Service--Winchester [32798]

Northwestern Community Services Board • Mental Health and Substance Abuse Svcs [49791]

Northwestern Counseling and Support Services [32678]
    Group Home [32679]

Northwestern Counseling & Support Services, Inc. [51410]

Northwestern Human Services--Edgewater Partial Hospitalization Program [32023]

Northwestern Human Services--Lafayette Hill [32032]

Northwestern Human Services of Montgomery County [32034]

Northwestern Human Services--Philadelphia [32094]

Northwestern Human Services of Philadelphia • Behavioral Health and Mental Retardation [8475]

Northwestern Human Services
    Specialized Supported Living [32095]
    Woodhaven Center [8476]

Northwestern Illinois Association [411]

Northwestern Illinois Association--Rockford Area [409]

Northwestern Lake Counseling [42671]

Northwestern Lake Forest Hospital • Cancer Program [5105]

Northwestern Medical Center [3566]

Cancer Program [6050]

Northwestern Medical Faculty Foundation Inc. [1995]

Northwestern Memorial Hospital [34792]
    Cancer Program [5073]

Northwestern Memorial Hospital/Northwestern University • Adult Cystic Fibrosis Center [7531]

Northwestern Memorial Hospital
    Palliative Care and Home Hospice Program [19503]
    Sleep Disorders Center [36925]

Northwestern Mental Health Center • East Grand Forks Branch Clinic [30675]

Northwestern Mental Health Center, Inc.
    Crookston [30673]
    Fosston [30679]

Northwestern Ohio Crisis Line, Inc. [10145]

Northwestern University
    Audiology Clinic [1996]
    Division of Rheumatology • Multidisciplinary Clinical Research Center [164]
    Feinberg School of Medicine
        Department of Obstetrics and Gynecology Division of Reproductive Genetics [12200]
        McGaw Medical Center Pain Management [35434]
    Infant Hearing Center [2032]

Northwestern University Medical Center • Department of Neurology • Galter Outpatient Facility • Multiple Sclerosis Clinic [34571]

Northwestern University
    Northwestern Center for Bleeding Disorders [12518]
    Speech Language Pathology Clinic [2033]

Northwind Lung Specialists and Sleep Center [37227]

Northwood Children Honors Home - Boys [34242]

Northwood Children Honors Home - Girls • Exceptional Children's Annex [34243]

Northwood Children's Home [34244]

Northwood Children's Services and Little Learners Enrichment Center. [34245]

Northwood Dialysis • DaVita [26176]

Northwood Health Systems [32943]
    Ash Avenue Clinic [32921]
    Wetzel Outpatient Center [32924]

Northwood West and Merritt Creek Academy - IDT [34246]

Northwoods Community Health Center--Hayward [7425]

Northwoods Guidance Center [32967]

Northwoods Women Inc. • New Day Shelter [10689]

Norton Audubon Hospital
    Cancer Program [5225]
    Sleep Disorders Center [37035]

Norton Cancer Institute • Cancer Program [5226]

Norton Family Practice [44532]

Norton Healthcare, Inc. • Cord Blood Storage Program [35052]

Norton Kosair Children's Medical Center [12524]

Norton Sleep Disorders Center • Old Brownsboro Crossing [37036]

Norton Sound Health Corporation • Behavioral Health Services [28111]

Norton Suburban Hospital • Cancer Center [5227]

Norwalk Clinic [33261]

Norwalk Hospital Rehabilitation [1484]

Norwalk Hospital
    Sleep Disorders Center [36748]
    Whittingham Cancer Center [4905]

Norwalk Regional Health Center [6331]

Norwell Visiting Nurse Association and Hospice [15530]

Norwell VNA and Hospice [19990]

Norwich Dialysis • DaVita [23177]

Norwood Dialysis [26048]

Norwood Dialysis Center [24789]

Norwood Health Center [32990], [50459]

Norwood Park Family Service [29631]

Nory's Home Services, Inc. [14098]

Notre Dame Hospice [20016]

Nova Care--Ardmore • Sports Medicine Inc. [38927]

Nova Care Outpatient Rehabilitation--Marmora [38738]

Nova Care Outpatient Rehabilitation--Minneapolis [38629]

Nova Care Outpatient Rehabilitation--Philadelphia [38967]

Nova Counseling Associates Inc [44671]

Oakland Peritoneal Dialysis Center • DaVita **[22846]**
Oakland Primary Health Services **[6856]**
Oakland Psychological Clinic **[44789]**, **[44795]**, **[44799]**, **[44876]**, **[44904]**, **[44921]**, **[45020]**
Oakland Sleep Disorder Center • Saint Joseph Mercy **[37190]**
Oaklawn **[33469]**
Oaklawn Center--Elkhart **[33452]**
Oaklawn Center--Goshen **[33470]**
Oaklawn Dialysis Center • Fresenius Medical Care **[24945]**
Oaklawn--Elkhart **[29715]**
Oaklawn--Goshen **[29732]**
Oaklawn Psychiatric Center Inc **[43026]**, **[43069]**
Oaklawn Psychiatric Center, Inc. **[33471]**
Oakmont Center **[39224]**
Oakridge Counseling Center **[44656]**
The Oaks Apartments **[29282]**
Oaks Behavioral Health Hospital **[33744]**
Oaks Rehabilitation Health Center **[47953]**
Oaks Rehabilitative Services Center **[47936]**
The Oaks Treatment Center **[34446]**
Oakshire House **[4053]**
Oakview Apartments **[32055]**
Oakwood Annapolis Hospital **[2664]**
Oakwood Center of the Palm Beaches **[33363]**
Oakwood Center of the Palm Beaches Inc • Panda Program **[41561]**
Oakwood Center of the Palm Beaches, Inc.--Belle Glade **[29107]**
Oakwood Center of the Palm Beaches, Inc.--West Palm Beach **[29319]**
Oakwood Center of the Palm Beaches
    Phoenix Residence II **[33364]**
    Synergy **[33365]**
    UMI Village **[33366]**
    Waldon Arms **[33367]**
Oakwood Clinical Associates Ltd **[50425]**, **[50501]**
Oakwood Dialysis & At Home • DaVita **[24500]**
Oakwood Healthcare System--Clinton Township **[22127]**
Oakwood Healthcare System--Dearborn • Center for Reproductive Medicine **[22128]**
Oakwood Hospital and Medical Center
    Cancer Center **[5370]**
    Genetics Division **[12251]**
Oakwood Hospital, Seaway Center **[2656]**
Oasis Behavioral Health Services LLC **[50281]**
Oasis of Care Home Health, Inc. **[14104]**
Oasis Center • Runaway and Homeless Youth Program **[36206]**
Oasis Clinical Services LP **[45984]**
Oasis Counseling **[41301]**
Oasis Counseling International **[45776]**
Oasis House • Community Healthlink, Inc. **[30487]**
OASIS, Inc. **[10016]**
Oasis Shelter Home, Inc. **[10232]**
Oasis Substance Abuse Clinic **[44434]**
Oasis Treatment Center **[39593]**
OASIS Women's Center **[9192]**
Oasis Women's Counseling Center **[27869]**
Oasis Womens Recovering Community **[40839]**
Oats Family Center **[42334]**
O'Berry Neuro-Medical Center **[8376]**
O'Brien House **[43813]**
Obycris Healthcare, Inc. **[18121]**
Ocala Hearing Center **[1684]**
Ocala Pulmonary Associates, PA • Sleep Disorders Center **[36800]**
Ocala Regional Kidney Center--East • DaVita **[23435]**
Ocala Regional Kidney Center North • DaVita **[23264]**
Ocala Regional Kidney Center--South • DaVita • Dialysis Facility **[23358]**
Ocala Regional Kidney Center--West • DaVita **[23436]**
Ocala Regional Kidney Centers - Home Dialysis • DaVita **[23437]**
Ocala Regional Medical Center • Cancer Program **[4974]**
Occupational Health Services • Driving Under The Influence Program **[40676]**
Occupations, Inc.
    Arthur H. Daddazio Rehabilitation Center **[31404]**
    Community Counseling **[31389]**
    Community Counseling at Scotchtown **[31390]**

Occusport Physical Therapy--Lockport **[38390]**
OccuSport Physical Therapy--Oak Lawn **[38399]**
OccuSport Physical Therapy--Orland Park **[38401]**
Occusport Physical Therapy--Palos Park **[38403]**
Ocean Breeze Infusion Care, Inc. **[16638]**
Ocean Breeze Recovery **[41900]**
Ocean County Medical Center--Brick • Dialysis Unit **[25408]**
Ocean Health Toms River Site **[6985]**
Ocean Medical Services Inc **[46185]**
Ocean Mental Health Services, Inc.--Bayville **[34299]**
Ocean Mental Health Services, Inc.--Manahawkin **[34302]**
Ocean Monmouth Care LLC **[45940]**
Ocean Recovery **[40263]**
Oceanaire Residential Eating Disorder Program for Women **[10977]**
Oceanhawk Counseling Alternatives LLC **[50534]**
Ocean's Harbor House • Runaway and Homeless Youth Program **[36081]**
Oceanside Counseling Center Inc • Medically Supervised **[46957]**
Ocha Home Health Services **[14105]**
Ochoco Community Clinic **[7144]**
Ochsner Addictive Behavior Unit **[43872]**
Ochsner Clinic Foundation Baton Rouge • Sleep Disorders Center **[37073]**
Ochsner Clinic Foundation
    Cancer Institute **[5258]**
    Ochsner Sleep Center **[37074]**
Ochsner Elmwood Medical Center **[22079]**
Ochsner Health Center--Covington • Sleep Disorders Center **[37075]**
Ochsner Home Health **[15281]**
Ochsner Home Health of Lutcher **[15321]**
Ochsner Multi-Organ Transplant **[24559]**
OCM BOCES Children's Village at Park Hill **[578]**
Ocoee Dialysis • DaVita **[23438]**
Oconee Adult Mental Health Clinic **[29473]**
Oconee Center **[29474]**
    Addictive Disease Services **[42135]**
Oconee Center Mental Retardation Services **[29475]**
Oconee Community Service Board • Wilkinson County Service Center **[29433]**
Oconee Dialysis Clinic Inc. • Fresenius Medical Care **[26767]**
Oconee Medical Center Home Health **[17619]**
Oconee Pain Clinic **[35409]**
Oconee Regional Library • Dublin Subregional Library • Library for the Blind and Physically Handicapped **[3777]**
Oconee Regional Medical Center • Sleep Evaluation Center **[36852]**
O'Connor Hospital
    Cancer Program **[4847]**
    Pain Clinic **[35320]**
Oconomowoc Developmental Training **[34491]**
Oconomowoc Developmental Training Center **[8627]**
Oconomowoc Memorial Hospital **[18613]**
Ocotillo Dialysis • DaVita **[22430]**
October Road Inc **[47217]**
O.D. Alsobrook Counseling Center **[28061]**
Odessa Kidney Dialysis Center **[27277]**
Odessa Mental Health/Mental Retardation Center **[32521]**
Odessa R--VII School District **[529]**
Odyssey Counseling **[41351]**
Odyssey Family Counseling Center **[42056]**
Odyssey Health Care of Conroe **[21421]**
Odyssey Health Care of Harrisburg **[21065]**
Odyssey Health Care of Houston **[21488]**
Odyssey Health Care of Philadelphia **[21057]**
Odyssey Health Care of Rhode Island **[21197]**
Odyssey HealthCare of Amarillo **[21380]**
Odyssey Healthcare of Arlington Virginia **[21741]**
Odyssey Healthcare of Athens **[19344]**
Odyssey Healthcare of Atlanta Inpatient **[19380]**
Odyssey Healthcare of Austin **[21391]**
Odyssey Healthcare of Bakersfield **[18890]**
Odyssey Healthcare of Beaumont **[21399]**
Odyssey HealthCare of Big Spring **[21405]**
Odyssey Healthcare of Birmingham, Inc. **[18687]**
Odyssey Healthcare of Central Indiana **[19612]**
Odyssey HealthCare of Charleston **[21212]**
Odyssey HealthCare of Chicago South **[19504]**
Odyssey HealthCare of Cincinnati **[20815]**
Odyssey Healthcare of Cleveland **[20865]**
Odyssey Healthcare of Colorado Springs **[19093]**

Odyssey Healthcare of Corpus Christi **[21424]**
Odyssey Healthcare of Dayton **[20835]**
Odyssey Healthcare of Detroit **[20123]**
Odyssey HealthCare of East Texas **[21582]**
Odyssey HealthCare of El Paso **[21452]**
Odyssey HealthCare-Flowood **[20234]**
Odyssey Healthcare of Fort Worth **[21462]**
Odyssey HealthCare of Georgia **[19352]**
Odyssey Healthcare of Gulf Coast **[20241]**
Odyssey HealthCare of Hampton Roads **[21710]**
Odyssey HealthCare, Inc. **[18938]**
Odyssey HealthCare of Kansas City **[20313]**
Odyssey Healthcare of Lake Charles **[19851]**
Odyssey Healthcare of Las Vegas **[20421]**
Odyssey HealthCare of Little Rock **[18862]**
Odyssey Healthcare of Los Angeles **[19078]**
Odyssey HealthCare of Lubbock **[21524]**
Odyssey HealthCare of Memphis **[21349]**
Odyssey HealthCare-Miami **[19257]**
Odyssey HealthCare of Milwaukee **[21826]**
Odyssey HealthCare-Milwaukee **[21857]**
Odyssey HealthCare of Mobile **[18740]**
Odyssey HealthCare of Nashville **[21361]**
Odyssey Healthcare of New Jersey **[20489]**
Odyssey Healthcare of New Mexico **[20521]**
Odyssey Healthcare of North Texas **[21435]**
Odyssey HealthCare of Northern California **[18898]**
Odyssey HealthCare of Omaha **[20400]**
Odyssey Healthcare of Orange County **[18934]**
Odyssey HealthCare-Pacific Northwest **[21032]**
Odyssey Healthcare of Palm Springs **[18996]**
Odyssey HealthCare of Pennsylvania **[21142]**
Odyssey Healthcare of Phoenix **[18813]**
Odyssey HealthCare of Phoenix-Mesa Inpatient **[18800]**
Odyssey HealthCare of Portland **[20987]**
Odyssey HealthCare of Richmond **[21727]**
Odyssey Healthcare of Riverside **[19010]**
Odyssey HealthCare of St. Louis **[20335]**
Odyssey Healthcare of San Antonio **[21557]**
Odyssey Healthcare of San Diego **[19017]**
Odyssey Healthcare of Savannah **[19417]**
Odyssey HealthCare of Shreveport **[19879]**
Odyssey HealthCare of South Texas **[21409]**
Odyssey HealthCare of Toledo **[20864]**
Odyssey Healthcare of Tucson **[18832]**
Odyssey HealthCare of Waxahachie **[21590]**
Odyssey Healthcare of Wilmington **[19186]**
Odyssey Hospice-Augusta **[19358]**
Odyssey Hospice of New Orleans **[19861]**
Odyssey Hospice-Ocala **[19275]**
Odyssey House Inc
    Adolescent Treatment Facility **[49690]**
    Adult Outpatient **[49691]**
    Adult Residential Treatment Program **[49692]**
    Eldercare Program **[46897]**
    Family Re-Entry Program **[46436]**
    Fathers with Children Residential **[49693]**
    Lafayette Program **[46437]**
    Leadership Center **[46898]**
    Mabon Adult Program **[46899]**
    Mabon Family Program **[46900]**
    Manor Adults **[46901]**
    Manor Family Center Program **[46902]**
    Mothers with Children Program **[49694]**
    Outpatient Services **[46438]**
    Transitional Services **[49695]**
Odyssey House • Inpatient Facility **[21422]**
Odyssey House Louisiana Inc **[43873]**
Odyssey House Texas **[49389]**
Odyssey Learning Center **[7800]**
O.E. Meyer Co. **[17035]**
Oesterlen Services for Youth, Inc. **[34387]**
Office of Maternal and Child Health **[36459]**
Office of Patricia Fodor, MD, PC • Multiple Sclerosis Center **[34543]**
Ogden Regional Medical Center ACT **[49647]**
Ogden Speech and Hearing Center **[3551]**
Ogeechee Area Hospice **[19421]**
Ogeechee Area Mental Health Clinic **[29495]**
Ogeechee Behavioral Health Clinic **[29505]**
Ogeechee Behavioral Health/Day Services **[29506]**
Ogeechee Behavioral Health Services **[29494]**, **[42163]**, **[42164]**, **[42184]**
Oglala Sioux Tribe • Runaway and Homeless Youth Program **[36199]**
Ogle County Hospice Association **[19552]**
Ohana Hearing Center of Hawaii **[1937]**

Ohana Makamae Inc [42192]
Ohel Children's Home and Family Services [34331]
Critical Care Residence [34332]
Group Home [34333]
Group Residence for Boys [34334]
Ohio County Hospital [15188]
Sleep Center [37037]
Ohio County Office [29811]
Ohio County Community Center [29973]
Ohio Department of Health • Child and Family
Health Services Bureau • SIDS Program [36530]
Ohio Domestic Violence Shelter [9156]
Ohio Eastern Star Community Services [17006]
Ohio Health Sleep Services--Grove City [37552]
Ohio Health Sleep Services--MacKenzie Drive,
Columbus [37553]
Ohio Health Sleep Services--Pickerington [37554]
Ohio Health Sleep Services--Westerville [37555]
Ohio Healthcare Plus, LLC [16915]
Ohio Home Care--Belpre [16852]
Ohio Northeast Health Systems, Inc. [7100]
Ohio Pike Dialysis • DaVita [26008]
Ohio Rainbow Babies and Children's Hospital •
Sickle Cell Center [36414]
Ohio Renal Care Group--North Randall • Fresenius
Medical Care • Dialysis Facility [26175]
Ohio School for the Deaf [652]
Ohio Sleep Disorders Center--Olentangy River
Road, Columbus [37556]
Ohio Sleep Disorders Center--Sleep Services
[37557]
Ohio Sleep Disorders Centers--Delaware [37558]
Ohio Sleep Disorders Centers--Dublin [37559]
Ohio Sleep Disorders Centers--Flint Road [37560]
Ohio Sleep Disorders Centers--Grant Medical Center
[37561]
Ohio Sleep Medicine and Neuroscience Institute Inc.
[37562]
Ohio Sports & Spine Institute, Ltd.--Boardman
[38855]
Ohio Sports & Spine Institute--Poland [38888]
Ohio State Adult Down Syndrome Clinic [10848]
Ohio State School for the Blind [3730]
Ohio State University
Arthur G. James Cancer Hospital and Richard J.
Solove Research Institute [4696]
Division of Infectious Disease • Adult AIDS Clini-
cal Trials Unit [28]
MDA/ALS Center [138]
Ohio State University Medical Center
Burn Unit [4606]
Hemophilia Treatment Center [12579]
MDA/ALS Clinic [34853]
Multiple Sclerosis Clinic [34675]
Pain Management [35614]
Rehabilitation Services [4374]
Sleep Disorders Center [37563]
Universities Hosp East/Talbot Hall [47728]
Ohio State University
Office for Disability Services [653]
Speech, Language and Hearing Clinic [3232]
Ohio State University--Suicide Prevention Services
[51207]
Ohio State University Transplant [26090]
Ohio State University Voice Institute [3233]
Ohio Valley Home Health Services Inc. [16933]
Ohio Valley Medical Center • Cancer Program
[6142]
OhioHealth [35615]
Ohitika Najin Win Oti [10381]
Ohlhoff Recovery Programs [10978]
Henry Ohlhoff House [40626]
San Francisco Outpatient Program [40627]
Skip Byron Primary [40628]
Ohlone College • Deaf Studies Division • Center for
Deaf Studies [276]
OHM HomeCare Network [17620]
OHSU Avel Gordly Center for Healing [48206]
OHSU, Eugene • Center for Health and Healing • In
Vitro Fertilization Program [22222]
OHSU Gabriel Park Sports Medicine Clinic [38920]
Okaloosa County Schools [348]
Okanogan Behavioral Healthcare [51455]
Okanogan Behavioral Healthcare Inc • Chemical
Dependency Services [50044]
Okc Area Inter-Tribal Health Board [48025]
Oklahoma Addiction Specialists • Incorporated
Services [47931]

Oklahoma Center for Bleeding Disorders • Pediatric
Hematology/Oncology [12582]
Oklahoma Center for Orthopaedic and Sports
Medicine [38909]
Oklahoma City Department of Mental Health • Teen-
line [51243]
Oklahoma City Orthopedics and Sports Medicine
[38910]
Oklahoma City Public Schools [670]
Oklahoma City Veterans Affairs Medical Center
[17151], [31904]
Oklahoma Cystic Fibrosis Center--Tulsa [7645]
Oklahoma Department of Human Services •
Runaway and Homeless Youth Program [36157]
Oklahoma Families First • Ada [47902]
Oklahoma Families First Inc [47942]
Seminole [48016]
Oklahoma Kidney Care Dialysis LLC [26283]
Oklahoma Library for the Blind and Physically
Handicapped [3830]
Oklahoma Lions Eye Bank [35171]
Oklahoma Mental Health Council Inc • DBA Red
Rock Behav Hlth Services [47990]
Oklahoma Psychological Center [3277]
Oklahoma Respiratory Care [17140]
Oklahoma School for the Blind [3731]
Oklahoma School for the Deaf [673]
Oklahoma Sports and Orthopedics Institute [38906]
Oklahoma State Department of Health • Family
Health Services • Maternal and Child Health Divi-
sion • SIDS Program [36532]
Oklahoma State University
Deaf Student Services [671]
Speech-Language Pathology Department [3285]
Oklahoma State University--Tulsa • Speech and
Hearing Clinic [3291]
Oklahoma Treatment Services LLC
Bartlesville Rightway Medical [47913]
Rightway Medical of Roland [48012]
Oklahoma University • Family Medicine Center -
Sports Medicine [38911]
Oklahoma University Medical Center
Cade Cancer Center [5780]
Cancer Center [4698]
Children's Dialysis [26284]
Okmulgee County Health Department • Speech and
Hearing Clinic [3280]
Okmulgee Safehouse [10207]
Oktibbeha County Hospital
Center for Sleep Medicine [37256]
Physical, Occupational and Speech Therapy
[2773]
Okuli Eagles Nest Foundation Inc • Okuli Counsel-
ing Services [39729]
Olalla Recovery Centers [50036]
Olathe Dialysis • DaVita [24341]
Olathe Medical Center • Cancer Program [5201]
Olathe Medical Center, Inc. • Sleep Disorders
Center [36999]
Olathe Medical Center • Pain Clinic [35456]
Old Baltimore Pike Group Home [29072]
Old Bridge Dialysis Center • DaVita [25492]
Old Colony Hospice [19997]
Old Dominion Eye Bank [35255]
Old Dominion Home Health Services, Inc.--
Petersburg [18348]
Old Dominion Home Health Services--Richmond
[18371]
Old Forge Dialysis • DaVita [26497]
Old Vineyard Youth Services [33745]
Older Adult Home care Services, Inc. [15848]
Older Women's League: Voice of Mid--Life and
Older Women [9701]
Oldham County Center [30039]
Olean Veterans Affairs Clinic [31442]
Olin E. Teague Veterans Affairs Medical Center
[32558]
Olive Crest RTC--Rosemead [33192]
Olive Crest Treatment Centers, Inc. [34023]
Oliver Headache and Pain Clinic/Advanced Pain
Care Clinic [35448]
Oliver--Payatt Centers • Eating Disorders Program
[11028]
Olives Home Health Care, Inc.--Dallas [17886]
Olives Home Health Care, Inc.--Rowlett [18131]
Olivia White Hospice Home [18791]
Olivias House [39225]
Olney Dialysis Center • DaVita [24058]

OLOM Home Care, Inc.--New York [16560]
OLOM Home Care, Inc.--Yonkers [16682]
Olson Huff Center for Child Development [8366]
Olympia Behavioral Health Clinic [32877]
Olympia Center/Preston Inc • Adolescent Treatment
Program [50319]
Olympia Dialysis Center • DaVita [27623]
Olympia Fields Dialysis Center & At Home • DaVita
[24034]
Olympia Psychotherapy Inc [50041]
Olympic Medical Center • Cancer Program [6108]
Olympic Medical Home Health [18445]
Olympic Peninsula Kidney Center [27598]
Olympic Peninsula Kidney Center--North [27629]
Olympic Peninsula Kidney Center--South Kitsap
[27628]
Olympic Personal Growth Center [50148]
Olympic View Dialysis Center & At Home • DaVita
[27637]
Olympic Wellness Center [49915]
Omada Behavioral Health Services • Northfield
[45251]
Omaha Central Dialysis • DaVita [25339]
Omaha Division • Veterans Affairs Nebraska
Western Iowa Health Care System [51601]
Omaha Hearing School [2859]
Omaha Public Schools [539]
Omaha South Dialysis • DaVita [25340]
Omaha Treatment Center [45799]
Omaha Tribe Alcohol Program [45768]
Omak Dialysis Center • Fresenius Medical Care
[27624]
OMART Inc [39536]
Omed Home Healthcare [15819]
Omega Centre [41585], [41661]
Omega Health Care of Georgia [19341]
Omega Health Care--Lees Summit [20316]
Omega Health Care of NW Georgia [19372]
Omega Health Care of SW Missouri, Inc. [20342]
Omega Home Care Services, Inc. [14106]
Omega Home Health Care--Brooklyn [16407]
Omega Home Health Care, Inc.--Evanston [14788]
Omega Home Healthcare--Oak Park [15762]
Omega Hospice of Cullman [18697]
Omega House [34415]
Omega Independent Living Services [47463]
Omegon Inc [45236]
OMH Hospice of the Foothills [21277]
Omicron Medical Equipment, Inc. [17483]
OMNI Behavioral Health--Beatrice [30974]
OMNI Behavioral Health--Columbus [30978]
Omni Behavioral Health • Eating Disorder Clinic
[11131]
OMNI Behavioral Health--Omaha [31009]
Omni Clinic [51503]
Omni Dialysis Center • DaVita [27166]
Omni Home Care, Inc. [15773]
Omni Home Health Inc. [13144]
Omni House, Inc. [30290]
Day Program [30291]
Omni Mental Health Clinic [30292]
Omni Youth Services [42426], [42966]
Arlington Heights Office [42391]
Ela Township Office [42739]
Runaway and Homeless Youth Program [35936]
Vernon [42427]
Omnicare of King of Prussia [17355]
OmniCare of Northern Illinois [14768]
Omnicare Pharmacy Services of Pittsburgh [17444]
Omnix Health Care Services, Inc. [17855]
On-Belay House [45265]
Eden Prairie [45141]
On-Call Home Health & Rehabilitation Services
[18102]
On-Call Medical Option Care [17719]
On Pointe Home Health Care [15839]
On With Life, Inc. [4054]
Oncology/Hematology Care, Inc. [16878]
One 2 One Mentors Inc • Stepping Stones to
Recovery [40915]
One Hope United--Centralia [33407]
One Hope United--Chicago [33415]
One on One Home Health Care [14107]
One Plus One Florida, Inc. [13764]
One Source Home care Services [16671]
One Source Nutrition [11005], [11006]
One Stop Medical Supplies [14392]
One World Speech and Language Consulting [2675]

Oneida Crisis Center [9179]
Oneida--Herkimer--Madison BOCES [591]
Oneida Nation Domestic Abuse Program [10728]
ONeill Valley Hope • Alcoholism Treatment Center [45806]
OneLegacy [34954]
OneWorld Community Health Center [6944]
Onida Clinic [7249]
Only Human Counseling Services LLP [47571]
Onslow Carteret Behavioral Healthcare Services [31552]
    Adult Development Activity Program [31553]
    Developmental Disabilities Services [31554]
Onslow Memorial Hospital • Sleep Disorders Lab [37477]
Onslow Women's Center, Inc. [10048]
OnTarget Speech and Language Consulting PLLC [1533]
Ontario Community Support Services [31333]
Ontario County Mental Health Center [8310], [31334]
Ontario Dialysis Inc. [22857]
Ontario Intensive/Supportive Apartments [31335]
Ontario Provincial Schools for the Deaf
    Deaf/Hard of Hearing Program [679]
    Robarts School for the Deaf [678]
Ontario-Yates Hospice [20569]
Ontrack Inc [48122], [48149]
    DADS Program [48150]
    Home Program [48151]
Onyx Home Health Care [15639]
Oonalaska Wellness Center • Behavioral Health Program [39355]
Opal Home Health Care Corporation [14108]
OPC Foundation [31515]
Opelousas Behavioral Health Clinic [43880]
Opelousas Developmental Center [8072]
Opelousas General Health System • Sleep Disorders Center [37076]
Opelousas General Hospital • Cancer Program [5261]
Opelousas Mental Health Center [33546]
Open Airways, Inc. [18345]
Open Arms • The Bridge • Runaway and Homeless Youth Program [35909]
Open Arms Care Speech-Language-Pathology Services [2775]
Open Arms Christian Counseling Inc. [3648]
Open Arms Domestic Violence Shelter [10147]
Open Arms Hospice • St. Francis Hospital [21279]
Open Arms Inc [44380]
    Chemical Depend Community Residence [46686]
    Supportive Living Facility [46687]
Open Arms Mens Center Inc [40144]
Open Arms Minnesota • Alcohol and Drug Program [45307]
Open Cities Health Center, Inc. [6873]
Open Door BMH Health Center • Open Door Health Center [6697]
The Open Door--Cherry Tree [51278]
Open Door Counseling at Mazzoni Center [48548]
Open Door Family Medical Centers, Inc. [7034]
Open Door Health Center [6866]
Open Door Inc [41514], [48322]
The Open Door Inc [48298], [48413]
The Open Door--Indiana [51285]
Open Door Mission • Mens Ministries [45800]
Open Door Missions • Lydia House [45801]
Open Door Recovery Center [43970]
Open House of Coastal Horizons Center, Inc. • Crisis Line [51180]
Open-Inn • Runaway and Homeless Youth Program [35796]
Open Lines Communication Center [3072]
Open Options Inc [47991]
Open Waters Home Health Care [14931]
Opening Doors Consulting [2416]
Operation Angel [36449]
Operation Care • Amador County Crisis Line [8823]
Operation Par Inc
    Cornerstone of Successful Achie [41919]
    COSA Developmental Center [41920]
    Detoxification Program [41597]
    Medication Assisted Patient Services [41573], [41598], [41821], [41905]
    Par Village [41745]
    Shirley Coletti Acad for Behav Chg [41921]

    Therapeutic Community [41746]
Operation Recovery [44168]
Operation Safehouse, Inc. • Runaway and Homeless Youth Program [35835]
Opiate Addiction Recovery Services [47664]
Opiate Replacement Therapy Centers of America Inc [43818]
Opiate Treatment Program • Portland VA Medical Center [48207]
Opp Nursing Facility [28010]
Opportunities and Self Help Program [31310]
Opportunities Unlimited [4055]
Opportunity Center • OCI [7870]
Opportunity Council [10632]
Opportunity Enterprises [8009]
Opportunity House [8648], [33125]
Optima Health Care Inc. [13046]
Optima Home Health Services [13192]
Optima Infusion Pharmacy [17526]
Optimae Life Services [29871]
Optimal Eating [10979]
Optimal Home Health [18994]
Optimal Home Health Care Services, Inc.--Miami Lakes [14215]
Optimal Hospice [19072]
Optimal Hospice Care-Bakersfield [18891]
Optimal Hospice Care-Bay Area [19039]
Optimal Hospice Care-Fresno [18931]
Optimal Hospice Care-Lake Isabella [18953]
Optimal Hospice Care-Modesto [18969]
Optimal Hospice Care-Ridgecrest [18999]
Optimal Hospice Care-Visalia [19073]
Optimal HospiceCare-Bay Area [19040]
Optimist Youth and Family Services [33993]
Optimum Care Home Health Services Inc. [12977]
Optimum Home Health Care [15723]
Optimum Home HealthCare Inc. [13456]
Optimum Plus Home Care [15849]
Optimum Professionals Home Health Care [14749]
Optimum Rehab and Learning Specialists [3625]
Option Care [14368]
Option Care Enterprises - Everett [18429]
Option Care/Missouri River Hospice [20291]
Option House, Inc. [8882]
Option, Inc.--Hobbs [9873]
Option One Home Medical Equipment, Inc [12957]
OPTIONCARE Enterprises--Ann Arbor [15578]
OPTIONCARE of Sparta [14940]
OptionCare Tampa Home Health [14423]
Options [32123]
Options Counseling [41087], [41308]
Options Counseling Center [46126]
Options Domestic Violence and Sexual Assault, Inc. [10095]
Options EAP [50871]
Options, Inc.--Monticello [8775]
Options, Inc.--Morganton [10065]
Options/Lynnwood [50015]
Options of Marion County [41836]
Options Recovery Services [39657]
Options for Recovery • Stork Club [40855]
Options Treatment Center [33475]
Options Unlimited of Mexico [30876]
Options With Learning [3002]
Oqirrh Ridge - East [32591]
Oqirrh View Community Health Center [7328]
Oral and Maxillofacial Surgery and Pain Management [35646]
Oralingua School for the Hearing Impaired [314]
Orange City Home Health Hospice [19720]
Orange Coast Memorial Health Care • Coast Pain Management Center [35321]
Orange Coast Memorial Medical Center • Cancer Care Program [4776]
Orange Community Health Center [6980]
Orange Community Services [31340]
Orange County Board of County Commissioners • Runaway and Homeless Youth Program [35898]
Orange County Care Providers Inc. [13092]
Orange County Deaf Equal Access Foundation [1091]
Orange County Department of Social Services • Adult Services Unit [31549]
Orange County Detox [39751]
Orange County Health Care Agency • Anaheim Alcohol and Drug Abuse Services [39594]
Orange County Healthcare Agency
    Alcohol/Drug Abuse Services/AlisoViejo [39586]

    Alcohol/Drug Abuse Services/Santa Ana [40718]
    Drug Court and DUI Unit [40719]
    West Alcohol and Drug Abuse Services [40949]
Orange County Library System • Talking Book Section [3766]
Orange County Rehab [39752]
Orange County Safe Homes Project, Inc. [9966]
Orange County Services [29798]
Orange County Vet Center [51885]
Orange Day Treatment Center [31341]
Orange Dialysis Facility [27532]
Orange/Durham Coalition for Battered Women, Inc. [10034]
Orange Grove Center [8514]
Orange Intensive Day Treatment Program [31324]
Orange Outpatient Services [32522]
Orange Park Kidney Center • Fresenius Medical Care [23443]
Orange Park Medical Center • Cancer Center [4975]
Orange Regional Family Program • Alcoholism and Chemical Dependency [46780]
Orange Regional Medical Center--Horton • Tucker Center for Cancer Care [5588]
Orangeburg Area Mental Health Center [32211]
Orangeburg Dialysis • Renal Advantage Inc. [26756]
Orangeburg District Four [728]
Orangevale Dialysis Center • DaVita [22863]
Orca House Inc [47697]
    Mens Program [47698]
    Womens Program [47699]
Orchard Hill ResCare [29900]
Orchard Park Dialysis Center [25751]
Orchard Place--Child Guidance Center [29855]
Orchard Place • Child Guidance Center [34140]
Orchard Place Child Guidence Center • PACE Juvenile Justice [43267]
Orchard Place • PACE Juvenile Center [33499]
Orchid LLC [41880]
Oregon Clinic • Sleep Disorders Center [37621]
Oregon Department of Education • Oregon Deaf-blind Project [3319]
Oregon Dialysis Services • Fresenius Medical Care [26319]
Oregon Headache Clinic [12461]
Oregon Health & Science University [140], [34857]
Oregon Health and Science Univ. Clinical Transplant Program [26344]
Oregon Health and Science University • Comprehensive Pain Center [35635]
Oregon Health and Science University Hospital • Cancer Institute [5801]
Oregon Health Science University • Multiple Sclerosis Center [34683]
Oregon Health and Science University
    Oregon Hemophilia Treatment Center [12583]
    Richmond Clinic [7141]
Oregon Health Sciences University
    Child Development and Rehabilitation Center • Genetics and Birth Defects Clinic [12323]
    Cystic Fibrosis Care, Teaching and Research Center [7647]
Oregon Pain Associates [35636]
Oregon Partnership [51263]
Oregon Reproductive Medicine [22223]
Oregon Research Institute • Ctr for Family and Adolescent Research [48208]
Oregon School for the Deaf [692]
Oregon Sleep Associates • Sleep Disorders Center [37622]
Oregon State Hospital [33793]
Oregon State Hospital--Portland [33792]
Oregon State Library • Talking Book and Braille Services [3831]
Orem Veterans Affairs Clinic [32604]
Organization for Recovery Inc [46137]
Organogenesis Inc. [35073]
Oriana House • Alcohol and Drug Crisis Center [47608]
Origami Brain Injury Rehabilitation Program [4180]
Orillia Solders' Memorial Hospital • Simcoe County Eating Disorders Service for Youth [11227]
Orion Academy [7794]
Orion Health--Calgary [35282]
OrionHealth--Canmore [35283]
OrionHealth--Temple [35284]
OrionHealth--Vancouver [35299]
Orlando Artificial Kidney Center • Fresenius Medical Center [23450]

Orlando Behavioral Healthcare [41753]
   Orlando Outpatient [41865]
Orlando Cancer Center • Sickle Cell Disease Center [36324]
Orlando Dialysis • DaVita [23451]
Orlando Downtown Dialysis • DaVita • Dialysis Facility [23452]
Orlando East Dialysis • DaVita [23453]
Orlando Home Training Dialysis • DaVita [23454]
Orlando Methadone Treatment Center [41866]
Orlando North Dialysis • DaVita [23455]
Orlando Park Dialysis • DaVita [23456]
Orlando Regional Medical Center
   Burn and Tissue Rehab Unit [4533]
   M.D. Anderson Cancer Center [4977]
Orlando Regional Outpatient Rehabilitation [3990]
Orlando Regional Rehabilitation Institute [3991]
Orlando Regional Rehabilitation Services--Kuhl Avenue, Orlando • Orthopedics and Sports Medicine [38268]
Orlando Regional Rehabilitation Services--Sligh Blvd., Orlando [38269]
Orlando Regional--Sand Lake Hospital [1700]
Orlando Southwest Dialysis • DaVita • Dialysis Facility [23457]
Orlando Speech and Language [1790]
Orlando Sports Medicine Group--Altamonte Springs [38214]
Orlando Sports Medicine Group--Orlando [38270]
Orlando VA Medical Center [14300]
Orlando Veterans Affairs Medical Center [51555]
   Kissimmee Clinic [29193]
   Leesburg Clinic [29207]
   Viera Clinic [29317]
   William V. Chappell, Jr., Veterans Affairs Outpatient Clinic [3992]
Orleans Essex Visiting Nurse Association and Hospice, Inc. [18235]
Ormond Beach Dialysis • DaVita [23458]
Oroville Dialysis Clinic • Dialysis Clinic Inc. [22864]
Oroville Hospital [1215]
Orsini Home Medical Equipment [14780]
Ortho Care Physical Therapy, Inc. • Prevention and Rehabilitation Clinic [38602]
Ortho Home Health Care, LLC [13823]
Ortho Montana Orthopedics and Sports Medicine [38676]
OrthoArkansas North [38068]
OrthoArkansas Orthopedics and Sports Medicine [38067]
OrthoCare Physical Therapy and Sports Rehabilitation [38776]
OrthoCarolina--Charlotte • Sports Medicine Center [38830]
OrthoCarolina Foot and Ankle Institute [38831]
OrthoCenter • Orthopedic Sports Medicine and Rehabilitation Center [38755]
Orthopaedic Associates of Portland [38512]
Orthopaedic and Fracture Clinic [38621], [38921]
The Orthopaedic Group, P.C. [38008]
Orthopaedic Hospital of Los Angeles • Hemophilia Program [12491]
Orthopaedic Institute of Henderson [38695]
Orthopaedic Institute of Western Kentucky [38487]
Orthopaedic Research Clinic of Alaska [38019]
Orthopaedic Specialists of Austin [39047]
Orthopaedic Specialty Group [38192]
Orthopaedic & Sports Medicine Center [38514]
Orthopaedic and Sports Medicine Center--Manhattan [38463]
Orthopaedic and Sports Medicine Center--Norman [38907]
Orthopaedic Sports Medicine Clinic of Alabama [37996]
Orthopaedic and Sports Medicine Clinic of Kansas City [38462]
Orthopaedics and Sports Medicine Clinic [38497]
Orthopedia Physical Therapy [39063]
Orthopedic Associates [38912]
Orthopedic Associates, Inc.--Evansville [38427]
Orthopedic Associates of Long Island, LLP [38823]
Orthopedic Associates, PC--Billings [38677]
The Orthopedic Clinic Association [38034], [38045]
Orthopedic Clinic and Sports Medicine • Ted Honghiran MD [38070]
Orthopedic Institute of New Jersey--Hackettstown [38728]
Orthopedic Institute of New Jersey--Vernon [38765]

Orthopedic Specialists, PC [38667]
Orthopedic Specialists of Southwest Florida • Sports Medicine Center of Excellence [38227]
Orthopedic Specialty Group • Pain Clinic [35365]
The Orthopedic Sports Clinic [39075]
Orthopedic and Sports Medicine Clinic [39023]
Orthopedic and Sports Medicine Institute of Las Vegas [38699]
Orthopedic and Sports Therapy of Metairie [38500]
Orthopedic and Sports Therapy of Westbank [38494]
OrthoPTic Rehabilitation Clinic of Metairie [38501]
ORTHOSPORT Physical Therapy [39012]
OrthosportsMed Physical Therapy [38561]
OrthoWest Orthopaedic and Sports Medicine [38691]
Osawatomie State Hospital [33512]
Osborne Treatment Services Inc • Outpt Drug Abuse Clinic/El Rio Program [46439]
Oscar G. Johnson VA Medical Center [15697]
Oscar G Johnson VAMC • Behavioral Health Service [44856]
Oscar G. Johnson Veterans Affairs Medical Center [30574], [51589]
Osceola Counseling Center • Center for Drug Free Living [41722]
Osceola Mental Health, inc. • DBA Park Place Behavioral Health Care [29194]
OSF Home Care [14905]
OSF HomeCare [19565]
OSF Hospice [20054]
OSF Hospice, Bloomington [19489]
OSF Hospice-Loves Park [19539]
OSF Hospice-Peoria [19562]
OSF Saint Anthony Medical Center
   Center for Cancer Care [5124]
   Sleep Disorders Center [36926]
OSF Saint Francis Home Health [15649]
OSF Saint Francis Medical Center • Cancer Program [5121]
OSF Saint Francis Medical Group Center • MDA Clinic [34793]
OSF Saint Joseph Medical Center • Cancer Program [5064]
OSF Saint Mary Medical Center • Speech Pathology Department [2042]
OSF SportsCare [38347]
Osiris Therapeutics Inc. [35064]
Oso Home Care, Inc. [13084]
OSPTA at Home [17281]
OSR Medical • IMSL Sleep Disorders Centre [37720]
OSR Medical Sleep Disorders Diagnostic Centre [37721]
Ossining Group Home [34344]
Osterlen Services for youth • Robert Hall Group Home [34388]
Oswego County Hospice [20594]
Oswego County Opportunities, Inc. [9923]
Oswego County Opportunities • Runaway and Homeless Youth Program [36118]
Oswego Hospital Home Aide Service [16585]
Oswego Industries [8317]
Oswego Veterans Affairs Clinic [31445]
OTA--Wakefield [2531]
Otero County Council on Alcohol Abuse and Alcoholism [46226]
Otis R Bowen Center for Human Services [43227]
Otis R. Bowen Center for Human Services [29688], [29801]
Otis R Bowen Center for Human Services Inc [43225]
   Huntington County Office [43081]
   Marshall County Office [43181]
   Whitley County Office [43009]
Otis R. Bowen Center for Human Services
   Russell House [29802]
   Shady Rest Home [29803]
   Wabash Office [29828]
   Warsaw Corporate Office [29829]
   Whitley County Office [29705]
Otsego County Community Services • Otsego Chemical Dependencies Clinic [46963]
Otsego Northern Catskills BOCES [582]
Ottagan Addictions Recovery Inc [44631], [44800], [44844]
   Chester A Ray Center [44845]
   Harbor House for Women [44846]

Ottawa Area Intermediate School District [491]
Ottawa County Community Mental Health Services • Crisis Intervention Services • Help-Line [51018]
Ottawa Dialysis • Fresenius Medical Care [24062]
Ottawa Hospital
   Multiple Sclerosis Clinic [34681]
   Regional Centre for the Treatment of Eating Disorders Outpatient Program [11228]
Ottawa Regional Hospital and Healthcare Center [14897]
Ottumwa Regional Health Center--Alta Vista Site [15100]
Ottumwa Regional Health Center • Cancer Program [5193]
OU Medical Center Sleep Disorders Center [37604]
Ouachita County Medical Center • Behavioral Health [28250]
Ouachita County Medical Center Hospice [18841]
Ouachita Medical Center • Chemical Dependency Unit [39525]
OUCH Sports Medical Center [38148]
Our Children First [29145]
Our Common Ground Inc [39793]
   Adolescent [40439]
Our Home Inc • Rediscovery Program [48999]
Our Hope Association [44812]
Our House, Inc. • Runaway and Homeless Youth Program [35976]
Our House/Nuestra Casa [8701]
Our Lady of Bellefonte Hospital [2255]
   Bellefonte Behavior Health Center [43523]
   Oncology Services [5210]
Our Lady of Confidence Day School [8493]
Our Lady of Consolation Geriatric Care Center [16658]
Our Lady of Fatima/Saint Joseph Health Services of Rhode Island • Cancer Program [5888]
Our Lady of the Lake Regional Medical Center • Cancer Program [5243]
Our Lady of the Lake University • Communication Disorders Program [3538]
Our Lady of Lourdes Dialysis Services • Renal Center of Sewell • Renal Ventures Management [25508]
Our Lady of Lourdes Hospital [20554]
Our Lady of Lourdes Medical Center--Camden • Lourdes Health System [25413]
Our Lady of Lourdes Medical Center
   Cancer Program [5505]
   Dialysis Unit [25414]
Our Lady of Lourdes Memorial Hospital, Inc. [16350]
Our Lady of Lourdes Memorial Hospital • Regional Cancer Center [5559]
Our Lady of Lourdes • Multiple Sclerosis Center [34588]
Our Lady of Lourdes Regional Medical Center [15313]
   ALS Clinic [117]
   Cancer Program [5249]
   Lourdes Sleep Disorders Center [37077]
Our Lady of Lourdes Rehabilitation Center [35469]
Our Lady of Peace [33527], [43693]
Our Lady of the Resurrection Medical Center [1998]
Our Lady's Haven Pain Management Program [35495]
Our Place Drug and Alcohol • Education Services Inc [43165]
Our Sister's Keeper [8959]
Our Sister's Place [9477]
Our Town Family Center • Runaway and Homeless Youth Services [35797]
Outagamie County Crisis Intervention Center [51501]
Outer Banks Hotline [51171]
Outer Banks Hotline, Inc. [10058]
Outfront Minnesota [9618]
Outpatient Center for Orthopedic Rehabilitation [3951]
Outpatient Center West [29234]
Outpatient New Horizons [46385]
Outpatient Rehab Center [4335]
Outpatient Services
   Wabash Valley Alliance [43160]
   Wabash Valley Alliance Inc [43015]
Outpatient Therapy Center [1036]
Outreach Development Corporation
   Greenpoint Clinic [46523]
      Outreach House I [47017]

Outreach Project Bellport/Day Program [46375]
Outreach Project Bellport/Evening Prog [46376]
Outreach Health Services, Inc. • Shubuta Medical Clinic [6896]
Outreach Home Health Services Inc. [12944]
Outreach Home Services [17136]
Outreach House II [46393]
Outreach Management Services LLC [47324]
Outreach Outpatient Services • Medically Supervised Subst Abuse Prog [47013]
Outreach Program [28984]
Outside In • Runaway and Homeless Youth Program [36173]
Outside in Pathway to Recovery Outpatient [48383]
Outstanding Home Health Care [14446]
Over the Mountain Speech, Language and Learning [904]
Overbrook School for the Blind [3733]
Overlake Hospital Medical Center [32807]
Cancer Program [6093]
Overlake Reproductive Health [22296]
Overlake Sleep Disorders Center [37921]
Overland Park Regional Medical Center • Sleep Disorders Center [37000]
Overlook Hospital
Atlantic Health Sleep Centers [37353]
Simon Cancer Center [5542]
Overlook Mobile Crisis Unit [51361]
Overlook VNA and Hospice--Charlton [19952]
Overlook VNA and Hospice--North Dartmouth [19987]
Overton Brooks VA Medical Center [15361]
Overton Brooks Veterans Affairs Medical Center [30173]
Cancer Program [5264]
PTSD Clinical Team [51742]
Overton Speech and Language Center [3495]
Owatonna Hospital [2724], [15924]
Owens Healthcare, Inc. [13256]
Owensboro Advanced Sleep Center [37038]
Owensboro Area Shelter and • Information Services [43738]
Owensboro Area Shelter and Information Services • OASIS [9397]
Owensboro Dialysis Center • DaVita [24432]
Owensboro Medical Health System Home Care [15240]
Owensboro Medical Health System
Sleep Laboratory [37039]
Speech and Audiology Clinic [2293]
Owensboro Mercy Health System • Cancer Program [5233]
Owensboro Veterans Affairs Clinic [30091]
Owl Rexall Drug [12964]
Owl's Nest Apartments [29283]
Owosso Medical Group Sleep Center [37191]
Owyhee Community Health Facility • Substance Abuse Program [45863]
Oxford City Schools [206]
Oxford County Mental Health Services [30236], [30244]
Oxford Health Care--Columbia [16003]
Oxford Health Care--Joplin [16018]
Oxford Health Care--National [16072]
Oxford Health Care--Sunshine [16073]
Oxford HealthCare--Broken Arrow [17108]
Oxford House • Lake Smith [49856]
Oxy-Med Homecare Equipment Corp. [16279]
Oxy Med, Inc. [16997]
Oxy Respiratory & Home Medical Equipment Specialist, Inc. [13419]
Oxycare of Tennessee [17654], [17757]
Oxygen One, Inc. [18638]
Oxygen Plus--Chattanooga [17652]
Oxygen Plus--Clarksville [17655]
Oxygen Plus, Inc.--Gaffney [17590]
Oxygen Plus--Jasper [17686]
Oxygen Plus--Manchester [17723]
Oxygen Plus--Murfreesboro [17747]
Oxygen Plus--Nashville [17758]
Ozanam [34269]
Ozanam Pathways [34270]
Ozark Center [51055]
Ozark Center - Community Placement Program [30855]
Ozark Center--Joplin [30856]
Turn Around Ranch [30857]
Ozark Center--Neosho [30881]

Ozark Center/New Directions
Neosho Office [45574]
New Directions/Lamar Office [45548]
Substance Abuse Unit [45509]
Virginia Street Site [45510]
Ozark Center/Ozark Oaks [30858]
Ozark Counseling Services, Inc. • Maple Corner [28280]
Ozark Counseling Services, Inc.--Marshall [28316]
Ozark Counseling Services, Inc.--Yellville [28364]
Ozark Dialysis Services--Monett • Cox Health [25246]
Ozark Dialysis Services--South • Cox Health [25292]
Ozark Guidance Center, Inc. • Assertive Community Treatment [33974]
Ozark Guidance Center, Inc.--Berryville [28246]
Ozark Guidance Center Inc.
Club of the Ozarks [33116]
Hemingway House [33126]
Ozark Guidance Center Inc.--Huntsville [33119]
Ozark Guidance Center Inc. • Miriam Enfield Center for Community Mental Health [33115]
Ozark Guidance Center, Inc.--Siloam Springs [28353]
Ozark Guidance Center, Inc.--Springdale [28354]
Ozark Guidance Center, Inc.
Watson Street Apartments [28269]
Williams Building [28355]
Ozark Home Dialysis and PD Services--Primrose • Cox Health [25293]
Ozark Mountain Alcohol Residental • Treatment Inc [39537]
Ozark Neuro Rehabilitation Center [4237]
Ozark Therapy Institute [2825]
Ozone House • Runaway and Homeless Youth Program [36023]
Ozone House Youth and Family Services [51006]
Ozzie Home Health Care [14109]

P

P-B Health Home Care Agency, Inc. [15421]
P J & M Home Care Services [14110]
P & M Home Health Services, LLC [14395]
PA Association LLC • DBA Mount Pocono [48477]
PA Treatment and Healing [48299], [48347], [48406], [48447], [48468], [48471], [48637], [48648], [48650], [48660], [48702]
PA02 Home Medical Equipment, Inc. [17374]
PAAR Center [40411]
PAAR East [40412]
PAAR West [40413]
Porterville Halfway House [40414]
PAC Program of the Bronx • CD Outpatient Clinic [46440]
Pace-Brantley Hall School [7890]
Pace Inc [41522]
PACE Juvenile Center [29856]
Pace School [32109]
Pace University • Speech and Hearing Center [3073]
Paces Counseling Associates Inc [41380]
Pachard Children's Hospital at Stanford [1218]
Pachuta Dialysis [25153]
Pacific Alcohol and • Drug Counseling Inc [48113], [48255]
Pacific Clinic [39893], [40373]
Pacific Clinic Center • Bonita Family Services [40405]
Pacific Clinics [28379], [28850], [40753]
Pacific Clinics--Bonita Family Center [28710]
Pacific Clinics Children's Services I [28697]
Pacific Clinics Children's Services II [28698]
Pacific Clinics Passageways Program [28699]
Pacific Coast Speech Services [1133]
Pacific Dialysis Services Inc. [22757]
Pacific Fertility Center [21929]
Pacific Gateway Dialysis, LLC • Innovative Dialysis Systems [22705]
Pacific Health Services Inc. [13145]
Pacific Hearing Inc. [1168]
Pacific Hearing Service [1177]
Pacific Hearing and Speech [3626]
Pacific Hills Treatment Center
Main Treatment Center and Mens Residential [40542]
Womens Residential [39683]

Pacific Home Health Care Inc. [13274]
Pacific Home Health and Hospice [20994]
Pacific Home Health Services, LLC [16916]
Pacific Hospice [19011]
Pacific Hospice Care Corp. [13146]
Pacific In Vitro Fertilization Institute [22028]
Pacific Lodge Youth Services [33211]
Pacific Pain Treatment Centers [35322]
Pacific Pulmonary Services [13498]
Pacific Pulmonary and Sleep Disorder Diagnostics Center [36871]
Pacific Reproductive Center [21930]
Pacific Respiratory Care Inc. [13475]
Pacific Rim Consulting LLC [42363]
Pacific Shores Hospital [33170]
Pacific Sleep Center [37922]
Pacific Sleep Disorders Center [36678]
Pacific Sleep Medicine Services, Inc. [36679]
Pacific Sleep Program [37623]
Pacific Sleep Tech [36872]
Pacific South Bay Dialysis Inc.
Beach Cities Dialysis--Gardena [22706]
Beach Cities Dialysis--Torrance [23037]
Coastal Dialysis Center [22898]
Pacific Speech and Language [3640]
Pacific Speech and Language Center [1265]
Pacific Sports Medicine [39152]
Pacific University - Psychological Service Center [31963]
Pacifica Hospital of the Valley • Pain Clinic [35323]
Pacifica Recovery Services [10980]
PacifiCord [34955]
PACS • Tri Hab Division of Gateway Healthcare [48868]
PACTS [41138], [41342]
Padre Behavioral Hospital [49271]
Padron Counseling Services LLC [42339]
Paducah Independent School District [445]
Paducah Professional Associates [43747]
Paducah Veterans Affairs Community Based Outpatient Clinic [30096]
Page Memorial Hospital, Inc. [18320]
Page Regional Domestic Violence Services [8704]
Pageland Dialysis • DaVita [26757]
Pagosa Recovery Center PC [41283]
Pahokee Community Clinic [6531]
Pahrump Dialysis Center • DaVita [25380]
Pahrump Mental Health Center [31042]
Pahrump Veterans Affairs Clinic [31043]
Pain Associates of Charleston [35665]
Pain Care Associates of Oklahoma [35622]
Pain Care Boise [35422]
Pain Care Center Inc. [35703]
Pain Care Center Katy [35704]
Pain Care Center Richmond [35705]
Pain Center [35623]
Pain Centers of America [35564]
Pain Clinic [35451]
Pain Clinic of Michigan [35508]
Pain Consultants of the Rockies [35778]
Pain Control and Rehabilitation Institute of Georgia [35410]
Pain Diagnostics Associates [35509]
Pain Evaluation and Rehabilitation Center [35420]
Pain Evaluation and Treatment Center--Macon, GA [35411]
Pain Evaluation and Treatment Center--Tulsa, OK [35624]
Pain Institute of Tennessee [35676]
Pain Management Association [35550]
Pain Management Center at Hamilton [35565]
Pain Management Center at Voorhees [35566]
Pain Management Clinic [35412]
Pain Management Consultants [12406]
Pain Management Group [35677]
Pain Management Institute of Santa Barbara [35324]
Pain Management and Rehab Center [35367]
Pain Management and Rehabilitation Center--Lewes [35368]
Pain Management and Rehabilitation Center-- Seaford [35369]
Pain Management and Rehabilitation Center-- Wilmington [35370]
Pain and Neurologic Care Institute [35366]
Pain and Rehab Services of the Southwest, LLC/ Rehabilitative Pain Management [35706]
The Pain and Rehabilitation Medical Group [35325], [38149]

Pain Research Institute [35744]
Pain Solutions [35556]
Pain Specialists of Southern Oregon [35637]
Pain Treatment Center [35525]
Pain Treatment Center of Baton Rouge [35470]
Paines Rosenberg and Associates PA [2412]
Painesville Veterans Affairs Clinic [31823]
Painnet Medical Group • Pain Clinic [35290]
Painsouth [35274]
Paintsville Professional Assoc LLC [43751]
Pajaro Valley Prevention and • Student Assistance [40938]
PAL Mission • Runaway and Homeless Youth Program [36148]
Palace Home Health Care [15820]
Palavra Tree • Central South West Teen Recovery Center [40571]
Palestine Dialysis Center • Fresenius Medical Care [27281]
Pali Momi Medical Center • Cancer Program [5044]
Palisades Medical Center • Sleep/Wake Center [37354]
Palladia Inc
    Comprehensive Treatment Institute [46903]
    Continuing Care Treatment [46904]
    Dreitzer Women and Children Treatment Center [46905]
    Parole Transition Program [46906]
    Starhill/Intensive Residential [46441]
Palliative Care Center and Hospice of Catawba Valley [20713]
Palliative Care/Lifeline of Hays Medical Center [19754]
Palliative Center for Caring [20603]
Palm Avenue Detox/Horizons Services Inc [40680]
Palm Bay Community Hospital • Health First Sleep Center [36801]
Palm Bay Kidney Center • Melbourne Kidney Centers [23460]
Palm Beach County Library Annex • Talking Books [3767]
Palm Beach County Public Health Department [6568]
Palm Beach ENT Associates [1793]
Palm Beach Fertility Center [22000]
Palm Beach Habilitation Center [7887], [29198]
Palm Beach Headache Center [12407]
Palm Beach Home Health Agency [13594]
Palm Beach Institute [41998]
Palm Beach Recovery Coalition • GW House [41733]
Palm Beach Vet Center [51921]
Palm Bluff Dialysis Center • DaVita [22699]
Palm Breeze Dialysis • DaVita [23433]
Palm Coast Dialysis • DaVita [23463]
Palm Desert [28176]
Palm Garden of Clearwater [1560]
Palm Garden of Largo [1631]
Palm Garden of North Miami [1677]
Palm Garden of Ocala [1685]
Palm Garden of Pensacola [1721]
Palm Garden of Port St. Lucie [1737]
Palm Garden of Tampa [1780]
Palm Health Agency [13837]
Palm House Inc • Residential Community Recovery Service [39691]
Palm Partners Recovery Centers [41636]
Palm Pediatric Therapy [1709]
Palm Springs Dialysis • DaVita [22868]
Palmdale Regional Dialysis Center • DaVita [22871]
Palmer Continuum of Care [48044]
Palmer Dialysis Center • DaVita [26423]
Palmer Program [30617]
Palmerton Dialysis Center & At Home • DaVita [26498]
Palmetto Addiction Recovery Center [43887]
Palmetto Artificial Kidney Center • Fresenius Medical Care [23465]
Palmetto Center [48933]
Palmetto Citizens Against Sexual Assault [10355]
Palmetto Coastal [21252]
Palmetto Family Healthcare Center [6534]
Palmetto Fertility Center of South Florida [22001]
Palmetto Health Baptist • Cancer Program [5903]
Palmetto Health Behavioral Care • Richland Springs [48921]
Palmetto Health Home Care & Hospice [17575]
Palmetto Health Hospice--Columbia [21222]

Palmetto Health Hospice--Newberry [21265]
Palmetto Health Hospice-Summerville [21283]
Palmetto Health Richland • Cancer Center [5904]
Palmetto Infusion Services [17615], [17626]
Palmetto Language and Speech Center LLC [3404]
Palmetto Lowcountry Behavioral Health [32210]
Palmetto Lowcountry • Behavioral Health [48912]
Palmetto Pain and Rehabilitation Physicians [35666], [39018]
Palmetto Place [29222]
Palms of Pasadena Homecare--Saint Petersburg [14369]
Palms of Pasadena Homecare--Tampa [14424]
Palms of Pasadena Hospital [14370]
    Cancer Program [4991]
Palms Pediatrics Gainesville [6467]
Palms Residential Care Facility • Mount Carmel Treatment Center [40145]
Palmyra Medical Centers [1802]
Palo Alto Center • Palo Alto Medical Foundation [22832]
Palo Alto County Office [29869]
Palo Alto Health Care System [51542]
Palo Alto Medical Foundation • Sleep Disorders Center [36680]
Palo Pinto General Hospital • Home Health Agency [18090]
Palo Verde Hospital • Palo Verde Mental Health Services [33110]
Palomar Medical Center [12994]
    Behavioral Health Services [28489]
Palos Community Hospital [14900], [42841]
    Cancer Program [5118]
Palos Community Hospital Hospice [19555]
Palos Community Hospital • Primary Care Center [42834]
Palouse Recovery Center LLC • Pullman [50069]
Palouse Regional Crisis Line [51459]
Palouse River Counseling [50070]
Panacea Services Inc • Drug and Alcohol Treatment [40496]
Panama City Dialysis Center • DaVita [23467]
Panhandle Community Services
    Panhandle Community Services Health Center [6940]
    Runaway and Homeless Youth Program [36066]
Panhandle Crisis Center [10498]
Panhandle Mental Health Center [30972], [45814]
    Chadron Community Clinic [30977]
    Substance Abuse Treatment Services [45812]
Panorama [8040]
Panorama Orthopedics • Sports Medicine Unit [38173]
Paoli Memorial Hospital
    Cancer Program [5848]
    Sleep Disorders Center [37680]
Paoli Sports Medicine Rehabilitation Center [38965]
Pape and Associates [42964]
Para-Pharm Inc. [13554]
Paraclete Counseling Center [11038]
Paradise Home Health Agency [17805]
Paradise Home Health Care Inc. [13203]
Paradise Home Health Care, LLC [13765]
Paradise Valley Hospital [13195]
Paragon Home Healthcare, Inc. [15781]
Parallax Center Inc • Chem Dependency Ambulatory Detox [46907]
Parallels [45762]
Paramos Counseling Center [42720]
Paramount Professionals Inc. [13425]
PARA's Peach Tree, Speech and Developmental Center [2050]
Parc Place [32907], [39375]
PARC Program • Penobscot Bay Medical Center [44050]
Parc West [32908]
Pardee Hospital [47379]
Parent Care Family Recovery Center [39959]
Parent--Child Center [9774]
Parent Education Infant Development Program [8586]
Parent & Infant Development Program • DC Department of Mental Health [29099]
Parenteral Infusion Associates [15540]
Parents Against Teen Suicide/T.E.A.C.H. [51163]
Parents and Children Together
    Family Peace Center, Dilligham Blvd. [9144]
    Family Peace Center, Linapuni Street [9145]

Parents' Partner Inc. [2598]
Parents Place/The Children's Center [30056]
Paris Dialysis • Dialysis Facility • DaVita [26500]
Parish of Ascension • Substance Abuse Center [43826]
Park Ave. Dialysis Center • Fresenius Medical Care Dialysis • Dialysis Center [25048]
Park Avenue Center on 24th • Mens [45222]
Park Avenue Center • Womens [45223]
Park Avenue Fertility and Reproductive Medicine [21971]
Park Avenue West Group Home [31800]
Park Bench Group Counseling LLC [46105]
Park Center Carew [29726]
Park Center Inc [43053]
    Decatur Counseling Services [43018]
Park Center Inc. [6686]
Park Center, Inc. [33447], [34125]
Park Center, Inc.--Bluffton [29702]
Park Center, Inc. • Drop In Center [33458]
Park Center, Inc.--Fort Wayne [29727]
Park Center, Inc.
    Harmony House [33459]
    Haven House [33460]
    Lee House [33461]
    Leslie House [33462]
    Noel House [33463]
    Quinn House [33464]
    Unity House [33465]
Park Center • Lifeplan--Employee Assistance Program [33466]
Park Cities Speech, Language and Hearing Center [3481]
Park County Mental Health Center [33037], [33059]
Park DuValle Community Health Center [6736]
Park Hill Dilaysis • Fresenius Medical Care [23113]
Park Hill Health Center [6416]
Park Nicollet Clinic [2679]
Park Nicollet Melrose Eating Disorders Institute [11109]
Park Nicollet Sports Medicine Center [38637]
Park Place [31005]
Park Place Center [42875]
Park Place Medical Center [7360]
Park Place Outreach and Counseling [39362]
Park Place Outreach Inc. • Runaway and Homeless Youth Program [35910]
Park Place Recovery Center [43539]
Park Place Residence [30417]
Park Plaza Dialysis • DaVita [24899]
Park Plaza Hospital • Cancer Program [6001]
Park Plaza Hospital and Medical Center • Sleep Center [37832]
Park Ridge Chemical Dependency Inc
    Adolescent Community Residence [47042]
    Womens Community Residence [47043]
Park Ridge Home Health [16726]
Park Ridge Hospital
    Cancer Program [5644]
    Dialysis Center [25765]
Park Ridge Hospital Inc • Unity Chemical Dependency [47044]
Park Ridge Hospital • Sleep Center [37478]
Park Ridge Youth Campus [33437]
Park Row Group Home [34109]
Park Slope Center for Mental Health, Inc. [31271]
Park Slope Safe Homes Project [9907]
Park West Medical Center, Inc. [6789]
Park West Men and Family Health Center [6790]
Parker Adventist Hospital [1440]
Parker Dialysis Center • DaVita [23135]
Parker Froyd and Associates • Mental Health Services [41007], [41241]
Parker Health Care services, Inc. [17887]
Parker Hearing Institute [1315]
Parker Hearing Institute of Beverly Hills [1068]
Parker Hearing and Speech Institute [1340]
Parker Jewish Institute for Health Care and Rehabilitation [16542]
Parker Valley Hope [41287]
Parkersburg Dialysis • DaVita [27686]
Parkersburg Treatment Center [50334]
Parkersburg and Wood County Public Library • Services for the Blind and Physically Handicapped [3853]
Parkland Health & Hospital System • Cancer Program [5976]

Pathways of Courage, Inc. [10709]
Pathways Day Support [32791]
Pathways • Delta County Site [30547]
Pathways - Dyer County Office [32306]
Pathways to Freedom [47557]
Pathways to Freedom LLC [41356]
Pathways--Gastonia [31534]
Pathways--Hampton [32746]
Pathways - Haywood County Office [32275]
Pathways to Healthy Living - Luce County [30612]
Pathways - Henderson County Office [32345]
Pathways Home Health and Hospice [13376]
Pathways Home Health and Hospice--Oakland [18982]
Pathways Home Health and Hospice--San Francisco [19024]
Pathways Home Health and Hospice--Sunnyvale [19058]
Pathways Home Health Services [14806]
Pathways Hospice - Community Care for Northern Colorado [19107]
    Care Center at McKee [19120]
Pathways House I [40209]
Pathways Inc [46238]
    Bath County Outpatient [43744]
    Boyd County Outpatient [43524]
    Carter County Outpatient [43608]
    Detox Plus [43525]
    Elliott County Outpatient [43777]
    Greenup County Outpatient [43611]
    Hillcrest Hall [43724]
    Lawrence County Outpatient [43672]
    Menifee County Outpatient [43598]
    Montgomery County Outpatient [43725]
    Morgan County Outpatient [43795]
    Rowan County Outpatient [43718]
Pathways, Inc.--22nd Street, Ashland [29965]
Pathways, Inc. of Ashland • Crisis Service [50928]
Pathways, Inc.--Bath Avenue, Ashland [29966]
Pathways, Inc.--Frenchburg [30018]
Pathways, Inc.--Grayson [30021]
Pathways, Inc.--Greenup [30023]
Pathways, Inc.--Greenwich [28997]
Pathways, Inc.--Louisa [30059]
Pathways, Inc.--Sandy Hook [30110]
Pathways, Inc.--West Liberty [30120]
Pathways - Lake County Office [32386]
Pathways--Marquette [30597]
Pathways--Mentor [31806]
Pathways MI • formerly Child and Family Services of Western MI [44632], [44801], [44847]
Pathways--Morehead [30082]
Pathways--Mount Sterling [30085]
Pathways--Owingsville [30094]
Pathways PA • Runaway and Homeless Youth Program [36182]
Pathways • Pathways - The Turning Point Program [32388]
Pathways Professional Counseling Inc [47992]
Pathways--Saint Helens [31973]
Pathways at Seifert Counseling Center [42613]
Pathways • The Start Program [32349]
Pathways of Tennessee Inc [49044], [49127], [49198]
    Substance Abuse Treatment Division [49092]
Pathways of Tennessee, Inc. [32319]
Pathways Therapy Center LLC [1400]
Pathways
    Tooele County Women's Shelter [10534]
    Touchstone Act [30548]
Pathways Treatment Center [49808]
    Kalispell Regional Medical Center [45706]
Patient Aids [15259]
Patient Care--Denville [16197]
Patient Care Home Health Services, LLC [13595]
Patient Care, Inc.--Mountain Lakes [16245]
Patient Care, Inc.--Passaic [16254]
Patient Care, Inc.--West Orange [16289]
Patient Care Pennsylvania, Inc.--Allentown [17235]
Patient Care Pennsylvania, Inc.--Wyomissing [17514]
Patient Care--Rochelle Park [16260]
Patient Choice Hospice and Palliative Care [19865]
Patient First Dialysis [22349]
Patient Home Health Services [15783]
Patient's Choice Home Health Care [15724]
Patient's Choice Hospice-Forrest City [18848]
Patient's Choice Hospice-Holiday Island [18855]

Patients First Health Care • Sleep Disorders Center [37278]
Patients First Home Health Agency Inc. [13394]
Patio Drugs [15329]
Patricia Ely and Associates [42818]
Patricia Kenney Counseling Services LLC [46205]
Patricia Neal Rehabilitation Center [4434]
Patrick B. Harris Psychiatric Hospital [33832]
Patrick Murphy [47235]
PATS Prevention and Treatment Svcs [42937]
Patti Hards Marriage and • Family Therapy Practice [43664]
Patti Solomon-Rice & Associates [1064]
Pattie A. Clay Regional Medical Center • Sleep Disorders Center [37040]
Patton Peer-Support Center [32281]
Patton State Hospital [33172]
Paul Booth MFT CADC NCACII [40911]
Paul J. Cooper Center for Human Services [31273]
Paul J Cooper Center for Human Services • Drug Abuse Outpatient Rehab Clinic [46524]
Paul J. Cooper Center for Human Services • Mental Health Clinic [31274]
Paul J Cooper Center for Human Services • Outpatient Alcohol/Substance Abuse Program [46525]
Paul J Kemberling LCPC [43959]
Paula J. Baber Hospice Home [19692]
Paulding County Hospital [17018]
Paulding County School District [371]
Paulding Dialysis • DaVita [23667]
Paulo Braga LCPC LCCS • Private Practice [44031]
Pauls Place [45150]
Paulson Rehabilitation Center [7976]
Paulson Rehabilitation LaGrange [2054]
Pauqette Center Reedsburg • Family Service Associates [50515]
Pauquette Center--Baraboo [32950]
Pauquette Center--Columbus [32963]
Pauquette Center for • Psychological Services [50364], [50505]
Pauquette Center--Portage [33008]
PAVE [10539]
Pavilion Behavioral Health System [33408]
The Pavilion Foundation [29575]
Pavillion • Intensive Outpatient [48947]
Pavillon [47416]
Pawnee Mental Health Services [8029], [43402]
    Belleville Office--Republic Co. Hospital [29909]
    Beloit Office [29910]
    Clay Center Office [29913]
Pawnee Mental Health Services Community Mental Health Center [29941]
Pawnee Mental Health Services
    Concordia [43329]
    Junction City [43371]
    Junction City Office [29935]
    Manhattan [43399]
    Mankato Office [29942]
    Marysville Office [29943]
    Washington Office [29960]
Pawtuxet Valley Infusion Care [17533]
Pax Christi Hospice [20586]
Payne County Drug Court [48020]
Payne County Youth Services Inc [48021]
Payne County Youth Services • Runaway and Homeless Youth Program [36158]
Paynesville Area Health Care System [2725]
Payson Regional Dialysis [27412]
Payson Regional Medical Center [12797]
Payson VA Health Care Clinic-Payson, AZ [3874]
PCC Community Wellness Center [6673]
PCC Inc/DBA Professional • Counseling Center of Delano [45121]
PCD Jacksonville [22359]
PCD Talladega • Fresenius Medical Care [22407]
PCH Home Health--Beckley [18495]
PCH Home Health--Princetone [18536]
PD Dialysis Center of Middle Tennessee • Dialysis Clinic Inc. [26909]
PDAP of Ventura County Inc [39675]
PDCI/Home Dialysis of Dayton [26097]
PDI--Ephrata • DaVita [26586]
Peabody Dialysis [27504]
Peabody Dialysis Center • Fresenius Medical Care [24792]
Peabody Health Center • AIDS Arms • AIDS Clinical Trials Unit [34]

Peace Counseling Inc [43055]
Peace for Families [8790]
Peace Harbor Hospice [21000]
Peace Harbor Hospital Home Health [17190]
Peace at Home • Battered Persons Advocacy [10256]
Peace at Home Family Shelter [8760]
Peace Hospice of Montana/Teton [20356]
Peace House [10528]
Peace Over Violence [8842]
Peace Place [9131]
Peace Rehabilitation Center • Roger C. Peace Rehabilitation Hospital [4426]
Peace River Center • Bartow Office [29106]
Peace River Center Crisis Line [50749]
Peace River Center
    Domestic Violence Shelter [9040]
    Lakeland Office [29199]
    Wauchula Office [29318]
Peace River Home Health--North Port [14272]
Peace River Regional Medical Center [1734], [14348]
Peaceful Choices [9433]
Peaceful Paths Domestic Abuse Network [9053]
Peaceful Solutions [41025]
Peaceful Solutions Counseling Services [43597]
Peacehealth • Center for Sleep Disorders [37923]
Peacehealth Dialysis Center [27616]
PeaceHealth Medical Group • Sleep Disorders Center [37924]
Peacekeepers • Domestic Violence Program [9883]
Peach State Therapy, Inc. [38320]
Peach Tree Clinic [6325]
Peachford Behavioral Health System [33370]
Peachford Behavioral Health Systems [42032]
Peachford Hospital [29353]
Peachtree Hospice, LLC-Texas [21512]
Peachtree Hospice, Poteau, LLC [20971]
Peachtree Orthopaedic Clinic [38312]
Peachtree Place Group Home [29485]
Peak Community Services, Inc. [7999]
Peak Health Services Inc [39922]
Peak Performance Physical Therapy and Sports Medicine [38648]
Peak Performance Therapy Services [1947]
PEAK Rehab Inc. [2422]
Peak Rehabilitation Group [2543]
Peak Respiratory & Sleep, Inc. [16220]
Peak Vista Community Health Centers, Inc. • Family Health Center [6392]
Peak Wellness Center [50577]
    Albany County Clinic [50588]
    Goshen County Clinic [50606]
Peak Wellness Center--Laramie [33053]
Peak Wellness Center--Seymour Avenue, Cheyenne [33035]
Peak Wellness Center • Substance Abuse Services [50607]
Peak Wellness Center--Torrington [33073]
Peak Wellness Center • Transitions Residential Program [50578]
Peak Wellness Center--W 29th Street, Cheyenne [33036]
Peak Wellness Center--Wheatland [33074]
Pear Lake Womens Program • Hope House [45166]
Pear Tree Dialysis Center • DaVita [23045]
Pearl Buck Center [8442]
Pearl Crisis Center [9610]
PEARL • Residential Program [41938]
Pearl River Dialysis [25156]
Pearl Speech Associates [2900]
Pearland Dialysis • DaVita [27286]
Pearsall Wellness Center [49482]
Peavy Switch Programs and Substance Abuse Services [32506]
PEC Inc [41999]
Pecan Valley Centers
    COPSD Program [49266]
    Stephenville Clinic [49546]
    Weatherford Clinic [49579]
Pecan Valley Mental Health and Mental Retardation Center--Stephenville [32553]
Pecan Valley Mental Health and Mental Retardation Clinic--Granbury [32471]
Pecan Valley Mental Health and Mental Retardation Clinic--Weatherford [32569]
Peconic Bay Medical Center Home Health Services [16612]

Pecos Valley Medical Center, Inc. [7002]
Pederson-Krag Center [31358]
Pederson/Krag Center Inc • Chemical Dependency
   Outpatient Program [46707], [47082], [47195]
PediaPsych • Eating Disorders Program [11295]
PediaSpeech Services for Children [1890]
PediaSpeech Services Inc. [1891]
PediaTalk LLC [2034]
Pediatria Health Care LLC [17248]
Pediatria HealthCare--Columbus [14505]
Pediatria HealthCare--Forsyth [14529]
Pediatria HealthCare--Savannah [14582]
Pediatria HealthCare--Shrewsbury [15542]
Pediatria HealthCare--Tucker [14599]
Pediatric and Adolescent Speech Therapy Associ-
   ates [1504]
Pediatric & Adult Therapy Services [3354]
Pediatric Center for Communication Feeding
   Deficiencies [1659]
The Pediatric Connection, Inc. [18261], [18372]
Pediatric Development Associates [1074]
Pediatric Development Center [8141]
Pediatric Diagnostic Center • Cystic Fibrosis Center
   [7477]
Pediatric Dialysis Unit at UCSF [22956]
Pediatric Ear, Nose and Throat of Atlanta [1827]
Pediatric Genetics Clinic • Department of Molecular
   and Human Genetics • Baylor College of Medicine
   [12352]
Pediatric Haematology • Sickle Cell Services
   Department [36398]
Pediatric Health Center [6393]
Pediatric Home Care 2000 [15317]
Pediatric Home Service [15933]
Pediatric Language Associates [2257]
Pediatric Nursing Specialists of Indiana, Inc.--
   Indianapolis [15003]
Pediatric Nursing Specialists of Indiana--Valparaiso
   [15057]
Pediatric Place, A Physiotherapy Associates
   Company [2062]
Pediatric Place--Naperville [2079]
Pediatric Place--Saint Charles [2105]
Pediatric Pulmonary Associates • Pediatric Cystic
   Fibrosis Center [7508]
Pediatric Rehabilitation Services Inc. [2896]
Pediatric Speech and Language [2731]
Pediatric Speech, Language and Learning Center
   LLC [2894]
Pediatric Speech-Language Pathologist, Inc. [1701]
Pediatric Speech and Language Services [1505]
Pediatric Speech & Language Specialists [983]
Pediatric Speech Language Therapy [2899]
Pediatric Speech Therapy Associates [1401]
Pediatric Therapies [1907]
Pediatric Therapy Associates--Dallas [3482]
Pediatric Therapy Associates--Searcy [1040]
Pediatric Therapy Center [1667]
Pediatric Therapy Connections Inc. [1999]
Pediatric Therapy of Forsyth [1805]
Pediatric Therapy Institute [1420]
Pediatric Therapy and Learning Center LLC [2319]
Pediatric Therapy Network [1341]
Pediatric Therapy Services Inc. [2704]
Pediatric Therapy Specialists [1444]
Pediatrics Dialysis Service at Wesley • Fresenius
   Medical Care [24356]
Pee Dee Coalition Against Domestic and Sexual As-
   sault [10350]
Pee Dee Dialysis Center • Fresenius Medical Care
   [26735]
Pee Dee Mental Health Center
      Adult Crisis Services [51327]
      Child Crisis Services [51328]
Pee Dee Regional Center [8503]
Pee Dee Speech and Hearing Center [3400], [3406]
Peece Keepers Inc • Peece Keepers Oak Park
   Community Center [40497]
Peekskill-Cortlandt Dialysis Center • DaVita [25647]
PEER Services Inc [42664], [42688]
Pegasus Dialysis, LLC [22597]
Pegasus-East • Psychiatric Day Treatment [28549]
Peggy Coloney's House at Hope Village • Center for
   Hope Hospice & Palliative Care [20495]
Pekin Memorial Hospital [14902]
Pelham Mental Health Center [28017]
Pelham MI Outpatient [27890]
Pelham Parkway Dialysis Center • DaVita [25596]

Pelican Bay Hearing Care [1674]
Pella Care [16408]
Pella Regional Health Center • Dialysis Unit [24295]
Pella Regional Home Health [15101]
Pelvic Pain and Reconstructive Surgery Center
   [35678]
Pembina Special Education Cooperative [639]
Pembroke Hospital [33580]
Pembroke Pines Artificial Kidney Center • KRU
   Medical Ventures [23470]
Pemi-Baker Home Health and Hospice [20453]
Pemiscot Memorial Health Systems [2790]
Pend Oreille County Counseling Center • Chemical
   Dependency Treatment [50031]
Pend Oreille County Mental Health [51452]
Pend Oreille Crime Victims Services [10630]
Pender Memorial Hospital [16701]
Pendleton Academies [34400]
Pendleton Community Care [7405]
Pendleton County Office • Northern Kentucky Com-
   munity Care [30009]
Pendleton Dialysis • DaVita [26759]
Penelope House, Inc. [8645]
Penelope's Place [9472]
Penfield Christian Homes Inc
      North Campus [42118]
      South Campus [42016]
Penfield Christians Homes Inc • Main Campus
   [42173]
Peniel Ministries • Drug and Alcohol Treatment
   Facility [48419]
Peninsula Addiction Services [44348]
Peninsula Associates [7792]
Peninsula Associates--Menlo Park [1178]
Peninsula Associates--San Mateo [1302]
Peninsula Community Health Services [7375]
Peninsula Community Mental Health Center [32846],
   [51457], [51468]
      Community Resource Center [32862]
      Substance Abuse Services [50057]
Peninsula Counseling Center • Chemical
   Dependence Treatment Services [47155]
Peninsula Counseling Center--Lawrence [31379]
Peninsula Counseling Center--Valley Stream [31486]
Peninsula Counseling Center--Woodmere [31495]
Peninsula Counseling Inc [49969]
Peninsula Dialysis Center • Dialysis Unit • DaVita
   [27520]
Peninsula Hospital [33848]
      Dual Diagnosis Program [49123]
Peninsula Lighthouse [49114]
Peninsula Medical Center • Behavioral Health
   Services [28421]
Peninsula NRH Regional Rehab [4122]
Peninsula Pharmacy [15746]
Peninsula Regional Health System • Cancer
   Program [5313]
Peninsula Regional Medical Center [6800]
      ALS Clinic [118]
Peninsula Sleep Center, Inc. [36681]
Peninsula Vet Center [51891]
Penn Care at Home [17356]
Penn Care at Home King of Prussia [17357]
Penn Foundation Inc • Recovery Center [48639]
Penn Home Infusion Therapy [17358]
Penn Presbyterian Medical Center [48552], [48553]
Penn Square Clinic [32465]
Penn State Milton S. Hershey Medical Center •
   Penn State Eating Disorder Program [11253]
Penn State University • Milton Hershey Medical
   Center • Pain Management [35647]
Penn Valley Dialysis Clinic • Fresenius Medical Care
   [25224]
Penndel Mental Health Center [32061]
Pennock Hospital Home Care Services [15682]
Pennock Hospital • Michigan Pain Consultants
   [35510]
Pennsauken Dialysis Center and At Home • DaVita
   [25497]
Pennsylvania Comprehensive Hemophilia and
   Thrombosis Program • University of Pennsylvania
   Hospital [12589]
Pennsylvania Counseling Services [48320]
      Carlisle [48317]
      Gettysburg Psychiatric [48381]
      Harrisburg [48397]
      Lancaster City [48431]
      Reading City [48628]

Reading Psychiatric [48629]
Renaissance [48444]
York [48713]
Pennsylvania Department of Health • Maternal Child
   Health Outreach [36534]
Pennsylvania Dialysis Clinic of Reading Inc. [26617]
Pennsylvania Hospital • Sleep Disorders Center
   [37681]
Pennsylvania School for the Deaf [707]
Pennsylvania State Milton S. Hershey Medical
   Center • Cancer Program [5831]
Pennsylvania State University
      Hershey Medical Center
         Cystic Fibrosis Center [7655]
         Multiple Sclerosis Diagnostic and Evaluation
            Center [34693]
      Milton S. Hershey Medical Center
         Division of Human Genetics, Growth and
            Development Down Syndrome Clinic
            [10857]
         Section of Neurology MDA Clinic [34868]
The Pennsylvania State University School of
   Medicine • Milton S. Hershey Medical Center •
   Department of Pediatrics • Cancer Genetics
   Program [12328]
Pennsylvania State University • Speech and Hearing
   Clinic [3383]
Pennsylvania Training and Technical Assistance
   Network • Pennsylvania Deafblind Initiative [709]
Penny Lane Centers [28444]
      Doctor Rose Jenkins Memorial Clinic [28652]
      Main Facility [34002]
      Satellite I [28653]
      Satellite II [28654]
      Satellite IV [28845]
      Satellite IX [28846]
      Satellite V [28655]
      Satellite VI [28520]
      Satellite VII [28658]
      Satellite VIII [28659]
Pennyroyal Center
      Adult Clinic [43631]
      Pennyroyal Childrens Services [43632]
Pennyroyal Hospice [19807]
Pennyroyal Mental Health Services
      Caldwell County Mental Health Center [43766]
      Muhlenberg County MH/MR Center [43613]
Pennyroyal MH/MR Board [43706]
Pennyroyal Regional Mental Health Center • Hop-
   kinsville Crisis Line [50934]
Penobscot Bay Medical Center • Cancer Program
   [5276]
Penobscot Community Health Center, Inc. [6767]
Penobscot County Metro Treatment Center [43932]
Penobscot Nation Counseling Services • Penobscot
   Nation Health Department [43988]
Penobscot Pediatrics [6768]
Penobscot Sports Associates [38505]
Penquis • Runaway and Homeless Youth Program
   [35984]
Penrod Counseling Center [42987], [43109]
Penrose Saint Francis Health Services • Regal
   Center for Behavioral Health [41067]
Pentacare Health Network [14111]
Pentech Health [17260]
People Acting To Help Inc [48554]
People Against A Violent Environment [10692]
People Against Domestic Abuse [10708]
People Against Rape [10359]
People Against Violent Environments [9199]
People Assuming Control of their Environment
   [2116]
People Care Inc.--Hicksville [16488]
People Care, Inc.--New York [16561]
People Care Inc.--Patchogue [16591]
People Care Inc.--White Plains [16672]
People Coord Services of Southern CA
      Castle Subst Abuse Prog/Residential [40146]
      Castle Substance Abuse Prog/Outpt [40147]
People Encouraging People Inc • Co-Occuring
   Disorders Program [44169]
People Helping People in Need [46071]
People Inc • Huss Recovery Services [45224]
People Inc of • Sequoyah County [48013], [48026]
People Incorporated [30659]
People Incorporated--Heather Ridge [30704]
People Incorporated • Upton House [30711]
People, Inc. of Virginia [10551]

People in Progress
  Outpatient Services [40148]
  Sun Valley Community Rehab Center [40834]
Peoplefirst Rehabilitation [19815]
People's Clinic • Broadway and San Juan Peoples Clinic [6388]
Peoples Community Addictions Program [44170]
People's Community Health Clinics [6715]
Peoples Health Center--Indianapolis [6692]
People's Health Center--Lincoln [6941]
People's Health Centers Inc.--Saint Louis [6920]
People's Hospice [21789]
Peoria Treatment Center [41008]
Pequot Health Center [1463]
Perception Programs Inc • Perception House [41497]
Perfect Solutions Inc [45051]
Performance Chiropractic and Sports Rehabilitation [38430]
Performance Physical Therapy [38256]
Performance Physical Therapy of Bridgeview [38349]
The Performance Place Sports Medicine [39122]
Perham Memorial Hospital and Home [15927]
Perinatal Services and Next Step Intensive Outpatient Treatment [40969]
Perinatal Treatment Services [50120]
Peritech Home Health Associates, Inc. [17302]
Peritoneal Dialysis Center of America, Inc. [22824]
Peritoneal Dialysis Center of Northwest Ohio • Innovative Dialysis Systems [26213]
Peritoneal Dialysis Concepts Inc. [26098]
Perkins Counseling Center [45282]
Perkins Medical Supply [14440]
Perkins School for the Blind [3714]
  Braille and Talking Book Library [3802]
  Deafblind Program [2534]
Permanente Medical Group • Sickle Cell Disease Center [36304]
Permian Basin Community Centers [51388]
Permian Basin Community Centers for Mental Health/Mental Retardation [32514]
Permian Basin Community Centers for MH/MR • Johnson Center [49466]
Permian Basin Community Centers • Turning Point [49472]
Permian Basin Dialysis Center • Fresenius Medical Care [27259]
Permian Regional Medical Center [17795]
Perris Valley Recovery Programs [40382]
Perry A. Klaassen Family Medical Center [7111]
Perry Behavioral Health Choices Inc [47825]
Perry Counseling Center [31818]
Perry County Counseling Center Inc
  Mental Health Services [42634]
  Outpatient Treatment Services [42635]
Perry County Medical Center, Inc. [7263]
Perry County Memorial Hospital [16039]
Perry County Services [29819]
Perry County Treatment Services [43623]
Perry Dialysis Center • DaVita [23770]
Perry Dialysis Centers • Fresenius Medical Care [25254]
Perry Dialysis • DaVita [23478], [24296]
Perry Human Services [48479]
Perry Point VA Medical Center [4123]
Perry Point Veterans Affairs Center [30304]
Perry's Place [30198]
Persad Center Inc [48602]
Persad • Runaway and Homeless Youth Program [36183]
Pershing County Domestic Violence Intervention [9795]
Person Family Medical Center, Inc. [7057]
Person to Person Consulting [42134]
Personal Best Speech Services [1540]
Personal Care Home Health Services, Inc. [17361]
Personal Consulting Services [46154]
Personal Counseling Services [42919]
Personal Crisis Service [51075]
Personal Development • An Affinity Inc Company [42357]
Personal Development Center--Marshfield [10716]
Personal Development Center--Neillsville [10727]
Personal Development • Foundations in Recovery [42315]
Personal Dialysis Inc. [24817]
Personal Enrichment through Mental Health

Services, Inc. [50782]
Personal Enrichment Through Mental Health [33354]
Personal Enrichment Through Mental Health Services [33349]
Personal and Family Counseling Services • Harbor House [47826]
Personal Frontiers Inc [50584]
Personal Growth Behavioral Health Inc [41575]
Personal HeomeCare, Inc. [18387]
Personal Home Care Skilled Services, Inc. [15756]
Personal Nursing Care [17152]
Personal Relationships Inc. [10883]
Personal Therapy PLC [1018]
Personal Touch Home Care and Hospice [21711]
Personal Touch Home Health Care [15640]
Personal Touch Home Healthcare, Inc. [15821]
Personalized Home Care Ltd. of Connecticut--Bridgeport [13514]
Personalized Home Care Ltd. of Connecticut--Stamford [13542]
Personalized Home Care Ltd. of Connecticut--West Haven [13552]
Personalized Home Care of New Jersey--Cliffside Park [16194]
Personalized Home Care of New Jersey--Newark [16250]
Personalized Nursing Light House Inc [44645], [44963]
Perspectives Counseling Center [45027]
Perspectives Counseling Services LLC • Adult Intensive Outpatient Program [39508]
Perspectives of Troy PC [45038]
Perth Amboy Dialysis Center • DaVita [25498]
Peru Dialysis • Fresenius Medical Care [24220]
Petaluma Health Care District • Petaluma Health Center [6340]
Petaluma Valley Hospital [13244]
Peterborough Regional Health Centre
  Adult Eating Disorder Program [11229]
  Youth Eating Disorder Program [11230]
Petersburg Health Care Alliance [7362]
Petersburg Mental Health Services [28115]
Petersburg Mental Health Services Inc [39347]
Peterson Hospice • Hill Country Memorial Hospice [21503]
Peterson Regional Medical Center [18026]
Pharmacist Home Medical [17660]
Pharmatrend Infusions [14577]
PharmHealth Infusion, Inc. [16615]
PHASE Inc [42410]
PHASE, Inc./WAVE Program [9248]
Phase Piggy Back Inc
  ARU [46908]
  Striver House [46909]
PHC of MI Inc/DBA Pioneer Counseling • Centers Farmington Hills [45058]
P.H.C. Services, LTD. [16683]
PHC Services LTD.--Bronx [16368]
PHC Services LTD.--Brooklyn [16409]
PHC Services LTD.--Hempstead [16481]
PHCS I, Inc. [18178]
Pheasant Run [28138]
Phelps County Regional Medical Center [2812]
  Delbert Day Cancer Institute [5457]
Phelps County Regional Medical Center Health Services, Inc. [16046]
Phelps Hospice, Phelps Memorial Hospital Center [20607]
Phelps Memorial Health Center [16104]
Phelps Memorial Hospital Center [16625]
  Alcohol Treatment Services [46966]
  CD Inpatient Rehabilitation Program [47080]
  Chem Dependency Outpatient Rehab [46967]
Phelps Regional Homecare [20331]
Phelps Threshold • Alcohol Outpatient Clinic [47128]
Phenix City Dialysis Center • DaVita [22391]
PHHC, LLC [16887]
Philadelphia Center for Human Development [33818]
Philadelphia District Health Center Number 10 [7178]
Philadelphia District Health Center Number 9 [7179]
Philadelphia Elwyn [32098]
Philadelphia Home Care Agency [17422]
Philadelphia Suicide and Crisis Center [51292]
Philadelphia VA Medical Center [4401]
  Addiction Recovery Unit [48555]
  Opioid Treatment Program [48556]

Philadelphia Veterans Affairs Medical Center [32099]
  Cancer Care Program [5853]
  VISN 4 Eastern Regional Sleep Center [37682]
Philhaven Behavioral Health [33810]
Philhaven--Elizabethtown [33803]
Philhaven--Harrisburg [33805]
Philhaven--Lancaster [33807]
Philhaven--Lebanon [33808]
Philhaven--Leola [33809]
Philio Inc • DBA New Concepts [47867]
Philip J. Bosha, MD [39068]
Philip J. Rock Center and School • Project Reach: Illinois Deaf--Blind Services [2044]
Philippians Management Company [14463]
Phillippi Cottage [19450]
Phillips City Domestic Violence Program [9755]
Phillipsburg Dialysis Center • Fresenius Medical Care [25499]
Phoebe Home Care--Albany [14470]
Phoebe Home Care--Americus [14472]
Phoebe Home Care--Edison [14527]
Phoebe Physical Medicine Center [1803]
Phoebe Putney Memorial Hospital [14471]
  Phoebe Cancer Center [5005]
Phoebe Sumter Hospice [19342]
Phoebe's Home [10449]
Phoenix Academy of Austin [49234]
Phoenix Associates Counseling Services [49217], [49340], [49350]
Phoenix Associates of Hancock Cnty LLC [43072]
Phoenix Behavioral Health Services LLC [50455]
Phoenix Center [29500], [48948]
The Phoenix Center [29515]
Phoenix Center Behavioral Health Services [42101]
Phoenix Center • Child and Family Counseling Center [29501]
Phoenix Center Crisis Stabilization [29502]
Phoenix Center Day Treatment Center [28454]
Phoenix Center • Peach County Office [29429]
Phoenix Children's Hospital [971]
  Adult Cystic Fibrosis Center [7461]
  Dialysis Center [22485]
  Hemophilia and Thrombosis Center [12482]
  Pediatric Cystic Fibrosis Center [7462]
Phoenix Children's Hospital Renal Transplant Center [22486]
Phoenix Counseling Center [47494]
Phoenix Counseling Center Inc [48175]
Phoenix Crisis Center [9231]
Phoenix East Valley Vet Center [51864]
Phoenix Health Center LLC [44294]
Phoenix Hickory [47384]
Phoenix Home [34024]
Phoenix Home Care [14703]
Phoenix Hospice • Home Care and Hospice Services, Mendocino County [19080]
Phoenix House [29833], [49442]
Phoenix House Academy of Dallas [49293]
Phoenix House Academy of Long Island [47156]
Phoenix House Academy of Los Angeles [39976]
Phoenix House Academy of San Diego [39780]
Phoenix House Academy of Westchester [47079]
Phoenix House/Arbour House [44485]
Phoenix House Career Academy [46526]
Phoenix House
  Carlsbad Teen Recovery Center [39684]
  Community Residential [46527]
Phoenix House Counseling Center • Phoenix Houses of the Mid-Atlantic [49763]
Phoenix House Day Services [29503]
Phoenix House
  Delaware County Center [47084]
  Domestic Violence/Sexual Assault Services [9324]
  Hauppauge Center [46683]
Phoenix House Inc [39297], [44833]
  Residential Substance Abuse Program [44686]
Phoenix House, Jack Aron Center • Riverside Community Residential [46910]
Phoenix House • Keene Center [45902]
Phoenix House of Long Island
  Brentwood Outpatient Program [46394]
  Lake Ronkonkoma Campus - Mens Program [46746]
  Mental Health Community Residential [47173]
Phoenix House • Mother and Child Program [46747]
Phoenix House of New England [48875]
  Dublin Center/Adult Residential [45895]

Phoenix House of New England Inc • Phoenix
House Academy of Maine [43920]
Phoenix House of New England
    Phoenix Academy at Dublin [45896]
    Phoenix Academy at Wallum Lake [48862]
    Phoenix House Exeter Center [48851]
    Sympatico [48884]
Phoenix House of New York • Outpatient and
Residential Programs [46442]
Phoenix House
    Orange County [40720]
    Outpatient Center [48890]
Phoenix House Outpatient Services of Western MA
[44585]
Phoenix House RISE II [49719]
Phoenix House
    RTC/Long Island City/Queens [46764]
    Short-Term Residential Program [46443]
Phoenix House of Texas [49391]
Phoenix House of Texas Inc [49211]
Phoenix House/Venice [40903]
Phoenix Houses of California • Santa Fe Springs
Center [40754]
Phoenix Houses of Florida [41588]
    Derek Jeter Center at Phoenix House [41969]
Phoenix Houses of New England
    Brattleboro/Rise Program [49729]
    Springfield Center [44586]
Phoenix Medical Supply, Inc. [15822]
Phoenix Neurological Associates • Multiple Sclerosis
Center [34516]
Phoenix Place [31652]
Phoenix Preferred Care [43717]
Phoenix Program • Phoenix Houses of the Mid-
Atlantic [49764]
Phoenix Programs Inc [45465]
Phoenix Recovery Center Inc [44249]
Phoenix Recovery Programs [45197]
Phoenix Recovery Services LLC [50024]
Phoenix Recovery Systems [43409]
Phoenix Residence I [29320]
Phoenix Residence II • Oakwood Center of the Palm
Beaches [29321]
Phoenix of Santa Barbara Inc [40732]
Phoenix Training Institute [48266]
Phoenix Union High School District • Hearing
Research Program [233]
Phoenix VA Healthcare System • Substance Abuse
Treatment Program [39444]
Phoenix Veterans Affairs Health Care System
[51532]
Phoenixville Hospital • Cancer Center [5857]
Phone-a-Friend Crisis Line [50904]
Physical Fitness Center [38313]
Physical Medicine at Phoebe Northwest [38301]
Physical Therapy Center [38200]
Physical Therapy Center of Elmbrook [39172]
Physical Therapy First, LLC [38517]
Physical Therapy Plus [38992]
Physical Therapy Services [39169]
Physical Therapy and Sports Injury Rehabilitation
[38348]
Physical Therapy & Sports Injury Rehabilitation--
Hazel Crest [38379]
Physical Therapy & Sports Injury Rehabilitation Ltd.--
Lansing [38387]
Physical Therapy & Sports Injury Rehabilitation--
Tinley Park [38414]
Physical Therapy and Sports Medicine [38508]
Physical Therapy and Wellness Institute [38978]
Physical Therapy & Wellness Institute--Lansdale
[38952]
Physician Alliance for Mental Health [47525]
Physician Diagnostics Sleep Program [37123]
Physician Hearing Center [2260]
Physician Preferred Home Health Services [17905]
Physician Support Associates [14545]
Physicians' Center for Sleep Disorders [37041]
Physicians Choice in Care, LLC [20963]
Physician's Choice Diagnostic Sleep Center [36983]
Physicians Choice Dialysis--East Montgomery •
DaVita [22377]
Physicians Choice Dialysis--Montgomery • DaVita
[22378]
Physicians Choice Dialysis--Prattville • DaVita
[22393]
Physician's Choice Hearing and Dizziness Center--
Sun City Center [1765]

Physician's Choice Hearing and Dizziness Center--
Tampa [1781]
Physician's Dialysis--Fitchburg • DaVita [24767]
Physicians Dialysis Inc. • DaVita [23180]
Physicians Dialysis of Lancaster • Dialysis Facility &
At Home • DaVita [26460]
Physicians Dialysis North Houston • DaVita [27167]
Physicians Dialysis South Houston • DaVita [27168]
Physicians Health Center [34902]
Physicians' Hearing Services--Laguna Hills [1143]
Physicians Hearing Services--Raleigh [3191]
Physicians' Pain and Rehabilitation Specialists
[35413]
Physicians Plus [38741]
Physician's Therapy Group [1010]
Physio, Inc. Physical and Occupational Therapy
[39076]
Physiotherapy Associates - Legacy [38696]
Physiotherapy Associates--Owings Mills [38530]
Physiotherapy Associates--Tampa [38292]
Physiotherapy Associates--Timonium • Merritt
Athletic Club [38535]
Physiotherapy Association--Birmingham [37997]
Physiotherapy Works, LLC [38299]
Pias Place [39457]
Piatt County Mental Health Center [29649], [42785]
Pickaway Area Recovery Services [47674]
Pickaway Dialysis Center • American Renal Associ-
ates [26058]
Pickhaven Centre • Private Care Facility for Eating
Disorders [10890]
Pickwick Dialysis • Dialysis Facility • DaVita [26919]
Piedmont Community Services [49812]
Piedmont Community Services--Martinsville [32767]
Piedmont Community Services--Rocky Mount
[32785]
Piedmont Community Services--Stuart [32790]
Piedmont Counseling Services [47349]
Piedmont Dialysis Center • Wake Forest University
[25980]
Piedmont Fayette Hospital • Cancer Center [4669]
Piedmont Geriatric Hospital [33898]
Piedmont Home Care [16746]
Piedmont Hospital • Cancer Program [5010]
Piedmont Hospital Transplant [23603]
Piedmont Medical Center • Cancer Center [5913]
Piedmont Mental Health Clinic [51338]
Piedmont Orthopaedic Complex [38322]
Piedmont Physical Medicine and Rehabilitation •
Pain Clinic [35667]
Piedmont Psychological Practice [50601]
Piedmont Regional Feeding and Oral--Motor Clinic
LLC [3596]
Piedmont Reproductive Endocrinology Group
[22202], [22244]
Piedmont School [8381]
Piedmont Sleep Center [37737]
Pierce and Agnew LLC [49476]
Pierce County Alliance [50213]
Pierce County Dept of Human Services • Alcohol
and Other Drug Abuse Services [50386]
Pierremonte Dialysis • Fresenius Medical Care
[24588]
Pierson Medical Center [6539]
Pike County Home Health and Hospice [20282]
Pike County Partnership Against Domestic Violence
[10182]
Pike County Recovery Council • Alcohol and Drug
Outpatient Treatment [47880]
Pike Street Clinic [6727]
Pikes Peak Behavioral Health Group
    Administrative & Business Office [28871]
    First Choice Counseling [28872]
Pikes Peak Center on Deafness [1389]
Pikes Peak Dialysis Center • DaVita [23103]
Pikes Peak Hospice and Palliative Care of Colorado
Springs, Inc. [19094]
Pikes Peak Mental Health Center [7834]
    Adult Services Network [28873]
    Child and Family Center [28874]
Pikesville Dialysis • DaVita [24712]
Piketon Family Health Centers [7096]
Piketon Regional Dialysis Center • American Renal
Associates [26184]
Pikeville Medical Center • Cancer Program [5235]
Pikeville Medical Center Home Health Agency
[15246]
Pikeville Medical Center

Sleep Center [37042]
    Sleep Related Breathing Disorders Lab [37043]
Pikeville Treatment Center [43758]
Pilgrim Psychiatric Center [33728]
    Buckman Center [33729]
    Peconic Center [33718]
    Progress House [33730]
    Western Suffolk Center [33731]
Pillars [42732], [42824]
Pillars Community Service [9253]
Pillars Community Services [42702]
Pilsen Inn Residential Program • Community Crisis
Center [29594]
Pilsen Little Village CMHC [42567]
Pilsen Little Village Community Mental Health
Center, Inc. [29595]
    Vocational/Psychosocial Program [29596]
Pilsen Wellness Center [42927]
Pilsen Wellness Center Inc [42568], [42776]
Pima Community College • Disabled Student
Resources [240]
Pima Lund & Sleep, PC [36631]
Pin Oak Dialysis • DaVita [27200]
Pinal County Domestic Violence Coalition [8681]
Pine Belt Mental Healthcare Resources [30779],
[45428]
    Greene County [45401]
    Marion County Office [45368]
    Oak Arbor [45381]
    Perry County Office [45416]
    Region 12 [45382]
Pine City Dialysis • DaVita [25061]
Pine Grove [33699]
Pine Grove Counseling Center of Meridian [30793]
Pine Grove Life Focus [30770]
Pine Grove Recovery Center [30771]
Pine Haven Boy's Center [34292]
Pine Heights Treatment Center [44171]
Pine Hills Family Health Center [6529]
Pine Island Kidney Center • DaVita [23483]
Pine Island Medical and Dental Office [6545]
Pine Manor Inc • Chemical Dependency Services
[45246]
Pine Medical Center [2745]
Pine Rest Christian Hospital • Health Services
[33596]
Pine Rest Christian Mental Health Services [33598],
[33604]
Pine Rest Christian Mental Hlth Services
    Caledonia Clinic [44685]
    Campus Clinic [44813]
    Hispanic Recovery Program [44814]
    Holland Clinic [44848]
    Kalamazoo Clinic [44871]
    Southwest Clinic [44826]
Pine Rest
    Demey Center [44815]
    Jellema House [44816]
    Jellema Treatment Center [44817]
Pine Rest--Zeeland Clinic [30657]
Pine Ridge Outpatient Center [40529]
Pine Ridge Treatment Center [40185], [40347],
[40477], [40916]
Pine Ridge Vet Center Outstation [52091]
Pine Street Dialysis • Fresenius Medical Care
[23746]
Pine Tree Hospice [19893]
Pine Tree Society [2349]
Pine Valley Day Treatment [28317]
Pine Valley Rehabilitative Day Services • Augusta
Inn [28235]
Pine View Apartments [27875]
Pine Woods • Crisis Stabilization, Respite Care
[29365]
Pinecrest [31775]
Pinecrest Dialysis Center • DaVita [27249]
Pinecrest Supports and Services Center [8073]
Pineland Area MH/MR/SA CSB
    Appling Counseling Center [29366]
    Appling- Jeff Davis Service Center [29367]
    Toombs Service Center [29462]
    Wayne Service Center [29446]
Pineland Mental Health [50810]
Pineland MH/MR/SA CSB • Womens Place [42158]
Pinellas County Schools [351]
Pinellas Emergency Mental Health Services [50787]
Pinellas Talking Book Library [3768]
Pinellas West Shore Dialysis • DaVita [23504]

Pines Behavioral Health Services [44715], [51012]
Pines and Cady Hills Chemical • Dependency Treatment Center [45370]
Pines Home Health Care Services, Inc. [13636]
The Pines Residential Treatment Center [34464]
Pines Treatment Center [43899]
Pineview Recovery Center [45186]
Pineville Community Hospital Association, Inc. • Home Health Agency [15247]
Pineywoods Hospice Inc [21427]
A Pineywoods Hospice, Inc. [21528]
Pinnacle Dialysis of Boca Raton • DaVita [23242]
Pinnacle Health Home Care [17335], [17458]
Pinnacle Health Hospitals - Polyclinic • Speech and Hearing Center [3336]
Pinnacle Health Rehab Options [35648]
Pinnacle Health System • Regional Cancer Center [5830]
Pinnacle Health Transplant Unit at Harrisburg Hospital [26441]
Pinnacle Physical Therapy [39069]
Pinnacle Pointe Hospital [33122]
Pinnacle Sports Medicine and Orthopaedics [38460]
Pinnacle Treatment • DBA State Line Medical [46133]
Pioneer Adult Counseling Tacoma • Pioneer Human Services [50214]
Pioneer Center Clay Group Home [29646]
Pioneer Center East [50178]
Pioneer Center of McHenry County [29647]
Pioneer Center North • Branch of Pioneer Human Services [50145]
Pioneer Counseling Center • Sterling Heights [45028]
Pioneer Counseling Services • Branch of Pioneer Human Srvs/Adult [50121]
Pioneer Counseling Services--Evanston [33039]
Pioneer Counseling Services--Farmington Hills [30549]
Pioneer Counseling Services--Lyman [33056]
Pioneer Counseling Services • Spokane Branch [50179]
Pioneer Counseling - Spanaway [50161]
Pioneer Family Medical of Hamilton • Sleep Disorders Center [37257]
Pioneer Medical, Inc. [17759]
Pioneer Medical Services--Beckley [18496]
Pioneer Medical Services--Man [18522]
Pioneer Memorial Home Health and Hospice [21003]
Pioneer Memorial Hospice-Prineville [21027]
Pioneer Memorial Hospital Home Care [17642]
Pioneer Recovery Center [45079]
Pioneer Valley Dialysis Center • Fresenius Medical Care [24812]
Pioneer Vocational/Industrial Services [8041]
Pioneer Youth Home [34280]
Pipestone Dialysis • DaVita [25062]
Pit River Health Service Inc • Substance Abuse Program [39671]
Pitt County Memorial Hospital
    Pain Management Center [35594]
    Regional Rehabilitation Center [8379]
Pitt County Memorial Hospital Transplant Program • University Health Systems [25880]
Pitt County Memorial Hospital • University Health Systems of Eastern Carolina • Leo W. Jenkins Cancer Center [5642]
Pittard Clinic [42172]
Pittsburg County Health Department [7108], [31891]
Pittsburgh Center for Sports Medicine • Shadyside Hospital [38973]
Pittsburgh County Health Department • Speech and Hearing Clinic [3272]
Pittsburgh Cryobank [35193]
Pittsburgh Dialysis & At Home • DaVita [26563]
Pittsfield Public Schools • Hearing Impaired Program [477]
Place of Hope Inc [49062]
Placentia/Yorba Linda Unified School District [289]
Placer County Mental Health Services [33128], [33177]
Placer County Mental Health Services--Auburn [28385]
Placer County Mental Health Services--Roseville [28726]
Placer Extends A Caring Environment for Families [8877]

Placer Hearing [1244]
Placerville Dialysis Center • DaVita [22882]
Places for People [45623]
Places for People, Inc. [30900]
Plainfield Dialysis Center & At Home • DaVita [25500]
Plainfield Health Care Center [2178]
Plains Area Mental Health Center [29847]
Plains Regional Dialysis Center • Fresenius Medical Care [25542]
Plains Regional Medical Center
    Home Health and Hospice [16308]
    Portales Home Healthcare [16323]
Plainview/Old Bethpage Youth Activity • DBA Reflection Counseling Center [46977]
Plainview Serenity Center Inc [49456]
    Mens Residential [49487]
Plan De Salud Del Valle, Inc. • SALUD Family Health Center [6405]
Planet Home HealthCare [13785]
Planned Parenthood of Alabama
    Birmingham Center [11313]
    Hattiesburg Health Center [11676]
    Mobile Center [11314]
Planned Parenthood of Arizona
    Archer Health Center [11320]
    Chandler Health Center [11321]
    Flagstaff Health Center [11322]
    Glendale Health Center [11323]
    Jean Hoffman Health Center [11324]
    Margaret Sanger Health Center [11325]
    Maryvale Health Center [11326]
    Mesa Health Center [11327]
    North East Phoenix Health Center [11328]
    Prescott Health Center [11329]
    Scottsdale Health Center [11330]
    Southwest Valley Health Center [11331]
    Tempe Health Center [11332]
    Yuma Health Center [11333]
Planned Parenthood of Arkansas and Eastern Oklahoma
    Broken Arrow Health Center [11867]
    Midtown Health Center--Family Planning [11868]
    Midtown Health Center--Pediatrics [11869]
    Midtown Health Center: Prenatal [11870]
    Pharmacy Center [11871]
    South Peoria Health Center [11872]
    Westside Health Center [11873]
Planned Parenthood Associates of Cameron and Willacy Counties
    Alice Family Planning Health Center [11951]
    Kingsville Family Planning Center [11952]
Planned Parenthood Association of Bucks County
    Bensalem Health Center [11896]
    Bristol Health Center [11897]
    Quakertown Health Center [11898]
    Warminster Health Center [11899]
Planned Parenthood Association of Cameron and Willacy Counties
    Brownsville Clinic [11953]
    Harlingen Clinic [11954]
    Southmost Clinic [11955]
Planned Parenthood Association of Hidalgo County [11956]
    Bruce Galloway Health Center [11957]
    Edinburg Health Center [11958]
    Progreso Community Center [11959]
    Rio Grande City Center [11960]
    San Carlos Community Center [11961]
    San Juan Community Center [11962]
    Weslaco Health Center [11963]
Planned Parenthood Association of Lubbock • Lubbock Health Center [11964]
Planned Parenthood Association of the Mercer Area
    College of New Jersey Health Center [11720]
    Hamilton Health Center [11721]
    Trenton Health Center--Unit 1 [11722]
    Trenton Health Center--Unit 2 [11723]
Planned Parenthood Association of Utah - Metro Health Center [12025]
Planned Parenthood Association of Utah • Salt Lake Clinic [12026]
Planned Parenthood of Austin Family Planning
    Downtown Austin Clinic--Express Clinic [11965]
    Downtown Austin Clinic--Teen Clinic [11966]
Planned Parenthood of Austin Surgical and Sexual Health Services
    North Austin Clinic [11967]

South Austin Clinic [11968]
Planned Parenthood of Central New Jersey
    Freehold Health Center [11724]
    Hazlet Health Center [11725]
    New Brunswick Center [11726]
    Perth Amboy Health Center [11727]
    Shrewsbury Health Center [11728]
    Spotswood Health Center [11729]
Planned Parenthood of Central North Carolina
    Chapel Hill Health Center [11824]
    Durham Health Center [11825]
    Fayetteville Health Center [11826]
Planned Parenthood of Central Ohio
    Athens Health Center [11833]
    Central Ohio Women's Center [11834]
    Circleville Health Center [11835]
    Delaware Health Center [11836]
    East Health Center [11837]
    Franklinton Health Center [11838]
    North/Campus Health Center [11839]
    Orchard Centre Health Center [11840]
Planned Parenthood of Central Oklahoma
    Central Oklahoma City Clinic [11874]
    Edmond Clinic [11875]
    Midwest City Clinic [11876]
    Norman Clinic [11877]
    South Oklahoma City Clinic [11878]
Planned Parenthood of Central Pennsylvania
    Chambersburg Health Center [11900]
    Gettysburg Health Center [11901]
    Hanover Health Center [11902]
    Red Lion Health Center [11903]
    York Health Center [11904]
Planned Parenthood of Central Texas
    Marlin Health Center [11969]
    Mary Ruth Duncan Women's Health Center [11970]
Planned Parenthood Choice • San Angelo Center [11971]
Planned Parenthood of Collier County
    Immokalee Health Center [11490]
    Naples Health Center [11491]
Planned Parenthood of the Columbia/Willamette
    Beaverton Health Center [11879]
    Central Oregon Health Center [11880]
    Clackamas Health Center [11881]
    Gresham Health Center [11882]
    McMinnville Clinic [11883]
    Northeast Portland Health Center [11884]
    Salem Health Center [11885]
    Salmon Creek Health Center [12054]
    Southeast Portland Health Center [11886]
Planned Parenthood of the Columbia/Williamette • Mount Hood Community College [11887]
Planned Parenthood of the Columiba/Willamette • Vancouver Center [12055]
Planned Parenthood of Connecticut • New Haven Health Center [11466]
Planned Parenthood of Delaware
    Dover Health Center [11484]
    Newark Delaware Health Center [11485]
    Rehoboth Beach Health Center [11486]
    Wilmington Health Center [11487]
Planned Parenthood of Georgia
    Atlanta Health Center [11514]
    Cobb Health Center [11515]
    Gwinnett Health Center [11516]
    Savannah Health Center [11517]
Planned Parenthood of the Great Northwest
    Anchorage Health Center [11315]
    Bellevue Health Center [12056]
    Boise Health Center [11522]
    Bremerton Health Center [12057]
    Centralia Health Center [12058]
    Everett Health Center [12059]
    Fairbanks Health Center [11316]
    Federal Way Health Center [12060]
    Forks Health Center [12061]
    Issaquah Health Center [12062]
    Juneau Health Center [11317]
    Kenmore North Shores Health Center [12063]
    Kent Valley Health Center [12064]
    Lynnwood Health Center [12065]
    Marysville Health Center [12066]
    Oak Harbor Health Center [12067]
    Olympia Health Center [12068]
    Port Angeles Health Center [12069]
    Puyallup Health Center [12070]

Seattle Northgate Health Center [12071]
Sequim Health Center [12072]
Shelton Health Center [12073]
Silverdale Health Center [12074]
Sitka Health Center [11318]
Soldotna Health Center [11319]
Tacoma Health Center [12075]
Twin Falls Health Center [11570]
University District Roosevelt Health Center [12076]
West Seattle Health Center [12077]
Planned Parenthood of Greater Memphis Region • Memphis Health Center [11944]
Planned Parenthood of Greater Northern New Jersey
Elizabeth Clinic [11730]
Englewood Clinic [11731]
Flemington Clinic [11732]
Hackensack Clinic [11733]
Manville Clinic [11734]
Morristown Clinic [11735]
Newton Clinic [11736]
Phillipsburg Clinic [11737]
Plainfield Clinic [11738]
Planned Parenthood of Greater Orlando [11492]
Planned Parenthood of Greater Orlando - Eastside Clinic [11493]
Planned Parenthood of Greater Texas - Dallas Surgical Health Services Center [11972]
Planned Parenthood of Greater Texas - North Dallas Shelburne Health Center [11973]
Planned Parenthood of Greater Washington and North Idaho
Ellensburg Health Center [12078]
Francis Clinic [12079]
Indiana Health Center [12080]
Kenenwick Health Center [12081]
Pasco Health Center [12082]
Pullman Health Center [12083]
Sunnyside Health Center [12084]
Valley Health Center [12085]
Walla Walla Health Center [12086]
Yakima Health Center [12087]
Planned Parenthood Gulf Coast [11974]
Bryan Health Center--Family Planning Services [11975]
Dickinson Health Center [11976]
Planned Parenthood Gulf Coast - Greenspoint Health Center [11977]
Planned Parenthood Gulf Coast
Huntsville Health Center [11978]
Lufkin Health Center [11979]
Planned Parenthood Gulf Coast - Prevention Park Dysplasia Clinic [11980]
Planned Parenthood Gulf Coast - Prevention Park Health Center - Family Planning [11981]
Planned Parenthood Gulf Coast • Rosenberg Health Center [11982]
Planned Parenthood Gulf Coast - Southwest Health Center [11983]
Planned Parenthood Gulf Coast • Stafford Health Center--Family Planning Center [11984]
Planned Parenthood of Hawaii
Honolulu Clinic [11519]
Kona Clinic [11520]
Maui Clinic [11521]
Planned Parenthood Health Systems
Asheville Health Center [11827]
Blacksburg Health Center [12044]
Charleston Health Center [11940]
Charlotte Health Center [11828]
Charlottesville Health Center [12045]
Columbia Health Center [11941]
Greensboro Health Center [11829]
Raleigh Health Center [11830]
Roanoke Health Center [12046]
Wilmington Health Center [11831]
Winston--Salem Health Center [11832]
Planned Parenthood of the Heartland
Ames Health Center [11571]
Ankeny Health Center [11572]
Cedar Falls Health Center [11573]
Council Bluffs Health Center [11574]
Creston Health Center [11575]
Family Practice Center [11576]
Fort Dodge Health Center [11577]
Planned Parenthood of the Heartland, Iowa • Cedar Rapids Health Center [11578]

Planned Parenthood of the Heartland • Iowa City Health Center [11579]
Planned Parenthood of the Heartland, Iowa
Dubuque Health Center [11580]
Fort Madison Clinic [11581]
Keokuk Clinic [11582]
Mount Pleasant Clinic [11583]
Planned Parenthood of the Heartland
Knoxville Health Center [11584]
Newton Health Center [11585]
Northwest Health Center [11706]
Quad Cities Health Center [11586]
Red Oak Health Center [11587]
Rosenfield Health Center [11588]
Sioux City Health Center [11589]
South Street Health Center [11707]
Southwest Center [11708]
Spencer Health Center [11590]
Storm Lake Health Center [11591]
Susan Knapp Health Center [11592]
West Health Center [11593]
Planned Parenthood of Hudson Peconic
Amagansett Health Center [11757]
Brewster Health Center [11758]
Huntington Health Center [11759]
Mount Vernon Health Center [11760]
New Rochelle Health Center [11761]
Patchogue Health Center [11762]
Riverhead Health Center [11763]
Smithtown Health Center [11764]
Spring Valley Health Center [11765]
West Islip Health Center [11766]
White Plains Health Center [11767]
Yonkers Health Center [11768]
Planned Parenthood of Idaho • Twin Falls Health Center [11523]
Planned Parenthood of Illinois
Aurora Health Center [11525]
Austin Health Center [11526]
Bloomington Health Center [11527]
Champaign Health Center--Family Planning and Abortion Services [11528]
Decatur Health Center [11529]
Effingham Health Center [11530]
Englewood Health Center [11531]
Loop Health Center--Family Planning and Abortion Services [11532]
Near North Center--Family Planning and Abortion Services [11533]
Orland Park Planned Parenthood Express [11534]
Ottawa Health Center [11535]
Pekin Health Center [11536]
Peoria Health Center [11537]
Rogers Park Health Center [11538]
Roseland Health Center [11539]
Wicker Park Health Center [11540]
Planned Parenthood of Indiana
Avon Health Center [11542]
Bedford Health Center [11543]
Bloomington Health Center [11544]
Castleton Health Center [11545]
Columbus Health Center [11546]
East Chicago Health Center [11547]
Elkhart Health Center [11548]
Evansville Health Center [11549]
Fort Wayne Health Center [11550]
Gary Health Center [11551]
Hammond Health Center [11552]
Planned Parenthood of Indiana and Kentucky [11553]
Planned Parenthood of Indiana and Kentucky - Indianapolis-Georgetown at 86th [11554]
Planned Parenthood of Indiana
Lafayette Health Center [11555]
Madison Health Center [11556]
Merrillville Health Center [11557]
Michigan City Health Center [11558]
Midtown Health Center [11559]
Mishawaka Health Center [11560]
Muncie Health Center [11561]
New Albany Health Center [11562]
Richmond Health Center [11563]
Scottsburg Health Center [11564]
Seymour Health Center [11565]
Southside Health Center [11566]
Terre Haute Health Center [11567]
Valparaiso Health Center [11568]

Warsaw Health Center [11569]
Planned Parenthood of Kansas and Mid Missouri • Columbia Health Center [11677]
Planned Parenthood of Kansas and Mid-Missouri
Comprehensive Health Center [11595]
Hays Health Center [11596]
Planned Parenthood of Kansas and Mid Missouri
Independence Health Center [11678]
Jefferson City Health Center [11679]
North Kansas City Health Center [11680]
Patty Brous Health Center [11681]
South Kansas City Health Center [11682]
Warrensburg Health Center [11683]
Planned Parenthood of Kansas and Mid-Missouri • Wichita Health Center [11597]
Planned Parenthood of Kentucky
Bluegrass Health Center [11598]
EKU Satellite Health Center [11599]
Louisville Health Center [11600]
Planned Parenthood League of Massachusetts [11617]
Central Massachusetts Health Center [11618]
Marlborough Health Center [11619]
Milford Health Center [11620]
Planned Parenthood Express Center [11621]
Western Massachusetts Health Center [11622]
Planned Parenthood of Los Angeles - Bixby Health Center [11336]
Planned Parenthood of Los Angeles
Burbank Medical Center [11337]
Canoga Park Health Center [11338]
Planned Parenthood of Los Angeles - Dorothy Hecht Health Center [11339]
Planned Parenthood of Los Angeles - East Los Angeles Health Center [11340]
Planned Parenthood of Los Angeles • El Monte Medical Center [11341]
Planned Parenthood of Los Angeles - Hollywood Health Center [11342]
Planned Parenthood of Los Angeles
Lakewood Health Center [11343]
Long Beach Health Center [11344]
Planned Parenthood of Los Angeles - Planned Parenthood Basics, Baldwin Hills/Crenshaw [11345]
Planned Parenthood of Los Angeles
Planned Parenthood of Basics, Lakewood [11346]
Pomona Health Center [11347]
Planned Parenthood of Los Angeles - S. Mark Taper Foundation Center for Medical Training [11348]
Planned Parenthood of Los Angeles
Santa Monica Health Center [11349]
South Bay Health Center [11350]
Van Nuys Medical Center [11351]
Whittier Health Center [11352]
Planned Parenthood of Louisiana and the Mississippi Delta
Baton Rouge Health Center [11601]
New Orleans Health Center [11602]
Planned Parenthood - Manchester Center [11467]
Planned Parenthood of Mar Monte
B Street Health Center [11353]
Bakersfield Health Center [11354]
Blossom Hill Health Center [11355]
Capitol Plaza Health Center [11356]
Eastland Plaza Health Center [11357]
Eastside Health Center [11358]
Family First Health Center [11359]
Fifth Street Health Center [11709]
Fruitridge Health Center [11360]
Fulton Street Health Center [11361]
Gilroy Health Center [11362]
Greenfield Health Center [11363]
Hayward Health Center [11364]
Madera Health Center [11365]
Manteca Health Center [11366]
Mar Monte Community Clinic [11367]
Merced Health Center [11368]
Modesto Health Center [11369]
Mountain View Health Center [11370]
North Highlands Health Center [11371]
North Stockton Health Center [11372]
Peckham Health Center [11710]
Roseville Health Center [11373]
Salinas Health Center [11374]
San Benito Planned Parenthood Health Center [11375]

Planned Parenthood Mar Monte • San Jose Health Center [11376]
Planned Parenthood of Mar Monte
Seaside Health Center [11377]
South Hayward Health Center [11378]
Sunnyvale Health Center [11379]
Tahoe City Health Center [11380]
Tracy Health Center [11381]
Visalia Health Center [11382]
Watsonville Health Center [11383]
Westside Health Center [11384]
Woodland Health Center [11385]
Yuba City Health Center [11386]
Planned Parenthood of Maryland • Annapolis Health Center [11607]
Planned Parenthood of Maryland - Baltimore City Health Center [11608]
Planned Parenthood of Maryland
Easton Health Center [11609]
Frederick Health Center [11610]
Owings Mills Health Center [11611]
Salisbury Health Center [11612]
Planned Parenthood of Maryland - Towson Health Center [11613]
Planned Parenthood of Maryland • Waldorf Health Center [11614]
Planned Parenthood of Massachusetts • Fitchburg Health Center [11623]
Planned Parenthood of Metropolitan New Jersey
Chubb Health Center [11739]
Gale Health Center [11740]
Ironbound Health Center [11741]
Montclair Health Center [11742]
Paterson Center [11743]
Pompton Lakes Clinic [11744]
Planned Parenthood of Metropolitan Washington, DC • Downtown Center [11488]
Planned Parenthood of Metropolitan Washington DC
Falls Church Health Center [12047]
Gaithersburg Health Center [11615]
Northeast Egypt Health Center [11489]
Silver Spring Health Center [11616]
Planned Parenthood of Mid--Hudson Valley
Goshen Health Center [11769]
Kingston Health Center [11770]
Middletown Health Center [11771]
Monticello Health Center [11772]
Newburgh Health Center [11773]
Poughkeepsie Health Center [11774]
Planned Parenthood of Mid and South Michigan
Ann Arbor Health Center [11624]
Ann Arbor--West Health Center [11625]
Benton Harbor Health Center [11626]
Brighton Health Center [11627]
Burton Health Center [11628]
Cherry Street Health Center--Irwin/Martin [11629]
Detroit Health Center [11630]
East Lansing Health Center [11631]
Flint Health Center [11632]
Jackson Health Center [11633]
Lansing Health Center [11634]
Livonia Health Center [11635]
Owosso Health Center [11636]
Saginaw Health Center [11637]
Warren Health Center [11638]
Ypsilanti Health Center [11639]
Planned Parenthood of Middle and East Tennessee • Knoxville Health Center [11945]
Planned Parenthood of Middle and East Tennessee - Nashville Health Center [11946]
Planned Parenthood of Minnesota, North Dakota and South Dakota [11652]
Planned Parenthood of Minnesota, North Dakota, South Dakota
Albert Lea Clinic [11653]
Alexandria Health Center [11654]
Apple Valley Clinic [11655]
Bemidji Clinic [11656]
Brainerd Clinic [11657]
Brooklyn Park Clinic [11658]
Centro de Salud Health Center [11659]
Duluth Clinic [11660]
Fairmont Clinic [11661]
Grand Rapids Clinic [11662]
Mankato Clinic [11663]
Minneapolis Clinic [11664]
Moorhead Clinic [11665]

Owatonna Clinic [11666]
PLAN Express Care [11667], [11668]
Planned Parenthood Minnesota, North Dakota, South Dakota • Rapid City Clinic [11942]
Planned Parenthood of Minnesota, North Dakota, South Dakota
Red Wing Clinic [11669]
Rochester Clinic [11670]
Saint Cloud Clinic [11671]
Saint Paul Clinic--Rice Street [11672]
Planned Parenthood Minnesota, North Dakota, South Dakota • Sioux Falls Clinic [11943]
Planned Parenthood of Minnesota, North Dakota, South Dakota
Thief River Falls Clinic [11673]
Virginia Clinic [11674]
Willmar Clinic [11675]
Planned Parenthood of Mohawk Hudson
Amsterdam Health Center [11775]
Clifton Park Center [11776]
Cobleskill Health Center [11777]
Glens Falls Center [11778]
Granville Health Center [11779]
Herkimer Health Center [11780]
Johnstown Health Center [11781]
Oneida Health Center [11782]
Rome Health Center [11783]
Saratoga Springs Health Center [11784]
Schenectady Health Center [11785]
Ticonderoga Health Center [11786]
Planned Parenthood Mohawk Hudson • Utica Health Center [11787]
Planned Parenthood of Montana
Planned Parenthood of Fort Benton [11694]
Planned Parenthood Great Falls [11695]
Planned Parenthood Heights [11696]
Planned Parenthood Helena [11697]
Planned Parenthood Missoula [11698]
Planned Parenthood of Plentywood Clinic [11699]
Planned Parenthood of Poplar [11700]
Planned Parenthood of Rosebud County [11701], [11702]
Planned Parenthood of Teton [11703]
Planned Parenthood West [11704]
Plentywood Rexall Drug [11705]
Planned Parenthood of Nassau County • Glen Cove Health Center [11788]
Planned Parenthood of Nassau County - Hempsted Center [11789]
Planned Parenthood of Nassau County • Massapequa Health Center [11790]
Planned Parenthood of New Mexico
Farmington Health Center [11751]
Nob Hill Medical Office [11752]
Northeast Heights Medical Office [11753]
Santa Fe Medical Office [11754]
Surgical Center [11755]
Westside Clinic [11756]
Planned Parenthood of New York City
Boro Hall Health Center [11791]
Bronx Health Center [11792]
Margaret Sanger Health Center [11793]
Planned Parenthood of the North Country, New York
Canton Center [11794]
Lowville Health Center [11795]
Malone Clinic [11796]
Ogdensburg Health Center [11797]
Planned Parenthood of North Country New York • Plattsburgh Clinic [11798]
Planned Parenthood of the North Country, New York
Saranac Lake Clinic [11799]
Watertown Health Center [11800]
Planned Parenthood of North Florida
3rd Street South Health Center [11494]
Gainesville Clinic [11495]
Planned Parenthood of North Florida - Jacksonville Health Center [11496]
Planned Parenthood of North Florida • Sally Bellamy Clinic [11497]
Planned Parenthood of North Texas
Addison Health Center [11985]
Arlington North Clinic [11986]
Arlington South Clinic [11987]
Burleson Clinic [11988]
Corsicana Health Services [11989]
Denton Clinic [11990]
Gainesville Health Services [11991]

Garland Clinic [11992]
Henderson Clinic [11993]
Irving Clinic [11994]
Lewisville Health Center [11995]
McKinney Health Center [11996]
Mesquite Clinic [11997]
Mesquite Health Services [11998]
Northeast Clinic [11999]
Northside Clinic [12000]
Paris Health Services [12001]
Plano Clinic [12002]
Plano Health Services [12003]
Powell Clinic--Red Bird [12004]
Sherman Clinic [12005]
Southeast Clinic [12006]
Terrell Health Services [12007]
Tyler Clinic [12008]
Waxahachie Clinic [12009]
West Clinic [12010]
Planned Parenthood of Northeast and Mid-Penn
Allentown Medical Center [11905]
Carlisle Medical Center [11906]
Easton Medical Center [11907]
Harrisburg Medical Center [11908]
Lancaster Medical Center [11909]
Reading Medical Center [11910]
Scranton Medical Center [11911]
State College Medical Center [11912]
Stroudsburg Medical Center [11913]
Wilkes-Barre Medical Center [11914]
Planned Parenthood of Northeast Ohio
Akron Health Center [11841]
Bedford Health Center [11842]
Canton Health Center [11843]
Cleveland Health Center [11844]
Cortland Health Center [11845]
Kent Health Center [11846]
Lorain Health Center [11847]
Mansfield Health Center [11848]
Medina Health Center [11849]
Old Brooklyn Health Center [11850]
Ravenna Health Center [11851]
Rocky River Health Center [11852]
Solon Express Center [11853]
Wooster Health Center [11854]
Youngstown Health Center [11855]
Planned Parenthood of Northern New England
Barre Health Center [12034]
Bennington Health Center [12035]
Biddeford Health Center [11603]
Brattleboro Health Center [12036]
Planned Parenthood of Northern New England - Burlington Health Center [12037]
Planned Parenthood of Northern New England
Claremont Health Center [11714]
Derry Health Center [11715]
Exeter Health Center [11716]
Hyde Park Health Center [12038]
Keene Health Center [11717]
Manchester Health Center [11718]
Middlebury Health Center [12039]
Newport Health Center [12040]
Portland Health Center [11604]
Rutland Health Center [12041]
Saint Albans Health Center [12042]
Sanford Health Center [11605]
Topsham Health Center [11606]
West Lebanon Health Center [11719]
Williston Health Center [12043]
Planned Parenthood of Northwest Ohio • Jefferson Avenue Health Center [11856]
Planned Parenthood of Orange and San Bernardino Counties
Anaheim Health Center [11387]
Mission Viejo Health Center [11388]
Planned Parenthood of Orange and San Bernardino Counties - Orange Health Center [11389]
Planned Parenthood of Orange and San Bernardino Counties
San Bernardino Health Center [11390]
Santa Ana Health Center [11391]
Upland Health Center [11392]
Westminster Health Center [11393]
Planned Parenthood of the Pacific Southwest [11394]
Carlsbad Isabella Center [11395]
Chula Vista Center [11396]
City Heights Express Center [11397]

Coachella Valley Health Center [11398]
El Cajon Health Center [11399]
Escondido Center [11400]
Euclid Avenue Francis Torbert Center [11401]
First Avenue Family Planning Michelle Wagner
Center [11402]
First Avenue Surgical Services Michelle Wagner
Center [11403]
Kearny Mesa Center [11404]
Mira Mesa Center [11405]
Mission Bay Parker Center [11406]
Mission Valley Express Center [11407]
Moreno Valley Center [11408]
Pacific Beach Express Mimi Brien Center
[11409]
Rancho Mirage Family Planning Center [11410]
Rancho Mirage Surgical Services Center
[11411]
Riverside Family Planning Center [11412]
Riverside Surgical Services Center [11413]
Planned Parenthood of Pasadena and San Gabriel
Valley
Alhambra Health Center [11414]
Eagle Rock Express Center [11415]
Pasadena Health Center [11416]
Planned Parenthood of Rhode Island • Providence
Health Center [11939]
Planned Parenthood of the Rochester/Syracuse
Region
Batavia Health Center [11801]
Canandaigua Health Center [11802]
Greece Health Center [11803]
Planned Parenthood of Rochester/Syracuse Region
• Rochester Health Center--University Avenue
[11804]
Planned Parenthood of the Rochester/Syracuse
Region • Syracuse Health Center [11805]
Planned Parenthood of the Rocky Mountains
Alamosa Health Center [11443]
Arvada Health Center [11444]
Aurora Health Center [11445]
Boulder Health Center [11446]
Casper Health Center [12117]
Colorado Springs Eastside Health Center
[11447]
Colorado Springs Westside Health Center
[11448]
Cortez Health Center [11449]
Denver Central Health Center [11450]
Denver Southeast (Glendale) Health Center
[11451]
Durango Health Center [11452]
Fort Collins Abortion Center [11453]
Fort Collins Health Center [11454]
Glenwood Springs Health Center [11455]
Granby Health Center [11456]
Greeley Health Center [11457]
La Junta Health Center [11458]
Lakewood Health Center [11459]
Las Vegas East Flamingo Health Center [11711]
Las Vegas North Martin Luther King Health
Center [11712]
Las Vegas West Charleston Health Center
[11713]
Littleton Health Center [11460]
Longmont Health Center [11461]
Parker Express Center [11462]
Pueblo Health Center [11463]
Salida Health Center [11464]
Steamboat Springs Health Center [11465]
Planned Parenthood of the Saint Louis Region
Central West End Health Center [11684]
Fairview Heights Health Center [11541]
North County Health Center [11685]
Reproductive Health Services [11686]
Saint Peters Health Center [11687]
South Grand Health Center [11688]
West County Health Center [11689]
Planned Parenthood of Santa Barbara, Ventura and
San Luis Obispo Counties • San Luis Obispo
Center [11417]
Planned Parenthood of Santa Barbara, Ventura, and
San Luis Obispo Counties - Santa Barbara Center
[11418]
Planned Parenthood of Santa Barbara, Ventura and
San Luis Obispo Counties
Santa Maria Center [11419]
Thousand Oaks Center [11420]

Ventura Center [11421]
Planned Parenthood Sexual Healthcare Services
Babcock Sexual Healthcare Services [12011]
Bandera Road Sexual Healthcare Services
[12012]
Northeast Sexual Health Center [12013]
Planned Parenthood of Shasta-Diablo • Concord
Health Center [11422]
Planned Parenthood Shasta Pacific [11423]
Antioch Health Center [11424]
Central Richmond Health Center [11425]
Chico Health Center [11426]
Clearlake Health Center [11427]
Costa Mesa Health Center [11428]
El Cerrito Health Center [11429]
Fairfield Health Center [11430]
Hilltop--Richmond Health Center [11431]
Mill Valley Health Center [11432]
Napa Health Center [11433]
Pittsburg Health Center [11434]
Redding Health Center [11435]
San Ramon Health Center [11436]
Santa Rosa Health Center [11437]
Vacaville Health Center [11438]
Vallejo Health Center [11439]
Walnut Creek Health Center [11440]
Planned Parenthood of South Central Michigan
Battle Creek Health Center [11640]
Coldwater Clinic [11641]
Kalamazoo Health Center [11642]
Sturgis Clinic [11643]
Three Rivers Clinic [11644]
Planned Parenthood of South Central New York
Binghamton Clinic [11806]
Norwich Clinic [11807]
Oneonta Clinic [11808]
Sidney Clinic [11809]
Walton Clinic [11810]
Planned Parenthood of South Florida and the
Treasure Coast
Boca Raton Health Center [11498]
Indian River (Vero Beach) Health Center [11499]
Jean Shehan Health Center [11500]
Kendall Health Center [11501]
Lake Worth Health Center [11502]
Martin County Health Center [11503]
North Miami Health Center [11504]
Pembroke Pines Health Center [11505]
Planned Parenthood of South Florida and Treasure
Coast • West Palm Beach Health Center [11506]
Planned Parenthood Southeast • Augusta Health
Center [11518]
Planned Parenthood of Southeast Iowa • Burlington
Clinic [11594]
Planned Parenthood of Southeast Texas Surgical
and Comprehensive Health Services
Bryan Health Center--Abortion Services [12014]
Prevention Park Health Center--Surgical and
Comprehensive Health Services/Vasectomy
Services [12015]
Stafford Health Center--Abortion Services
[12016]
Planned Parenthood of Southeastern Pennsylvania
Ambler Health Center [11915]
Avondale Health Center [11916]
Castor Avenue Health Center [11917]
Coatesville Health Center [11918]
Collegeville Health Center [11919]
Elizabeth Blackwell Health Center [11920]
Far Northeast Health Center [11921]
Far Northeast Surgical Center [11922]
Locust Street Health Center [11923]
Locust Street Surgical Center [11924]
Media Health Center [11925]
Norristown Abortion Center [11926]
Norristown Health Center [11927]
Pottstown Health Center [11928]
Saint Davids Health Center [11929]
West Chester Health Center [11930]
West Chester Surgical Center [11931]
Yeadon Health Center [11932]
Planned Parenthood of Southeastern Virginia
Hampton Health Center [12048]
Newtown Medical Center [12049]
Planned Parenthood of the Southern Finger Lakes
Corning Health Center [11811]
Elmira Health Center [11812]
Planned Parenthood of Southern Finger Lakes •

Hornell Health Center [11813]
Planned Parenthood of the Southern Finger Lakes
Ithaca Clinic [11814]
Watkins Glen Clinic [11815]
Planned Parenthood of Southern New England
Bridgeport Health Center [11468]
Danbury Health Center [11469]
Danielson Health Center [11470]
Enfield Health Center [11471]
Hartford North Health Center [11472]
Meriden Health Center [11473]
New Britain Health Center [11474]
New London Health Center [11475]
Norwich Health Center [11476]
Old Saybrook Health Center [11477]
Shelton Health Center [11478]
Stamford Health Center [11479]
Torrington Health Center [11480]
Waterbury Health Center [11481]
West Hartford Health Center [11482]
Willimantic Health Center [11483]
Planned Parenthood of Southern New Jersey
[11745]
Atlantic City Health Center [11746]
Bellmawr Health Center [11747]
Edgewater Park Health Center [11748]
Hammonton Health Center [11749]
Stockton College [11750]
Planned Parenthood of Southwest and Central
Florida
Fort Myers Health Center [11507]
Lakeland Health Center [11508]
Manatee Health Center [11509]
Pinellas Health Center [11510]
Planned Parenthood of Southwest and Central
Florida - Sarasota Health Center [11511]
Planned Parenthood of Southwest and Central
Florida
Tampa Health Center [11512]
Winter Haven Health Center [11513]
Planned Parenthood of Southwest Missouri
Joplin Health Center [11690]
Springfield Health Center [11691]
Planned Parenthood of Southwest Ohio Region •
Clermont Health Center [11857]
Planned Parenthood of Southwest Ohio Region -
Elizabeth Campbell Medical Center [11858]
Planned Parenthood of Southwest Ohio Region -
Elizabeth Campbell Surgical Center [11859]
Planned Parenthood of Southwest Ohio Region •
Fairborn Health Center [11860]
Planned Parenthood of Southwest Ohio Region -
Jean K. Spritz Center [11861]
Planned Parenthood of Southwest Ohio Region •
Kettering/Phillips Health Center [11862]
Planned Parenthood of Southwest Ohio Region -
Mary M. Yeiser Health Center [11863]
Planned Parenthood of Southwest Ohio Region
Mary Stark Health Center [11864]
Middletown Health Center [11865]
Springfield Health Center [11866]
Planned Parenthood of Southwestern Oregon
Ashland Health Center [11888]
Bethel Express Center [11889]
Cottage Grove Outreach Clinic [11890]
Eugene Clinic [11891]
Florence Outreach Clinic [11892]
Grants Pass Health Center [11893]
Medford Health Center [11894]
Springfield Health Center [11895]
Planned Parenthood Surgical Health Services of
North Texas
Fort Worth Health Center [12017]
North Texas Health Center [12018]
Planned Parenthood of Utah
Logan Clinic [12027]
Ogden Clinic [12028]
Park City Clinic [12029]
Saint George Clinic [12030]
South Jordan Health Center [12031]
Utah Valley Clinic [12032]
West Valley Clinic [12033]
Planned Parenthood of Waco Family Planning and
Surgical Services • Audre Rapoport Women's
Health Center [12019]
Planned Parenthood of West and Northern Michigan
Big Rapids Health Center [11645]
Evenson Health Center [11646]

Ionia Health Center [11647]
Marquette Health Center [11648]
Muskegon Center [11649]
Petoskey Health Center [11650]
Traverse City Center [11651]
Planned Parenthood of West Texas
Abilene Perini Center [12020]
Abilene Perini Center--Planned Parenthood Choice [12021]
Midland Byerley Center--Planned Parenthood Choice [12022]
Midland Byerley Health Center [12023]
San Angelo Health Center [12024]
Planned Parenthood of West Virginia • Vienna Health Center [12089]
Planned Parenthood of Western New York
Buffalo Medical Center [11816]
Niagara Falls Office [11817]
North Tonawanda Office [11818]
West Seneca Medical Center [11819]
Wheatfield Office [11820]
Planned Parenthood of Western Pennsylvania [11933]
Bridgeville Health Center [11934]
Johnstown Health Center [11935]
Moon Township Health Center [11936]
Pittsburgh Family Planning Health Center [11937]
Somerset Health Center [11938]
Planned Parenthood of Western Washington [12088]
Planned Parenthood of Wisconsin
Appleton Central Health Center [12090]
Appleton North Health Center [12091]
Beaver Dam Health Center [12092]
Planned Parenthood of Wisconsin - Capitol Drive Health Center [12093]
Planned Parenthood of Wisconsin
Chippewa Falls Health Center [12094]
Delavan Health Center [12095]
Eau Claire Health Center [12096]
Fond du Lac Health Center [12097]
Green Bay Health Center [12098]
Johnson Creek Health Center [12099]
Kenosha Health Center [12100]
Madison East Health Center [12101]
Madison South Health Center [12102]
Manitowoc Health Center [12103]
Planned Parenthood of Wisconsin • Milwaukee-Jackson Center Health Center [12104]
Planned Parenthood of Wisconsin • Milwaukee--Lincoln Plaza Health Center [12105]
Planned Parenthood of Wisconsin - Milwaukee-Northwest Health Center [12106]
Planned Parenthood of Wisconsin - Milwaukee-Wisconsin Avenue Health Center [12107]
Planned Parenthood of Wisconsin - Mitchell Street Health Center [12108]
Planned Parenthood of Wisconsin
Oshkosh Health Center [12109]
Portage Health Center [12110]
Racine Health Center [12111]
Shawano Health Center [12112]
Sheboygan Health Center [12113]
Waukesha Health Center [12114]
West Bend Health Center [12115]
Wisconsin Rapids Health Center [12116]
Plano Dialysis Center • DaVita [27292]
Plano Orthopedics and Sports Medicine Center [39091]
Plant City Dialysis • DaVita [23480]
Plant City Family Care Center [6540]
Plantation Dialysis • DaVita [23484]
Plateau Mental Health Center [32301], [49064]
Platinum Care Home Health Inc. [13377]
Platinum Care Home Health Services, Inc. [15840]
Platinum Homecare [15641]
PlatinumOne Home Health Services [14216]
Platte County Home Care [18666]
Platte Woods Dialysis • DaVita [25225]
Plattsburgh Veterans Affairs Clinic [31449]
Play On Words Therapy Services [2819]
Playa Azul Home Health Care [14112]
Playtime Children's Therapies [1041]
Playworks [1235]
Plaza Community Center • Esperanza Program [40149]
Plaza Medical Center of Fort Worth • Cancer Program [5989]

Plaza Rehabilitation Service [31964]
Pleasant Counseling [42619]
Pleasant Grove Health Care Center [28025]
Pleasant Point Health Center • Wolipomawsu Behavioral Health Program [44022]
Pleasant Run Dialysis • Fresenius Medical Care [27043]
Pleasant Valley Dialysis [27687]
Pleasant Vallley Home Health, Hospice and Private Duty [18535]
Pleasant View Dialysis • University Health Care [27411]
Pleasanton Dialysis Center • DaVita [22884]
Pleasanton Road Dialysis Facility • US Renal Care [27339]
Plex [39077]
Plumas Rural Services [40417]
Plumas Rural Services, Inc. • Domestic Violence Services [8871]
Plumas Street Dialysis Center [23083]
Plumfield Farm [34025]
Plumfield, Inc. • Administrative Office [34026]
Plumfield Ranch [33194]
Plumfield Villa [34027]
A Plus Athlete Sports Medicine [38757]
A Plus Children's Therapy Inc. [1570], [1745]
Plus DUI Services LLC [42920]
A Plus Hearing Service Inc. [1027]
A Plus Home Health Care [15713]
PLUS NeuroRehabilitation [4294]
Plus One Holdings Inc. [38801]
Plus One Physical Therapy [38802]
A Plus Professional Therapy--Speech/Language Services [1033]
A Plus Speech Services Inc. [1903]
Plymouth Bay Orthopedics and Sports Therapy [38551]
Plymouth Ears, Nose and Throat [2516]
Plymouth Ears, Nose and Throat at Bourne [2463]
Plymouth Kidney Center • Fresenius Medical Care [25925]
PM Sleep Medicine [37951]
PMA Sleep Wellness Center [37683]
PMS--Carlsbad Family Health Center [6991]
PMS--Ortiz Mountain Health Center [6992]
Pneu-Med Inc. [17186]
Po'Ailani Inc • Dual Diagnosis Program [42234]
Po'ailani Inc • Outpatient Clinic [42235]
Pocahontas Community Hospital Hospice [19727]
Pocahontas County Schools • Deaf and Hard of Hearing Program [874]
Pocatello Clinic [6643]
Pocatello Veterans Affairs Clinic [29549]
Pocatello Veterans Center [29550]
Pocomoke City Veterans Affairs Clinic [30306]
Pocono Dialysis Center • DaVita [26421]
Pocono Medical Center • Dale and Frances Hughes Cancer Center [5824]
Pocono Speech Center [3382]
Pod House [33427]
POEM Human Services [45062]
POH Regional Medical Center [44966]
A Point of Change LLC [43752]
Pointe Coupee Hospice [19868]
Pokagon Band of Potawatomi Indians • Tribe/Keepers of the Fire Behav Hlth [44770]
Pola Tenenbaum Center for Renal Care • Dialysis Facility [25570]
Polish American Association • Starting Point [42569]
Polk County Mental Health • Alcohol and Drug Treatment Program [48096]
Polk County Office [21515]
Polk County ResCare [29857]
Polk County Women's Shelter [9097]
Polk Sleep disorders LLC [36803]
Polyclinic Sleep Medicine Center [37925]
Pomaikai Elementary School [385]
Pomeroy Crisis Recovery House • The Brien Center [30448]
Pomona Alcohol and Drug Recovery Center [40406]
Pomona Community Crisis Center Inc [40407]
Pomona Dialysis • DaVita [22886]
Pomona Valley Hospital Medical Center • Lewis Family Cancer Care Center [4823]
Pomona Valley Hospital Sleep Disorders Center [36682]
Pompano Beach Vet Center [51916]
Ponca Tribe of Nebraska [45777]

Ponce de Leon Center • AIDS Clinical Trials Unit [10]
Ponce Regional Hospital • Dialysis Center [26646]
Ponce Veterans Affairs Outpatient Clinic [17530]
Pooler Dialysis • DaVita [23771]
Pooser Communication Services [1757]
Pope Field • ADAPT Program [47448]
Poplar Bluff Mental Health Center [30886]
Poplar Bluff Regional Medical Center • Danny Bell Cancer Treatment Center [5456]
Poplar Bluff Veterans Affairs Medical Center [30887]
Poplar Outpatient Clinic [32100]
Poplar Springs Hospital [33906]
Port Angeles Kidney Center • Dialysis Facility • Northwest Kidney Center [27627]
Port Charlotte Artificial Kidney Center • DaVita [23488]
Port Charlotte Veterans Affairs Primary Care Clinic [29267]
Port Chester Dialysis and Renal Center • DaVita [25757]
Port Colborne General Hospital • Niagara Eating Disorder Outpatient Program [11231]
Port Counseling Center Inc • Outpatient Drug Abuse Clinic [46991]
Port Gamble S'Klallam Recovery Center [49988]
Port Gardner Bay Recovery [49955]
Port of Hope Centers Inc
Nampa Treatment Center [42358]
Region I [42331]
PORT Human Services [47362]
Port Human Services [31588]
PORT Human Services
Aberdeen [47202]
Adolescent Substance Abuse [47363]
Adult Program [47364]
Facility Based Crisis Services [47365]
FBC Facility Based Crisis [47203]
Methadone/IV Programs [47366]
New Bern [47432]
Port Huron ENT [2637]
Port Huron Hospital • Cancer Center [5393]
Port Huron Hospital Medical Equipment [15780]
Port Jefferson Speech and Hearing [3097]
Port Jervis Mental Health Clinic [31456]
Port Lavaca Dialysis Facility • DaVita [27294]
Port Saint Lucie Children's Health Center [6542]
Port Washington Dialysis Center • DaVita [25759]
Portage Area Senior Services • Day Treatment Program • Coleman Professional Services [31784]
Portage County Health Center [7088]
Portage County Kidney Center • Fresenius Medical Care [26141]
Portage Dialysis • DaVita [24224]
Portage Health Dialysis [24913]
Portage Health Sleep Disorders Center [37192]
Portage Hearing Services [2601]
Portage Hospital Home Health [15680]
Portage Orthopedic and Sports Physical Therapy [39188]
Portage Path Behavioral Health [31648], [31659]
Psychiatric Emergency Services [31649]
Portage Path Community Mental Health Center [51195]
Portals House, Inc.
Corporate Headquarters [28607]
Portals Mariposa Clubhouse [28608]
Portals Partners [28609]
Portals Twin Peaks Transitional Residence [28610]
Porter Adventist Hospital [36729]
Cancer Care Center [4873]
The Centre for Behavioral Health [41139]
Porter Dialysis--Dundalk • Fresenius Medical Care [24678]
Porter Dialysis--Pikesville • Fresenius Medical Care [24713]
Porter Dialysis--Rosedale • Fresenius Medical Care [24722]
Porter Dialysis--White Marsh • Fresenius Medical Care [24739]
Porter-Leath Children's Center • Runaway and Homeless Youth Program [36207]
Porter Starke Services Inc [43127], [43182], [43219], [43220]
Porter-Starke Services, Inc. [29824]
Porter-Starke Services, Inc.--Knox [29758]
Porter-Starke Services, Inc.--Portage [29804]
Porterville Developmental Center [7809]

Porterville Hemodialysis Facility [22887]
Porterville Women's Shelter [8870]
Portia Bell Hume Behavioral Health [28455]
Portland Community College • Disability Access Services [689]
Portland Community Health Center [6782]
Portland Dialysis Center • Innovative Dialysis Systems [26345]
Portland Habilitation Center [8445]
Portland Help Center [34165]
Portland Home Dialysis Clinic • Peritoneal Dialysis Center • Innovative Dialysis Systems [26346]
Portland Metro Treatment Center [48209]
Portland VA Clinic [44032]
Portland VA Medical Center SATP [48210]
Portland Veterans Affairs Medical Center [34684]
    Portland Campus [31965]
    Vancouver Campus [32879]
Portland Veterans Affairs Medical Center - Vancouver Division [18477]
Portland Women's Crisis Line [10249]
Portner Counseling Group LLC [41901]
Portneuf Medical Center [14669]
    Cancer Program [5055]
    Southeast Idaho Sleep Disorders Center [36881]
Portrero Hill Neighborhood House • ZAP Project [40629]
Portsmouth Behavioral Healthcare Services [32774]
Portsmouth Community Health Center [7363]
Portsmouth Dialysis Center • DaVita [27538]
Portsmouth House [32167]
Portsmouth Public Schools [855]
Portsmouth Veterans Affairs Clinic [31091]
Positive Adjustments [49607], [49711], [49717]
Positive Adjustments Corporation [49648]
Positive Alternative Inc [50122]
Positive Alternatives, Inc. • Teen Care Crisis Intervention • Runaway and Homeless Youth Program [36270]
Positive Behavioral Strategies Inc [48046]
Positive Change [41068]
Positive Connections [42380]
Positive Directions • Center for Prevention and Recovery [41494]
Positive Education Program • Main Office and DAS [31720]
Positive Images [44757]
Positive Images Residential [44758]
Positive Pathways [11002]
Positive Progression Inc [40663]
Positive Reflections [11003]
Positive Solutions Counseling [47572]
Positive Steps Inc [39981]
Post Falls Dialysis Unit • Fresenius Medical Care [23886]
Postgraduate Center for Mental Health [31425]
Postgraduate Center for Mental Health--John Gutheil Residence [31426]
Postgraduate Center for Mental Health--Residence No. 1 [31427]
Postgraduate Center for Mental Health--Residence No. 2 [31428]
Postgraduate Center for Mental Health--Richard Dicker Residence [31429]
Poteau Dialysis Center [26289]
Potentials LLC [48066]
Potomac Behavioral Solutions [11296]
Potomac Center [8093]
Potomac Highlands Guild [32914]
Potomac Highlands Mental Health Center • Cottage Highland House [32928]
Potomac Highlands Mental Health Center--Franklin [32903]
Potomac Highlands Mental Health Center--New Creek [32923]
Potomac Highlands Mental Health Center--Petersburg [32929]
Potomac Highlands Mental Health Center--Romney [32934]
Potomac Highlands Mental Health Guild Crisis Unit--Franklin [51486]
Potomac Highlands Mental Health Guild Crisis Unit--New Creek [51492]
Potomac Highlands Mental Health Guild Crisis Unit--Petersburg [51493]
Potomac Highlands Mental Health Guild Inc [50329], [50338]

Hampshire County Adolescent Substance AbuseServices [50341]
Mineral County Substance AbuseServices [50318]
Pendleton County Office [50304]
Potomac Home Health Care [15461]
Potomac Hospital • Cancer Program [6090]
Potomac Ridge Behavioral Health [33567]
Potomac Valley Psychotherapy Associates • Group Therapy for Compulsive Overeaters and Binge Eaters [11082]
Potter's Clay Women and Children in Crisis Shelter [8766]
Potters House [42112]
Pottstown Memorial Medical Center [26569]
    Cancer Program [5864]
Poudre Valley Hospital [4880]
    Sleep Disorders Center [36730]
Powell Recovery Center • Site I [44172]
Powell Veterans Affairs Clinic [33060]
POWER Halfway House [48603]
Power House Services Inc [43827]
POWER Outpatient Program [48604]
Power Stuttering Center [1197]
Powerhouse • Mount Rogers Community Services Board [32738]
Poweshiek County Mental Health Center [29873]
Poynette Counseling and • Psychotherapy Associates Inc [50506]
PPC Violence Free Network [10277]
PPEP Behavioral Health Services [39361], [39509]
PQN Inc. [14217]
Practical Hearing [1120]
Practical Recovery [39955]
Practical Rehabilitation Services, Ltd. [1954]
Prairie Band Potawatomi Nation • Family Violence Prevention Program [9371]
Prairie Center Health Systems Inc
    Hill Street Unit [42453]
    Killarney Street Unit [42938]
    Outpatient Services [42614]
Prairie du Chien Memorial Hospital Association, Inc. [18619]
Prairie Community Services [30703]
Prairie Counseling Services [50538]
Prairie Haven Hospice Alliance
    Regional West Health Services--Alliance [20375]
    Regional West Health Services--Scottsbluff [20403]
Prairie Home Hospice [20179]
Prairie House [45238]
Prairie Lakes Area Education Agency • Special Education Division • Hearing Department [2206]
Prairie Lakes Healthcare System • Dialysis Facility [26801]
Prairie Ridge • Addiction Treatment Services [43289]
Prairie Saint John's [33608], [33746]
Prairie Saint John's Day Treatment [33607], [33611]
Prairie Saint Johns LLC [47573]
Prairie View Inc
    Hillsboro [43362]
    Hutchinson [43366]
    McPherson [43405]
    Newton [43415]
Prairie View, Inc. [29933]
Prairie View Inc.--Hutchinson [33473]
Prairie View Inc.--McPherson [33508]
Prairie View, Inc.--Newton [33510]
Prairie View Inc.--Wichita [33515]
Prairie View at Legacy Park [29961]
Prairie View at McPherson [29944]
Prairie View Mental Health Center • Wichita at Legacy Park [43502]
Prairie View at Newton • Harvey County Community Mental Health Center [29945]
Prairie View at Reflection Ridge [29962]
Prairieview Hospice [20795]
Pratt Dialysis Center • DaVita [24345]
Prattville Baptist Hospital • Sleep Disorders Center [36595]
Praxair Healthcare Services [16580]
Praxair Healthcare Services--Feasterville Trevose [17321]
Praxair Healthcare Services, Inc.--Austin [17816]
Praxair Healthcare Services, Inc.--Cedar City [18195]

Praxair Healthcare Services, Inc.--Chandler [12786]
Praxair Healthcare Services Inc.--Colorado Springs [13467]
Praxair Healthcare Services, Inc.--Cuyahoga Falls [16921]
Praxair Healthcare Services, Inc.--Denver [13476]
Praxair Healthcare Services Inc.--Fort Collins [13487]
Praxair Healthcare Services, Inc.--Hingham [15500]
Praxair Healthcare Services, Inc.--Lindon [18202]
Praxair Healthcare Services, Inc.--Livingston [18046]
Praxair Healthcare Services, Inc.--Logan [18204]
Praxair Healthcare Services Inc.--Loouisville [13502]
Praxair Healthcare Services, Inc.--Ogden [18208]
Praxair Healthcare Services Inc.--Price [18212]
Praxair Healthcare Services Inc.--Pueblo [13509]
Praxair Healthcare Services, Inc.--Rochester [15931]
Praxair Healthcare Services, Inc.--Saint George [18217]
Praxair Healthcare Services, Inc.--Salt Lake City [18225]
Praxair Healthcare Services, Inc.--San Antonio [18149]
Praxair Healthcare Services, Inc.--Tooele [18228]
Praxair Healthcare Services, Inc.--Vernal [18229]
Preble County Counseling Center Hotline [51216]
Preble County Regional Dialysis, Inc. [26106]
Preble Domestic Violence Program [10146]
Preble Street Resource Center • Runaway and Homeless Youth Program [35985]
Precious Home Health Care [15862]
Precision Allograft Solutions [35238]
Precision Care Home Health Services, Inc. [13673]
Precision Health Care Services [47401]
Precision Physical Therapy of Collegeville [38936]
Preferred Behavioral Health--Barnegat [31102]
Preferred Behavioral Health--Brick [31106]
Preferred Behavioral Health--Howell [31139]
Preferred Behavioral Health--Lakewood [31142]
Preferred Behavioral Health of New Jersey [46031]
Preferred Care Home Health Services [14113]
Preferred Choice Home Care [18502]
Preferred Choice Home Health Care Services [15725]
Preferred Counseling Services [41159]
Preferred Excellent Care [13013]
Preferred Family HC Inc/Adol/Adult • Family Recovery [43323]
Preferred Family Healthcare • Family Recovery Wichita [43503]
Preferred Family Healthcare Inc [45485], [45507], [45523], [45552], [45567], [45624]
    Adolescent CSTAR/Kirksville Office [45544]
    Adult CSTAR [45625]
    Brookfield Adult Program [45444]
    Chillicothe Adult Program [45456]
    Jefferson City Adolescent CSTAR [45508]
    Joplin Adolescent CSTAR [45511]
    Kahoka Site [45512]
    Kirksville Adult CSTAR Program [45545]
    Liberty Office [45559]
    Moberly Adult Program [45570]
    Saint Charles Adolescent Program [45605]
    Saint Joseph Adolescent Program [45609]
    Trenton Adult Program [45658]
    Troy Adolescent [45660]
Preferred Home Care [15422]
Preferred Home Care Services, Inc. [15652]
Preferred Home Health [18501]
Preferred Home Health Agency [14447]
Preferred Home Health Provider [13251]
Preferred Home Health Services, Inc.--Bluefield [18251]
Preferred Home Health Services, Inc.--Richlands [18357]
Preferred Hospice of Missouri Central [20292]
Preferred Pain and Rehab Center [35291]
Preferred Pediatric Home Health Care, Inc.--Oklahoma City [17153]
Preferred Pediatric Home Health Care, Inc.--Tulsa [17167]
Pregnant Substance Abusing Women [41929]
PREHAB of Arizona • Center for Family Enrichment [28164]
Premier Care [44721]
Premier Care of Indiana Inc [43148]
Premier Community HealthCare Group [6455]

Premier Community HealthCare Group--West Pasco [6516]
Premier Diagnostics, Inc.--Oxnard • Sleep Disorders Center [36683]
Premier Diagnostics Inc.--Thousand Oaks • Sleep Disorders Center [36684]
Premier Diagnostics Inc.--Ventura • Sleep Disorders Center [36685]
Premier Dialysis North County [25201]
Premier Dialysis West County [25183]
Premier Home Care, LLC [16917]
Premier Home Health Care [16829]
Premier Home Health Care Services--Bronx [16369]
Premier Home Health Care Services--Brooklyn [16410]
Premier Home Health Care Services--Charlotte [16713]
Premier Home Health Care Services of Florida [14255]
Premier Home Health Care Services--Hempstead [16482]
Premier Home Health Care Services--Kew Gardens [16504]
Premier Home Health Care Services--New York [16562]
Premier Home Health Care Services--Poughkeepsie [16602]
Premier Home Health Care Services--Ronkonkoma [16623]
Premier Home Health Care Services--Staten Island [16639]
Premier Home Health Services Inc.--Madison [13529]
Premier Home Health Services Inc.--Stamford [13543]
Premier Home Healthcare, LLC--Okemos [15765]
Premier Hospice & Palliative Care [18814]
Premier Medical Corp. [13477]
Premier Orthopaedics and Sports Medicine Associates--Folsom [38943]
Premier Orthopaedics and Sports Medicine Associates--Havertown [38948]
Premier Orthopedic Center [38302], [38305]
Premier Physical Therapy--Cordele [38315]
Premier Physical Therapy--East Windsor [38720]
Premier Services of Michigan [45043]
Premier Sleep Disorders Center of Kosciusko [37258]
Premier Sleep Disorders Center of Victoria [37833]
Premier Sleep Medicine Center [37078]
Premier Speech and Language [1636]
Premier Therapy Services Inc. [2798]
Premier Visiting Nurse and Home Health Services [15863]
Premiere Chiropractic & Sports Medicine [38118]
Premiere Rehab LLC [2163]
Premium Home Health Care [14114]
Presbyterian Child Welfare Agency • Buckhorn Children's Center [34149]
Presbyterian Children's Village Services [34425]
Presbyterian Ear Institute [554]
Presbyterian Healthcare Services [16304]
Presbyterian Healthcare Transplant [25537]
Presbyterian Homes Hospice, Inc. [20201]
Presbyterian Hospice [20522]
Presbyterian Hospice of Mid-America [20295]
Presbyterian Hospice and Palliative Care [20635]
Presbyterian Hospital • Adult Sickle Cell Program [36406]
Presbyterian Hospital--Albuquerque • Cancer Program [5550]
Presbyterian Hospital--Charlotte • Cancer Center [5635]
Presbyterian Hospital of Dallas [17888]
   Comprehensive Cancer Center [5977]
Presbyterian Hospital Dallas • Eating Disorders Program [11281]
Presbyterian Hospital of Dallas • Sleep Medicine Institute [37834]
Presbyterian Hospital • Pediatric Sickle Cell Program [36407]
Presbyterian Hospital of Plano
   Seay Behavioral Health Center [32532]
   Seay Behavioral Healthcare Center [49491]
Presbyterian Hospital Speech Pathology [3170]
Presbyterian Hospitality House [28090], [35790]
Presbyterian Hospitals of Dallas/Plano • In Vitro Fertilization Program [22265]

Presbyterian Intercommunity Hospital--Arcadia • Arcadia Home Nursing and Health Services [12895]
Presbyterian Intercommunity Hospital--La Mirada • Home Health Services [13093]
Presbyterian Intercommunity Hospital • Ruby L. Golleher Comprehensive Cancer Program [4866]
Presbyterian Intercommunity Hospital--Whittier [13449]
Presbyterian Kaseman Hospital [16305]
Presbyterian Medical Center [17423]
Presbyterian Medical Services
   Artesia Health Resources [46248]
   Crisis Response of Santa Fe [51131]
   Cuba Health Center [46259]
Presbyterian Medical Services Home Care [16326]
Presbyterian Medical Services
   Questa Health Center [46294]
   Rio Rancho Family Health Center [46297]
   San Juan County Adolescent RTC [46268]
Presbyterian Medical Services--Santa Fe Community Guidance Center [31215]
Presbyterian Medical Services
   Santa Fe Community Guidance Center [46305]
   Totah Behavioral Health Authority [46269]
   Valley Community Health Center [46263]
   Western New Mexico Medical Group BH [46273], [46316]
Presbyterian Service Agency [28177], [28204]
Presbyterian Sleep Lab--Ballantyne [37479]
Presbyterian Sleep Lab--Huntersville [37480]
Preschool Center for the Sensory Impaired [201]
Prescott House Inc [39458]
Prescott Speech Language Services, Inc. [975]
Prescott Unified School District [234]
Prescott Valley Health [6246]
Present Women's Support Services [9004]
Presidio Sport & Medicine [38129]
Pressing Toward the Mark [46100]
Pressley Ridge of Delaware [33271]
Pressley Ridge School for the Deaf [710]
Pressure Management Resources, LLC [17739]
Prestera Center - Boone Satellite Office [32896]
Prestera Center - Kanawha County [32893]
Prestera Center • Lincoln County Office [32889]
Prestera Center for Mental Health [32909]
   Cornerstones [32910]
   Rehabilitation and Support Services [32911]
Prestera Center for Mental Health Services, Boone County • Crisis Helpline [51485]
Prestera Center for Mental Health Services, Cabell County • Crisis Helpline [51488]
Prestera Center for Mental Health Services, Clay County • Crisis Helpline [51484]
Prestera Center for Mental Health Services Inc [50296], [50309], [50339], [50355]
   Addiction Services [50310]
   Hopewell Place [50317]
   Innerchange [50291]
   Lincoln County [50287]
   Pinecrest Short-Term Residential Tx [50311]
   Prestera Addict Rec Center (PARC)/Detox [50312]
Prestera Center for Mental Health Services, Kanawha County • Crisis Helpline [51482]
Prestera Center for Mental Health Services, Lincoln County • Crisis Helpline [51481]
Prestera Center for Mental Health Services, Mason County • Crisis Helpline [51494]
Prestera Center for Mental Health Services, Putnam County • Crisis Helpline [51499]
Prestera Center for Mental Health Services • Safe Quarters Homelss Program [50313]
Prestera Center for Mental Health Services, Wayne County • Crisis Helpline [51497]
Prestera Center - Next Step [32897]
Prestera Center - Viewpoint [32895]
Prestera Center - Wayne [32940]
Prestera Crisis Unit • Kanawha Street Center [32935]
Presteras Addiction Recovery Centers [50297]
Prestige Care, Inc. [16563]
Prestige Home Care Agency [17424]
Prestige Home Health Care--Detroit [15642]
Prestige Home Health Care--Hialeah [13767]
Prestige Home Health Care, Inc.--Canton [16867]
Prestige Home Health Services [14115]
Preston Counseling [42367], [42376]
Preston-Taylor Community Health Centers, Inc. •

Medical Center of Taylor County [7406]
Prestonsburg Veterans Affairs Primary Care Clinic [30102]
Prevail, Inc. [9302]
Prevent of Brevard County Inc • Chris Sanok [41760]
Prevention Classes Inc [42570]
Prevention Counseling Services [43607]
Prevention Physical Therapy [38277]
Prevention and Recovery Center • Mount Auburn Hospital [44437]
Prevention and Training Services [44890]
Preventive Medicine and Clinical Genetics [12164]
PRG Assessment and Counseling Center [47542]
PRI Counseling Services [47491], [47499]
Pride Health Services Inc
   Outpatient [39946]
   Substance Abuse Treatment [40150]
Pride Institute [30676], [45142]
   Outpatient Program [45225]
Pride of North Carolina [47236]
Pride Place [4082]
Pride Program [43665]
Prima Home Health, LLC [13853]
Primacare [39083]
Primary Care Health Services, Inc. [7183]
Primary Care Medical Services--Poinciana [6482]
Primary Care and Pain Relief Center [35679]
Primary Care Service [33347]
Primary Care Services [32838]
Primary Care Sports Medicine [38630]
   Encino Sports Medicine and Pediatric Orthopedics [38086]
Primary Care Systems [7402]
Primary Children's Care Transplant [27423]
Primary Childrens Medical Center • Adolescent Residential and Day Treatment [49696]
Primary Children's Medical Center • Down Syndrome Clinic [10872]
Primary Children's Speech, Language and Hearing Center [3557]
Primary Connection Health Care, Inc. • Bridge Community Health Clinic [7442]
Primary Health Services Center [6753]
Primary Home Care Specialties [15519]
Primary Home Health Care [15607]
Primary Screening Center for Gloucester County • Newpoint Behavioral Health Care, Underwood Memorial Hospital [51126]
Primary Screening Center for Hudson County
   Christ Hospital [51104]
   Jersey City Medical Center [51105]
   Palisades Medical Center [51117]
Primary Screening Center for Hunterdon County • Hunterdon Medical Center [51102]
Primary Screening Center for Mercy County • Capital Health System at Fuld [51124]
Primary Screening Center for Monmouth County • Monmouth Medical Center [51107]
Primary Screening Center for Morris County • Saint Clare's Hospital [51097]
Primary Screening Center for Ocean County • Kimball Medical Center [51106]
Primary Screening Center of Passaic County • Saint Joseph's Hospital & Medical Center [51119]
Primary Screening Center of Salem County • Healthcare Commons, Inc. at Memorial Hospital of Salem County [51095]
Primary Screening Center of Somerset County • Somerset County PESS [51123]
Primary Screening Center of Sussex County • Newton Memorial Hospital [51116]
Primary Screening Center of Union County • Trinitas Hospital [51099]
Primary Screening Center of Warren County • Family Guidance Center of Warren County [51121]
Prime Care Health Agency, Inc.--Miami [14116]
Prime Care Health Agency--Lauderhill [13858]
Prime Care Home Health Agency Inc. [13183]
Prime Care Hospice, LLC [18815]
Prime Care Medical Supply, Inc. [16491]
Prime HealthCare Sleep Disorders Center [36749]
Prime Home Care [15763]
Prime Home Health Services [14117]
Prime Homecare Agency, LLC--Bloomfield Hills [15592]
Prime Homecare Agency--Southfield [15823]
Prime Medical Care, Inc. [14118]

Prime Medical Supply Corp. [16411]
Primecare Northwest [6664]
Primecare Pain Clinic [35599]
Primis Healthcare Systems, Inc. [15864]
Primrose Center [7902]
Prince Georges County Dialysis • Fresenius Medical Care [24699]
Prince Georges County Health Dept
  Addictions/Northern Region [44219]
  Addictions/Southern Region [44222]
Prince George's County Hotline and Suicide Prevention Center [50977]
Prince George's County Public Schools [463]
Prince William County Community Services Board [32762]
  Adult Day Treatment Program [32763]
Prince William County Dialysis • Dialysis Center • Fresenius Medical Care [27510]
Prince William County Schools • Hearing Impaired Program [854]
Prince William Hospital • Cancer Program [6067]
Prince William Speech and Hearing Center Inc. [3617]
Princeton Baptist Medical Center • Gordon L. Ross Cancer Center [4724]
Princeton Child Development Institute [8270]
Princeton Community Hospital • Cancer Program [6141]
Princeton Dialysis • DaVita [24226]
Princeton Headache Clinic [12444], [35567]
Princeton Healthcare System Home Care Services [16258]
Princeton Home Health, LLC [12634], [12679]
Princeton House Behavioral Health [46144]
Princeton Orthopaedic Associates [38752]
Princeton Spine & Sports Medicine, P.C. • Richard Levandowski, MD [38734]
Principal Knox, LLC [15013]
Principles Alcohol and Drug Program [40874]
Principles Inc [40378]
Printers Place Dialysis Center • DaVita [23104]
Priority Healthcare Services Inc [39730]
Priority Home Care--New York [16564]
Priority Home Care--Sleepy Hollow [16626]
Priority Home Care--White Plains [16673]
Priority Home Care--Yonkers [16684]
PRISM Center of Crystal Lake [42608]
PRISM Physical Therapy, PA • Rider University [38729]
Private Clinic North [42148]
Private Duty Home Care [15111]
Private Nursing Inc. [12826]
Privilege Home Health Care Inc. [13089]
PRN Home Health and Hospice-Wamego [19783]
PRN Physical and Hand Therapy [38085]
Pro-Care Home Health [15189]
Pro--Care Home Health--Madisonville [15227]
Pro--Care Home Health--Owensboro [15241]
Pro--Care Home Health--Russellville [15251]
Pro Health Advocates Inc [42602]
Pro Health Care Neuroscience Center • Multiple Sclerosis Center [34745]
Pro of Kennett Inc. [2803]
Pro--Life Home Health Services [14119]
PRO Physical Therapy--Newark [38206]
  Hand and upper Extremity Center [38207]
PRO Physical Therapy--West Chester [38989]
PRO Physical Therapy--Wilmington [38209]
Pro-Speech [1266]
Pro--Speech and Language LLC [2914]
Pro Vita Home Care [14750]
Proaction Behavioral Health Alliance
  Life Guidance Services [44818]
  Life Guidance Services/Outpatient [44819]
  Project Rehab/Mens Recovery Center [44820]
ProActive Physical Therapy [38080]
Proactive Resources • Berg Counseling Services Inc [43005], [43171]
Procare Centers/Resurrection • Behavioral Health at Procare Centers [42959]
ProCare Homecare [15643]
ProCare Medical Associates, LLC [38735]
Proceed Inc • Addiction Services [45985]
Proctor Hospital [14906]
  Sleep Disorders Center [36927]
Prodex Home Health Agency [13103]
Prodigious Health Services LLC [47375]
Prodigy Dialysis, LLC--Ebensburg [26425]

Prodigy Dialysis LLC--Franklin Street [26454]
Prodigy Dialysis, LLC--Meyersdale [26478]
Prodigy Dialysis, LLC--Osborne St. [26455]
Prodigy Dialysis, LLC--Richland Square [26456]
Prodigy Dialysis, LLC--Somerset [26583]
Productive Rehabilitation Institute of Dallas for Ergonomics [35707]
Professional Audiology Associates [1619]
Professional Care Home Health Agency [13685]
Professional Care Home Health Services [13356]
Professional Care Services [32302]
Professional Care Services of • West Tennessee [49065], [49073], [49178], [49191]
Professional Center for Child Development [8106]
Professional Communications Care, P.C. [2164]
Professional Community Services Counseling Center [28482]
Professional Consultations Inc [42401], [42609], [42685], [42956]
  All Alcohol/Substance Abuse Progs on Site [42405]
Professional Counseling and • Consulting Services PC [47954]
Professional Counseling Associates [46108]
Professional Counseling Associates - Cabot Clinic [28249]
Professional Counseling Associates, Inc.--Hazen [28282]
Professional Counseling Associates--Jacksonville [28289]
Professional Counseling Associates • Lonoke Clinic [28310]
Professional Counseling Associates--North Little Rock [28334]
Professional Counseling Associates--Sherwood [28352]
Professional Counseling Associates • Southwest Little Rock Clinic [28305]
Professional Counseling Center [44978], [45097]
Professional Counseling Services [46574]
Professional Counseling Services of • Ruston [43888]
Professional Counseling Solutions [47937]
Professional Foot Care Specialists [38364]
Professional Health Care Services, LLC [12660]
Professional Healthcare Resources [19915], [21674]
Professional Hearing Center [2841]
Professional Hearing Healthcare Centers [961]
Professional Hearing Management Inc. [2193]
Professional Hearing Services--Hillsdale [2604]
Professional Hearing Services--Jackson [2611]
Professional Hearing Services--Pasadena [1223]
Professional Home Care Service [13147]
Professional Home Care Service, Inc. [17455]
Professional Home Health Care--Albuquerque [16306]
Professional Home Health Care--Dearborn [15623]
Professional Home Health Care Inc.--Los Angeles [13148]
Professional Home Health Care, Inc.--Taylor [15850]
Professional Home Health Care--Las Vegas [16322]
Professional Home Health Care--Santa Fe [16327]
Professional Home Health Services of Baton Rouge [15273]
Professional Home Health Services of Caddo [15362]
Professional Home Hospice [20945], [20972]
Professional Homecare, Inc. [15747]
Professional Imaging LLC [3510]
Professional Medical Home Health [13768]
Professional Medical Home Healthcare, Inc. [14588]
Professional Medical Supply [12980]
Professional Mental Health Associates [11115]
Professional Nurses Homecare, Inc. [14326]
Professional Nurses Service, Inc. [18240]
Professional Pharmacy Services, Inc. [17589]
Professional Plus Home Health [14120]
Professional Psychology Associates PC • Center for Lifestyle Change [39445]
Professional Services Corporation [49649]
Professional Sleep Diagnostics, Inc. [37952]
Professional Speech Services Inc. [3238]
Professional Therapy Solutions Inc. [2837]
Professional Training Associates/Comprehensive Addiction and Rehabilitation Education • Eating Disorder Program [11029]
Professional Training Association • CARE/Outpatient [41827]

Professional Treatment Services [43388]
Proficient Healthcare Services [14848]
Progenics Cord Blood Cryobank [35179]
Program for Addictions • Consultation and Treatment [46135]
Program for Assertive Community Treatment [33932]
Program for Deaf/Hard of Hearing [508]
Program for Women and Families [10261]
Programa Ley 22 - San Juan [48819]
Programa SER/Renton • Sole Prop under Miguel Orozco Delgado [50085]
Programs for Peaceful Living [10609]
Progress Foundation
  Administrative Office [28762]
  Cortland House [28763]
  Dorine Loso House Transitional Program [28764]
  La Amistad [28765]
  La Posada [28766]
  Laurel House [28646]
  Progress House [28767]
  Progress Place [28647]
  Shrader House [28768]
  Supported Living Program [28769]
Progress at Home, LLC [15877]
Progress House Inc • Progress House Counseling Center [40394]
Progress Valley I [45226]
Progress Valley II [45272]
Progressive Health Care Services, Inc. [17308]
Progressive Health of Pennsylvania, Inc. [4402]
Progressive Home Care Services [15726]
Progressive Home Health Care, Inc. [13827]
Progressive Home Health Services, Inc. [16565]
Progressive HomeCare Services, Inc. [15004]
Progressive Life Center [29100]
Progressive Living Program [28416]
Progressive Medical Specialists Inc [40573], [48407], [48605]
Progressive Physical Therapy and Sports Medicine Clinic [38524]
Progressive Rehabilitation Associates [4381], [35638]
Progressive Speech Corporation [1293]
Progressive Speech and Language PC [3074]
Progressive Speech & Voice [2180]
Progressive Step Rehabilitation Services [3454]
Progressive Therapeutic Home Health Care [15753]
Progressive Therapy [1856]
Progressive Therapy Inc. [1185]
ProHealth Care, Inc. • Cancer Program [6177]
ProHealth Care Sleep Disorders Center • Waukesha Memorial Hospital [37974]
ProHealth Home Care [18575]
ProHealth Primary Care Clinic [7268]
ProHealth Sleep Center [36750]
ProHEALTH Sleep Disorders Center [37411]
Project Achieve--Bronx • HIV Vaccine Trials Unit [88]
Project Achieve--Union Square • HIV Vaccine Trials Unit [89]
Project ADAM [10489]
Project Adam • Community Assistance Center Inc [42185]
Project Adapt [40630]
Project COPE • Outpatient Substance Abuse Services [44508]
Project CURE [47743]
Project DOVE • Domestic Violence Eliminated [10242]
Project Eden • A Program of Horizon Services Inc [39914]
Project Free Catholic Charities [46079]
Project Hope at Quin Rivers [10580]
Project Horizon, Inc. [10576]
Project Hospitality Inc • Chemical Dependence Outpatient [47096]
Project Lighthouse • Runaway and Homeless Youth Program [36195]
Project Linden [47729]
Project LOVE, Inc. [9116]
Project Ninety Inc
  Elliott Center [40818]
  O'Toole Center [40681]
  Simmons House [40682]
Project Oz • Runaway and Homeless Youth Services [35937]
Project PATCH Ranch [29545]
Project PAVE [8954]

PRS, LLC [23988]
Prudence Crandall Center for Women [8999]
PSC for Safe Babies • Runaway and Homeless
   Youth Program [36271]
PSCH--48th Street Residence [31275]
PSCH--ACT Team [31276]
PSCH--Bridger/ICM Program [31277]
PSCH--Horizon I & II [31278]
PSCH, Inc. [31307]
PSE&G Children's Specialized Hospital [4295]
PSI Health Care--Aberdeen [17628]
PSI Health Care--Pierre [17632]
PSI Health Care--Rapid City [17635]
PSI Health Care--Sioux Falls [17639]
PSI Health Care--Yankton [17643]
PSI Healthcare--Gillette [18652]
PSN Health Care Corporation--Hialeah [13769]
PSN Health Care Corporation--Miami [14122]
Psycare Associates Inc • Psycare Intensive
   Outpatient Program [40574]
Psychesoma Center [10981]
Psychiatric Care Center [40426]
Psychiatric Crisis Services [33941], [50998]
Psychiatric Hospital at Vanderbilt [33852]
Psychiatric Institute of Washington [33284]
Psychiatric Intervention Center [30593]
Psychiatric and Psychological Services [47756]
Psychiatric Rehabilitation Services [30297]
Psychiatric Services • East Alabama Medical Center
   [28007]
Psycholinguistic Associates Inc. [2484]
The Psychological Center [30404]
The Psychological Center Inc [44497]
Psychological Center
   Pegasus [44498]
   Womens View [44499]
Psychological Consultants of MI PC • DBA Chemical
   Dependency Resources [44657], [44836], [44872]
Psychological Services [42788], [48300]
Psychological Services Clinic [48337], [48652]
Psychological Services Inc [42782]
Psychological Trauma Center [50677]
Psychology Services of Idaho [11042]
Psychotherapeutic Services [30275], [47237]
Psychotherapeutic Services--Alachua County
   [29174]
Psychotherapeutic Services, Inc. [29060]
   Felton Group Home [29063]
   Georgetown Transitional Housing [29064]
Psychotherapeutic Treatment Services [30255]
Psychotherapeutic Treatment Services, Inc.
   Mobile Crisis [31511]
   Together House [31512]
PsychSolutions, Inc. [29223]
PsychStrategies [10982]
Public Hlth Dayton and Montgomery Cnty • Alcohol-
   ism and Drug Addiction Services [47744]
Public School Intensive Counseling Program [34166]
Pueblo Community Health Center [6417]
Pueblo Dialysys • Fresenius Medical Care [23137]
Pueblo of Nambe [46306]
Pueblo of San Felipe • Behavioral Health Program
   [46246]
Pueblo South Dialysis • Fresenius Medical Care
   [23138]
Pueblo Suicide Prevention Center, Inc. [50720]
Pueblo West Dialysis • Fresenius Medical Care
   [23139]
Puente House [39763]
Puente de Vida/Bridge of Life: A Center for Caring
   and Individualized Eating Disorder Treatment
   [10983]
Puerto Rican Family Institute • Queens Mental
   Health Clinic [31462]
Puerto Rico Addiction Medical Services • (PRAMS)
   [48805]
Puerto Rico Department of Education • Deaf and
   Hard of Hearing Education Program [716]
Puerto Rico Department of Public Health [36537]
Puerto Rico Regional Library for the Blind and
   Physically Handicapped [3834]
Puget Sound Blood Center • Northwest Tissue
   Services [35260]
Puget Sound Blood Center and Program •
   Hemophilia Program [12610]
Puget Sound Home Health, LLC [18437]
Puget Sound Kidney Center • Dialysis Facility
   [27604]

Puget Sound Kidney Center--Smokey Point [27592]
Puget Sound Kidney Center--South [27619]
Puget Sound Kidney Center--Whidbey Island
   [27620]
Puget Sound Spine Institute [39153]
Pulaski Center [32776]
Pulaski Child and Adolescence Services [30114]
Pulaski Child and Adolescent Services [43784]
Pulaski Community Hospital • Cancer Center [6077]
Pulaski County Mental Retardation Service Center
   [29439]
Pulaski County Special School District [248]
Pulaski Memorial Hospital [15062]
Pulmonary Associates of Northern New Jersey •
   Sleep Disorders Center [37355]
Pulmonary Associates and Sleep Center [37953]
Pulmonary Associates • Sleep Disorders Center
   [37892]
Pulmonary Clinic of the Carolinas--Huntersville
   [37481]
Pulmonary and Critical Care Consultants, PC •
   Sleep Disorders Center [37412]
Pulmonary and Critical Care Services • Sleep
   Disorders Center [37413]
Pulmonary Home Care - West Virginia [18509]
Pulmonary Medicine Associates Sleep Center
   [37320]
Pulmonary Medicine Associates • Sleep Disorders
   Center [36686]
Pulmonary Physicians Sleep Center [37564]
Pulmonary Prescription Providers [14316]
Pulmonary and Sleep Associates • Sleep Center
   [37002]
Pulmonary and Sleep Center of Lake City [36804]
Pulmonary and Sleep Center of the Valley [37835]
Pulmonary and Sleep Disorders of New York
   [37414]
Pulmonary and Sleep Medicine--Dalton • Sleep
   Disorders Center [36853]
Pulmonary and Sleep Medicine--Ocean Springs •
   Sleep Laboratory [37259]
Pulmonary and Sleep Specialists • Sleep Disorders
   Center [36854]
Pupil Appraisal Center [2335]
Purcell Clinic [31913]
Purcellville Dialysis Center & At Home • DaVita
   [27541]
Purdue University
   Audiology Clinic [2195]
   Department of Audiology and Speech Services
   [2196]
Purdy Farm House [33428]
Purity Dialysis--Brookfield [27705]
Purity Dialysis--Fort Atkinson [27716]
Purity Dialysis--Germantown [27717]
Purity Dialysis--Menomonee Falls • Dialysis Center
   [27741]
Purity Dialysis--Mukwonago [27761]
Purity Dialysis--Oconomowoc [27765]
Purity Dialysis--Watertown [27793]
Purity Dialysis--Waukesha [27795]
Purity Dialysis--Waukesha South [27796]
Purity Home Health Services [13336]
Pushmataha Counseling Services Inc [48010]
Putham County Ambulatory Care • Dialysis Center
   [26128]
Putnam Behavioral Healthcare • Residential and
   Detoxification [41871]
Putnam Community Medical Center [1705]
Putnam County Comprehensive Services Inc. [7991]
Putnam County Family Support Services [9278]
Putnam County HomeCare & Hospice [20879]
Putnam County Hospital • Cancer Program [5151]
Putnam Family and Community Services Inc •
   Chemical Dependency Outpatient [46585]
Putnam Hospital Center • Cancer Care Program
   [5573]
Putnam Hospital Center Home Care [16432]
Putnam Hospital • Sleep Center [37415]
Putnam/North Westchester Women's Resource
   Center [9943]
Pu'uhonua - The Domestic Violence Drop-in-Center
   [9146]
Pu'ukama • Kid Behavioral Health of Hawaii [34093]
Puyallup Behavioral Health Clinic [32848]
Puyallup Dialysis Center • DaVita [27631]
Puyallup Tribal Treatment Center [50216]
PYR Services LLC [2000]

Pyramid Alternatives Inc [40343]
Pyramid Educational Consultants [1481]
Pyramid Healthcare Inc
   Tradition House [48275]
   Transitions/Detox [48698]
   Womens Facility [48345]
   York Pharmacotherapy Services [48714]
PYRYSYS Psychology Group • Supporting ME
   (Moderate Eating) Program [10984]

Q

Q. A. Nursing Services [14123]
Q-Care Home Health [14124]
QA Health Services [14125]
QSA Inc/CD Outpatient Program • DBA The PAC
   Program of Queens [46627]
Quaboag Valley Hospice [19993]
Quad Cities Kidney Center - Bettendorf LLC [24251]
Quad Cities Kidney Center--Davenport [24262]
Quad Cities Kidney Center - Geneseo [23997]
Quad Cities Kidney Center Ltd. [24044]
Quad Cities Kidney Center--Rock Island, LLC
   [24072]
Quad Cities Kidney Center Silvis LLC [24084]
Quad Cities Vet Center [51950]
Quad Counties Dialysis Center • Diversified
   Specialty Institutes [24114]
Quad County Treatment Center [41837]
QuadMed Subst Abuse Counseling Service [50409],
   [50440], [50561]
QuadMed Substance Abuse Counseling • Service
   [50541]
Qualicenters Albany • Dialysis Center • Fresenius
   Medical Care [26311]
Qualicenters Bend • Dialysis Center • Fresenius
   Medical Care [26315]
Qualicenters Coos Bay • Dialysis Center • Fresenius
   Medical Care [26317]
Qualicenters Eugene/Springfield • Dialysis Center •
   Fresenius Medical Care [26357]
Qualicenters Salem • Dialysis Center • Fresenius
   Medical Care [26354]
Quality Addiction Management [50370], [50404],
   [50451], [50526], [50551]
   Narcotic Treatment Program [50512]
   West Milwaukee [50484]
Quality Behavioral Health [49929]
Quality Behavioral Health Inc [44759]
Quality Care Dialysis Center • Fresenius Medical
   Care [24816]
Quality Care Dialysis Center--North County • Fres-
   enius Medical Care [25207]
Quality Care Dialysis Center--Saint Louis • Fres-
   enius Medical Care [25178]
Quality Care Dialysis Center--Saintn Clair Shores •
   Fresenius Medical Care [24968]
Quality Care Dialysis--Hammond • Fresenius Medi-
   cal Care [24503]
Quality Care Dialysis--Southern Maryland • Fres-
   enius Medical Care [24664]
Quality Care Home Services [14126]
Quality Community Health Care, Inc. [7180]
Quality Concept, Inc. [17789]
Quality Dialysis Two Inc. [27364]
Quality First Home Health Care [13406]
Quality Health Care Group Inc. [17425]
Quality Health Care Providers [13770]
Quality Healthcare Services [16188]
Quality Hearing Center [3532]
Quality Home Care Providers, Inc. [16232]
Quality Home Care Solutions [14218]
Quality Home Care Solutions Corporation [13771]
Quality Home Health Care [15644]
Quality Home Health Care of Columbus, LLC
   [16918]
Quality Home Health Care Services of Michigan
   [15824]
Quality Home Health Services, Inc. [15851]
Quality Homecare of Nevada, Inc. [16157]
Quality Hospice Care, Inc. [20259]
Quality Life Health Care, LLC [14939]
Quality of Life Health Services [6189]
Quality Life Home Agency Corporation [13610]
Quality Life Home Care Corporation [13772]
Quality Life Hospice [20964]
Quality Living Center Inc [39549]
Quality Living, Inc. [4261]

Quality Plus Care [14839]
Quality Renal Care--Carpentersville [23910]
Quality Renal Care, LLC--Marengo [24028]
Quality Resources LLC [50258]
Quality Service Home Health [13773]
QUANADA [9244]
Quantah Assessment and • Counseling Services [50123]
Quantum Homecare [15727]
Quapaw Counseling Services [47959], [47993]
Quapaw House Inc [39540]
    DG Dunston Adolescent Center [39560]
Quapaw Tribal Substance Abuse Services [47960]
Queen Annes County Health Dept • Alc and Drug Abuse Treatment and Prev Services [44214]
Queen City Sports Medicine and Rehabilitation [38863]
Queen City Treatment Center [47265]
Queen Elizabeth II Health Sciences Centre
    Burn Unit [4602]
    Eating Disorders Program [11191]
Queen of Peace Center at Cathedral • Cathedral Tower [45628]
Queen of Peace Hospital [15921]
Queen of the Universe Day Center [8470]
Queen of the Valley Hospital • Cancer Program [4810]
Queens Artificial Kidney Center • Renal Research Institute [25687]
Queens Centers for Progress [8324]
Queens Children's Psychiatric Center [31241]
Queens College [3020]
Queens Community Living Program [31364]
Queens Dialysis Center • DaVita [25688]
Queens Dialysis Unit, Inc. [23070]
Queens Hospital Center
    Cancer Program [5584]
    Center for Child Development [12297]
Queens Hospital Center for Hearing and Speech [3035]
Queens-Long Island Renal Institute [25711]
Queen's Medical Center [29523]
    Cancer Institute [5047]
Queens Medical Center • Day Treatment Services [42214]
Queen's Medical Center/Department of Health • Hawaii Community Genetics [12194]
The Queen's Sleep Center [36873]
Queens Vet Center [52047]
Queens Village Comm for Mental Health
    JCAP Inc [47061]
    JCAP/Residential Re-Entry Unit [46726]
Queens Village Committee for Mental • Health/JCAP [46727]
Queens Village Dialysis Center • Dialysis Facility • DaVita [25761]
QueensCare Family Clinic, Eagle Rock [6319]
Quentin Price MD • Crisis Residential Unit [42089]
Quest [4231]
Quest Center for Intergrated Health [48213]
Quest Counseling Center Inc [41557]
Quest Counseling and Consulting [45871]
Quest for Excellence/WINGS [9288]
Quest Health Care--Bend [17181]
Quest Health Care--Eugene [17187]
Quest Health Care--Fife [18431]
Quest Health Care--Portland [17219]
Quest Health Care--Redmond [18449]
Quest Home Health Services Inc. [13214]
Quest Recovery House/Wilson Hall • Mens Residential Facility [47806]
Quest Recovery and Prevention Services [47638], [47807]
    Quest Deliverance House [47639]
Quest Recovery Services • Alliance Division [47612]
Quest Services Inc [48287], [48576], [48577]
Questhouse Inc [43540]
Quigley House, Inc. [9070]
Quinault Indian Nation • Chemical Dependency Program [50223]
Quinco Behavioral Health Systems [29707]
Quinco Community Mental Health Center [49041]
Quinco Consulting Associates of Southern Indiana [29754]
Quinco Mental Health Center
    Chester County Center [49080]
    Decatur County Center [49069]
    Hardin County Center [49181]

Henderson County Center [49120]
Madison County Center [49093]
McNairy County Center [49183]
Quincy Dialysis • DaVita [23495]
Quincy Medical Center • Cancer Center [5353]
Quincy Medical Group • Peritoneal Dialysis Center [24071]
Quincy Mental Health Center [33581]
Quincy School for the Handicapped [7967]
Quincy Sports Medicine [38566]
Quincy Veterans Affairs Clinic [29669]
Quinebaug Day Treatment Center [33263], [41464]
Quinn-Miller Group, Inc. [13565]
Quotidian Dialysis [22739]

R

R & A Home Health Service, Inc. [13047]
R House • Speers Facility [40785]
R & M Health Care [14127]
R P H Home Health Care, Inc. [14128]
R P Home Care [13563]
R Quest [40397]
R and R Hearing Center LLC--Windsor [1443]
R and R Hearing Center--Longmont [1433]
R & R Home Care, Inc.--Metairie [15330]
R & R Home Care--Mandeville [15323]
R and R Outpatient LLC [1686]
Raceland Dialysis Center [24571]
Rachel Coalition/Jewish Family Service [9835]
Rachell Home Health Services--Miami [14129]
Racine Community Health Center [7438]
Racine Psychological Services Inc [50513]
Rader Programs/Pacific Shores Hospital [10985]
Radford Dialysis & At Home • DaVita [27543]
Radius Foundation Inc [42842]
Radnor Dialysis & At Home • DaVita [26573]
Rady Children's Hospital of San Diego [22946]
Rady Children's Hospital of San Diego
    Children's Home Care [13300]
    Developmental Services--Audiology [1267]
Rady Children's Hospital of San Diego • Pediatric Down Syndrome Center [10778]
Rady Children's Hospital San Diego/University of California, San Diego • Cystic Fibrosis Center [7478]
RAFT Recovering Adolescents and • Families Together Treatment Center LLC [48354]
Raging River Recovery Center • Snoqualmie Tribe [50032]
Rago and Associates [11054]
RAI Bancroft • Renal Advantage Inc. [22847]
RAI--Broadway--Chula Vista • Renal Advantage Inc. [22635]
RAI Care Center--Ames Ave. • Renal Advantage Inc. [25341]
RAI Care Center--Center Street • Renal Advantage Inc. [25342]
RAI Care Center--Fremont • Renal Advantage Inc. • Dialysis Facility [25321]
RAI Care Centers--Charlotte • Renal Advantage Inc. [25842]
RAI Care Centers--Fort Pierce • Renal Advantage Inc. [23307]
RAI Care Centers--Goldsboro • Renal Advantage Inc. [25873]
RAI Care Centers--Haines City • Renal Advantage Inc. [23314]
RAI Care Centers--Lake Wales • Renal Treatment Center • Dialysis Facility [23361]
RAI Care Centers--Largo • Renal Advantage Inc. • Dialysis Facility [23367]
RAI Care Centers--Port Saint Lucie • Renal Advantage Inc. [23493]
RAI--Centinela--Inglewood • Renal Advantage Inc. [22735]
RAI Ceres Ave Chico • Renal Advantage, Inc [22628]
RAI Cesar Chavez • Renal Advantage Inc. [22957]
RAI Chadbourne • Renal Advantage Inc. [22685]
RAI--Corporate Way--Palm Desert • Renal Advantage Inc. [22867]
RAI E. 14th • Renal Advantage Inc. [22981]
RAI-East Bay-Oakland • Renal Advantage Inc. [22848]
RAI--East First Street--Tustin • Renal Advantage Inc. [23044]

RAI--East Olympic--Los Angeles • Renal Advantage Inc. [22787]
RAI Elk Grove Blvd. • Renal Advantage Inc. [22675]
RAI Fairway Rocklin • Renal Advantage Inc. • Comprehensive Renal Services [22909]
RAI--Foothill Blvd.--Glendora • Renal Advantage Inc. [22712]
RAI--Garden Grove Blvd.--Garden • Renal Advantage Inc. [22703]
RAI--Goldenwest--Westminster • Renal Advantage Inc. [23073]
RAI Greenville Ave--Winchester • Renal Advantage Inc. [24247]
RAI Haight • Renal Advantage Inc. [22958]
RAI-Harbor Blvd.--Garden Grove • Renal Advantage Inc. [22704]
RAI Harding Blvd. • Renal Advantage Inc. [22912]
RAI Hemlock St.--Macon • Renal Advantage Inc. [23747]
RAI--Hospital Circle--Westminster • Renal Advantage Inc, [23074]
RAI--Indiana Court--Redlands • Renal Advantage Inc. • Dialysis Center [22897]
RAI--Juniper Ave--Fontana • Renal Advantage Inc. [22688]
RAI Kings Way--Valdosta • Renal Advantage Inc. [23822]
RAI--Laguna Canyon--Irvine • Renal Advantage Inc. [22736]
RAI Lincoln Dialysis • Renal Advantage Inc. [22750]
RAI Medical Center Dr.--Swainsboro [23804]
RAI--Monroe--Indio • Renal Advantage Inc. [22728]
RAI North California • Renal Advantage Inc. [23023]
RAI--North Riverside--Rialto • Renal Advantage Inc. [22901]
RAI North St--Muncie • Renal Advantage Inc. • Dialysis Unit [24211]
RAI Oakland Home Program 1 • Renal Advantage Inc. [22849]
RAI Ocean Avenue • Renal Advantage Inc. [22959]
RAI Peach Orchard Rd.--Augusta [23615]
RAI Peralta • Renal Advantage Inc. [22850]
RAI-S Courtenay--Merritt Island • Renal Advantage Inc. [23386]
RAI S Harris St.--Sandersville [23782]
RAI Secret Ravine Pkwy. • Renal Advantage Inc. [22913]
RAI West March • Renal Advantage Inc. [23024]
Railbelt Mental Health and Addictions [39346]
Railbelt Mental Health & Addictions
    Healy Office [28094]
    Nenana Office [28110]
Rainbow Babies and Children's Hospital • Down Syndrome Clinic [10849]
Rainbow Center • Day School [8194]
Rainbow Center of Michigan Inc [44840]
    Monroe [44925]
Rainbow Home Health Care Agency Inc. [13113]
Rainbow Hospice Care Inc. [21843]
Rainbow Hospice Inc. [19557]
Rainbow House [30028], [30927], [35911]
Rainbow House--Chicago [9212]
Rainbow House Columbia • Runaway and Homeless Youth Program [36057]
Rainbow House Domestic Abuse Services, Inc. [10715]
Rainbow House--Rockingham [10077]
Rainbow Industries Production Company/RIPCo [4181]
Rainbow Kids Therapy Inc. [1748]
Rainbow Lodge, Inc. [34397]
Rainbow Mental Health Facility [33506]
Rainbow Recovery Center [48467]
Rainbow Recovery Resources [43016]
Rainbow Rehabilitation Centers, Inc.
    NeuroRehab Campus Northmeadow [4182]
    Ypsilanti Center [4183]
Rainbow Rehabilitation Centers
    Livonia [4184]
        Rainbow Oakland Center [4185]
Rainbow Services, Ltd. [8900]
Rainelle Medical Center [7413], [32932]
Raines Dialysis • Fresenius Medical Care • Dialysis Center [26320]
Rainforest Recovery Center • Bartlett Regional Hospital [39337]
Rainrock Treatment Center [11251]
Raintree Clinic [47312]

Raise the Bottom Training and • Counseling Services [42316]
Raleigh Dialysis Clinic Inc. • Fresenius Medical Care [25928]
Raleigh General Hospital • Sports Medicine Department [39158]
Raleigh Methadone Treatment Center • (RMTC) [47464]
Raleigh Neurology Associates • Multiple Sclerosis Center [34664]
Raleigh Neurology • Sleep Medicine Program [37482]
Raleigh Orthopaedic Clinic [38836]
Raleigh Professional Associates [49142]
Raleigh Regional Resource Center for the Deaf and Hard of Hearing • Division of Services for the Deaf and Hard of Hearing [3192]
Raleigh Veterans Affairs Clinic [31582]
Ralph D Raphael PhD PA [44173]
Ralph H Johnson VA Medical Center • Substance Abuse Treatment Center [48913]
Ralph H. Johnson Veterans Affairs Medical Center [17568]
        Cancer Program [5900]
        Multiple Sclerosis Center [34707]
        PTSD Clinical Team [51812]
Ralph McGill Dialysis • DaVita [23604]
Ram Clinic [48214]
Ramak Home Health Agency Corporation [13674]
Ramapo Ridge Psychiatric Hospital [33666]
RAMAS Counseling Center [46222]
Ramey Nutrition [11305]
Ramona VNA & Hospice [18940]
Ramsey County Adult Mental Health Services • Crisis Center [51045]
Ramsey County Receiving Center [45308]
Ramsey House--People Incorporated [30726]
Ranch [49171]
The Ranch [11271]
Ranch at Dove Tree [49457]
Ranch Recovery Centers Inc
        DBA The Ranch [39781]
        Hacienda Valdez [39782]
Rancho Los Amigos Medical Center • Communication Disorders [1095]
Rancho Los Amigos National Rehabilitation Center [3914]
        MDA Clinic [34761]
Rancho Los Amigos School [7774]
Rancho Valmora [34318]
Randall G. Lynch Middle School [1005]
Randi Massey [46106]
Randolph Children's Home [34347]
Randolph County Family Crisis Center [10013]
Randolph County Satellite Office [28027]
Randolph County Schools [871]
Randolph Helpline [51157]
Randolph Hospital [16690]
        Cancer Care Program [5626]
Randolph Hospital Cardiopulmonary Rehabilitation Program [38827]
Randolph W. Evans, MD [12470]
Range Center Inc. [2681]
Range Mental Health Center [30686], [30731]
Range Mental Health Center, Inc. [30732]
Range Treatment Center [45176]
Range Women's Advocates [9642]
Rangely Victim Services [8981]
Rangeview Counseling Center [41021], [41189]
Ranier School [8599]
Ranken Jordan Pediatric Rehabilitation Center [8205]
Ransom Memorial Hospital [15145]
RAP Inc/Regional Addiction Prevention • Residential Treatment Facility [41546]
Rape and Abuse Crisis Center of Fargo-Moorhead [10112]
Rape and Abuse Crisis Service [9686]
Rape, Child and Family Abuse Crisis Council [10080]
Rape Crisis Center [10357]
Rape Crisis Center of Central Massachusetts, Inc. [9508]
Rape Crisis Council of Pickens County [10349]
Rape Crisis Intervention Center [9824]
Rape Crisis Program [10005]
Rape/Domestic Abuse Program, Inc. [9779]
Rape and Domestic Violence Crisis Center [9806]

Rape and Domestic Violence Information Center, Inc. [10679]
Rape Prevention/Crisis Intervention [9930]
Rape Response and Crime Victims Center [9175]
Rape and Sexual Assault Program [9331]
Rape Victim Advocacy Program [9337]
Rape and Violence End Now [9722]
Rapha Treatment Center [39211]
Raphael House of Portland [10250]
Rapid City Area Schools [744]
Rapid City CBOC • Outpatient Treatment Program [49009]
Rapid City Mobile Vet Center [52092]
Rapid City Regional Hospital - Home Care Services [17636]
Rapid City Regional Hospital - Home Care Services - Custer [17637]
Rapides Drug Court Treatment [43804]
Rapides Parish Schools [446]
Rapides Parish Vet Center [51967]
Rapides Regional Medical Center • Cancer Program [5239]
Rapids Counseling Services Inc [45167]
Rappahannock Area Community Serv Board
        Caroline Clinic [49838]
        King George Clinic [49804]
        North Stafford Clinic [49845]
        Spotsylvania Clinic [49844]
        Substance Abuse Services [49788]
        A Womans Place Clinic [49789]
Rappahannock Council Against Sexual Assault [10567]
Rappahannock Council on Domestic Violence [10568]
Rappahannock General Hospital [18314]
Rappahannock General Hospital--Behavioral Health [32752]
Raritan Bay Medical Center
        Cancer Program [5534]
        Center for Sleep Medicine [37356]
        Methadone Treatment Program [46132]
Rathdrum Counseling Center LLC [42368]
Rational Alternatives [45179]
Rational Steps [41641]
Rational Treatment Services Inc • (RTS) [49893]
Raton Dialysis • Dialysis Clinic Inc. [25555]
RAVE - Ionia/Montcalm/Domestic and Sexual Violence Program [9545]
Ravenna Veterans Affairs Clinic [31828]
Ravenswood Clinic [50485]
Ravenwood Mental Health Center [31680], [31807]
        Drug and Alcohol Treatment Services [47644]
Ravinder N Agarwal Renal Center • Renal Center [25747]
Ray Graham Association for People with Disabilities [7949]
Raymond G. Murphy Veterans Affairs Medical Center [31183]
Raymond Naftali Center for Rehabilitation [3075]
Rays of Hope Unlimited [45309]
Rays of Sonshine [43861]
RB Home Health Service [14130]
R.C. Goodman Institute for Pain Management [35278]
RC Ward Addiction Treatment Center • Inpatient Rehabilitation Unit [46781]
RCA-Cabot [39524]
RCG--Ft Walton Beach • Fresenius Medical Care • Dialysis Facility [23309]
RCG--Sacred Heart Adult Dialysis • Fresenius Medical Care [23473]
RCI [8287]
Re-Enter Inc [48557]
Re-Entry Inc • Re-Entry Residential [40972]
Re Entry Mental Health Services • Addiction Services [44388]
REACH Beyond Domestic Violence [9506]
REACH of Clay County [10043]
REACH of Haywood County, Inc. [10096]
REACH Inc • Comprehensive Menth Health Clinic [50396]
REACH of Jackson County, Inc. [10089]
REACH of Macon County, Inc. [10038]
Reach Out [28411]
REACH Project Inc [39609]
        Reach Brentwood [39667]
Reach for Speech [2936]
Reaching Across Illinois Library System

Mid-Illinois Talking Book Center [3787]
        Voices of Vision Talking Book Center [3788]
Reaching Out Against Eating Disorders [11165]
REACHOUT of Saint Lawrence County, Inc. [51149]
Reading Dialysis Center [26574]
Reading Hospital and Medical Center [48424]
        Regional Cancer Center [5868]
Reading and Language Learning Center [3614]
Reading and Speech Clinic Inc. [3305]
Reading Therapy Center [2752]
Real Care [16412]
REAL Crisis Intervention, Inc. [51168]
Real House Inc [46064]
Real Life Nutritional Counseling [11070]
Reality Counseling Services [44891], [45066]
Reality Health Care [18043]
Reality House Inc • Chemical Dependence Outpatient Service [46765]
Reality House Programs Inc • PMI [45466]
Reality Inc
        Continuing Care Facility Male/Female [44305]
        Intermediate Care Facility ICF [44306]
Realization Center Inc/Licensed Outpatient • Addictions Treatment Program [46528], [46913]
Reasonable Choices [47861]
Reasonable Service [42620]
Rebecca Vinson Center [9364]
Rebecca's House • Eating Disorders Treatment Program [10986]
Rebeccas Residence [45320]
Rebekah Children's Servies [28515]
Rebos Chris Farley House [50452]
Rebound Sports Medicine • Morton Hospital and Medical Center [38572]
Rebuild [40315]
Recco Home Care Service--Eat Quogue [16437]
Recco Home Care Service--Forest Hills [16466]
Recco Home Care Service, Inc.--Massapequa [16517]
Recco Home Care Service--New Rochelle [16543]
Recco Home Care Service--Smithtown [16627]
Reconnect With Food • Inner Door Center [11100]
Recover at Baptist Health • Medical Center/Little Rock [39550]
Recovering Spirit LLC [41140]
Recovery 4 Life [42317]
Recovery Assoc of the Palm Beaches • Outpatient/Intensive Outpatient Prog [41734]
Recovery Associates [47475], [47500]
Recovery Associates of Southern Maine [43992], [44033], [44055], [44068]
Recovery Center [47786]
Recovery Center of Cameron County
        Brownsville [49252]
        Harlingen [49355]
Recovery Center of Crozer Chester • Medical Center [48323]
Recovery Center at Mercy Hospital [44084]
Recovery Center of Northern Virginia [49802]
Recovery Center at Nyack Hospital
        Chemical Dependency Acute Care Prog [46955]
        Chemical Dependency Inpatient Rehab [46956]
Recovery Center at Valley General Hosp [50019]
Recovery Center--Warrensburg [30912]
Recovery Centers of Arkansas [39551], [39566]
        Williamsburg [39552]
Recovery Centers Inc [47891]
Recovery Centers of King County [50124]
        Detoxification Facility [50125]
Recovery Centers of King County/Kent • Outpatient [49986]
Recovery for the City International • T/A Recovery for Life [49857]
Recovery in Community [44174]
Recovery Concepts [42700]
        Addiction Counseling Services Inc [48284]
Recovery Concepts of the Carolina • Upstate [48928]
Recovery Concepts Inc • Indian Alcoholism Treatment Services [43504]
Recovery Concepts LLC [48971]
Recovery Connection [39313]
Recovery Connections Treatment Services LLC • Recovery Connections Residential Treatment [40740]
Recovery Consultants Inc [44669], [45052]
Recovery Counseling Services • Raymond Smith [43199]

Recovery Dynamics [47410]
Recovery First Inc [41692]
    Outpatient [41611]
Recovery Healthcare Corporation [49294]
Recovery Home Health Care Systems [17807]
Recovery Home Health Services [13420]
Recovery House Inc [45371]
    Serenity House [49748]
Recovery Innovations Inc [46183]
Recovery Innovations of NC [47376]
Recovery Journey Inc [43027]
Recovery Management Services Inc • Crossroads Treatment Center I [39740]
Recovery Network • Halfway Houses Program [44175]
Recovery Network of Programs Inc • Regional Adolescent Program [41367]
Recovery Options Northwest Inc. [50126]
Recovery Outreach Services LLC [45650]
Recovery Physical Therapy--Lexington Avenue, New York [38803]
Recovery Physical Therapy--Wall Street, New York [38804]
Recovery Place [41658]
Recovery Place Inc
    Intensive Outpatient Program [42153]
    Womens Residential Treatment [42154]
Recovery Plus--Del Nor Center [31290]
Recovery Plus--Elmwood • Wellness Center [31291]
Recovery Plus--Lakeside [31328]
Recovery Plus--Lancaster [31378]
Recovery Plus--Miller Broadway [31292]
Recovery Plus--North Buffalo [31293]
Recovery Plus--North Tonawanda [31439]
Recovery Plus--Ransomville [31461]
Recovery Plus--Zoar Valley [31308]
Recovery Pointe [50090]
Recovery and Prevention Resources [47748], [47821]
Recovery Program [28985]
Recovery Resource Center [45227]
Recovery Resources [40922], [47350], [47700], [47701]
Recovery Resources Enterprises Inc [41828]
Recovery Resources Group Inc [44287]
Recovery Resources • West Side Office [47783]
Recovery Resources Winsted LLC [45353]
Recovery Resources • Women/Family Services Program [47702]
Recovery Response Center [47377]
Recovery Revolution Inc [48282]
Recovery Road Medical Center [40733]
Recovery Rx [39446]
Recovery Services Center • Ottawa [43429]
Recovery Services Council [43505]
Recovery Services of New Jersey Inc • DBA Lighthouse at Mays Landing [46054]
Recovery Services of New Mexico [46239]
Recovery Services of North West Ohio [47629], [47747], [47759], [47824], [47879]
Recovery Systems PC [41069]
Recovery Unlimited Counseling Services [44930], [45009]
Recovery Unlimited Treatment Center [44790]
Recovery Unlimited West Douglas [43506]
Recovery Ways • Mountainview Center LLC [49640]
Recovery Works Drug and Alcohol • Rehabilitation Center LLC [43601]
Recovery Zone [42880]
Red Ball Medical Supply Inc. [15363]
Red Bluff Dialysis • DaVita [22893]
Red Bud Regional Hospital, LLC [14911]
Red Cedar Clinic [44892]
Red Cliff Family Violence Prevention Program [10691]
Red Cliff Tribe • Red Cliff AODA Program [50367]
Red Lodge Mental Health Center [30961]
Red Moon Dialysis [25371]
Red Oak Counseling Ltd [50387]
Red River Home Care--Antlers [17098]
Red River Home Care--Reno [18115]
Red River Hospital [33890], [49588]
Red River Mental Health Clinic [30135]
Red River Recovery Center [45125], [49589]
Red River Valley Sports Medicine Institute [38842]
Red Rock Behavioral Health--Charles Allen [31878]
Red Rock Behavioral Health Services--Chandler [31877]

Red Rock Behavioral Health Services--Oklahoma City [31905]
Red Rock Behavioral Health--W Choctaw Avenue [31879]
Red Rock Canyon School [49674]
Red Rock Fertility Center [22153]
Red Rock North [31906]
Red Rock West Behavioral Health Services--Clinton [31881]
Red Rock West Behavioral Health Services--Elk City [31884]
Red Rock West Behavioral Health Services--Watonga [31926]
Red Springs Dialysis Center • Fresenius Medical Care [25933]
Red Top Meadows Residential Treatment Center [34505]
Red Wing Dialysis • DaVita [25067]
Redbank Village Dialysis • DaVita [26049]
Redbird Dialysis Center • Fresenius Medical Care [27037]
Redco Group Behavioral Health Services--Pottsville • Turning Point [32112]
Redding Dialysis Center & At Home • DaVita [22895]
Redding Dialysis Center • DaVita [22896]
Redding Hearing Institute [1234]
Redding Outpatient Clinic • Outpatient Program [40427]
Redding Treatment Network Inc • Cedar Rose Programs AOD Abatement Srvs [40428]
Redeemed Inc [41912]
Redeemed Recovery Services [40429]
Redefine U LLC [48027]
Redevelopment Opportunities for Women, Inc. [9723]
Redford Counseling Center [44984]
Redi-American Nursing Care [15044]
REDI Clinic [11307]
REDI Clinic in Dealfield [11308]
Redington-Fairview General Hospital • Cancer Program [5278]
ReDiscover [45553]
    Alt Care [45524]
    Catherines Place [45525]
ReDiscover Mental Health Services [30867]
ReDiscover • Psychiatric Rehabilitation Services [45526]
ReDiscover - South [30863]
ReDiscover
    Substance Abuse [45527]
    Women and Children [45528]
Redlands Community Hospital [1236], [13258]
Redlands Speech and Language [1237]
Redmond Regional Medical Center • Cancer Program [5036]
Redwood Area Hospital Hospice [20195]
Redwood Coast Medical Services, Inc. [6305]
Redwood Community Action Agency • Runaway and Homeless Youth Program [35836]
Redwood Dialysis • DaVita [26321]
Redwood Falls Dialysis • DaVita [25068]
Redwood Family Institute [28493]
Redwood Memorial Hospital • Cancer Program [4774]
Redwood School and Rehabilitation Center [8043]
Redwood Sleep Center [36687]
Reed Academy [34194]
Reedsburg Area Medical Center • Sleep Disorders Laboratory [37975]
Reeves County Hospital • Dialysis Center [27288]
Reeves County Mental Health Center [32525]
Referral Center for Alcohol and • Drug Services of Central Oklahoma Inc [47994]
Reflections Eating Disorders Clinic [11297]
Reflections Family Services Inc [39510]
Reflections • Mens Residence [44520]
Reflective Treatment Center [44176]
Reflex Home Care, LLC [15879]
Refuah Health Center [7042]
Refuge A Healing Place [41838]
Refuge Domestic Violence Shelter, Inc. [9128]
Refuge House, Inc. [9082]
The Refuge Network [9590]
The Refuge North [9624]
Refugee Women's Alliance [10651]
Regal Healthcare, Inc. [17841]
Regence Health Network, Inc. [7304]

Regency of Boro Park LHCSA [16413]
Regency Dialysis Center • DaVita [23351]
Regency Homecare [15841]
Regency Hospice--Aiken [21201]
Regency Hospice-Augusta [19359]
Regency Hospice-Columbia [21223]
Regency Hospice--Hiawassee [19392]
Regency Hospice, LLC--Cartersville [19373]
Regency Hospice-Myrtle Beach [21237]
Regency Hospice of Northwest Florida [19229]
Regency Hospice-Rock Hill [21274]
Regency Provider Services, Inc. [18086]
Regenerative Medicine Institute [35109]
ReGenesis Community Health Center [7243]
Regent Home Care, Inc. [15825]
Reggie White Sleep Disorders Center--Southaven [37260]
Reggie White Sleep Disorders Center--Tupelo [37261]
Regina General Hospital • South Saskatchewan Firefighters Burn Unit [4630]
Regina Public Schools [724]
Reginald S. Lourie Center [2432]
Region 8 Mental Health Services • New Roads [45364]
Region 8 • Residential Treatment Center [45402]
Region Care [16472]
Region Care Nursing Agency [16483]
Region I Mental Health Center
    Alcohol and Drug Services [45366]
    Fairland Center [45375]
    Sunflower Landing [45376]
Region I Mental Health Emergency Service • W. George Moody Health Center [50821]
Region I Mental Health - Kellogg/Wallace [50823]
Region I Mental Health Services [29546]
Region II Human Services [45749], [45770], [45780]
Region II--North Central Human Service Center [31636]
Region III Chemical Dependency Service [45422]
Region III--Lake Region Human Service Center [31624]
Region III Mental Health Center [30816]
    Monroe County [30740]
Region IV Mental Health Center • Boise Emergency Line [50819]
Region IV MH/MR Commission [45372]
    Booneville Extension Office [45362]
Region IV Timber Hills Mental Health Services
    Children's Services [30775]
    Rainbow Clubhouse [30746]
Region Six Alcohol and Drug Abuse • (RESADA) [41248]
Region Ten Community Services Board [32754], [49774]
Region V Delta Community Mental Health Services [30810]
    Work Activity Center - Level 1 [30763]
Region V Mental Health Center • Twin Falls Emergency Service [50826]
Region V Mental Health Services • Department of Health and Welfare [29537]
Region V Services [8225]
Region V--Southeast Human Service Center [31628]
Region VI Life Help Mental Health Center • Lexington Office, Holmes County [30781]
Region VI Mental Health Center • Life Help [30764]
Region VI--South Central Human Service Center [31634]
Region VII Community Counseling Services [30739]
    Macon PSR [34261]
Region VII Mental Health Center [50822]
Region VII--West Central Human Service Center [31623]
    Satellite Office [31620]
Region VIII--Badlands Human Service Center [31626]
Region VIII Mental Health Services [30747]
Region X Community Services Board [32720]
    Blue Ridge House [32721]
Region X Weems Community Mental Health Center [30794]
    Clark County [30808]
    Jasper County - Bay Springs [30742]
    Kemper County [30754]
    Pinnacle House [30795]
Region XI Southwest Mississippi
    Adams County Lifeskills Center [30798]

Adams County Mental Health Center [30799]
Amite County Mental Health Center [30782]
Claiborne County Mental Health and Pathway
House [30805]
Franklin County Mental Health Center [30790]
Jefferson County Mental Health Center/New
Hope [30759]
Lawrence County Mental Health Center [30796]
Lincoln County Mental Health Center [30748]
Region XI Southwest Mississippi Mental Health
Complex [30787]
Region XI Southwest Mississippi Mental Health •
Lincoln County Life Skills Center [30749]
Region XI Southwest Mississippi
New Haven Recovery Center [30750]
Pike Country Lifeskills Center [30788]
Summit House [30814]
Walthall County Mental Health Center [30817]
Wilkinson County Mental Health Center [30826]
Region XI Southwest MS • Train Clubhouse [30761]
Region XII Pine Belt Mental Health
Covington County [30751]
Jeff Davis County Mental Health Center [30806]
Marion County [30752]
Region XII Pine Belt Mental Health Resources
[30772]
Region XII Pine Belt Mental Health--Richton [30809]
Region XII Pine Belt Mental Health--Waynesboro
[30823]
Region XII Pine Belt Mental Health • Work Activity
Program [30807]
Region XIII Gulf Coast Mental Health Center [30766]
Friendship House [30822]
Hancock County Office [30741]
Live Oaks [30767]
New Hope House Group Home [30768]
Pearl River County Office [30804]
Stone County Office [30824]
Venture House [30783]
Region XIII RDSPD [769]
Region XIV Singing River Mental Health/Mental
Retardation Services [30760]
Region XIV Singing River Services [30801]
Eden House [30802]
Singing Pines Program [30785]
Stevens Center [30803]
Region XV RDSPD [814]
Region XV Warren-Yazoo Mental Health Service
[30818], [30827]
Chemical Dependency Center [30819]
Warren County Group Home [30820]
Regional Access and Mobilization Project • Center
for Independent Living [2104]
Regional Action Phone, Inc. [51134]
Regional Center of Orange County [7824]
Regional Center for Sleep Medicine [37565]
Regional Day School Program for the Deaf [770]
Regional Dialysis--Bay City [24838]
Regional Dialysis Center [26794]
Regional Dialysis Center--Spearfish [26799]
Regional Dialysis--Gladwin [24904]
Regional Dialysis--Midland [24946]
Regional Dialysis--West Branch [24991]
Regional Economic Comm Action Program
RECAP CD Community Residence [46942]
RECAP Outpatient Rehab Program [46782]
Regional Evaluation and Counseling [47584]
Regional Family Crisis Center [9709]
Regional Home Care Inc. [15508]
Regional Hospice • Hayward Team [21841]
Regional Hospice Services Inc.--Ashland [21821]
Regional Hospice Services-Ironwood Team [20073]
Regional Hospice - Spooner Team [21867]
Regional Hospice of Western Connecticut, Inc.
[19140]
Regional Institute for Children and Adolescents -
Baltimore [34173]
Regional Institute for Children and Adolescents -
Southern Maryland [34176]
Regional Kidney Center Inc. • Kidney Care of Santa
Paula [23006]
Regional Kidney Center, inc. • Kidney Center of
Sherman Oaks, Inc. [23012]
Regional Kidney Center Inc. • Kidney Center of
Thousand Oaks, Inc. [23034]
Regional--KRU Medical Ventures • Hallandale
Artificial Kidney Center [23326]
Regional Medical Center [43958], [44008], [44011]

Regional Medical Center--Bayonet Point • Cancer
Program [4948]
Regional Medical Center Calais [6771]
Regional Medical Center of Hopkins County Home
Health [15228]
Regional Medical Center of Hopkins County • Merle
M. Mahr Cancer Center [5230]
Regional Medical Center at Lubec [6780]
The Regional Medical Center of Orangeburg & Cal-
houn Counties [17617]
Regional Medical Center of Orangeburg and Cal-
houn County • Cancer Program [5912]
Regional Medical Center of San Jose [13318]
Regional Medical Clinic • Sports Medicine [39024]
Regional Mental Health Center [43156], [43157]
Regional Mental Health Services • 24-Hour Crisis
Line [50825]
Regional Nephrology Inc.--Blackthorn [24237]
Regional Nephrology Inc.--Elkhart [24135]
Regional Nephrology Inc.--LaPorte [24189]
Regional Network of Programs Inc
Center for Human Services [41476]
Kinsella Treatment Center/Detox [41368]
Regional Counseling Services /(RCS)/OP/DF
[41369]
Regional Pain Treatment Center [35327]
Regional Physical Therapy at Center IMT Bloomfield
[38187]
Regional Rehabilitation Hospital [923]
Regional Rehabilitation Institute • MDA Clinic
[34876]
Regional Sleep Management [37749]
Regional Tissue Bank, QEII Health Sciences [35153]
Regional West Medical Center [16131]
Cancer Treatment Center [5486]
Regions Alcohol and Drug Abuse Program [45310]
Regions Hospital [20207]
Burn Center [4573]
Cancer Program [5418]
CRISIS Program [51046]
Health and Wellness Program Serving Dear and
Hard of Hearing People [2744]
Regions Hospital/New Connections Prog
Eden Prairie Outpatient Treatment [45143]
Outpatient Program Hastings [45175]
Regions Hospital • Sleep Health Center [37228]
Regis House [41798]
Rehab After Work [41576], [41930], [42000],
[46049], [48414], [48493], [48558], [48580]
Rehab Center [3245]
The Rehab Group [35708]
Rehab at Home [15491]
Rehab Management Inc • DBA Rehab After Work
[48432]
Rehab Matters Home Health, Inc.--Lutz [13868]
Rehab Matters Home Health--Tampa [14425]
Rehab Medicine Center of New Jersey • Pain
Center [35568]
Rehab New England/Physiotherapy Associates
[3392]
REHAB Programs Inc. [3102]
Rehab Unlimited Inc. [1169]
Rehab Without Walls [1361]
Rehab Without Walls (RWW)--A Gentiva Company
[3875]
Rehab Without Walls (RWW)--Bay Area [3915]
Rehab Without Walls (RWW)--Sacramento [3916]
Rehab Without Walls (RWW)--Southern California
[3917]
Rehabilitation Achievement Center [2121]
Rehabilitation Associates, Inc. [1458]
Rehabilitation Center [8339], [31796]
The Rehabilitation Center [2142]
Rehabilitation Center for Children and Adults [1707]
Rehabilitation Center of Sheboygan • Early Interven-
tion Program [8628]
Rehabilitation Centers of Charleston [39013]
Rehabilitation Consultants [3616]
Rehabilitation Consultants Inc.--Amherst [38851]
Rehabilitation Consultants, Inc.--Wilmington [38210]
Rehabilitation Counseling Associates [45988]
Rehabilitation Equipment, Inc. [16370]
Rehabilitation and Health Inc • East Boston [44453]
Rehabilitation Hospital of Indiana, Inc. [4039]
Rehabilitation Hospital of the Pacific [35421]
Rehabilitation Hospital of Tinton Falls [38761]
Rehabilitation Institute of Chicago [7942]

Midwest Regional Spinal Cord Injury Care
System [4028]
The Rehabilitation Institute of Kansas City [2799],
[4238]
Rehabilitation Institute of Michigan [4186]
Center for Spinal Cord Injury Recovery [4187]
Rehabilitation Institute of Michigan--Novi Center
[4188]
Rehabilitation Institute of Michigan
Speech-Language Pathology Department [2574]
Variety Myoelectric Center [8170]
Rehabilitation Institute of Saint Louis [38669]
Rehabilitation Institute of Southern California [7799]
Rehabilitation Institute of Washington [35757]
Rehabilitation One Home Health, LLC [15625]
Rehabilitation and Pain Management Associates
[35482]
The Rehabilitation Service of North Central Ohio
[8419]
Rehabilitation Services [1485]
Rehabilitation Services Inc. [2418]
Rehabilitation Services Network [38365]
Rehabilitation Services of North Central Ohio • Deaf
Services [3246]
Rehabilitation Services Speech Therapy Center
[2313]
Rehabilitation Services of Tifton Inc. [1919]
Rehabilitation Solutions, Cambridge [35629]
Rehabilitation Solutions, Mississauga [35630]
Rehabilitation Solutions, Toronto [35631]
Rehabilitation Specialists [4296]
Rehabilitation Specialists--Allison Park [3320]
Rehabilitation Specialists--DeVoe [4297]
Rehabilitation Specialists--Haledon Ave. [4298]
Rehabilitation Specialists--Park Avenue [4299]
Rehabilitation Specialists--Pittsburgh [3368]
Rehabilitation Support Services Inc • Chemical
Dependence Comm Residence [47070]
Rehabilitation Support Services, Inc. [31343]
Rehability Center [39138]
Rehoboth McKinley Christian Healthcare Services
[16318]
Rehoboth McKinley Christian • Healthcare Services
Behavioral Health [46274]
Rehoboth McKinley Christian Hospital
Dialysis Center [25546]
Dialysis Facility [25565]
Reid Hospital and Health Care Services [15045]
Cancer Program [5172]
Reid Hospital and Health Care Services Hospice
[19646]
Reidsville Dialysis • DaVita [25934]
Reiss--Davis Child Study Center [33994]
Relapse Prevention Counseling Center [42626]
Reliable Community Care, Inc [16566]
Reliable Home Care Services [16297]
Reliable Medical Supply [15915]
Reliable Nurses, LLC [12834]
Reliance Home Health Care [14924]
Reliance House, Inc. [29035]
Bozrah House [28971]
Reliance House, Inc.--Bridge Program [29003]
Reliance House, Inc.
Community Apartment Program [29036]
Montville Home [29012]
Penobscot Place [29037]
Respite Program [29038]
Teamworks Clubhouse [29039]
TLC I and II [29040]
Reliance Medical Group [17927]
Reliant Dialysis • DaVita [27169]
Reliant Healthcare, LLC [27871]
Reliant Renal Care--Colorado Springs • Dialysis
Facility [23105]
Reliant Renal Care--East Fort Worth [27089]
Reliant Renal Care--Flint [24900]
Reliant Renal Care--Marlette [24943]
Reliant Renal Care--Trinidad [23142]
REM Medical Scottsdale • Sleep Disorders Center
[36632]
REM Medical West Phoenix [36633]
REM Sleep Center [37836]
REM Sleep Diagnostics • Sleep Disorders Center
[36688]
ReMed/Devon Road [4403]
ReMed--Gibsonia House [4404]
ReMed--Harvey La. [4405]
ReMed--Malvern Apartments [4406]

ReMed--Manor Ave. [4407]
ReMed--Monument House [4408]
ReMed--New Street [4409]
ReMed--Paoli [4410]
ReMed--Paoli Apartments [4411]
ReMed--Pittsburgh [4412]
Remedial Specialists--Chalmette [2310]
Remedial Specialists--New Orleans [2334]
REMEDIES [9249]
Remedy Addictions Counselors Inc • Remedy
 Behavioral Systems [49295]
Remedy Home Health Agency, Inc. [17889], [18132]
Remedy Sleep Disorders Center [37566]
Remuda Ranch Center for Anorexia & Bulimia
 [28226]
Remuda Ranch • Programs for Anorexia and Bu-
limia [10904]
Renacer Latino Inc [42689], [42704], [42798],
 [42953]
Renaissance Center [29188]
Renaissance Challenge Conquerors • Training
 Center [46101]
Renaissance Club, Inc. [30409]
Renaissance Home Health Care [16414]
Renaissance Home Health Services [13149]
Renaissance House • Womens Transition Project
 Inc [39366]
Renaissance LLC [13301]
Renaissance Project Inc
  Ellenville Residential Facility [46620]
  Mount Vernon Outpatient Clinic [46797]
  New Rochelle Center [46801]
  Outpatient [46975]
Renaissance Project Inc/Port Chester • Chem
 Dependency Treatment Facility [46984]
Renaissance Ranch [49597]
Renaissance Recovery Resources PC [48135]
Renaissance Treatment Center [49493]
Renaissance West • Swope Parkway Site [45529]
Renal Advantage Hamacher--Waterloo [24102]
Renal Advantage Inc--Roanoke • Roanoke Dialysis
 Clinic [22396]
Renal Advantage Inc--Talladega [22408]
Renal Advantage Inc.--Airline Portsmouth • Dialysis
 Facility [27539]
Renal Advantage Inc.--Barbourville [24361]
Renal Advantage Inc.--Beaumont [22603]
Renal Advantage Inc.--Beltsville • Dialysis Facility
 [24658]
Renal Advantage Inc. Care Centers--Bancroft
 [22851]
Renal Advantage Inc. Care Centers--Broadway--
 Chula Vista [22636]
Renal Advantage Inc. Care Centers--Chico [22629]
Renal Advantage Inc. Care Centers - Clearwater
 [23268]
Renal Advantage Inc. Care Centers--East Bay--
 Oakland [22852]
Renal Advantage Inc. Care Centers--Old
 Alexandria--Clinton [24669]
Renal Advantage Inc. Care Centers--Snow St.--
 Oxford [22385]
Renal Advantage Inc. Care Centers--Winter Haven
 [23561]
Renal Advantage Inc. Care Centers--Zeeland
 [24997]
Renal Advantage Inc.--Centre West Springfield
 [24092]
Renal Advantage Inc.--Charleston West • Dialysis
 Facility [26692]
Renal Advantage Inc.--Chesapeake Avenue [27521]
Renal Advantage Inc.--Chillum--Hyattsville • Dialysis
 Center [24695]
Renal Advantage Inc.--Churchland - Chesapeake •
 Dialysis Facility [27474]
Renal Advantage Inc.--Clyde Park • Dialysis Facility
 [24994]
Renal Advantage Inc.--Colton [22642]
Renal Advantage Inc. Crossroads--Augusta [23753]
Renal Advantage Inc.--Dickson • Dialysis Clinic
 [26831]
Renal Advantage Inc.--Fletcher Parkway, El Cajon
 [22668]
Renal Advantage Inc.--Fountain Valley • Dialysis
 Center [22691]
Renal Advantage Inc.--Fredericktown [25208]
Renal Advantage Inc.--Frontenac [25209]
Renal Advantage Inc.--Georgetown [24382]

Renal Advantage Inc.--Goode Way--Portsmouth •
 Dialysis Facility [27540]
Renal Advantage Inc. • Gray Dialysis Center
 [23710]
Renal Advantage Inc.--Hampton Ave.--St. Louis
 [25275]
Renal Advantage Inc.--Holland [24917]
Renal Advantage Inc.--Jackson • Dialysis Center
 [24922]
Renal Advantage Inc.--Jacobs Point Blvd.--Ravenel
 [26761]
Renal Advantage Inc.--John Tyler Highway Williams-
 burg [27585]
Renal Advantage Inc.--Kansas City [24327]
Renal Advantage Inc. • Manchester Dialysis Clinic
 [26877]
Renal Advantage Inc.--MCV Turnpike • Dialysis
 Center [27553]
Renal Advantage Inc.--Mission Gorge San Diego
 [22947]
Renal Advantage Inc.--Moncks Corner • Dialysis
 Facility [26745]
Renal Advantage Inc. • Mount Pleasant Dialysis
 Center [26748]
Renal Advantage Inc.--New Castle [24216]
Renal Advantage Inc.--North Waterman • San
 Bernardino Dialysis Center [22931]
Renal Advantage Inc.--Oceanside [22854]
Renal Advantage Inc.--Oxon Hill • Dialysis Facility
 [24709]
Renal Advantage Inc.--Palmetto [23769]
Renal Advantage Inc.--Potosi [25257]
Renal Advantage Inc.--Punta Gorda • Dialysis Facil-
 ity [23494]
Renal Advantage Inc.--Richmond • Dialysis Facility
 [27554]
Renal Advantage Inc. • Riverside Dialysis Center--
 Gloucester [27496]
Renal Advantage Inc.--Rockford Park [24961]
Renal Advantage Inc. Royal Park--Zeeland [24998]
Renal Advantage Inc.--Saint Petersburg [23505]
Renal Advantage Inc.--Savannah • Dialysis Facility
 [23786]
Renal Advantage Inc.--Silver Hill • Dialysis Facility
 [24676]
Renal Advantage Inc.--South Church--Smithfield
 [27563]
Renal Advantage Inc.--Summerville [26776]
Renal Advantage Inc.--Thimble Shoals • Dialysis
 Facility [27522]
Renal Advantage Inc.--Valdosta [23823]
Renal Advantage Inc.--West Norton [24951]
Renal Associates of Boca Raton, Inc. [23243]
Renal Care of Bowie • DaVita [24662]
Renal Care of Buffalo & At Home • Dialysis Facility •
 DaVita [25803]
Renal Care Center--Belle Glade • Fresenius Medical
 Care [23238]
Renal Care Center--Okeechobee • Fresenius Medi-
 cal Care • Dialysis Facility [23439]
Renal Care Center--Sebring • Fresenius Medical
 Care [23515]
Renal Care Center--Vero Beach • Fresenius Medical
 Care • Dialysis Facility [23550]
Renal Care Center--Wellington • Fresenius Medical
 Care • Dialysis Facility [23362]
Renal Care of Clarion • Dreiling Medical Manage-
 ment [26405]
Renal Care Group--AK-Chin • Dialysis Facility
 [22452]
Renal Care of Lanham & At Home • DaVita •
 Dialysis Facility [24700]
Renal Care of Northern New York, LLC [25801]
Renal Care of Oil City Inc. • Dreiling Medical
 Management [26409]
Renal Care Partners--Hapeville [23716]
Renal Care Partners Home Program [23279]
Renal Care Partners Inc.--Philadelphia [26532]
Renal Care Partners at Memorial West, LLC [23327]
Renal Care of Rockland, Inc. [25796]
Renal Care of Seat Pleasant • DaVita [24726]
Renal Care of White Oak • Dreiling Medical
 Management [26608]
Renal Carepartners--Amarillo [26940]
Renal CarePartners - Arlington/Alexandria [27461]
Renal Carepartners--Dahlonega [23666]
Renal Carepartners--Delray Beach [23291]
Renal Carepartners of Dunwoody [23605]

Renal Carepartners--Fairfax [27485]
Renal Carepartners--Prince Frederick [24715]
Renal Carepartners of Reston LLC [27544]
Renal Carepartners--Woodbridge [27589]
Renal Center of Carrollton • Renal Ventures
 Management [26989]
Renal Center of Midland--Odessa • Renal Ventures
 Management [27278]
Renal Center of Moorefield LLC • Renal Ventures
 Management [27682]
Renal Center of Newton • Renal Ventures Manage-
 ment [25489]
Renal Center of North Denton • Renal Ventures
 Management [27049]
Renal Center of North Jersey, LLC • Renal Ventures
 Management LLC [25454]
Renal Center of Passiac • Renal Ventures Manage-
 ment [25418]
Renal Center of Philadelphia • Dialysis Facility
 [26533]
Renal Center of Storm Lake, LLC • Dialysis Facility
 [24302]
Renal Center of Trenton • Renal Ventures Manage-
 ment [25520]
Renal Center of Tyler • Renal Ventures Managment
 • Dialysis Center [27381]
Renal Center--Westwood • Renal Ventures Manage-
 ment [25527]
Renal Centers of Guam [23840]
Renal Centers of North Jersey • Renal Ventures
 Management [25455]
Renal Institute of Central Jersey--Toms River • Fres-
 enius Medical Care [25517]
Renal Research Institute
  Beth Israel Medical Center
    Dialysis Center [25732]
    Dialysis Unit [25733]
  Strong Health Dialysis • Inpatient Unit [25766]
  University of Michigan Dialysis Clinics--Livonia
   [24938]
Renal Solutions Dialysis Services [27170]
Renal South of St. Tammany [24527]
Renal Treatment Center--Derby • DaVita • Dialysis
 Facility [24314]
Renal Treatment Center--Marianna • DaVita [23381]
Renal Treatment Centers--Garden City • DaVita
 [24318]
Renal Ventures Management--Bayonne • Dialysis
 Center [25403]
Renal Ventures Management--Brick • Renal Center
 [25409]
Renal Ventures Management of Frisco [27098]
Renal Ventures Management of the Hills [27274]
Renal Ventures Management of Waterton [27382]
Renew Center of Florida [11030]
Renew Eating Disorder Recovery [11064]
RENEW--Gillette • Brain Injury Program [4497]
Renew, Inc. [8943]
Renew Integrated Program 2 Inc [40037]
RENEW--Newcastle • Brain Injury Program [4498]
RENEW--Sheridan • Brain Injury Program [4499]
Renewal House [9501]
Renewal House Inc [49161]
Renewed Hope Community Services [42571]
Renfrew Center of Connecticut [11007]
Renfrew Center of Florida [11031]
Renfrew Center Foundation [11254]
Renfrew Center of Maryland [11083]
Renfrew Center of New Jersey [11146]
Renfrew Center of New York [11166]
Renfrew Center of North Carolina [11175]
Renfrew Center of Philadelphia [11255]
Renfrew Center of Radnor [11256]
Renfrew Center of Tennessee [11272]
Renfrew Center of Texas [11282]
Reno Alcohol Drug Services Hutchinson [43367]
Reno Dialysis Center & At Home • DaVita [25383]
Reno Sparks Indian Colony • Drug and Alcohol
 Program [45872]
Renovados En Cristo Inc • Institutos [48737]
Renovation Health Care [13774]
Renovation Home Health Care, Inc. [14131]
Renown Institute for Neurosciences • Multiple
 Sclerosis Center [34626]
Renown Regional Medical Center • Cancer Center
 [5490]
Renown Regional Medical Center Home Care
 [16164]

Renton Area Youth and Family Services [50086]
Renton Public Health Center [7383]
ReNu Life Extended Inc. [4336]
Renville County Hospice [20187]
Renwick Recovery Inc • Residential Supportive Living Facility [46943]
Renz Addiction Counseling Center [42898], [42928]
    All Alcohol/Substance Abuse Progs on Site [42658]
Repay, Inc.--Lenoir [31556]
Repay, Inc.--Morganton [31564]
Repay, Inc.--Newton [31574]
Reproductive Biology Associates--Atlanta [22019]
Reproductive Biology Associates--Fayetteville [22020]
Reproductive Biology Associates--Lawrenceville [22021]
Reproductive Biology Associates • North Crescent Medical Center [22022]
Reproductive Care Center [22276]
Reproductive Care of Indiana [22060]
Reproductive Endocrinology Associates--Indianapolis [22061]
Reproductive Endocrinology Associates--Springfield [22044]
Reproductive Genetics In Vitro [21961]
Reproductive Genetics Institute [12201]
Reproductive Genetics Institute-Oakbrook [12202]
Reproductive Gynecology Labs, LLC • In Vitro Fertilization/Andrology Center [22217]
Reproductive Health Associates, PA [22002]
Reproductive Health Center [21899]
Reproductive Health Center, Inc. [21900]
Reproductive Health and Fertility Center [22045]
Reproductive Health Specialists [22046]
Reproductive Medicine Associates of Connecticut [21972]
Reproductive Medicine Associates of New Jersey [22164], [22165]
Reproductive Medicine Associates of New York [22191]
Reproductive Medicine Associates of New York--Garden City [22192]
Reproductive Medicine Associates of New York--New York [22193]
Reproductive Medicine Associates of New York--White Plains [22194]
Reproductive Medicine Associates of Texas--Austin [22266]
Reproductive Medicine Associates of Texas--Medical Drive, San Antonio [22267]
Reproductive Medicine Associates of Texas--Stone Oak Parkway, San Antonio [22268]
Reproductive Medicine and Fertility Center [21962], [22174]
Reproductive Medicine Group [22003]
The Reproductive Medicine Group--Brandon [22004]
The Reproductive Medicine Group--Clearwater [22005]
Reproductive Medicine and Infertility Associates [22140]
Reproductive Partners Medical Group [21931]
Reproductive Resource Center [22069]
Reproductive Resource Center of Greater Kansas City [22070]
Reproductive Science Center [22112]
Reproductive Science Center of New England--Milford [22113]
Reproductive Science Center of New England--Providence [22240]
Reproductive Science Center of the San Francisco Bay Area [21932]
Reproductive Science Institute [22234]
Reproductive Specialty Center [22300]
ReproTech, Ltd., Fort Lauderdale [35004]
ReproTech, Ltd.--Reno, NV [35110]
ReproTech, Ltd.--Saint Paul, MN [35087]
Res Med Sup Withdrawl Loyola Recovery [46372]
ResCare HomeCare [15198], [15225]
ResCare Premier--Downers Grove [4029]
ResCare Premier--Fort Lauderdale [3993]
ResCare Premier--Town Program [4457]
Rescue Incorporated [47868]
Rescue Mental Health Services [51233]
Rescue Mission of Trenton [46193]
Rescue Mission of Utica Inc • Addictions Crisis Center [47152]
The Research & Education Group • Community

Program for Clinical Research on AIDS [67]
Research Institute on Addictions • Clinical Research Center [46567]
Research Medical Center [2800]
Research Medical Center, Brookside Campus [2801], [37279]
Research Medical Center
    Cancer Program [5447]
    Dialysis Unit [25226]
Research Medical Center Transplant Institute • HCA Midwest Health System [25227]
Research Psychiatric Center • Millcreek Outpatient Clinic [30884]
Reseda Substance Abuse Treatment [40267]
Residence Hospice Care, Inc. [20270]
Residence XII for Women [49993]
Residencial Tratamiento • Mujeres Adultas San Juan [48820]
Residential Care Crossroads [27915]
Residential Care Home [27906]
Residential Re-Entry Center [33160]
Residential Services Mental Health Clinic [33702]
Residential Support Services • Steps to Recovery [49783]
Residential Treatment Facility • Dwight D Eisenhower Mem Hospital [42098]
Residential Treatment Services of Alamance Inc [47238]
Residential Treatment Unit • Highland Rivers Community Service Board [29386]
Residential Youth Services, Inc., Alexandria • Runaway and Homeless Youth Program [36246]
Resolutions Hospice-Austin [21392]
Resolutions Hospice-Houston [21489]
Resolutions Hospice-Katy [21502]
Resolve Community Counseling Center Inc [46157]
Resource Care Corp. Austin [17817]
Resource Center for Women and Their Families [9832]
The Resource Connection [8881]
Resource Treatment Center [34129]
Resources for Human Development [32101]
Resources for Independent Living • Deaf and Hard of Hearing Program [3605]
Resp-I-Care, Inc.--Bristol [17646]
Resp-I-Care, Inc.--Kingsport [17696]
Resp-I-Care, Inc.--Knoxville [17710]
Respect My Wishes • Saint Francis Medical Center Hospice [20383]
RespiCare of Central Florida [13886]
RespiCare of South Florida [13644]
Respiratory Home Care Specialists, Inc. [14622]
Respiratory and Medical Homecare Unlimited, Inc. [17913]
Respiratory Physicians of Southwest Washington • Sleep Disorders Center [37928]
Respiratory Services of Northwest Florida, Inc. [13631]
Respiratory Specialists Sleep Health Center [37684]
Respiratory Therapy Home Care [12909]
Respite Center • Provena Behavioral Health [29576]
Respitek Medical Services [14426]
RESPOND [9503]
Response: Help for Survivors of Domestic Violence and Sexual Assault [8933]
Response Inc. [10601]
Response to Sexual and Domestic Violence [9804]
Response of Suffolk County, Inc. [51152]
Responsibility House Residential Treatment [43828]
Responsive Solutions, Inc. [17610]
RESTA Sleep Disorders Center [36689]
Restart Inc [47367]
reStart, Inc. • Runaway and Homeless Youth Program [36058]
Reston Dialysis Center • DaVita [27545]
Reston Hospital Center • Rodriguez Cancer Center [6078]
Reston Speech and Language Center [3588]
Restor III Kansas City [43379]
Restoration Center Inc JC [43372]
Restoration Center Manhattan [43400]
Restoration of Hope [8786]
Restoration House [41675]
Restoration MBS Center Inc • RMBS [42960]
Restorative Management Corp [46988]
Restorative Management Corporation
    Outpatient Drug/Alcohol Abuse Clinic [46944]
    Outpatient Substance Abuse Clinic [46783]

Restore Community Living Program [4006]
Restore FX [35709]
Restore Health and Counseling LLC [41141]
Restore Health Group [4007]
Restore House Inc [45085]
Restored Paths [42332]
RESULTS Speech Therapy Services [1916]
Resurrection Addiction Services
    Chicago Loop [42572]
    Downers Grove [42633]
    Lincoln Park Professionals Program [42573]
Resurrection Behavioral Health [33443]
Resurrection Behavioral Health--Broadview [34098]
Resurrection Behavioral Health Center • Palos Heights [42843]
Resurrection Behavioral Health • Lake Bluff [42736]
Resurrection Behavioral Health--Melrose Park [34115]
Resurrection Behavioral Health • Procare Recovery Center [42777]
Resurrection Health Care • Cancer Program [5074]
Resurrection Medical Center
    Outpatient Dialysis Center [23954]
    Speech Pathology and Audiology [2001]
Resurrection Sports Medicine Center [38366]
Reto Juvenil de Puerto Rico [48725]
Retreat Healthcare [32645]
Retreat Hospital • Wound Healing Center • Burn Program [4645]
Retreat, Inc.--East Hampton [9919]
Retreat, Inc.--Wainscott [9999]
Revere Counseling Center [30458]
Revival Home Health Care Agency, Inc. [18296]
Rewind Inc [45259]
Rex Healthcare
    Cancer Center [5656]
    Sleep Disorders Center [37483]
Rex Hospital Inc. Home Services [16770]
Rexburg Home Health and Hospice [19476]
Reynolds Army Community Hospital • Pain Clinic [35625]
Reynolds Memorial Hospital, Inc. [18514]
RG Care Home Health Corporation [14132]
RGA Home Health Services Inc. [13499]
RHC, LLC [17373]
RHD Nova III [48559]
Rhea County School System [750]
Rhema Medical--Houston [18004]
Rhema Medical--Webster [18187]
Rhinelander Dialysis Center [27777]
Rhinelander Veterans Affairs Clinic [33012]
RHJ Medical Center Inc [48409]
    Vandergrift [48666]
Rhode Island College • Paul V. Sherlock Center on Disabilities • Rhode Island Services to Students with Dual Sensory Impairments [721]
Rhode Island Department of Health • Division of Family Health [36538]
Rhode Island/Hasbro Children's Hospital • Audiology and Speech Pathology [3389]
Rhode Island Hospital
    Burn Center [4629]
    Child Development Center • MDA Clinic [34871]
    Cystic Fibrosis Center • Brown University Medical School [7657]
    Dialysis Unit [26667]
    Division Of Hemotology-Oncology [5891]
    George Clinic • Hemophilia Center of Rhode Island [12591]
Rhode Island Hospital/Hasbro Children's Hospital
    Child Development Center [8498]
    Sickle Cell Disease Center [36423]
Rhode Island Hospital
    Hearing and Speech Center [3390]
    Louise Wilcox ALS Center [147]
    Multiple Sclerosis Center [34704]
    Pain Clinic [35657]
    Sleep Disorders Center of Lifespan Hospitals [37727]
Rhode Island School for the Deaf [722]
Rhode Island SIDS Alliance [36539]
Rhode Island Youth Guidance Center, Inc. [32166]
RIC and Loyola [2122]
Rice Hospice - Appleton [20141]
Rice Hospice - Benson [20146]
Rice Hospice - Dawson [20154]
Rice Hospice - Granite Falls [20167]
Rice Hospice - Montevideo [20182]

Rice Hospice - Ortonville/Graceville [20189]
Rice Hospice - Paynesville [20191]
Rice Hospice--Willmar [20216]
Rice Memorial Hospital [15948]
    Dialysis Facility [25096]
    Willmar Cancer Center [5422]
Rich Square Dialysis Center • Fresenius Medical
    Care [25850]
Richard Colligan LCADC CSW [45934]
Richard H. Young Hospital [33644]
Richard Hall CMHC • Outpatient and Intensive
    Outpatient [45948]
Richard Hall Community Mental Health Center
    [31107]
Richard L Parris MI Residential Home [27879]
Richard L. Rosenthal Hospice Residence [19166]
Richard L. Roudebush VAMC, Bloomington [4040]
Richard L. Roudebush VAMC, Indianapolis [4041]
Richard L. Roudebush VAMC, Terre Haute [4042]
Richard L. Roudebush Veterans Affairs Medical
    Center [29746]
    Cancer Program [5156]
    PTSD Clinical Team [51729]
Richard P. Stadter Psychiatric Center [33747]
Richardson Counseling Center LLC [42406]
Richardson Medical Center Home Care, LLC
    [15354]
Richardson Regional Medical Center • Sleep
    Disorders Center [37837]
Richford Dental Clinic [7336]
Richland Community Health Care Association [7227]
Richland County Coalition Against Domestic
    Violence [9762]
Richland County Health and Human Services
    [50520]
Richland County School District One [726]
Richland Memorial Hospital • Children's Hospital •
    Sickle Cell Disease Center [36426]
Richland Mental Health Center [30171]
Richland Sleep Disorders Center [37929]
Richland Therapy Services Inc. [3247]
Richmond AIDS Consortium • Community Program
    for Clinical Research on AIDS [75]
Richmond Behavioral Health Authority [32780]
    Substance Abuse Services [49829]
The Richmond Center--Ames [29838]
The Richmond Center--Boone [29842]
Richmond Center for Fertility and Endocrinology •
    IVF Program [22289]
Richmond Community Hospital [32781]
Richmond County Hospice/Hospice Haven [20724]
Richmond Eating Disorders Center [10918]
Richmond IOP PLC • Recovery Resources [49830]
Richmond Private Methadone Clinic • (RPMC)
    [49831]
Richmond Road Diagnostic and Treatment Centre •
    Calgary Eating Disorder Program [10891]
Richmond Southside Treatment Center [49832]
Richmond State Hospital [8004], [33488], [43187]
Richmond State School [8563]
Richmond Treatment Center LLC [43188]
Richmond University Medical Center
    Bayley Seton Hosp Alcohol Acute Care Unit
        [47097]
    Cancer Care Program [5616]
    Chemical Dependence Crisis Center [47098]
Richmond Veterans Affairs Community Based
    Outpatient Clinic [29810]
Richton Dialysis [25130]
Richton Dialysis Unit • Hattiesburg Clinic [25158]
Riddle Dialysis Center • DaVita [26477]
Riddle Memorial Hospital
    Riddle Cancer Center • Jefferson Radiation On-
        cology Center [5843]
    Sleep Center [37685]
Rideout Memorial Hospital • Fremont-Rideout
    Cancer Center [4805]
Ridgaway Philips Co. [17484]
Ridge Area -ARC [7879]
Ridge Audiology [1625]
Ridge Behavioral Health System [33525], [43666]
Ridge House Inc [45873]
    Vine [45874]
Ridgecrest Regional Hospice [19000]
Ridgecrest Regional Hospital [13264]
RidgeGate Hearing Clinic [1428]
Ridgeland Dialysis • DaVita [26763]
Ridgeview [33853]

Ridgeview Home Care [20213]
Ridgeview Hospice [20211]
Ridgeview Institute [11039], [33392]
    Adult Addiction Medicine Services [42155]
Ridgeview Medical Center [15945]
    Cancer Program [5421]
    Ridgeview Sleep Disorders Center [37229]
Ridgeview Pediatric Rehabilitation [2750]
Ridgeview Psychiatric Hospital and Center [33847]
Ridgeview Psychiatric • Hospital and Center [49174]
Ridgeview Psychiatric Hospital and Center
    Quest Psychosocial Program [33855]
    Scott County Outpatient Clinic [33856]
    Stepping Stones Psychosocial Program [33854]
Ridgeview Ranch [39588]
Ridgewood Dialysis Center [25762]
Ridgewood Recovery Inc • DBA The Superior Treat-
    ment Center [45135], [50540]
Ridgewood Speech and Language Center [2950]
Riel House [50275]
Riggs Community Health Clinic [6693]
Right Avenue Counseling [41042]
Right Choice Counseling Serv Inc [49916]
Right Choice of Orange County [49474]
Right Choice Port Arthur [49494]
Right Choice Vancouver [50241]
RIGHT Program [40151]
Right Road Recovery Programs Inc [39602]
Right Step [49239], [49392], [49393]
The Right Step Inc [49997]
Right Step • Solutions Plus [49394]
Right Turn of Maryland [44321]
Rightcare Home Health Services Inc. [13048]
Rightway Medical [47995]
Riley Center [8889]
Riley Children's Hospital • Center for Youth and
    Adults with Conditions of Childhood • Down
    Syndrome Clinic [10799]
Riley Hospital for Children
    Ann Whitehill Down Syndrome Program [10800]
    Sleep Disorders Center [36959]
Rim Family Services Inc [40803]
Rim Guidance Center [28170]
RIM Novi [4189]
RIM Sterling Heights [4190]
Rimrock Foundation [45682]
Rimrock Trails ATS
    Bend Outpatient [48080]
    Prineville Residential [48224]
Rimrock Trails • Redmond Outpatient [48227]
Rincon Rural Health Initiative Program [7210]
Rinehart Center for Reproductive Medicine [22047]
Rinehart--Coulam Center [22048]
Ringer Center [47351]
Ringgold County Hospital • Dialysis Unit [24288]
Rio Grande • Alcoholism Treatment Program
    [46285]
Rio Grande Health Center of El Paso, Inc. dba • Rio
    Grande Rehab Center [35710]
Rio Grande Intensive Outpatient Treatment [46313]
Rio Grande State Center [32473]
    South Texas Health Care System [33868]
Rio Grande Valley Council Inc [49484]
Rio Grande Valley Outpatient • Serving Children and
    Adol in Need [49253]
Rio Grande Valley Sleep Centers [37838]
Rio Hondo Mental Health Services [28431]
Rio Rancho dialysis • Dialysis Clinic, Inc. [25558]
Rio Rancho Public Schools [562]
Rio Vista CARE [40453]
Ripley County Counseling Center [29797]
Risch Home Health Care, Inc. [16960]
RISE [7728]
Rita Ranch Dialysis • DaVita [22520]
Rita and Stanley H. Kaplan House [31430]
RITAS Ministry/Restoring Inmates • to Americas
    Society [42813]
Rite Choice Home Health Care [15608]
Rite Surgical Supplies Inc. [16415]
RiteCare Childhood Language Clinic [2692]
Rivendell Behavioral Health Service--Bowling Green
    [33518]
Rivendell Behavioral Health Services [43541]
Rivendell Behavioral Health Services--Benton
    [33114]
River Bend Christian Counseling Inc [42783]
River Bend Dialysis • Saint Charles Parish Hospital
    • Dialysis Center [24526]

River Centre Clinic [11198]
River City Dialysis • DaVita [25090]
River City Recovery Center Inc • Mens South
    Campus [39927]
River City Rehabilitation Center Inc [49529]
River City Rehabilitation Center • New Braunfels
    [49470]
River Crest Hospital [33881], [49508]
River District Counseling Center [30497]
River District Hospital • Speech Language Pathology
    [2578]
River East Community Health Center [7097]
River Edge Behavioral Health Center [29463]
    Addictive Disease Outpatient Program [42126]
    Forensic Services Division [29464]
    Peer Support [29465]
River Edge Project Connect [42127]
River Edge Recovery Center [42128]
River Falls Area Hospital • Rivers Cancer Center
    [4719]
River Hills Community Health Center [6712]
River Hills House--People Incorporated [30668]
River Hills School [8010]
River House Shelter [9539]
River Landings OB/GYN [6444]
River Oak Center for Children, Inc. [34015]
River Oaks Hospital [30166]
    Admission and Referral Service [50951]
    Eating Disorders Treatment Center [11071]
River Oaks Psychiatric Hospital [33545]
River Parishes • Addictive Disorders Clinic [43837]
River Parishes Dialysis • DaVita [24517]
River Parishes Mental Health Center [30147]
River Park Dialysis • DaVita [27004]
River Park Hospital [33918]
River Psychological Services • Eating Disorders
    Program [11074]
River Region Hospice, LLC [19872]
River Region Human Services Inc [41708]
    Dual Diagnosis Program [41709]
    Outpatient Services [41710]
River Regional Health System • Cancer Center of
    vicksburg [5435]
River Ridge Program • Learning Services
    Residential Rehabilitation • Raleigh North Carolina
    [4337]
River Ridge Treatment Center [45102], [45237]
River School [343]
River Source Treatment Center [39372]
River Stone Health Clinic [6925]
River Valley Behavioral Health [43618]
    Crisis and Information Line [50938]
River Valley Behavioral Health--Henderson •
    Therapeutic Rehabilitation Program [33520]
River Valley Behavioral Health Hospital [30092]
    Psychiatric Residential Treatment [33531]
River Valley Behavioral Health--Industrial Drive,
    Owensboro [33532]
River Valley Behavioral Health • Therapeutic
    Rehabilitation Program [30032]
River Valley Behavioral Health--Walnut Street,
    Owensboro [33530]
River Valley Behavioral Health • Webster County
    Office [30103]
River Valley Behavioral Healthcare [43531], [43627],
    [43721], [43768]
    Outpatient Clinic [43739]
    Regional Chemical Dependency Program
        [43740]
River Valley Counseling Inc • Outpatient Services
    [39535]
River Valley Medical Center [28262]
River Valley Services • Mobile Crisis Team [50731]
River Valley Shelter for Battered Women [8782]
River View Kidney Center • Renal Advantage Inc.
    [26753]
Rivera Health Center [6694]
Riverbend Center for Mental Health [27921]
    Evergreen Place [27922]
    Franklin Street Home II [28051]
    Franklin Street House [27923]
    Huntsville Road Home [27924]
    Substance Abuse Services [39244]
Riverbend Children's Intervention Program [31056]
Riverbend Community Mental Health--Admissions
    [31057]
Riverbend Community Mental Health Inc. [31058]

Riverbend Community Mental Health Services [51081]

Riverbend Community Support Program--Pillar House [31059]

Riverbend Contoocook Valley Counseling Center [31072]

Riverbend Elders Program [31060]

Riverbend Emergency and Assessment Services [31061]

Riverbend Russellville [28030]

Riverbend Twitchell House [31062]

RiverBend Youth Center [34399]

Riverbrook Residence [8150]

Rivercenter Dialysis • DaVita [27340]

Rivercrest Treatment Center [50242]

Rivercross Hospice--Bartlesville [20923]

Rivercross Hospice--Wichita [19789]

Riverdale Dialysis Center • DaVita [25597]

Riverdale Mental Health Assoc Inc • CD Outpatient [46449]

Riverdale Mental Health Association [31252]

Riverdale Mental Health Association Community Residence [31253]

Rivereast Day Hospital & Treatment Center [33265]

Riveredge Hospice [20150]

Riveredge Hospital [33420]

Riverhead Mental Health Clinic [31465]

Riverpark Hospital [50314]

Riverplace Counseling Center
   Elk River Inc [45147]
   Mens Program [45074]

Riverpoint Dialysis • DaVita [24268]

RiverRidge Center [4083]

Rivers Bend PC [45039]

Rivers Edge Dialysis • DaVita [26014]

Rivers of Hope [9622]

Riverside Behavioral Center [33350]

Riverside Behavioral Health Center [32743], [49799]

Riverside Care Inc [48348]

Riverside Center for Behavioral Health [33175]

Riverside Center for Behavioral • Medicine [40462]

Riverside Cnty Latino Comm on Alcohol and • DA Services Inc/Casa Las Palmas II [39965]

Riverside Community Care [30363], [50995]
   Brook Street [30387]
   Family and Social Support [30368]
   Milton Street [30364]
   Neponset River House [30438]

Riverside Community Care - Osborne Path [30429]

Riverside Community Care • Unity Place [30365]

Riverside Community Care--Urgent Care Center [30330]

Riverside Community Center [44007]

Riverside Community Hospital [1242]
   Cancer Care Center [4826]

Riverside Community Hospital Transplant Center [22907]

Riverside Counseling Services LLC [41761]

Riverside County Department of Mental Health [28538], [28722]
   Hemet/San Jacinto Mental Health Services [28533]
   Milestones Residential Facility [28539]
   Substance Abuse Program [28459], [28540]

Riverside County Drug Court • Recovery Opportunity Center [40463]

Riverside County Latino Commission on Alcohol/ Drug Abuse Casa Las Palmas [39936]

Riverside County Latino Commission on Alcohol Drug Services • Casa Cecilia Recov Home [40848]

Riverside County Regional Medical Center • Inpatient Treatment Facility [28723]

Riverside County Substance Abuse • Outpatient Drug Free [40464]

Riverside County Substance Abuse Prog [39663], [39744], [39937], [40846]
   Cathedral Canyon Clinic [39694]
   Hemet [39923]

Riverside Dialysis Center [27171]

Riverside Early Intervention [30423]

Riverside General Hospital • Houston Recovery Campus [49395]

Riverside Group Home [34016]

Riverside Hospice [21709]

Riverside Hospital and Madison Center QuietCare [33496]

Riverside Hospital and Treatment Center [33285]

Riverside Medical Center [29635]
   Multiple Sclerosis Center [34527]
   Rush-Riverside Cancer Center [5103]
   Sleep Center [36929]

Riverside Methodist Hospital • Riverside Cancer Institute [5711]

Riverside Outpatient Center • at Wakefield [44593]

Riverside Outpatient Center at Newton [30430]

Riverside Outpatient Center • Newton [44525]

Riverside Outpatient Center - Norwood [30439]

Riverside PD Central • DaVita [22908]

Riverside Recovery [42343]

Riverside Recovery-Orofino [42359]

Riverside Recovery Resources
   First Step House [39924]
   Omega Program [39975], [40383]
   Our House [39925]

Riverside Recovery • Riverside House [42344]

Riverside Regional Medical Center • Virginia Oncology Associates • Cancer Services [6071]

Riverside Rehabilitation Institute [4479]
   ALS Center [155]

Riverside Resolve Center [42758]

Riverside Respite Program - Norwood [30440]

Riverside San Bernardino County • Indian Health [39642]

Riverside San Bernardino County Indian • Health Inc/San Manuel Clinic [40530]

Riverside San Bernardino County
   Indian Health/Pechanga [40847]
   Indian Health/Torres Martinez Clinic [40849]

Riverside Sleep Disorders Center [37893]

Riverside Tappahannock Hospice [21740]

Riverside Walter Reed Hospice [21700]

Riverside Walter Reed Hospital [18305]

Riverside Williamsburg Neurology, PC • Sleep Disorders Center [37894]

Riverstone Clinic [7149]

Riverstone Counseling and Personal Development [51175]

Riverstone Health Hospice Services [20351]

Riverton Community Health Center [7455]

Riverton Place [50127]

Riverton Veterans Affairs Clinic [33063]

Rivertown Community Health Center [6437]

Rivertowne Dialysis Center • DaVita [24710]

Riverview Center--Galena [9228]

Riverview Center, Inc.--Dubuque [9332]

Riverview Foot and Ankle Specialists [6445]

RiverView HealthCare [2686]

Riverview Hearing, Speech and Language Centers [1123], [1156]

Riverview Hospital [2176], [15037]

Riverview Hospital for Children and Youth [33253]

Riverview Medical Center
   Addiction Recovery Services [46163]
   Dialysis Unit [25502]
   Helpline - Crisis Unit [51122]

Riverview Medical Center Hospice-Redbrook Cancer Center [20492]

Riverview Psychiatric Center [33550]

Riverview Regional Medical Center
   Behavioral Health [27933]
   Sleep Lab [36597]

Riverview Rehabilitation and Fitness [2177]

Riverview Rehabilitation and Fitness Center of Carmel [2132]

Riverview Sleep Laboratory • Aspirus Sleep Disorders Center [37976]

Riverways Home Health, Hospice and Support Services [16082]

Riverwood Center [30614]
   Barrien Mental Health Authority [30515]

Riverwood Center--Residential Home [30532]

Riverwood Mental Health Services [32180]

RJ Blackley • Alcohol and Drug Abuse Treatment Center [47240]

R.J. Reynolds Patrick County Memorial Hospital • Hospice of Patrick County [21738]

RM Home Care [15714]

RMA of New York [35141]

RMA of Philadelphia [22235], [22236]

Road Called STRATE [41009]

Road to Freedom Inc [43110]

Road to Recovery [42033], [49296], [49396]

Road to Recovery Inc [42304], [42345], [42346], [42364], [42365]
   Residential [42366]

Road to Recovery LLC [43411]

Roadback Inc/Helen Holliday Home • Female Halfway House [47949]

Roadback Inc • Outpatient [47950]

Roads Inc [49010]

Roane County Family Health Care [7416]

Roane County Schools [753], [882]

Roane Home Care [18541]

Roanoke Chowan Community Health Center [7045]

Roanoke-Chowan Human Services Center [51156]

Roanoke - Chowan SAFE [10012]

Roanoke Health Care Center [28028]

Roanoke Neurological Associates, Inc. • MDA Clinic [34900]

Roanoke Public Library • Talking Book Services [3848]

Roanoke Valley Regional Program for Deaf and Hard of Hearing [857]

Roanoke Valley Speech and Hearing Center Inc. [3610]

Robbins Headache Clinic [12422]

Robbins Speech, Language and Hearing Center [2462]
   Nursery/Emerson College [470]

Robert A Moylan LCPC [42753]

Robert A. Teitge, MD [38583]

Robert E Howe Ltd [47574]

Robert F. Kennedy Children's Action Corps, Inc. [34184]

Robert J. Dole Medical and Regional Office Center • Veterans Affairs Medical Center [51573]

Robert J. Dole VA Medical Center [15157]

Robert J. Dole Veterans Affairs Medical Center [29963]
   PTSD Clinical Team [51736]

Robert J Wilson House • Residential [48869]

Robert M. Greer Center/Liberty of Oklahoma Corp. [8435]

Robert Packer Hospital
   Cancer Program [5870]
   Dialysis Center [26576]
   Towanda Satellite Unit [26590]

Robert Parker Hospital [17469]

Robert Swain Recovery Center [47223]

Robert W Dail Memorial • Treatment Center [42061]

Robert W. Johnson University Hospital at Hamilton • Cancer Program [5516]

Robert Wood Johnson Center for Multiple Sclerosis [34635]

Robert Wood Johnson Hospital at Rahway [16259]

Robert Wood Johnson Medical School
   Bristol-Myers Squibb Children's Hospital
      Adult Cystic Fibrosis Center [7604]
      Pediatric Cystic Fibrosis Center [7605]

Robert Wood Johnson University Hospital [36382]
   Cancer Program [5526]
   Comprehensive Sleep Disorders Center [37357]
   Division of Hematology • New Jersey Regional Hemophilia Program [12558]
   Rahway Hospital Hospice [20491]
   Transplant Center [25481]

Robert Young Center [29648], [50859]

Robert Young Center for Community Health [50840]

Roberta's Place, Inc. [9872]

Roberts Catherine A [47547]

Roberts Home Medical and Home IV Care [15442]

Roberts Home Medical, Inc.--Ashland [18248]

Roberts Home Medical, Inc.--Charlottesville [18262]

Roberts Home Medical, Inc.--Harrisonburg [18311]

Roberts Home Medical, Inc.--Lynchburg [18324]

Roberts Home Medical, Inc.--Newport News [18337]

Roberts Hospice Care Center [19284]

Robeson Healthcare [47368]

Robeson Healthcare Corp
   Cambridge Place [47498]
   Our House [47441]

Robinson Memorial Hospital [17026]
   Cancer Program [5747]

Robinwood Dialysis Facility • Fresenius Medical Care [24693]

Robley Rex Veterans Affairs Medical Center [51576]
   PTSD Clinical Team [51739]

Robs Road to Recovery Ranch [48011]

Rochelle House [33202]

Rochelle Medical Center [6601]

Rochester City School Number One [596]

Rochester/Finger Lakes Eye and Tissue Bank [35142]

Rochester General Hospital
Addiction Services [47046]
Dialysis Unit [25767]
Lipson Cancer Center [5612]
Speech and Pathology Department [3112]
Rochester Hearing and Speech Center [3144]
Rochester Hills Dialysis • DaVita [24960]
Rochester Institute of Technology
National Technical Institute for the Deaf [597]
Audiology Speech and Language Department [3113]
Rochester Multiple Sclerosis Center [34651]
Rochester Pediatrics Services [3433]
Rochester Psychiatric Center [33719]
Rochester Rehabilitation Center [3114]
Rochester VA Outpatient Clinic [16616]
Rochester Veterans Affairs Clinic [30713], [31466]
Rock Bottom Recovery Place LLC [41188]
Rock Brook School [8271]
Rock Hill Orthopaedic Clinic/Carolina Ortho Surgery Association [39016]
Rock Island Cnty Council on Addictions • All Alcohol/ Substance Abuse Progs on Site [42639]
Rock Landing Psychological Group [49815]
Rock Recovery [11298]
Rock Springs Veterans Affairs Clinic [33064]
Rock Valley Community Programs [50371]
Rock Valley Community Programs Inc [50421]
Rockaway Community Life Skills Center [31320]
Rockaway CSS Screening [31321]
Rockaway Mental Health Services [31322]
Rockaway Outreach Mobile Crisis Team [31323]
Rockbridge Area Hospice [21704]
Rockcastle Home Health Agency [2291]
Rockcastle Hospital Home Health [15236]
Rockcastle Hospital and Respiratory Care Center Inc. [2296]
Rockdale Center • GRN Community Services Board [29396]
Rockdale House for Men [42066]
Rockdale Kidney Center • Fresenius Medical Care [27299]
Rockdale Medical Center [14509]
Cancer Program [5020]
Rockdale Mental Health Center [42067]
Rockford Center [33275]
Rockford Dialysis
DaVita [24074]
Dialysis Center of America, Inc. [24075]
Rockford Meld, Inc. • Runaway and Homeless Youth Program [35938]
Rockford Memorial Hospital • Cancer Center [5125]
Rockingham County Schools [615]
Rockingham Kidney Center • Fresenius Medical Care [25935]
Rockingham Memorial Hospital • Center for Sleep Medicine [37895]
Rockingham Memorial Hospital Hospice [21702]
Rockingham Memorial Hospital
Regional Cancer Center [6063]
Rehabilitation Services [39124]
Rockingham VNA & Hospice [20434]
Rockland Children's Psychiatric Center [33712]
Rockland County BOCES--Itinerant Program [606]
Rockland County Department of Mental Health [31453]
Rockland County Dept of Mental Health • Methadone Treatment Program [46983]
Rockland Family Shelter [9946]
Rockland Intensive Day Treatment Program [31490]
Rockland Psychiatric Center [33713]
Rockport Dialysis • DaVita [27301]
Rockside Dialysis • DaVita [26137]
Rockville Center Narcotics/Drug Abuse • Confide/ Outpatient Drug Free [47057]
Rockville General Hospital [1496]
Rockwall Dialysis Center • DaVita [27303]
Rockwell Continuing Day Treatment Program [31279]
Rockwood Clinic • Rockwood Multiple Sclerosis Center [34736]
Rocky Mount Treatment Center [47478]
Rocky Mountain Behavioral Health Inc [41032]
Rocky Mountain Center for Reproductive Medicine [21963]
Rocky Mountain Deaf School [324]

Rocky Mountain Dialysis • Fresenius Medical Care [23114]
Rocky Mountain Ear Center [1409]
Rocky Mountain Fertility Center [21964]
Rocky Mountain Hospice--Billings [20352]
Rocky Mountain Hospice-Butte [20355]
Rocky Mountain Hospice-St. George [21637]
Rocky Mountain Lions Eye Bank [34973]
Rocky Mountain Multiple Sclerosis Center [34544]
Rocky Mountain Multiple Sclerosis Clinic [34723]
Rocky Mountain Offender Management Sys [41081], [41343]
Golden [41200]
Lakewood [41242]
Rocky Mountain Sleep Disorders Center, Butte [37299]
Rocky Mountain Sleep Disorders Center, Helena, Inc. [37300]
Rocky Mountain Sleep Disorders Center, LLC, Great Falls [37301]
Rocky Mountain Tissue Bank [34974]
Rocky Mountain Treatment Center [45700]
Rocky River Dialysis • DaVita [26189]
ROCMND Area Youth Services Inc [48053]
RocVALE Children's Home [7969]
Rodgers Speech, Hearing and Educational Services [3548]
Roger C. Peace Rehabilitation Hospital [4427]
Speech Pathology Department [3401]
Roger Williams Home Care [17552]
Roger Williams Medical Center
Addiction Medical Treatment Center [48880]
Cancer Data Center [5892]
Rogers Counseling Center [10613], [32816], [51432]
Rogers County Drug Abuse Program Inc [47921]
Rogers Memorial Hospital--Kenosha [51507]
Child and Adolescent Day Treatment [33930]
Rogers Memorial Hospital--Madison • Eating Disorders Program [11309]
Rogers Memorial Hospital--Milwaukee [33942]
Eating Disorders Program [11310]
Rogers Memorial Hospital--Oconomowoc [33944]
Rogers Memorial Hospital • Oconomowoc [50496]
Rogers Memorial Hospital--Oconomowoc • Eating Disorders Program [11311]
Rogosin Institute • Dialysis Center [25734]
Rogosin Institute--Queens • Dialysis Center [25807]
Rogosin Kidney Center--Brooklyn • Dialysis Unit [25627]
Rogue Valley Dialysis Services • DaVita [26331]
Rogue Valley Home Care and Hospice [17205]
Rogue Valley Medical Center
Cancer Program [5794]
Sleep Disorders Center [37628]
Rolling Hills Hospital [31866], [47903]
Rolling Hills Hospital LLC [49076]
Rolling Hills School-Based Day Treatment [33998]
Rolling Meadows Counseling Center [42893]
Rolling Plains Memorial Hospital [18168]
Romano Woods Kidney Clinic [27172]
Rome Dialysis • DaVita [23777]
Rome Memorial Hospital/Community • Recovery Center Alcohol/Drug Outpatient Clinic [47058]
Rome Veterans Affairs Clinic [31468]
Romeo Medical Clinic Inc. [38153]
Romero Chiropractic Health Center [38135]
Ronald Sockolov, MD [38121]
Ronat Home Health Care [14133]
Rondo ECSE [518]
Roosevelt Ed Alcohol Counseling Treatment Center • Outpatient Clinic [47060]
Roosevelt Warm Springs Institute for Rehabilitation • Speech-Language Pathology & Audiology Department [1924]
Roper Hospital
Cancer Center [5901]
Sleep/Wake Disorders Center [37738]
Roper Saint Francis Home Care [17569]
Roque Center [39882]
Rosa Parks Elementary School [512]
Rosalie House [8890]
Rosary Hall [47703]
Rose Academy [29737]
ROSE Advocates [9190]
Rose Arbor-Residential Hospice Facility [20079]
Rose Basaraba Counseling Services [47558]
Rose Briear at Astoria Pointe [48067]
Rose Brooks Center [45530]

Rose Brooks Center, Inc. [9691]
Rose Garden Dialysis Center • El Camino Hospital [22971]
Rose Haven • Center for Domestic Violence [8642]
Rose Hill Center [30568]
Rose Home Health Services [18005]
Rose Medical Association Inc/Peoria [42866]
Rose Medical Center • Cancer Center [4874]
Rose Quarter Dialysis • Fresenius Medical Care [26349]
Rose Rock Recovery Center [48054]
Rose Speech and Academic Center [1774]
Rose Street Community Center • Runaway and Homeless Youth Program [35994]
Rosebud Dialysis • DaVita [26795]
Rosebud Sioux Tribe • Indian Child Welfare Office • Runaway and Homeless Youth Program [36200]
Rosebud Sioux Tribe Piya Mani Otipi [49002]
Roseburg/Mercy Dialysis & At Home • DaVita [26351]
Roseburg Veterans Affairs Medical Center [31971]
Rosecrance Inc [42676]
Griffin Williamson Adolescent Campus [42890]
Harrison Adult Campus/Health Center [42891]
Monarch Homes/Outpatient [42892]
Rosedale Kidney Disease Clinic • Dialysis Facility • Fresenius Medical Care [27341]
Rosehill School [8452]
Rosel Home Equipment Care, Inc [14134]
Roseland Christian Health Ministries [6665]
Rosemead Dialysis Center [22911]
Rosemont Center [31723]
Rosemoor Assessment • Substance Abuse Program Inc [42574]
Rosenberg Dialysis Facility • Fresenius Medical Care [27305]
Rosenblum Mental Health Center [30140]
Rosenthal Collins Group L.P. [23955]
Roses Home Care Services [16199]
Roseville Speech and Language [1176]
Rosewood Center for Eating Disorders [39515]
Rosewood Center • Programs for the Mentally Retarded [8095]
Rosewood Centers for Eating Disorders [10905]
Rosewood Outpatient Center [10906]
Ross County Coalition Against Domestic Violence [10132]
Ross County Home Health Agency [16870]
Ross Dialysis--Englewood • Fresenius Medical Care [23956]
Roswell Addiction Treatment [43380]
Roswell Hospice HomeCare and Hospice • Family HomeCare Services, Inc. [20542]
Roswell Independent School District [563]
Roswell Park Cancer Institute
Cancer Program [5570]
Comprehensive Cancer Center [4690]
Roswell Refuge for Battered Adults [9881]
Rotech--Berwick [17256]
Rotech--Clarks Summit [17286]
Rotech--Columbia [17576]
Rotech Home Medical Care--Christianburg [18272]
Rotech Home Medical Care--Danville [18171]
RoTech Home Medical Care, Inc.--Roanoke [18378]
Rotech Home Medical Care--Pearlsburg [18346]
Rotech Home Medical Care--Staunton [18391]
Rotech--Minersville [17388]
Rotech Oxygen and Medical Equipment [14453]
Roudebush VA Medical Center • Substance Abuse Treatment Section [43111]
Round Rock Clinic • Capital Nephrology Associates [27307]
Round Valley Residential [28171]
Roundup Mental Health Center [30963]
Route 2 Language [1303]
Routt County Alcohol Council [41314]
Rowan Medical Facilities [16777]
Rowan Regional Medical Center • Lifeworks Behavioral Health Division [47488]
Rowan--Salisbury School System [630]
Rowan Trees [42575]
Roxboro Dialysis • DaVita • Dialysis Center [25940]
Roxboro Dialysis--Philadephia • DaVita [26534]
Roxbury [48318]
Roxbury Comp Comm Health Center Inc • Methadone Services [44493]
Roxbury Comprehensive Community Health Center • RoxComp [6824]

Roxbury Dialysis Center & At Home • DaVita [24076]
Roxbury Treatment Center [48321], [48642]
Roxie Avenue Center • Substance Abuse Services [47313]
Roy Maas' Youth Alternatives • The Bridge • Runaway and Homeless Youth Program [36231]
Royal Alexandra Hospital • Capital Health Edmonton Area Eating Disorders Nutrition Counseling Center [10892]
Royal C. Johnson Sioux Falls Veterans Affairs Medical Center [17640]
Royal C. Johnson Veterans Affairs Medical Center [32247], [51649]
Royal C. Johnson Veterans Medical Center • Multiple Sclerosis Center [34710]
Royal Care [16416]
The Royal Care [16461]
Royal Care Home Health Services [13786]
Royal Home Care [13448]
Royal Home Health Network [15826]
Royal Home Healthcare Agency Inc. [13049]
Royal Jubilee Hospital • Burn Unit [4512]
Royal Oaks Hospital [33639], [45676]
Royal Palm School [7889]
Royal University Hospital • Burn Unit [4631]
Royal Victoria Hospital of Barrie--Collingwood • Youth Eating Disorders Program [11232]
Royal Victoria Hospital of Barrie • Simcoe County Eating Disorders Service [11233]
Royal Victoria Hospital • Burn Unit [4628]
Royale Home Health Care, Inc. [15827]
Royalty Home Health Care [13775]
Roybal Family Mental Health Services [28611]
Royce Centers Pain Medicine [35414]
Roze Room Hospice--Los Angeles [18960]
Roze Room Hospice of the Valley, Inc. [13150]
Roze Room Hospice of Ventura [18961]
RPK Associates [46181], [46206]
RRC--Davison [24860]
RRC Lapeer [24934]
RRC--Mt. Morris [24948]
RS Eden Womens Program [45228]
RSA Schertz [27361]
RTC Columbia Dialysis & At Home • DaVita [25188]
RTI Biologics Inc. [35005]
RTI Donor Services--Middleton [35267]
RTI Donor Services, Texas Division/Corpus Christi [35239]
RTI Donor Services, Texas Division/Dallas [35240]
RTI Donor Services, Texas Division/El Paso [35241]
Ruan Neurology Multiple Sclerosis Center [34581]
Rubal Home Health Care [14135]
Rubicon Inc
    Outpatient Services [49833]
    Womens Treatment Community [49834]
RUMC Silberstein Clinic Med Sup Outpatient [47099]
Rumford Group Homes • Runaway and Homeless Youth Program [35986]
Rumford Veterans Affairs Clinic [30237]
Runaway-Youth and Shelter Services [50900]
Runnells Specialized Hospital of Union County [33654]
Runnels County Mental Health Center [32572]
Running Creek Counseling Service [41288]
Rural Clinics Community Mental Health Center [31026]
Rural Health Corp. of Northeastern Pennsylvania [7163]
Rural Health Services Consortium, Inc. • Roan Mountain Medical Center [7270]
Rural Human Services • Harrington House [8807]
Rural Iowa Center [9325]
Rural Medical Services [7269]
Rural Resources Community Action Agency • Youth. Dot.Com • Runaway and Homeless Youth Program [36256]
Rush Children's Hospital • Section of Pediatric Hematology/Oncology [12519]
Rush--Copley Center for Reproductive Health [22049]
Rush-Copley Medical Center • Cancer Care Center [5061]
Rush County Dialysis • DaVita [24228]
Rush County Services • Centerstone of IN Inc [43194]

Rush Foundation Hospital • Pain Treatment Center [35526]
Rush Presbyterian-St. Luke's Medical Center • Department of Orthopedic Surgery • Section of Sports Medicine [38367]
Rush-Presbyterian-Saint Luke's Medical Center • Department of Pediatrics • Genetics Clinic [12203]
Rush Presbyterian-Saint Luke's Medical Center
    Multiple Sclerosis Center [34572]
    Rush Center for Advanced Reproductive Care • In Vitro Fertilization Program [22050]
Rush University Medical Center [2002]
    Adult Cystic Fibrosis Center [7532]
    AIDS Clinical Trials Unit [11]
Rush University Medical Center-Aurora • Genetics Clinic [12204]
Rush University Medical Center
    Cancer Program [5075]
    Centers for AIDS Research [51]
    Department of Communicative Disorders and Sciences [2003]
Rush University Medical Center-Hoffman Estates • Genetics Clinic [12205]
Rush University Medical Center-Joliet • Genetics Clinic [12206]
Rush University Medical Center-Kankakee • Genetics Clinic [12207]
Rush University Medical Center
    MDA Clinic [34794]
    Pain Management [35435]
    Pediatric Cystic Fibrosis Center [7533]
    Pediatric Dialysis Unit [23957]
Rushford Center Inc
    ACE Program [41422]
    Intensive Treatment Program [41423]
    Intermediate Residential Unit [41463]
    Outpatient [41424]
    Positive Step/Glastonbury [41385]
Rushville Dialysis • DaVita [24079]
Rushville Health Center, Inc. [7040]
Rusk Institute of Rehabilitation Medicine • Brain Injury Rehab [4315]
Rusk Outpatient Services/Howard A. Rusk Rehabilitation Center [35529]
Rusk State Hospital [33880]
Russell Center for Chiropractic & Sports Medicine [38539]
Russell County Child Day Treatment • Russell County Schools [28035]
Russell County Counseling Center [28023]
Russell County Day Services [28024]
Russell County Medical Center [18316]
Russell County Public Schools • Hearing Impaired Program [853]
Russell E Blaisdell • Addiction Treatment Center [46964]
Russell House • Phelps County Family Crisis Services [9712]
Russell Medical Center • Sleep Disorders Center [36598]
Russell-Murray Hospice [20932]
Russellville Hospital [12719]
Russellville Transitional Crisis Unit [28348]
Ruston Addictive Disorders Clinic [43889]
Ruston Developmental Center [8074]
Ruth Cooper Center [50758]
Ruth Cooper Center Campus [29162]
Ruth Cooper Center • Drug Abuse Treatment and Education [41662]
Ruth Dykeman Children's Center [34470]
Ruth Dykeman Children's Center--Youth and Family Services [34466]
Ruth Dykeman Youth and Family Service [49919]
Ruth Ellis Center • Runaway and Homeless Youth Program [36024]
Ruth Hospice • Village at Manor Park [21858]
Ruth House--People Incorporated [30727]
Ruth Levisohn and Associates [1402]
Ruth Meiers Adolescent Center [31632]
Ruthe B. Cowl Rehabilitation Center [8554]
Ruthe Feilbert Willis [41466]
Rutherford Hospital • Cancer Program [5658]
Rutherford Hospital, Inc. [16776]
Rutherford Internal Medicine Associates [37484]
Ruth's Cottage [9126]
Rutland Area Community Service [32676]
    Group Home [32677]

Rutland Area Visiting Nurse Association and Hospice [18236]
Rutland Area VNA & Hospice [21666]
Rutland County Women's Network and Shelter [10547]
Rutland Mental Health Services [49742]
Rutland Regional Medical Center
    Community Cancer Center [6049]
    Sleep Center [37879]
RV Counseling Services [43507]
RV Somerville Dialysis Center • Renal Ventures Management [25511]
RVM-Renal Center of Mountain Home [22563]
Rx Solutions, Inc. [14846]
Rye Hospital Center [33722]
Ryther Child Center [34471]
    Adolescent Chem Dependency Treatment Prog [50128]

S

2nd Chance Counseling and Management Services [43707]
2nd Chance Ministries Inc [43082]
2nd Chance Recovery Center of • Washington [49918]
2nd Chance for Recovery Inc [40887]
75 Medical Group/SGOWS • ADAPT [49615]
7th Avenue Family Health Center [6460]
S & A Unified Home Care, Inc.--Brooklyn [16417]
S & A Unified Home Care--Staten Island [16640]
S L Hunter and Associates [3297]
A S Martin Orthopedics • Sports Medicine and General Orthopedics [38700]
S and S Counseling Service [44392]
S and S Counseling Services and Assc Inc
    Fort Bend Recovery Zone [49497]
    Northeast Recovery Zone [49397]
    Residential [49398]
S & S Health Care Management [14136]
S & Y Home Health Care [14137]
SAAFE House [10477]
Sabine Valley Center [8555]
Sabine Valley Regional Mental Health/Mental Retardation Center
    Marshall Family Services [32508]
    Panola County Family Services [32425]
    Rusk County [32477]
    Sabine Valley Center [32501]
    Sabine Valley Counseling [32469]
Sable House [10228], [51251]
Sabra Sanctuary [8652]
Sabrina L West LCSW • Counseling Service [43617]
Sacajawea Substance Abuse Counseling [47567]
Sacheen H. Mehta, MD, PA [39094]
Saco River Health Services [44074]
Sacramento Area Emergency Housing Center
    34th Street Facility [40499]
    Family Shelter [40500]
Sacramento Black Alcoholism Center • Sobriety Brings a Change [40501]
Sacramento Children's Home [34017]
Sacramento Community Clinic at Del Paso [6347]
Sacramento Community Clinic at Southgate [6348]
Sacramento County Mental Health Treatment Center [33180]
Sacramento County Probation • Adult Drug Court Treatment Center [40502]
Sacramento Native American • Health Center Inc [40503]
Sacramento Pathway • Pathways Recovery [39714]
Sacramento Recovery House Inc [40504]
Sacramento Scottish Rite Language Center [1250]
Sacramento Veterans Affairs Medical Center [13167]
    Chico Outpatient Clinic [28434]
    Fairfield Outpatient Clinic [28494]
    Martinez Outpatient Clinic [28621]
    Mather Mental Health Clinic [28622]
    Oakland Mental Health Clinic [28680]
    Redding Outpatient Clinic [28712]
Sacramento Veterans Resource Center [40505]
Sacred Circle [10382]
Sacred Health [14138]
Sacred Heart Children's Hospital • Sickle Cell Disease Center [36325]
Sacred Heart Dialysis • Saint Joseph Hospital [27707]
Sacred Heart Health System-Pensacola • Center for

Cancer Care [4982]
Sacred Heart Home Pain Management Program [35496]
Sacred Heart Hospice-Allentown [21045]
Sacred Heart Hospital--Allentown • Cancer Program [5811]
Sacred Heart Hospital Dialysis [27712]
Sacred Heart Hospital--Eau Claire • Cancer Program [6148]
Sacred Heart Hospital • Sleep Disorders Center [37686]
Sacred Heart Medical Center • Burn Program [4648]
Sacred Heart Medical Center - Home Care Services [17188]
Sacred Heart Medical Center
    Inland Northwest Genetics Clinic [12368]
    MDA Clinic [34859]
    Oregon Rehabilitation Center [4382]
Sacred Heart Medical Center--Spokane • Cancer and Research Center [6122]
Sacred Heart Medical Center--Spokane, WA • Sleep Institute of Spokane [37930]
Sacred Heart Medical Center--Springfield, OR • Sleep Disorders Center [37629]
Sacred Heart Medical Center Transplant [27651]
Sacred Heart • New Life Home for Recovering Women Inc [44760]
Sacred Heart Pediatric Dialysis • Fresenius Medical Care [23474]
Sacred Heart Pediatric • Fresenius Medical Care [23475]
Sacred Heart Rehabilitation [1715]
Sacred Heart Rehabilitation Center Inc [44630], [44791], [44917], [44941], [45044]
    BASIS [44662]
    Clearview Substance Abuse Services [44979]
Sacred Heart Rehabilitation Institute [4495]
    Columbia St. Mary's • Pediatric Program [8624]
Sacred Heart Visiting Nurses [17236]
Sacred Heart • Women's Shelter [10367]
Sacred Shield WRIR [10762]
Sacro Veterans Affairs Clinic [30241]
Saddle Rock Counseling [41043]
Saddleback Dialysis • DaVita [22744]
Saddleback Memorial Medical Center [13095]
    Cancer Program [4789]
Saddleback Rehabilitation System [3918]
Sadler Health Center [7154]
Safe Alternatives for Abused Families [10109]
Safe Avenues [9644]
Safe Center [9573]
The SAFE Center [9773]
Safe Embrace [9799]
Safe and Fear Free Environment [8659]
SAFE Foundation Inc • CD Outpatient [46529]
Safe Harbor [10987]
Safe Harbor--Aberdeen [10364]
Safe Harbor--Ashland • Domestic Violence Shelter [9384]
Safe Harbor Children's Shelter • Runaway and Homeless Youth Program [35912]
Safe Harbor Crisis House [28849]
Safe Harbor Domestic Abuse Program [10735]
Safe Harbor Family Crisis Center [9229]
Safe Harbor--Greenville [10352]
Safe Harbor Hospice, Inc. [20298]
Safe Harbor Inc • Kingman [43383]
Safe Harbor Inc.--Mandeville [9413]
SAFE Harbor, Inc.--Poison [9761]
SAFE Harbor--Pablo [9759]
Safe Harbor Recovery Center/Beacon of • Hope Port Townsend [50067]
Safe Harbor Retreat • The Dunes [46612]
Safe Harbor--Richmond [10589]
Safe Harbor Treatment Center for Women Inc [39753]
Safe Harbour [30706]
Safe Harbour Domestic Violence Shelter, Inc. [10170]
S.A.F.E. of Harnett County, Inc. [10054]
A Safe Haven [42576]
Safe Haven [42577], [42578], [42579]
Safe Haven Crisis and Recovery Center [10410]
Safe Haven of Greater Waterbury [9007]
SAFE HAVEN, Inc. [9649]
Safe Haven Ministries [9537]
Safe Haven of Pender, Inc. [10019]
Safe Haven--Person County [10079]

Safe Haven of Pike County [10299]
Safe Haven of Racine, Inc. • Runaway and Homeless Youth Program [36272]
Safe Haven Shelter for Battered Women [9595]
Safe Haven of Tarrant County [10440]
Safe at Home [9301]
Safe Home [9365]
A Safe Home for Everyone [10049]
Safe Home Health Care, Inc. [14775]
Safe Home Program [30346]
Safe Homes of Augusta, Inc. [9090]
Safe Homes • Rape Crisis Coalition [10362]
Safe Horizon
    Crime Victim's Center--Sexual Assault Project [9956]
    Runaway and Homeless Youth Program [36119]
Safe Horizons [9570]
SAFE House [32331]
Safe House [44177]
The Safe House [9819]
SAFE House--Albuquerque [9857]
SAFE House, Inc.--Henderson [9792]
Safe House, Inc.--Kingsport [10408]
Safe House--Lake Monroe [9060]
Safe House/Sexual Assault Services, Inc. [10748]
Safe House for Women, Inc. [9666]
Safe House--Yuma [8747]
Safe In Hunterdon [9826]
SAFE, Inc.--Blairsville [9091]
SAFE Inc. of Schenectady • Runaway and Homeless Youth Program [36120]
Safe, Inc. of Transylvania County [10017]
Safe Journey [10321]
SAFE in Lenoir County, Inc. [10050]
Safe Passage Domestic Violence--Moberly • Crisis Intervention Services [9704]
Safe Passage, Inc.--Dekalb [9221]
Safe Passage, Inc.--Johnson City [10407]
Safe Passage, Inc.--Northampton [9497]
Safe Passage, Inc.--Rock Hill [10361]
Safe Passage--Melbourne [8773]
Safe Passage • Runaway and Homeless Youth Program [35837]
Safe Passages, Inc.--Batesville [9265]
A Safe Place [8859], [9260], [9815]
The Safe Place [8776]
SAFE Place--Battle Creek [9516]
A Safe Place to Heal [11283]
A Safe Place, Inc. [9492]
Safe Place, Inc.--Dumas [10458]
A Safe Place • Lake County Crisis Center [9257]
Safe Place Ministries [9161]
Safe Place and Rape Crisis Center--Sarasota [9079]
SAFE Project [10755]
SAFE Shelter [10114]
Safe Shelter, Inc.--Benton Harbor [9519]
Safe Shelter of Saint Vrain Valley [8975]
Safe and Sound Medical Clinic [7127]
Safe Space--Butte [9742]
Safe Space, Inc. [31431]
Safe Space, Inc.--Louisburg [10056]
Safe Space, Inc. • Spa West [31432]
Safe Space--Sevierville [10432]
Safe Step LLC [45063]
SAFE: Supporters of Abuse Free Environments, Inc. [9748]
SafeHarbor HealthCare Services [16641]
Safehaven Community Homes [27984]
SafeHaven of Kansas City, Inc. [9692]
SafeHaven of Tarrant County [10461]
SAFEHOME, INC. [9374]
Safehome Systems, Inc. [10560]
Safehouse of Bullhead City, Inc./Westcare [8678]
Safehouse Crisis Center--Coffeyville [9352]
SafeHouse Denver [8955]
SafeHouse of the Desert • Runaway and Homeless Youth Program [35838]
Safehouse Inc.--Meeker [8977]
SAFEHOUSE, Inc.--Pittsburg [9375]
SafeHouse of Shelby County [8649]
Safeline [10542]
SafeNest [9794]
SafeNet [10274]
SafeNet Home Health Services [12820]
SafePlace: Domestic Violence and Sexual Assault Survival Center [10441]
Safeplace--Florence [8641]
Safeplace--Olympia [10634]

SafePlace of the Permian Basin [10490]
SafeQuest Solano, Inc. [8812]
SafeSpace Domestic Violence Services, Inc. [9051]
SafeSpace Inc.--Stuart [9081]
Safety Consultant Services [40038], [40152], [40953]
Safety Consultant Services Inc [40260], [40807]
Safety Council of Greater Saint Louis • Kirkwood - Best Western Inn WIP [45629]
Safety Education Center [40443], [40944]
Safety Net for Abused Persons [9418]
Safety Net Academy [27974]
Safetycord Inc. [35196]
SafetyNet Montgomery [28001]
Safford Clinic [6247]
Sagamore Children's Psychiatric Center [8312]
Sagamore Children's Psychiatric Center--Dix Hills [33692]
Sagamore Children's Psychiatric Center • Waverly Clinic [33715]
SAGE Institute [41022]
SAGE Project Inc [40631]
Sagebrush Center - Children's [28395]
Sagebrush Treatment Inc [49796]
Saginaw Chippewa Indian Tribe • Behavioral Health Programs [44931]
Saginaw Chippewa Indian Tribe - Victims of Crime Program [9560]
Saginaw City Mental Health Center • Crisis Intervention Services [51028]
Saginaw County Community Mental Health Authority [30629]
Saginaw County Youth Council/Innerlink Transitional Living and Emergency Shelter • Runaway and Homeless Youth Program [36025]
Saginaw Dialysis Clinic • DaVita [24967]
Saginaw Intermediate School District • Hearing Impaired Program [500]
Saginaw Odyssey House [45002]
Saginaw Psychological Services Inc [45003]
Saginaw Valley Hearing Clinic [2641]
Sagrado Corazon de Jesus Home Care [14139]
Saguaro Home Health Services, Inc. [16158]
Saint Aemilian-Lakeside [34488]
Saint Agatha Home • Runaway and Homeless Youth Program [36121]
Saint Agnes HealthCare • Cancer Program [5289]
Saint Agnes Hospice [18932]
St. Agnes Hospital [37977]
Saint Agnes Hospital
    Behavioral Health Services [50393]
    Department of Audiology and Speech-Language Pathology [2380]
Saint Agnes Hospital Domestic Violence Program [10702]
Saint Agnes Medical Center [13010]
    Cancer Program No. 345 [4779]
Saint Agnes Medical Center Hospice • Inpatient Unit - VITAS [21132]
Saint Albans Dialysis Center • Renal Research Institute [25689]
Saint Alexius Home Care and Hospice [20775]
Saint Alexius Medical Center--Bismarck • Cancer Program [5669]
Saint Alexius Medical Center • Department of Speech-Language Pathology [3201]
Saint Alexius Medical Center-Hoffman Estates • Cancer Program [5099]
Saint Alexius Medical Center Home Care & Hospice [16807]
Saint Alexius Medical Center
    Kidney Care Center • Dialysis Center [25987]
    Sleep Center [37500]
Saint Alexius Medical • Partial Hospitalization Program [47559]
Saint Alphonsus • Addiction Recovery Center [42318]
Saint Alphonsus Behavioral Health Services [29541]
Saint Alphonsus Cancer Care Center • Cancer Genetics Program [12195]
Saint Alphonsus Medical Center • Nampa Sleep Laboratory [36882]
Saint Alphonsus Regional Medical Center
    Cancer Treatment Center [5050]
    Pain Center [35423]
    Sleep Disorders Center [36883]
Saint Alphonsus Rehabilitation Unit [4014]
Saint Ambrose Health Center [6812]

Saint Anne Mercy Hospital • Cancer Center [5753]
Saint Annes Home Inc [39226]
Saint Anne's Hospital • Harold K. Hudner Oncology
Center [5332]
Saint Anne's Hospital/May Institute • Fernandes
Center for Children and Families [8124]
Saint Anne's Hospital • Outpatient Rehabilitation
[2477]
Saint Ann's Home [34201]
Saint Anthony Central Hospital [1403]
    Oncology Services [4875]
    Regional Mountain Cancer Center [4664]
Saint Anthony Hospital [17211]
Saint Anthony Hospital--Oklahoma City • Frank C.
Love Cancer Institute [5781]
Saint Anthony Hospital--Pendleton • Cancer
Program [5797]
St. Anthony Hospital--Transplant [26285]
Saint Anthony Medical Center • Burrell Cancer
Institute [5140]
Saint Anthony Memorial Health Centers • Cancer
Center [5167]
Saint Anthony Regional Hospice [19669]
Saint Anthony School Programs [8490]
Saint Anthony Sleep Disorders Center [37931]
Saint Anthony's Health Center [1955]
    Cancer Program [5058]
Saint Anthony's Healthcare Center of Morrilton
[28325]
Saint Anthony's Hospice-Dixon [19797]
Saint Anthony's Hospice--Henderson [19806]
Saint Anthony's Hospice--Morganfield [19820]
Saint Anthony's Hospice--Saint Louis [20336]
Saint Anthony's Hospital • Cancer Program [4992]
Saint Anthonys Hospital • Start Recovery and Treat-
ment Program [47996]
Saint Anthony's Medical Center [16060]
    Cancer Center [4682]
    Sleep Disorder Center [37280]
Saint Anthony's Memorial Hospital [14773]
    Cancer Program [5087]
Saint Anthony's North Hospital [1442]
Saint Anthony's Regional Hospital • Dialysis Unit
[24252]
Saint Anthony's Rehabilitation Hospital [3994]
Saint Augustine Artificial Kidney Center • KRU Medi-
cal Ventures [23500]
Saint Augustine Plantation In-Home Care [14401]
Saint Augustine VA Community Based Outpatient
Clinic [14364]
Saint Augustine Youth Services [34082]
    Transitional Independent Living Program [33353]
Saint Barnabas Behavioral Health Center [33663]
Saint Barnabas Fordham Tremont Family Violence
Crisis Service [9904]
Saint Barnabas Hospice and Pall Care Ctr at
Newark Beth Israel Medical Center [20511]
Saint Barnabas Hospice and Palliative Care Center
at Monmouth Medical Center [20477]
Saint Barnabas Hospice and Palliative Care Center--
West Orange [20512]
Saint Barnabas Hospital
    Chem Dependence Medically Mngd Detox
    [46450]
    Chemical Dependence Outpatient Service
    [46451]
    Dialysis Center [25598]
    Methadone Substance Abuse Treatment [46452]
    Multiple Sclerosis Center [34636]
    Speech and Hearing Center [2983]
Saint Barnabas Medical Center
    Burn Center [4587]
    Cancer Program [5519]
    Center for Sleep Disorders [37358]
    Cystic Fibrosis Center [7606]
St. Barnabas Medical Center--Transplant • St.
Barnabas Health Care System [25460]
Saint Barnabus Medical Center • Valerie Fund
Children's Center • Sickle Cell Disease Center
[36383]
St. Benedict Hospice • Avera St. Benedict Health
Center [21296]
Saint Bernard Battered Women's Program, Inc.
[9402]
Saint Bernard Mental Health Center [30134]
Saint Bernardine Care Provider Inc. [13426]
Saint Bernardine Medical Center • Cancer Program
[4832]

Saint Bernard's Behavioral Health [33120]
Saint Bernard's Community Hospital Corporation
[12885]
Saint Bernards Counseling Center [28295]
Saint Bernard's Home Health Care [12861]
Saint Bernard's Hospice--Jonesboro [18859]
Saint Bernard's Medical Center • Sleep Disorders
Center [36649]
Saint Bernards Regional Medical Center [12862]
    Dialysis Center [22548]
Saint Bernard's - Wynne [22580]
Saint Cabrini Home Inc • Chemical Dependency
Program [47176]
Saint Cabrini Home, Inc. [31491]
Saint Camillus Speech and Hearing [3132]
Saint Catherine Home Care Services [19753]
Saint Catherine Hospital [2140]
St. Catherine Hospital [15124]
Saint Catherine Hospital • Saint Catherine Neurodi-
agnostic and Sleep Disorders Center [37003]
St. Catherine of Siena Hospital [20608]
Saint Catherine of Siena Medical Center • Dialysis
Center [25776]
Saint Catherine's Center for Children [34320]
    Brady House [34321]
    Group Residence [34322]
    Hubbard House [34323]
    Marrillac Shelter [34324]
Saint Catherine's Kidney Center • United Hospital
System [27771]
Saint Charles Center for Health Promotions [3251]
Saint Charles Community Health Center, Inc. [6751]
Saint Charles Community Health Center • Kenner
Pediatrics [6749]
Saint Charles County Dialysis • Fresenius Medical
Care [25286]
St. Charles Dialysis • DaVita • Dialysis Facility
[25262]
Saint Charles Educational and Therapeutic Center
[3122]
Saint Charles Habilitation Center [8207]
Saint Charles Hospital
    Cancer Program [5609]
    Chemical Depend Inpatient Program [46985]
    Hearing and Speech Center [3098]
Saint Charles Hospital and Rehabilitation Center •
MDA Clinic [34840]
Saint Charles Medical Center-Bend [17182]
Saint Charles Medical Center • Cancer Program
[5786]
Saint Charles Mercy Hospital
    [5744]
    Sleep Disorders Center [37567]
Saint Charles Parish Hospital • Psychiatric Unit
[43849]
Saint Charles Rehabilitation Center • Speech-
Language Pathology Department [3306]
Saint Charles Sleep Disorders Center [37416]
Saint Charles Veterans Affairs Clinic [30890]
Saint Christopher's Hospital for Children
    Department of Pediatrics • Section of Clinical
    Genetics [12329]
    Pediatric Burn Center [4623]
    Sleep Center for Children [37687]
    Transplant/Dialysis Center [26535]
Saint Christopher's, Inc. [31313], [31483]
Saint Christophers Inn Inc • Saint Anthonys
Outpatient Clinic [46649]
Saint Christopher's-Jenny Clarkson Child Care
Services, Inc. [34337]
Saint Clair County Community Mental Health
Services [51027]
Saint Clair County Library for the Blind and Physi-
cally Handicapped [3812]
Saint Clair Memorial Hospital [17445]
    Cancer Center [5859]
Saint Claire Home Care/Hospice [19819]
Saint Claire Home, Inc. [8810]
Saint Claire Medical Center Home Health [15235]
Saint Claire Regional Medical Center
    Cancer Program [5231]
    Sleep Lab [37044]
Saint Claire's Home Health [13076]
Saint Clair's Home Health Inc. [13080]
Saint Clare Center • Saint Clare Hospital [50365]
St. Clare Dialysis Center [27699]
Saint Clare Hospital--Baraboo • Sleep Disorders
Laboratory [37978]

Saint Clare Hospital--Lakewood
    Cancer Program [6103]
    Sleep Disorders Clinic [37932]
Saint Clare's Behavioral Health Center [31108]
Saint Clare's Hospital [14678]
Saint Clare's Hospital--Denville • Cancer Program
[5507]
Saint Clare's Hospital • Dialysis Unit [25735]
Saint Clare's Hospital--Dover • Center for Sleep
Medicine [37359]
St. Cloud Dialysis • DaVita [23501]
St. Cloud Hospital [15943]
Saint Cloud Hospital • Coborn Cancer Center [5416]
Saint Cloud Hospital Hospice/Homecare [20203]
Saint Cloud Hospital
    Recovery Plus [45295]
    Regional Centracare Dialysis [25075]
    Sleep Disorders Program [37230]
Saint Cloud Orthopedic Associates Ltd. [38635]
Saint Cloud State University • Department of Com-
munication Disorders • Speech-Language and
Hearing Clinic [2734]
Saint Cloud VA Medical Center [15936]
Saint Cloud Veteran Affairs Medical Center [30718]
Saint Cloud Veterans Affairs Health Care System •
Women's Stress Disorder Treatment Team
Outpatient [51758]
Saint Coletta Day School [8625]
Saint Coletta of Greater Washington [8576]
Saint Coletta School [8614]
Saint Croix Education Complex School Health
[7342]
Saint Croix Falls Dialysis • DaVita [27780]
Saint Croix Family Medical Clinic [6875]
Saint Croix Regional Family Health Center [6783]
Saint Croix Tribal • Mental Health/AODA Clinic
[50560]
Saint Croix Veterans Affairs Community Based
Outpatient Clinic [32691]
Saint David's Center for Child and Development
[2718]
Saint David's Medical Center • Cancer Program
[5962]
Saint David's Pavilion [33858]
Saint David's Round Rock Medical Center • Cancer
Program [6021]
Saint David's South Austin Hospital • Cancer
Program [5963]
Saint Dominic Behavioral Health Services [45396]
Saint Dominic-Jackson Memorial Hospital • Cancer
Center [5429]
Saint Edward Mercy Medical Center [12848]
    Cancer Program [4751]
Saint Edward Mercy Medical Center Hospice
[18853]
Saint Elizabeth Alcohol and Drug Treatment [43587]
Saint Elizabeth/American Nursing Care Inc. [15177]
Saint Elizabeth Community Health Center • Regional
Burn Center [4583]
Saint Elizabeth Community Hospital [13252]
Saint Elizabeth-Falmouth [43588]
Saint Elizabeth Health Center • Cancer Center
[5769]
St. Elizabeth Health Center • Humility of Mary
Health Partners [26242]
Saint Elizabeth Healthcare--Covington • Sports
Medicine [38473]
Saint Elizabeth Healthcare--Florence • Sports
Medicine [38476]
Saint Elizabeth Hospice--Lafayette [19623]
Saint Elizabeth Hospice--Red Bluff [18997]
Saint Elizabeth Hospice • St. Elizabeth Regional
Medical Center--Lincoln [20391]
Saint Elizabeth Hospital • Comprehensive Cancer
Center [6144]
Saint Elizabeth Hospital, Inc. • Sleep Disorder
Center [37045]
Saint Elizabeth Hospital Medical Center • Dean
Martin Neuromuscular Clinic • MDA Clinic [34854]
Saint Elizabeth Hospital West • Sleep Disorders
Center [37046]
Saint Elizabeth • Intensive Outpatient Program
[43592]
Saint Elizabeth Medical Center
    Behavioral Health Center [43576]
    Crisis Evaluation Team [51153]
Saint Elizabeth Medical Center--Edgewood KY •
Sleep Disorders Center [37047]

Cancer Program [5462]
Dialysis Facility [25276]
Multiple Sclerosis Center [34619]
St. John's Mercy Rehabilitation Center [4239]
Saint John's Multiple Sclerosis Center [34661]
Saint John's Queens Hospital • Dialysis Unit [25654]
Saint John's Queens Rehabilitation Center [3107]
St. John's Regional Center/St. John's Pleasant Valley Hosp. [3919]
Saint John's Regional Health Center
MDA Clinic [34824]
Midwest Sports Medicine Center [38672]
Sleep Disorders Center [37282]
Saint John's Regional Health Center--Springfield • C. H. O'Reilly Cancer Center [5466]
Saint John's Regional Medical Center Home Health [16019]
Saint John's Regional Medical Center--Joplin • Cancer Center [5445]
Saint John's Regional Medical Center
MDA Clinic [34825]
Pain Clinic [35328]
Sleep Disorders Center [37283]
Saint John's Rehabilitation Hospital and Nursing Center [13854]
Saint Johns Riverside Hospital
Archway Outpatient Alcohol and Substance AbuseTreatment Prog [46798]
Greenburgh Addiction Treatment Service [47187]
Inpatient Rehabilitation [47196]
MMTP Behavioral Health Services [47197]
New Focus Center [47198]
Outpatient Rehabilitation [47188]
Park Care Pav/Chemical Dep Detox Prog [47199]
Saint John's Sleep Disorders Center [37988]
Saint John's Sleep Disorders Center, Berryville [36650]
Saint John's Specialty Clinic • Outreach Clinic • Cystic Fibrosis Center [7592]
Saint John's University • Speech and Hearing Center [3105]
Saint Johns Well Child and Family Center [6320]
St. Johnsbury Dialysis • Fresenius Medical Care [27445]
Saint Jones Center for Behavioral Health [33272]
Saint Joseph/American Nursing Care Inc. [15210]
Saint Joseph At Home [15017]
Saint Joseph Behavioral Health • Chemical Dependency Services [43056]
Saint Joseph Center [28837]
Saint Joseph Center for Special Learning [8482]
Saint Joseph County Community Mental Health [51029]
Saint Joseph Dialysis & At Home • DaVita [25263]
Saint Joseph Dialysis Center--Gig Harbor • Franciscan Health System West [27606]
Saint Joseph Health Center
Audiology Department [3258]
Cancer Program [5757]
New Start Treatment Center [47876]
Saint Joseph Health Center/Saint Joseph Hospital West • Cancer Program [5452]
Saint Joseph Health Center • Sleep Disorders Laboratory [37284]
St. Joseph Health Center/St. Joseph Hospital West [16047]
Saint Joseph Health System • Home Health Agency [13174]
St. Joseph Health System Home Health Agency [13226]
Saint Joseph Health System LLC • Saint Joseph Hospital [43057]
Saint Joseph Home Care Network [13272]
Saint Joseph Home Care Network--Humboldt County [13003]
Saint Joseph Home Health [13319]
Saint Joseph Home Health & Hospice [15843]
St. Joseph Hospice [19886]
Saint Joseph Hospital [2885]
St. Joseph Hospital [14984]
Saint Joseph Hospital--Bellingham [18418]
Community Cancer Center [6094]
Saint Joseph Hospital--Breese [14700]
Saint Joseph Hospital Center for Life • Speech Pathology/Audiology [1834]

Saint Joseph Hospital--Cheektowaga • Sleepcare [37420]
Saint Joseph Hospital--Chicago • Cancer Center [5076]
Saint Joseph Hospital--Chippewa Falls • Marshfield Clinic • Sleep Disorders Center [37980]
Saint Joseph Hospital • Detox and Rehabilitation Services [48560]
St. Joseph Hospital Dialysis Center--Santa Ana [22994]
Saint Joseph Hospital--Eureka [12996]
Cancer Program [4772]
Saint Joseph Hospital Home & Hospice Care [16177]
Saint Joseph Hospital Kidney Dialysis Denter • St. Joseph Health System [22859]
Saint Joseph Hospital--Kokomo • Sleep Disorders Center [36963]
Saint Joseph Hospital--Lexington • Cancer Center [5220]
Saint Joseph Hospital/Marshfield Clinic • Cancer Care [6160]
Saint Joseph Hospital and Medical Center • Children's Hospital • Sickle Cell Disease Center [36384]
Saint Joseph Hospital Medical Center • Dialysis Unit [25495]
Saint Joseph Hospital--Nashua • Cancer Program [5499]
Saint Joseph Hospital--Orange [13227]
Regional Cancer Center [4815]
Sleep Disorders Center [36691]
Saint Joseph Hospital Palliative Care [20448]
Saint Joseph Hospital--Polson [16093]
Saint Joseph Hospital • Trinity House [43128]
Saint Joseph Institute for the Deaf [525]
Saint Joseph Institute Inc [48618]
Saint Joseph Medical Center--Fort Wayne • Sleep Disorders Center [36964]
Saint Joseph Medical Center--Kansas City • Cancer Care Program [5448]
Saint Joseph Medical Center
Nephrology Services [27654]
Pain Clinic [35483]
Saint Joseph Medical Center--Reading • Cancer Program [5869]
Saint Joseph Medical Center--Tacoma • Cancer Center [6126]
Saint Joseph Medical Center • Tacoma Chronic Pain Management Program [35758]
Saint Joseph Medical Center--Towson
Cancer Program [5316]
Sleep Disorders Center [37108]
Saint Joseph Memorial Hospital • Sleep Disorders Center [36931]
Saint Joseph Mercy Ann Arbor • Pain Clinic [35511]
Saint Joseph Mercy Behavioral Services [30522]
Saint Joseph Mercy Behavioral Services--Brighton [44681]
Saint Joseph Mercy Health System
Behavioral Health/Greenbrook Recovery [44646]
Saint Joseph Mercy Hospital • Joyce M. Massey Traumatic Brain Injury Day Treatment Service [4191]
Saint Joseph Mercy Home Care [15887]
St. Joseph Mercy Hospice [20137]
Saint Joseph Mercy Hospital • Dialysis Center [24830]
Saint Joseph Mercy Hospital Health Systems • Sleep Disorder Center [37194]
Saint Joseph Mercy Hospital-Ypsilanti • McAuley Cancer Care Center [5402]
Saint Joseph Mercy Livingston Home Care & Hospice [15688]
Saint Joseph Mercy Oakland [5391], [15775]
Saint Joseph Mercy--Oakland [2567]
Saint Joseph Mercy--Oakland Auburn Hills [2556]
Saint Joseph Mercy Oakland Hospital [2636]
Saint Joseph Metro Treatment Center [45610]
Saint Joseph Pain Management Center [35616]
Saint Joseph Regional Health Center [17835]
Saint Joseph Regional Health Center--Bryan • Cancer Center [5970]
Saint Joseph Regional Medical Center [14662]
Cystic Fibrosis Center [7542]
Genetics and Risk Assessment Center [12214]
Saint Joseph Regional Medical Center-Lewiston • Cancer Program [5054]
Saint Joseph Regional Medical Center--Mishawaka •

Cancer Institute [5168]
Saint Joseph Regional Medical Center • Sleep Disorder Center [36884]
Saint Joseph Safety and Health Council • WIP [45611]
Saint Joseph School for the Deaf [572]
Saint Joseph Sleep Disorders Center [37332]
Saint Joseph Veterans Affairs Clinic [30893]
Saint Joseph VNA Home Care [15030]
Saint Josephs Addiction Treatment Center • Josephs House Supportive Living [47002]
Saint Josephs Addiction Treatment
Elizabethtown Outpatient Clinic [46619]
Malone Outpatient Clinic [46770]
Saint Josephs Addiction Treatment and Recovery Centers [47066]
Saint Josephs Addiction Treatment • Saranac Lake Outpatient Clinic [47067]
Saint Joseph's Area Health Services [15925]
Saint Joseph's Behavioral Health Center [33197]
Saint Josephs Behavioral Health Center [40826]
Saint Joseph's/Candler Health System [1908]
Saint Joseph's/Candler Health Systems • Cancer Program [5038]
Saint Joseph's/Candler Sports Medicine [38327]
Saint Joseph's Center [8483]
Saint Joseph's Children's Home [34504]
Saint Joseph's Children's Hospital • Cystic Fibrosis Center [7607]
Saint Joseph's Children's Hospital of Tampa • MDA Clinic [34782]
Saint Joseph's Community Hospital • Washington County Mental Health Center [33026]
Saint Joseph's Cortland • Liberty Dialysis [25646]
Saint Joseph's Healthcare Hamilton • Eating Disorders Program [11234]
Saint Joseph's Home for Children [34252]
Saint Joseph's Home Health Agency [12855]
Saint Joseph's Home Health & Hospice [21828]
St. Joseph's Hospital [18563]
Saint Josephs Hospital • Addiction Services [45311]
Saint Joseph's Hospital of Atlanta • Specialty Center for Cancer Care and Research [5011]
Saint Joseph's Hospital of Buckhannon, Inc. [18500]
Saint Joseph's Hospital • Burn Unit [4594]
Saint Josephs Hospital • CD Service Coordination [45312]
Saint Joseph's Hospital • E Trammell Voice and Swallowing Center [1828]
Saint Joseph's Hospital--Eagan • HealthEast Sleep Care [37231]
Saint Joseph's Hospital--Elmira • Sleep Disorders Center [37421]
Saint Joseph's Hospital--Fayetteville • Northeast Sleep Laboratory [37422]
Saint Joseph's Hospital and Health Center--Dickinson [16809]
Saint Joseph's Hospital Health Center • Sleep Laboratory [37423]
Saint Joseph's Hospital Health Center--Syracuse [16648]
Saint Joseph's Hospital and Health Center--Yonkers • Dialysis Unit [25808]
St. Joseph's Hospital of Huntingburg, Inc. [14990]
Saint Joseph's Hospital and Medical Center • MDA/ALS Center • Barrow Neurological Institute [34754]
Saint Joseph's Hospital and Medical Center-Phoenix • Cancer Program [4744]
Saint Joseph's Hospital
Methadone Maintenance Treatment Prog [47189], [47200]
New Dawn/Stars ARU [46629]
O'Reilly Care Center [39511]
Outpatient Rehabilitation [47201]
Saint Joseph's Hospital • Regional Dialysis Center • Liberty Dialysis [25788]
Saint Joseph's Hospital--Savannah [14583]
Cancer Program [5039]
Sleep Disorders Center [36855]
Saint Josephs Hospital • Southern Tier Addiction Rehab Services [46630]
Saint Joseph's Hospital • Speech/Language Pathology Department [3015]
Saint Joseph's Hospital Sports Medicine [39167]
Saint Joseph's Hospital-Tampa • Cancer Institute [4997]
Saint Joseph's Hospital--Wisconsin Rapids • Dialysis

Center [27807]
Saint Joseph's Hospital--Yonkers [16685]
Saint Josephs Hospital/Yonkers • Methadone Treatment Queens Clinic II [46728]
Saint Joseph's House [21790]
St. Joseph's Kidney Center [25656]
St. Joseph's Medical Center [15892]
Saint Joseph's Medical Center--Brainerd • Cancer Care Program [5403]
St. Joseph's Medical Center • Burn Center [4545]
Saint Joseph's Medical Center • Firefighter's Burn Center [4649]
Saint Josephs Medical Center
  Focus Unit [45092]
  OTC [47190]
Saint Joseph's Medical Center of Stockton [13371]
Saint Joseph's Medical Center-Stockton • Sister Mary Pia Regional Cancer Center [4855]
Saint Joseph's Mercy Health Center--Hot Springs • Mercy Cancer Center [4753]
Saint Joseph's Mercy Health Center • Sleep Disorders Center [36651]
Saint Joseph's Northeast Dialysis Center • Liberty Dialysis [25659]
Saint Joseph's Regional Health Center [12856]
Saint Joseph's Regional Medical Center [2185]
  Feeding and Swallowing Center [2942]
Saint Joseph's Regional Medical Center--Paterson • Cancer Program [5533]
Saint Joseph's Rehabilitation Center [4043]
Saint Joseph's Satellite--Paterson • Outpatient Dialysis Center [25496]
Saint Joseph's School for the Blind • Concordia Learning Center [3721]
Saint Joseph's Villa • Harmony Place • Eating Disorders Program [11167]
Saint Joseph's Villa of Rochester [34352]
  Group Home [34353], [34361]
  Group Home Program [34354]
Saint Josephs Villa of Rochester Inc • Chemical Dependency Services [47047]
Saint Jude Centers for Rehabilitation and Wellness [3920]
St. Jude Children's Research Hospital [4706]
Saint Jude Children's Research Hospital
  Comprehensive Sickle Cell Center [36344], [36429]
    Hemophilia Treatment Center [12595]
    Pediatric Hematology Center of Memphis [36430]
Saint Jude Continuing Rehabilitation Center • Synergy Fitness Center [3921]
Saint Jude Health Care [14140]
Saint Jude Home Care, Inc. [17536]
St. Jude Hospice--Cambridge [20151]
St. Jude Hospice-Tupelo [20271]
St. Jude Hospital and Rehabilitation Center [7779]
Saint Jude House, Inc. [9269]
Saint Jude Medical Center
  Cancer Program [4781]
  Chronic Pain Management Center [35329]
  Rehabilitation Center [3922]
  Sleep Disorders Institute [36692]
Saint Jude Womens Recovery Center [43694]
Saint Judes Recovery Center Inc [42034]
  Day Outpatient Program [42035]
Saint Katherine Day School [8495]
Saint Landry Home Care [15349]
Saint Lawrence Addiction Treatment Center • CD Inpatient Rehab Program [46958]
Saint Lawrence County • Chemical Dependency Services [46580]
Saint Lawrence County Comm Services Board • Chemical Depd Outpatient Clinic/Ogdensburg [46959]
Saint Lawrence Psychiatric Center--Ogdensburg [33710]
  Hamilton Hall [33711]
Saint Lawrence Renewal House for Victims of Family Violence [9914]
Saint Louis Association for Retarded Citizens [8214]
Saint Louis Behavioral Medicine Institute--Chesterfield • Eating Disorders Program [11123]
Saint Louis Behavioral Medicine Institute • Chronic Headache Program [12440]
Saint Louis Behavioral Medicine Institute--Saint Louis • Eating Disorders Program [11124]
Saint Louis Center [8167]

Saint Louis Children's Hospital
  Burn Center [4579]
  Dialysis Center [25277]
Saint Louis Children's Hospital/Washington University School of Medicine • Pediatric Cystic Fibrosis Center [7587]
Saint Louis Circuit Attorney's Victim Services [9667]
Saint Louis Community College, Florissant Valley • Access Office • Disability Support Services [532]
Saint Louis Cord Blood Bank [35098]
Saint Louis Developmental Disabilities Treatment Center [8215]
St. Louis Dialysis Center • DaVita • Dialysis Facility [25278]
Saint Louis High School [504]
Saint Louis Metro Treatment Center [45443]
Saint Louis Orthopedic Rehabilitation and Sports Injury Clinic [38657]
Saint Louis Park Dialysis • DaVita [25078]
Saint Louis Psychiatric Rehabilitation Center [33637]
Saint Louis Renal Care--Des Peres • Dialysis Center [25279]
St. Louis Renal Care--Forest Park • Fresenius Medical Care [25280]
Saint Louis University
  Cardinal Glennon Children's Hospital • John Bouhasin Center for Children with Bleeding Disorders [12550]
  Department of Communication Sciences and Disorders • International Adoption Clinic [2820]
Saint Louis University Hospital • Cancer Program [5463]
Saint Louis University Hospital Transplant Unit [25281]
Saint Louis University • Multiple Sclerosis Center [34620]
Saint Louis University School of Medicine • Division of Medical Genetics [12264]
Saint Louis University
  School of Medicine • HIV Vaccine Trials Unit [86]
  SLUCare Sleep disorders Center [37285]
  Speech/Language/Pathology and Audiology Clinic [2821]
Saint Louis Valley Hope [45630]
Saint Louis Veterans Affairs Medical Center
  Jefferson Barracks Division [30901]
    PTSD Clinical Team [51765]
  John Cochran Division [30902]
  Multiple Sclerosis Center [34621]
Saint Louis West Dialysis • DaVita [25282]
Saint Louis West PD Dialysis • DaVita [25192]
Saint Louise Behavioral Medicine Institute • Pain Clinic [35531]
St. Lucie Hospice House [19225]
Saint Lucie Medical Center • Cancer Program [4986]
Saint Luke Hospitals East • Cancer Program [5216]
Saint Lukes Behavioral Health Center [39409], [39447]
Saint Lukes Behavorial Health Center • Outpatient [39448]
Saint Luke's Burn Center [4546]
Saint Luke's Canyon View Behavioral Health Services [29552]
Saint Luke's Children's Special Health Program • Cystic Fibrosis Clinic [7524]
Saint Luke's Children's Specialty Center • Genetics Clinic [12196]
Saint Luke's Cornwall Hospital [3084]
Saint Luke's-Cornwall Hospital • Cancer Program [5601]
Saint Luke's Cornwall Hospital--Newburgh • Dialysis Center [25741]
Saint Luke's Dialysis Center • Diversified Specialty Institutes [25228]
Saint Luke's Episcopal Hospital
  Texas Cancer Institute [6002]
  Transplant Center [27173]
Saint Luke's Health Center [15105]
Saint Luke's Home Care/Hospice--McCall [14663]
St. Luke's Home Care Services [15067]
Saint Luke's Home Health Services [15995]
St. Luke's Hospice-Bethlehem [21052]
Saint Luke's Hospice--Bosie [19451]
Saint Luke's Hospice, Duluth [20156]
Saint Luke's Hospice--Kansas City [20314]
Saint Luke's Hospital [1282]

Saint Luke's Hospital--Allentown • Sleep Disorders Center [37688]
Saint Luke's Hospital--Bethlehem • Sleep Disorders Center [37689]
Saint Luke's Hospital • Cancer Center [4673]
Saint Luke's Hospital Center New York City • Dialysis Center [25736]
Saint Luke's Hospital--Chesterfield
  Center for Cancer Care [5439]
  Medicine and Research Center [37286]
Saint Luke's Hospital • Dialysis Center [26382]
Saint Luke's Hospital-Duluth • Regional Trauma Center • Cancer Center [5405]
Saint Luke's Hospital and Health Network--Bethlehem [5814]
Saint Luke's Hospital Hospice [19673]
Saint Luke's Hospital • Infertility Center of Saint Louis [22146]
Saint Luke's Hospital of Kansas City [2802]
  Cancer Institute [5449]
Saint Luke's Hospital--Kansas City • Sleep Disorders Center [37287]
Saint Luke's Hospital Kidney Transplant Unit • Saint Luke's Health System [25229]
Saint Luke's Hospital--Maumee
  Cancer Program [5737]
  Sleep Disorders Center [37569]
Saint Luke's Hospital
  Multiple Sclerosis Center [34694]
  Outpatient Rehabilitation [2199]
  Outreach Clinic • Cystic Fibrosis Center [7656]
Saint Luke's Hospital and Regional Trauma Center Home Care [15901]
Saint Luke's Hospital South • Sleep Disorders Center [37004]
Saint Luke's Hospital--West Dialysis Unit • Saint Luke's Health System [25184]
Saint Luke's Hospitals--Meritcare • Coordinated Treatment Center • Down Syndrome Outpatient Service [10842]
Saint Luke's House, Inc. [30301]
  Parkwood House [30296]
  Southport Residential [30268]
Saint Luke's Magic Valley Regional Medical Center [14676]
  Southern Idaho Regional Cancer Center [5056]
Saint Luke's McCall • Sleep Medicine Institute [36885]
Saint Luke's Medical Center--Bertner Avenue, Houston • Sleep Center [37839]
Saint Luke's Medical Center--Braeswood, Houston • Sleep Center, Kirby Glen [37840]
Saint Luke's Medical Center--Greenfield • Aurora Sleep Disorders Center [37981]
Saint Luke's Medical Center--Milwaukee • Cancer Center [6167]
Saint Luke's Medical Center POB • Advanced Institute of Fertility [22301]
Saint Luke's Medical Center • Roosevelt Hospital Center • Pain Management [35583]
Saint Luke's Memorial Hospital • Rome Dialysis Clinic [25771]
Saint Luke's Meridian Medical Center • Sleep Medicine Institute [36886]
Saint Luke's Miners Memorial Home Care [17492]
Saint Luke's Miners Memorial Hospital [17288]
Saint Luke's North Dialysis Center, LP [26383]
Saint Luke's Quakertown Hospital
  Cancer Program [5867]
  Dialysis Facility [26572]
Saint Luke's Regional Medical Center [14650]
Saint Luke's Regional Medical Center-Boise • Mountain States Tumor Institute [5051]
Saint Luke's Regional Medical Center • Sleep Medicine Institute [36887]
Saint Luke's Rehabilitation Center [3645]
Saint Luke's Rehabilitation Institute [4484]
  Valley Medical Center [4485]
St. Luke's Renal Transplant Center [27758]
Saint Lukes/Roosevelt Hospital Center
  Addiction Institute/Halfway House [46914]
  The Addiction Institute of NY/Day Treatment [46915]
  The Addiction Institute of NY/Outpatient [46916]
  Addiction Institute/Outpatient Clinic [46917]
Saint Luke's - Roosevelt Hospital Center • Cancer Care Program [5599]
Saint Lukes/Roosevelt Hospital Center • CARES /

CAPA [46918]
Saint Luke's Roosevelt Hospital Center •
Comprehensive Sickle Cell Program [36399]
Saint Luke's/Roosevelt Hospital Center
Outpatient Drug Abuse Clinic [46919]
Sub Acute Inpatient Detox Service [46920]
Saint Luke's Sleep Disorders Center--Duluth [37232]
Saint Luke's Sleep Disorders Center--Quakertown
[37690]
Saint Luke's South Shore • Behavioral Health
[32965]
Saint Lukes'Rehabilitation Institute • MDA Clinic
[34904]
Saint Margaret Mercy--Dyer • Sleep Disorders
Center [36965]
Saint Margaret Mercy--Hammond • Sleep Disorders
Lab [36966]
Saint Margaret Mercy Healthcare Centers • Oncol-
ogy Center [5153]
Saint Margaret's Hospice [19575]
Saint Margaret's Hospital [2111]
Saint Margaret's Sports Medicine Center [38974]
Saint Mark's Hospital • Cancer Support Center
[6043]
Saint Mark's Institute [31433]
Saint Marks Institute for Mental Hlth • DBA Unitas
Chemical Dependence Outpatient [46921]
Saint Martha's Hall [9724]
Saint Martin Parish School District [449]
Saint Martins Hospitality Center [46240]
Saint Mary Addictive Disorders Clinic [43864]
Saint Mary-Corwin Medical Center • Dorcy Cancer
Center [4886]
Saint Mary--Corwin Medical Center • Pain Clinic
[35353]
Saint Mary Home Care [17370]
Saint Mary Hospital [2620]
St. Mary Medical Center [13114]
Saint Mary Medical Center-Apple Valley • Cancer
Program [4756]
Saint Mary Medical Center • Cancer Program [5837]
Saint Mary Medical Center--Langhorne • Sleep
Disorders Center [37691]
Saint Mary Medical Center-Long Beach • Cancer
Program [4793]
Saint Mary Medical Center--Walla Walla • Kathryn
Severyns Dement Sleep Disorders Center [37934]
Saint Mary Mercy Hospital
Dept of Behavioral Medicine [44905]
Our Lady of Hope Cancer Center [5384]
Saint Mary Parish • Office of Special Services
[2315]
Saint Mary's At Home [14978]
Saint Marys Center • Recovery 55 [40305]
Saint Marys Dialysis Center • West Pennsylvania
Alleghany Health System [26575]
St. Mary's Dialysis • DaVita [23781]
Saint Mary's/Duluth Clinic • Comprehensive Multiple
Sclerosis Program [34612]
Saint Mary's Health Care--Grand Rapids • Sleep
Disorders Center [37195]
Saint Mary's Health Care System--Athens • Saint
Mary's Hospital • Sleep Disorders Center [36856]
Saint Mary's Health Care System, Inc. [14478]
Saint Mary's Health Center • Sleep Disorders Center
[37288]
Saint Mary's Healthcare Center [17633]
Dialysis Facility [26792]
St. Marys Healthcaretransportationnsplant [24910]
Saint Mary's Home for Boys [34392]
Saint Mary's Home Care Services--Jefferson City
[17689]
Saint Mary's Home Care Services--Knoxville [17711]
Saint Mary's Home Care Services--La Follette
[17716]
Saint Mary's Home Care Services--Maynardville
[17729]
Saint Mary's Home Care Services - North [17712]
Saint Mary's Home for Children [27985]
Saint Mary's Home for Disabled Children [8592]
Saint Mary's Home Health--Ada [15888]
St. Mary's Hospice of Northern Nevada [20428]
St. Mary's Hospice and Palliative Care-Grand
Rapids [20166]
Saint Mary's Hospice--Pierre [21297]
Saint Mary's Hospice--Saint Paul [20208]
Saint Mary's Hospice Services • Mercy Health
Partners--Knoxville [21343]

St. Mary's Hospice=Watkinsville [19435]
Saint Marys Hospital
Alcoholism Inpatient Rehab Program [46358]
Behavioral Healthcare Services [41492]
Saint Mary's Hospital • Center for Physical
Rehabilitation [2357]
Saint Mary's Hospital-Centralia • Cancer Program
[5066]
Saint Marys Hospital
Chemical Dependency Outpatient Clinic [46359]
Chemical Dependency Outpatient Rehab
[46666]
Saint Mary's Hospital for Children [8296]
Saint Mary's Hospital • Dialysis Unit [23557]
Saint Mary's Hospital -Home Health Services
[14948]
Saint Mary's Hospital--Huntington • Saint Mary's
Regional Sleep Center [37955]
Saint Mary's Hospital--Leonardtown • Cancer
Program [5308]
Saint Mary's Hospital and Medical Center--Grand
Junction • Cancer Center [4881]
Saint Mary's Hospital Medical Center • Sleep
Disorders Center [37982]
Saint Marys Hospital • MMTP Clinic [46360]
Saint Mary's Hospital Ozaukee, Inc. [18590]
Saint Mary's Hospital • Regional Burn Center [4653]
Saint Mary's Hospital--Rogers • Mercy Sleep
Disorders Center [36652]
Saint Mary's Hospital-Saginaw • Regional Cancer
Treatment Center [5396]
Saint Mary's Hospital of Saint Mary's County
[15451]
Saint Mary's Hospital • Speech and Hearing Service
[2113]
St. Marys Hospital Transplant • Mayo Clinic [25072]
Saint Mary's Hospital-Waterbury • Harold Leever
Regional Cancer Center [4910]
Saint Mary's Hospital--Waterbury • Sleep Disorders
Laboratory [36752]
St. Mary's Medical Center [19595]
Saint Mary's Medical Center
Burn Trauma Intensive Care Unit [4568]
CHW Cancer Center [4662]
Cystic Fibrosis Center [7509]
Saint Mary's Medical Center--Duluth • Duluth
Regional Sleep Center [37233]
Saint Mary's Medical Center of Evansville • Oncol-
ogy Program [5145]
Saint Mary's Medical Center Home Health Services
[17024], [18519]
Saint Mary's Medical Center--Huntington • Tumor
Conference [6137]
Saint Mary's Medical Center--Knoxville
Cancer Program [5938]
Sleep Disorders Center [37777]
St. Mary's Medical Center-Langhorne [21108]
Saint Mary's Mercy Medical Center [15678]
Saint Mary's Mercy Medical Center-Grand Rapids •
The Lacks Cancer Center [5378]
Saint Mary's Pain Center [35532]
Saint Marys Pharmacy Home Health Care [17468]
Saint Mary's Regional Health Center [15896]
Saint Mary's Regional Medical Center [12882]
Behavioral Health Services [30218]
Saint Mary's Regional Medical Center • Chemical
Dependency Service [43998]
Saint Mary's Regional Medical Center Home Care
Services [16165]
Saint Mary's Regional Medical Center--Lewiston •
Center for Cancer & Blood Disorders [5272]
Saint Mary's Regional Medical Center • RehabCare
Program [4378]
Saint Mary's Regional Medical Center--Reno •
Cancer Care Program [5491]
Saint Mary's Regional Medical Center • Sleep
Disorders Center [37093]
Saint Mary's Rehabilitation Center [1037]
Saint Mary's Rehabilitation Center for Children •
Speech Therapy Services [3151]
St. Mary's Residential Training School [8063]
Saint Mary's School for the Deaf [577]
Saint Mary's Sleep Disorders Center [36967]
Saint Marys Treatment Center [42621]
Saint Mary's Villa for Children and Families [34405]
Saint Mary's Women's Center [9457]
Saint Mary's Women's and Children Center [6813]
St. Michael Hospital [18598]

Saint Michael's Hospice [20209]
St. Michael's Hospice Corporation [21436]
Saint Michael's Hospital [33014]
Multiple Sclerosis Center [34682]
Saint Michael's Hospital--Stevens Point • Dialysis
Center [27788]
Saint Michael's Medical Center
Cancer Center [5530]
Dialysis Unit [25488]
Saint Monicas • Project Mother Child [45763]
Saint Nicholas Hospice • Matthews Oncology As-
sociation [21866]
St. Nicholas Hospital [18628]
Saint Nicholas Hospital
Cancer Program [6175]
Comprehensive Rehabilitation Inpatient Unit •
Center for Pain and Work Rehabilitation
[35776]
Dialysis Facility [27784]
Saint Patrick--Butte Dialysis Center • Saint James
Community Hospital [25307]
Saint Patrick Center [45631]
Saint Patrick Hospital and Health Sciences Center •
Montana Cancer Center [5471]
Saint Patrick Hospital - Missoula Dialysis Center
[25313]
Saint Patrick Hospital • Sleep Center [37302]
Saint Patrick's Psychiatric Hospital [33542]
Saint Paul Capital Dialysis, At Home & PD • DaVita
[25084]
St. Paul Dialysis • DaVita [25085]
Saint Paul Domestic Abuse Intervention Project
[9638]
St. Paul Elder Services [21844]
Saint Paul Health Center [39348]
Saint Paul Metro Treatment Center [45287]
Saint Paul Street Group Home [32665]
Saint Paul Vet Center [52001]
Saint Paul's Dialysis Center • DaVita [25942]
Saint Paul's Hospital • Eating Disorders Center
[10919]
Saint Peter Area Hospice/ Immanuel-Saint Joseph's
Mayo HS Program [20178]
Saint Peter Home Health Care Agency, Inc. [14141]
Saint Peters Addiction Rec Center • Alcoholism
Inpatient Rehab Center [46672]
Saint Peters Addiction Recovery Center [46749]
Acute Care Unit [46337]
Alcoholism Outpatient Clinic [47075]
Ballston Spa Substance Abuse Clinic [47068]
Cohoes Outpatient Clinic [46596]
Day Rehabilitation and Outpatient [46338]
Mens Halfway House [46339]
Outpatient Chem Dependency [46340]
Saint Peters Community Hospital • Pain Manage-
ment Services [35537]
St. Peters Dialysis • DaVita [25287]
Saint Peter's Hospital [16090]
Saint Peter's Hospital--Albany • Cancer Program
[5556]
Saint Peter's Hospital • Dialysis Unit [25310]
Saint Peter's Hospital--Helena • Cancer Program
[5470]
Saint Peter's Hospital Home Care [16336]
Saint Peters Hospital • Lewis Golub MDA/ALS Clinic
[34841]
Saint Peter's Hospital
Sleep Center [37424]
Speech Pathology and Audiology Department
[3120]
Saint Peter's Regional Treatment [33609]
Saint Peter's University Hospital
Cancer Program [5527]
Institute for Genetic Medicine [12278]
Sickle Cell Disease Center [36385]
Sleep Center [37361]
Saint Petersburg College • Office of Services for
Students with Disabilities [354]
Saint Petersburg Dialysis • DaVita • Dialysis Facility
[23506]
St. Petersburg South Dialysis • DaVita • Dialysis
Facility & At Home [23507]
Saint Petersburg Veterans Affairs Primary Care
Clinic [29284]
Saint Pius Homeless Shelter [9169]
St. Raphael Dialysis Center--New Haven • Hospital
of St. Raphael [23169]
Saint Regis Mohawk Health Services

Alcoholism Chem Depend Outpatient Prog [46698]
    Partridge House [46699]
Saint Rita Medical Center • Audiology Unit [3244]
St. Rita School for the Deaf [647]
St. Rita's Dialysis Center • Kidney Services of West Central Ohio [26149]
Saint Rita's Hospice [20853]
Saint Rita's Medical Center [35617]
Saint Ritas Medical Center • Addiction Services [47789]
Saint Rita's Medical Center • Cancer Program [5732]
St. Ritas Medical Center ESRD Unit [26150]
Saint Rita's Medical Center Home Care [16965]
Saint Rita's Medical Center
    Pediatric and Adolescent Rehabilitation Center [8418]
    Saint Rita's Sleep Disorders Laboratory [37570]
Saint Rose Dominican Hospitals Home Health & Hospice [16140]
St. Rose Dominican Hospitals-Rose de Lima Campus [20411]
Saint Rose Hospital • Cancer Program [4785]
Saint Simons By-The-Sea Hospital [33389]
Saint Simons by the Sea [42151]
Saint Stephen's Health Center [7083]
Saint Tammany Parish Hospital [15282]
    Cancer Program [5246]
    Sleep Disorders Center [37079]
Saint Tammany Parish Schools [450]
St. Theresa's Hospice and Palliative Care [19850]
Saint Thomas Community Health Center [6758]
Saint Thomas East End Medical Center [7343]
St. Thomas Hospice [19530]
Saint Thomas Hospital [16830]
    Dan Rudy Cancer Center [5949]
    Ignatia Hall Summa Health System [47609]
Saint Thomas More Dialysis • Dialysis Corporation of America [24696]
Saint Thomas Neurosciences Institute • Center for Multiple Sclerosis Treatment [34714]
Saint Thomas Sleep Center [37880]
Saint Thomas Veterans Affairs Clinic [32692]
Saint Vincent Carmel Hospital • Sleep Disorders Center [36968]
Saint Vincent Catholic Medical Centers--Brooklyn • Home Health Agency [16418]
Saint Vincent Catholic Medical Centers--Islandia • Home Health Agency [16495]
Saint Vincent Catholic Medical Centers--New York • Home Health Agency [16567]
Saint Vincent Catholic Medical Centers--Rego Park • Home Health Agency [16607]
Saint Vincent Catholic Medical Centers--South Ave. Staten Island • Home Health Agency [16642]
Saint Vincent Catholic Medical Centers--Tompkins Ave., Staten Island • Home Health Agency [16643]
Saint Vincent Charity Hospital • Cancer Program [5704]
Saint Vincent De Paul Society of Waterbury [29049]
Saint Vincent DePaul Society of SF • Ozanam Reception Center [40632]
Saint Vincent Dialysis Center, Inc. [22788]
Saint Vincent Doctors Hospital • Behavioral Health Services [28306]
Saint Vincent Family Centers
    Deaf Services [654]
    Main Campus [34376]
Saint Vincent Health Center
    Sleep Center [37692]
    Speech Pathology/Audiology Department [3331]
Saint Vincent Health System • Cancer Care Center [5828]
Saint Vincent Healthcare
    Cancer Care Program [5467]
    New Hope Rehabilitation Center [2830]
    Sleep Center [37303]
Saint Vincent Home Care [15005]
Saint Vincent Home Health--Veedersburg [15058]
St. Vincent Hospice Indianapolis [19613]
Saint Vincent Hospice New Hope [19614]
Saint Vincent Hospital [2544]
St. Vincent Hospital [18571]
Saint Vincent Hospital--Green Bay
    Regional Cancer Center [6152]
    Sleep Disorders Center [37983]
Saint Vincent Hospital and Health Center • Burn

Care Unit [4581]
Saint Vincent Hospital and Health Services
    Cancer Center [5158]
    Sleep Disorders Center [36969]
Saint Vincent Hospital
    MDA Clinic [34912]
    Medical Genetics • Down Syndrome Clinic [10801]
    Pain Center [35572]
    Regional Rehabilitation Program [4496]
Saint Vincent Hospital--Santa Fe • Cancer Program [5554]
St. Vincent Hospital Transplant Services [24180]
Saint Vincent Hospital-Worcester • Worcester Medical Center • Cancer Center [5361]
Saint Vincent Hospital--Worcester • Worcester Medical Center • Sleep Disorders Institute of Central New England [37124]
St. Vincent Infirmary • Dialysis Center [22556]
Saint Vincent Infirmary Health System • Sleep Disorders Center [36653]
Saint Vincent Jennings Home Care [15038]
Saint Vincent Medical Center • Cancer Program [4800]
St. Vincent Medical Center--Renal TX [22789]
Saint Vincent Mercy Hospital • Cancer Program [5143]
Saint Vincent Mercy Medical Center [17056]
    Dialysis Unit [26214]
    Sleep Disorders Center [37571]
Saint Vincent Out-Patient Rehabilitation/Sports Medicine [38941]
Saint Vincent de Paul Society, Waterbury [6427]
Saint Vincent de Paul Village • Runaway and Homeless Youth Program [35839]
Saint Vincent Quadrangle/St. John Dialysis Network [26068]
Saint Vincent Regional Medical Center • Sleep Disorders Center [37369]
Saint Vincent Rehabilitation Hospital • Sleep Center [36654]
Saint Vincent - Sarah Fisher Center [34223]
Saint Vincent Sports Medicine [38425]
Saint Vincent Stress Center [43113]
Saint Vincents Catholic Med Center of NY • Alcoholism Inpatient Rehab Program [46679]
Saint Vincent's Catholic Medical Center of New York [3077]
Saint Vincent's Catholic Medical Centers Brooklyn & Queens [16568]
Saint Vincents Catholic Medical Centers • Methadone Treatment Queens Clinic II [46729]
Saint Vincent's East • Cancer Program [4725]
Saint Vincent's Group Home [34190]
Saint Vincent's Home [34191]
Saint Vincent's Home for Children [34234]
Saint Vincent's Hospital Birmingham • Bruno Cancer Center [4726]
Saint Vincent's Hospital
    Burn Center [4607]
    Cystic Fibrosis Center [7703]
    Hemodialysis Unit [24820]
Saint Vincents Hospital MC Alcoholism • Outpatient Clinic/The Maxwell Institute [47140]
Saint Vincent's Hospital and Medical Center of New York • Cystic Fibrosis Center [7621]
Saint Vincent's Hospital and Medical Center • New York Medical College • Pain Management [35584]
Saint Vincent's Hospital--New York • Comprehensive Cancer Center [5600]
Saint Vincent's Hospital
    Regional Dialysis Center [27722]
    Sleep Disorders Center [36599]
Saint Vincent's Medical Center • Behavioral Health [28977]
Saint Vincents Medical Center • Behavioral Health Service/Westport [41495]
Saint Vincent's Medical Center East • East Sleep Center [36600]
Saint Vincent's Medical Center
    Elizabeth Pfriem SWIM Center for cancer Care [4889]
    Mary Virginia Terry Cancer Center [4953]
Saint Vincent's Orthopedics [37998]
Saint Vincents Outpatient Addiction • Recovery Service [46680]
Saint Vincent's Outreach Program • Cystic Fibrosis Center [7593]

Saint Vincent's School of Boys [33191]
Saint Vincents Services Inc • Outpatient Chemical Dependence Program [46530], [46730], [47100]
Saint Vincent's Special Needs Services [7858]
Saint Vincent's Vinhaven [34192]
Saints Home Health Care LLC [13568]
Saints Mary and Elizabeth Medical Center • Cancer Care Center [5077]
Saints Medical Center • Cancer Center [5342]
Saints Medical Center Dialysis [24774]
Saints Memorial Medical Center [19974]
    Merrimack Valley Dialysis Center--Methuen [24780]
Sakakawea Hospice [20784]
Sakhi for South Asian Women [9957]
Sakowitz Counseling [46037], [46211]
Salem Area Visiting Nurse Association [17032]
Salem Chest Specialists • Southeastern Sleep Disorders Center [37485]
Salem Christian Home for the Handicapped [7798]
Salem County Women's Services [9846]
Salem Dialysis Center • Fresenius Medical Care • Dialysis Center [25506]
Salem Family Health Center [6826]
Salem Hospital • Cancer Center [5806]
Salem Hospital Home Care [17223]
Salem Hospital • Sleep Disorders Center [37630]
Salem Kidney Center • Wake Forest University [25981]
Salem Medical Center [6676]
Salem Memorial Hospital • Dialysis Facility [25288]
Salem North Dialysis • DaVita [26355]
Salem Northeast Dialysis • DaVita • Dialysis Center [24797]
Salem Veterans Affairs Clinic [30904], [31976]
Salem Veterans Affairs Medical Center [32787]
Salina Family Healthcare Center [6720]
Salina Regional Health Center • Cancer Program [5204]
Salina Veterans Affairs Clinic [29952]
Salinas Day Treatment Center [28738]
Salinas Dialysis Center • DaVita [22926]
Salinas Valley Memorial Hospital • Comprehensive Cancer Center [4831]
Salinas Women's Crisis Center [8879]
Saline County Dialysis--Junction City • Dialysis Facility [24326]
Saline County Dialysis--Salina [24347]
Saline County Safe Haven, Inc. [8750]
Saline Memorial Hospital [997]
Salisbury Dial Help [51176]
Salisbury Physical Therapy & Sportsmedicine [38532]
Salisbury Visiting Nurse Association, Inc. [19161]
Salmon Hospice [19985]
Salmon Hospice Care-Northbridge [19989]
Salmon Mental Health Clinic PA [42372]
Salmon River Central School [31327]
Salt Lake County Youth Services [49669]
    Runaway and Homeless Youth Program [36237]
Salt Lake Regional Medical Center • Rehabilitation Department [3558]
Salt River Community Health Center [6904]
Saltville Medical Center [7368]
Salud Integral en la Montana, Inc. [7206]
Salud Para La Gente, Inc. [6377]
Salud Y Provecho [9167]
Saluda Behavioral Health Systems [48974]
Saluda Mental Health Center [32214]
Saluda School District [735]
Salvation Army [41211]
The Salvation Army [43814]
Salvation Army Addiction Treatment Services • Continuum of Care Program [42215]
Salvation Army
    Adult Rehab Center Alcohol Abuse HH Care [41142]
    Adult Rehabilitation Center [47997]
    Adult Rehabilitation Program [45862]
Salvation Army--Baltimore, Maryland [9445]
Salvation Army Bell Shelter • Wellness Center [39647]
Salvation Army Brevard County • Domestic Violence Program [9044]
The Salvation Army--Buffalo • Emergency Shelter [9912]
Salvation Army • Clitheroe Center [39314]
The Salvation Army--Dallas • Family Violence

Program [10455]
The Salvation Army Depot • Family Crisis Center [40210]
Salvation Army--Des Moines [6708]
Salvation Army Elmira Citadel • Our House Community Residence [46631]
Salvation Army--Elmira, New York • Safehouse [9920]
Salvation Army Family Treatment Services--Honolulu [9147]
The Salvation Army Family Treatment Services • Kula-Kokua Pohai [29524]
Salvation Army Family Treatment Services • Womens Way [42216]
Salvation Army • First Choice [49341]
The Salvation Army--Greenville • Domestic Violence Shelter [9650]
Salvation Army--Harbor Light [6355]
Salvation Army Harbor Light Center [43114]
Salvation Army • Harbor Light Center [42580], [45632], [48606]
Salvation Army Harbor Light Center • Monroe County Center [44926]
Salvation Army Harbor Light • Multi Service Center Beacon Program [45229]
Salvation Army • Harbor Light Recovery Program [43381]
Salvation Army Harbor Light System • Subst Abuse Center/ Women/Children/Men [44761]
Salvation Army
    Harbor Light Treatment Center [41547]
    Haven [40153]
Salvation Army Hawaiian and Pacific Islands Division • Runaway and Homeless Youth Program [35918]
The Salvation Army, Hollywood CA • Runaway and Homeless Youth Program [35840]
Salvation Army Hospitality House [6364]
Salvation Army--Hudson, Florida • Domestic Violence Shelter [9054]
The Salvation Army--Indianapolis • Social Service Center [9289]
Salvation Army--Interim Care Program [6349]
Salvation Army--Jamestown, New York • Domestic Violence Program [9936]
Salvation Army Lighthouse Recovery Center • Lot Naval Air Station 19 [42186]
Salvation Army • Macomb Harbor Light [44713]
Salvation Army--Miami [6509]
Salvation Army • MO Shield of Service [45531]
Salvation Army Northeast Family Resource Center--Nashville, Tennessee [10427]
Salvation Army Outreach [7251]
The Salvation Army--Panama City • Domestic Violence Program [9074]
Salvation Army--Pascagoula, Mississippi • Domestic Violence Shelter [9657]
The Salvation Army--Roanoke • Turning Point [10591]
The Salvation Army, Rochester NY • Genesis House • Runaway and Homeless Youth Program [36122]
Salvation Army of Santa Maria [6365]
Salvation Army--Savannah [6603]
Salvation Army Shelter--Knoxville, Tennessee [10411]
Salvation Army--Syracuse, New York • Syracuse Area Services [9989]
The Salvation Army, Syracuse NY • Runaway and Homeless Youth Program [36123]
Salvation Army • Turning Point Programs [44821]
The Salvation Army--Warner Robins • Safe House [9129]
Salvation Army's Elim House [8717]
Sam Chwat Speech Center [3078]
Sam Rayburn Memorial Veterans Center • Domiciliary Substance Abuse Program [49250]
Samara Hospital • Northeastern Center Inc. [33444]
Samara House • CYWA [48331]
Samaritan Albany General Hospital [17174]
Samaritan Behavioral Health-- Crisis Care [51211]
Samaritan Behavioral Health • Howard S. Gray Educational Program [7746]
Samaritan Behavioral Health--Preble County [51217]
Samaritan Behavioral Health--Youth Resources [51212]
Samaritan Care Hospice [19280]
Samaritan Center [43228]
Samaritan Center Chem Dependency Services • Samaritan Center Inc [43224]

Samaritan Center • Pike County Office [43176]
Samaritan Colony [47476]
Samaritan Counseling Center [33001]
Samaritan Counseling Center--Menasha [32992]
Samaritan Counseling Center--Oshkosh [33004]
Samaritan Dialysis--Corvallis • Good Samaritan Regional Medical Center [26318]
Samaritan Dialysis--Lebanon • Dialysis Facility • Good Samaritan Regional Medical Center [26329]
Samaritan Healthcare [14681]
Samaritan Home Care--Ashland [16839]
Samaritan Home Care--Clinton [17112]
Samaritan Home Care Services [17154]
Samaritan Home Health Agency Inc. [13205]
Samaritan Homeless Interim Program [46171]
Samaritan Hospice [20479]
Samaritan Hospice Inpatient Center [20483]
Samaritan House [44098]
Samaritan House and Safe Harbor [10597]
Samaritan Inns [41548]
Samaritan Medical Center • Addiction Services [47167]
Samaritan Medical Center/Adolescent Health Associates • Cystic Fibrosis Center [7622]
Samaritan Medical Center
    Sleep Disorders Center of Northern New York [37425]
    Speech Pathology Department [3143]
Samaritan Memorial Hospital • Dialysis Unit [25242]
Samaritan North Lincoln Hospital [17202]
Samaritan North Sports Medicine Center [38875]
Samaritan Outreach [8757]
Samaritan Pacific Communities Hospital [17208]
Samaritan Pacific Dialysis • Samaritan Health Services [26334]
Samaritan Recovery Community Inc [49162]
Samaritan Sleep Disorders Center [37631]
Samaritan Village Inc
    Admission and Assessment Unit [46731]
    Drug Free Outpatient [46732]
    Drug Free Residential [46621]
    Drug Free Residential Unit [46922]
    Drug Residential Treatment Program [46923]
    Ed Thompson Veterans Center [47014]
    MTA/Residential [47015]
    Residential Drug Free Program [46453], [46733]
Samaritans [51084]
Samaritans of Boston [50985]
Samaritans on Cape Cod and the Islands, Inc. [50988]
Samaritans of Fall River/New Bedford [50987]
Samaritans of Merrimack Valley [50993]
The Samaritans of New York [51146]
Samaritans of Rhode Island [51311]
Samaritans, Suburban West [50989]
The Samaritans of The Capital Region [50728]
SAMHC Behavioral Health Services [50656]
Samish Indian Nation Wellness Program • Anacortes Branch [49878]
Samland Health Care [14751]
Sampson Regional Medical Center [16714]
Samuel S. Stratton VA Medical Center [16337]
Samuel U. Rodgers Health Center, Inc. • Samuel U. Rodgers Community Health Center [6908]
San Agustin Home Health Services [18038]
San Angelo Community Medical Center • Cancer Program [6022]
San Angelo Intermediate School District [815]
San Angelo State School [8539]
San Antonio College • Deaf and Hard of Hearing Services [820]
San Antonio Community Hospital • Cancer Program [4860]
San Antonio Eye Bank [35242]
San Antonio Intermediate School District [821]
San Antonio Orthpaedic Group • Sports Medicine Institute [39095]
San Antonio Sleep Centers [37841]
San Antonio State Hospital [33884]
San Antonio State School [8567]
San Augustine Dialysis Clinic [27352]
San Benito County Behavioral Health [39929]
San Benito County Mental Health [28534]
San Benito Dialysis • US Renal Care [27353]
San Benito Health Foundation [6306]
San Bernardino Cnty Dept of Behav Hlth • Barstow Counseling/Behavioral Health [39646]
San Bernardino County Department of Behavioral

Health [28718]
San Bernardino County • Rialto Behaviroal & Addiction Treatment Serv [40446]
San Bernardino CSS--West End [291]
San Bernardino Valley Home Dialysis Center [22932]
San Carlos Apache Tribe • San Carlos Apache Wellness Center [39464]
San Diego American Indian Health Center [40575]
San Diego Blood Bank--El Cajon [34956]
San Diego Blood Bank--El Centro • Imperial Valley Blood Services [34957]
San Diego Blood Bank--Escondido [34958]
San Diego Blood Bank--Murrieta • Valley Blood Services [34959]
San Diego Blood Bank--National City [34960]
San Diego Blood Bank--San Diego [34961]
San Diego Blood Bank--Vista [34962]
San Diego Center for Children [34019]
San Diego Community College District • Brain Injury Program [1268]
San Diego Community College District--ECC [1269]
San Diego Community College District--Mesa College [1270]
San Diego County Mental Health Service [28756]
San Diego County Mental Health Services
    Central Regional Mental Health Services [28757]
    North Inland Mental Health Center [33142]
San Diego County Psychiatric Hospital [28745]
San Diego Eye Bank [34963]
San Diego Fertility Center [21933]
San Diego Freedom Ranch Inc [39678]
San Diego Guild for Infant Survival [36455]
San Diego Health Alliance • West Office [40576]
San Diego Hospice and The Institute for Palliative Medicine [19018]
San Diego KidSpeak [1137]
San Diego Mesa College • Disability Support Program and Services [299]
San Diego Regional Center for the Developmentally Disabled [7815]
San Diego Rescue Mission Inc • Mens Recovery Program [40577]
San Diego Sports Medicine and Family Health Center [38125]
San Diego Youth and Community Services • Runaway and Homeless Youth Program [35841]
San Diego Youth Services • Teen Options [40578]
San Dimas Dialysis Center Inc. [22951]
San Fernando Mental Health Services [28521]
San Fernando Valley Community Mental Health Center [33208]
San Fernando West Kidney Center [23071]
San Francisco AIDS Foundation • The Stonewall Project [40633]
San Francisco Bay Counseling/Education [40634]
San Francisco Department of Public Health • HIV Vaccine Trials Unit [79]
San Francisco Dialysis Center • Dialysis Center & At Home • DaVita [22960]
San Francisco General Hospital [6356]
San Francisco General Hospital Medical Center • Cancer Program [4843]
San Francisco General Hospital
    Opiate Treatment Outpatient Prog/Methadone Detox [40635]
    Renal Center [22961]
    Stimulant Treatment Outpatient Program [40636]
    Substance Abuse Services /Meth Maintenance [40637]
San Francisco Headache Clinic [12388]
San Francisco Hearing and Speech Center [1283]
San Francisco Medical Clinic for Treatment • Pain Clinic [35330]
San Francisco Public Library • Library for the Blind and Print Disabled [3754]
San Francisco Senior Center • Deaf Seniors Program [1284]
San Francisco Sport and Spine Physical Therapy--Battery Street, San Francisco [38130]
San Francisco Sport and Spine Physical Therapy--Buchanan Street, San Francisco [38131]
San Francisco Sport and Spine Physical Therapy--Market Street, San Francisco [38132]
San Francisco Sports Medicine [38133]
San Francisco Suicide Prevention [50694]
San Francisco VA Medical Center [13311]

San Francisco Veterans Affairs Medical Center • Multiple Sclerosis Center [34528]
San Francisco Womens Rehab Foundation • Stepping Stone [40638]
San Gabriel Dialysis • Fresenius Medical Care [22582]
San Gabriel Nephrology Services LLC [22966]
San Gabriel Regional Dialysis Training Center [22828]
San Gabriel Valley Peritoneal Dialysis • Fresenius Medical Care [22583]
San Gabriel Valley YWCA [8927]
San Jacinto Methodist Hospital • Cancer Care Program [5968]
San Joaquin Community Hospital [12905]
San Joaquin County Behavioral Health Services [28823], [50703]
San Joaquin County
    Chemical Dependency Counseling Center [40827]
        Recovery House [39837]
San Joaquin Valley Dialysis Center [22700]
San Joaquin Valley Rehabilitation [1116]
San Jose At Home • DaVita [22972]
San Jose Chiropractic Center [38136]
San Jose State University • Disability Resource Center [1294]
San Juan Capistrano South Dialysis • DaVita [22979]
San Juan Counseling [49596]
San Juan County Program • Gentle Ironhawk Shelter [10521]
San Juan Dialysis Center • Fresenius Medical Care [26654]
San Juan Home Health Care [16317]
San Juan Mental Health [32574]
San Juan Regional Medical Center • Cancer Program [5553]
San Juan/Rio Pedros Vet Center [52086]
San Juaquin County • SJC Family Ties [39838]
San Lazaro Home Health [14142]
San Leandro Dialysis • Renal Advantage Inc. Care Centers [22982]
San Luis Obispo Addiction Recovery Center [40672]
San Luis Obispo County • Drug and Alcohol Services [39615], [39900], [40673]
San Luis Obispo County Mental Health • Atascadero Clinic [28382]
San Luis Obispo County Mental Health Department [28787]
San Luis Obispo County Office of Education [300]
San Luis Obispo County • Office of Education [7821]
San Luis Valley Comprehensive [28951]
San Luis Valley Comprehensive Community Mental Health Center [7833], [28937]
San Luis Valley Comprehensive Mental • Health Center/ [41046]
San Luis Valley Mental Health Center [41227], [41311]
San Luis Valley • Mental Health Center [40978], [40980]
San Luis Valley Mental Health Center • Rio Grande Outpatient [41272]
San Marcos Clinic • Capital Nephrology Associates [27356]
San Marcos Dialysis Center • DaVita [22985]
San Marcos Treatment Center [34454]
San Marino Home Health, Inc. [13326]
San Martin Counseling Center [39996]
San Mateo Medical Center • Methadone Treatment Program [40212]
San Miguel Resource Center [8986]
San Pablo Dialysis Center • DaVita [22988]
San Pablo Sleep Disorders Center [37718]
San Pedro Mental Health Services [28789]
San Saba Downtown Kidney Center • Innovative Dialysis Systems [27342]
San Ysidro Health Center [6352]
Sanco Industries [30535]
Sanctuary in Abused Family Emergencies [8918]
Sanctuary East Ltd • Chemical Dependency Outpatient [46613]
Sanctuary for Families [9958]
Sanctuary Hospice House, Inc. [20272]
Sanctuary, Inc.--Harrison [8762]
Sanctuary, Inc.--Hopkinsville [9389]
Sanctuary, Inc. • Runaway and Homeless Youth

Program [35916]
Sanctuary at the Lake • Lake Chelan Community Hospital [49927]
Sanctuary Psychiatric Centers • Casa del Mural [28800]
Sanctuary Psychiatric Centers of • Santa Barbara/ Outpatient [40734]
Sandcastle Dialysis LLC [27376]
Sanders County Coalition for Families [9763]
Sandhills Center [31608]
Sandhills Center for Mental Health/Developmental Disability/Substance Abuse [31503]
    Randolph County Archdale Trinity Center [31502]
Sandhills Center for MH, MR, SA Service [10099]
Sandhills Crisis Intervention Program [9780]
Sandhills Medical Foundation, Inc. • Jefferson Medical Center [7235]
Sandhills Mental Health Center
    Anson County Outpatient Unit [31603]
    Hoke County Outpatient Unit [31580]
    Montgomery County Outpatient Unit [31602]
    Moore County Outpatient Unit [31578]
    Richmond County Outpatient Unit [31587]
Sandhills Sleep Disorder Center [37486]
Sandra A Carlson Counseling [46152]
Sandra Sands-Arnaez Home Care [18006]
Sandrow and Keyes, MD, PA [38253]
Sandusky Dialysis Center • DaVita [26196]
Sandusky Veterans Affairs Clinic [31833]
Sandweiss Biofeedback Institute • Headache Clinic [12389]
Sandwich Dialysis LLC • Fresenius Medical Care [24080]
Sandy Center [7148], [31978]
Sandy Counseling Center • DBA Humanistic Counseling [49706]
Sandy Counseling • West Unit [49698]
Sandy Pines Hospital [34086]
Sandy Shores Crisis Residential [29226]
Sandy Valley Abuse Center [9399]
Sandys Place Inc [39212]
SANE Solutions and Family Violence Prevention Program [9162]
Sanford Bemidji Medical Center [4225]
Sanford Chamberlain Dialysis Unit [26785]
Sanford Children's Specialty Clinic
    Genetics Clinic [12336]
    South Dakota Center for Blood Disorders [12593]
Sanford Dialysis--Bemidji • Sanford Health [25002]
Sanford Dialysis--Canby [25010]
Sanford Dialysis • DaVita [23509]
Sanford Dialysis Detroit Lakes [25017]
Sanford Dialysis--Fargo • Sanford Health [25991]
Sanford Dialysis Morris [25055]
Sanford Dialysis Red Lake [25066]
Sanford Dialysis--Sioux Falls • Sanford Health [26796]
Sanford Dialysis--Thief River Falls [25091]
Sanford Health [4226]
Sanford Health Neuroscience • ALS Clinic [137]
Sanford Health • Orthopedics and Sports Medicine [38843]
Sanford Health System • Sleep Disorders Center [37501]
Sanford HealthCare [16810]
Sanford Home Care--East Grand Forks [15903]
Sanford Home Care--Fargo [16811]
Sanford Home Care--Lisbon [16816]
Sanford Home Care--Mahnomen [15910]
Sanford Home Care--Pelican Rapids [15926]
Sanford Home Health and Hospice-Sheldon [19729]
Sanford Hospice [21304]
Sanford Hospital • Luverne Outpatient Program [45189]
Sanford NeuroScience • Multiple Sclerosis Center [34668]
Sanford Pediatric Associates [38258]
Sanford Regional Hospital--Worthington • Dialysis Facility [25099]
Sanford Transplant--Fargo • Sanford Health [25992]
Sanford Treatment Center LLC [47492]
Sanford University Medical Center • Cancer Center [5919]
Sanford University • Pediatric Neurology [34762]
Sanford University of South Dakota Medical Center •

Sioux Valley Hospital • Cystic Fibrosis Center [7661]
Sanford USD Medical Center • Sleep Disorders Center [37750]
Sanford Women's Health [11269]
    Sanford Clinic Fertility and Reproductive Endocrinology [22246]
Sanger Sequoia Dialysis Center • DaVita [22990]
Sangre de Cristo Hospice and Palliative Care [19125]
Sangre De Cristo Hospice & Palliative Care-South Office [19130]
Sangre De Cristo Hospice- West [19090]
Sanilac County Community Mental Health Service Program [30634]
Sanilac County Health Department • Sanilac County Counseling Services [45010]
Sanrose Home Health Services Inc. [13232]
Santa Ana Social Services Domestic Violence Program [9877]
Santa Ana Veterans Affairs Medical Center • Bristol Medical Center [28797]
Santa Anita Family Service [28465]
    Chemical Dependency Programs [40236]
    Pathways [39764]
Santa Anita Family Services [28640]
Santa Barbara Artificial Kidney Center LLC [22997]
Santa Barbara Cottage Hospital [1308]
    Cancer Program [4850]
    COPE and Acute Detox Program [40735]
    Cottage Residential Center [40736]
Santa Barbara County Education Office [301]
Santa Barbara County Mental Health Services [28801]
    Lompoc Clinic [28565]
    Psychiatric Health Facility [28802]
    Santa Maria Clinic [28812]
Santa Barbara Rescue Mission
    Bethel House [40737]
    Santa Barbara Outpatient Services [40738]
Santa Barbara School District--Special Ed [302]
Santa Clara Cnty Dept of A/D Programs • Central Treatment and Recovery Center [40665]
Santa Clara Cnty Dept of Alcohol/Drug Serv
    Central Valley Methadone Clinic [40666]
    Family/Children/Community Services Div [40667]
Santa Clara County Dept of Alcohol and • Drug Services/South County Clinic [40678]
Santa Clara County Mental Health Department
    Central Community Mental Health Center [28778]
    Downtown Community Mental Health Center [28779]
    East Valley Community Mental Health Center [28780]
    South County Community Mental Health Center [28516]
Santa Clara County Suicide and Crisis Service [50695]
Santa Clara Sports Therapy [38139]
Santa Clara Valley Health and Hospital System • Mental Health Department [28781]
Santa Clara Valley Medical Center [3923]
    Pain Management Center [35331]
    Regional Burn Center [4518]
Santa Clara Valley Renal Care Center [22973]
Santa Clarita Kidney Center • Innovative Dialysis Systems [23050]
Santa Clarita Valley Battered Association [8855]
Santa Cruz Community Counseling Center [28809]
    Alto Counseling Center [40748]
    Runaway and Homeless Youth Services [35842]
    Si Se Puede [40939]
    Youth Services [40940]
    Youth Services North County [40749]
Santa Cruz County Vet Center [51874]
Santa Cruz Family Guidance Center Division [8702]
Santa Cruz Residential Recovery [40750]
Santa Fe Mobile Vet Center [52030]
Santa Fe Recovery Center • Residential [46307]
Santa Maria Hostel Inc [49399]
Santa Maria Valley Youth and Family • Family Treatment Center [40763]
Santa Monica Dialysis • DaVita [23004]
Santa Monica Fertility Specialists [21934]
Santa Monica Inc [45802]
Santa Monica Orthopaedic and Sports Medicine

Group [38141]
Santa Rosa Memorial Hospital • Cancer Program [4853]
Santa Rosa Nutrition [10988]
Santa Rosa Rancheria [39999]
Santa Rosa Speech & Language Services [1312]
Santa Rosa Treatment Program Inc [40786]
Santa Rosa Veterans Affairs Clinic [13342]
Santa Teresita Medical Center [1096]
Santa Ynez Band of Chumash Mission • Indians [40790]
Santan Dialysis • Fresenius Medical Care [22435]
Sante Center [10907]
Sante Center for Healing [11284], [49213]
Sante Fe Springs Regiona Dialysis Center [23001]
Santee Dialysis • DaVita [26766]
Santram House • Community Healthlink, Inc. [30488]
Sanz Health Services, Inc. [13776]
Sapulpa Dialysis • DaVita [26309]
Sara Hightower Regional Library • Northwest Georgia Talking Book Library [3778]
Sarah A. Reed Children's Center [34412]
Sarah A Thacher LADC LCSW [43952]
Sarah Anne Kelleher • Eating Disorders Treatment [11182]
Sarah and Benjamin Lincow Pain Foundation [35649]
Sarah Bush Lincoln Health Center [14855]
   Regional Cancer Center [5108]
Sarah Inc, [7848]
Sarah's House [8693]
Sarah's Inn [9239]
Sarah's Refuge Inc. [10094]
Sarasota Clinic • Outreach Clinic • Cystic Fibrosis Center [7510]
Sarasota County DUI/Drug Court [41931]
Sarasota Family YMCA • Youth and Family Services • Runaway and Homeless Youth Program [35899]
Sarasota Home Health Care Agency [14378]
Sarasota Memorial Hospital
   Cancer Care Services [4993]
   Sleep Disorders Center [36805]
Sarasota Migraine Clinic [12408]
Sarasota Physicians Dialysis Center [23511]
Sarasota Veterans Affairs Primary Care Clinic [29290]
Saratoga County Alcohol and • Substance Abuse Services [47069]
Saratoga Hospital • Cancer Center [4691]
Saratoga Mental Health Center [31471]
Saratoga Speech Center [3116]
Saratoga Street Mental Health Support Center [32792]
SARP Substance Abuse • Rehabilitation Program [41390]
Sasha Bruce Youthwork • Runaway and Homeless Youth Services [35873]
Sasha Bruce Youthworks [9037]
Satellite Dialysis--Central Modesto • Satellite Healthcare [22816]
Satellite Dialysis • Cupertino Dialysis Center [22654]
Satellite Dialysis--East San Jose [22974]
Satellite Dialysis--Gilroy [22707]
Satellite Dialysis--Greenbrae • Satellite Healthcare [22715]
Satellite Dialysis--Merced • Satellite Health [22807]
Satellite Dialysis--Milpitas • Satellite Healthcare [22808]
Satellite Dialysis--Modesto • Satellite Health [22817]
Satellite Dialysis of Orange • Satellite Healthcare [22860]
Satellite Dialysis--Ortonville [25059]
   Satellite Health [26802]
Satellite Dialysis--Redwood City [22899]
Satellite Dialysis--Santa Cruz • Satellite Healthcare [22999]
Satellite Dialysis--Santa Rosa • Satellite Healthcare [23009]
Satellite Dialysis--Santa Teresa • Satellite Health [22975]
Satellite Dialysis--Sonora • Satellite Healthcare [23016]
Satellite Dialysis--South San Francisco • Satellite Healthcare [23019]
Satellite Dialysis--South San Jose • Satellite Healthcare [22976]

Satellite Dialysis of Stockton • Satellite Healthcare [23025]
Satellite Dialysis--Sunnyvale • Satellite Healthcare [23029]
Satellite Dialysis--Tracy • Satellite Healthcare [23039]
Satellite Dialysis--Turlock • Satellite Healthcare [23043]
Satellite Dialysis--Watsonville • Satellite Healthcare [23067]
Satellite Dialysis--White Road • Satellite Health [22977]
Satellite Dialysis--Windsor • Satellite Healthcare [23078]
Satilla Center for Rehabilitation [38333]
Satilla Community Services
   Charlton Behavioral Health [29425]
   Clinch Behavioral Health [29442]
   Coffee Behavioral Health [29411]
   Mental Hlth and Substance Abuse Services [42087]
Satilla Regional Medical Center [1929]
Sauget Dialysis Center • DaVita [24081]
Sauk County Department of Human Services [32951]
Sauk County Dept of Human Services • Substance Use Treatment Outpatient Services [50366]
Sauk-Suiattle Indian Tribe • Departments of Health and Social Srvs [49933]
Sault Area Hospital • Eating Disorder Program [11235]
Sault Saint Marie Tribe of Chippewa Indians • Victim Service Program [9575]
Sault Tribe Health and Human Services • Behavioral Health Program [44911], [45014]
Savannah Area Family Emergency, Inc. • SAFE [9123]
Savannah Primary Care Clinic [14584]
Savannah Rehabilitation and Nursing Center [1909]
Savannah Sleep Disorders Center [36857]
Savannah Speech and Hearing Center [1910]
Save the Family [8699]
Saving Grace [10223]
Savio House [41143]
Savoy Medical Center • New Horizons [43850]
Savvy Speech LLC [977]
Sawtooth Mountain Clinic, Inc. [6865]
Sawyer County Information and Referral • Center on Alcohol and Other Drug Abuse [50412]
Say It Please Inc. [1661]
Say 'n' Play Summer Speech Camp [1090]
SBFHC--Inglewood [6308]
SBFHC--Redondo Beach [6344]
SBH Medical, LTD [17084]
SCAN Emergency Youth Shelter • Runaway and Homeless Youth Program [36232]
SCAN Inc • RGV Youth Recovery Home [49534]
SCAN/NY Making Choices Treatment Center • Chemical Dependence Outpatient [46454]
SCAR/Jasper Mountain [34396]
Scarsdale Physical Therapy and Sports Rehabilitation Services [38818]
Scattered Site Transitional Apartment Program [9489]
SCCD/Crossroads of Sanford [41925]
Scenic Bluffs Health Center [7421]
Scenic Rivers Health Services [6863]
Scharome Cares [16419]
Schaumburg Dialysis Center • Diversified Specialty Institutes [24082]
Schaumburg Interventions and • Counseling Center LLC [42905]
Schenectady Family Health Services [7041]
Schenectady Veterans Affairs Clinic [31473]
Schexnayder Accent Modification [2306]
Schick Shadel Hospital • Substance Abuse Program [50129]
Schiefelbusch Speech--Language--Hearing Clinic [2226]
Schmidt & Sons Pharmacy of Tecumseh, Inc. [15852]
Schneck Medical Center • Cancer Program [5173]
Schneck Medical Center Hospice [19649]
Schneider Children's Hospital
   Department of Pediatrics • Division of Human Genetics [12298]
   Development and Behavioral Pediatrics • Down Syndrome Center [10834]

   Developmental and Behavioral Pediatrics [8327]
Schneider Children's Hospital at North Shore [8330]
Schneider Children's Hospital • Sickle Cell Clinic [36400]
Schneider Hospital Saint Thomas • Dialysis Center [27449]
Schneider Speech Pathology [3042]
Schoharie Cnty Chem Dependency Clinic [47076]
School Based Services [30069]
School Board of Polk County [344]
School and Community Support [3043]
School for Contemporary Education • Phillips School [8577]
School District of La Crosse [886]
School District Number 22--Vernon • Deaf/Hard of Hearing Program [258]
School District of Palm Beach County ESE [359]
School District of Superior • Hearing Impaired Program [892]
School District of Waukesha [898]
School of the Holy Childhood [8349]
School and Home--based Consultation Services [8144]
School Ten [39595], [40323]
   Drinking Driver Unit [39596]
   Main Street Unit [40721]
Schreiber Pediatric Rehab Center [8468]
Schuyler Counseling and • Health Services [42896]
Schuylkill Health Counseling Center • North [48375]
Schuylkill Medical Center--E Norwegian Street, Pottsville • Cancer Program [5865]
Schuylkill Medical Center--Jackson Street, Pottsville • Cancer Program [5866]
Schuylkill Medical Center - South Jackson Street [17459]
Schuylkill Women in Crisis [10311]
Schwab Rehabilitation Hospital and Care Network [2004]
Schwartz Center for Children [8120]
Science Care of Colorado [34975]
ScienceCare Anatomical Body Donation Services [34926]
Scioto-Paint Valley Mental Health Center--Chillicothe [31682]
Scioto-Paint Valley Mental Health Center • Chillicothe Crisis Center [51203]
Scioto-Paint Valley Mental Health Center--Circleville • Pickaway County [31699]
Scioto Paint Valley Mental Health Center
   Fayette County Office [47878]
   Highland County Office [47779]
Scioto Paint Valley Mental Health Center--Hillsboro • Highland County Satellite [31778]
Scioto Paint Valley Mental Health Center
   Martha Cothrill Clinic [47645]
   Pickaway County Office [47675]
   Pike County Office [47881]
Scioto Paint Valley Mental Health Center--Waverly [31857]
SCO Family of Services--Dix Hills [31312]
SCO Family Services--Glen Cove [31337]
SCO Family Services
   Morning Star Community [46608]
   Morning Star II [46609]
Scotland County Dialysis • Fresenius Medical Care [25898]
Scotland County Schools [622]
Scott County Clinic [28360]
Scott County Comprehensive Care Center • Bluegrass Regional MH/MR Board Inc [43602]
Scott County Dialysis
   DaVita [25087]
   Fresenius Medical Care [24233]
Scott County Mental Health Center [32739]
Scott House--People Incorporated [30665]
Scott and White Alcohol and Drug • Dependence Treatment Program [49552]
Scott and White Artificial Kidney Unit [27370]
Scott and White Clinic
   Department of Obstetrics and Gynecology • In Vitro Fertilization Program [22269]
   Sleep Disorders Center [37842]
Scott & White Home Care and Hospice Agency [21573]
Scott and White Hospital • Sleep Center [37843]
Scott and White Memorial Hospital
   Killeen Dialysis Unit [27206]
   Killeen Dialysis West [27207]

Round Rock Dialysis **[27308]**
Vasicek Cancer Treatment Center **[6030]**
Scottish Rite Center **[7878]**
Scottish Rite Center for Child Language Disabilities
• Children's Hospital **[1534]**
Scottish Rite Center for Childhood Language
Disorders **[3646]**
Scottish Rite Childhood Language Center--Richmond
[3606]
Scottish Rite Childhood Language Center--San
Diego **[1271]**
Scottish Rite Childhood Language Clinic--Cheyenne
[3691]
Scottish Rite
Children's Healthcare of Atlanta
Cystic Fibrosis Center **[7522]**
Sleep Disorders Center **[36858]**
Scottsbluff Dialysis Center • DaVita • Dialysis Facil-
ity **[25345]**
Scottsdale Behavioral Health • Addiction Program
and Counseling **[39470]**
Scottsdale Dialysis Center • Diversified Specialty
Institutes **[23958]**
Scottsdale Health Center **[6698]**
Scottsdale Healthcare--Osborn **[4745]**
Scottsdale Healthcare--Shea • Cancer Program
[4746]
Scottsdale Healthcare Sleep Disorders Center
[36634]
Scottsdale Hearing Center **[984]**
Scottsdale Pain Center **[35292]**
Scottsdale Sleep Center **[36635]**
Scottsdale Sports Medicine Institute **[38049]**
Scottsdale Treatment Institute PLC **[39471]**
Scottsdale Unified School District Number 48 **[235]**
Scranton Counseling Center **[8484]**, **[32117]**
Scranton Dialysis • DaVita **[26578]**
Scranton Primary Health Care Center, Inc. **[7184]**
Scranton State School for Deaf and Hard of Hearing
Children **[694]**
Scribner Kidney Center • Northwest Kidney Center
[27638]
Scripps Clinic Carmel Valley **[1272]**
Scripps Clinic • Department of Audiology/Speech
Language Pathology **[1138]**
Scripps Clinic Fertility Center **[21935]**
Scripps Clinic Sleep Center **[36693]**
Scripps Clinic • Sports Medicine Department
[38091]
Scripps Green Hospital • Cancer Program **[4786]**
Scripps Health • Cancer Care Program **[4835]**
Scripps Home Care Services **[13302]**
Scripps McDonald Center **[39956]**
Scripps Memorial Hospital **[1139]**
Scripps/Memorial Hospital Encinitas **[12988]**
Scripps Memorial Hospital--Encinitas • Cancer
Program **[4771]**
Scripps Memorial Hospital, Encinitas • Rehabilitation
Center **[3924]**
Scripps Memorial Hospital - La Jolla **[13090]**
Scripps Memorial Hospital--La Jolla • Thomas T.
Stevens Cancer Center **[4787]**
Scripps Memorial Hospital • Pain Center **[35332]**
Scripps Memorial Hospital Rehabilitation Center
[1102]
Scripps Mercy Hospital
Cancer Program **[4836]**
Sleep Disorders Center **[36694]**
Scurry County Mental Health Center **[32552]**
SE Council on Alcohol and Drug Dependence Inc
[41447]
Altruism House Female **[41448]**
Altruism House/Male **[41458]**
Detox **[41449]**
Outpatient Program **[41459]**
SE Missouri Behavioral Health **[45637]**
Aquinas Center **[45475]**
Potosi Office **[45593]**
Salem Center **[45638]**
Sea Haven, Inc. • Runaway and Homeless Youth
Program **[36196]**
Sea Haven, Inc.--Transitional Living • Runaway and
Homeless Youth Program **[36197]**
Sea Island Medical Centers, Inc. **[7236]**
Sea Mar Behavioral Health
Aberdeen **[49874]**
Bellingham **[49902]**
Lynnwood **[50016]**

Puyallup **[50074]**
Tacoma **[50217]**
Sea Mar Community Health Center **[18454]**, **[49957]**
Sea Mar Community Health Center--15th Avenue,
Seattle **[7387]**
Sea Mar Community Health Center--Henderson,
Seattle **[7388]**
Sea Mar Community Healthcare Centers • Monroe
Branch **[50020]**
Sea Mar Olympia Branch • Outpatient Substance
Services **[50232]**
Sea Mar Renacer Youth Treatment Center **[50130]**
Sea Mar Residential Alcohol/Drug Treatment • Des
Moines **[49937]**
Sea Mar Residential Alcohol Drug Treatment •
Inpatient **[50218]**
Sea Mar Substance Abuse • Outpatient Services/
Mount Vernon **[50025]**
Sea Mar Visions Female Youth Treatment Center
[49903]
Seacliff Recovery Center **[39932]**
Seacoast Dialysis Center • Fresenius Medical Care
[25398]
Seacoast Language Services **[2365]**, **[2880]**
Seacoast Mental Health Center, Inc.--Exeter **[31069]**
Seacoast Mental Health Center, Inc.--Portsmouth
[31092]
Seacoast Mental Health Services **[51088]**
Seacoast Orthopedics and Sports Medicine **[38711]**
Seafarers • Addiction Rehabilitation Center **[44377]**
Seafield Center Inc • Alc and Subst Abuse Inpt
Rehab Unit **[47182]**
Seafield Services Inc
Alcoholism and Substance Abuse Services
[46776], **[46786]**, **[47022]**
CD Outpatient Clinic **[46354]**
Outpatient Drug Abuse Clinic **[46974]**
Seafield Amityville Clinic/CD OP Rehab **[46355]**
Seaford Audiology **[1516]**
Seaford Group Home **[34356]**
Seal's Healthcare **[12960]**
Search for Change, Inc. **[31403]**, **[31493]**
Search for Change, Inc.--Wyndover Woods **[31494]**
Search Day Program **[8264]**
Searcy Behavioral **[28349]**
Searcy Family Health Center **[6279]**
Searcy Hospital **[33092]**
Searcy Outreach **[28350]**
Sears Methodist Hospice **[21376]**
Searsport Counseling Associates **[44012]**
Belfast Center **[43944]**
Holly Duesenberry **[43971]**
Irene Laney LADC MSW **[43972]**
Kirsten Webb LADC MED **[43945]**
Maxine Wolph Johnson LSW LADC **[44070]**,
[44081]
Seashore Family Services of New Jersey **[45941]**,
[45942]
Seasons Center for Community Mental Health
Buena Vista County **[29899]**
Clay County **[29896]**
Dickinson County **[29897]**
Lyon County **[29891]**
O'Brien County **[29892]**
Osceola County **[29893]**
Seasons Counseling Inc **[48242]**, **[48249]**, **[48251]**,
[48260]
Seasons Hospice **[20198]**
Seasons Hospice, Inc.--Des Plains **[19512]**
Seasons Hospice & Palliative Care of California,
LLC--Pasadena **[18991]**
Seasons Hospice & Palliative Care of California-San
Diego, LLC **[19074]**
Seasons Hospice & Palliative Care-Dallas **[21437]**
Seasons Hospice and Palliative Care, Inc-
Randallstown **[19938]**
Seasons Hospice and Palliative Care, Inc. - Willow-
brook Office **[19584]**
Seasons Hospice and Palliative Care of Mas-
sachusetts, LLC **[19983]**
Seasons Hospice and Palliative Care of Michigan,
Inc. **[20089]**
Seasons Hospice and Palliative Care-Newark
[19181]
Seasons Hospice & Palliative Care--Orange **[18984]**
Seasons Hospice and Palliative Care of
Pennsylvania **[21104]**
Seasons Hospice & Palliative Care of Texas **[21463]**

Season's Hospice and Palliative Care of Wisconsin,
Inc. **[21872]**
Seasons Hospice and Palliative of Indiana LLC
[19615]
Seasons of Life Hospice Home • Ministry Home
Care **[21874]**
SeaTac Kidney Center • Northwest Kidney Center
[27634]
Seattle Behavioral Health Clinic **[32858]**
Seattle Central Community College • Disability Sup-
port Services **[865]**
Seattle Children's Home **[34472]**
Seattle Childrens Hospital **[50131]**
Seattle Children's Hospital
Division of Nephrology • Dialysis Center **[27639]**
Hemophilia Treatment Center **[12611]**
MDA Clinic **[34905]**
Pediatric Sleep Disorders Center **[37935]**
Seattle Counseling Service for Sexual • Minorites
[50132]
Seattle Counseling Service for Sexual Minorities
[51466]
Seattle Indian Health Board **[7389]**, **[10652]**
Alcohol Drug Outpatient/Assessment **[50133]**
Seattle Kidney Center • Northwest Kidney Center
[27640]
Seattle Mental Health--Rainbow Creek **[32808]**
Seaview Community Services **[8672]**, **[28118]**,
[39350]
Seaview Dialysis Center • DaVita **[27614]**
Seaview Sports Medicine--Brick **[38714]**
Seaview Sports Medicine--Freehold **[38725]**
Seaview Sports Medicine--Lakewood **[38733]**
Seaview Sports Medicine--Ocean **[38750]**
Sebastian Dialysis • DaVita **[23512]**
Sebastian River Home Health--Barefoot Bay **[13584]**
Sebastian River Home Health--Sebastian **[14381]**
Sebastian River Medical Center **[14382]**
Sebring Veterans Affairs Primary Care Clinic **[29291]**
Second Chance **[8636]**, **[45405]**
Second Chance Hayward Recovery Center **[39915]**
Second Chance Inc • Recovery Services **[39966]**
Second Chance, Inc. **[8853]**, **[50682]**
Second Chance Newark Center **[40257]**
Second Chance Recovery • Frazier Marion **[47479]**
Second Chance Substance Abuse Services **[44857]**
Second Change Recovery Center **[39569]**
Second Genesis Inc
Mellwood House **[44376]**
Residental TC and Co-occurring TC **[44234]**
Therapeutic Community **[41549]**
The Second Step, Inc. **[9495]**
Second Step Shelter **[8874]**
Second Street • Community Healthlink, Inc. **[30489]**
Second Street House **[28887]**
Second Wind Inc **[44349]**
Second Wind Respiratory Care **[17453]**
Secret Harbor School **[34467]**
Secu Hospice House-Smithfield **[20738]**
Securacell Inc. **[35167]**
Security--Winter Haven Square • Renal Advantage
Inc. • Dialysis Facility **[23562]**
Seeds of Hope **[9335]**
Seeds of Hope--Bustleton, Philadelphia • Adult/
Adolescent Eating Disorders Program **[11257]**
Seeds of Hope--Exton • Adult/Adolescent Eating
Disorders Program **[11258]**
Seeds of Hope--Haddonfield • Adult Eating
Disorders Program **[11147]**
Seeds of Hope--Jenkintown • Adult Eating Disorders
Program **[11259]**
Seeds of Hope--Lansdale • Adult Eating Disorders
Program **[11260]**
Seeds of Hope--Marlton • Adult Eating Disorders
Program **[11148]**
Seeds of Hope--Media • Adult/Adolescent Eating
Disorders Program **[11261]**
Seeds of Hope--Paoli • Adult/Adolescent Eating
Disorders Program **[11262]**
Seeds of Hope--Walnut St., Philadelphia • Adult/
Adolescent Eating Disorders Program **[11263]**
SEEDS/National Advocacy and Training Network
[8718]
SEEDS of the Willistons Inc. **[3149]**
Seekers of Serenity **[30979]**
Seekers of Serenity Place **[45733]**
Seekhaven **[10525]**
Seeking Peaceful Solutions Inc **[40154]**

Selah Hospice Care, Inc. [21534]
Selah House [11063]
A Select Group Home Health Care [14285]
Select Physical Therapy [38947]
Self Concepts Clinical Counseling Inc [47325]
Self Help Addiction Rehab
    East [44762]
    Main [44763]
Self-Help Center Inc [50571]
Self-Help HomeCare and Hospice [19025]
Self Help Movement Inc [48561]
Self Inc [48562]
Self Regional Healthcare • Cancer Program [5909]
Self Support Personal Care, LLC [16831]
Selfcare Mediquip, Inc. [16223]
Selfrefind [43542], [43558], [43574], [43719],
    [43741], [43748]
Selinsgrove Dialysis • Dialysis Center & At Home •
    DaVita [26580]
Sellati and Co Inc
    Virginia Beach Methadone Clinic [49858]
    Woodbridge Methadone Treatment Center
        [49810]
Sellersville Dialysis Center • DaVita [26581]
Selma Dialysis Center • DaVita [23011]
Selmer Dialysis • Dialysis Center • DaVita [26920]
Semi-Supervised Living Project [28758]
Seminole Community Mental Health Center [29152]
    Group Home [29286]
Seminole County Crisis Stabilization [29287]
Seminole County Mental Health [29410]
Seminole County Victims Rights Coalition/Safe-
    House of Seminole [9061]
Seminole Dialysis Center [23516]
Seminole Intermediate School District [824]
Seminole Nation Domestic Violence [10218]
Semoran Treatment Center [43064]
Senator Garrett W. Hagedorn Psychiatric Hospital
    [33657]
Seneca Behavioral Health Center [51489]
Seneca Center for Children and Families [28785]
Seneca Community Residence [31488]
Seneca County Addictions Program [47162]
Seneca County Dialysis • Davita [26207]
Seneca Health Services Inc [50321], [50324],
    [50343], [50348]
Seneca Health Services, Inc.--Lewisburg [32916]
Seneca Health Services, Inc.--Marlinton [32917]
Seneca Health Services, Inc.--Summerville [32938]
Seneca Health Services, Inc.--Webster Springs •
    Conway House [32941]
Seneca Highlands Intermediate Unit Number 9 [713]
Seneca Sleep Disorders Center [37693]
SENICA LLC [45022]
Senior Helpers [14357]
Senior Home Health Agency [14865]
Senior Home Health Care Inc.--Glendale [13050]
Senior Hope Counseling Inc • Alcoholism Outpatient
    Clinic [46341]
Senior Independence of Akron/Canton [20799]
Senior Independence-Canfield [20807]
Senior Independence-Dayton [20836]
Senior Link Home Health Care--Dearborn [15626]
Senior Link Home Health Care, Inc.--Troy [15865]
Senior Nursing Care Services, Inc. [15684]
Senior Recovery Program [45313]
Senior Solutions Home Health Care [14284]
Senior Support Program of Tri Valley [40398]
Senior's Home Health [14143]
Seniors Home Health Care [15828]
Seniors Home Health Services [15728]
Seniors, Inc.--Canon City [13461]
Seniors! Inc.--Denver [13478]
Seniors, Inc.--Trinidad [13510]
Sensible Recovery Systems [49500]
Sentara Bayside Hospital • Sleep Disorders Center
    [37896]
Sentara Careplex Hospital • Cancer Services [6062]
Sentara Healthcare System • Cancer Program
    [6073]
Sentara Home Care & Hospice [21744]
Sentara Home Care & Hospice-Hampton [21701]
Sentara Home Care and Hospice Services [21712]
Sentara Home Care Services [18270]
Sentara Hospice Program [21681]
Sentara Hospice Program-Covington [21685]
Sentara Leigh Hospital • Cancer Center [4715]
Sentara Norfolk General Hospital

Eastern Virginia Medical School • Burn Trauma
    Unit [4646]
Sentara Cancer Institute [6074]
Sentara Norfolk General Hospital Transplant
    Program [27529]
Sentara Obici Hospital • Sleep Disorders Center
    [37897]
Sentara Virginia Beach General Hospital
    Coastal Cancer Center [6087]
    Sleep Disorders Center [37898]
Sentara Williamsburg Regional Medical Center
    Community Cancer Center [6088]
    Sleep Wellness Center [37899]
Sepulveda Rehabilitation Center [40897]
Sepulveda VA OPC and Nursing Home
    Addictive Behaviors Clinic [40795]
    OTP Treatment/Maintenance [40796]
Sequel TSI of Tuskegee [28058]
Sequel Youth and Family Services [28011]
Sequoia Adolescent Treatment Center [34309]
Sequoia Health Services • Sleep Disorders Center
    [36695]
Sequoia Mental Health [48075]
Sequoia Recovery Services LLC [44967]
Sequoyah County Clinic [7114]
Serendipity I [46531]
Serendipity II [46532]
Serene Center Long Beach [40039]
Serene Harbor, Inc. [9073]
Serenidad Recovery Home [49498]
Serenidad Womens Recovery Home [49499]
Serenity Acres Treatment Center LLC [44235]
Serenity Adult Recovery Dynamics [49200]
Serenity Behavioral Health Systems [42046]
    Crisis Line [50796]
    McDuffie/Wilkes Outpatient CLinic [42169]
Serenity Bridges LLC [42789]
Serenity Counseling Advocates Inc [39580]
Serenity Counseling Center [43075]
Serenity Counseling and DWI [47440]
Serenity Counseling Services [41942], [49964]
Serenity Counseling Services LLC [43172]
Serenity Education and Therapy [41243]
Serenity Foundation of Texas • Outpatient Program
    [49201]
Serenity Health Care, Inc. [13061]
Serenity Health LLC [44092]
Serenity Home Health Care--Miami Dade County
    [14144]
Serenity Home Inc/Substance Abuse ICF • Halfway
    Treatment Services [49790]
Serenity Hospice Care-Vidalia [19430]
Serenity Hospice-Fowler [19601]
Serenity Hospice-Lafayette [19624]
Serenity Hospice, LLC--Magnolia [18864]
Serenity Hospice and Palliative Care [18816]
Serenity Hospice-Texarkana [21577]
Serenity Hospice-Tyler [21583]
Serenity House [49650]
Serenity House of Clallam County • Runaway and
    Homeless Youth Program [36257]
Serenity House Counseling Services Inc
    Halfway House/Administration/Outpt [42382]
    Womens Recovery Home [42807]
Serenity House • DBA Serenity Park Inc [39553]
Serenity House--Gallipolis [10149]
Serenity House of Gary Inc [43065]
Serenity House Inc [44034]
Serenity House--Mountain Home [8777]
Serenity House--Phoenix [8817]
Serenity House--Santa Barbara [19036]
Serenity Knolls • Chemical Dependency Recovery
    Program [39831]
Serenity Lane [48062], [48081], [48107], [48215],
    [48233], [48243], [50243]
    New Hope [48108]
Serenity Mental Health Services [32221], [32258]
Serenity Palliative Care and Hospice [21026]
Serenity Partnerships [47297]
Serenity Path [45258]
Serenity Place [41503]
    NCADD Affiliate [45911]
    Womens Residential Treatment Program
        [48949]
Serenity Point Counseling Services [50252]
Serenity Recovery Centers Inc [49143]
Serenity Services [9530]
Serenity Shelter [10412]

Serenity at Stout Street Foundation [41076]
Serenity Treatment Center Inc [44273]
Serento Gardens • Alcohol and Drug Services
    [48403]
Sertoma Centre, Inc. [29556]
SERV Behavioral Health System Inc [45962]
SERV Home Health Inc. [12979]
Service First Outpatient Program [40828], [40829]
Service League of San Mateo County • Hope House
    [40440]
Service Net • Emergency Service of Northampton
    [50994]
ServiceNet Inc
    Beacon House for Men Recovery House
        [44480]
    Beacon House for Women [44481]
ServiceNet, Inc. [30434]
    Emergency Services [30435]
    Greenfield Shelter [30392]
    Outpatient Clinic [30436]
    Runaway and Homeless Youth Program [36003]
Services to Abused Families, Inc. [10561]
Services to Aid Families [9972]
Services Empowering the Rights of Victims [9827]
Services de Sante Mentale Communautaire [11137]
Services United Inc • Joshua House Recovery
    Home [40771]
Servicios Ambulatorio • Alcohol Y Drogas Adultos
    [48787]
Servicios de Hospicio de Adjuntas [21184]
Servicios Ninos Adolescentes de Salud • Mental
    Drogas Y Alcohol Ambulatorio [48738]
Servicios de la Raza [8956]
Servicios Suplementarios De Salud, Inc. [21187]
Serving Children/Adolescents In Need (SCAN) Inc.
    Stand Outpatient Program [49439], [49591]
    Youth Recovery Home [49440]
Servy Institute for Reproductive Endocrinology
    [22023]
Set Free DAT Center [49400]
Seton Addiction Services at • Saint Marys Hospital
    [47137]
Seton Drive Dialysis • DaVita [24653]
Seton Health Addiction Services • Acute Care
    [47138]
Seton Health System • Home Health Care Agency
    [16651]
Seton Healthcare Network • Shivers Cancer Center
    [5964]
Seton Highland Lakes [17837]
Seton Highland Lakes Hospice [21415]
Seton Home Health [15213]
Seton House, Inc. • Runaway and Homeless Youth
    Program [36247]
Seton Medical Center [12973]
Seton Medical Center Austin • Cancer Center [5965]
Seton Medical Center • Cancer Program [4769]
Seton Northwest Hospital • Cancer Program [5966]
Seton Shoal Creek Hospital [33859]
Settlement Health and Medical Services, Inc. [7031]
Settlement Home for Children [34447]
Seven 12 House • Youth and Shelter Services
    [43235]
Seven Counties Services [43780]
Seven Counties Services, Inc. [30070]
Seven Counties Services Inc. • Crisis and Informa-
    tion Center [50936]
Seven Counties Services
    Jefferson Alcohol/Drug Abuse Center [43695]
    LANSAT Program [43696]
    Lighthouse Adolescent Recovery Center [43697]
    Spencer [43789]
Seven Direction Inc [43508]
Seven Hills Behavioral Health Inc [44457]
    Methadone Services [44521]
Seven Hills Behavioral Health, Inc.--Chelmsford
    [30358]
Seven Hills Behavioral Health, Inc.--Marion [30413]
Seven Hills Behavioral Health, Inc.--New Bedford
    [30426]
Seven Hills Behavioral Institute [45832]
Seven Hills Foundation • Mental Health Services
    [30372]
Seven Lakes Recovery Program [41353]
Seven Rivers Regional Medical Center [13633]
Seventh Step Foundation Inc [39916]
Seventh Street Medical Supply Inc. [17322]
Sevier Valley Dialysis [27417]

Seward Medical Center [7185]
Sewickley Valley Hospital • Speech Pathology Department [3381]
Sexual Assault Crisis Team [10538]
Sexual Assault and Domestic Violence Center [8929]
Sexual Assault/Domestic Violence Center, Inc. [9360]
Sexual Assault and Family Violence [10751]
Sexual Assault Prevention and Awareness Center [9514]
Sexual Assault Program of Child and Family Services [9571]
Sexual Assault Resource Agency [10558]
Sexual Assault Resource Center [10222]
Sexual Assault Response and Awareness [10592]
Sexual Assault Services of Calhoun County [9517]
Sexual Assault Services • Central Michigan University [9561]
Sexual Assault/Spouse Abuse Resource Center, Inc. [9448]
Sexual Assault Support Services/Crisis Call Center [9800]
Sexual Assault Support Services--Eugene [10229]
Sexual Assault Support Services--Portsmouth [9816]
Sexual Trauma and Counseling Center [10354]
Sexual Trauma Services of the Midlands [10347]
SF Chinatown Dialysis Center • DaVita [22962]
Shades of Hope Treatment Center [11285]
Shadow Mountain Behavioral Health [33787]
Shady Grove Adventist Hospital • Cancer Program [5312]
Shady Grove Fertility Center--Annapolis [22092]
Shady Grove Fertility Center--Baltimore [22093]
Shady Grove Fertility Center--Bel Air [22094]
Shady Grove Fertility Center--Frederick • Patriot Medical Center [22095]
Shady Grove Fertility Center--Rockville • Reproductive Science Center [22096]
Shady Grove Fertility Center--Towson [22097]
Shady Grove Fertility--Leesburg [22290]
Shady Grove Fertility--Washington [21985]
Shaffer House [47666]
Shaker Square Dialysis • DaVita [26069]
Shalom Bayit--Atlanta • Jewish Family and Career Services of Atlanta [9089]
Shalom Bayit--Oakland [8860]
Shalom Bayit--San Francisco [8891]
Shalom House Inc. [30230]
Shalom Inc [48563]
SHALVA [9213]
Shamar Hope Haven [49401]
Shamrock Dialysis • DaVita [23687]
Shamrock Group Inc [50134]
Shamrock Visiting Nurse and Home Health Aide Agency [13525]
Shandin Hills Behavioral Therapy Center [28741]
   Shandin Hills Adolescent Center [33184]
Shands Comprehensive Pediatric Sickle Cell Center [36326]
Shands Home Care [13712]
Shands Hospital • MDA Clinic [34783]
Shands Jacksonville [1614]
   Dialysis Clinics Inc. • ESRD [23352]
Shands Jacksonville Medical Center [13821]
   Cancer Center [4954]
Shands Jacksonville Medical Center, Inc. • Comprehensive Multiple Sclerosis Center [34559]
Shands Rehab Hospital • Spinal Cord and Brain Injury Services [3995]
Shands Rehabilitation Hospital [1588], [38230]
Shands Sleep Disorders Center [36806]
Shands at the University of Florida • Cancer Program [4945]
Shands at Univ. of Florida Outpatient Dialysis • Adult Dialysis [23312]
Shands at University of Florida • Sleep Disorders Center [36807]
Shands at Vista [33304]
Shannon Medical Center • Cancer Program [6023]
Shannon Medical Center Outpatient Dialysis Center [27311]
Shannon Medical Center - Saint John's Campus [18134]
Shapiro Developmental Center [7958]
SHARE House, Inc. [9107]
SHARE of Idaho [36472]
SHARE, Inc. [8963]

SHARE National Office [36500]
ShareHouse [47575]
ShareHouse Stepping Stones [45250]
ShareHouse Wellness Center [45241]
Sharon Community Health Center [7187]
Sharon Ear, Nose and Throat [1489]
Sharon Hospital [1490]
   Cancer Program [4907]
Sharon Regional Health System [21157]
   Cancer Program [5874]
Sharon Regional Health System Home Health Agency [17478]
Sharon Regional Health System Hospice and Palliative Care [21096]
Sharon Wermut, PT [38143]
Sharp Chula Vista Medical Center • Cancer Program [4765]
Sharp Grossmont Hospital [13091]
   David & Donna Long Center for Cancer Treatment [4788]
SHARP Grossmont Hospital • Grossmont Hospital Sleep Disorders Center [36696]
Sharp Hospice Care [19019]
Sharp HospiceCare [18949]
Sharp Memorial Hospital [13303]
   Cancer Program [4837]
Sharp Memorial Hospital Renal Transplant [22948]
Sharp Memorial Rehabilitation [3925]
Sharp Mesa Vista Hospital • Chemical Dependency Program [40579]
Sharp Vista Pacifica [40580]
Sharpe Health School • Special Education, Division 6 [1535]
SHARPP • University of New Hampshire [9808]
Shasta Community Health Center [6343]
Shasta County Alcohol and Drug Program [40430]
Shasta County Health and Human Service • Shasta County Perinatal Treatment Serv [40431]
Shasta County Mental Health Services [28713]
Shasta County Women's Refuge, Inc. [8872]
Shasta Options [40432]
Shasta Treatment Center • Shasta Treatment Center Drug and Alc [40433]
Shasta View Speech Center [3312]
Shaughnessy-Kaplan Rehabilitation • In/Out-patient Rehabilitation Services • Communication and Swallowing Disorders [2520]
Shaw House • Runaway and Homeless Youth Program [35987]
Shaw Regional Cancer Center [4877]
Shawano Community Hospice [21865]
Shawano County Dept of Community Progs • Outpatient Services [50522]
Shawano Medical Center [18626]
Shawnee County Health Agency • Hillcrest Clinic [6722]
Shawnee Health Service and Development Corporation [6649]
Shawnee Library System • Southern Illinois Talking Book Center [3789]
Shawnee Mental Health Center, Inc. [31826]
   Adams County Clinic [31858]
Shawnee Mission Home Health Care--North Kansas City [16033]
Shawnee Mission Home Health Care--Shawnee Mission [15151]
Shawnee Mission Medical Center [2241]
   Addiction Recovery Unit [43461]
   Behavioral Health Unit [29956]
   Cancer Program [5205]
   Sleep Laboratory [37005]
SHCC Centers for Neurology and Pain Management--Boca Raton [12409]
SHCC Centers for Neurology and Pain Management--Delray Beach [12410]
SHCC Centers for Neurology and Pain Management--Pembroke Pines [12411]
SHCC Centers for Neurology and Pain Management--Tamarac [12412]
SHCC Centers for Neurology and Pain Management--West Palm Beach [12413]
Sheboygan County Health and Human Serv • Mental Health and SAT Center [50527]
Shedden Pain Relief and Sports [38004]
Sheehan Memorial Hospital • CD Outpatient Rehabilitation Service [46568]
Sheepshead Bay Renal Care Center • DaVita [25628]

Shelby Baptist Medical Center • Cancer Program [4721]
Shelby Center for Mental Health [30965]
Shelby County Community Services Inc [42909]
Shelby County Community Services, Inc. [29676]
Shelby County Counseling Center Inc [47855]
Shelby County Treatment Center [39203]
Shelby Medical Associates • Sleep Laboratory [37487]
Shelby Memorial Hospital [14925]
Shelbyville Community Dialysis [24083]
Shelter for Abused Women and Children [9067]
Shelter Against Violent Environments [8813]
Shelter Agencies for Families in East Texas, Inc. [10492]
Shelter and Assistance in Family Emergencies, Inc. [9659]
Shelter Care, Inc. • Safe Landing Youth Shelter • Runaway and Homeless Youth Program [36149]
Shelter of Gaston County [10039]
Shelter for Help in Emergency [10559]
Shelter Home of Caldwell County, Inc. [10052]
Shelter House, Inc. [9052]
Shelter, Inc. [9512]
The Shelter, Inc. [10414]
Shelter Our Sisters [9829]
Shelter Outreach Plus [8846]
Shelter Services for Women, Inc. [8903]
Shelter Services for Women: Santa Maria [8906]
Shelter from the Storm--La Grande • Domestic Violence and Sexual Assault Service [10236]
Shelter from the Storm--Palm Desert [8865]
Shelter for Victims of Domestic Violence [9865]
Shelter from Violence, Inc. [10150]
Shelter Women of Long Beach [8833]
Sheltered Aid For Families in Emergencies, Inc. [10101]
Sheltering Wings Center for Women [9270]
Shelton Dialysis • DaVita [23181]
Shenandoah Dialysis • DaVita [24297]
Shenandoah Valley Medical Systems, Inc. • Shenandoah Migrant Services [7409]
Shenandoah Women's Center, Inc. [10678]
Shepherd Care Hospice [21266]
Shepherd Center [4008]
Shepherd Center, Inc.
   Multiple Sclerosis Center [34566]
   Spinal Cord Injury Model Systems [4009]
Shepherd Home Health Care Inc. [13151]
Shepherd House • Learning Services Residential Rehabilitation • Durham, North Carolina [4338]
Shepherd Pathways [4010]
Shepherd's Crossing [4192]
Shepherd's Gate [8829]
Shepherds House Inc [43667]
Sheppard Pratt • Center for Eating Disorders [11084]
Sheppard Pratt at Ellicott City • Taylor Manor Hospital [33562]
Sheppard Pratt Health System [33556]
Sher Institute for Reproductive Medicine--Las Vegas [22154]
Sher Institutes for Reproductive Medicine--Bedminster [22166]
Sher Institutes for Reproductive Medicine--Chino Hills [21936]
Sher Institutes for Reproductive Medicine--Creve Coeur [22147]
Sher Institutes for Reproductive Medicine--Dallas [22270]
Sher Institutes for Reproductive Medicine--Greater Lehigh Valley [22167]
Sher Institutes for Reproductive Medicine--Long Island [22195]
Sher Institutes for Reproductive Medicine--New York [22196]
Sher Institutes for Reproductive Medicine--Peoria [22051]
Sher Institutes for Reproductive Medicine--Sacramento [21937]
Sher Institutes for Reproductive Medicine--Westchester [22197]
Sheridan Home Healthcare, Inc. [13799]
Sheridan Memorial Hospice [20370]
Sheridan Veterans Affairs Medical Center [33068]
Sheriff's Youth Program of Austin [34240]
Sheriffs Youth Programs of Minnesota [34251]
Sherman Hospital • Oncology Services [5089]

Sherman Intermediate School District • Deaf Education Program [825]
Sherwood Center for the Exceptional Child [8200]
Sherwood Clinic--Cartersville [14500]
Sherwood Clinic--Demorest [14518]
Sherwood Clinic--Thomaston [14593]
Sherwood Dialysis Center • DaVita [26356]
Shiawassee RESD [498]
Shield Institute • Aug Communication Center [3021]
Shields for Families
    Ark [40188]
    Eden Dual Diagnosis [40189]
    Exodus [39731]
    Genesis Family Day Treatment Program [40155]
    Revelation [39732]
Shingle Springs Tribal Health Program [40799]
Shining Star DaVita Bricktown Dialysis Center [25410]
Shining Star DaVita Middletown Dialysis Center [25503]
Shining Star DaVita Somerset Dialysis [25510]
Shining Star Neptune Dialysis Clinic [25479]
Shipowick Smith Counseling and • Positive Living Center [50259]
Shiprock Dialysis • DaVita [25562]
Shirley Goodman/Himan Brown Residence [20587]
Shoals Treatment Center [39292]
Shoalwater Bay Indian Tribe • Shoalwater Bay Counseling/CD Program [50224]
Shodair Children's Hospital [33640]
    Medical Genetics Clinic [10822]
    Medical Genetics Program [12268]
Shodair Residential Treatment Center [33641]
Shoemaker Center [44363]
Sholom Care and Johnson Hospice [20205]
Shore Behavioral Health Services [44247]
Shore Health Services, Inc. [18332]
Shore Health System • Cancer Center [5301]
Shore Home Care and Hospice [19922]
Shore Memorial Hospital [7357]
Shore Memorial Hospital--Nassawadox • Cancer Program [6070]
Shore Memorial Hospital--Somers Point • Cancer Program [5540]
Shore Rehabilitation at Denton • Balance Center [2397]
Shore Rehabilitation at Easton [2410]
Shorefront Jewish Geriatric Center [16420]
Shorehaven Behavioral Health Inc [50374]
Shoreline Behavioral Health Services [48925]
Shoreline Center for Eating Disorder Treatment [10989]
Shoreline Dialysis Center • Avantis Renal Therapy [23149]
Shoreline Hearing Program [866]
Shoreline Inc [49548]
Shorkey Center [8534]
Short Term Rehabilitation System at Willow Pond [4413]
Shoshone/Bannock Tribe • Victims of Crime Services [9172]
Shoshone House [28888]
Shoulder [39237]
Show Low VA Health Care Clinic-Show Low Arizona [3876]
Show Low Veterans Affairs Healthcare Clinic [28201]
Shrader House Crisis Program [28770]
Shreveport Home Dialysis • DaVita [24585]
Shreveport Mental Health Center [30174]
Shriners Hospital for Children [34906]
    Burns Institute, Galveston [35243]
Shriners Hospital for Children--Houston [8553]
Shriners Hospital for Children, Northern California • Burn Care Unit [4519]
Shriners Hospital for Children--Portland [8446]
Shriners Hospital for Children--Spokane [8606]
Shriner's Hospital for Crippled Children--Portland [3318]
Shriners Hospital--Erie [8459]
Shriners Hospital--Philadelphia [8477]
Shriners Hospital--Saint Louis [8216]
Shriners Hospitals for Children-Boston • Burn Center [4562]
Shriners Hospitals for Children--Chicago [7943]
Shriners Hospitals for Children-Cincinnati • Shriners Burn Hospital - Cincinnati [4608]
Shriners Hospitals for Children-Galveston • Burn Care Unit [4638]

Shriners Hospitals for Children--Los Angeles [7789]
Shriners Hospitals for Children--Sacramento [7813]
Shriners Hospitals for Children--Shreveport [8077]
Shring Home Care, Inc. [15829]
Shuman HealthCare of Brunswick [14495]
Shuman HealthCare Specialty Pharmacy [14606]
Shuree Home Healthcare, Inc. [14752]
Sibley Memorial Hospital [1536]
    Cancer Program [4924]
    Sleep Disorders Center [36764]
Side by Side Counseling [47369]
Sidney Health Center
    Audiology and Hearing Aid Services [2839]
    Sleep Lab [37304]
Sidney Kimmel Comprehensive Cancer Center at Johns Hopkins [4676]
SIDS Alliance • Greater Houston Chapter [36546]
SIDS Alliance of Northern California [36456]
SIDS Foundation of Southern California • SIDS Alliance Affiliate [36457]
SIDS Mid-Atlantic [36552]
SIDS Network, Inc. [36460]
SIDS Network of Kansas, Inc. [36483]
SIDS Network of Kentucky, Inc. [36485]
SIDS of Pennsylvania [36535]
SIDS Resources [36536]
SIDS Resources, Inc. [36501]
SIEDA Substance Abuse Services • Chariton Office [43246]
Siemsen Dialysis Facility • Liberty Dialysis [23852]
Siena/Francis House [45803]
Siena Residence [31239]
Sierra Council on Alcoholism and
    Drug Depend/South Placer Res Treatment Prog [39623]
    Drug Dependence [39624]
    Drug Dependence Roseville Service Center [40475]
Sierra Council on Alcoholism and Drug • Dependence [40000]
Sierra County Human Services • Alcohol and Drug Department [40184]
Sierra Family Health Center [6946]
Sierra Family Services
    Roseville [40476]
    Tahoe [40841]
Sierra Hospice [18902]
Sierra Medical Center • Cancer Program [5984]
Sierra Nevada Memorial Hospital [13067]
    Cancer Center [4783]
Sierra Providence Physical Rehabilitation Hospital [4458]
Sierra Pulmonary and Sleep Consultants • Sleep Disorders Center [37321]
Sierra Recovery Center • Vitality Unlimited [40809]
Sierra Rehabilitation Services [1190]
Sierra Rose Dialysis Center • DaVita [25384]
Sierra Speech and Language Group [2872]
Sierra Tribal Consortium Inc • Turtle Lodge Recovery Home [39866]
Sierra Tucson [10908]
Sierra Tucson Inc [39512]
Sierra Tucson, Inc. [28221]
Sierra Tucson Pain Management Program [35293]
Sierra View District Hospital Dialysis Center [22888]
Sierra Vista [7832]
Sierra Vista Children's Center [34001]
Sierra Vista Community Based Outpatient Clininc [3877]
Sierra Vista Dialysis • DaVita [22500]
Sierra Vista Hospital [33181], [40506]
    Counseling Center [46318]
Sierra Vista Regional Health Center [12823]
Sievers Sports Medicine • Eastern Medical Associates [38774]
SightLife [35261]
Sigma Center for Counseling [41711]
Sigma House [45652]
Sigma House/DOC [45653]
Signature Health [47884]
Signature Healthcare Brockton Hospital [5326]
Signature Home Health Care [14145]
Signature Hospice--Beaverton [20989]
Signature Hospice-Eugene [20999]
Signature Hospice-Tigard [21036]
Signature Hospice-Wilsonville [21039]
Signs of Communication [972]

Sigourney House • Community Healthlink, Inc. [30490]
Sikeston Jaycee Regional Dialysis Center [25290]
Sikora Center Inc [45953]
Silas Home Care Services [15742]
Silence Speaks [8861]
Siletz Tribal • Alcohol and Drug Program [48216]
Silo Mision Cristiana Inc [48838]
Silva Clinic [3489]
Silver Age Home Health Care Agency Inc. [13152]
Silver City Dialysis • Dialysis Clinic, Inc. [25563]
Silver Creek Dialysis [25161]
Silver Cross Hospital [24013]
    Cancer Program [5114]
    Chemical Dependency Unit [42722]
Silver Cross Renal Center Morris [24046]
Silver Cross Renal Center West [24014]
Silver Dialysis--Cherry Hill • Fresenius Medical Care [25417]
Silver Hill Hospital [33255]
Silver Lake Support Services Inc • Chemical Dependence Outpatient Clinic [47101]
Silver Leaf [45683]
Silver Lightning Home Health Care, LLC [14274]
Silver Lining Public Relations and Community Resources [13153]
Silver Spring Health and Rehabilitation Center [3667]
Silver Spring Vet Center [51979]
Silver Springs Martin Luther School [34423]
Silver Springs Mental Health Center [31046]
Silver Years Home Health Services [14327]
Silverado Hospice of Houston [21571]
Silverado Hospice-Houston [21490]
Silverado Hospice of San Diego [19020]
Silverado Hospice-San Juan Capistrano [19030]
Silverado Hospice--Simi Valley [19048]
Silverado Hospice of Utah-Salt Lake City [21652]
Silverage Home Health Care Services, Inc. [17932]
Silverleaf Hospice [19345]
Silverman and Associates Inc [45898]
Silverton Dialysis & Home Training • DaVita [26050]
Simi Dialysis Center LLC [23014]
Simi Valley Hospital [1322]
    Cancer Services [4854]
    Child Development Center [7829]
Simi Valley Hospital and Health Care Services [13357]
Simi Valley Mental Health Clinic • Ventura County Mental Health Center [28819]
Simi Valley Unified School District Hearing Impaired Program [305]
Simmerman Hearing and Speech Associates [3653]
Simone Physical Medicine [38169]
Simple Choice LLC [43398]
Simply Speaking Speech and Language Center [2994]
Sims Counseling PC [44764]
Sims/Kemper Clinical Counseling and Recovery Services [43467]
Sinai--Grace Audiology [2577]
Sinai-Grace Hospital • Sleep Disorders Center [37196]
Sinai Hospital of Baltimore • Center for Pain Management and Rehabilitation [35650]
Sinai Hospital • Baltimore Crisis Line [50969]
Sinai Hospital of Baltimore
    Lapidus Cancer Institute [5290]
    Sinai Rehabilitation Center [4124]
Sinai Hospital
    Pain Center [35484]
    Sleep Disorders Center [37109]
Sinclair Community College • Office of Disability Services [655]
Singing River Dialysis • DaVita • Dialysis Center [25154]
Singing River Hospital System • Regional Cancer Center [5433]
Singing River Services • Region 14 [45378]
Singing Trees Recovery Center [39879]
Singleton Housing Project Inc [40156]
Sinnissippi Centers Inc [42791], [42832], [42879], [42926]
    All Alcohol/Substance Abuse Progs on Site [42629]
Sioux City Veterans Affairs Clinic [29894]
Sioux Falls Treatment Center LLC [49023]
Sioux Falls VAMC [49024]

Williamsville [37437]
Sleep Medicine Services of Western Massachusetts, LLC [37135]
Sleep Medicine Specialists--Eastern Parkway, Louisville • Sleep Disorders Center [37051]
Sleep Medicine Specialists--Greenwood Road, Louisville [37052]
Sleep Medicine West Virginia, Inc./dba Charleston Sleep Solutions [37957]
Sleep On Call, Inc. [16240]
Sleep Partners of Acadiana [37081]
Sleep and Pulmonary Care Center [36603]
Sleep Resolutions • Sleep Disorders Center [37006]
Sleep Solutions [37785]
Sleep Solutions of Lafayette • Sleep Disorders Center [37082]
Sleep Solutions of Mississippi • Sleep Disorders Center [37263]
Sleep Solutions of New Iberia [37083]
Sleep Solutions of Smithtown [37438]
Sleep Source Kentucky [37053]
Sleep Specialty Center [36861]
Sleep Therapy and Research Center [37855]
Sleep Unlimited, Inc.--Cordova [37786]
Sleep Unlimited, Inc.--Corinth [37264]
Sleep Unlimited, Inc.--Southaven [37265]
Sleep Wake Disorder Center [36816]
Sleep Well Centers--Ann Arbor [37203]
Sleep Well Centers, LLC--Twinsburg [37580]
Sleep Well Centers--Willoughby Hills • Sleep Disorders Center [37581]
Sleep Wellness Center of Pottstown [37699]
Sleep Wellness Institute [37984]
SleepCare Diagnostics, Eastgate [37582]
Sleepcare Diagnostics, Inc., Mason • Sleep Disorders Center [37583]
Sleepcare Diagnostics, Mason [37584]
Sleepcare Diagnostics--Sarasota • Sleep Disorders Center [36817]
SleepCare Diagnostics--West [37585]
SleepCare • Mid-State Medical Center [36753]
SleepMed [37856]
SleepMed of Central Georgia [36862]
SleepMed of Niles [36933]
SleepMed of South Carolina [37740]
SleepMed of West Columbia [37741]
Sleepwell Center [36734]
Sleepwell Partners LLC • Sleep Disorders Center [37874]
SleepWise Sleep and Behavioral Medicine Center [36701]
Sleepworks, Inc. [37084]
Slidell Addictive Disorder Clinic • FPHSA/ADS [43903]
Slidell Memorial Hospital [2343], [15369]
Slidell Memorial Hospital and Medical Center Regional Cancer Center [5265]
    Sleep Disorder Lab [37085]
Slidell Veterans Affairs Outpatient Clinic [30175]
Slidell/Youth Serv/Bureau of • Saint Tammany [43904]
Slife Treatment Group Home [34290]
SLV Family and Addiction Counseling [40979]
Small Steps [1621]
SMART Care Link Inc. [13243]
SMART Rehabilitation [38957]
SMDC Cancer Center [5406]
SMDC Hospice & Palliative Care-Duluth/Superior Hospice [20157]
SMH Care 1 Corporation [12965]
Smith Assessment and Treatment Service • Incorporated [47425]
Smith Counseling Centers [44670]
Smith House/Villa De Fidelis V [8722]
Smith Phayer Hospice House • Hospice of the Carolina Foothills [21256]
Smithfield Kidney Center • Fresenius Medical Care [25868]
SMKC Biloxi Home Dialysis • Fresenius Medical Care [25103]
SMOC
    Sage House [44473]
    Serenity House [44487]
SMOC/South Middlesex Opport Council • Behavioral Health Services [44474]
Smokey Mountain Dialysis • DaVita [25917]
Smokie Mountain Dialysis Center [26853]

Smoky Hill Foundation for Chemical Dep [43359], [43417]
Smoky Mountain Home Health & Hospice, Inc. • Corporate Office [21362]
Smoky Mountain Home Health & Hospice-Morristown [21353]
Smouse Opportunity School [8014]
Smyrna Pulmonary and Sleep Associates • Sleep Center [37787]
Smyth County Community Hospital [18327]
    Audiology Department [3595]
Snellville Dialysis Center [23791]
SNI Home Care, Inc. [17371]
Snohomish County Center for Battered Women [10620]
Snohomish County Mental Health Services • Crisis Intervention and Referral • Care Crisis Response Services [51440]
Snoqualmie Ridge Kidney Center • Northwest Kidney Centers [27647]
Snow Sleep Center PC [36604]
Snowline Hospice of El Dorado County, Inc. [18917]
Snyder Charleson Therapy Services [2860]
So Many Roads Recovery [48082]
So Others Might Eat Inc [41550]
SOAR [48564]
Sobaks Home Medical [15768]
Sober Living By The Sea [40264], [40265]
    Sunrise Recovery Ranch [40465]
Sober Roads Inc [39804]
SOBOBA [40648]
Sobriety First [45296]
Sobriety House Inc [41145], [44765]
    Phoenix Concept [41146]
    Stepping Stone [41147]
Sobriety Through Outpatient Inc [48565]
Sobriety Works [39611]
Social Advocates for Youth • Runaway and Home-less Youth Program [35843]
Social Model Recovery Systems
    River Community [39625]
    River Community Covina [39765]
Social Science Services Inc
    Cedar House Rehabilitation Center [39661]
    Maple House [39662]
Social Solutions Inc [41934]
Social Strides Speech, Language and Social Therapies [1241]
Social Treatment Opportunity Programs [49875], [50180], [50181]
Social Treatment Opportunity Programs II Inc • Shelton [50151]
Social Treatment Opportunity Programs
    Puyallup [50075]
    Tacoma [50219]
Society for Rehabilitation [8423]
Socorro General Hospital Home Health Care & Hospice [16330]
Socorro Mental Health Inc [46312]
SODAT Delaware Inc [41523]
SODAT of New Jersey Inc [46075], [46156], [46224]
SOFHA Sleep Center [37788]
Soft Landing Interventions [42827]
Soft Touch Medical, LLC [14551]
Softcare Home Health Services [14148]
Soifer Center for Learning and Child Development [3145]
Sojourn House Inc [42679], [42681]
Sojourn Services for Battered Women and Their Children [8907]
Sojourn Shelter and Service [9250]
Sojourner Adolescent Services • Residential [47771]
Sojourner Center [8719]
Sojourner Home [47772]
    Herland Family Center [47773]
Sojourner House [48607]
Sojourner House, Inc.--Providence [10337]
Sojourner House--Youngstown [10185]
Sojourner Project, Inc. [9602]
Sojourner Recovery Services [47774]
Sojourner Recovery Services Inc [47800]
Sojourner Recovery Services • Opiate Treatment [47667]
Sojourner Truth House, Inc. [10724]
Sojourners Care Network • Runaway and Homeless Youth Program [36150]
Sokaogan Chippewa Tribe [10696]
Sol Stone Center [11168]

Solace • Center for the Treatment of Eating Disorders [11273]
Solace Counseling Assoicates PLLC [49297]
Solace Counseling Services [41244]
Solace Health Care [19465]
SolAmor Hospice--Albuquerque [20523]
SolAmor Hospice-Allegiance Hospice-South Portland [19901]
Solamor Hospice--Bourne [19948]
Solamor Hospice--Colorado Springs [19095]
SolAmor Hospice-Manchester [20443]
Solamor Hospice-Middleton [19978]
SolAmor Hospice--Milford [19152]
Solamor Hospice--Muskogee [20946]
Solamor Hospice-North Hampton [20452]
Solamor Hospice-Oklahoma City [20965]
Solamor Hospice-Shrewsbury [20000]
Solamor Hospice-Toms River [20505]
Solano County Economic Opportunity Council • Domestic Violence Program [8915]
Solano County Mental Health Children's Mental Health Services [28495]
Solara Hospice & Palliative Care [19049]
Solari Hospice Care [20422]
Solaris Hospice-Abilene [21377]
Solaris Hospice-Charleston • National HealthCare Corporation [21259]
Solaris Hospice-Graham [21473]
Solaris Hospice-Greenville • National HealthCare Corporation [21244]
Solaris Hospice Inc-Bowie [21406]
Solaris Hospice Inc-Breckenridge [21407]
Solaris Hospice Inc-Mineral Wells [21533]
Solaris Hospice Inc-Olney [21541]
Solaris Hospice Inc-Springtown [21568]
Solaris Hospice Inc-Wichita Falls [21593]
Solaris Hospice, Inc. [21411], [21443]
Solaris Hospice Myrtle Beach • National HealthCare Corporation [21228]
Solaris Hospice-West Columbia • National Health-Care Corporation [21287]
Soledad Dialysis Center • DaVita [23015]
Soledad Enrichment Action Program • Atlantic Recovery Services [40157]
Solid Foundation
    Keller House [40306]
    Mandela II [40307]
Solid Ground [10653]
Solidarity Fellowship Inc • Mission House [40683]
Solita Road Group Home [34010]
Solleys Place [42667]
Solomon Therapeutics and Resource Specialists [2953]
Solomon Valley Hospice [19746]
Solution for Life [42301]
The Solutions Alcohol and Drug • Recovery Founda-tion [40158]
Solutions Behavioral Healthcare • Consultants [41747]
Solutions Behavioral Healthcare Inc [47812]
Solutions Center [10703]
Solutions Counseling and • Consultation Services PC [48295]
Solutions Counseling & Consultation Services [31994]
Solutions Counseling and DUI Services [42921]
Solutions Counseling Services LLC [43548], [43742]
Solutions FPC Inc [39705]
Solutions Home Health [13675]
Solutions for Life [50591]
Solutions for Life, Inc. [33044]
Solutions for Life • Substance Free Solutions [50581]
Solutions Outpatient Services [49298]
Solutions for Recovery [40670]
Solutions to Recovery [44968], [44969], [44970], [44971]
Solutions Recovery Inc [45850]
Solutions of Savannah [49182]
Solvay Hospice House [20158]
Someplace Safe--Fergus Falls [9597]
Someplace Safe--Warren [10181]
Somerset Counseling Center [50091]
Somerset County Behavioral Health [44390]
Somerset Dialysis Center • DaVita [26584]
Somerset Home for Temporarily Displaced Children • Runaway and Homeless Youth Program [36082]

Somerset Medical Center, Hillsborough • Sleep for Life [37364]
Somerset Medical Center • Steeplechase Cancer Center [5541]
Somerset Treatment Services [46172]
Somersworth Veterans Affairs Clinic [31095]
Somerville Dialysis • DaVita [26925]
Somerville Mental Health Association [30462]
Something 2 Talk About Inc. [2437]
SomiTech Inc. Sleep Disorders Center, Lee's Summit [37290]
SomiTech Inc. Sleep Disorders Center, Northland [37291]
Sommer Group • Eating Disorders Program [11199]
Sommer Sports Chiropractic [38144]
SomniTech Inc. Sleep Disorders Center [36985]
somniTech, Inc. • Sleep Disorders Center [37007]
Somnos Sleep Disorders Center [37318]
Somnus Sleep Clinic of Central Mississippi [37266]
Somos Familia [9876]
Somos Familia San Antonio Mental Health Services [28403]
Sonno Sleep Center East [37857]
Sonno Sleep Center of New Mexico [37372]
Sonoma Cnty Indian Health Project Inc • Behavioral Health Department [40787]
Sonoma Developmental Center [7776]
Sonoma Valley Community Health Center [6368]
Sonoma Valley Health Care District [13359]
Sonora Behavioral Health Hospital [28207], [39513]
Sonora Hearing Care [992]
Sonora Regional Home Health & Hospice of the Sierra [19052]
Sonora Regional Medical Center [13360]
Sonoran Sports and Family Medicine [38028]
Sooner Dialysis Center--Norman • Fresenius Medical Care [26272]
Sooner Dialysis--Lawton • Liberty Dialysis [26263]
Sooner Hospice [20966]
Sor Juana Ines Services for Abused Women [8899]
SORCC Grants Pass West [17193]
Sorensons Ranch School Inc [49618]
Soroptimist House of Hope Inc [39643], [39783]
SOS Counseling [42981]
SOS Counseling Services • Substance Abuse Treatment Services [44822]
SOS Crisis Center [51032]
SOS, Inc. [9355]
SOS Shelter, Inc. [9921]
SOSPT, Inc. • Spine Orthopaedic Sport Physical Therapy [38573]
Souhegan Home and Hospice Care [16175]
Soujourner Recovery Services • Adult Services [47775]
Soulistic Hospice [18824]
Sound Alternatives [28082], [50631]
Sound Alternatives Behavioral • Health Clinic [39322]
Sound aSleep • Sleep Diagnostic Lab [37204]
Sound Center [2089]
Sound Community Services, Inc. [29025]
Sound Counseling Inc [50076]
Sound Hearing Audiology [3039]
Sound Mental Health [49886], [51467]
Sound Mental Health--Auburn Way N [32803]
Sound Mental Health Counseling Services [32849]
Sound Mental Health • Counseling Services - Northgate [50135]
Sound Mental Health--S Center Boulevard [32876]
Sound Mental Health--Seattle [32859]
Sound Practices LLC [1750]
Sound Shore Dialysis Center • Renal Research Institute [25712]
Sound Shore Medical Center of Westchester Alcoholism Acute Care Program [46802]
Goldstein Cancer Center [5593]
Sound Sleep Centers--Burnsville [37234]
Sound Sleep Centers--Maple Grove [37235]
Sound Sleep Centers--Willmar [37236]
Sound Sleep Health--Kirkland [37936]
Sound Sleep Health--Seattle [37937]
Sound Solutions Inc. • Audiology and Hearing Aid Center [1011]
Soundingboard Services [1849]
Soundview Dialysis Center • DaVita [25599]
Soundview Healthcare Network [7012]
Source One Rehabilitation [35711], [35712]
South Albany Medical Center [6579]

South Anthony Dialysis Center • Diversified Specialty Institutes [24146]
South Antonio Dialysis Center • DaVita [27343]
South Arkansas Regional Health Center [28263]
Camden Division [28251]
Community Support Program [28264]
El Dorado Connections [28265]
Hope House [28266]
Magnolia Division [28311]
Recovery Center [28267]
South Arlington Dialysis Center [26945]
South Asian Women's Empowerment and Resource Alliance [10251]
South Atlanta Kidney Care Dialysis Facility LLC [23775]
South Augusta Dialysis Center • Renal Advantage Inc. [23616]
South Austin Dialysis • DaVita [26958]
South Baldwin Regional Medical Center [12666]
South Barrington Dialysis Center • American Renal Associates [24087]
South Bay Alcoholism Services • Building Blocks [39692]
South Bay Community Services
Casa Segura [8803]
Runaway and Homeless Youth Program [35844]
South Bay Drug Abuse Coalition [40856]
South Bay Early Intervention [30352]
South Bay Guidance Center [28442]
South Bay Home Health Care [13396]
South Bay Mental Health Center [30325]
South Bay Mental Health Services [28526]
South Bay Sports Medicine Physical Therapy [38150]
South Beach Acute Day Treatment Program • Sheepshead Bay Day Hospital [33684]
South Beach Addiction Treatment Center • Addiction Inpatient Rehab Program [47102]
South Beach Clinic [31980]
South Beach Dialysis • DaVita [23410]
South Beach Psychiatric Center [33725]
Baltic Street Outpatient Clinic & Day Hospital [33685]
Bensonhurst Outpatient Clinic & Day Hospital [33686]
South Beach Psychiatric Center--Coney Island • Sheepshead Bay Day Hospital [33687]
South Beach Psychiatric Center • Fort Hamilton Outpatient Clinic [33688]
South Beach Psychiatric Center--Heights • Heights Hill Outpatient Clinic [33689]
South Bend Orthopedics Sports Medicine and Rehabilitation [38448]
South Bend Veterans Affairs Clinic [29817]
South Boston Community Health Center [6808]
South Broad Street Counseling Services [46194]
South Broad Street Dialysis • DaVita [26536]
South Bronx Dialysis Center • DaVita [25600]
South Bronx Mental Health Council Inc • CMHC Alcoholism Outpatient Clinic [46455]
South Bronx Mental Health Council, Inc.
Adult Outpatient Services [31254]
Community Mental Health Center [31255]
Community Support Systems [31256]
Triple Jeopardy Center [31257]
South Brooklyn Medical Admin Services • MMTP Clinic [46533]
South Brooklyn Nephrology Center • DaVita • Dialysis Facility [25629]
South Broward Artificial Kidney Center • DaVita [23328]
South Broward Home Care, Inc. [14328]
South Brunswick Dialysis • DaVita [23629]
South Carolina Department of Health and Environment • Division of Perinatal Systems/MCH • SIDS Information and Counseling Program [36540]
South Carolina Primary Health Care Association [7228]
South Carolina School for the Deaf and Blind [3409]
South Carolina School for the Deaf and the Blind [3735]
South Carolina School for the Deaf and Blind • Midlands Regional Outreach Center [727]
South Carolina School for the Deaf and Blind/Spartanburg Technical College • Cooperative Program for Deaf/Hard of Hearing • Adult Postsecondary Program [736]
South Carolina Sleep Medicine [37742]

South Carolina Sports Medicine and Orthopaedic Center [39006]
South Carolina State Hospital/William S. Hall Psychiatric Institute [33834]
South Carolina State Library • Talking Book Services [3836]
South Central Alabama Community Mental Health Center
Andalusia Manor [27825]
Coffee County Training Center [27908]
Covington County Day Treatment [27826]
Early Intervention Program [27827]
South Central Alabama Community Mental Health Clinic • Covington Substance Abuse/Prevention [27828]
South Central Alabama Genetics and Birth Defects Clinic [12118]
South Central Area Special Education Cooperative [428]
South Central Behavioral Services
Hastings Clinic [45745]
Holdrege Clinic [45746]
South Central Behavioral Services, Inc. [30992], [30993]
ACT Program [30987]
Hastings Office [30988]
Rehabilitation Services [30989]
Unity House [30994]
South Central Behavioral Services • Kearney Clinic [45748]
South Central BOCES [326]
South Central Community Services, Inc. [29597]
South Central Counseling Center [50628]
South Central Family Health Center [6321]
South Central Fulton Community Mental Health Center [29355]
South Central Fulton Mental Health Center [7911]
South Central Health and Rehabilitation Program--Los Angeles [28612]
South Central Health and Rehabilitation Program (SHARP)--Lynwood [28617]
South Central Human Relations [30707]
South Central Human Relations Center [30690]
South Central Human Relations • Dual Recovery Program [45256]
South Central Human Service Center [51191]
Chemical Dependency Program [47588]
South Central Kansas Foundation on Chemical Dependency Inc [43448]
South Central Mental Health [29906]
South Central Mental Health Counseling Center--Andover [50910]
South Central Mental Health Counseling Center--Augusta [50912]
South Central Mental Health Counseling Center--El Dorado [50914]
South Central Mental Health • Counseling Center Inc [43317], [43321], [43339]
South Central Montana Regional Mental Health Center • Addiction Services Program [45684]
South Central Primary Care Center [6599]
South Central Regional Medical Center [30780], [45400]
Sleep Disorders Center [37267]
South Central Vet Center [52104]
South Central Veterans Affairs Clinic [30719]
South Charlotte Clinical Associates [11176]
South Chico Dialysis Center • DaVita [22630]
South Coast Counseling Inc [39754]
South Coast Counseling and Psych Services [39755]
South Coast Hospice [20995]
South Coast Medical Center [10990], [13094]
South Coast Medical Center--Behavioral Health [28554]
South Columbia Dialysis • Fresenius Medical Care [26702]
South Community Inc [47745]
South County Clinic [28903]
South County Creative Living Center [28504]
South County Dialysis Center & At Home • DaVita [25283]
South County Dialysis Center • Fresenius Medical Care [24810]
South County Habilitation Center [8217]
South County Hospital
Cancer Program [5895]
Sleep Disorders Laboratory [37729]

South County Mental Health Center [29150]
South County Orthopedics and Sports Medicine [38998]
South County Pediatric Speech [1183]
South County Psychotherapy • Athletic Program [38092]
South County Speech and Language Center Inc. [3388]
South County Surgical Supply [17545]
South Dade Health Center [6476]
South Dakota Braille and Talking Book Library [3837]
South Dakota Department of Education • Program for Deaf--Blind Children and Youth [743]
South Dakota Department of Health • South Dakota Infant Loss Center [36541]
South Dakota Developmental Center [8507]
South Dakota Human Services Center
  Gateway Chem Dependency Treatment Center [49036]
  State Psychiatric Hospital [33837]
South Dakota Lions Eye Bank [35204]
South Dakota School for the Blind and Visually Impaired [3736]
South Dakota School for the Deaf [745]
South Denver Anesthesiologists • Pain Clinic [35354]
South Denver Dialysis • DaVita [23115]
South Denver Valley Hope Outpatient [41044]
South East Alcohol and • Drug Abuse Center [42583]
South East Texas Council on A/D Abuse • Unity Treatment Center [49240]
South East Texas Management Network
  Jefferson County COADA Right Choice [49241]
  Land Manor Inc/Adams House Adol Prog [49242]
  Land Manor Inc/Franklin South [49243]
  Spindletop MH/MR Services [49244], [49495], [49540]
  Spindletop MH/MR Services/Tejas [49475]
South End Community Health Center [30347]
South Florida Evaluation and Treatment Center [33301]
South Florida Home Care Services [14219]
South Florida Home Health Care, Inc. [14149]
South Florida Institute for Reproductive Medicine--Miami [22006]
South Florida Institute for Reproductive Medicine--Naples [22007]
South Florida Orthopaedics and Sports Medicine • Center for Neurology [38273]
South Florida Orthopaedics & SportsMedicine [38289]
South Florida Provider [41799]
South Florida Pulmonary Care, Inc. [14220]
South Florida State Hospital [33337]
South Fulton Dialysis • DaVita [23606]
South Fulton Medical Center • Oncology Services [5024]
South Gaston Dialysis • Fresenius Medical Care [25871]
South Georgia Medical Center • Pearlman Comprehensive Cancer Center [5043]
South Georgia Regional Library • Valdosta Talking Book Center [3779]
South Georgia Treatment [42110]
South Hampton Hospital [25676]
South Harvard Medical [17170]
South Haven Community Hospital [15796]
South Hayward Dialysis Center • DaVita [22723]
South Henry Dialysis Center [23755]
South Hill Dialysis • DaVita • Dialysis Facility [24447]
South Jersey Drug Treatment Center [45945]
South Jersey Fertility Center--Egg Harbor Township [22168]
South Jersey Fertility Center--Forked River [22169]
South Jersey Fertility Center--Marlton [22170]
South Jersey Healthcare HomeCare [16263]
South Jersey Healthcare Hospice • Inpatient Center [20461]
South Jersey Healthcare • Scarpa Regional Cancer Pavillion [5547]
South Jersey Speech Pathology Services [2890]
South Kendall Home Care, Inc. [14150]
South Laburnum Dialysis • American Renal Associates [27555]

South Lake Family Health Center [6468]
South Lake Home Health [13619]
South Lake Tahoe Outpatient Clinic [28820]
South Lake Tahoe Women's Center [8913]
South Las Vegas Dialysis • DaVita [25372]
South Lincoln Dialysis • DaVita [25331]
South Main Street Group Home [32631]
South of Market Mental Health Clinic [28771]
South Meadows Dialysis Center • DaVita [25385]
South Metro Speech Services LLC [2746]
South Miami Audiology Consultants [1758]
South Miami Hospital [14151]
  Addiction Treatment Program [41800]
  Cancer Program [4968]
  Child Development Center [1662]
South Middlesex Opportunity Council [30384]
  Rhodes to Recovery [44513]
South Mississippi Kidney Center North Gulfport • Fresenius Medical Care • South Mississippi Kidney Center • Dialysis Facility [25127]
South Mississippi Regional Center [8188]
South Mississippi State Hospital [33625]
South Mountain Dialysis • Liberty Dialysis [27429]
South Nassau Communities Hospital [3088]
  Cancer Care Center [5604]
  Center for Sleep Medicine [37439]
South Nassau Community Hospital • Acute Dialysis Unit [25744]
South Nassau Outpatient Dialysis Center [25745]
South Neighborhood Family Service Center [31029]
South Norwalk Dialysis • DaVita [23176]
South Oak Cliff Dialysis Center • Fresenius Medical Care [27038]
South Oaks Hospital [33674]
South Ogden Veterans Affairs Clinic [32598]
South Oregon Regional Services for Low Income Disabled [684]
South Peninsula Haven House [8662]
South Peninsula Mental Health Association, Inc. [28095]
South Philadelphia Dialysis Center • DaVita [26537]
South Plains Educational Cooperative [804]
South Plains Rural Health Services [7299]
South Plains Rural Health Services, Inc. • Levelland Primary Health Clinic [7300]
South Platte Community Counseling [41318]
South Pointe Hospital • Cancer Program [5758]
South Queens Dialysis Center • Renal Research Institute [25690]
South Rainbow Dialysis • Fresenius Medical Care [25373]
South Ranch, Marshall [30872]
South Riding Speech Therapy Inc. [3576]
South Seminole Hospital [1638]
South Shore Child Guidance Center • CARE [46644]
South Shore Dialysis & At Home • DaVita [27225]
South Shore Dialysis Center [25680]
South Shore Dialysis Center II [25577]
South Shore Home Health Services, Inc. [16581]
South Shore Hospital
  Chemical Dependency [42584]
  Medical Detox Services [42585]
  Oncology Program [5355]
South Shore Mental Health [30452]
South Shore Mental Health--Bayview Associates [30349]
South Shore Mental Health Cape Services [30399]
South Shore Mental Health Center [30453]
South Shore Mental Health Center-Addictions Program [32142]
South Shore Mental Health Center
  Community Support Program [30454]
  Discovery Day/Evening Treatment Program [30455]
South Shore Mental Health Center, Inc. [32178]
South Shore Mental Health Centers [8143]
South Shore Mental Health Centers Inc • Addictions Program [48844]
South Shore Mental Health • Quitting Time [44548]
South Shore Neurologic Associates, PC • Comprehensive Multiple Sclerosis Care Center [34652]
South Shore Recovery Home [44549]
South Shore Sleep Diagnostics [37136], [37137]
South Shore Speech [2558]
South Shore Visiting Nurse and Health Services [15478]

South Shore Women's Center [9499]
South Side Community Health Center [7098]
South Sound Clinic of Evergreen Treatment Services [50042]
South Street Community Health Center [6809]
South Suburban Council on Alcoholism and Substance Abuse [42636]
South Suburban Dialysis Facility • Fresenius Medical Care [24795]
South Suburban Family Shelter, Inc. [9234]
South Suburban YWCA [9216]
South Texas Acute Dialysis Center • Diversified Specialty Institutes [27011]
South Texas Behavioral Health Center [49316]
South Texas Blood and Tissue Center [35244]
South Texas Comprehensive Hemophilia Center • Christus Santa Rosa Children's Hospital [12601]
South Texas Council on Alcohol/Drug Abuse [49356], [49441], [49501], [49583], [49592]
South Texas Dialysis Center • Fresenius Medical Care [27264]
South Texas Health Care [18073]
South Texas Rehabilitation Hospital [3474]
South Texas Rural Health Services Inc
  Substance Abuse Program [49276]
  Uvalde Unit [49565]
South Texas Rural Health Services, Inc./Presidio County Health Services [7281]
South Texas Subst Abuse Recovery Services [49502]
  (STSARS) [49272]
South Texas Transplant Center [27253]
South Texas Veterans Affairs Health Care System • Kerrville Division [51660]
South Texas Veterans Affairs Healthcare System • Frank M. Tejeda Outpatient Clinic • PTSD Clinical Team [51829]
South Texas Veterans Health Care System [18150]
  Audie L. Murphy Memorial Veterans Hospital • Spinal Cord Injury Service [4459]
  Audie Murphy Veterans Affairs Hospital [51661]
South Texas Veterans Health Care System - HBPC [18151]
South Texas Veterans Healthcare System • Villa Serena [49530]
South Towne Square Dialysis Clinic • Renal Advantage Inc. [25284]
South Tucson Dialysis • Fresenius Medical Care [22521]
South Valley Dialysis Center [27428]
South Valley Dialysis • DaVita [22679]
South Valley Sanctuary [10536]
South Washington Street Physical Therapy [39150]
South Western Indiana Mental Health Center, Inc. • Chestnut Home [29719]
South Wind Hospice [19774]
South Windsor Public Schools [332]
Southampton Memorial Hospice [21695]
Southbay Physical and Industrial Rehabilitation [38109]
Southbury Training School [7856]
Southcentral Foundation
  Dena A Coy [39315]
  Runaway and Homeless Youth Program [35791]
Southcoast Audiology Services [2505]
Southcoast Hospice [19959]
Southcoast Hospital Group
  Charlton Memorial Hospital [2478]
  Saint Luke's Hospital [2500]
Southcoast Hospitals Group [5333], [15492]
SouthCoast Rehab Associates [1062]
Southcross Dialysis Center • DaVita [27344]
Southeast Addictions Institute and • Learning Center [47266]
Southeast AK Regional • Health Consortium/Ravens Way [39353]
Southeast Alabama Home Care [12655], [12658]
Southeast Alabama Medical Center [12652]
  Cancer Program [4732]
  Dothan Sleep Disorders Center [36605]
  Enterprise Sleep Clinic [36606]
Southeast Alabama Rural Health Assoc., Inc. [6201]
Southeast Alaska Regional Health [28102]
Southeast Arkansas Behavioral Healthcare
  Star City Clinic [28356]
  Stuttgart Clinic [28357]
Southeast Arkansas Human Development Center [7763]

Southeast Colorado Hospital [19127]
Southeast Counseling Services [31742]
Southeast County Mental Health Center [28759]
Southeast Family Center • DC Department of Mental Health [29101]
Southeast Family Health Care Center [6446]
Southeast Georgia Regional Medical Center [35415] Cancer Program [5016]
Southeast Georgia Treatment Center LLC [42094]
Southeast Hospice [20287]
Southeast Hospice Network [18734]
Southeast Hospice Network, LLC--Marshall County [18671]
Southeast Hospice Network-Montgomery [18746]
Southeast Hospice Network-Pelham [18752]
Southeast Houston Dialysis Center [27174]
Southeast Human Service Center • Alcohol and Drug Abuse Unit [47576]
Southeast Inc [47730], [47731]
Southeast, Inc.--Carrollton [31678]
Southeast, Inc.--Columbus [31743]
Project Work [31744]
Southeast, Inc.--Hopedale [31779]
Southeast, Inc.--New Philadelphia [31820]
Southeast Island School District [222]
Southeast Kansas ESC [433]
Southeast Kansas Mental Health Center [43324], [43348], [43369]
Southeast Kansas Mental Health Center Alcohol and Drug Abuse Program [43353]
Southeast Kansas Mental Health Center • Pleasanton [43447]
Southeast Kansas Mental Health Services • Emergency Line [50918]
Southeast Kidney Center • Fresenius Medical Care [27175]
Southeast Kidney Disease Center • Dialysis Facility • Fresenius Medical Care [27345]
Southeast Lancaster Health Services, Inc. [7169]
Southeast Louisiana Hospital [33541]
Southeast Louisiana Veterans Health [43874]
Southeast Louisiana Veterans Health Care System [4067]
Southeast Louisiana Veterans Healthcare System • New Orleans Veterans Affairs Outpatient Clinic • PTSD Clinical Team [51741]
Southeast Lung and Critical Care Specialists • Southeast Sleep Lab Hardeeville [37743]
Southeast Mental Health Center Inc • Alcohol and Drug Abuse Program [49144]
Southeast Mental Health Center, Inc. [32357]
Orange Mound Location [32358]
Pauline Location [32359]
Summer Location [32360]
Southeast Mental Health Services [28919], [28952]
Southeast Michigan Kidney Center • Greenfield Health Systems [24840]
Southeast Mississippi Rural Health Initiative, Inc. • Minor Care Clinic [6882]
Southeast Missouri Behavioral Health [45470], [45503], [45583], [45586], [45589], [45655], [45666]
CSTAR [45590]
Houston Office [45499]
Park Hills [45584]
Rolla Office [45600]
Southeast Missouri Community Treatment [45471]
Southeast Missouri Family Violence Council • New Way Shelter [9662]
Southeast Missouri Hospital Home Health [15990]
Southeast Missouri Hospital
Outreach Clinic • Cystic Fibrosis Center [7588]
Regional Cancer Center [5438]
Sleep Diagnostic Center [37292]
Southeast Missouri Mental Health Center [33629]
Southeast Missouri (SEMO) Health Network [6913]
Southeast Missouri State University • Center for Speech and Hearing [2779]
Southeast Nassau Guidance Center [47077]
Drug Abuse Treatment Unit 1 [47160]
Southeast Oklahoma Services for Family Violence Intervention [10199]
Southeast Regional Pain Center [35416]
Southeast Regional Sleep Disorders Center--Easley [37744]
Southeast Regional Sleep Disorders Center--Greenville [37745]
Southeast Spouse Abuse Program [9407]

Southeast Texas Hospice [21542]
Southeast Texas RDSPD [773]
Southeast Tissue Alliance, Inc. [35006]
Southeast Tucson Community Based Outpatient Clinic [28222]
Southeast VA Health Care Clinic-Mesa, Arizona [3878]
Southeastern Alabama Genetics and Birth Defects Clinic • Wiregrass Rehabilitation/Children's Rehabilitation Service [12119]
Southeastern Arizona Behavioral Health Services, Inc.
Benson Office [28131]
Bisbee Clinic [28132]
Clifton Clinic [28139]
Douglas Clinic [28144]
Nogales Outpatient [28168]
Safford Outpatient [28195]
Southeastern AZ Behavior Health Services [39363], [39376], [39412], [39462], [39477], [39516]
Psychiatric Health Facility [39364]
Southeastern Behavioral Healthcare
Canton Office [32222]
Center House [32248]
Community Support Services [32249]
Judy House [32250]
Klondike House [32251]
Parker Office [32239]
Sioux Falls Office [32252]
Solar House [32253]
Solar House 2 [32254]
Southeastern Dialysis & At Home • DaVita [25974]
Southeastern Dialysis--Burgaw • DaVita [25823]
Southeastern Dialysis Center & At Home--Jacksonville • DaVita [25889]
Southeastern Dialysis DaVita • DaVita [25972]
Southeastern Dialysis--Elizabethtown • DaVita [25860]
Southeastern Dialysis Kenansville • DaVita [25892]
Southeastern Dialysis--Shallotte • DaVita [25946]
Southeastern Family Violence Center [10057]
Southeastern Fertility Center--Charleston [22245]
Southeastern Health Services of Pennsylvania, Inc.--Bristol [17266]
Southeastern Health Services of Pennsylvania, Inc.--Downingtown [17296]
Southeastern Health Services of Pennsylvania, Inc.--New Britain [17395]
Southeastern Health Services of Pennsylvania, Inc.--Telford [17493]
Southeastern Home Care [16845]
Southeastern Home Health Services • Lawndale Bldg. [17426]
Southeastern Home Oxygen Service, Inc. [14507]
Southeastern Hospice • Southeastern Region Medical Center [20700]
Southeastern IL Counseling Centers Inc
Alcohol Outpatient Services [42828]
Clay Family Counseling Center [42669]
Crawford Family Counseling Center [42877]
Lawrence Family Counseling Center [42744]
Wabash Family Counseling Center [42790]
Wayne Family Counseling Center [42668]
Southeastern Illinois Counseling Centers, Inc.--Albion [29555]
Southeastern Illinois Counseling Centers, Inc.--Flora [29621]
Southeastern Louisiana University [2317]
Southeastern Lung Care
Sleep Disorder Center of South Atlanta [36863]
Sleep Disorders Center, Decatur [36864]
Southeastern Massachusetts Dialysis Clinic [24762]
Fresenius Medical Care [24787]
Southeastern Mental Health Center • Wayne Dahl Transition House [32255]
Southeastern New Hampshire Services
AMCCC [45892]
Outpatient Services [45893]
Turning Point Halfway House [45894]
Southeastern New Mexico Kidney Center Inc. • Fresenius Medical Care • Dialysis Center [25559]
Southeastern Ohio Regional Medical Center [16861]
Cambridge Regional Cancer Center [5685]
Southeastern Oklahoma 211 Helpline [51239]
Southeastern Oklahoma Family Services [47924]
Southeastern Oklahoma • Social Services Inc [47955]
Southeastern Regional Medical Center • Gibson

Cancer Center [5650]
Southeastern Regional Medical Center Home Care Services [16750]
Southeastern Regional Mental Health Center [34364]
Southeastern Regional Mental Health, Developmental Disabilities and Substance Abuse Services [8385]
Southeastern Renal Dialysis--Fort Madison [24273]
Southeastern Renal Dialysis LC--Lee County • Dialysis Facility [24282]
Southeastern Renal Dialysis LC--Mount Pleasant [24289]
Southeastern Renal Dialysis LC--West Burlington [24309]
Southeastern Renal Dialysis,L.C.--Fairfield [24271]
Southeastern Virginia Training Center [8581]
Southeastern Youth/Family Services Inc • Noah House [50552]
Southern Adamsville Dialysis • DaVita [23607]
Southern Alberta Organ and Tissue Program [34921]
Southern Arizona Anesthesia Services • Pain Clinic [35294]
Southern Arizona VA Health Care System [12835]
Southern Arizona Veterans Affairs Health Care System [3879]
Multiple Sclerosis Center [34517]
Sierra Vista Community Based Outpatient Clinic [28202]
Southern Arizona Veterans Affairs Healthcare System • Yuma Community Based Outpatient Clinic [28229]
Southern Assured Home Health, LLC [17818], [18152]
Southern CA Alcohol and Drug Progs Inc [40385]
Angel Step II [39653]
Awakenings/Outpatient Program [40954]
Awakenings/Residential Treatment [40955], [40956]
Casa Libre [39650]
Foley House [40957]
Heritage House [39756]
Heritage House North [39597]
Heritage Village [39598]
La Casita for Women and Children [39787]
Paramount Counseling Services [40359]
Positive Steps [39788]
Youth and Family Services [39789]
Southern California reproductive Center--Lancaster [21938]
Southern California Coalition for Battered Women [8908]
Southern California Counseling Center [28613]
Southern California Pulmonary and Sleep Disorders Medical Center [36702]
Southern California Rehabilitation Services [3926]
Southern California Reproductive Center--Beverly Hills [21939]
Southern California Reproductive Center Medical Group [21940]
Southern California Reproductive Center--San Luis Obispo [21941]
Southern California Reproductive Center--Santa Monica [21942]
Southern California Reproductive Center--Valencia [21943]
Southern California Reproductive Center--Ventura [21944]
Southern California Sleep Disorders Specialists [36703]
Southern Christian Services • Runaway and Homeless Youth Program [36044]
Southern CO Comprehensive Court Services [41303]
Southern Colorado Comprehensive Court • A Better Choice Counseling [41038]
Southern Community Hospice Inc. • Community Hospice [19431]
Southern Connecticut State University • Center for Communication Disorders [1478]
Southern Consortium for Children • Runaway and Homeless Youth Program [36151]
Southern Cord [34917]
Southern Dominion Health Systems, Inc. [7372]
Southern Eye Bank [35060]
Southern Hearing Associates [924]
Southern Highlands Comm Mental Health Center Inc [50333], [50340]

Southern Highlands • Community Medical Health Center [50352]
Southern Highlands Community Mental Health Center--12th Street, Princeton [51495]
Southern Highlands Community Mental Health Center • Mental Health Council [32930]
Southern Highlands Community Mental Health Center--Mercer Street, Princeton • Crisis Respite Unit [51496]
Southern Highlands Community Mental Health Center--Mullens [32922]
    Mullens Clinic [51491]
Southern Highlands Community Mental Health Center • Welch Clinic [32942]
Southern Highlands Community Mental Health Center--Welch • Welch Clinic [51498]
Southern Highlands Mental Health Center--Princeton [32931]
Southern Hills Alcohol/Drug Ref Center [48996]
Southern Hills Counseling Center [29747], [43191]
Southern Hills Counseling Center Inc [43120], [43211]
    Orange County Services [43174]
Southern Hills Dialysis Center • DaVita [25374]
Southern Hills Medical Center • Cancer Center [5951]
Southern Hills Therapy Services [3260]
Southern Home Care Services: Stork Watch Program [17255]
Southern Home Health [15318], [18113]
Southern Home Health--Dequincy [15287]
Southern Home Medical Supply, LLC [12874]
Southern Homecare, Inc. [17914]
Southern Idaho Pain Institute [35424]
Southern IL Regional Social Services • (SIRSS) [42439]
Southern Illinois Healthcare Foundation [6677]
Southern Illinois Home Care & Hospice [14771]
Southern Illinois Region [403]
Southern Illinois Regional Social Service [29570]
Southern Illinois Regional Social Services [50834]
Southern Illinois Regional Social Services, Inc. • Runaway and Homeless Youth Program [35939]
Southern Illinois Surgical Appliance Co. [14955]
Southern Illinois University
    Down Syndrome Clinic [10795]
    School of Medicine
        Cystic Fibrosis Center [7535]
        Department of Pediatrics Clinical and Metabolic Genetics Division [12208]
Southern Indian Rehabilitation Hospital [4044]
Southern Indiana Rehab Hospital [38486]
Southern Indiana Resource Solutions [7981]
Southern Iowa Economic Development • Association/Substance Abuse Services [43295]
Southern Iowa Mental Health Center [29890]
Southern Jersey Family Medical Centers, Inc. [6973]
Southern Maine Medical Center [2352]
Southern Maine Medical Center--Biddeford • Visiting Nurses [15386]
Southern Maine Medical Center • Cancer Program [5270]
Southern Maine Medical Center--Kennebunk • Visiting Nurses [15393]
Southern Manhattan Dialysis Center • Fresenius Medical Care [25737]
Southern Maryland Hospital Center • Cancer Program [5297]
Southern Michigan Pain Consultants [35512]
Southern Nevada Adult Mental Health Services [33648]
Southern Nevada Child and Adolescent Mental Health Services [31034]
Southern Nevada Division of Child & Family Services [31035]
Southern New England Anesthesia and Pain Associates [35658]
Southern New Hampshire Medical Center [6963]
    Cancer Program [5500]
Southern New Hampshire Sports Medicine [38704]
Southern New Jersey AIDS Clinical Trials • Community Program for Clinical Research on AIDS [58]
Southern New Mexico Human Development [46247]
Southern Ocean County Hospital • Cancer Program [5521]
Southern Ocean Hospice [20478]
Southern Ohio Medical Center [17022]
    Cancer Care Program [5746]

LIFE Center [38889]
Southern Ohio Task Force on Domestic Violence, Inc. • Southern Ohio Shelter [10168]
Southern OK Treatment Services Inc [47998]
Southern Oklahoma Treatment Services [47956]
    DBA Ardmore [47911]
Southern Oregon Adolescent Study and Treatment Center [34395]
Southern Oregon Child Study & Treatment Center [31928]
Southern Orthopedic Specialists [38274], [38329]
Southern Pines Dialysis Center • DaVita [25953]
Southern Plains Behavioral Health Services--Gregory [32226]
Southern Plains Behavioral Health Services--Mission [32235]
Southern Plains Behavioral Health Services--Winner [32263]
Southern Quality Home Health Care [15300]
Southern Region Community Health Center [6612]
Southern Regional Homecare [14574]
Southern Regional Medical Center [1895]
    Cancer Program [5034]
    Pain Center [35417]
Southern Sleep Clinics--Andalusia [36607]
Southern Sleep Clinics--Donalsonville [36865]
Southern Sleep Clinics--Dothan • Sleep Disorders Center [36608]
Southern Sleep Clinics--Enterprise [36609]
Southern Sleep Clinics--Eufaula [36610]
Southern Sleep Clinics--Ozark [36611]
Southern Star Community Services [42019]
    Crisp Outpatient Services [42068]
    New Beginnings [42020]
    Serenity Farm [42021]
Southern Tier Drug Abuse Treatment Center • Outpatient Methadone Treatment Clinic [46386]
Southern Tier Hospice and Palliative Care [20565]
Southern Utah Hospice--Cedar City [21602]
Southern Utah Hospice-Hildale [21610]
Southern Utah Hospice--Hurricane [21611]
Southern Utah Hospice--Kanab [21612]
Southern Utah Hospice--Saint George [21638]
Southern Valley Alliance for Battered Women [9584]
Southern Virginia Mental Health Institute [33901]
Southern Virginia Regional Medical Center [18288]
Southern West Virginia • Fellowship Home Inc [50284]
Southern Westchester BOCES [609]
Southern Westchester Dialysis Center • Renal Research Institute [25809]
Southern Wisconsin Center [8629]
Southfield West Dialysis • DaVita [24978]
Southgate Dialysis • Dialysis Clinic Inc. [22921]
Southhampton Dialysis Center • Fresenius Medical Care [27489]
Southlake Center for Mental Health Inc • Regional Mental Health Center [43134]
Southlake Center for Self Discovery • Eating Disorders Program [11177]
Southland Outpatient Recovery Center • Southland Outpatient Services [39733]
Southlight Inc [47318]
    Lifeplus [47465]
    Wakeview Clinic [47466]
Southmountain Children and Family Services [31569]
Southport Dialysis Center • DaVita [25954]
Southside Behavioral Lifestyle • Enrichment Center [42036]
Southside Community Health Clinic [7256]
Southside Community Health Services, Inc. • Southside Community Medical/Dental Clinics [6872]
Southside Community Hospital [18297]
Southside Community Services Board • Halifax County [49843]
Southside Family Health Center [6530]
Southside Hospital • Cancer Center [5558]
Southside Kidney Disease Clinic • Fresenius Medical Care [27346]
Southside Medical Center [14481]
Southside Medical Center, Inc. [6584]
Southside Medical Center, Inc. Home Health [14482]
Southside--Norcross Clinic [6598]
Southside Regional Medical Center • Renal Dialysis Unit [27536]
Southside Virginia Training Center [8594]
Southview Acres Health Care Center [2751]

Southwest Alabama Behavioral Health Care System--Brewton [50611]
Southwest Alabama Behavioral Health Care System--Evergreen [50613]
Southwest Alabama Behavioral Health Care System--Grove Hill [50615]
Southwest Alabama Behavioral Health Care System--Monroeville [50619]
Southwest Alabama Medical Center • Behavioral Medicine Center [27901]
Southwest Alabama Mental Health Center [50620]
Southwest Alabama Mental Health/Mental Retardation Board, Inc. [27990]
Southwest Alabama Regional School--Mobile County [202]
Southwest Arkansas Counseling [39539]
Southwest Arkansas Counseling Mental Health Center [39578]
Southwest Arkansas Counseling • Mental Health Center [28358]
Southwest Arkansas Counseling Mental Health Center • River Ridge Treatment Center [39579]
Southwest Arkansas Crisis Center [8758]
Southwest Arkansas Dialysis--Magnolia [22558]
Southwest Atlanta Dialysis Center • DaVita [23608]
Southwest Audiology [973]
Southwest Behavioral Care Inc [48656]
Southwest Behavioral Health [28178]
    Brookside Residential [28165]
Southwest Behavioral Health Center [49595]
    Horizon House West [49603]
Southwest Behavioral Health
    Community Counseling Services [28199]
    Crisis Recovery Unit [28179]
    Crisis Recovery Unit II [28180]
    Harvard Independent Living [28181]
    Mesa Clinic [28166]
    Northern Landing Transitional Living [28182]
Southwest Behavioral Health Service [50647]
Southwest Behavioral Health Services Inc
    Methadone Maintenance [39449]
    Payson Division [39414]
Southwest Behavioral Health • Villa Agave [28183]
Southwest Behavioral Systems Inc [49299]
Southwest Carolina Treatment Center LLC [48903]
Southwest Center [49657]
    Behavioral Health Services [49676]
    Horizon House East [49604]
    Outpatient [49616]
Southwest Chemical Dependency Program [45709]
Southwest Christian Care Hospice [19427]
Southwest Collegiate Institute for the Deaf [774]
Southwest Colorado Mental Health Center, Inc. • Crossroads [28895]
Southwest Community Health Center [6366]
Southwest Community Health Center, Inc. [6419]
Southwest Community Services for the Deaf [993]
Southwest Connecticut Mental Health System • Greater Bridgeport Community Mental Health Center [28978]
Southwest Counseling Center--Downtown Mall, Las Cruces [31200]
Southwest Counseling Center Inc [46282]
    Casa de Carinos [46283]
    Serenity Center [46284]
Southwest Counseling Center--Philadelphia [32102]
Southwest Counseling Center--S Main, Las Cruces [31201]
Southwest Counseling Center--W Griggs Avenue, Las Cruces [31202]
Southwest Counseling Service [50596]
Southwest Counseling Service--Green River [33045]
Southwest Counseling Service--Rock Springs [33065]
Southwest Crisis Center--Cottonwood County [9645]
Southwest Crisis Center--Jackson County [9603]
Southwest Crisis Center--Luverne [9607]
Southwest Crisis Center--Nobles County [9647]
Southwest Crisis Center--Pipestone County [9629]
Southwest Dallas Family Medical Center/dba Family Physical Therapy and Rehabilitation [35713]
Southwest Family Life Center--Hondo [10471]
Southwest Family Life Center--Uvalde [10515]
Southwest Family Services [41045]
Southwest Fertility Center--Mesa [21901]
Southwest Fertility Center--Phoenix [21902]
Southwest Fertility Services [22175]
Southwest Florida Addiction Services

Detoxification [41663]
Outpatient [41664]
Residential Level II [41665]
Southwest Florida Dialysis Center • Renal Carepartners [23255]
Southwest Florida Fertility Center [22008]
Southwest Florida Pain Center [12414]
Southwest Fort Worth Dialysis Center • Fresenius Medical Care [27090]
Southwest General Health Center • Ireland Cancer Center [5740]
Southwest General Health Center/Oakview • Behavioral Health Center/Alcohol/Drug Add Treatment [47815]
Southwest General Health Center • Speech-Language Therapy Division [3249]
Southwest Georgia Dialysis [23808]
Southwest Georgia Regional Library • Bainbridge Subregional Library for the Blind and Physically Handicapped [3780]
Southwest Guidance Center, Inc. • Sublette Medical Clinic [29957]
Southwest Health Center--E Side Road, Platteville [33005]
Southwest Health Center--N Elm Street, Platteville [33006]
Southwest Hearing Care Inc. [994]
Southwest Houston Dialysis Facility • Fresenius Medical Care [27176]
Southwest Idaho ENT [1941]
Southwest Indiana Mental Health Center, Inc. • Chandler Home [29720]
Southwest Louisiana Center for Health Services [6750]
Southwest Louisiana Developmental Center [8067]
Southwest Louisiana Education and Reference Center [50946]
Southwest Louisiana Primary Health Care Corp. [6760]
Southwest Medical Center • Integris Sleep Disorders Center of Oklahoma [37607]
Southwest Medical Group • Vancouver Neurologists, PS • Sleep Disorders Center [37938]
Southwest Memorial Hospital [13470]
Southwest Mental Health Center [32543]
Southwest Mental Health Center, Inc. • Whitehaven [32361]
Southwest Michigan Center for Orthopedics and Sports Medicine [38605]
Southwest Montana Therapy Works [2829]
Southwest NU Stop [48566]
North [48567]
Southwest Ohio Developmental Center [8399]
Southwest Ohio Dialysis • DaVita [26240]
Southwest Orthopaedic Group [39048]
Southwest Orthopaedic • Sports Medicine Center [38057]
Southwest Orthopaedics & Sports Medicine [38905]
Southwest Rehabilitation Hospital • Speech and Hearing Department [2559]
Southwest Speech and Hearing Center [3484]
Southwest Speech Pathology & Orofacial Myology [956]
Southwest Speech Services Inc. [938]
Southwest Sports Medicine & Orthopedics [38050]
Southwest Sports and Spine [39058]
Southwest Sports and Spine at Velocity [39059]
Southwest Sullivan School Corporation [2186]
Southwest Teller County Hospital • Cripple Creek Rehab and Wellness Center [41084]
Southwest Utah Public Health Department • Southwest Utah Community Health Center [7326]
Southwest Virginia Community Health [7369]
Southwest Wake Dialysis • Fresenius Medical Care [25930]
Southwest Washington Medical Center [18478]
Cancer Center [6128]
Southwest Women Working Together [9214]
Southwest Youth and Family Services Inc [47906], [47918]
Southwest Youth and Family Services • Runaway and Homeless Youth Program [36159]
Southwestern Behavioral Health Center [33774]
Southwestern Behavioral Healthcare Inc [43037], [43162]
Gibson Regional Services [43184]
Warrick Regional Services [43000]
Southwestern Colorado Mental Health Center, Inc. •

Pagosa Springs Counseling Center [28940]
Southwestern Home Health Care [17502]
Southwestern Indiana Mental Health Center [29721]
Southwestern Indiana Mental Health Center, Inc. [50886]
Gibson Regional Center [29806]
Moulton Center [29722]
Posey Regional Office [29785]
Riverside Home [29723]
Robert M. Spear Building [29724]
Southwestern Indiana Mental Health Center • Warrick Regional Center [29725]
Southwestern Medical Center
Cancer Program [5773]
Sleep Services [37608]
Southwestern Mental Health Center, Inc.--Luverne [30693]
Southwestern Mental Health Center, Inc.--Pipestone [30709]
Southwestern Mental Health Center, Inc.--Windom [30734]
Southwestern Mental Health Center, Inc.--Worthington [30737]
Southwestern Mental Health Unity House [30738]
Southwestern Regional Medical Center • Oncology Program [5785]
Southwestern Sleep Center [37373]
Southwestern State Hospital [7920], [33393]
Gateway Dual Diagnosis Comm Res Prog [42168]
Southwestern Vermont Medical Center • Cancer Program [6046]
Southwestern Vermont Renal Center • Fletcher Allen Dialysis Services, LLC [27439]
Southwestern Veterans Center [17446]
Southwestern Virginia Mental Health Institute [33904]
Southwestern Virginia Training Center [8589]
Southwestern Youth Services Inc [47905]
Southwestern Youth Services • Runaway and Homeless Youth Program [36160]
Southwood Psychiatric Hospital Inc. [33819]
Sovereign Health of California [40543]
Space Coast Sleep Disorders Center [36818]
Spalding County Dialysis [23714]
Spalding Regional Center for Rehabilitation [1868]
Spalding Regional Medical Center • Cancer Program [5027]
Spalding Rehabilitation Hospital [1378], [4141]
Brain Injury Program [3940]
Spalding Unit at P/SL • Brain Injury Program [3941]
Spanish Action League • Domestic Violence Program [9990]
Spanish Clinic LLC [41148], [41149]
Spanish Oaks Hospice [19418]
Spanish Peaks Mental Health Center [28945], [41304], [41305], [41306]
Chaurtard House [28946]
Community Support Program/Geriatrics [28947]
Lavilla De Evans [28948]
Spanish Peaks Apartments [28949]
Trinidad Office [28957]
Walsenburg Office [28959]
Sparks Dialysis Facility • DaVita [25386]
Sparks Home Health [12849]
Sparks Regional Medical Center [12850]
Cancer Program [4752]
Sparks Regional Medical Center - Home Health Department [17158]
Sparrow Behavioral Health Services [30586]
Sparrow Dialysis--Saint Lawrence Campus [24932]
Sparrow Dialysis--Sparrow Campus [24933]
Sparrow Health Services - SANE Program [9552]
Sparrow Health System
Audiology Center and Pediatric Rehabilitation [2618]
Regional Cancer Center [5383]
Sparrow Fertility Services [22129]
Sparrow Sleep Center [37205]
Sparrow Hearing Services [2619]
Sparrow Regional Pain Management Center [35513]
Sparrow Rehabilitation [1930]
Spartan Sleep Studies [37293]
Spartanburg Alcohol and DA Commission [48977]
Detoxification [48978]
Spartanburg County Hearing Impaired Program [737]
Spartanburg District Six [734]

Spartanburg Neurological Services [34874]
Spartanburg Regional Healthcare System • Community Clinical Oncology Program [5914]
Spartanburg Regional Home Care Services [17621]
Spartanburg Regional Medical Center • Sleep Center [37746]
Spartanburg Treatment Associates [48979]
Spaulding Braintree [4142]
Spaulding Brighton [4143]
Spaulding Cambridge [4144]
Spaulding Downtown Crossing [4145]
Spaulding Framingham [4146]
Spaulding Lexington [4147]
Spaulding Medford [4148]
Spaulding Wellesley [4149]
Spaulding Youth Center [34296]
Program for Neurobehavioral Disorders and Autism [8241]
Speak Easy Solutions [1704]
Speak Easy! Speech and Language Services [1239]
Speak Out New York [3146]
Speak Right Now [1180]
Speak Right NOW Pediatric Therapy Services [2676]
Speak Your Mind [1224]
SpeakEasy Speech Services SLP [3036]
Speaking of Speech [3106]
Spearfish Regional Hospital [3418]
Special Care Home Health Agency [14152]
Special Care Pharmacy Services, Inc. [17531]
Special Communications LLC [1589]
Special Education [717]
Special Education Service Agency • Alaska Dual Sensory Impairment Services [935]
Special Education Services, Liberal [434]
Special Health Resources of East Texas • East Texas Adolescent Treatment Prog [49447]
Special Kids [3444]
Special Medical Services [8234]
Special Needs Schools of Gwinnett Inc. [1877]
Special Needs Specialists, Inc. [14698]
Special Service for Groups Inc • HOP/ICS [40159]
Special Services Clinic Inc [41150]
Special Services for Groups Inc
HOP/ICS Family Center [40160]
Pacific Asian Alcohol and Drug Program [40161]
Special Touch Home Care Services, Inc. [16421]
Special Treatment Education and Prevention Services [39636]
Special Treatment Education and Prevention Services Inc [39637]
Special Tree Rehabilitation System
Arbor Court Community Residence [4193]
Beverly Hills Community Residence [4194]
Cottage Community Residence [4195]
Greenbriar Community Residence [4196]
Mid-Michigan Rehabilitation Center • Head Injury Therapy Service [4197]
River Ridge Community Residence [4198]
Riverview Community Residence [4199]
Romulus [4200]
Royal Oak Community Residence [4201]
Saginaw [4202]
Special Tree Rehabilitation System--Student Center [4203]
Special Tree Rehabilitation System
Trevino Community Residence [4204]
Troy Neuro Skills Center • Therapeutic Activity Program and Day Treatment Center [4205]
Tyler I Community Residence [4206]
Tyler II Community Residence [4207]
Special Tree Rehabilitation System--Wabash Center • Romulus Neuro Skills Center [4208]
Special Tree Rehabilitation System
Webster Court Apartments - Semi Independent Living [4209]
Westwoods Community Residence [4210]
Williams House Community Residence [4211]
Special Tree Rehabilitation Systems [2660]
Specialists in Reproductive Medicine and Surgery [22009]
Specialized Alternatives for Youth • Runaway and Homeless Youth Program [36152]
Specialized Assistance Services NFP
Branden House [42759]
Outpatient [42586]
Specialized Health Care Services Inc. [13051]
Specialized Home Nursing, Inc. [17171]

Specialized Hospital [2049]
Specialized Medical Devices, Inc. [12685]
Specialized Orthopedic Physical Therapy [39003]
Specialized Outpatient Services Inc [47999]
Specialized Therapy Services [3455]
Specialized Treatment Educ/Prevt Services Inc • Substance Abuse Day and Night Services [41604]
Specialized Treatment Education and Prevention Services Inc [41867]
Specialized Treatment Out-Patient • Services LLC - STOPS [41245]
Specialized Treatment Services Inc [45230], [45231]
Specialty Care for Women [21945]
Specialty Therapeutic Care [18007]
Spectracare--Barbour County Clinic [33087]
Spectracare--Dale County Clinic and Day Treatment [33095]
SpectraCare--Dallas [27833]
SpectraCare • Geneva Co IOP [39253]
Spectracare--Geneva County [33089]
SpectraCare
    The Haven [39242]
    Henry Co IOP [39202]
Spectracare--Henry County Clinic [33077]
Spectracare--Houston County • Rehabilitation Day Program [33102]
Spectracare Mental Health System [27902]
    Kornegay Street Foster Home [27903]
Spectracare--Webb Group Home Number One [33103]
Spectracare--Webb Group Home Number Two [33104]
Spectrum Care Academy, Inc. [29991]
Spectrum Consulting Services [11192]
Spectrum Counsleing PLLC [41151]
Spectrum Health [5379]
Spectrum Health Care Inc [46025]
Spectrum Health Continuing Care [4212]
Spectrum Health • Genetics Services [12252]
Spectrum Health Hospice and Palliative Care [20064]
Spectrum Health
    Kent Community Hospital [2599]
    Michigan Pain Consultants [35514]
Spectrum Health Neuro Rehabilitation Services [4214]
Spectrum Health
    Neuro Rehabilitation Services [4213]
    Regional Burn Center [4569]
    Sleep Disorders Center [37206]
Spectrum Health Systems Inc [44475], [44576]
    Outpatient Services [44620], [44621]
    Primary Care [44598]
    Project Turnabout [44605]
    Residential Recovery Program [44599]
    Spectrum Outpatient Services [44512]
    Transitional Support Services [44600]
Spectrum Healthcare Services [14379]
Spectrum Home Health Agency [12686]
Spectrum Home Health Care and Hospice [15510]
Spectrum Home Health and Hospice Care [19972]
Spectrum Human Services--Buffalo [31294]
Spectrum Human Services
    Chemical Dependency Outpatient [46570]
    New Alternatives [46571]
Spectrum Human Services--Orchard Park [31444]
Spectrum Human Services • Southtowns Counseling Services [46965]
Spectrum Nurses, Inc. [14694]
Spectrum Orthopedics [38884]
Spectrum Programs Inc • South Florida Provider Coalition [41801]
Spectrum of Supportive Services [31721]
Spectrum Therapy Services [1597]
Spectrum Youth and Family Services [49735]
    Runaway and Homeless Youth Program [36240]
Speech 4 Kids PC [2037]
Speech Advantage--Madison [3676]
Speech Advantage--Middleton [3680]
The Speech Arc [3124]
Speech CARE Specialists Inc. [1886]
Speech Castle [1946]
The Speech Center [1342]
Speech Center of Texas PC [3527]
Speech Clinic [1938]
The Speech Clinic, Inc. [1521]
Speech and Communication Professionals [2971]
Speech Communication Therapies Inc. [3490]

Speech Connections [2876]
Speech Connections LLC [3405]
Speech Enhancement Diagnostic and Treatment Services [2096]
Speech Fun at CSUN [1201]
The Speech Garden [3171]
Speech and Hearing Associates--Avenel [2891]
Speech and Hearing Associates--Clifside Park [2903]
Speech and Hearing Associates--Elizabeth • General Medicine at Elizabeth [2910]
Speech and Hearing Associates Inc.--Edmond [3267]
Speech and Hearing Associates--Martinsville [2928]
Speech and Hearing Associates--Park Ridge [2940]
Speech and Hearing Associates--Randolph [2944]
Speech and Hearing Associates--Seacaucus [2946]
Speech and Hearing Associates--South Orange [2947]
Speech and Hearing Associates--Westfield [2957]
Speech and Hearing Associates--Woodland Park [2958]
Speech & Hearing Center [3424]
Speech and Hearing Clinic--Plattsburgh [3095]
Speech and Hearing Clinic • University of Iowa Hospital [2207]
Speech Hearing and Counseling [2271]
The Speech, Hearing and Learning Center [3402]
Speech, Hearing and Neurosensory Center [1273], [12492]
Speech Improvement Group [2401]
The Speech Key [1809]
Speech for Kids [3571]
Speech and Language Associates of Greater Cincinnati [3222]
Speech and Language Associates Inc. [3471]
Speech Language and Auditory Learning [3545]
The Speech and Language Center [2503]
Speech and Language Center LLC [1584]
Speech and Language Center of Northern Virginia [3597]
Speech and Language Center at Stone Oak [3539]
Speech and Language Connection--Houston [3511]
Speech and Language Connections--Bloomington [1968]
Speech and Language Connections--Maple Grove [2706]
Speech and Language Connections--Normal [2082]
Speech and Language Consultant LLC [1450]
Speech and Language Consulting [3442]
Speech Language Consulting Services Inc. [2326]
Speech and Language Development Center [1070]
Speech Language Fundamentals [2057]
Speech and Language Group [1170]
Speech--Language and Hearing Associates of Greater Boston [2494]
Speech, Language, Hearing Clinic [2250]
Speech, Language and Hearing Services Inc. [3462]
Speech & Language Institute [1470]
Speech Language Learning Associates [1251]
Speech Language Learning Center Inc. [2586]
Speech Language and Learning Place [2845]
Speech, Language and Learning Service of Marin-Sonoma [1304]
Speech Language and Learning Services [3525]
Speech/Language and Learning Services [3621]
Speech, Language, and Learning Solutions Inc. [2040]
Speech Language Learning Systems Inc./Language Pathways [2822]
Speech-Language Partners, Inc. [1917]
Speech--Language Pathology Consultants Inc. [1915]
Speech--Language Pathology Inc. [2090]
Speech-Language Pathology Rehabilitation Services • Saint Luke's Regional Medical Center [1942]
Speech-Language Pathology Services [1349]
Speech and Language Pathology Services, PC [2097]
Speech Language Pathology Unlimited [3087]
Speech and Language Professional Services [1130]
Speech, Language and Reading Services Inc. [2602]
Speech & Language Rehabilitation Services, Ltd.--Bloomington [1969]
Speech & Language Rehabilitation Services, Ltd.--Peoria [2099]
Speech and Language Remediation Center Inc. [3512]

Speech and Language Resources [2481]
Speech and Language Services [3544]
Speech--Language Services [3278]
Speech and Language Services of South Texas [3477]
Speech and Language Solutions LLC [2919]
Speech Language Specialists, Inc. [2320]
Speech and Language Specialists PC--Bronxville [2985]
Speech and Language Specialties [2523]
Speech and Language Stimulation Center [1413]
Speech and Language Therapy Associates Inc.--Citrus Heights [1081]
Speech and Language Therapy Associates--Raleigh [3193]
Speech and Language Therapy Associates--Staten Island [3125]
Speech/Language Therapy Services [2270]
Speech and Learn SLP [3152]
Speech and Learning Center [2328]
Speech and Learning Services [1056]
Speech and Literacy Center Inc. [2114]
Speech Management Services Inc. [1326]
Speech Masters Therapy Services Inc. [3194]
Speech and Neurorehabilitation Center Inc. [1722]
Speech Partners Inc. [2895]
Speech Path [3660]
The Speech Path [1186]
Speech Path LLC [1894]
Speech Patherapy [2864]
Speech Pathology Associates [2755], [3261]
Speech Pathology Associates Inc. [1134]
Speech Pathology Center of Louisiana [2307]
Speech Pathology Consultants [3328]
Speech Pathology Consultants LLC [2013]
Speech Pathology and Educational Center Inc. [1663]
The Speech Pathology Group [1359]
Speech Pathology Service--Columbia [2784]
Speech Pathology Services--Billings [3697]
Speech Pathology Services--Carmel [2133]
Speech Pathology Services, Inc.--Atlanta [1829]
Speech Pathology Services--Texarkana [3543]
Speech Pathology Services of West County Inc. [2780]
Speech Paths [3513]
Speech Pathways [2438]
Speech Pathways PLLC [3263]
Speech Pathways at the Shafer Center [2426]
Speech Plus--Dexter [2355]
Speech Plus PC--Frankfort [2039]
Speech Ptahology Services of East Tennessee LLC [3437]
Speech and Reading Solutions [2035]
The Speech Solution [2486]
Speech Solutions LLC [1479]
Speech Station [1077]
Speech Success [3523]
Speech Therapists of Old Town [3569]
Speech Therapy Associates--Beaverton [3303]
Speech Therapy Associates--Las Vegas [2867]
Speech Therapy Associates--Lodi [1148]
Speech Therapy Associates of North Texas [3485]
Speech Therapy Center of Excellence Inc. [2868]
Speech Therapy Clinic of Hattiesburg [2760]
Speech Therapy Enterprises [3310]
Speech Therapy Group LLC--Beverly [2451]
Speech Therapy Group--Los Angeles [1171]
Speech Therapy and Learning Interventions [2550]
Speech Therapy and Rehabilitation Services [2036]
Speech Therapy Services--Bainbridge [1838]
Speech Therapy Services Inc.--Provo [3553]
Speech Therapy Services--Montgomery [919]
Speech Therapy Solutions PC [2889]
Speech Time Inc. [1664]
Speech and Voice Clinic of WNC [3156]
The Speech Works [1371]
SpeechCare Inc. [3348]
Speechcenter Inc. [3158]
SpeechSouth Inc. [3172]
Speechtree Therapy LLC [2402]
SpeechWorks Inc.--Columbia [3398]
SpeechWorks Inc.--Long Beach [1157]
Speechworks LLC--Chardon [3214]
SpeedyCare Medical Distributors, Inc. [13154]
Spencer County Hospice [19648]
Spencer County Services [29813]
Spencer House [31112], [33434]

Mens Recovery Center [47828]
Spencer Recovery Centers Inc • Spencer Recovery Center [39970]
Spencer's Place [31571]
The Sperm Bank of New York Inc. [35143]
Sperm and Embryo Bank of New Jersey [35123]
Sphinx Home Health Care [15842]
SPHS Behavioral Health [48333]
    Alle Kiski Area Office [48484]
    Greensburg Area Office [48384]
    Latrobe Area Office [48440]
    Mon Valley Drug and Alcohol Program [48472]
SPHS Care Center [48681]
Spiller Park Apartments [4084]
Spinal Cord Injury Service Line [4240]
SpinalGraft Technologies, LLC [35211]
Spindletop Mental Health/Mental Retardation Services [32411]
    Community Psychiatric Center [32412]
    Orange [32523]
    South County Outpatient Services [32533]
Spindletop MHMR Services [8535]
Spine and Brain Neurosurgical Center--Lexington [35462]
Spine and Brain Neurosurgical Center--London [35463]
Spine and Brain Neurosurgical Center--Pikeville [35464]
Spine Care and Pain Management [35418]
Spine, Orthopedic, & Sports Physical Therapy [39106]
Spine and Pain Clinic [35600]
Spine and Sports Center of Connecticut [38201]
Spine and Sports Institute [38623]
Spinecare Medical Group • Pain Clinic [35333]
SpineOne • Colorado Spine and Orthopedic Rehabilitation Center [38178]
Spirit Home Health Care [14153]
Spirit Lake Tribal Health Services • Youth Healing and Wellness Center [47577]
Spirit Lake Veterans Affairs Clinic [29898]
Spirit Lodge [49541]
Spirit Mind and Body • Behavioral Health Services PLLC [49402]
Spirit of Woman of California [39867]
Spirits of Hope Coalition [10195]
SPIRITT Family Services • Share Program [39964]
A Spiritual Abode Inc [40764]
Spivey Peritoneal, Home Dialysis Center & At Home • DaVita [23727]
Spofford Home [34271]
Spokane Addiction Recovery Centers [50182], [50183]
    Outpatient Services [50184]
Spokane Kidney Center • Fresenius Medical Care [27652]
Spokane Mental Health [32865]
Spokane Mental Health Elder Services [32866]
Spokane Mental Health • First Call for Help [51470]
Spokane Public Schools [867]
Spokane Regional Health District • Treatment Services [50185]
Spokane Tribal of Indians Substance • Spokane Tribe Substance Abuse Program [50255]
Spokane Veterans Affairs Medical Center [32867]
    Multiple Sclerosis Center [34737]
SPORT Clinic [38233], [38284]
Sport Clinic [38254]
The SPORT Clinic [38119]
Sport Clinic of Greater Milwaukee [39190]
S.P.O.R.T. Physicians, PC [38607]
SportONE-Orthopaedics Northeast [38429]
Sports Care [38898]
Sports Injury Center [38458]
Sports Medicine Associates [38580]
Sports Medicine Atlantic Orthopedic [38710]
The Sports Medicine Center of Northern Arizona [38032]
Sports Medicine Center • Washington Hospital Healthcare System [38088]
Sports Medicine Clinic of Green Bay [39175]
Sports Medicine Clinic
    Howard Beach [38787]
    Phoebe Family Care Center [38303]
Sports Medicine Consultants [38670]
Sports Medicine and Injury Center [38832]
Sports Medicine Institute • Glendale [38035]

Sports Medicine Institute of Indiana--Indianapolis [38439]
Sports Medicine Institute of Indiana at Muncie [38442]
Sports Medicine Institute of Indiana at Noblesville [38445]
Sports Medicine Institute of Memorial Hospital [38449]
Sports Medicine Institute • Saint Vincent Hospital [38678]
Sports Medicine, Ltd. [38368]
Sports Medicine North Orthopaedic Surgery, Inc. [38565]
Sports Medicine and Orthopaedic Center [38736]
Sports Medicine & Orthopaedics [39041]
Sports Medicine Performance Center [39186]
Sports Medicine and Performance Center at CHOP • Specialty Care Center [38950]
Sports Medicine Rehab [39171]
Sports Medicine and Rehabilitation Therapy Inc.--Malden [38557]
Sports Medicine and Rehabilitation Therapy Inc.--Reading [38568]
Sports Medicine South [38321]
Sports Medicine Specialists [38850]
Sports Medicine & Therapy Services • Cypress Fairbanks Medical Center Hospital [39078]
Sports Medicine and Training Center [38673]
Sports Medicine at Winters Run • Winters Run Family Medical Center • Hartford Primary Care [38522]
Sports and Occupational Medicine Rehabilitation Center [38107]
Sports and Orthopaedic Rehabilitation Center [39113]
Sports and Orthopaedic Therapy Services [38534]
Sports Performance International [39049]
Sports Performance & Orthopaedic Rehabilitation Team • Southcoast Hospitals Group [38564]
Sports & Physical Therapy Associates
    Charles River Park Health & Swim Club [38545]
    Wellesley [38574]
Sports Physical Therapy Institute [38753]
Sports and Physical Therapy of Seminole Heights [38293]
Sports Plus [38440]
Sports Podiatry Resources Inc. [38547]
Sports Rehabilitation and Physical Therapy Associates Inc. [38465]
Sports Rehabilitation and Physical Therapy Associates--Kansas City [38660]
Sports Rehabilitation and Physical Therapy Associates--Overland Park [38466]
Sports & Spine Associates, PA [39050]
Sports Therapy and Advanced Rehabilitation [39051]
Sports Therapy Associates [38078]
SportsCare and Rehabilitation [39092]
SportsClinic • Fairfield Medical Center [38883]
SportsFocus Physical Therapy [38811]
SportsMed Physical Therapy & Spine Clinic, Inc. [38182]
SportsMed Wheaton Orthopaedics [38352]
SportsMedicine of Atlanta [38328]
SportsMedicine Fairbanks [38022]
SportsMedicine Grant [38871]
SPOT Kids [1140]
Spotted Bull Treatment Center [45720]
Spousal Abuse/Sexual Assault Crisis Center [9772]
Spouse Abuse/Sexual Assault Victims Emergency Services [9754]
Sprain Brook Audiology--New York [3079]
Sprain Brook Audiology--Riverdale [3108]
Sprain Brook Audiology--Scarsdale [3117]
Spring Branch Community Health Center [7297]
Spring Branch Dialysis • DaVita [27177]
Spring City Veterans Affairs Outpatient Clinic [17485]
Spring Dialysis Inc. [27178]
Spring Grove Hospital Center [33559]
Spring Harbor Hospital [33555], [44085]
Spring Hill Apartments [27916]
Spring Hill Manor Nursing Home • Mobile Community Mental Health Center [27986]
Spring House • Female Halfway House [46115]
Spring Meadows Home Health Care, LLC [14860]
Spring Mountain Treatment Center [31036]
Spring River Mental Health and Wellness Inc [43327]

Spring River • Mental Health and Wellness Inc [43449]
The Spring of Tampa Bay [9083]
Spring Valley Hearing Center [1537]
Spring Valley Hospice, LLC [20255]
Spring Villa Home--MR [28008]
Springbrook [8340]
SpringBrook Behavioral Health System [33835]
Springbrook Hospital [33293]
Springdale Treatment Center [39577]
Springfield Center for Independent Living [2112]
Springfield Central Dialysis & At Home • DaVita [24093]
Springfield City Schools [661]
Springfield Dialysis Center--Massachusetts [24803]
Springfield Dialysis Center--New York [25691]
Springfield Hospital Center [33568]
Springfield Hospital • Pain Management Center [35749]
Springfield Internal Medicine [7338]
Springfield Montvale Dialysis • DaVita [24094]
Springfield Neurology Associates • Multiple Sclerosis Center [34602]
Springfield Outpatient Clinic and Community Care Center [15549]
Springfield Public Schools District Number 186 [412]
Springfield Regional Medical Center • Springfield Regional Cancer Center [5749]
Springfield Shriners Hospital [8148]
Springfield Veterans Affairs Community Based Outpatient Clinic [31840]
Springfield Veterans Affairs Outpatient Clinic [29678], [30469]
SpringHaven Inc. [9387]
Springhill Home [27896]
Springhill Memorial Hospital • Southeast Regional Center for Sleep/Wake Disorders [36612]
Springhurst Dialysis Center • DaVita [24420]
Springs Hospice • Avera Weskota Memorial Medical Center [21306]
Springs Memorial Hospital [17601]
Springtime Counseling Center Inc [43115]
Springwoods Behavioral Health [28270]
Spruce Run [9428]
Spurwink Clinic [34167]
Spurwink School [8083], [34168]
Spurwink Services, Inc. • Auburn Day Treatment Program [30179]
Spurwink Services, Lewiston [30219]
Spurwink Services, South Portland [30247]
Square One Redmond [50078]
Squaxin Island Tribe Behavioral Health • Outpatient Program [50152]
SRI Sleep Disorders Center [37700]
SRS Recovery Services [40415], [40923]
SSM DePaul Health Center • Cancer Program [5436]
SSM Dialysis--Madison Station [27732]
SSM Rehabilitation Hospital
    St. Joseph Health Ctr. [4241]
    St. Mary's Health Center [4242]
SSM Saint Joseph Hospital West • Cancer Care [4683]
SSM Saint Mary's Health Center • Cancer Program [5464]
SSQ Home Health Care, Inc. [17928]
SSTAR Lifeline Program [44458]
SSTAR of Rhode Island Inc
    Residential Alcohol/Drug Detox [48861]
    SSTAR Birth [48848]
SSTAR Women's Center [9478]
St Vincents Hospital Westchester • A Division of St Josephs Medical Center [46534]
Staff Mates Homecare [13527]
Staffing Home Care [13366]
Stafford Dialysis [27365]
Stafford Family Services [41470]
Stairways Behavioral Health [32019]
Stamford Dialysis • DaVita [23182]
Stamford Health System • Carl and Dorothy Bennett Cancer Center [4908]
Stamford Hospital
    Connecticut Center for Sleep Medicine [36754]
    Reproductive Endocrinology and Infertility [21973]
STAND! Against Domestic Violence [8806]
STAND Inc [42081]
Standing Together Against Rape [8655]

Stanford Children's Hospital • Sickle Cell Disease Center [36305]
Stanford Hospital & Clinics Transplant Services [23021]
Stanford Hospital • Multiple Sclerosis Center [34529]
Stanford School of Medicine • Sports Medicine Center [38145]
Stanford Sleep Medicine Center [36704]
Stanford University
    Adult Cystic Fibrosis Center [7479]
    Audiology Department [1327]
Stanford University Hospital/Lucile Salter Packard Children's Hospital • Department of Pediatrics • Genetics Clinic [12165]
Stanford University • Lucile Packard Children's Hospital • Down Syndrome Clinic [10779]
Stanford University Medical Center
    Clinical Cancer Center [4663]
    Pediatric Cystic Fibrosis Center [7480]
    School of Medicine • Division of Infectious Diseases Adult AIDS Clinical Trials Unit [2]
Stanford University
    Neurology Clinic [34763]
    Pain Management Center [35334]
    Reproductive Endocrinology and Infertility Clinic [21946]
Stanislaus Cnty Behavioral Health and • Recovery Services/Turlock Regional [40866]
Stanislaus County Behavioral Health
    Eastside Regional Services [28663]
    Garden Gate Respite--Turning Point [28630]
    Health/Mental Health Team [28428]
    Integrated Forensics Team [28631]
    Kirk Baucher Day Treatment [28632]
    Leaps and Bounds Program [28633]
    Oakdale Community Care Center for Children [28664]
Stanislaus County Behavioral Health & Recovery Services [28634]
Stanislaus County
    Genesis Narcotic Replacement Therapy [40233]
    Modesto Recovery Services [40234]
Stanislaus County Office of Education [285]
Stanislaus Recovery Center • Adult Treatment Programs [39696]
Stanislaus Sleep Disorders Center [36705]
Stanley Dialysis Center • Saint Joseph's Hospital • Ministry Dialysis [27787]
Stanley Street Treatment and Resources
    Alcoholism/Drug Detox Program [44459]
    Chemical Dependency Services/Outpt [44460]
Stanly Memorial Hospital [33733]
Star Care Home Health Inc. [13173]
Star Center Inc [44766]
Star Choice Home Health, Inc. [18112]
STAR Clinic Physical Therapy [38108]
STAR Council on Substance Abuse [49267], [49547], [49580]
    Adult Program [49305]
Star Home Care Services [15729]
Star Home Health Care Services [14154]
Star of Hope/New Hope Program • Transitional Living Center [49403]
Star Hospice [21540]
Star Hospice of Vista Health [19582]
Star Light Health Agency [14155]
Star Med Home Health Care [13407]
Star Multi Care Services [14329]
Star Multi Care Services, Inc. • Extended Family Care of Allentown [17237]
STAR Physical Therapy, Inc. [38105]
STAR Professional Therapy, Inc. • Sports Training and Rehabilitation, Inc. [38142]
A STAR Professionals, LLC [937]
Star Shine Hospice of Children's Hospital [20816]
STAR View Adolescent Center [28828]
Star World Health Care Services Inc. [13421]
Starbright Home Health Services Inc. [13358]
Starfish Family Services [8174], [30594]
    Lifespan Clinical Services [30572]
    Runaway and Homeless Youth Program [36026]
Starke Center • Southlake Community Mental Health Center [43021]
Starlight Community Services [28782]
Starlite Recovery Center [49263]
Starr Battle Creek [30510]
Starr Columbus [34377]

Starr Commonwealth [30496]
Starr Hospice [20536]
Starr My Place [34378]
Starry: A Children at Heart Ministry • Runaway and Homeless Youth Program [36233]
STARS Behavioral Health Group [28681]
    Oasis Rehabilitation Center [28541]
STARS Community service [28786]
STARS Liberty Location [4015]
Starting Place Inc • Plantation [41898]
Starting Point [9807], [44205]
Starting Point of Florence Inc [48934]
Starting Point Inc [39316], [39359]
    Longview Branch [50009]
    Mill Plain Clinic [50244]
StarVista • Runaway and Homeless Youth Program [35845]
StaRX, Inc. [18065]
STAT Home Health--Baton Rouge [15274]
STAT Home Health--New Orleans [15343]
STAT Home Health--Paulina [15350]
STAT Medical, Inc. [14623]
State 27 Home Health Services [14156]
State of Alaska
    Alaska Genetics Clinic-Division of Public Health • Women's, Children's and Family Health [12122]
    Bethel Public Health Center [12123]
    Cordova Public Health Center [12124]
    Craig Public Health Center [12125]
    Delta Junction Public Health Center [12126]
    Dillingham Public Health Center [12127]
    Fort Yukon Public Health Office [12128]
    Galena Public Health Center [12129]
    Haines Public Health Center [12130]
    Homer Public Health Center [12131]
    Juneau Public Health Clinic [12132]
    Kenai Public Health Center [12133]
    Ketchikan Public Health Clinic [12134]
    Kodiak Public Health Center [12135]
    Mat-Su Public Health Center [12136]
    Petersburg Public Health Center [12137]
    Seward Public Health Center [12138]
    Sitka Public Health Clinic [12139]
    Tanana Valley Clinic [12140]
    Tok Public Health Center [12141]
    Valdez Public Health Center [12142]
    Wrangell Public Health Center [12143]
State of Connecticut Department of Public Health • Family Health Division • SIDS Program [36461]
State Fair Dialysis Center [24885]
State of the Heart Home Health and Hospice [19643], [20844]
State Hospital North [33402]
State of Iowa Human Rights • Deaf Services Commission of Iowa [2203]
State Library of Louisiana • Talking Books and Braille Library [3799]
State Library of North Carolina • North Carolina Library for the Blind and Physically Handicapped [3827]
State of Mind Mental Health and
    Consultation Services PC [42701]
    Consultations Services PC [42587]
State Street Clinic [31280]
State Street House [33429]
State of Tennessee Rehabilitation Services • Services for the Blind and Visually Impaired/ Services for the Deaf and Hard of Hearing [3448]
State University College • Psychological Counseling Center [51144]
State University of New York, Buffalo • Department of Communication Disorders • Speech--Language and Hearing Clinic [3001]
State University of New York • Department of Communicative Disorders • Harold Starbuck Memorial Fluency Enhancing Clinic [3025]
State University of New York Health Science Center at Brooklyn • University Hospital • Department of Pediatrics • Division of Clinical Genetics [12299]
State University of New York
    Health Science Center • Communication Disorders Unit [3133]
    Health Sciences Center • Department of Neurology • MDA/ALS Center [34842]
    Jacobs Neurology Institute • Pediatric Center of Excellence • Pediatric Multiple Sclerosis Center [34653]

    Pediatrics/Child Development • Down Syndrome Clinic [10835]
    Sickle Cell Center [36401]
State University of New York, Stony Brook • Department of Neurology • Comprehensive Multiple Sclerosis Care Center [34654]
State University of New York at Stony Brook
    Pain Management [35585]
    School of Social Welfare • Health Sciences Center • New York State Center for Sudden Infant Death [36525]
    University Hospital
        Cystic Fibrosis Center [7623]
        Genetics Clinic [12300]
State University of New York, Stony Brook • University Medical Center Burn Unit [4595]
State University of New York Upstate Medical University
    Adult Cystic Fibrosis Center [7624]
    Pain Management [35586]
    University Hospital • Robert C. Schwartz Cystic Fibrosis Center [7625]
Staten Island Developmental Disabilities Service Office [8357]
Staten Island Dialysis Clinic--AKC • Dialysis Clinic Inc. [25782]
Staten Island Pulmonary • Sleep Disorders Centers of Staten Island [37440]
Staten Island University Hospital
    Alcoholism Outpatient Clinic [47103]
    Behavioral Sciences Department [47104]
    Chemical Dependency Rehab Unit [47105]
    Institute of Sleep Medicine [37441]
    Methadone Treatment Clinic [46535]
    OTP [47106]
    Outpt Methadone Treatment Program [46536]
    Sanford R. Nalitt Institute for Cancer and Blood-Related Diseases [5617]
Staten Island YMCA Counseling Service [47107]
Staunton Public Library • Talking Book Center [3849]
Stay Well Health Care, Inc. [6428]
Steadfast Home Care Health Services, Inc. [14898]
Steadman Clinic [38183]
Steam Dialysis • DaVita [25395]
Steamboat Mental Health Center [50722]
Steele House [49634]
Stein Hospice Service Inc. [20890]
Stein Wellness Center [6413]
Steindler Orthopedic Clinic [38453]
Steininger Behavioral Care Services, Inc. [31104], [31117]
Steininger Behavioral Care Srvs Inc [45958]
Steinway Child and Family Services, Inc. [31381]
Steljes Cardiology • Steljes Health Heart Sleep Facility [37322]
Stella Maris [47704], [47705]
Stellar Home Health [13184]
Stemcyte, Inc. [34964]
STEP [33348]
Step Ahead Inc [46178]
Step Ahead Pediatric Rehab Inc. [2696]
Step Ahead Program of KHI Services [44279]
Step By Step • Health and Family Services LLC [46020]
Step By Step Inc [48267]
Step Forward Inc [44178]
A STEP Inc [40416]
STEP Inc [44421]
STEP Med [49300]
Step O.N.E. [10546]
Step One [46622], [46745]
Step One Inc [45875]
Step One Recovery Center • Community Mental Health of Middle GA [42090]
Step Out Transitional Age Youth Program [28448]
Step Two
    Lighthouse of the Sierra [45876]
    Transitional House Residential [45877]
A Step Up [28461], [39759]
Step Up Support Center [39554]
Stephen Center Inc [45804]
Stephen F. Austin State University • Speech and Hearing Clinic [3526]
Stephen Ratcliffe Community Health Center [7329]
Stephens County Mental Health/Substance Abuse Center [29498]

Stephens Memorial Hospital • Cancer Program [5273]
Stephenville Clinic [32554]
Stepping Stone Center for Recovery [41712]
Stepping Stone Manor [31611], [47526]
Stepping Stone Program [34394]
Stepping Stone Recovery [40219]
Stepping Stone of San Diego Inc • Residential [40581]
Stepping Stone Shelter for Women [9299]
Stepping Stone • Southwestern Behavioral Health-care Inc [43038]
A Stepping Stone to Success [42010]
Stepping Stones [8404], [28519]
Stepping Stones Agencies [8723]
Stepping Stones • Dakota Counseling Institute Inc [49003]
Stepping Stones Home [39766], [39767]
Stepping Stones Inc [42723]
    Conference Center [42724]
    Mens Recovery Home [42725]
    Womens Recovery Home [42726]
Stepping Stones, Inc. [10717]
Stepping Stones Intensive Outpatient Program [11286]
Stepping Stones • Residential Facility [39317]
Stepping Stones Therapy LLC [2394]
Stepping Stones Unit at Meadville Medical Center [48462]
Stepping Stones Wellness Center Inc [47228]
Steppingstone Inc
    Mens Program [44461]
    Therapeutic Community [44462]
    Transition House [44463]
    Womens Program [44522]
Steppingstones to Recovery [42047]
STEPS to End Family Violence [9959]
Steps Forward LLC [1754]
Steps to Hope [10029]
STEPS at Liberty Center Inc [47888]
    Beacon House [47889]
Steps Recovery Center [49659]
    Muhlenberg Campus [46138]
Steps Ultimate Solutions [39610]
StepStone [9380]
Stepworks Addiction Resources [43583]
Sterling Area Health Center [6858]
    Behavioral Health Care Services [45025]
Sterling Healthcare Services Inc. [15364]
Sterling Ranch [7747]
Sterling Sharpe Pediatric Center [7229]
Steuben County Alcoholism and
    Substance Abuse Services [46373]
    Substance Abuse Services /Outpt Clinic [46599]
Steuben County CD Outpatient Clinic [46702]
Steuben County Community Mental Health Center--Bath [31236]
    Clinic & Continuing Treatment Center [33676]
Steuben County Community Mental Health Center--Corning [31309]
Steuben County Community Mental Health Center--Hornell [31352]
Steuben County Office • Northeastern Center Inc [42983]
Steven E. Roberts, MD [38115]
Stevens Avenue [30231]
The Stevens Center [32001]
Stevens Center of Singing River Services [45411]
Stevens Children's Home, Inc. • Transitional Living Program [34193]
Stevens County Crisis Center [9625]
Stevens Hospital • Puget Sound Tumor Institute [6098]
Stevens Inc [46038], [46173]
Stevens Treatment Programs [34216]
Stevenson Waplak and Associates • Eating Disorders Treatment [11236]
Steward Good Samaritan/NORCAP/ATS [44468]
Steward Saint Elizabeth/SECAP/ATS [44427]
Stewart Community Center [7139]
Stewart Home School [8045]
Stewart-Marchman-Act Behavioral Healthcare [29254]
Stewart Marchman Act/Behavioral
    Healthcare Adolescent Residential [41616]
    Healthcare Adult Detox [41617]
    Healthcare Flagler County Outpatient [41581]
    Healthcare Four Towns Care Center [41618]

    Healthcare Outpatient and Gen Intervention [41872]
Stewart Memorial Community Hospital • Community Hospice [19706]
Stewart Webster Rural Health Clinic [6600]
STHS Sleep Center [37789]
Stigler Health and Wellness Center, Haskell County [7115]
Stigler Health and Wellness Center • McIntosh County Clinic [7104]
Stiles Corporation • Melody Stiles [43116]
Stillmeadow Counseling Center • DUI Center [42922]
Stillriver Centre for Wellness [41310]
Stillwater Domestic Violence Service, Inc. [10215]
Stillwater Public Schools [672]
Stillwater Sleep Laboratory [37237]
Stilwell Dialysis Facility • DaVita [26297]
Sto-Rox Family Health Council, Inc. [7170]
Stockbridge Dialysis Clinic LLC [23798]
Stockbridge Munsee Health/Wellness Center • Behavioral Health Department [50372]
Stockley Center [7865]
Stockton Home Dialysis Center • DaVita [23026]
Stockton Kidney Clinic • DaVita [23027]
Stockwell Center • Southwestern Behavioral Health-care Inc [43039]
Stokes County Schools [614]
Stokes Task Force on Domestic Violence, Inc. [10031]
Stone Belt Arc [7980]
Stone County Abuse Prevention [8778]
StoneCrest Medical Center
    Sarah Cannon Cancer Center [5955]
    Sleep Center [37790]
Stonewall Institute [39450]
Stonewall Jackson Memorial Hospital [18548]
Stoney Brook Physicians [7359]
Stonington Institute [41452]
Stonington Institute--Groton [28999]
Stonington Institute--North Stonington [29030]
Stonington Public Services [331]
Stony Brook Kidney Center • Dialysis Clinic, Inc. [25651]
Stony Brook Orthopedic Associates, P.C. [38785]
Stony Brook University Hospital
    Long Island Cancer Center [5618]
    Speech, Language and Hearing Department [3012]
Stony Brook University Medical Center • Sleep Disorders Center [37442]
Stony Creek Community Health Center [7370]
Stony Creek Dialysis • DaVita [24054]
Stony Island Dialysis • DaVita [23960]
Stony Lodge Hospital--Elmsford • Partial Hospitaliza-tion Program [33694]
Stony Lodge Hospital Inc.--Ossining [33714]
Stony River clinic [12775]
Stonybrook Center Inc [42968]
STOP [43509]
Stop Abuse for Everyone, Inc. [10269]
Stop Abusive Family Environments, Inc. [10682]
Stop Domestic Violence [10007]
STOP Domestic Violence Program • Los Angeles Gay and Lesbian Center [8843]
STOP Program • East Location [43510]
Stopover • Runaway and Homeless Youth Program [35952]
Stopover Services of Newport County • Runaway and Homeless Youth Program [36191]
Stopping Women Abuse Now, Inc. [9240]
Stork Medical [35013]
Storm Lake Area Hospice • Buena Vista Regional Medical Center [19735]
Stormont Vail Health Care • Stormont Sleep Center [37008]
Stormont-Vail Healthcare • Cotton-O'Neal Cancer Center [5207]
Stormont Vail West Substance Abuse [43468]
Stoughton Hospital [18631]
    Substance Abuse Services [50535]
Stout Street Foundation [41077]
Stowe Family Practice [7340]
Strafford County Dialysis • Fresenius Medical Care [25399]
Strafford Guidance Center, Inc. • Emergency Crisis Team [51083]
Straight and Narrow Inc [46128]

Straight Talk • Gerry House [40722]
Straight Talk Speech Therapy [1782]
Strategies for Change [40507], [40508]
Strategies Therapy Group [2761]
Stratford Program [8579]
Stratford Visiting Nurse Association, Inc. [13545]
Straub Clinic and Hospital
    Burn Unit [4539]
    Sleep Disorders Center of the Pacific [36875]
    Tumor Registry [5048]
Streamwood at Saint Mary's [33440]
Streetwork Harlem Drop-In Center • Runaway and Homeless Youth Program [36124]
Strength Through Emotions Management [9674]
Strengthen Our Sisters [9831]
Stress Management and Mental Health Clinic [33022]
Stress Management and Mental Health Clinics [50553]
Stride Learning Center [8632]
Strides LLC [41010]
Stringfellow Sleep Diagnostics Center [36613]
Stroger Hospital - Cook County Children's Hospital • Department of Pediatric Hematology/Oncology • Hemophilia Treatment Center [12520]
Stroke Comeback Center [3615]
Strong Behavioral Health
    Strong Recovery Chemical Dependency [47048]
    Strong Recovery Methadone Maintenance [47049]
Strong Health Dialysis--Brighton [25768]
Strong Health Dialysis--Clinton Crossing • Renal Research Institute [25769]
Strong Health Dialysis--Fingerlakes • New York Dialysis Services [25800]
Strong Health Dialysis--Highlands Living Center • Renal Research Institute [25754]
Strong Health Outpatient Rehabilitation Center [4316]
Strong Memorial Hospital--Ambulatory Care • Dialysis Unit [25770]
Strong Memorial Hospital of the University of Rochester • Cystic Fibrosis Center [7626]
Strong Memorial Hospital • University of Rochester • Kessler Burn and Trauma Center [4596]
Strong Mothers • IOP Services [46174]
Strong Speech Consulting Inc. [2580]
Strong University, Rochester • Golisano Children's Hospital • Comprehensive Sickle Cell Clinic [36402]
Strongsville Dialysis & At Home • DaVita [26206]
Stroudsburg Hospice [21160]
Structure House [11178]
Stuart F. Meyer Hospice House [19288]
Stuart Meyer Hospice and Home Health [14309]
Student Assistance Program [32323]
Studio 12 Private Alcohol and Drug • Treatment Prog/Detox/Male/Female [40274]
Sturdy Memorial Hospital [2445]
    Cancer Program [5318]
Stuttering Center of Western Pennsylvania • Com-munication Science and Disorders [3369]
Stutzman Addiction Treatment Center • Chemical Dependent Inpt Rehab Program [46572]
Su Casa Family Crisis and Support Center [8834]
Su Casa Health Care Services of New Mexico, LLC [16328]
Su Clinica Familiar • Su Clinica Familiar - Dental [7293]
Sublette County Sexual Assault and Family Violence Task Force [10759]
Substance Abuse Counseling Center [42268]
    Marine and Family Services Center [40582]
Substance Abuse Evaluation • Resource Center [40583]
Substance Abuse Foundation of • Long Beach Inc [40040]
Substance Abuse Guidance and Education • (SAGE) [49436], [49581]
Substance Abuse Operations [42771]
Substance Abuse Program [29637]
Substance Abuse Recovery Center • Adult Mental Health [42072]
Substance Abuse Rehabilitation Program [41713], [49273]
    Naval Health Clinic [44324]
    Naval Health Clinic New England [48859]
Substance Abuse Services Center Inc [43271]

Substance Abuse Services Inc [48047]
Outpatient Services [47869]
Substance Abuse Treatment Unit [33259]
Evaluation and Treatment [41445]
Substance Use Disorder Clinic • Robert J Dole VA Medical Center [43511]
Substance Use Disorder Services • (SUDS) [43900]
Suburban Dialysis Center [25568]
Suburban Home Care [15866]
Suburban Home Dialysis • Fresenius Medical Care [26228]
Suburban Hospital and Audiology and Speech Pathology [2395]
Suburban Hospital of Audiology and Speech Pathology [2381]
Suburban Hospital • Behavioral Health Services [44204]
Suburban Hospital Healthcare System • Comprehensive Cancer Program [5296]
Suburban Schools' Program for Deaf and Hard of Hearing Students [540]
Suburban Therapy Center [38715]
Success Counseling Services Inc • Outpatient AOD Clinic [46456]
Success Rehabilitation, Inc. [4414]
Successful Alternatives for Addiction Counseling Services Inc
Hayward [39917]
Vallejo [40883]
Successfully Speaking [2424]
Sudbury Regional Hospital • Regional Eating Disorders Program [11237]
Sudden Infant Death Network of Ohio [36531]
Sudden Infant Death Services of Illinois, Inc. [36475]
Sudden Infant Death Syndrome Center of New Jersey • Hackensack University Medical Center • CJ Foundation for SIDS [36512]
Suffolk Center for Myofunctional Therapy and Speech Rehabilitation [3127]
Suffolk Cnty Div of Com Mental Hygiene • North County MMTP [46684]
Suffolk County Department of Health • Alcohol and Substance AbuseServices Huntington/MMTP [46710]
Suffolk County Dept of Health Services • Div of Comm Mental Hyg Riverhead MMTP [47023]
Suffolk County Hauppauge • Div of Comm Mental Hyg/MM/KEEP [46685]
Suffolk Hearing and Speech Center [3010]
Suffolk Jewish Community Center [38780]
Suffolk Kidney Center [25678]
Sugar Land Dialysis [27366]
Sugarhouse Health Center • Community Rehabilitation Services [4470]
Sugarloaf Dialysis • DaVita [23733]
Suicide Anonymous [51050]
Suicide and Crisis Center--Dallas [51377]
Suicide and Crisis Center--Honolulu [50815]
Suicide--Crisis Center, Inc. [51423]
Suicide and Crisis Control--Denver [50716]
Suicide and Crisis Intervention Service [50763]
Suicide and Crisis Service of Alamance County [51159]
Suicide Education and Support Services of Weld County [50719]
Suicide Prevention Action Network [50748]
Suicide Prevention Center of Clark County, Inc. [51077]
Suicide Prevention Center--Dayton [51213]
Suicide Prevention Center--Gila Bend [50643]
Suicide Prevention Center--Lanham [50978]
Suicide Prevention--Clarendon [51374]
Suicide Prevention and Community Counseling Service of Marin [50698]
Suicide Prevention and Crisis [50689]
Suicide Prevention and Crisis Center [50684]
Suicide Prevention--Crisis Center, Salt Lake City [51405]
Suicide Prevention - Crisis Intervention Service [50868]
Suicide Prevention/Crisis Line of Volunteer Center of Napa County [50681]
Suicide Prevention and Crisis Service of Tompkins County [51141]
Suicide Prevention--Crisis Services, Sacramento [50688]
Suicide Prevention Hotline [50953]
Suicide Prevention--Juneau [50635]

Suicide Prevention Partnership [50714]
Suicide Prevention Service of the Central Coast [50702]
Suicide Prevention Service--Zeeland [51034]
Suicide Prevention Services--Columbus [51208]
Suicide Prevention Services, Inc.--Batavia • Crisis Line of the Fox Valley [50830]
Suicide Prevention Services of Santa Cruz County [50668]
Suicide Prevention Services--Toksook [50641]
Suicide Prevention--Wisconsin Rapids • Crisis Intervention and Referral Service [51522]
Suicide Prevention of Yolo County [50670]
Suicide Resource Center of Larimer County [50717]
The Suite at St. Antoine [21193]
Sullivan Center of Holston Valley [39033]
Sullivan County Alcohol and Drug Abuse Services • Outpatient Clinic [46751]
Sullivan House [44494]
Sumic Care, Inc. [18008]
Summa Barberton Hospital • Cancer Program [5680]
Summa Health System • Akron City Hospital • Cooper Cancer Center [5677]
Summa Sleep Medicine Centers--White Pond [37586]
Summa Western Reserve Sleep Medicine Centers--Hudson [37587]
Summa's Home Infusion [16832]
Summer Fluency Camp [2337]
Summer House [41824]
Summerhill Counseling Center [49557]
Summerlin Dialysis Center • DaVita [25375]
SummerSmith Inc. [10909]
Summit Achievement [44071]
Summit Behavioral Healthcare [33752]
Summit Care and Wellness [45764]
Summit County Health District • Counseling Services [47610]
Summit Dialysis Center • DaVita [25474]
Summit Dialysis • DaVita [27179]
Summit Eating Disorders and Outreach Program [10991]
Summit Home Health & Hospice [21622]
Summit Medical Care [23961]
Summit Medical Center
Cancer Program [5932]
Summit Center for Sleep Health [37791]
Summit Medical Services [48608]
Summit Nursing Services [13874]
Summit Oaks Center [34441]
Summit Oaks Hospital [33662], [46180]
Summit Pain Management Clinic [35745]
Summit Physical Therapy [38054]
Summit Physical Therapy West [38039]
Summit Respiratory Services [13468]
Summit Sleep Disorder Center, PA • Sleep Disorders Center [37493]
Summit Sleep Disorders Center--Winston Salem [37494]
Summit Sleep Services [37792]
Summit Speech and Rehab LLC [1436]
Summitview Child and Family Servies [28475]
Sumner Dialysis • DaVita [26840]
Sumner Mental Health Center/Wellington [43473]
Sumner Regional Medical Center • Cancer Program [5930]
Sumter Behavioral Health Services [48981], [48982]
Sumter County Office [27965]
Sumter School District Number 17 [738]
Sumter Speech and Language Therapy Center [1552]
Sun City Center • DaVita [23497]
Sun City Dialysis Center
American Renal Associates [23521]
DaVita [27074]
Sun City Hearing Service [1331]
Sun Coast Hospital • Center for Speech and Hearing [1632]
Sun Coast Hospital, Inc. [13850]
Sun Coast Hospital • Sleep Laboratory [36819]
Sun Country Medical, Inc. [17915]
Sun Crest Home Health [12639]
Sun Health Inc. • Dialysis Facility [24015]
Sun Life Family Health Center [6226]
Sun Life Home Care [14448]
Sun Ray Addictions Counseling/Educ [39926]
Sun Ray Court • Adult Male Branch [50186]

Sun Ray Dialysis • DaVita [25086]
Sun Street Centers
Residential Recovery Program [40516]
Sun Street Centers Recovery Services [40517]
Sun Valley Pain Management [35425]
Sunbelt Homecare - Jellico [17690]
Sunbridge Clinic [12843]
Sunbright Home Health Agency, Inc. [13637]
Suncoast ALS Clinic • ALS Center [109]
Suncoast Center Inc • Forensic Focused Outreach [41922]
Suncoast Community Health Centers, Inc. • Ruskin Health Center [6543]
Suncoast Dialysis Center [23536]
Suncoast Hospice--Clearwater [19206]
Suncoast Hospice House Brookside [19289]
Suncoast Hospice--Largo [19248]
Suncoast Hospice • North Community Center--Palm Harbor [19290]
Suncoast Rehabilitation Center [41936]
Sundance Center [39472]
Sundance Methadone Treatment Center [42588]
Sundance Rehabilitation [2826]
Sundown M Ranch [50276]
Sundown Ranch Inc [49260]
Sunflower Diversified Services • Early Education Center [8024]
Sunflower Health Care, Inc-Stilwell [19778]
Sunflower Health Care, Inc.--Lansing [19760]
Sunglo Home Health Services, Inc.--Brownsville [17832]
Sunglo Home Health Services, Inc.--Harlingen [17946]
Sunglo Home Health Services, Inc.--McAllen [18074]
Sunglo Home Health Services, Inc.--Rio Grande City [18122]
SunHealth Behavioral Health System for Boise [33399]
Sunland Center at Marianna [7891]
Sunlight Recovery LLC [41621]
Sunmount Developmental Disabilities Service Office [8360]
Sunny Hills Children's Garden [34018]
Sunny Hills Services [28739]
Sunny Hills Services Braun Day Treatment [28792]
Sunny Hills Services
Simmons Day Treatment [28660]
Sutro Day Treatment [28661]
Vivian Court Day Treatment [28662]
Sunny Lakes Home Health Care, Inc. [14221]
Sunnybrook Health Sciences Centre • Ross Tilley Burn Centre [4617]
Sunnyside Renal Center • Diversified Specialty Institutes • Dialysis Services [26332]
Sunnyside Village [29276]
Sunnyview Hospital and Rehabilitation Center [4317], [8353]
Sunpath LLC [47326]
Sunrise, A Speech Pathology Corp. [1117]
Sunrise Alcohol and Drugs Rehab Center [40244]
Sunrise Canyon Hospital [33878]
Sunrise Centers [50136]
Sunrise Centre [44635]
Sunrise Community [7897]
Sunrise Community Counseling Center [40162]
Sunrise Community Dialysis Center • DaVita [22889]
Sunrise Community Health Center [6403]
Sunrise Counseling Westport [50260]
Sunrise Detox II [46177]
Sunrise Detoxification Center LLC [41735]
Sunrise Family Dental Clinic [6410]
Sunrise Family Health Care, LLC [16919]
Sunrise Home Health Agency [13430]
Sunrise Home Health Care--Miami [14157]
Sunrise Home Health Services [17933]
Sunrise Hospital and Medical Center
Cancer Program [5488]
Regional Center for Sleep Disorders [37323]
Sunrise House [32666]
Sunrise House Foundation Inc • Detoxification and Residential Treatment [46029]
Sunrise House/Halfway House [45997]
Sunrise Inc • Larned [43384]
Sunrise Lodge • Substance Abuse Treatment Center [39289]
Sunrise Medications & Infusion Pharmacy [17603]
Sunrise Oxygen and Home Medical Products, Inc. [14488]

Sunrise of Pasco County, Inc. [9045]
Sunrise Place [31006]
Sunrise Recovery Center [41319]
Sunrise Recovery Services [49958]
Sunrise Sleep Diagnostics • Sleep Disorders Center [36820]
Sunrise Speech Services Inc. [1971]
Sunset Community Health Center [6255]
Sunset Community Health Center, Inc. [6248]
Sunset Dialysis Center • DaVita [22890]
Sunset Healthcare Group [13676]
Sunset Home Health Services, Inc. [13611]
Sunset Home Services [15702]
Sunset Hospice, Inc-Tomball [21580]
Sunset House Inc [41876]
Sunshine Cottage School for Deaf Children [822]
Sunshine Gold Care [14271]
Sunshine Home Health Care [14158]
Sunshine Inc. of Northwest Ohio [8421]
Sunshine Orthopedic Sports Physical Therapy--Commack [38781]
Sunshine Orthopedic Sports Physical Therapy--Dix Hills [38783]
Sunshine Social Club [31393]
Sunshine Speech-Language Therapy Services Inc. [985]
Sunshine Suicide Prevention • Hooper Bay Native Village [50634]
Sunshine Treatment Institute PLLC [44767]
SUNY Downstate Medical Center • MDA Clinic [34843]
SUNY Health Science Center at Syracuse [25789]
SUNY Parkside Dialysis Center [25630]
SUNY Upstate Medical University
    Center for Children with Cancer and Blood Disorders [12566]
    Department of Neurology • Multiple Sclerosis Center [34655]
    Regional Oncology Center • Adult Program [12567]
Super Care, Inc. [12945]
Superior DME, Inc. [17916]
Superior Health Services, Inc. [17304]
Superior Home Health Care Services Inc. [13185]
Superior Home Health Group [14222]
Superior Home Nursing and Hospice [20037]
Superior Hospice-Murray [21623]
Superior Mobility, Inc. [13397]
Superior Psychology Services [44858]
Superior Therapy Services Inc. [1563]
Superstition Mountain Mental Health Center [28129]
Supervised Group Homes • LifeLinks, Inc. [29577]
The Support Center [10635]
Support Center Against Domestic Violence and Sexual Assault [9811]
Support Center Inc
    Substance Abuse Outpatient Program [46989]
    Substance Abuse Residential Treatment Prog [46990]
Support for Harbor Area Womens Lives • Shawl House [40697]
Support Inc [47327]
Support, Inc. • Family Crisis Center [9789]
Support Network for Battered Women [8851]
Supportive Home Health [14685]
Supportive Home Health Care Corporation [13155]
Supportive Living Adaptive Group Residence [29331]
SUPRA Home Care of Mansfield [15325]
SUPRA Home Care of Shreveport [15365]
SUPRA Home Care of Tulsa [17172]
SUPRA Home Care of Tulsa - Bartlesville Office [17104]
SUPRA Home Care of Tulsa - Okmulgee Office [17156]
Supra Home Health [14330]
Supreme Home Healthcare, LLC [14753]
Suquamish Tribe Wellness Center [50196]
Sure Help Line Center [50672]
Surgical Biologics • MiMedx Group [35014]
Surry Counseling Services [32794]
Surry County Domestic Violence Center [10032]
Surry Domestic Violence Program [10066]
Survival Adult Abuse Center [9733]
Survivor Project [10252]
Survivors Against Violent Environments [10428]
Survivors Inc. [10278]
Surya K Challa [47543]

Susan B. Allen Dialysis Center • Fresenius Medical Care [24316]
Susan B. Allen Memorial Hospital [2214], [15119]
Susan B. Anthony Project [9006]
Susan B Anthony Recovery Center [41888]
Susan B. Krevoy Eating Disorders Program for Adults and Adolescents [10992]
Susan Weston McMillan MS LMHC CAP [41697]
Susanna Wesley Family Learning Center [9675]
Susanna Wesley House [9446]
Susanville Indian Health Center [40837]
Susie Bowling Lawrence Hospice • Johnson County Healthcare Center [21875]
Susquehanna Health System
    Cancer Program [5882]
        Sports Medicine Center [38991]
Susquehanna HomeCare & Hospice [21173]
Susquehanna Valley Women in Transition [10293]
Sussex Counseling Services [32796]
Sussex County Sexual Trauma Resource Center [9843]
Sutter Auburn Faith Hospice [18887]
Sutter Auburn Faith Hospital [12897]
    Cancer Care Program [4759]
Sutter Center for Psychiatry [33182]
Sutter Coast Home Care [17183]
Sutter Coast Hospital [12967]
Sutter Counseling Center [33183]
Sutter East Bay Physicians Medical Group • Multiple Sclerosis Clinic [34530]
Sutter General Hospital • Cancer Center [4829]
Sutter Lakeside Community Service [8828]
Sutter Lakeside Hospital [13097]
Sutter Maternity and Surgery Center [13333]
Sutter Medical Center • Cystic Fibrosis Center [7481]
Sutter Medical Center Transplant • Sutter Health [22922]
Sutter Rehabilitation Institute [3927]
Sutter Roseville Medical Center • Cancer Program [4827]
Sutter Sleep Disorders Center--Roseville [36706]
Sutter Sleep Disorders Center--Sacramento [36707]
Sutter Solano Medical Center • Cancer Center [4862]
Sutter Visiting Nurse Association and Hospice [13398]
Sutter VNA and Hospice--Concord [18912]
Sutter VNA and Hospice--Emeryville [18919]
Sutter VNA and Hospice--Roseville [19005]
Sutter VNA and Hospice--Sacramento [19006]
Sutter VNA and Hospice--San Francisco [19026]
Sutter VNA and Hospice--San Mateo [19034]
Sutter VNA and Hospice--Santa Rosa [19045]
Sutter-Yuba Mental Health Crisis Clinic [50708]
Sutter Yuba Mental Health Services • Options for Change [40973]
Sutton Place Behavioral Health Inc [42013]
Suwannee River Kidney Center • Fresenius Medical Care [23545]
SUWS of the Carolinas [31575]
Suzanne Lawrence BS LADC [43973], [44072]
SVH Neuroscience Center • Multiple Sclerosis Center [34623]
SW Sports Medicine [39097]
Swain/Qualla SAFE, Inc. [10018]
Swallowing Diagnostics [1445]
Swallowing Diagnostics Inc. [1633]
Swallowing Disorders Center of Connecticut [1491]
Swan Communication Therapies [2521]
Swank Institute [3463]
Swannanoa Dialysis Center • DaVita [25960]
Swansea Wood School [8152]
Swanson Center [29759]
Swanson Center LaPorte County • Comprehesive Mental Health Council Inc [43129]
Swanson Center--Shorewood Place Residential [29781]
Swanson Center--Ventures [29782]
Swedish American Health System • Sleep Disorders Center [36934]
Swedish American Hospital [14915]
    Regional Cancer Center [5126]
Swedish Covenant Hospital
    Cancer Program [5078]
    Sleep Disorders Center [36935]
Swedish Health Services • Cancer Program [6115]
Swedish Home Care Services [18455]

Swedish Medical Center [1410], [18456]
Swedish Medical Center/Ballard • Addiction Recovery Services [50137]
Swedish Medical Center • Division of Perinatal Medicine [12369]
Swedish Medical Center--Edmonds [37939]
Swedish Medical Center--Englewood • Sleep Disorders Center [36735]
Swedish Medical Center
    Neuroscience Institute [12475]
    Radiation Oncology Program [4878]
Swedish Medical Center Transplant Services [27641]
Swedish Visiting Nurse Services [21762]
Sweeney, Gendel and Associates [2108]
Sweet Angels Health Services [14159]
Sweet Care Home Health Agency, Inc. [14160]
Sweet and Gentle Home Health Care [13677]
Sweet Home Care, Inc. [16468]
Sweet Home Health Agency [14161]
Sweetser [8084], [34170]
Sweetser Affiliate [43953], [43954], [43999], [44035]
    Charlene Barton [43984]
Sweetser - Affiliate • David Appell LCSW LADC CCS [43963]
Sweetser Affiliate
    David Prichard [44036]
    Deborah Jo Landry [44056]
    Gordanna Hassett [43933]
    Greg Stine [44047]
    Jennifer Fowler Greaves [44037]
Sweetser - Affiliate
    Kary Laban LCPC LADC CCS [43977]
    Lorrie Roberts LADC [43981]
Sweetser Affiliate
    Marlene Silva [44038]
    Mary C Kennedy LCSW LADC CCS [44053]
    Mary Ellen Ostherr [44048]
    Rachel Davis LADC [44000]
Sweetser - Affiliate • Ruth DeWitt [44001]
Sweetser Affiliate
    Stephanie Beck/Julia Orr [44002]
    Susan Managan MS LADS CCS [43949]
    Tanya Dunton LADC [43934]
    Timothy Ericson [43993]
    Tracy Hutch [44054]
Sweetser Affilitate • Greg Ford [44039]
Sweetser Children's Home and Community Residence [34171]
Sweetser Children's Services • Crisis Intervention and Stabilization [50962]
Sweetwater Dialysis • DaVita [23734]
Sweetwater Hospital Association [17775]
Swigert and Associates [2276]
Swinomish Wellness Program Chemical • Dependancy Services [49995]
Swiss Avenue Dialysis Center • Fresenius Medical Care [27039]
Switchboard, Inc. [50887]
Switchboard of Miami, Inc. [50775]
Switzer School and Clinical Services [1343]
Switzerland County Counseling Center [29826]
    Community Mental Health Center Inc [43222]
Swope Health Independence [6905]
Swope Health Services [45532]
    Behavioral Health Services [30864]
Swope Health Services Central [6909]
Swope Health Services • Imani House [45533]
Swords to Plowshares • Residential Program [40639]
Sycamore Dialysis & At Home • DaVita [24097]
Sycamore Medical Office Building [12794]
Sycamore Sports Medicine [38450]
The Sycamores [34011]
Sylva Dialysis Center • DaVita [25961]
Sylvia's House [19276]
Sylvia's Place [9511]
Symbii Home Health and Hospice--Layton [21614]
Symbii Home Health and Hospice-Salt Lake City [21656]
Sympatico [51313]
Synergy Counseling Services [32962]
Synergy Group Services Inc [41877]
Synergy Healthcare Services [15427]
Synergy Home Healthcare, Inc. [14870]
Synergy Recovery at the • William L Bundy [47438]
Synergy Services, Inc./Safe Haven [9708]
Synergy Services • Runaway and Homeless Youth

Program [36059]
Synergy Treatment Centers [49145]
Syosset Speech and Hearing Center [3128]
Syracuse Behavioral Health • Syracuse Brick House [47119]
Syracuse Behavioral Healthcare
 Outpatient Services [47120]
 Syracuse Brick House Inc [47121]
Syracuse Brick House Inc
 Alcoholism Supportive Living Facility [47122]
 Mens Halfway House [47123], [47124]
Syracuse City School District [605]
Syracuse Community Health Center Inc • Alcohol and Drug Treatment Outpatient [47125]
Syracuse Community Health Center, Inc. [7043]
Syracuse Outpatient Office • The Bowen Center [43209]
Syracuse Recovery Services LLC [47126]
Syracuse University • Gebbie Speech-Language-Hearing Clinics [3134]
Syracuse Veterans Affairs Medical Center [4318], [31479]
Syringa General Hospital • Hospice Program [19461]
Syzygy Associates--Hampton Road, Dallas [35714]
Syzygy Associates LP--Fort Worth [35715]
Syzygy Associates LP--North Central Expressway, Dallas [35716]

T

12 Palms Recovery Inc • 12 Palms Recovery Center [41715]
12 and 12 Inc [48032]
12th St. Covington Dialysis • DaVita [24371]
13th Place, Inc. [50614]
2-1-1 Big Bend [50788]
2-1-1 Brevard [50753]
2-1-1 Fingerlakes [51151]
2-1-1 Tampa Bay Cares [50769]
2001 State Street Center [6670]
21st Century Rehabilitation [38478]
24 Seven Health Care Services, Inc. [14716]
24-7 Quality Infusion and Home Health, Inc. [13445]
25 Judicial District Youth Services [43349]
25th Street Dialysis Inc. • DaVita [24625]
281-CARE: Crisis Care Center [51204]
3 RS/Nuway Counseling Center Inc [45201]
310 Info [50947]
360 Physical Therapy [38027]
3HC - Goldsboro [20669]
3rd Step Mental Health Program [41644]
T. J. Samson Community Hospital [15182]
T K Consulting Inc [42037]
T W Neumann and Associates [49820]
TAAP • Women's Resource Center [10593]
Table Rock Dialysis Center • DaVita [23868]
Tacachale Children and Families [7883]
Tacoma Behavioral Health Clinic [32874]
Tacoma Dialysis and At Home • DaVita [27655]
Tacoma General Hospital • MultiCare Sleep Disorders Center [37940]
Tacoma Home Health Services [17674]
Tacoma Pierce County Health Department • Treatment Services Unit 1 [50220]
Tacoma Public Schools
 Deaf and Hard of Hearing Program [868]
 Special Education Department [8607]
Tacoma Treatment Solutions [50002]
Taconic Developmental Disabilities Service Office [8362]
Tadiso Inc [48609]
Tahana Whitecrow Foundation [48244]
Tahlequah City Hospital [7117]
Tahlequah Health Center [7118]
Tahoe Forest Hospice [19065]
Tahoe Safe Alliance [8825]
Tahoe Spine and Pain Care [35551]
Tahoe Turning Point Inc • Treatment Center Main Office [40810]
Tahoe Women's Services [9793]
Tahoe Youth and Family Services [40811], [45829]
 Runaway and Homeless Youth Program [35846]
Take Back Control LLC [43117]
Taking Control [42814]
Taking It to the Street Ministries [41896]
Takoma Park Dialysis • DaVita [24697]
Talbert House [31696]

ADAPT for Men [47668]
 Adult Services/Outpatient [47669]
 Alternatives for Young Men [47670]
 The Bridge [47671]
 Passages for Young Women [47672]
 RHH Expansion [47673]
Talbot County Addictions Program [44248]
Talbot Hospice Foundation [19923]
Talbott Recovery Campus [29356]
Talk to Kelly LLC [3080]
Talk to Me Speech, Language Therapy [3549]
Talk Shoppe [1949]
Talk SLP Services [3629]
TALK--Teaching and Assessing Language for Kids [1071]
Talk Time for Kids Inc. [1830]
Talk-Time Speech and Language Center [3352]
Talk Time Speech and Language Services [1688]
Talk Time Therapy Inc. [1582]
Talking Books Plus [3835]
Talking with Technology Camp • The Children's Hospital of Denver [1404]
Talkline Help Lines Inc. [50844]
Talktime Speech Therapy [3323]
Tall Oaks Apartments [28009]
Talladega Health Care Center [28048]
Talladega Satellite Office [28049]
Tallahassee Dialysis • DaVita • Dialysis Facility [23522]
Tallahassee Memorial HealthCare [14402]
Tallahassee Memorial Healthcare • Cancer Treatment Center [4995]
Tallahassee Memorial Hospital • Chemical Dependency Program [41950]
Tallahassee Neurological Clinic • MDA Clinic [34784]
Tallahassee South Dialysis • DaVita • Dialysis Facility [23523]
Tallgrass Sleep Center [37009]
Tallulah Mental Health Center [30176]
Tamarac Artificial Kidney Center • DaVita [23525]
Tamarac Kidney Center • Fresenius Medical Care [23526]
Tamarack Behavioral Health Center [50456]
Tamarack Center [34473]
Tamarack Treatment and Counseling Center [42375]
Tamayo House • Runaway and Homeless Youth Program [35847]
Tamcare Home Health, Inc. [18077]
Tampa Bay Academy [34079]
Tampa Bay Hearing and Balance Center [1783]
Tampa Bay Home Health Care, Inc.--Safety Harbor [14361]
Tampa Bay Home Health Care--Tampa [14427]
Tampa Bay Pulmonary Sleep Disorders Center [36821]
Tampa Bay Sleep Center [36822]
Tampa Bay Sleep Disorders Center at New Tampa [36823]
Tampa Cares 211 [50770]
Tampa Clinic • Outreach Clinic • Cystic Fibrosis Center [7511]
Tampa Crossroads [29309]
Tampa Crossroads Inc [41971]
 Rose Manor Residential Program [41972]
Tampa Family Health Center--E Columbus [6558]
Tampa Family Health Center--N Dale Mabry [6559]
Tampa Family Health Center--N Mitchell [6560]
Tampa Family Health Center--N Sheldon [6561]
Tampa Family Health Center--W Waters [6562]
Tampa General Hospital
 Adult Cystic Fibrosis Center [7512]
 Headache and Pain Center [12415]
 Pediatric Dialysis [23537]
Tampa General Hospital Rehabilitation Center • Pain Management Clinic [35397]
Tampa General Hospital
 Sleep Disorders Center Program [36824]
 Tampa Bay Regional Burn Center [4534]
Tampa General Hospital Transplant Center [23538]
Tampa General Rehabilitation Center [3996]
Tampa Health Center--SW Shore [6563]
Tampa Hearing Services [1784]
Tampa Help Line/Christian Helpline Network [50792]
Tampa (James A. Haley) Veterans Hospital [51556]
Tampa Metro Treatment Center [41973]
Tampopo Speech Clinic [1344]
Tanager Place [34139]

Tanaka House [31722]
Tanana Chiefs Conference [28091]
Tangipahoa Parish School [2336]
Tangipahoa Parish School District [453]
Tangu Inc [42038]
Tanner Center for Multiple Sclerosis [34506]
Tanner Hospice Care [19369]
Tanner Medical Center, Inc. [14499]
Tantaglio Home [31990]
Tanya Dunton [43935]
Taos Dialysis • Dialysis Clinic, Inc. [25564]
Taos Municipal Schools [565]
TAP Resources Inc [42865]
Tapestry Comprehensive Eating Disorder Treatment for Women [11179]
Tapestry LLC [45314]
Tappahannock Dialysis Center • Fresenius Medical Care [27575]
Tar Heel Human Services [47221]
Tar River Speech & Language Services [3185]
Tara Treatment Center Inc [43061], [43062], [43169]
Tarrant County Campus Dialysis • Fresenius Medical Care [27091]
Tarrant County Medical Education and • Research Foundation/Outpatient [49342]
Tarrant County Vet Center [52116]
Tarrant Dialysis Center--Arlington • US Renal Care [26946]
Tarrant Dialysis Center--Central • US Renal Care [27092]
Tarrant Dialysis Center--Fort Worth • US Renal Care [27093]
Tarrant Dialysis Center--Grand Prairie • US Renal Care [27112]
Tarrant Dialysis Center--Mansfield • US Renal Care [27245]
Tarrant Dialysis Center--North Richland Hills • US Renal Care Inc. [27275]
Tarrant Dialysis Center--Tarrant County • US Renal Care [27094]
Tarrant Dialysis Center--Weatherford • US Renal Care [27390]
Tarrant Dialysis Cleburne • US Renal Care [26997]
Tarzana Treatment Center Inc [39989], [40843]
 Antelope Valley [39990]
 Long Beach [40041]
 Tarzana Treatment Center [40844]
 Tarzana Treatment Center/Long Beach [40042]
 Tarzana Treatment Center/Reseda [40444]
 TTC Youth Services/Lancaster [39991]
Tarzana Treatment Centers
 Antelope Valley [28558]
 Atlantic Avenue, Long Beach [28576]
 Lancaster Boulevard, Lancaster [28559]
 Magnolia Avenue, Long Beach [28577]
 N 10th Street W, Lancaster [28560]
 Reseda [28717]
 Tarzana [28826]
Task Force on Family Violence • REACH, Inc. [10067]
Tasks Unlimited, Inc. [30700]
Tate Foundation Chesapeake Hospice House [19933]
Taunton Kidney Center • Fresenius Medical Care [24807]
Taunton Regional Dialysis Center [24808]
Taunton State Hospital [33583]
Tavarua Health Services • Rehab Services [40386]
Taylor County Clinic [29263]
Taylor County Dialysis • Davita [24367]
Taylor County • Human Services Department [50461]
Taylor County Mental Health Center [29987]
Taylor County Vet Center [52100]
Taylor Dialysis • DaVita [27369]
Taylor Hardin Secure Medical Facility [33101]
Taylor Home Health Supply--Beaumont [17825]
Taylor Home Health Supply--Tyler [18179]
Taylor Hospital • Crozer Keystone Sleep Disorders Center [37701]
Taylor House [19688]
Taylor House Battered Women's Program [9414]
Taylor Life Center/Owosso [44953]
Taylor Psychological Clinic [30553]
Taylor Psychological Clinic PC [44792]
Taylor Regional Hospital--Hawkinsville [14535]
Taylor Regional Hospital • James G. Brown Cancer Center [5213], [15167]

Taylormayd Inc • CD Outpatient Services [46457]
Taylorville Dialysis • DaVita [24098]
Tazewell Community Health [7361]
Tazewell Community Home Health Services [18394]
Tazewell Community Hospital [18395]
Tazwood Mental Health Center [29659]
Tazwood Mental Health Center Inc [42643], [42644], [42750], [42854]
Tazwood Mental Health Center--Pekin [50866]
Tazwood Mental Health Center--Peoria [50869]
TBI Solutions LLC [4215]
TC Home Health Care [13777]
T.C. Thompson Children' Hospital • Sickle Cell Center [36431]
T.C. Thompson Children's Hospital • Pediatric Cystic Fibrosis Center [7663]
TCC Allakaket Counseling Center [39329]
TCN Behavioral Health Services Inc [47758] Christopher House [47892]
TCN Behavioral Health Services, Inc. [31766]
TDS Speech Pathology Associates Inc. [2447], [2490]
TEA Healthcare Services Inc. [13442]
TEACH, Inc. • Modoc Crisis Center [8789]
Teaching Alternative Strategies and Knowledge Inc [47239]
The T.E.A.M. Approach [3514]
Team Coordinating Agency Inc • Ambulatory Services Division [44482]
Team Management 2000 Inc [46216]
Team Therapy Inc. [2117]
Team-Work Rehabilitation, Inc.--Mexico [38661]
Team-Work Rehabilitation, Inc.--Saint Charles [38662]
TeamBuilders Counseling Services, Inc.--Alamogordo [31181]
TeamBuilders Counseling Services, Inc.--Clayton [31188]
TeamBuilders Counseling Services, Inc.--Clovis [31189]
TeamBuilders Counseling Services, Inc.--Espanola [31193]
TeamBuilders Counseling Services, Inc.--Fort Sumner [31196]
TeamBuilders Counseling Services, Inc.--Mescalero [31208]
TeamBuilders Counseling Services, Inc.--Portales [31210]
TeamBuilders Counseling Services, Inc.--Raton [31211]
TeamBuilders Counseling Services, Inc.--Rio Rancho [31213]
TeamBuilders Counseling Services, Inc.--Ruidoso [31214]
TeamBuilders Counseling Services, Inc.--Santa Rosa [31216]
TeamBuilders Counseling Services, Inc.--Taos [31221]
TeamBuilders Counseling Services, Inc.--Tucumcari [31222]
Teaming for Success LLC [50253]
Teamwork Therapies Inc. [1069]
Tech Med, Inc. [16178]
Teche Action Board, Inc. • Tech Action Clinic [6745]
Teche Action Clinic at Dulac [6746]
Teche Regional Medical Center [15337]
Technology and Language Center, Inc. [2109]
Ted R. Montoya Hemophilia Program • University of New Mexico [12559]
Teen Challenge [40584] Bayamon 1 [48739]
Teen Challenge International • Teen Challenge Mens Ranch [40797]
Teen Challenge Philadelphia Mens Home [48568] Philadelphia Womens Home [48569]
Teen Challenge Training Center Inc [48630]
Teen Challenge of Western Pennsylvania [48633]
Teen Challenge Wisconsin • Robbie Dawson Home for Women [50486]
Teen Challenge Women Center [48744]
Teen Focus Recovery Center [45288]
Teen Lifeline [50648]
Teen Line [50678]
Teen Living Programs, Inc. • Foundation House • Runaway and Homeless Youth Program [35940]
Teen Solutions [40223]
Teens Living Clean [39638]

Teens Need Teens Hotline [50870]
Teens Talk To Teens [50645]
Tehama County Health Services Agency Drug and Alcohol Division [40424] Drug and Alcohol Division/South County [39741]
Tehama County Special Schools and Services [292]
Tejas Recovery and Counseling Services [49531]
Tel Huron Waterford Dialysis • DaVita [24989]
Telecare Corporation Alameda STRIDES [40308] La Casa Mental Health Rehab Center [40043] Solano STRIDES [40509]
Telecare Recovery Access Center • Homeless Outreach Program [28635]
Telephone Equipment Distribution Program [2735]
Telephone FIRST • Free Information and Referral System [51296]
Telesis [41201]
Temada Associates [46186]
Temenos Institute, Inc. [29051]
Tempe Valley Hope Outpatient • Rio Sureno Medical Plaza [39481]
Temple City Dialysis Facility, Inc. [23031]
Temple Kidney Center • Dialysis Facility • Fresenius Medical Care [27371]
Temple Physical Therapy [38195]
Temple Regional Day School • Program for the Deaf [828]
Temple Terrace Dialysis • DaVita • Dialysis Facility [23541]
Temple University Hospital Cancer Program [5854] Pain Management [35372] Temple Burn Center [4624] Temple Sleep Disorders Center [37702]
Temple University Hospital Transplant Unit [26538]
Temple University Marlton Sports Medicine Center [38737] School of Medicine • Temple HIV Programs • Community Program for Clinical Research on AIDS [68] Speech, Language, Hearing Center [3361] Sports Medicine Center [38968] Western Pennsylvania Hospital • Pain Management [35651]
Templeton Developmental Center [8109]
Templum House [10137]
Tempo Group Inc • Outpatient Drug Treatment Program [47193]
Temporary Lodging for Children • Runaway and Homeless Youth Program [35963]
Ten Broeck Hospital of Jacksonville [33310]
Ten Broeck Hospital - Kentucky [33528]
Ten Sixteen Recovery Network [44672], [44698], [44798], [49919], [44932] Mount Pleasant Detox Center [44933] Outpatient Counseling Services [44920]
Tenbroeck Hospital at KMI Campus [33529]
Tenbrook • Sligo Woods Preschool [8104]
Tender Care Home Health Services--Davie [13638]
Tender Care Home Health Services--Miami [14162]
Tender Heart Home Health, LLC [17808]
Tender Heart Hospice Care-Arlington [21384]
Tender Home Health Care--Farmington [15653]
Tender Home Health Care--Pontiac [15776]
Tender Love Health Services [13605]
Tender Loving Care Home Care and Hospice-Franklinton • Amedisys Home Health Services [20665]
Tender Loving Care Home Care and Hospice-Garner • Amedisys Home Health Services [20667]
Tender Loving Care Home Care and Hospice--Morgantown • Amedisys Home Health Services [21808]
Tender Loving Care Home Care and Hospice--Saint Clairsville • Amedisys Home Health Services [20888]
Tender Loving Care Home Care and Hospice--Wheeling • Amedisys Home Health Care [21816]
Tender Loving Care Home Hospice [13191]
Tender Loving Care Home Hospice--Moorpark [18974]
Tender Texas Heart, LLC [18075]
Tender Touch Therapy [3668]
Tendercare Clinic, Inc. [6594]
Tennessee Community • Counseling Services Inc [49054]
Tennessee Community Health Services Inc [49186]

Alfred E Watts Recovery Center [49169]
Blount County [49129]
Cocke County [49170]
Jefferson County [49067]
Tennessee Comprehensive Lung and Sleep Center [37793]
Tennessee Department of Health • Maternal and Child Heath [36542]
Tennessee District 12-0 Lions Eye Bank and Sight Service [35212]
Tennessee Donor Services--Chattanooga [35213]
Tennessee Donor Services--Gray [35214]
Tennessee Donor Services--Knoxville [35215]
Tennessee Donor Services--Nashville [35216]
Tennessee Home Medical, Inc. [17760]
Tennessee Infant Parent Services School [3434]
Tennessee Orthopaedic Alliance [39038]
Tennessee Quality Hospice--Camden [21312]
Tennessee Quality Hospice--Jackson [21340]
Tennessee Quality Hospice--Waynesboro [21373]
Tennessee School for the Blind [3737]
Tennessee School for the Deaf [755]
Tennessee SIDS Alliance [36543]
Tennessee State Library and Archives • Tennessee Library for the Blind and Physically Handicapped [3838]
Tennessee Temple University • School of Deaf Studies and Interpreter Training Program [749]
Tennessee Valley Dialysis Center • DaVita [26854]
Tennessee Valley Family Services • Runaway and Homeless Youth Program [35783]
Tennessee Valley Health Care System • Nashville Campus [4435]
Tennessee Valley Healthcare System Alvin C. York, Murfreesboro Campus [4436] Alvin C. York Veterans Affairs Medical Center [51652] Charlotte Avenue Clinic [4437] Chattanooga Outpatient Clinic [4438] Clarksville Outpatient Clinic [4439] Cookeville Veterans Primary Clinic [4440] Nashville Women Veterans Healthcare Center [4441] Veterans Affairs Medical Center • Nashville Campus [51653]
Tennessee Valley Veterans Affairs Health Care System PTSD Clinical Team Outpatient [51821] Women's Stress Disorder Treatment Team [51822]
Tennessee Valley Veterans Affairs Healthcare System Nashville Campus [32369] PTSD Clinical Team [51823]
Tensas Community Health Center [6762]
Teras Interventions and Counseling Inc [48217]
Terence Cardinal Cooke Health Care Center [8336]
Terence Cardinal Cooke Health Center • Dialysis Unit [25738]
Terra Firma Diversion • Educational Services [39918]
Terra Nova Counseling [40510]
Terre Haute Regional Hospital • Cancer Care Program [5175]
Terre Haute Veterans Affairs Clinic [29821]
Terrebonne Addictive Disorders Clinic [43831]
Terrebonne General Medical Center [2318] Mary Bird Perkins Cancer Center [5247]
Terrebonne Mental Health Center [30143]
Terrell County Mental Health Center [29404]
Terrell Dialysis Center • Fresenius Medical Care [27373]
Terrell State Hospital [33885]
Terrio-Therapy Fitness Inc. [1063]
Terros Inc [39451], [39452]
Terry Children's Psychiatric Center [34061]
Terry County Mental Health Center [32417]
Terry Reilly Health Services [6639]
Tesca Hospice, Inc. [18894]
TESSA [8942]
Teton Orthopaedics Afton Start Valley Medical Center [39192] Driggs 4 Peaks Clinic [38341] Green River Castle Rock Medical Center [39193] Jackson Hole [39194] Marbleton/Big Piney Marbleton Clinic [39195] Pinedale Clinic [39196]

Rawlins Clinic [39197]
Rock Springs Clinic [39198]
Wilson Medical [39199]
Teton Youth and Family Services [34500]
Teton Youth & Family Services--Jackson [33048]
Teton Youth & Family Services • Runaway and
Homeless Youth Program [36281]
Teton Youth & Family Services--Wilson [33075]
Tewksbury Public Schools [2529]
Tewksbury State Hospital [33584]
Texana Center [32540]
Texana Mental Health & Retardation Center [8569]
Texarkana Home Care [18174]
Texarkana RDSPD [829]
Texas Alcoholism Foundation Inc • Texas House
Treatment Program [49404]
Texas Back Institute--Arlington [35717]
Texas Back Institute--Denton [35718]
Texas Back Institute--Flower Mound [35719]
Texas Back Institute--Fort Worth [35720]
Texas Back Institute--Mansfield [35721]
Texas Back Institute--McKinney [35722]
Texas Back Institute--McKinney North [35723]
Texas Back Institute--North Denton [35724]
Texas Back Institute--Odessa [35725]
Texas Back Institute--Plano [35726]
Texas Back Institute--Rockwall [35727]
Texas Back Institute--Trophy Club [35728]
Texas Back Institute--Tyler [35729]
Texas Back Institute--Wichita Falls [35730]
Texas Child and Family Institute [49236]
Texas Children's Hemophilia and Thrombosis Center
[12602]
Texas Children's Hospital
Children's Sleep Center [37858]
Clinical Care Center • Metabolic Clinic [12353]
Meyer Center for Developmental Pediatrics •
Down Syndrome Clinic of Houston [10871]
Transplant Services [27180]
Texas Choice Healthcare Services, Inc. [18125]
Texas Christian University • Miller Speech and Hear-
ing Clinic [3496]
Texas City Dialysis LLP [27377]
Texas Clinic
Fulton [49405]
Westview [49406]
Texas Council on Problem and Compulsive
Gambling [51390]
Texas Department of Health Services • Bureau of
Children's Health • SIDS Information Program
[36547]
Texas Education Agency • Texas Deaf--Blind Project
[3464]
Texas Fertility Center--Austin [22271]
Texas Fertility Center--Rock Round [22272]
Texas Headache Associates--Garland [12471]
Texas Headache Associates--San Antonio [12472]
Texas Health Harris Methodist Hospital Fort Worth •
Klabzuba Cancer Center [5990]
Texas Health Presbyterian Hospital Denton [37859]
Texas Health Presbyterian Hospital Plano • Cancer
Care Program [6018]
Texas Home Health Hospice--Austin [21393]
Texas Home Health Hospice--Beaumont [21400]
Texas Home Health Hospice--College Station
[21419]
Texas Home Health Hospice--Houston [21491]
Texas Home Health Hospice--Longview [21519]
Texas Home Health Hospice--Quincy [21588]
Texas Human Biologics [35245]
Texas Medical Center • Memorial Hermann Hospital
• Sleep Disorders Center [37860]
Texas Medical Clinic [39096]
Texas Medical Diagnostics • Sleep Disorders Center
[37861]
Texas Neuro Rehab Center [8531]
Texas Neurology • MDA Clinic [34889]
Texas Neurology Sleep Disorders Center [37862]
Texas NeuroRehab Center [33860]
Texas Orthopaedic Specialists, PA [39061]
Texas Panhandle Mental Health Authority [51370]
Texas Panhandle Mental Health/Mental Retardation
[32400]
Texas Premier Care Services, Inc. [18009]
Texas Prevention Network Inc [49407]
Texas Pulmonary Sleep Center [37863]
Texas Renal Ventures • Dialysis Facility • Renal
Ventures Management [27095]

Texas School for the Blind and Visually Impaired
[3738]
Texas School for the Deaf [771]
Texas Scottish Rite Hospital for Children [8542]
Texas Sleep Medicine [37864]
Texas Sports Rehab [39060]
Texas State Library and Archives Commission •
Talking Book Program [3839]
Texas State Technical College • Deaf/Disabled
Student Services [830]
Texas State University, San Marcos • Office of Dis-
ability Services [823]
Texas Tech Health Sciences Center • Texas Tech
Medical Center [22273]
Texas Tech Univ Health Sciences Center • Dept of
Psychiatry SW Institute [49458]
Texas Tech University Health Sciences Center •
Cystic Fibrosis Center [7677]
Texas Tech University • Health Sciences Center •
Department of Pediatrics • Genetics Clinic [12354]
Texas Tech University Health Sciences Center •
MDA Clinic [34890]
Texas Tech University • Health Sciences Center •
Speech and Hearing Clinic [3522]
Texas Tech University, Lubbock • Pain Management
[35731]
Texas Treatment Centers Inc [49408]
Texas Women's University • Speech-Language-
Hearing Clinic [3486]
TexasHealth, LLC [35732]
Texoma Council of Governments • Advocacy Sup-
port Network Project [3540]
Texoma Medical Center [17894]
TMC Behavioral Health Center [49539]
Texoma Neurology Associates • MDA Clinic [34891]
TGI Care Brain Injury Program [3928]
TGR Home Health Care [14163]
THA Group--Island Health Care [14587]
Thalia House [11065]
Thames Hearing Services [1457]
Thames Valley Programs [33262]
Theda Care Behavioral Health at • Theda Clark
Medical Center [50491]
Theda Care Behavioral Health • Midway [50463]
Theda Care Hospitals • Siekman Cancer Center
[6145]
Theda Clark Medical Center • Sleep Disorders
Center [37985]
ThedaCare Behavioral Health [33023]
ThedaCare at Home [21820]
ThedaCare at Home--Appleton [18556]
ThedaCare at Home--Neenah [18608]
ThedaCare at Home--New London [18612]
ThedaCare at Home--Oshkosh [18615]
ThedaCare at Home--Shawano [18627]
ThedaCare at Home--Waupaca [18640]
THEE Hospice • Home Health Hospice [21454]
Thelma McMillen Center [40857]
TheraCom, Inc. [15462]
TheraKids Inc. [1687]
Therap-Ease, Inc. [15535]
Therapeak Inc. [2869]
Therapeutic Alternatives Inc [47447]
Therapeutic Associates, Inc. [1482]
Therapeutic Center at Fox Chase • AKA The Bridge
[48570]
Therapeutic Connections [1567]
Therapeutic Health Services
Central Youth and Family Services [50138]
Eastside Branch [49894]
Therapeutic Health Services - Kent Ann [49987]
Therapeutic Health Services
Rainier Branch South [50139]
Seneca Branch [50140]
Shoreline Branch [50155]
Therapeutic Health Services/Snohomish • Everett
[49959]
Therapeutic Health Services • Summit Branch
[50141]
Therapeutic Interventions of Georgia Inc. [1835]
Therapeutic Nursery Programs [34169]
Therapeutic Resources, Inc. [38222]
Therapies of The Rockies [1405]
Therapies To Grow On [1298]
Theraplay Institute [7977]
Therapro, Ltd. [2100]
Therapy Associates [2697]
Therapy Associates of the Ozarks Inc. [2827]

Therapy Care Ltd. [1961]
Therapy Center of Ann Arbor • Center for Eating
Disorders [11101]
Therapy Center, Sebring [1756]
A Therapy Connection [3533]
Therapy Connections for Kids--Coon Rapids [2685]
Therapy Connections for Kids--Little Canada [2700]
The Therapy House [2290]
Therapy In Your Face [49699]
Therapy Innovations [1761]
Therapy--Learning Clinic [1975]
Therapy Playhouse [1831]
Therapy Plus Speech and Language Services
[2995]
Therapy Rehab Ltd. [2017]
Therapy Relief Inc. [2781]
Therapy Resources, Inc. [1194]
Therapy Services Burlington [43322]
Therapy Solutions of Georgia Inc. [1926]
Therapy Solutions of NEA Inc. [1019]
Therapy Solutions--Philadelphia [3362]
Therapy Solutions--Tulsa [3293]
Therapy and Sports Center [38282]
Therapy Spot [2518]
Therapy Support, Inc.--Cincinnati [16879]
Therapy Support, Inc.--Springfield [16075]
Therapy Team [3340]
Therapy Zone [2772]
TheraSolutions Inc. [1860]
Theratalk Speech/Language Pathology [3147]
Therese M Reynolds MA LMHC NCC [41666]
Thibodaux Addictive Disorders Clinic [43907]
Thibodaux Regional Medical Center
Cancer Center [5266]
Sleep Disorders Center [37086]
Third Avenue Clinic Member of CRC • Health Group
[39711]
Third Avenue Group Home [29332]
Third Level Crisis Center [51030]
Third Level Crisis Intervention Center • Youth and
Family Services • Runaway and Homeless Youth
Program [36027]
Third Street Community Clinic • Third Street Family
Health Services [7094]
Third Way Center [28889]
Third Way Center Inc. [34045]
Third Way Center Inc.--Pontiac [33217]
Thirteenth Place, Youth and Family Services Inc. •
Runaway and Homeless Youth Program [35784]
Thomas B. Finan Center [33561]
Thomas Cnty Alcohol/Drug Abuse Council [43326],
[43355]
Thomas E. Creek Veterans Affairs Medical Center
[32401]
Thomas E Hand and Professional Assoc • AKA
IDRC Counseling Associates [46001]
Thomas E. Langley Medical Center [6551]
Thomas Home Health [12661]
Thomas Hospital
Adult and Pediatric Speech Therapy [909]
Thomas Hospital Sleep Services [36614]
Thomas J Bumpas M Divinity [43698]
Thomas Jefferson University • Comprehensive
Multiple Sclerosis Center [34695]
Thomas Jefferson University Hospital • Cancer
Program [5855]
Thomas Jefferson University Hospital Transplant
Unit [26539]
Thomas Jefferson University
Jefferson Pain Center [35652]
Narcotic Addiction Rehab Program [48571]
Thomas Memorial Hospital [18540]
Behavioral Health Services [50342]
Sleep Disorder Center [37958]
Thomas Peeples and Associates PSC [43603],
[43680]
Thomas Street Residence [4085]
Thomaston Dialysis • DaVita [23806]
Thomaston Hospice, Inc. [19424]
Thomasville City Schools [214]
Thomasville Dialysis Center • Wake Forest
University [25963]
Thomasville Mental Health Rehabilitation [33097]
Thompkins Child & Adolescent Services, Inc.
[34381]
Thompson Child and Family Focus [31559]
Thompson Counseling Services [42796]

Top Rank Youth • Permian Basin Community Centers MHMR [49247]

Topeka and Shawnee County Public Library • Talking Books [3796]

Topeka Veterans Affairs Medical Center [29958]

Toro School for the Deaf and Hard of Hearing [297]

Torrance Memorial Home Health and Hospice [19061]

Torrance Memorial Medical Center [1345]
    Burn Center [4520]
    Cancer Center [4859]
    Sleep Disorders Center [36708]

Torrance State Hospital [33821]
    Mental Retardation Unit [8488]

Torrence Memorial Medical Center • Medical Stabilization Program for Patients with Eating Disorders [10993]

Torrey House • CareLink Community Support Services [32024]

Torrington Board of Education [333]

Torrington Dialysis • DaVita [23183]

Total Care Home Health Agency [13271]

Total Care Home Health Services Inc. [13115]

Total Child Speech and Learning Center [2657]

Total Communication--Alhambra • Alhambra Community Hospital [1052]

Total Communication--Arcadia [1059]

Total Communication--Austin [3465]

Total Family Support Clinic [40044], [40840]

Total Health and Fitness Chiropractic Clinic • Pain Center [35335]

Total Health Service of West Virginia, Inc. [18506]

Total Healthcare Inc • Substance Abuse Services [44179]

Total Home Care--Abingdon [18243]

Total Home Care--Bluefield [18252]

Total Home Care--Clintwood [18277]

Total Home Care--Richlands [18358]

Total Home Care--Vansant [18396]

Total Home Health Care--Hallandale [13717]

Total Home Health Care, Inc.--Miami [14165]

Total Home Health, Inc.--Culver City [12970]

Total Home Health, Inc.--Elgin [14776]

Total Learning and Therapy Center [1495]

Total Life Counseling Foundation [48000]

Total Patient Care [14166]

Total Rehab Services [41806]

Total Rehabilitation and Athletic Conditioning Center [38598]

Total Rehabilitation Care at Robinwood [4126]

Total Renal Care--Fairfax • Dialysis Center • DaVita [27486]

Total Renal Care--Georgetown on the Potomac • DaVita [23226]

Total Results LLC [48234]

Total Sleep Apnea Care [37959]

Total Solution Home Health [13787]

Total Source for Hearing Loss and Access [3294]

Total Speech and Language Services [2645]

Total Therapy--Margate [1643]

Total Therapy--Riverview [1742]

Total Therapy--Tampa [1785]

Total Wellness Health Center [38081]

Totalcare Homecare and Nursing Services [13535]

Totally Kids Specialty Healthcare [7785]

Totem Lake Kidney Center • Northwest Kidney Center [27611]

A Touch of Grace Hospice [19493]

Touchette Regional Hospital [14709]

Touchpoint Autism Services [8218]

Touchstone Behavioral Counseling [29843]

Touchstone Behavioral Health, Inc. [28153]

Touchstone Counseling Center [41246], [41274]

Touchstone Counseling, Inc. [28705]

Touchstone Hall [46155]

Touchstone Innovare [44823]

Touchstone Ranch Recovery Center [49358]

Touchstone Short Term Residential • Substance Abuse Treatment Program [45765]

Touchstones [40324]

Touro College Speech and Rehabilitation [2996]

Touro Infirmary • Cancer Program [5259]

Touro Rehabilitation Center [4068]
    Pain Management Center [35471]
    Rehabilitation Services [35472]

Tower Recovery Center [39720]

Tower Sleep Medicine [36709]

Towers Healthcare Center [6447]

Town of Babylon Div of Drug and Alcohol Services [46356]

Town Center Chiropractic [39098]

Town Center Sports Injury Clinic [39129]

Town of East Hartford Department of Youth Services [28991]

Town Gate Dialysis Center • Fresenius Medical Care [27105]

Town Hall Center • Wedgwood Christian Services [34236]

Town of Islip Dept of Human Services
    Acceso [46395]
    Access [46716]

Town of Smithtown/Horizons Counseling and Educational Center [47083]

Townhall II [47782]

Townhall II Helpline [51221]

Townhall II • Horizon Halfway House [47844]

Townhouse Creative Living Center [28682]

Towns Counseling Services PSC [43584]

Townsend Center for Mental Health [30969]

Towson Addictions Center [44180]

Towson Ear, Nose and Throat LLC [2382]

Towson University
    Counseling Center [44374]
    Speech, Language and Hearing Center [2436]

Toxicology Associates Inc [49274], [49409], [49410], [49411], [49434]

Toxicology Associates of North Georgia [42132]
    Carrollton Villa Rica Highway [42055]
    Gwinnett Inc [42122]

John Tracy Clinic [1159]

Tracy Dialysis Center • DaVita [23040]

Trade Winds Rehabilitation Center, Inc. [7990]

Traditional Home Health Care--Clarks Summit [17287]

Traditional Home Health Care--Dunmore [17303]

Traffic School of Behavior Change [42727]

Trafford Speech Language and Literacy Services [2504]

Training Room Sports [38567]

Tralee Crisis Center for Women, Inc. [10495]

Tranquil Haven [11010]

Tranquility Counseling Services [47332]

Tranquility Home Health Services [14167]

Transcultural Health Development [40960]

Transformation House • For Men [45075]

Transformation House I • For Women [45076]

Transformations House II • For Women [45156]

Transformations Treatment Center Inc [41637]

Transformations Wellness Center [48139]

Transition Hospice Care [19413]

Transition House • Domestic Violence Program [9474]

Transition House Inc [41937]

Transition and Recovery • A Counseling Agency [41152]

Transitional Age Youth FSP Drop-In Center [28544]

Transitional Alternative • Re Entry Initiative [42404]

The Transitional Learning Center at Galveston • Regency Care Center [4460]

Transitional Learning Center at Lubbock [4461]

Transitional Lifestyles Community [44793]

Transitional Living Center [33788]

Transitional Living Centers, Inc. [28561]

Transitional Living Inc [47776]

Transitional Living, Inc.--Middletown [31810]

Transitional Living, Inc.--Park Avenue, Hamilton [31776]

Transitional Living, Inc.--Princeton Road, Hamilton [31777]

Transitional Living Services [46241]

Transitional Living Services, Inc. • Crisis Resource Center [51514]

Transitional Ministry of Christ • Helping Hands Recovery Center [40163]

Transitional Youth Program [29019]

Transitioning Lives Inc [44181], [44182]

Transitions [10186], [28290]

Transitions Center LLC [50519]

Transitions Counseling Services [43382]

Transitions Family Counseling andMediation Center [50572]

Transitions Family Violence Services [10572]

Transitions Inc
    Outpatient Services [43567]
    Womens Res Addiction Prog [43568]

Transitions of Long Island [3047]

Transitions Recovery Program [41825]

Transitions of Western Illinois • Suicide Prevention and Crisis Service [50872]

Transmountain Dialysis • DaVita [27075]

Transylvania Community Hospital [3159]

Transylvania Community Hospital Home Care [16700]

Transylvania Regional Hospital Hospice [20625]

Tratamiento Ambulatorio Adultos • Humacao [48773]

Traumatic Brain Injury Network • Alcohol/Drug Outpatient Treatment [47732]

Trautz Associates [46062]

Travco Behavioral Health Inc [47633]

Travelers Aid of Puerto Rico [10329]

Traverse Bay Intermediate School District [505]

Traverse City Outpatient Clinic [15856]

Traverse City Vet Center [51998]

Travis County Health and Human Services • Travis County Services for the Deaf and Hard of Hearing [3466]

TRC Counseling [47352]

Treasure Coast Community Health [6565]
    Fellsmere Medical Center [6459]

Treasure Coast Counseling Center Inc [41908]

Treasure Coast Forensic Treatment Center [33308]

Treasure Coast Hospice North [19304]

Treasure Coast Hospice - Saint Lucie Hospice House [19226]

Treasure Coast Hospices--Fort Pierce [19227]

Treasure Coast Hospices--Okeechobee [19278]

Treasure Coast Hospices-South [19314]

Treasure Coast Kidney Center--North • Fresenius Medical Care • Dialysis Facility [23520]

Treasure Coast Speech and Language/Center for Successful Students [1764]

Treasure Valley Dialysis Center • DaVita [23877]

Treasure Valley Speech and Language [1943]

Treasured Memories Hospice [21880]

TREAT Services [3530]

Treat Speech, Language, and Myofunctional Clinic [3355]

Treatment Assessment Screening Center Inc • (TASC) [39396], [39453]

Treatment Associates [49570]

Treatment Associates Inc • Sacramento Treatment Clinic [40511]

Treatment Associates • McAllen [49462]

Treatment Center [41265]

Treatment Center of Brunswick [42053]

Treatment Center of Fayette [42096]

Treatment Center of Kennesaw [42115]

Treatment Center of Newnan [42138]

The Treatment Center of the Palm Beaches [41736]

Treatment Center of Valdosta [42176]

Treatment Center of Waycross [42182]

Treatment Centers of Illinois
    Bolingbrook Treatment [42421]
    Deerfield Treatment [42622]
    Hanover Park Treatment [42906]

Treatment Centers of Illinois LLC • Lombard Treatment [42754]

Treatment Centers of Illinois • Palatine Treatment [42839]

Treatment Centers LLC • Rowan Treatment Associates [47489]

Treatment Centers XL • Aminokit Labs [41153]

Treatment Dynamics [45993]

Treatment Homes, Inc. [28307]

Treatment and Learning Centers [2433], [8100]

Treatment Resources for Youth [44183]

Treatment Services Northwest LLC [48218], [48219]

Treatment Solutions Inc [40164]

Treatment Trends Inc
    Confront Program [48268]
    Halfway Home of Lehigh Valley [48269]
    Keenan House [48270]

Treatment Works [41667], [41814]

Tree City Dialysis • Fresenius Medical Care [24158]

Trellis Mental Health and Development Services--Kitchener [11241]

Trellis Mental Health and Developmental Services--Fergus • Regional Eating Disorders Program [11242]

Trellis Mental Health and Developmental Services--Orangeville • Regional Eating Disorders Program [11243]

Trellis Services Inc. [2383]

Trend Home Health Services [14194]

Trenton Program for the Hearing Impaired [506]
Trenton Psychiatric Hospital [33664]
Trenton Vet Center [52022]
Tressler Brandywine Program Center of Delaware [50746]
Trevor Project [50707]
TRHS Caldwell Clinic [6635]
TRI Center Inc
    Chemical Dependency Treatment/New York [46924]
    Drug Abuse Treatment [46537]
    Drug Abuse Treatment/New York [46458]
Tri-Cities Chaplaincy [21756]
Tri Cities Dialysis LLC [23998]
Tri-City Audiology, LLC [957]
Tri-City Comprehensive Community Mental Health Center, Inc.--Geminus [29714]
Tri-City Family Services [29626]
Tri City Institute
    Pajo Corporation [39695]
    South [40165]
Tri-City Medical Center [13222]
    Cancer Program [4814]
Tri-City Mental Health Center [28711]
Tri-City Mental Health/Mental Retardation Center, Inc. [30411]
Tri City Substance Abuse Center Inc [48017]
Tri City Youth and Family Center Inc [47919]
Tri-Community Counseling Safe Home [8703]
Tri County Alcohol and Drug Services LLC • Outpatient Treatment Services [42640]
Tri County Commission on Alcohol and Drug Abuse [48967]
Tri-County Communication Services [3666]
Tri County Community Action Prog Inc
    Friendship House Residential [45888]
    Step One [45887]
Tri County Community Health [47282]
Tri-County Community Health Council, Inc. • Tri-County Community Health Center [7049]
Tri-County Community Mental Health Center [32188]
Tri County Community Services Inc [46255]
    Alcohol and Drug Program [46314]
    Detoxification Center [46315]
    Raton Alcohol and Drug Program [46295]
Tri County Council on Domestic Violence and Sexual Assault [10731]
Tri-County Council on Domestic Violence and Sexual Assault [10699]
Tri County Counseling and Life • Skills Center [41829]
Tri--County Crisis Intervention, Inc. [10113]
Tri County Dialysis Facility • US Renal Care [27242]
Tri-County Group Home [34501]
Tri-County Health Clinic, Inc. [7414]
Tri-County Health System, Inc. [6608]
Tri-County Home Care, LLC [15645]
Tri-County Home Care Services, Inc. [16341]
Tri County Home Health--Batesburg [17563]
Tri County Home Health--Columbia [17577]
Tri County Home Health--Sumter [17622]
Tri-County Homecare Services, LLC [17507]
Tri County Hospice [21146]
Tri-County Hospice--London [19811]
Tri-County Hospice--Wadena [20214]
Tri-County Hospital [15946]
Tri-County Hospital Hospice [20387]
Tri-County Human Services Center [32048]
Tri County Human Services Inc
    Highlands Outpatient Clinic [41559]
    Lakeland Outpatient Services [41685]
    RASUW Center for Women [41560]
    Wauchula Outpatient Clinic [41987]
    Winter Haven Outpatient [42003]
Tri County Medical Center [6185]
Tri-County Mental Health & Counseling--Athens [31657]
Tri County Mental Health and Counseling Services • Careline [51196]
Tri County Mental Health/Mental Retardation Services [32427]
Tri-County Mental Health/Mental Retardation Services [32430]
Tri County Mental Health Service • Crisis Intervention Unit [50958]
Tri County Mental Health Services [30252], [45534]
Tri-County Mental Health Services [8079]
Tri-County Mental Health Services--Bridgton [30200]

Tri-County Mental Health Services • Crisis Intervention [30220]
Tri-County Mental Health Services--Farmington [30211]
Tri-County Mental Health Services • Group Home [30221]
Tri-County Mental Health Services--Lewiston [30222]
Tri County Mental Health Services • Main Office [45535]
Tri-County Mental Health Services • Oxford Hills Clinic [30229]
Tri-County Mental Health Services--Rumford [30238]
Tri--County Orthopedics [38744]
Tri--County Pain Consultants [35515]
Tri--County Pain Management Centre [35734]
Tri-County Protective Agency [9113]
Tri-County Psych Services Inc [45564]
Tri-County Resource Center [8978]
Tri-County Respite • Newvitae, Inc. - Mount Trexler Manor [32039]
Tri-County Sleep Center [37138]
Tri-County Speech Associates Inc. [3223]
Tri County Treatment [40335]
Tri County Treatment Center [39227]
Tri-County Treatment • Outpatient [40336]
Tri-County Youth Services, Paterson • Runaway and Homeless Youth Program [36083]
Tri-Development Center of Aiken County [8500]
Tri-Flexsi Home Health Care [18011]
Tri Hab Inc
    Div of Gateway Healthcare Counseling [48894]
    King House [48895]
    Mens Residence [48896]
Tri-Lakes Relational Center--Springfield [11125]
Tri-Life Center, LLP [35601]
Tri-Parish Community Home Care, LLC [15347]
Tri--Rivers Planned Parenthood • Lake Ozark Clinic [11692]
Tri-Rivers Planned Parenthood • Rolla Clinic [11693]
Tri-Services Military
    Adult Cystic Fibrosis Center [7678]
    Pediatric Cystic Fibrosis Center [7679]
Tri--Star Home Health Care [15589]
Tri-State Coalition Against Domestic and Sexual Abuse [9338]
Tri-State Community Health Center, Inc. [6796]
Tri-State Dialysis Center [23875]
Tri--State Dialysis • DaVita [26266]
Tri-State Dialysis--Dubuque [24269]
    Dubuque Internal Medicine [24270]
Tri-State Dialysis--Manchester [24283]
Tri State Dialysis--Platteville [27770]
Tri-State Home Care, Inc. [17447]
Tri State Hospital Home Health and Hospice [21751]
Tri-State Medical, LLC [18545]
Tri-State Memorial Hospital [18424]
    Sleep Diagnostic Services [37941]
Tri--State Sleep Disorders Center • Center for Research in Sleep Disorders [37591]
Tri-State Tristate Memorial Hospital Inc. • Dialysis Unit [27600]
Tri--Town [7217]
Tri Town Community Action Agency [48854]
Tri-Trax Therapy, Inc. [18012]
Tri-Valley Haven Shelter [8830]
Tri-Wil Porta Cras School [7713]
Triad Associates PC/Clarkston [44702]
Triad Dialysis Center • Wake Forest University [25886]
Triad Home Care [15670]
Triad Psychiatric and • Counseling Center [47353]
Triad Therapy Mental Health Center LLC [47206]
Triality [2810]
Triangle Aphasia Project [3154]
Triangle Family Services [47467]
Triangle Speech Services [3175]
Tricon Counseling Centers [42445]
TriCounty Homecare [16440]
Trident Medical Center • Cancer Program [5902]
Trident United Way's 211 Hotline [51336]
TriHealth • Cancer Care Services [5699]
Trillium Family Services [31938]
Trillium Family Services--Corvallis [34393]
Trillium Family Services--Portland [34403]
Trillium Family Solutions [47613]
Trillium Family Solutions Inc [47640]
Trillium Home Care Solutions [15657]
Trillium Treatment Center [50058]

Trilogy [29601]
Trilogy Center for Women [43633]
Trilogy Evanston [29620]
Trilogy Inc [42589]
Trinitas Hospital
    Dialysis Unit [25429]
    Sleep Disorders Center [37365]
    Substance Abuse Services [45986]
Trinitas Livingston Street • Dialysis Unit [25430]
Trinitas Regional Medical Center
    Cancer Program [5511]
    Comprehensive Sleep Disorders Center [37366]
Trinitas Satellite--Linden [25456]
Trinity Addiction Services [47594]
Trinity Alliance of the Capital Region • Homer Perkins Center Inc [46342]
Trinity Behavioral Care [48927], [48961]
Trinity Care Hospice [18901]
Trinity Children and Family Services--Colton [33984]
Trinity Children and Family Services--Ukiah [33204]
Trinity Children and Family Services--White Water [33210]
Trinity Children's and Family Services--Yucaipa [34038]
Trinity Dialysis Clinic [23692]
Trinity Health • Cancer Program [5674]
Trinity Health Care Services [14454]
Trinity Health Care Services, Inc. [14248]
Trinity Health Services [14168]
Trinity Health System [17048]
Trinity Health System Behav Med Center [47863]
Trinity Health System • Tony Teramana Cancer Center [5750]
TRINITY Home Medical Equipment [17120]
Trinity Home Services-Aiken • Center for Hospice and Palliative Care [21202]
Trinity Hospice [19693]
Trinity Hospice Agency [20790]
Trinity Hospice-Augusta [19360]
Trinity Hospital at Saint Joseph's • Dialysis Center [25997]
Trinity Iowa Health • Home Care and Hospice [15096]
Trinity Lifecare Home Health • INTEGRIS Grove General Hospital [17121]
Trinity Medical Center Behavioral Health [29108]
Trinity Medical Center--Birmingham • Teaching Hospital Cancer Program [4727]
Trinity Medical Center--Rock Island • Cancer Program [5123]
Trinity Mental Health Services • Minot Suicide Prevention Service [51192]
Trinity Mother Frances Health System • Cancer Program [6034]
Trinity Mother Frances Rehabilitation Hospital [18180]
Trinity Mother Frances Sleep Center [37865]
Trinity Mother Francis Rehabilitation Hospital/Healthsouth [39101]
Trinity Muscatine New Horizons • Outpatient Substance Abuse Program [43292]
Trinity Orthopaedics [38400]
Trinity Outpatient Rehabilitation Services [35436]
Trinity Pain Center [35602]
Trinity Pathway Hospice [19667]
Trinity Plus Healthcare Services • Trinity Plus Alcohol and Drug Treatment [40166]
Trinity Regional Medical Center [24272]
    Cancer Center [5189]
Trinity Regional Medical Center Dialysis--Webster City [24308]
Trinity Rehabilitation Services [35437]
Trinity Senior Care [13678]
Trinity Services Inc. [33423]
Trinity Services, Inc.--Joliet [29634]
Trinity Services--Lockport [29639]
Trinity Sports Medicine--Minot [38846]
Trinity Sports Medicine--Steubenville [38896]
Trinity Treatment Center Inc [42129]
Trinity Visiting Nurse and Homecare Association-Moline [19545]
TrinityCare [13215]
TrinityCare Extended Care [13189]
TrinityCare Hospice [19062]
TrinityValley RDSPD [805]
Triple Alliance Health Services, Inc. [17890]
Triple R Behavioral Health, Inc. [28184]
    Carol Ann [28154]

Fairmount [28185]
Greenway [28186]
Palm Desert [28187]
Palm Desert LTS [28188]
Palm Lane [28189]
Phoenix Clubhouse [28190]
Raiven Gardens [28191]
Tonopah [28155]
Villages East [28205]
Tripler Army Medical Center
Audiology and Speech Pathology Clinic [1935]
Cancer Program [5049]
Department of Obstetrics and Gynecology •
Reproductive Endocrinology Infertility [22029]
Tripler Army Medical Center MCHK/PST • Tri Serv
Addictions Recovery Facility [42285]
Tripler Army Medical Center
Pediatric and Adult Cystic Fibrosis Center [7523]
Sickle Cell Disease Center for Adults [36338]
Tristate Dialysis • Fresenius Medical Care [26035]
Triumph Home Health Care [15730]
Triumph LLC [47468]
Triumph Treatment Services Inc • Community Drug
and Alcohol Center [50277]
TriWest Healthcare Alliance [50649]
Tropical Health & Homecare Services, Inc. [13695]
Tropical Texas Behavioral Health • Mid-Valley
[32570]
Tropical Texas Center for Mental Health/Mental
Retardation [32450]
Harlingen [32474]
TROSA Transitional House [47298]
TROSA Triangle Residential Options • For
Substance Abusers Inc [47299]
Trover Foundation Regional Medical Center • Sleep
Disorders Center [37054]
Troy Doctors Hospital, LLC [12729]
Troy Regional Medical Center • Sleep Disorders
Center [36615]
Troy Sleep Center [37207]
Troy Veterans Affairs Clinic [31480]
TRS Behavioral Care Inc
Right Step [49412], [49413], [49545], [49590]
The Right Step [49301], [49532], [49542]
Right Step and The Next Step [49326]
TRS Behavioral Care • Right Step-Solutions Plus
[49480]
Tru--Care Home Health [14840]
Truckee Clinic [28829]
Trude Weishaupt Memorial Dialysis Center [25668]
True Health Center [6791]
True North Student Assistance and
Treatment Service System [50279]
Treatment Services [50153]
Treatment Services/Grays Harbor [49876]
Treatment Services/Lewis [49926]
True North Student Assistance Center [50233]
True North The Shelter [9673]
True Star Behavioral Health Services [50059]
True To Life Children's Services & Orchid House
[34028]
Truman Medical Center [16023]
Truman Medical Center Behavioral Hlth • Outpatient
Treatment and Recovery [45536]
Truman Medical Center
Comprehensive Adult Sickle Cell Center [36370]
Comprehensive Adult Sickle Cell Disease Center
[36371]
Truman Medical Center--Hospital Hill • Cancer
Program [5450]
Truman Medical Center Lakewood Medical • Detox
Services/ FKA Addiction Recovery [45537]
Truman Neurological Center Community [8201]
Trumbull 2aa [51235]
Trumbull Counseling Center [50737]
Trumbull County Council for Mentally Retarded
Citizens • Fairhaven Program [8428]
Trumbull Memorial Hospital • Genetics Clinic
[12319]
Trumbull Public Schools [334]
Trunnell and Assoc Counseling Center [43781]
Trussville Health Care Center [28053]
Trust Care Home Health Services, Inc. [14169]
Trust Home Health Care, Inc. [13052]
Trust The Process Inc [47314]
Trust Us Home Health Services, Inc. [18013]
Trust USA Home Health, LLC [14396]
Trusted Home Healthcare, LLC [16888]

Truth 180 Inc [43821]
TRW Associates [44199]
Tu Casa, Inc. [8932]
Tuality Home Health [17191]
Tuba City Outpatient Treatment Center • Behavioral
Health Services/DBHS [39484]
Tubman [9619]
DBA Chrysalis [45232]
Tubman Family Alliance [9604]
Tucker Dialysis • DaVita [23815]
Tucker Maxon Oral School [690]
Tucson Cystic Fibrosis Center • Adult and Pediatric
Clinic [7463]
Tucson Ear, Nose, and Throat [995]
Tucson Medical Center [33111]
Tucson Medical Center Hospice [18833]
Tudor House [33700]
Tuerk House
Alcohol and Drug Treatment Program [44184]
Outpatient Clinic [44185]
Tuesday's Child [2005]
Tufts Medical Center
Cystic Fibrosis Center [7570]
Department of Obstetrics and Gynecology •
Division of Reproductive Endocrinology and
Infertility [22114]
Floating Hospital for Children • Genetics Clinic
[12246]
TUFTS New England Medical Center • Center for
Children with Special Needs [8111]
TUFTS - New England Medical Center • Center for
Sleep Medicine [37139]
TUFTS New England Medical Center • Department
of Physical Medicine and Rehabilitation [8112]
Tufts New England Medical Center • Sleep Center in
Wellesley [37140]
Tufts University School of Medicine
Baystate Medical Center • Pain Management
[35497]
Lahey Clinic-- Transplant [24757]
Tug River Health Association, Inc. [7411]
Tug Valley Recovery Shelter [10684]
Tulalip Tribal Family Services • Chemical
Dependency Program [50230]
Tulane Adolescent Drop--In Clinic [6759]
Tulane Institute of Sports Medicine • Tulane
University Hospital & Clinic [38502]
Tulane Medical Center • Cancer Center [5260]
Tulane Sports Physical Therapy [38503]
Tulane University • Adult Cystic Fibrosis Center
[7556]
Tulane University Health Sciences • Louisiana Com-
munity AIDS Research Program [52]
Tulane University Hospital and Clinic • Fertility Clinic
[22080]
Tulane University Hospital Transplant [24560]
Tulane University Medical Center
Comprehensive Sleep Medicine Center [37087]
Neurology Department • Headache Clinic
[12429]
Tulane University--New Orleans • Dialysis Clinic Inc.
[24561]
Tulane University
School of Medicine
Hayward Genetics Center [12224]
Pediatric Cystic Fibrosis Center [7557]
Tulane University School of Medicine • Sickle Cell
Center [36353]
Tulare Community Health Clinic [6371]
Tulare Dialysis • DaVita [23041]
Tulare Local Healthcare District [13399]
Tullahoma CONTACT Life Line [51367]
Tully Hill Corporation
Chemical Dependency Inpatient Rehab [47141]
Chemical Dependency Outpatient [47142]
Inpatient Withdrawal Unit [47143]
Tulsa Bone and Joint Associates [38914]
Tulsa Boys Home [48014]
Tulsa Center for Behavioral Health [31923]
Tulsa Center for Fertility & Women's Health [22221]
Tulsa Community College • Resource Center for the
Deaf and Hard of Hearing [674]
Tulsa Helpline [51245]
Tulsa Outpatient Clinic [48048]
Tulsa Rightway Medical [48049]
Tulsa Scottish Rite Center • Language Disorders
Clinic [3295]
Tulsa Women and Childrens Center • Palmer

Continuum of Care [48050]
Tumbleweed Center for Youth Development •
Runaway and Homeless Youth Program [35798]
Tumbleweed Runaway • Runaway and Homeless
Youth Program [36063]
Tundra Women's Coalition [8657]
Tunkhannock Dialysis • DaVita [26591]
Tuolumne Inn [33203]
Tuolumne County Behavioral Health Dept [40804]
Tuomey Healthcare System Home Care [17623]
Tuomey Medical Park • Speech-Language Pathol-
ogy/Audiology Department [3411]
Tuomey Rehabilitative Services/Sports Medicine
[39019]
Turfway Dialysis & PD • DaVita [24379]
Turlock Regional Services [28832]
Turn About Inc of Tallahassee [41951]
Turn About Ranch [32584]
Turn Around Recovery Residences [42086]
TurnAround, Inc.--Baltimore [9447]
TurnAround, Inc.--Towson [9463]
Turning Corners Inc [44186], [44200]
A Turning Point [41033], [49543]
Turning Point [30591]
Turning Point, 8th St. [28412]
Turning Point
Acacia Lane [40788]
Aftercare [39868]
Turning Point Battered Women's Program [9401]
Turning Point Behavioral Health Center [29677]
Turning Point Behavioral Health Group [47328]
Turning Point Center For Youth/Famly [41180],
[41181], [41182]
Turning Point Centers [49707]
Turning Point of Central CA Inc • Turning Point
Youth Services [40924]
Turning Point
Chemical Dependency Outpatient Program
[46538]
Chemical Dependency Treatment Center
[48377]
Turning Point Clinic [44187]
A Turning Point of Colorado Springs Inc [41070]
Turning Point--Columbus • Domestic Violence
Services [9267]
Turning Point Community Programs • Fifth Street
Center [28636]
Turning Point Community Programs, Inc. [28735]
Turning Point Counseling/Consulting • Outpatient
Services [41916]
Turning Point Counseling Inc [44950]
Turning Point Counseling Services [31863], [39330]
Turning Point Counseling Services Inc [47896]
Turning Point Counseling Services • Struthers Office
[31843]
Turning Point Crisis Center [28686], [40316]
Turning Point for Families [9136]
Turning Point • Freedom Center for Women at Turn-
ing Point [48378]
Turning Point Home of San Diego [40585]
Turning Point Hospital [29478]
Turning Point II [48678]
Turning Point Inc [49414]
Fort Bend [49504]
Male Inpatient Program [45233]
Outpatient [46200]
South Office [49415]
Turning Point Inc.--Amesbury • Mainstream Housing
Program [9465]
Turning Point--Kemmerer • Lincoln County Self-Help
Center [10754]
Turning Point, King St. [28413]
Turning Point--Knoxville [9339]
Turning Point of Lehigh Valley, Inc. [10262]
Turning Point--Marion [10160]
Turning Point Mental Health Services [41154]
Turning Point--Mount Clemens [9559]
Turning Point • Outpatient Services [48379]
Turning Point Recovery Center • Extended Care
Unit [44972]
Turning Point Services, Inc. [31565]
Turning Point South [48001]
Turning Point of Tampa [11032]
Turning Point of Tampa Inc [41974]
Turning Point--Tuscaloosa • Domestic Violence/
Sexual Assault Services [8653]
Turning Point of Union County [10062]
Turning Point Violence Intervention Program [8759]

Turning Point--Warrenton [9734]
Turning Point of Washington County, Inc. [30295]
Turning Point--Woodstock [9259]
Turning Pointe Domestic Violence Services [10656]
Turning Points Counseling Center [34037]
Turning Points Network [9805]
Turningpoint for Victims of Domestic and Sexual Violence, Inc. [10733]
Turnings • Ontario Cnty Substance Abuse AB Services [46577]
Turtle Creek Manor Inc [49302]
Turtle Creek Valley Mental Health/Mental Retardation, Inc.--Braddock [31995]
Turtle Creek Valley Mental Health/Mental Retardation, Inc.--Maple Avenue, Homestead [32028]
Turtle Creek Valley Mental Health/Mental Retardation, Inc.--Turtle Creek [32125]
Turtle Creek Valley Mental Health/Mental Retardation Services--E 18th Avenue, Homestead [32029]
Turtle Creek Valley Mental Health/Mental Retardation Services--Rankin [32114]
Turtle Creek Valley Mental Health/Mental Retardation Services--Wilmerding [32133]
Turtle Creek Valley MH/MR Inc • Alternatives [48610], [48661]
Tuscaloosa Nephrology Associates • Home Dialysis [22412]
Tuscaloosa Treatment Center [39298]
Tuscaloosa VA Medical Center [12731]
Tuscaloosa Veterans Affairs Medical Center [3857]
    Residential Rehabilitation Program Intensive/Inpatient • PTSD Clinical Team [51681]
Tuscany Hills Health Care Services Inc. [12958]
Tuscany House [19315]
Tuscarawas County • Alcohol and Addiction Program [47750]
Tuscarawas County Kidney Center • Fresenius Medical Care • Dialysis Facility [26171]
Tuscola Behavioral Health Systems [30523]
    Pineland Behavioral Home [30524]
Tustin Hearing Center [1350]
TW Ponessa and Associates • Counseling Services Inc [48433]
TWB Speech Language Pathology Services Inc. [2359]
Twelfth Step House Inc [45335]
Twelfth Step House of San Diego I • DBA Heartland House [40586]
Twelve Oaks Alcohol/Drug Treatment Center [41816]
Twelve Step Programs of California [40641], [40642], [40643]
Twiggs County Even Start [7914]
Twin Boro Physical Therapy Associates--Somerset [38759]
Twin Boro Physical Therapy Associates--Toms River [38763]
Twin Boro Physical Therapy Associates--Union [38764]
Twin Boro Physical Therapy--Westfield [38768]
Twin Care Services [13053]
Twin Cities Pain Clinic [35522]
Twin City Counseling Center [47544]
Twin City Medical Center [7351]
Twin County Dialysis Center • Fresenius Medical Care [27495]
Twin County Hospice • Twin County Regional Healthcare [21698]
Twin County Recovery Services Inc
    Alcoholism Outpatient Clinic [46703]
    Outpatient Drug Treatment Program [46587]
    The Red Door Community Residence [46704]
    Riverside Recovery Residence [46588]
Twin County Regional Hospital [18304]
Twin Creeks Hospital • Traumatic Brain Injury Therapy Program [4462]
Twin Falls Dialysis Center • DaVita • Dialysis Center & At Home [23889]
Twin Falls Veterans Affairs Clinic [29553]
Twin Lakes Center for • Drug and Alcohol Rehabilitation [48285], [48420], [48646]
Twin Lakes Contact-Help [50898]
Twin Lakes Educational Cooperative [432]
Twin Lakes Hospice [20289]
Twin Lakes Hospice-Warsaw [20346]
Twin Lakes Regional Medical Center [15200]
Twin Palms Recovery Center [39715]
Twin Rivers Counseling Associates [31070]
Twin Rivers Regional Medical Center [45543]

Twin Town Treatment Centers [40052]
    Twin Town/North Hollywood [40275]
    Twin Town/Orange [40325]
    Twin Town/Torrance [40858]
Twin Town West Hollywood • West Hollywood [40945]
Twin Valley Psychiatric System
    Columbus Campus [33754]
    Dayton Campus [33755]
    Psychiatric Unit for the Deaf [3234]
Twinber Hospice Care [21441]
Twinber, Inc. [17896]
Twins Quality Home Health Care Inc. [13054]
Two Rivers Behavioral Health System [45538]
Two Rivers Counseling & Consulting PC [44982]
Two Rivers Psychiatric Hospital [33631]
Tyler Home Dialysis • Fresenius Medical Care [27383]
Tyler Home Health Services, Inc. [17495]
Tyler Institute [1573]
Tyler Medical Clinic • In Vitro Fertilization Program [21947]
Tyler Veterans Affairs Primary Care Clinic [32563]
Tylertown Dialysis Unit • Hattiesburg Clinic [25166]
Tyrone Apartments [29285]
Tyvola Assessment and Counseling [47267]

U

U-CARE [10028]
U-Mass Memorial Health Care Systems [24821]
U of MN Med Center--Fairview • Dialysis Center [25049]
U R First, LLC [16159]
U S VETS • Las Vegas [45851]
U Turn Alcohol and Drug Education Prog [40167]
UAB Center for Palliative Care [18688]
UAB Highlands • Sleep/Wake Center [36616]
UAB Medical West [27841]
UAHSC Transplant [22522]
UALR/UAMS Speech and Hearing Clinic [1028]
UAMS Subsance Abuse Treatment Clinic [39555]
UBA Hospital Center for Psychiatric Medicine [29109]
Ubieta Health Systems [14170]
UC Chronic Dialysis--Mount Zion [22963]
UC Davis Hospice [19007]
UC Davis Medical Center Transplant [22923]
UCA Speech Language Hearing Center • University of Central Arkansas [1003]
UCH Home Health of Pasco [13845]
UCI Medical Center,Renal TX • UC Irvine Healthcare [22861]
UCI Renal Dialysis Center [22862]
UCLA [40168]
UCLA Hospital • Down Syndrome Clinic [10780]
UCLA Intervention Program for Handicapped Children [7790]
UCLA Medical Center [13156]
UCLA Medical Center--Pediatrics, Renal TX • UCLA Health System [22790]
UCLA Neuropsychiatric Institute and Hospital [7791]
UCP of Central California • Parent/Child Development Center [7781]
UCP of Greater Birmingham [7708]
UCP of Greater Houston [8536]
UCP of Greater Kansas City [8202]
UCP of Metropolitan Dallas [8543]
UCP of New York City [8337]
UCP of Northeastern Maine [8081]
UCP of Putnam and South Dutchess Counties • Hudson Valley Health Services [3094]
UCP of South Florida [7885]
UCP of Ulster County [8326]
UCPC Behavioral Healthcare • Addiction Services [46139]
UCSD Co-Occurring Disorders • Treatment and Research Program [40587]
UCSD Medical Center • Dialysis Program [22949]
UCSD Medical Center--Renal Transplant [22950]
UCSF Center on Deafness [40644]
UCSF Kidney Transplant Center [22964]
UCSF Medical Center [13312]
UHHS Bedford Medical Center • Cancer Program [5682]
UHHS Geauga Regional Hospital • Cancer Program [5688]
UHHS Laurelwood Hospital and Counseling Centers

• Eating Disorder Programs [11200]
Uhlich Children's Advantage Network • Uhlich Children's Home [33416]
UHS Binghamton General Hospital • Speech--Language Pathology [2978]
UHS KeyStone Center [48324]
UHS Keystone Center • Key Recovery Outpatient [48278]
UHS Recovery Foundation Inc [48306]
UHSH Blood Disorders Center • UHS Wilson Hospital [12568]
Uintah Basin Dialysis Center [27418]
Uintah Basin Hospice [21635]
Uintah School District [842]
Ujima Family Recovery Services
    La Casa Ujima [40206]
    The Rectory Womens Recovery Center [40687]
    Ujima East Intensive Day Treatment [40390]
    Ujima West Intensive Day Treatment [40450]
Ujima House, Inc. [10429]
Ullucci Sports Medicine [38997]
Ulster County Crime Victim Assistance [9938]
Ulster County Dept of Mental Hlth Serv • Chemical Dependency Clinic [46743]
Ulster Intensive Day Treatment Program [31455]
Ultima Home Healthcare, Inc. [14171]
Ultimate Angels Home Health Care [13596]
Ultimate Care, Inc. [16422]
Ultimate Health Sleep Disorders Center--Hauppauge [37443]
Ultimate Health Sleep Disorders Center--New Hyde Park [37444]
Ultimate Healthcare professional Services, Inc. [13157]
Ultimate Home Health Care, Inc. [14754]
Ultimate Lifestyle Center [40169]
Ultimate Nursing Care [13634]
Ultimate Solutions Inc [44906]
Ultimate Treatment Center [43526]
Ulysses Area Mental Health Center [50925]
UMass Memorial Health Care • Pediatric Pulmonary, Asthma and Cystic Fibrosis Center [7571]
UMASS Memorial Hospice [20017]
UMASS Memorial Hospital, Inc. Home health & Hospice [15566]
UMass Memorial Medical Center • Cancer Center [5362]
UMASS Memorial Medical Center • Multiple Sclerosis Clinic [34603]
Umatilla County Human Services [48127], [48152], [48173]
Umbagog Kidney Center • Fresenius Medical Care • Dialysis Services [24619]
Umbrella, Inc. [10549]
The Umbrella Program [8989]
UMD New Jersey • University of Pain Care Center • University Headache Center [12445]
UMDNJ University Hospital • Cancer Program [5531]
UMESD Program for Deaf and Hard of Hearing [686]
Umma Community Clinic [6322]
UMOM Shelter [8720]
Umpqua Community Health Center, Inc. [7145]
John Umstead Hospital [33735]
UNA • Psychological and Psycotherapy Assoc [47354]
Unadilla Health Care Center, Inc. [6606]
Unalaskans Standing Against Family Violence [8674]
UNC Comprehensive Transplant Center • North Carolina Children's Hospital [25829]
UNC Department of Psychiatry [47247]
    Alcohol and Substance Abuse Program [47248]
UNC Hospice--Chapel Hill [20633]
UNC Hospice--Pittsboro [20716]
Uncompahgre Medical Center • Norwood Medical Clinic [6415]
Underground Railroad, Inc. [9572]
Understanding U [1590]
Underwood Memorial Hospital Homecare Services, Inc. [16298]
Unicare Home Health Services [14172]
Unicare Home Health System, Inc. [15833]
Unicoi County Memorial Hospital, Inc. [17667]
Unicorn Inn • Community Healthlink, Inc. [30491]
Unidad Emergencia y Detox de Alcoholismo [48806]
Unified Community Services [32985], [50378], [50439]

Unik Home Health Care Services Inc. [13055]
Unio Recovery Center
    Drug and Alcohol Treatment Center [48163]
    Mommy and Me [48164]
Union City Dialysis Center • DaVita [23046]
Union City Dialysis • DaVita [23816]
Union City Renal Center [25522]
Union County Commission on Alcohol and Drug
    Abuse [48983]
Union County Counseling [29559]
Union County Counseling Service [50827]
Union County Dialysis--Georgia [23626]
Union County Dialysis--North Carolina • DaVita •
    Dialysis Center [25910]
Union County Drug Court • DBA South Arkansas
    Substance Abuse [39528]
Union County Mental Health Clinic [50798]
Union County Office [30083]
Union County Public Schools [625]
Union County Schools [739]
Union Gap Dialysis Center • DaVita [27656]
Union Hospital • Altru Home Services and Outreach
    Therapy [16818]
Union Hospital Cecil County • Pain Clinic [35485]
Union Hospital Clinton [6681]
Union Hospital--Elkton • Cancer Program [5302]
Union Hospital, Inc. [2190]
Union Hospital, Inc.-Terre Haute • Hux Cancer
    Center [5176]
Union Memorial Hospital • Cancer Center [5291]
Union Memorial Hospital Dialysis Unit [24655]
Union Memorial Hospital • Dialysis Unit [24654]
Union Memorial Hospital Palliative Care [19916]
Union Memorial Sports Medicine at Bel Air [4127]
Union Memorial Sports Medicine, Bel Air [2389]
Union Memorial Sports Medicine at Lutherville
    [4128]
Union Memorial Sports Medicine at Stadium Place
    [4129]
Union Mental Health Center [32215]
Union Mental Health/Substance Abuse Clinic
    [29368]
Union Plaza Dialysis Center • DaVita [23227]
Union Street Clubhouse [29761]
Union Street School for the Deaf [546]
Uniontown Family Doctors [7189]
Uniontown Health Center [6203]
The Uniontown Hospital [17496]
Unique Home Health [18153]
Unique Med Home Health Care Services [14455]
UniqueAid [17280]
Unison Behavioral Health Group • Dual Recovery
    Program [47870]
Unison Behavioral Health Group--E Woodruff, Toledo
    [31845]
Unison Behavioral Health Group--Starr Avenue,
    Toledo [31846]
United Action for Youth • Runaway and Homeless
    Youth Program [35958]
United American Indian Involvement [40170]
United American Indian Involvement Inc [39639]
United Backcare, Inc.--Everett [35759]
United Backcare, Inc.--Puyallup [35760]
United Backcare, Inc.--Redmond [35761]
United Behavioral Health--Access and Crisis Line
    [50692]
United Bronx Parents Inc
    Chemical Dependence Outpatient Services
        [46459]
        La Casita 1/Mother and Child Program [46460]
        La Casita 3 [46461]
United Care Home Healthcare Agency [13158]
United Cerebral Palsy Association of Orange County
    [7782]
United Cerebral Palsy Delrey School [8094]
United Cerebral Palsy of Nassau • Treatment and
    Rehabilitation Center [8351]
United Community Action Program Inc [48006]
United Community and Family Services • Southern
    New London County [41460]
United Community Health Center, Inc. [6233]
United Community Health Center of Storm Lake
    [6714]
United Community Services [43268]
United Counseling Service of Bennington County
    [8572], [32639]
United Counseling Service of • Bennington County
    Inc [49720]

United Family Services--Cabarrus County •
    Domestic Violence Program [10025]
United Family Services Inc [39570]
United Family Services • Shelter for Battered
    Women [10026]
United Family Services--Union County • Domestic
    Violence Program [10063]
United General Hospital • North Puget Cancer
    Center [6119]
United Hands Hospice [20149]
United Health Centers of the San Joaquin Valley,
    Inc. [6338]
United Health Services • Dialysis Unit [25579]
United Health Services Hospital, Inc. • Renal Care
    Center [25580]
United Health Services Hospitals [3040]
United Health Services Hospitals Inc • New
    Horizons CD Inpt Rehab Unit [46387]
United Health Services Hospitals • Wilson Memorial
    Regional Medical Center • Cancer Program [5586]
United Health Systems, Inc. [13639]
United Hebrew Geriatric Center • Long Term Home
    Health Care Program [16544]
United Home Care--Atlanta [14567]
United Home Care--Blue Ridge [14493]
United Home Care--Cleveland [14501]
United Home Care--Cobb [14552]
United Home Care--Cumming [14513]
United Home Care--Gainesville [14533]
United Home Care--Griffin [14534]
United Home Care--Monroe [14556]
United Home Care--Newnan [14561]
United Home Care--Rome [14578]
United Home Care--Warm Springs [14602]
United Home Health Agency Inc. [13374]
United Home Health Care [15661]
United Hospice of Rockland, Inc. [16537], [20582]
United Hospice Service [20090]
United Hospital Center [18507]
    Cancer Center [4717], [6134]
    Sleep Disorders Center [37960]
United Hospital District [15891]
United Hospital • Oncology Care Center [5419]
United Hospital System--Saint Catherine's • Cancer
    Program [6172]
United Indian Health Services [39613]
United in Jesus Outreach Ministries [42436]
United Medical Associates • Sleep and Neurodiag-
    nostic Center [37445]
United Medical Care, Inc. [14932]
United Medical Center Hospice [21877]
United Medical Centers, Inc. [7286]
United Methodist Behavioral Hospital [33123]
The United Methodist Children's Home [34390]
United Methodist Children's Home • Treatment/
    Foster Care [34379]
United Methodist Western Kansas Mexican-
    American Ministries, Inc. • UMWKMAM-Garden
    City [6717]
United Methodist Youthville Inc • Newton Chem
    Depend Treatment Program [43416]
United Neighborhood Health Services [49163]
United Northwest Recovery Center Inc [50146]
United Pain Center [35523]
United Progress Inc • Trenton Treatment Center
    [46195]
United Regional Health Care System • Cancer
    Program [6037]
United Services Child Guidance Center [7847]
United Services, Inc.--Columbia [28981]
United Services, Inc.--Dayville [28988]
    Domestic Violence Program [8992]
United Services, Inc.
    The Lighthouse [29053]
    Passages [29054]
        Social Rehabilitation Services [29043]
        Stepping Stones [29055]
United Services, Inc.--Wauregan [29050]
United Services, Inc.--Willimantic [29056]
United Services • Runaway and Homeless Youth
    Program [35865]
United Services--Willimantic • Domestic Violence
    Program [9008]
United Sleep Center LLP [37238]
United Sleep Centers LLC [36710]
United Sleep Diagnostics • Sleep Disorders Center
    [36825]
United Sleep Medicine on Fairview [37495]

United State Home Health Services [13788]
U.S. Air Force Medical Genetics Center • 81 MDOS/
    SGOU [12260]
United States Army Community Service • Family
    Advocacy Program [9680]
U.S. Army Institute of Surgical Research • Burn Unit
    [4639]
U.S. Department of Health and Human Services
    National Human Genome Research Institute •
        Medical Genetics Branch [12230]
    National Institutes of Health • National Institute
        of Diabetes and Digestive and Kidney
        Diseases [7564]
U.S. Home Health Care [15027]
U.S. Hospice and Home Health Corporation [14755]
United States Veterans Initiative Inc [40045]
    Veterans in Progress Program [40046]
United States Virgin Islands Department of Public
    Health [36551]
United Summit Center [50294]
    Braxton County Office [50345]
United Summit Center Crisis Line [51483]
United Teen Equality Center • Runaway and Home-
    less Youth Program [36004]
United Treatment and Therapy [49895]
United Way 211 in Rhode Island [51312]
United Way of Connecticut /INFOLINE [50736]
United Way Helpline, Inc. [51240]
United Way of the Midlands [51325]
United Way of San Antonio • Information and Refer-
    ral Department [51393]
United Way of Westchester and Putnam [10010]
United Women in Transition • Outpatient [40171]
Unity 1 Home Health Care, LLC [17023]
Unity Chemical Dependency [47050]
    Formally Park Ridge Chem Dependency [47051]
Unity Counseling Services [50052]
Unity Family Home Care & Hospice [20175]
Unity Healing Center [47269]
Unity Health Care • Home Care & Hospice [19717]
Unity Health Care, Inc. • DC General [6433]
Unity Health Center • Cancer Program [5782]
Unity Health Hospice • Saint John's Mercy Hospice
    [20337]
Unity Health System [4319]
    Cancer Program [5613]
    Comprehensive Rehabilitation Center [4320]
    Department of Psychiatry and Behavior [31467]
    Sleep Disorders Center [37446]
Unity Hlth System Park Ridge Hosp Inc
    Chemical Dependency Outpatient [47052]
    Inpatient Rehabilitation [47053]
Unity Home Health Agency [13056]
Unity Home Health, Inc. [15344]
Unity Hospice [21830]
Unity Hospice Care--Batesville [20221]
Unity Hospice Care, Inc-Grenada [20239]
Unity Hospice Care, Inc.--Greenwood [20238]
Unity Hospice Care, LLC-Germantown [21334]
Unity Hospice Care, LLC--Oxford [20257]
Unity Hospice Care, LLC--Southaven [20263]
Unity Hospice Care, LLC-Starkville [20265]
Unity Hospice Care LLC--West Memphis [18883]
Unity Hospice Care-Tupelo [20273]
Unity Hospice-Marinette [21829]
Unity Hospital • Cancer Care Center [5408]
Unity Hospital Dialysis at Spencerport [25777]
Unity Hospital
    Outpatient Services [45157]
    Substance Abuse Services [45234]
Unity House of Cayuga County Inc • Grace House
    Supportive Living [46365]
Unity House Inc. • Emergency Services for
    Domestic Violence [9994]
Unity Medical Center • Altru Home Services [16813]
Unity Place [45959]
Unity Recovery Center [41687]
Universal Community Behavioral Health [32038]
Universal Counseling Services Inc [44188]
Universal Health Care [18014]
Universal Health Care Hospice [21570]
Universal Hlth Network and Systems Inc [39869]
Universal Home Health Care, Inc. [15830]
Universal Home Health and Hospices Services
    [21464]
Universal Home Healthcare of Indiana, Inc. [14985]
Universal Homecare [15658]
Universal Hospice Care Inc. [20124]

Universal Kidney Center of Boynton Beach [23251]
Universal Kidney Center of Davie [23280]
Universal Kidney Center, Inc. • Dialysis Facility [23302]
Universal Kidney Center of Margate--Coral Springs • Fresenius Medical Care [23379]
Universal Kidney Centers--Pembroke Pines Miramar [23329]
University of Akron • Speech and Hearing Center [3210]
University of Alabama • Adult Cystic Fibrosis Center [7458]
University of Alabama at Birmingham • Addiction Recovery Program [39228]
University of Alabama, Birmingham
    Adult Down Syndrome Clinic [10771]
    AIDS Outpatient Clinic • Adult AIDS Clinical Trials Unit [1]
    Burn Center [4501]
    Center for Pediatric-Onset Demyelinating Disease [34507]
    Centers for AIDS Research [38]
University of Alabama at Birmingham • Children's Hospital • Sports Medicine Program [37999]
University of Alabama, Birmingham
    Civitan International Research Center • Down Syndrome Clinic [10772]
    Comprehensive Cancer Center [4655]
    Comprehensive Headache Clinic [12378]
University of Alabama at Birmingham • Department of Medicine • Division of Infectious Diseases • AIDS Vaccine Research Clinic [77]
University of Alabama, Birmingham • Department of Medicine/Rheumatology • Multidisciplinary Clinical Research Center [158]
University of Alabama at Birmingham
    Department of Obstetrics and Gynecology • In Vitro Fertilization Program [21887]
    Department of Pathology • Musculoskeletal Disorders Core Center of Research [159]
University of Alabama, Birmingham
    Division of Hematology/Oncology [36287]
    Division of Medicine/Rheumatology • Rheumatic Diseases Core Center [160]
University of Alabama • Birmingham Hospital • MDA Clinic [34750]
University of Alabama, Birmingham
    Neurology Department [34508]
    Preventive Medicine Clinic [38000]
University of Alabama Birmingham • Spinal Cord Injury Model Systems [3858]
University of Alabama at Birmingham • UAB Substance Abuse Programs [39229]
University of Alabama • Brewer-Porch Children's Center [7729]
The University of Alabama Hospital at Birmingham [12635]
University of Alabama Hospital at Birmingham • UAB Comprehensive Cancer Center [4728]
University of Alabama Hospital • Laboratory of Medical Genetics • Genetics Laboratory [12120]
University of Alabama Medical Center • Pain Management [35275]
The University of Alabama Speech and Hearing Center [928]
University of Alberta Hospital
    Burn Care Unit [4507]
    Capital Health Edmonton Area Eating Disorder Program [10893]
    Comprehensive Tissue Centre [34922]
University Anesthesiologists • Pain Care [35659]
University of Arizona
    Cord Blood Bank [34927]
    Disability Resource Center [241]
University of Arizona Health Science Center • Arizona Hemophilia and Thrombosis Center [12483]
University of Arizona Pain Institute [35295]
University of Arkansas • IVF Program [21904]
University of Arkansas, Little Rock • Department of Audiology & Speech Pathology [1029]
University of Arkansas Medical Sciences [1030]
University of Arkansas for Medical Sciences
    Adult Cystic Fibrosis Center [7465]
    Arkansas Lions Eye Bank and Laboratory [34928]
    Arkansas Reproductive Genetics Program [12147]

    Department of Pediatrics • Clinical Genetics [12148]
    Kid's First [1031]
    MDA/ALS Clinic [34756]
University of Arkansas for Medical Sciences/ • SAT Clinic [39556]
University of Arkansas for Medical Sciences--Transplant • Kidney/Nephrology [22557]
University of Arkansas for Medical Sciences • Winthrop P. Rockefeller Cancer Institute • Clinical Cancer Genetics [12149]
University of Arkansas Medical Services • Adult Medical Genetics • Down Syndrome Clinic [10773]
University of Arkansas Speech & Hearing Clinic [1012]
University Artificial Kidney Center LLC • Regional KRU Medical Ventures [23281]
University Behavioral Center [29251]
University Behavioral Health Center--Cherry Hill [31118]
University Behavioral Health Center--New Brunswick [31154]
University Behavioral Health Center--Piscataway [31162]
University Behavioral Health of Denton [32445]
University Behavioral Healthcare [46083]
University of British Columbia • Multiple Sclerosis Clinic [34522]
University of Buffalo • Pain Management [35587]
University of Calgary • Multiple Sclerosis Center [34512]
University of California, Davis [10994]
    Fertility Center [21948]
University of California, Davis Health System [13286]
University of California at Davis • Hemophilia Program [12493]
University of California • Davis Medical Center • Adult Cystic Fibrosis Center [7482]
University of California, Davis Medical Center • Cancer Program [4830]
University of California Davis Medical Center • Pediatric Cystic Fibrosis Center [7483]
University of California, Davis Medical Center
    Regional Burn Center [4521]
    School of Medicine • Department of Obstetrics and Gynecology Prenatal Diagnosis [12166]
University of California Davis Medical Center
    Sickle Cell Disease Center [36306]
    UCDHS Sleep Disorders Center [36711]
University of California at Davis • Sacramento Medical Center • PM&R Muscular Dystrophy Clinic [34764]
University of California, Irvine • Center for Sleep Medicine [36712]
University of California, Irvine Healthcare • Headache Center [12390]
University of California, Irvine Medical Center
    Chao Family Comprehensive Cancer Center [4816]
    Department of Pediatrics • Division of Human Genetics and Birth Defects [12167]
    Pain Management Center [35336]
    Regional Burn Unit [4522]
University of California, Irvine/Medical Center • UCI Family Health Center-Santa Ana [6363]
University of California, Irvine • Multiple Sclerosis Clinic [34531]
University of California, Los Angeles [1311]
    Audiology & Speech Pathology Clinic [1172]
    CARE Center • AIDS Clinical Trials Unit [3]
    Centers for AIDS Research [40]
University of California, Los Angeles Medical Center • Medical Genetics Division [12168]
University of California, Los Angeles • Medical Center, Olive View • MDA Clinic [34765]
University of California, Los Angeles Medical Center • Santa Monica Sleep Disorders Laboratory and Center [36713]
University of California, Los Angeles
    Neurological Services • MDA/ALS Center [34766]
    Neuropsychiatric Hospital [33161]
University of California, Los Angeles School of Medicine • Jules Stein Eye Institute [34967]
University of California, Los Angeles • Sickle Cell Disease Center [36307]
University of California Medical Center, Davis

    Pain Management [35337]
    Transplant Center [34968]
University of California Medical Center, Irvine • Sickle Cell Disease Center [36308]
University of California Medical Center, La Jolla • Pain Management [35338]
University of California Medical Center, Los Angeles • David Geffen School of Medicine • Pain Management [35339]
University of California Medical Center, San Francisco • Pain Management Center [35340]
University of California, San Diego [1275]
    AIDS Research Institute • Centers for AIDS Research [41]
    ALS Center [102]
    Department of Medicine • Division of Medical Genetics-MC0639 [12169]
    Department of Pediatrics/Infectious Disease • Pediatric AIDS Clinical Trials Unit [4]
    Division of Family Medicine • La Jolla Family and Sports Medicine [38126]
    Eating Disorder Treatment Center [10995]
    MDA/ALS Clinic [103]
University of California San Diego Medical Center [13304]
University of California • San Diego Medical Center • Hemophilia Treatment Center [12494]
University of California, San Diego Medical Center
    Rebecca and John Moores Cancer Program [4838]
    Regional Burn Center [4523]
University of California, San Diego Medical Center--Thornton [7484]
University of California San Diego • Pain Management Medical Group [35341]
University of California, San Diego • University Hospital • Sickle Cell Disease Center for Children [36309]
University of California, San Francisco
    Adult Cystic Fibrosis Center [7485]
    AIDS Clinical Trials Unit [5]
    Center on Deafness [1285]
    Center for Reproductive Health [21949]
    Centers for AIDS Research [42]
    Department of Medicine • Multidisciplinary Clinical Research Center [161]
    Department of Pediatrics • Division of Medical Genetics [12170]
    East Bay Outreach Clinic • Cystic Fibrosis Center [7486]
    Hemophilia Program [12495]
    MDA/ALS Clinic [104]
University of California, San Francisco Medical Center • Cancer Program [4844]
University of California at San Francisco Medical Center • Down Syndrome Clinic • Pediatric Disabilities Clinic [10781]
University of California, San Francisco
    Northern California Comprehensive Sickle Cell Center [36310]
    Pediatric Center of Excellence • Pediatric Multiple Sclerosis Center [34532]
    Pediatric Cystic Fibrosis Center [7487]
    Sleep Disorders Center [36714]
    Tissue Bank [34969]
University of Central Florida • Communications Disorders [1702]
University of Central Missouri • Welch--Schmidt Center for Communication Disorders [2828]
University of Chicago
    Adult Cystic Fibrosis Center [7536]
    ALS Center [114]
University of Chicago Burn Center [4542]
University of Chicago
    Child and Adolescent Psychiatry Clinic [7944]
    Developmental and Behavioral Pediatrics • Down Syndrome Clinical Program [10796]
University of Chicago Hospital • Pain Management [35438]
University of Chicago Hospitals [2006]
    Head & Neck Surgery [2007]
    Pritzker School of Medicine • Department of Human Genetics [12209]
    Reproductive Endocrinology and Infertility [22052]
The University of Chicago Hospitals • Sleep Disorders Center [36936]
University of Chicago Hospitals • The University of

Chicago Children's Hospital • Pediatric Cystic Fibrosis Center [7537]
University of Chicago Medical Center • Cancer Program [5080]
University of Chicago
    Multiple Sclerosis Clinic [34573]
    Sonia Shankman Orthogenic School [33417]
University of Chicago--Woodlawn [23962]
University of Cincinnati
    AIDS Clinical Trials Unit [29]
    Communication Disorders Clinic [3224]
    Comprehensive Sleep Medicine Center [37592]
University of Cincinnati Hospital • Burn Unit [4609]
University of Cincinnati Medical Center [34855]
    Hemophilia Treatment Center [12580]
    University of Cincinnati College of Medicine • Pain Management [35618]
University of Cincinnati • Speech, Language, Hearing Clinic [3225]
University City Counseling Center [32103]
University of Colorado
    Advanced Reproductive Medicine [21965]
    Anschultz Cancer Center [4868]
    Anschutz Medical Campus • Multiple Sclerosis Center [34545]
    Colorado Sickle Cell Treatment and Research Center [36312]
    Cord Blood Bank [34976]
University of Colorado at Denver and Health Sciences Center • Clinical Genetics and Metabolism Section [12172]
University of Colorado at Denver • Psychiatry Service [28856]
University of Colorado • Health Sciences Center • Adult Cystic Fibrosis Center [7490]
University of Colorado Health Sciences Center
    Adult Medical Genetics Program [12173]
    Advanced Reproductive Medicine [21966]
University of Colorado • Health Sciences Center • MDA/ALS Center [105], [34771]
University of Colorado Hospital Audiology Services [1379]
University of Colorado Hospital • Burn Center [4529]
University of Colorado Hospital--Dialysis [23094]
University of Colorado
    MDA Clinic [34772]
    Pain Management [35355]
University Community Hospital • Center for Cancer Care [4998]
University Community Hospital Home Health Care [14428]
University of Connecticut Dialysis Center [23157]
University of Connecticut Health Center--Farmington • The Center for Advanced Reproductive Services [21974]
University of Connecticut Health Center--Hartford • Center for Advanced Reproductive Services [21975]
University of Connecticut Health Center
    Sleep Disorders Center [36755]
    University Cancer Center • Hemophilia Treatment Center [12497]
University of Connecticut Speech & Hearing Clinic [1494]
University of Dayton • Research Institute • Ohio Center for Deafblind Education [3259]
University Dialysis Center at Oswego • Dialysis Clinic Inc. [25752]
University Dialysis Center--Sacramento • DaVita [22924]
University Dialysis Center--Shrewsbury • Fresenius Medical Care [24799]
University Dialysis Southeast [27347]
University Dialysis--West San Antonio [27348]
University Emergency Medicine Foundation • Center for Sports Medicine [39002]
University Family Medicine Center [38181]
University Fertility Associates [22010]
University of Florida [38288]
    Adult Cystic Fibrosis Center [7513]
    College of Medicine • Genetics Institute [12183]
University of Florida Dialysis • Dialysis Clinic Inc. [23313]
University of Florida
    Division of Genetics and Metabolism [12184]
    ENT at Ayers [1591]
    Florida Outreach Project for Children and Young Adults Who Are Deaf--Blind [1592]

University of Florida, Gainesville • Sickle Cell Disease Center [36327]
University of Florida Health Science Center • Pain Management [35398]
University of Florida
    Orthopedics and Sports Medicine [38231]
    Pediatric Cystic Fibrosis [7514]
    Shands Burn Center [4535]
    Shands Hospital • Women's Health, Magnolia Parke In Vitro Fertilization Program [22011]
University of Florida/Shands Jacksonville • ALS Multispecialty Clinic [110]
University of Florida Speech and Hearing Center [1593]
University of Georgia • Disability Resource Center--Student Affairs [361]
University of Georgia Speech & Hearing Clinic [1810]
University of Hawaii at Manoa • Pacific Partnerships for Technical Assistance Services for Children Who Are Deaf--Blind • Center on Disability Studies [1936]
University Headache Center [35570]
University Health Care System • Cancer Program [5013]
University Health Center--Saint Antoine [6842]
University Health Services [14489]
University Health System • Cancer Program [6027]
University Health Systems of Eastern Carolina
    Pitt County Memorial Hospital
        Regional Rehabilitation Center [4339]
        Sleep Center [37496]
University Health Systems Home Health and Hospice [20750]
University Health Systems Hospice Care [20618]
University Healthcare Hospital and Clinics - Main Site [18226]
University Hearing and Speech Clinic [3647]
University High School Deaf/Hard of Hearing Program [278]
University Home Care [16735]
University Home Care of Cashie [16802]
University Home Health Services-- [14590]
University Home Health Services - Edgefield [17583]
University Home Health Services--Martinez [14554]
University Home Health Services - North Augusta [17611]
University Home Health Services--Sandersville [14579]
University Home Health Services - Wagener [17625]
University Home Health Services--Waynesboro [14608]
University Hospice [20609]
University Hospital--Albuquerque • Cancer Program [5551]
University Hospital of Brooklyn • Cancer Program [5568]
University Hospital--Cincinnati
    Barrett Cancer Center • Adult Sickle Cell Program [36415]
    Charles M. Barrett Cancer Center [5700]
University Hospital Cincinnati • Dialysis Center [26051]
University Hospital • Clark Burn Center [4597]
University Hospital--Indianapolis • Department of Obstetrics and Gynecology • In Vitro Fertilization Program [22062]
University Hospital Loyola • Dialysis Center [24037]
University Hospital • MDA Clinic [34828]
University Hospital--Newark, New Jersey • Headache Clinic [12446]
University Hospital--Newark • Sickle Cell Disease Center [36386]
University Hospital Renal Transplant Services • University of Texas Health Science Center [27351]
University Hospital--San Antonio • Renal Unit [27349]
University Hospital • Speech and Hearing Center [1836]
University Hospital Transplant ESRD • Nebraska Medical Center--Transplant Center [25343]
University Hospitals of Cleveland
    Dialysis Center [26070]
    Ireland Cancer Center [5705]
    Rainbow Babies and Children's Hospital • Leroy Matthews Cystic Fibrosis Center [7642]
    Sleep Center [37593]
    University Pain Center [35619]

University Hospitals Health System
    MacDonald Fertility and IVF Program [22218]
    Pediatric Hematology [12581]
University Hospitals Home Care Services, Inc. [17065]
University of Houston • Speech-Language-Hearing Clinic [3515]
University of IA Hospitals and Clinics • Chemical Dependency Service [43281]
University of Illinois--Chicago • Children's Habilitation Clinic [7945]
University of Illinois at Chicago • College of Medicine • Genetics Clinic [12210]
University of Illinois at Chicago Counseling Center • In-Touch Hotline [50836]
University of Illinois, Chicago • Department of Medicine • HIV Vaccine Trials Unit [81]
University of Illinois--Chicago • Division of Specialized Care for Children [7972]
University of Illinois at Chicago • Eating Disorders Clinic [11056]
University of Illinois--Chicago • Institute for Juvenile Research [7946]
University of Illinois, Chicago • MDA Clinic [34795]
University of Illinois at Chicago Medical Center
    Cancer Program [5081]
    Sports Medicine and Human Performance Center [38369]
University of Illinois, Chicago • Reproductive Endocrinology and Infertility [22053]
University of Illinois
    College of Medicine
        Pain Management [35439]
        Sickle Cell Disease Center [36340]
University of Illinois Hospital Dialysis [23963]
University of Illinois • MDA/ALS Center [115]
University of Illinois Medical Center
    Adult Pediatric Comprehensive Sickle Cell Center [36341]
    Mile Square Health Center • Near West Family Center [6666]
    Pediatric Comprehensive Sickle Cell Center [36342]
University of Illinois
    Speech and Hearing Clinic [1977]
    UAP Family Clinic [10797]
University of Iowa • Adult Cystic Fibrosis Center [7545]
University of Iowa Community HomeCare [19702]
University of Iowa
    Cord Blood Bank [35043]
    Department of Orthopaedic Surgery • Specialized Center of Research in Osteoarthritis [165]
    Department of Pediatrics • Division of Medical Genetics [12216]
University of Iowa Hospital & Clinics Dialysis [24278]
University of Iowa Hospital and Clinics--Grinnell [24274]
University of Iowa Hospital and Clinics • Iowa Regional Hemophilia Center [12522]
University of Iowa Hospital and Clinics--Muscatine • Muscatine Outreach Dialysis [24290]
University of Iowa Hospital and Clinics--North Liberty • Outreach Dialysis Unit [24292]
University of Iowa Hospital and Clinics • Transplant/Dialysis Center [24279]
University of Iowa Hospital and Clinics--Washington • Dialysis Unit [24304]
University of Iowa Hospitals and Clinics • Center for Disabilities and Development [10802]
University of Iowa Hospitals and Clinics--Davenport • Reproductive Endocrinology and Infertility Clinic [22065]
University of Iowa Hospitals and Clinics
    Department of Pediatrics • Iowa Neonatal Metabolic Screening Program [12217]
    Holden Comprehensive Cancer Center [5191]
University of Iowa Hospitals and Clinics--Iowa City • Reproductive Endocrinology and Infertility Clinic [22066]
University of Iowa Hospitals and Clinics
    MDA Clinic [34798]
    Pain Management [35452]
    Pediatric Cystic Fibrosis Center [7546]
The University of Iowa Hospitals and Clinics • Sleep Disorders Center [36986]
University of Iowa Hospitals and Clinics • University of Iowa Burn Center [4547]

University of Minnesota Hospital and Clinic •
University Ear, Nose and Throat Center [2714]
University of Minnesota Medical Center, Fairview
ALS Center [128]
Hemophilia and Thrombosis Center [12546]
University of Minnesota Medical Center • Sleep
Center [37239]
University of Minnesota
Multiple Sclerosis Center [34613]
School of Medicine • Pediatric Cystic Fibrosis
Center [7582]
Sickle Cell Disease Center [36367]
University of Mississippi Medical Center • Adult
Cystic Fibrosis Center [7583]
University of Mississippi • Medical Center for Com-
municative Disorders [2765]
University of Mississippi Medical Center
Department of Pediatric Nephrology [25139]
Department of Preventive Medicine • Medical
Genetics Clinic [12261]
In Vitro Fertilization Program [22143]
MDA Clinic [34823]
Pain Management [35527]
Pediatric Hematology/Oncology • Clinic for
Bleeding and Clotting Disorders [12547]
Sickle Cell Disease Center [36368]
Sleep Disorders Center [37268]
University Hospitals and Clinics
Cancer Program [5430]
Pediatric Cystic Fibrosis Center [7584]
University of Mississippi
Multiple Sclerosis Center [34616]
Speech and Hearing Center [2774]
University of Mississippi Sports Medicine [38645]
University of Missouri • Children's Hospital • Sickle
Cell Disease Center [36372]
University of Missouri-Columbia • Children's Hospital
• Cystic Fibrosis Center [7589]
University of Missouri Health Care
Department of Child Health • Division of Medical
Genetics [12265]
Hemophilia Treatment Center [12551]
University of Missouri Hospital • Sleep Disorders
Center [37294]
University of Missouri Health System • Sports
Medicine Service [38654]
University of Missouri Hospital and Clinics
Communication Disorders Unit [2785]
Ellis Fischel Cancer Center [5441]
Transplant/Dialysis Center [25189]
University of Missouri Hospitals and Clinics •
George David Peak Memorial Burn Center [4580]
University of Missouri, Kansas City • Children's
Mercy Hospital • Cystic Fibrosis Center [7590]
University of Missouri • Speech and Hearing Clinic
[2786]
University of Moncton • Eating Disorders Program
[11138]
University of Montana • Rural Institute on Disabilities
[10823]
University of Nebraska, Kearney • Speech,
Language & Hearing Clinic [2847]
University of Nebraska Medical Center
Adult Cystic Fibrosis Center [7594]
ALS Center [131]
College of Medicine • Pain Management
[35545]
Department of Orthopedic Surgery and
Rehabilitation [38692]
Eppley Cancer Center [4686]
Lions Eye Bank of Nebraska [35102]
Multiple Sclerosis Clinic [34625]
Munroe-Meyer Institute [8230]
Munroe-Meyer Institute for Genetics and
Rehabilitation [12269]
Nebraska Regional Hemophilia Treatment
Center [12552]
Pediatric Cystic Fibrosis Center [7595]
Physical & Occupational Therapy [34827]
University of Nebraska—Lincoln • Speech Produc-
tion Laboratory [2852]
University Neurologists [12460]
University of Nevada, Reno • Nevada Dual Sensory
Impairment Project [2873]
University of Nevada
School of Medicine
Adult Cystic Fibrosis Center [7597]
Genetics Program [12271]

Sickle Cell Disease Center for Adults
[36375]
University of New Hampshire
Institute on Disability • Down Syndrome Clinic
[10826]
Speech/Language/Hearing Center [2882]
University of New Mexico
Addictions and Substance Abuse Progs [46242]
Agora Crisis Center [51127]
Carrie Tingley Hospital [8288]
Pain Management Center for Adults [35573]
Center for Development and Disability's Project
for New Mexico Children and Youth Who are
Deafblind [2964]
University of New Mexico Children's Psychiatric
Center [33668]
University of New Mexico
Children's Psychiatric Center [8289]
Health Sciences Center
MDA/ALS Center [132]
Multiple Sclerosis Specialty Clinic [34639]
Office of the Medical Investigator Grief
Services Program [36515]
University of New Mexico Health Sciences Center •
Sleep Disorders Center [37374]
University of New Mexico Hospice Department
[20524]
University of New Mexico Hospital
MDA Clinic [34831]
Milagro Program [46243]
University of New Mexico Pediatric Dialysis [25538]
University of New Mexico Psychiatric Center [33669]
Psychosocial Rehabilitation Program [31184]
University of New Mexico
Regional Burn Center [4588]
School of Medicine
Adult Cystic Fibrosis Center [7608]
Department of Obstetrics and Gynecology
Prenatal Diagnosis and Genetics Unit
[12280]
University of New Mexico School of Medicine • Pain
Management [35574]
University of New Mexico • School of Medicine •
Pediatric Cystic Fibrosis Center [7609]
University of North Carolina
AIDS Clinical Trials Unit [25]
Carolinas Medical Center • MDA/ALS Clinic
[136]
University of North Carolina at Chapel Hill • Adult
Cystic Fibrosis Center [7632]
University of North Carolina, Chapel Hill
Centers for AIDS Research [65]
Comprehensive Sickle Cell Program [36408]
Department of Medicine • Thurston Arthritis
Research Center • Multidisciplinary Clinical
Research Center [173]
Eating Disorders Program [11180]
University of North Carolina at Chapel Hill
Hemophilia Diagnostic and Treatment Center
[12570]
School of Medicine
Department of Pediatrics Carolina Center for
Genome Sciences [12310]
Pediatric Cystic Fibrosis Center [7633]
University of North Carolina
Clinical Center for the Study of Development
and Learning [8371]
HIV Vaccine Trials Unit [91]
University of North Carolina Hospitals • Anesthesiol-
ogy and Pain Management Center [35596]
University of North Carolina Hospitals Home Health
[16705]
University of North Carolina Hospitals
Lineberger Comprehensive Cancer Center
[5630]
North Carolina Jaycee Burn Center [4599]
School of Medicine • Department of Neurology
MDA Clinic [34848]
University of North Carolina • Sleep Disorders
Center [37497]
University of North Carolina Sports Medicine Depart-
ment [38828]
University of North Dakota
Counseling Center [47585]
Division of Sports Medicine [38845]
School of Medicine • Department of Pediatrics
Division of Medical Genetics [12312]
University of North Texas • Speech and Hearing

Center [3487]
University of Oklahoma Health Science Center •
John W. Keys Speech and Hearing Clinic [3279]
University of Oklahoma • Health Sciences Center •
Child Study Center [8439]
University of Oklahoma Health Sciences Center •
University of Oklahoma Hospital • Pain Manage-
ment [35626]
University of Oklahoma Medical Center • Health Sci-
ences Center • Genetics Clinic [12321]
University of Oklahoma • Oklahoma Deafblind
Technical Assistance Project [3276]
University Orthopaedic Group [38747]
University Orthopaedic Sports Medicine Clinic
[38886]
University Orthopedics [38999]
University Pain Clinic [35517]
University Park Dialysis Center • DaVita [22791]
University Pediatric Hospital • Pediatric Renal
Center, Department de Salud • Dialysis Center
[26655]
University of Pennsylvania/Children's Hospital of
Philadelphia/Wistar Institute • Centers for AIDS
Research [69]
University of Pennsylvania
Department of Psychiatry • Center for
Psychotherapy Research [32136]
Department of Radiology • Computational
Breast Imaging Group [5856]
University of Pennsylvania Health System
Penn Sleep Center at Hilton Homewood Suites
[37703]
Penn Sleep Center at Sheraton University City
Hotel [37704]
Penn Sleep Centers [37705]
University of Pennsylvania • HIV Vaccine Trials Unit
[92]
University of Pennsylvania Hospital • Pain Manage-
ment [35653]
University of Pennsylvania Hospital System •
Comprehensive Multiple Sclerosis Care Center
[34696]
University of Pennsylvania Medical Center
Hamot Sports Medicine Center [38942]
Swallowing Disorders Center [3370]
University of Pennsylvania • School of Medicine •
Neurology Department • Laboratory for Cognition
and Neural Stimulation [4415]
University of Pennsylvania Sports Medicine Center
[38969]
University Physicians Healthcare • Department of
Orthopedic Surgery • Arizona Institute for Sports
Medicine [38058]
University Physicians Healthcare Hospital • MDA/
ALS Center [96], [34755]
University Physicians Inc. [996]
University of Pittsburgh
ALS Center [146]
Arthritis Institute • Rheumatic Diseases Core
Center [178]
Auditory Research Group [3371]
Cleft Palate--Cranio Center [3372]
University of Pittsburgh Medical Center
Comprehensive Adult Sickle Cell Program
[36422]
Division of Infectious Diseases • AIDS Clinical
Trials Unit [30]
University of Pittsburgh Medical Center Health
System • Western Psychiatric Institute and Clinic
[33820]
University of Pittsburgh Medical Center
Magee-Womens Hospital • Dan Berger Cord
Blood Program [35194]
MDA/ALS Center [34869]
MDA/ALS Clinic [34870]
Multiple Sclerosis Center [34697]
Pain Management [35654]
University of Pittsburgh
Model System on Spinal Cord Injury [4416]
Sleep Medicine Center [37706]
Spine Biomechanics Research Laboratory
[4417]
Sports Medicine Center [38975]
University of Puerto Rico
Escuela Elementary [718]
Pediatric Hospital • AIDS Clinical Trials Unit [31]
School of Medicine • Puerto Rico Hemophilia
Treatment Center [12590]

University of Rochester • Department of Orthopaedics • Center of Research Translation [172]
University of Rochester Medical Center
    Centers for AIDS Research [63]
    Department of Infectious Diseases
        Adult AIDS Clinical Trials Unit [22]
        AIDS Vaccine Evaluation Unit [90]
    Department of Pediatrics • Division of Pediatric Genetics • Genetic Consultation Clinic [12301]
    MDA/ALS Clinic [134]
    MDA Clinic [34844]
    Pain Management [35588]
    Steven Strong Memorial Hospital • James P. Wilmot Cancer Center [5614]
    Strong Center for Developmental Disabilities • Down Syndrome Clinic [10836]
    Strong Memorial Hospital • Spinal Cord Injury System [4321]
University of Rochester • Strong Memorial Hospital • Audiology and Speech Pathology Department [3115]
University of Rochester/Strong Memorial Hospital • Strong Sleep Disorders Center [37447]
University Services--Lansdale • North Penn Sleep Center [37707]
University Services--Philadelphia • Network I Sleep Center [37708]
University Services Sleep Diagnostic and Treatment Centers • Pottstown Sleep Laboratory [37709]
University Services--Warrington • Warrington Sleep Center [37710]
University Services--West Chester • Sleep Diagnostic and Treatment Centers • West Chester Sleep Center [37711]
University of South Alabama Burn Center • Regional Burn and Wound Center [4502]
University of South Alabama
    Cystic Fibrosis Center [7459]
    Department of Medical Genetics • Genetics/Birth Defects Center [12121]
    Department of Obstetrics and Gynecology • Reproductive Endocrinology Division In Vitro Fertilization Program [21888]
University of South Alabama Health System • Comprehensive Sickle Cell Center--Adult Care [36288]
University of South Alabama Medical Center • Cancer Program [4737]
University of South Alabama
    Pediatric Comprehensive Sickle Cell Center [36289]
    USA Speech and Hearing Center [916]
University of South Carolina
    Department of Exercise Science • Preventive Exercise Program [39008]
    School of Medicine • Department of Obstetrics and Gynecology • Division of Genetics [12335]
    Speech and Hearing Center [3399]
University of South Dakota
    Center for Disabilities [3420]
    Sanford School of Medicine • Center for Disabilities • South Dakota Deaf--Blind Program [3417]
    School of Medicine • Birth Defects Genetics Center [12337]
University of South Florida
    ALS Clinic [111]
    College of Medicine
        Department of Pediatrics Division of Genetics [12187]
        Pain Management [35399]
University of South Florida Dialysis Center [23539]
University of South Florida
    James A. Haley Veterans Affairs Hospital • Adult Hemophilia Treatment Center [12505]
    Pediatric Cystic Fibrosis Center [7517]
    Sickle Cell Disease Center [36331]
University of Southern Alabama • Headache Center [12379]
University of Southern California
    Adult AIDS Clinical Trials Unit [6]
    Comprehensive Sickle Cell Center [36311]
    Hospital of the Good Samaritan • Neuromuscular Center [34767]
    Keck School of Medicine • Internal Medicine, Inc. Cystic Fibrosis Center [7488]
University of Southern California and Los Angeles County • Southern California Burn Center [4525]

University of Southern California
    Multiple Sclerosis Comprehensive Care Center [34533]
    Norris Cancer Center and Hospital [4801]
    Pain Management [35342]
    School of Medicine • USC Neuromuscular Center Jerry Lewis MDA/ALS Clinical and Research Center [34768]
University of Southern Mississippi
    DuBard School for Language Disorders [2762]
    Payne Center [38643]
University Specialty Hospital [4130]
    Maryland ALS Center [119]
University Sports Medicine [38046]
    Kernan Hospital [38518]
    Kernan Physical Therapy and Spine Center [38519]
University Sports Medicine of Rochester [38817]
University Sports Medicine of Syracuse, PC [38821]
University Substance Abuse Clinic [44873]
University Suburban Sleep Center [37594]
University Suburban Sports Medicine Center [38895]
University Surgical Associates [2287]
University of Tennessee
    Boling Center for Speech--Language Pathology and Audiology [760]
    Center on Deafness [756]
University of Tennessee College of Medicine • Le Bonheur Children's Medical Center • Pediatric Cystic Fibrosis Center [7664]
University of Tennessee
    Department of Medical Genetics [12338]
    Department of Medicine • Rheumatic Diseases Core Center [180]
    Developmental and Genetics Center [36432]
University of Tennessee Health Science Center • Boling Center for Developmental Disabilities [8521]
University of Tennessee
    Hearing and Speech Center [3435]
    Le Bonheur Children's Medical Center • College of Medicine Adult Cystic Fibrosis Center [7665]
University of Tennessee Medical center • Cancer Program [5939]
University of Tennessee Medical Center
    Genetics Center [12339]
    MDA Clinic [34879]
University of Tennessee • Medical Center/Rehabilitation Services [3436]
University of Tennessee, Memphis • Center for Health Sciences • Division of Genetics • Boling Center for Developmental Disabilities [12340]
University of Tennessee-Memphis • College of Medicine • Hemophilia Treatment Program [12596]
University of Tennessee, Memphis • Scottish Rite Clinic for Childhood Language Disorders [3443]
University of Texas, Austin
    Department of Communication Science and Disorders • Speech and Hearing Center [3467]
    Services for Students with Disabilities [772]
University of Texas, Dallas • Callier Center • Preverbal Communication Project [3483]
University of Texas--El Paso • Speech, Hearing and Language Center [3491]
University of Texas • Harris County Psychiatric Center [33872]
University of Texas, Harris County • Psychiatric Center Behavioral Health Services [33873]
The University of Texas Health Center at Tyler [18181]
University of Texas Health Center, Tyler • Cystic Fibrosis Center [7680]
University of Texas Health Center Tyler • NeuroRestorative Special Services [4463]
University of Texas Health Center, Tyler • Sleep Disorders Center [37866]
University of Texas Health Science Center
    Allograft Resources, San Antonio [35246]
    Division of Rheumatology • Department of Internal Medicine Specialized Center of Research Translation in Scleroderma [182]
University of Texas Health Science Center at Houston • Multiple Sclerosis Clinic [34719]
University of Texas Health Science Center • MDA/ALS Clinic [151], [34892]
University of Texas Health Science Center at San Antonio • Department of Cellular and Structural

Biology [12355]
University of Texas Health Science Center, San Antonio • Pain Management [35735]
University of Texas, Houston • Houston AIDS Research Team • Community Program for Clinical Research on Aids [74]
University of Texas M.D. Anderson Cancer Center • Cancer Care Program [6003]
University of Texas
    M.D. Anderson Cancer Center • Cord Blood Bank [35247]
    MD Anderson Cancer Center • Pain Management [35736]
University of Texas Medical Branch
    Blocker Burn Center [4641]
    Center for Audiology and Speech Pathology [3497]
University of Texas Medical Branch--Dickinson • Department of Obstetrics and Gynecology • In Vitro Fertilization Program [22274]
University of Texas Medical Branch at Galveston • Genetics Clinic [12356]
University of Texas Medical Branch Hospitals
    Cancer Program [5991]
    Pain Clinic [35737]
University of Texas Medical Branch Transplant [27101]
University of Texas Medical Branch • Transplant/Dialysis Center [27102]
University of Texas Medical Center--Dallas • Department of Obstetrics and Gynecology • In Vitro Fertilization Program [22275]
The University of Texas Medical School at Houston • Department of Pediatrics • Medical Genetics Program [12357]
University of Texas Medical School, Houston • Houston AIDS Research Team • AIDS Clinical Trials Unit [35]
University of Texas Mental Sciences Institute [32488]
University of Texas
    Southwest Medical Center at Dallas • MDA/ALS Center [152], [34893]
    Southwestern Medical Center • Department of Internal Medicine Center of Research Translation in Genetic Dissection of SLE-From Mouse to Man [183]
University of Texas Southwestern Medical Center Multiple Sclerosis Center [34720]
    Transplant Services [27040]
University of Texas Southwestern Medical School
    John Peter Smith Hospital • Pain Management [35738]
    North Texas Comprehensive Hemophilia Center, Adult Program [12603]
    Pain Management [35739]
University of Texas Southwestern Saint Paul Hospital • Cancer Care Program [5978]
University of Texas Transplant Services Center [35248]
University of TN Medical Center Home Care Services--Knoxville [17713]
University of TN Medical Center Home Care Services--La Follette [17717]
University of TN Medical Center Home Care Services--Maryville [17728]
University of Toledo Medical Center • Cancer Program [5754]
University of Toledo
    Office of Accessibility [662]
    University Medical Center • Coghlin Rehabilitation Center [4375]
University of Utah • ALS Center [153]
University of Utah Dialysis Program [25377]
University of Utah
    Dialysis Program [27424]
        Gem State Regional Dialysis Center [23874]
    Health Care Rehabilitation Center [4471]
University of Utah Health Sciences Center
    Intermountain Cystic Fibrosis Center • Adult Cystic Fibrosis Center [7681]
    Intermountain Pediatric Cystic Fibrosis Center [7682]
    Pain Management [35746]
University of Utah Hospital • Burn Center [4642]
University of Utah Hospital and Clinics • Department of Pediatrics • Medical Genetics Clinic [12358]
University of Utah Hospitals and Clinic • Sleep/Wake

Center [37875]
University of Utah Hospitals and Clinics • Huntsman Cancer Institute [6044]
University of Utah • Huntsman Cancer Institute • Comprehensive Cancer Center [4713]
University of Utah--Kolff Dialysis Center • Kolff Dialysis Center [27425]
University of Utah Medical Center • Alcohol and Drug Abuse Clinic [49700]
University of Utah • Neuropsychiatric Inst Recovery Works [49701]
University of Utah Neuropsychiatric Institute [32619]
University of Utah • Pain Management Center [35747]
University of Utah Palliative Care [21653]
University of Utah Provo Dialysis Center [27416]
University of Utah Rehabilitation Services [8571]
University of Utah
    Reproductive Endocrinology and Infertility Division [22277]
    School of Medicine • Department of Neurology MDA/ALS Center [34895]
University of Utah School of Medicine • MDA/ALS Clinic [154]
University of Utah
    School of Medicine • Multiple Sclerosis Center [34724]
    Speech-Language-Hearing Clinic [3559]
    Utah Eating Disorder: Salt Lake City [11292]
University of Vermont
    Burn Center [4643]
    Center on Disability and Community Inclusion
        Down Syndrome Clinic [10873]
        University Center for Excellence in Developmental Disability Education [3562]
    College of Medicine
        Fletcher Allen Health Care Adult Down Syndrome Center [10874]
        Vermont Human Genetics Initiative Down Syndrome Clinic [10875]
    E.M. Luse Center [3563]
    Fletcher Allen Health Care • Pain Management [35750]
    Vermont Genetics Network [12359]
University of Virginia
    Adult Cystic Fibrosis Center [7689]
    Children's Hospital [3577]
    Children's Medical Center
        Kluge Children's Rehabilitation Center [8580]
        Eating Disorders Program [11299]
University of Virginia Health Sciences Center • De-Camp Burn Center [4647]
University of Virginia Health System [18263]
    Cancer Program [6055]
    James Q. Miller Consultative Multiple Sclerosis Clinic [34731]
    Pain Management [35754]
    Pediatric Cystic Fibrosis Center [7690]
    Richard R. Dart ALS Center [156]
University of Virginia Hospital
    Adult Hemophilia Program [12607]
    MDA Clinic [34901]
University of Virginia Medical Center
    Hemophilia Treatment Center [12608]
    Renal Services • Transplant/Dialysis Center [27469]
University of Virginia
    School of Medicine
        Department of Pediatrics Genetics Clinic [12362]
        Division of Hematology and Oncology [36441]
University of Virginia School of Medicine - Division of Rheumatology • Multidisciplinary Clinical Research Center [184]
University of Virginia • Speech, Language, Hearing Center [3578]
University of Washington
    Department of Medicine and Health Services • Multidisciplinary Clinical Research Center [185]
    Experimental Education Unit [8603]
University of Washington /Fred Hutchinson Cancer Research Center • HIV Vaccine Trials Unit [94]
University of Washington Hall Sports Medicine [39148]
University of Washington

Harborview Medical Center
    Burn Center [4650]
    Centers for AIDS Research [76]
University of Washington Medical Center
    Adult Cystic Fibrosis Center [7695]
    Cancer Program [6116]
University of Washington • Medical Center • Cystic Fibrosis Center [7696]
University of Washington Medical Center
    Department of Medicine • Medical Genetics Clinics [12370]
    Prenatal Genetics and Fetal Therapy Program • Department of Obstetrics and Gynecology [12371]
    Rehabilitation Medical Clinic • MDA/ALS Center [34907]
University of Washington Medical Center Transplant Services [27642]
University of Washington Medical Center • Western Multiple Sclerosis Center • Rehabilitation Unit [34738]
University of Washington, Roosevelt • Medical Center [35762]
University of Washington School of Medicine • Center for Pain Medicine [35763]
University of Washington, Seattle • Harborview Medical Center • AIDS Clinical Trials Unit [37]
University of Washington • Speech and Hearing Clinic [3641]
University of Wisconsin
    Adult Cystic Fibrosis Center [7704]
    Hospital and Clinics [3677]
University of Wisconsin Hospital and Clinics
    Burn Center [4654]
    Sports Medicine Center [39181]
University of Wisconsin Hospitals and Clinics
    Comprehensive Program for Bleeding Disorders [12618]
    Voice and Swallow Service [3678]
University of Wisconsin--Madison • MDA/ALS Clinical Research Center [34913]
University of Wisconsin, Madison
    Pediatric Cystic Fibrosis [7705]
    Waisman Center • Developmental Disabilities Clinic [10880]
University of Wisconsin, Milwaukee • Deaf and Hard of Hearing Program [889]
University of Wisconsin • Pain and Headache Clinic [12477]
University of Wisconsin Transplant [27759]
University of Wisconsin
    Waisman Center • Clinical Services Unit [8620]
    Women's Endocrinology & Reproductive Clinic • In Vitro Fertilization Program [22302]
University of Wisconsin—Madison
    Department of Communication Sciences and Disorders • Auditory Behavioral Research Laboratory [887]
    School of Medicine and Public Health • Department of Surgery Colon and Rectal Surgery Laboratory [6158]
Unlimited Care Inc.--Bronx [16371]
Unlimited Care Inc.--Clifton [16195]
Unlimited Care Inc.--East Orange [16200]
Unlimited Care Inc.--Englewood [16210]
Unlimited Care Inc.--Forest Hills [16467]
Unlimited Care Inc.--Garden City [16469]
Unlimited Care Inc.--Hauppauge [16476]
Unlimited Care Inc.--Hudson [16493]
Unlimited Care Inc.--Kingston [16508]
Unlimited Care Inc.--Middletown [16524]
Unlimited Care Inc.--Newburgh [16575]
Unlimited Care Inc.--Peekskill [16592]
Unlimited Care Inc.--Poughkeepsie [16604]
Unlimited Care Inc.--Rhinebeck [16608]
Unlimited Care Inc.--Rochester [16617]
Unlimited Care Inc.--West New York [16287]
Unlimited Care Inc.--White Plains [16674]
Unlimited Home Care [13778]
Unlimited Home Health Services [13704]
Unlimited Visions Aftercare Inc [49237], [49416], [49481]
UNS Group [13679]
UPC Jefferson Avenue Research Clinic [44769]
Upland Community Counseling [28835]
Upland Dialysis Center • DaVita [26593]
Upland Dialysis • DaVita [23047]
Upland Hills Dialysis Center [27709]

Upland Hills Home Care [18565]
Uplands Hills Home Care and Hospice [21831]
Uplift Comprehensive Services [47533]
UPMC Health System
    John Merck Program [8481]
    Presbyterian Renal Unit [26564]
UPMC Home Medical Equipment [17448]
UPMC Horizon • Greenville Regional Hospital • Cancer Program [5829]
UPMC Institute for Rehabilitation and Research
    UPMC Horizon [4418]
    UPMC McKeesport [4419]
    UPMC Northwest [4420]
    UPMC St. Margaret [4421]
UPMC Institute for rehabilitation and Research • UPMC Montefiore [4422]
UPMC/Jefferson Regional Home Health, LP [17449]
UPMC/Jefferson Regional Home Health, LP - Horizon [17342]
UPMC/Jefferson Regional Home Health Ohio Subunit [16955]
UPMC Mercy • Institute for Rehabilitation and Research [4423]
UPMC Northwest
    Cancer Center [5873]
    Sleep Center [37712]
UPMC Passavant • Cancer Center [4703]
UPMC Presbyterian--Transplant • Thomas E Starzl Transplantation Institute [26565]
UPMC Saint Margaret Memorial Hospital • Cancer Program [5860]
UPMC Shadyside • Cancer Program [5861]
UPMC/South Hills Health System Home Health, LP [17475]
UPO Comprehensive Treatment Center [41551]
Upper Bay Counseling and Support Services [30283]
Upper Chesapeake Medical Center • Cancer Center [5294]
Upper Chesapeake Sleep Disorders Center • Harford Memorial Hoapital [37112]
Upper Connecticut Valley Mental Health and Developmental Services [31054]
Upper Eastside Dialysis Facility [25739]
Upper Hudson Planned Parenthood
    Albany Health Center [11821]
    Hudson Health Center [11822]
    Troy Health Center [11823]
Upper Manhattan Mental Health Center
    Alcoholism Halfway House/ABLE House [46925]
    Chemical Dependence Services [46926]
Upper Mississippi Mental Health Center [30708]
    Program for Addictions Recovery [45086]
Upper Peninsula Home Health, Hospice, and Private Duty [20092]
Upper Shore Community Mental Health Center [33560]
Upper Tanana Alcohol Program [39354]
Upper Valley Community Health Service [6644]
Upper Valley Dialysis • DaVita [27076]
Upper Valley Help For Family Violence • Family Crisis Center [9186]
Upper Valley Medical Center [17060]
    Cancer Care Center and Infusion Services [5755]
Upper Valley Neurology Neurosurgery • Multiple Sclerosis Clinic of New Hampshire [34630]
Upper Valley Resource and Counseling [29551], [42377]
Upson County Counseling Center [29496]
Upstate Dialysis Center & At Home • DaVita [26724]
Upstate Medical Center • Center for Neuropsychiatric Genetics [12302]
Upstate Medical University
    Center for Genetic Communicative Disorders [12303]
    Development, Behavior and Genetics Clinic [12304]
    Genetics Clinic [12305]
    University Hospital • Cancer Program [5621]
Upstate New York Transplant Services Inc. [35144]
Upstate New York VA Health Care Network at Canandaigua [16431]
Upstate Sleep Disorders Center • A Division of Carolina Lung & Sleep Center [37747]
Upton County Mental Health Center [32509]
Uptown Chicago Dialysis • Fresenius Medical Care [23964]

Upward Foundation [7742]
Urban Family Ministries [49146]
Urban Health Plan, Inc. [7013]
Urban League of Rhode Island • Runaway and Homeless Youth Program [36192]
Urban Ministries • Safehouse [10395]
Urban Ounce of Prevention Services • Exodus Program [47611]
Urban Peak--Colorado Springs • Runaway and Homeless Youth Program [35857]
Urban Peak--Denver • Runaway and Homeless Youth Program [35858]
Urban Peak--Denver Shelter • Runaway and Home-less Youth Program [35859]
Urban Res Inst/Marguerite T Saunders • Urban Center for Alcohol/Addiction Services [46539]
Urban Women's Retreat [9960]
URDC Human Services Corporation • CHOICES [40379]
Uriel Treatment Center [46014]
Urra Home Health Corporation [14173]
Urton Associates [47480]
US Bioservices [17761]
US Grant Dialysis • DaVita [26127]
US Healthworks [38219]
US Home Health Care Services 2 [14460]
US Marine Corps • Substance Abuse Counseling Center [47397]
US Naval Hospital Guantanamo Bay [12886]
US Renal Care--Baylor Scott Street [27181]
US Renal Care of Bowling Green [26023]
US Renal Care--Canton HD and Home [26986]
US Renal Care--Delta [27077]
US Renal Care--Edinburg [27058]
US Renal Care--Home Therapies [27182]
US Renal Care Inc.--Boerne [26975]
US Renal Care of Kenwood [26052]
US Renal Care Kidney Center of McGehee [22560]
US Renal Care--Kingwood [27210]
US Renal Care--McAllen [27254]
US Renal Care of Northeastern Arkansas - Paragould [22567]
US Renal Care of Norwood Dialysis [26053]
US Renal Care Pine Bluff Dialysis Center [22569]
US Renal Care--Rio Grande [27297]
US Renal Care of SEA [22577]
   Pine Bluffs Dialysis [22570]
US Renal Care
   Tarrant Dialysis Center--North Fort Worth [27096]
   Tarrant Dialysis Center--South Fort Worth [26985]
USA Home Care Solution Agency--Coral Gables [13625]
USA Home Health Care Agency [14223]
USA Home Health Care Solution Agency--Miami [14174]
USAccent [2493]
USC Fertility [21950]
USC University Hospital, Renal TX [22792]
USPHS Phoenix Indian Medical Center • Native American or Alaska Native Only [39454]
Ussery - Roan Texas State Veterans Home [17794]
UT Health Houston • CNRA [49417]
UT MD Anderson Sleep Center [37867]
UT Medical Group--Germantown • Clinical Genetics [12341]
UT Medical Group--Jackson • Clinical Genetics [12342]
UT Medical Group--Memphis • Clinical Genetics [12343]
UT Southwestern - Child and Adolescent Psychiatry [11287]
Uta Halee Girls Village [34286]
Utah Cord Bank [35250]
Utah County Crisis Line [51402]
Utah County Div of Substance Abuse • Foothill Residential Treatment Center [49708]
Utah County Division of Substance Abuse Outpatient Services [49667]
Utah Department of Health • Maternal and Child Health Bureau • Child, Adolescent and School Health Program [36548]
Utah Dialysis Lab [27426]
Utah Lions Eye Bank • University of Utah Health Sciences Center • John A. Moran Eye Center [35251]
Utah School for the Deaf and the Blind [3739]

Utah Schools for the Deaf and the Blind [839]
   Utah Project for Children and Young Adults with Deafblindness [3552]
Utah SIDA Alliance [36549]
Utah Sleep Medicine Center [37876]
Utah State Developmental Center [8570]
Utah State Hospital [33895]
Utah State Library Division • Program for the Blind and Disabled [3840]
Utah State University
   Department of Communication Disorders and Deaf Education • Speech-Language-Hearing Center [3550]
   Disability Resource Center [838]
Utah Valley Family Practice and Sports Medicine--N 400 W, Provo [39107]
Utah Valley Family Practice and Sports Medicine--N 500 W, Provo [39108]
Utah Valley Regional Medical Center [3554]
   Cancer Program [6040]
Ute Mountain • Ute Tribe • Sunrise Youth Shelter • Runaway and Homeless Youth Program [35860]
Ute Mountain Ute Tribe • Ute Counseling and Treatment Services [41330]
Utica Avenue Dialysis Clinic • DaVita [25631]
Utica Supportive Living [47153]
UVA Altavista Dialysis • University of Virginia Health System [27456]
UVA Amherst Dialysis [27458]
UVA Augusta Dialysis [27488]
UVA Page Dialysis [27569]
Uvalde Memorial Home Health & Hospice Services [21584]
UVMC Dialysis Services • Outpatient Dialysis Center [26220]
UWM--MCFI Augmentative Communication Clinic [3685]
Uznis Physical Therapy & Rehabilitation Center [38585]

V

VA Ann Arbor Healthcare System [15579], [44648]
VA Black Hills Health Care System [4430]
VA Black Hills Healthcare System • Addictive Disorders Services [48997]
VA Boston Health Care System • Jamaica Plain Campus [15504]
VA Boston Health Care System--West Roxbury [15559]
VA Boston Health Care System • Worcester Outpatient Clinic [15567]
VA Caribbean Healthcare System [48821]
VA Central California Health Care System [13011]
VA Central California Hlthcare System • Chemical Dependency Treatment Program [39870]
VA Central Iowa Health Care System [15078]
VA Central Iowa Healthcare System [43269]
VA Community Based Outpatient Clinic--Hilo [14615]
VA Community Based Outpatient Clinic--Kahului [14630]
VA Community Based Outpatient Clinic--Kailua Kona [14633]
VA Community Based Outpatient Clinic • VA Montana Health Care Center [4256]
VA Community Living Center [14624]
VA Connecticut Health Care System [13553]
VA Connecticut Healthcare System [3945]
VA Connecticut Healthcare System--Newington Campus [13536]
VA Consolidated Mail Outpatient Pharmacy [13159], [15137]
VA Eastern Colorado Healthcare System [13479]
VA Eugene Community Based Outpatient Clinic [17189]
VA Greater LA Healthcare System [40172]
VA Greater Los Angeles Healthcare System [13160]
VA Gulf Coast Healthcare System • Mobile Outpatient Clinic [39277]
VA Gulf Coast Veterans Health Care System [15954]
VA Gulf Coast Veterans Healthcare System [4232]
VA Healthcare Network Upstate New York at Bath Elmira CBOC [16445]
VA Healthcare Network Upstate New York at Syracuse [16649]
VA Healthcare Systems of Connecticut • Substance Abuse Treatment Program [41493]
VA Hudson Valley HCS Montrose Campus [46794]

VA Hudson Valley Health Care System [16527], [20561]
VA - Illiana Health Care System [14760]
VA Illiana Healthcare System • Substance Abuse Rehab Program [42615]
VA Iowa City Health Care System [15091]
VA Long Beach Health Care System [13116]
VA Los Angeles Ambulatory Care Center [13161]
VA Maryland Health Care System [4131], [15423]
VA Maryland Health Care System BRECC and Home Care Services [15424]
VA Maryland Health Care System--Perry Point Campus [15457]
VA Maryland Healthcare System
   Addiction Treatment Program [44191]
   Perry Point Division/SARRTP [44325]
VA Medical Center [4376]
VA Medical Center and Ambulatory Care Clinic [4257]
VA Medical Center - Atlanta [14516]
VA Medical Center--Bath [16344]
VA Medical Center--Battle Creek [15582]
VA Medical Center--Birmingham [12636]
VA Medical Center--Boise [14651]
VA Medical Center • Cancer Center [4699]
VA Medical Center - Carl Vinson [14523]
VA Medical Center • Department of Infectious Diseases • Washington Regional AIDS Program • Community Program for Clinical Research on AIDS [46]
VA Medical Center--Durham [16718]
VA Medical Center • Evansville Outpatient Clinic [14851]
VA Medical Center Fargo, North Dakota [4358]
VA Medical Center - G.V. (Sonny) Montgomery [15967]
VA Medical Center--Hot Springs [26788]
VA Medical Center, HPHC-Indianapolis [19616]
VA Medical Center • Jack C. Montgomery VAMC [4700]
VA Medical Center - James A. Haley [14429]
VA Medical Center • Jefferson Barracks Division [16062]
VA Medical Center Jerry L. Pettis Memorial [13108]
VA Medical Center - John Cochran Division [16063]
VA Medical Center Leestown Division [15211]
VA Medical Center--Lexington [15212]
VA Medical Center--Louisville [15226]
VA Medical Center--Manchester [16174]
VA Medical Center--Miami [14175]
VA Medical Center/Michael E DeBakey • Substance Dependence Treatment Program [49418]
VA Medical Center - Minneapolis [15916]
VA Medical Center--N College Ave., Fayetteville [12844]
VA Medical Center--New Orleans [15345]
VA Medical Center Northport [16577]
VA Medical Center--Pineville [15351]
VA Medical Center--Ramsey St., Fayetteville [16725]
VA Medical Center - Richard L. Roudebush VAMC [15006]
VA Medical Center--Richmond Campus [15046]
VA Medical Center--Shreveport [15366]
VA Medical Center--Spokane [18466]
VA Medical Center Transplant--Iowa City [24280]
VA Medical Center - Wade park Division [16889]
VA Medical Center--Washington DC [13576]
VA Medical Center - West Palm Beach, Florida [14456]
VA Medical Center--Wilmington [13569]
VA Medical and Regional Office Center [16812]
VA Mental Health Clinic [40309]
VA Montana Health Care System [16086]
VA Nebraska-Western Iowa Health Care System [16126]
VA New Jersey Health Care System [16201]
VA New Jersey Healthcare System • Lyons Campus [46041]
VA New York Harbor Health Care System [16423]
VA New York Harbor Health Care System--New York Campus [16569]
VA New York Harbor Health Care System--Saint Albans Campus [16501]
VA New York Harbor Healthcare [46540]
VA Northern California Health Care System [13166]
VA Northern Indiana Health Care System [14986]
   Fort Wayne Campus [4045]
   Goshen CBOC [4046]

VA Northern Indiana Health Care System Marion [15025]
VA Northern Indiana Health Care System
    Muncie CBOC [4047]
    South Bend CBOC [4048]
VA Northern Indiana Healthcare [43058], [43149]
VA Northern Kentucky Healthcare Associates--CBOC [15162]
VA Northwest Tucson Clinic [3881]
VA Outpatient Clinic [50597]
VA Outpatient Clinic-Ft. Myers [3997]
VA Pacific Islands Health Care System [14625]
VA Palo Alto Health Care System [13234]
VA Pittsburgh Healthcare System • Center for Treatment of Addictive Disorders [48611]
VA Primary Care Clinic [14349]
VA Puget Sound Health Care System [18457]
VA Puget Sound Healthcare System • Seattle Division [50143]
VA Roseburg Healthcare System [48235]
VA San Diego Healthcare System [13305]
VA Sierra Nevada Health Care System [16166]
VA South Oregon Rehab Center and Clinics [48259]
VA Southern Nevada Healthcare System [16160]
VA Southern NV Healthcare System [20425]
VA Tennessee Valley Healthcare System [49164]
VA Western New York Health Care System [16430]
VA Western NY Healthcare System • Substance Abuse Program [46573]
VAC Substance Abuse Services [49254]
Vacaville Dialysis Clinic • DaVita [23049]
Vacherie Dialysis Center [24596]
VACO Domestic Violence Prevention [9961]
Vail Valley Medical Center [13511]
Vail Valley Medical Center--Edward Campus [13484]
Val Verde Regional Medical Center Hospice [21444]
Val Verde Renal Care Center • Dialysis Facility [27047]
Valdese General Hospital • Cancer Program [5662]
Valdese General Hospital, Inc. [16790]
Valdosta City Schools [1923]
Valencia Counseling Services • Belen Office [34310]
Valencia Counseling Services Inc [46264], [46276], [46290]
Valencia Counseling Services, Inc. • Casa Manzana [34314]
Valencia Shelter for Victims of Domestic Violence [9861]
Valeo Behavioral Healthcare • Stepping Stones [43469]
Valeo Recovery Center • Topeka [43470]
Valerie Fund Children's Center • Sickle Cell Disease Center [36387]
Valhalla Place [45357]
Valir Hospice, LLC [20967]
Valle Del Sol Inc
    Behavioral Health Program [39455]
    East Clinic [39482]
Valle del Sol [39410]
Valle Vista Counseling Center [29611]
Valle Vista Health System [33472], [43076]
Valle Vista Hospital Access Center [50890]
Vallejo City Unified School District [309]
Vallejo Dialysis Center • DaVita [23052]
Valley Alliance Treatment Services Inc [50331]
Valley Audiology [1084]
Valley Baptist Home Health [17833]
Valley Baptist Medical Center [27119]
    MDA Clinic [34894]
Valley Baptist • Raymondville Dialysis Center [27295]
Valley Bridge House Inc [44192]
Valley Center of the Deaf [974]
Valley Children's Hospital of Central California • Pediatric Neurology • MDA Clinic [34769]
Valley Children's Hospital • Department of Genetic Medicine and Metabolism [12171]
Valley Cities Counseling & Consultation [32804]
Valley City Dialysis • Fresenius Medical Care [26162]
Valley Clinical Services • YETC [39473]
Valley Community Clinic [6330], [40276]
Valley Community Health Centers [7072]
Valley Community Health Centers Larimore [7070]
Valley Community Mental Health Center [32920]
    Garden Towers [32915]
Valley Community Services Board • Substance Abuse Outpatient Services [49846]

Valley Community Support Center & Children's Outpatient Services [28706]
Valley Community Treatment Center [39681]
Valley Comprehensive Community Mental Health Center, Inc. [32904]
Valley Counseling Group [48296]
Valley Counseling Services--Warren [31853]
    Children's Office [31854]
Valley Counseling Services--Youngstown [31864]
Valley Creative Living Center [28707]
Valley ENT Associates PC [2642]
Valley Enterprises [29762]
Valley--Fairlawn Dialysis Center • Outpatient Dialysis Facility [25433]
Valley Family Health Care, Inc. • Valley Family Medical and Dental Clinic [6640]
Valley Forge Medical Center and Hosptial [48490]
Valley General Hospital • Cancer Care Program [6105]
Valley Health Associates [39898], [40242], [40518]
Valley Health Care [32901]
Valley Health Care, Inc. [7410]
Valley Health Systems, Inc. [7407]
Valley Health Team, Inc. • San Joaquin Health Center • Valley Smiles Mobile Dental Clinic [6357]
Valley HealthCare System [51490]
Valley Healthcare System [6588], [50300], [50305], [50320], [50332]
    ACT Unit [50301]
    New Beginnings Program for Women [50302]
Valley Hemodialysis Center • Fresenius Medical Care [26981]
Valley Home Care--Front Royal [18303]
Valley Home Care--Glendale [12792]
Valley Home Care--Paramus [16253]
Valley Home Care--Warrenton [18405]
Valley Home Care--Winchester [18408]
Valley Home Care--Woodstock [18411]
Valley Home Health Care Agency Inc. [13378]
Valley Home Health, Inc. [13206]
Valley Home Medical--Layton [18201]
Valley Home Medical--Midvale [18205]
Valley Home Medical--Orem [18211]
Valley Home Medical--Vernal [18230]
Valley Hope Association • Boonville Valley Hope [45440]
Valley Hope
    Atchison [43320]
    Mission [43410]
    Norton [43418]
    Outpatient Substance Abuse Treatment [48002]
    Wichita [43512]
Valley Hospice--Paramus [20487]
Valley Hospice--Steubenville [20894]
Valley Hospice--Wheeling [21817]
Valley Hospital • Community Hospital Comprehensive Cancer Program [5539]
Valley Hospital and Medical Center • Cancer Program [6123]
Valley Hospital Renal Care Center [25504]
Valley Hospital Sports Institute [38756]
Valley Infusion Care [14877]
Valley Lutheran Hospital [958]
Valley Medical Center
    Cancer Program [6110]
    Sleep Center [37942]
Valley Medical Supply, Inc. [13523]
Valley Mental Health Center
    Adolescent Day Care Program [32620]
    Adult Day Treatment Program [32621]
Valley Mental Health Center--Ansonia [28968]
Valley Mental Health Center
    Children's Behavior Therapy Unit [32622]
    North Valley Unit [32623]
Valley Mental Health Center--Salt Lake City [32624]
Valley Mental Health Center
    South Valley Unit [32592]
    Summit County Office [32606]
Valley Mental Health - Community Treatment Program [32596]
Valley Mental Health Crisis Service--Salt Lake City [51406]
Valley Mental Health--Midvale [51400]
Valley Mental Health--Murray [51401]
Valley Mental Health--Park City [51403]
Valley Mental Health--Tooele [51407]
Valley Mental Health • Tooele [49712]
Valley Mental Health--Tooele County Office [32627]

Valley Neurological Headache and Research Center [12382]
Valley Organization for Improved Communication and Equality [2643]
Valley Oximetry Sleep Disorders Center [36641]
Valley Oximetry • Sleep Disorders Center [36640]
Valley Regional Enterprises [18409]
Valley Regional Hospital [33650]
Valley Regional Sleep Disorders Center [36715]
Valley Ridge Mental Health Center [32338]
Valley Speech, Hearing and Rehabilitation Services [2308]
Valley Speech and Language Associates [1314]
Valley Sports & Arthritis Surgeons [38925]
Valley Star Children and Family Services [28742]
Valley Therapy Services--Alamosa [1372]
Valley Therapy Services--Montrose [1437]
Valley Therapy Services • Pain Clinic [35296]
Valley View 365U [410]
Valley View Hospital [1414]
Valley View Regional Hospital [17094]
    Cancer Program [5771]
Valley View Speech Pathology Services [1083]
Valley Vista [49724]
Valley Wide Counseling • A Program of MFI Recovery Center [40649]
Valley-Wide Health Services, Inc. [6382]
Valley Women's Resource Center [8671]
Valley Youth House • 8th Avenue Shelter • Runaway and Homeless Youth Program [36185]
Valley Youth House Committee • Runaway and Homeless Youth Program [36186]
ValleyCare Medical Center • Cancer Program [4822]
Valleyhead, Inc. [34200]
Valleyview Recovery [47599]
Valliant House LLC [48052]
Valor Hospice Care and Palliative Care [18793]
Valor Hospice Care--Sierra Vista [18822]
Valor Hospice Care--Tucson [18834]
Value Health Care Service [13518]
Valuecare, Inc. [16424]
Vamana Inc. in Texarkana [22578]
VAMC: Aleda E. Lutz VA Medical Center [20112]
VAMC Alexandria VA Medical Center [19871]
VAMC: Cincinnati [20817]
VAMC: Franklin Deleno Roosevelt Campus of the VA Hudson Valley Healthcare System [20580]
VAMC: Northern Indiana Health Care System-Marion Campus [19629]
VAMC at Syracuse [47127]
VAMC: VA Ann Arbor Healthcare System [20030]
VAMC: VA Butler Healthcare [21063]
Van Buren/Cass District Health Dept • Substance Abuse Services [44834]
Van Buren County CMHSP [30618]
    Center for Crisis Stabilization [30589]
    Hope Center [30563]
Van Buren County Community Mental Health Service Program
    MTI [30508]
    South Haven Outpatient Clinic [30635]
Van Buren Intermediate School District [494]
Van Dyke Addiction Treatment Center [46970]
Van Dyke Hospice & Palliative Care Center [20506]
Van Hoose and Associates [43669]
Van Horn Counseling Center [28724]
Van Matre Healthsouth Rehabilitation Hospital [4030], [38408]
Van Ness Recovery House [40173]
Van Veck House [34502]
Van Wert Dialysis • Fresenius Medical Care [26223]
VanArk Behavioral Mangement Inc [43759], [43765]
Vance Air Force Base • Substance Abuse Program [47932]
Vance County Dialysis • DaVita [25882]
Vance, Granville, Franklin, Warren Area Authority--HQ/Vance [31543]
Vancouver Behavioral Health Clinic [32880]
Vancouver Dialysis Center • DaVita [27659]
Vancouver General Hospital • Burn and Plastic Surgery Unit [4513]
Vancouver Island Health Authority • North Island Regional Eating Disorder Program [10921]
Vandalia Dialysis • DaVita [24100]
Vanderbilt Addiction Center • Vanderbilt Psychiatric Hospital [49165]
Vanderbilt Dialysis Clinic East • Fresenius Medical Care [26910]

Vanderbilt Dialysis Clinic • Fresenius Medical Care [26911]
Vanderbilt--Ingram Comprehensive Cancer Center [4707]
Vanderbilt Sports Medicine Center [39039]
Vanderbilt Stallworth Rehabilitation Hospital [39040]
Vanderbilt University Children's Hospital • Down Syndrome Clinic [10864]
Vanderbilt University
    Department of Medicine • Department of Pediatrics/Infectious Diseases • Vanderbilt HIV Vaccine Program [93]
    Mama Lere Hearing School [761]
Vanderbilt University Medical Center
    Adult Cystic Fibrosis Center [7666]
    Cancer Program [5952]
    Children's Hospital • Pediatric Sickle Cell Program [36433]
    Department of Medicine • Division of Infectious Diseases • Centers for AIDS Research [71]
    Hearing and Speech Department [3449]
    Hemostasis and Thrombosis Clinic [12597]
    MDA/ALS Center [34880]
    Meharry Medical College • Centers for AIDS Research [72]
    Sleep Disorders Center [37794]
    Therapeutics Clinical Research • AIDS Clinical Trials Unit [32]
    Vanderbilt Regional Burn Center [4635]
Vanderbilt University
    Peabody College • Project TREDS--Tennessee Technical Assistance and Resources for Enhancing Deaf--Blind Supports [3450]
    Pediatric Cystic Fibrosis Center [7667]
    Susan Gray School for Children [8525]
Vange John Memorial Hospice [21004]
VanNess Orthopedics and Sports Medicine [38656]
Vanregieva Home Health Services, Inc. [13800]
Vans House [47933]
Vantage Health System [45968]
Vantage Health System--Dumont [31122]
Vantage Health System--Englewood [31127]
VAPAHCS San Jose Clinic [13320]
Variety Care Family Health [7112]
Vascular Transplant Services--Millington [35217]
Vascular Transplant Services--Schaumburg [35028]
Vashon Youth and Family Services [50248]
Vashti Center Inc. [29497]
Vassar Brothers Center for Sleep Medicine [37448]
Vassar Brothers Medical Center [3104]
    Dyson Center for Cancer Care [5611]
Vaughan Regional Medical Center • Sleep Laboratory [36617]
VCP Home Healthcare [14828]
VCPHCS IV LLC • Behavioral Health Group Medical Center [48003]
VCPHCS VIII LLC • DBA The Memphis Center for Research/AT [49147]
VCUHS Center for Sleep Medicine [37904]
Venado Middle School [279]
Venice Kidney Center • Fresenius Medical Care [23548]
Ventura College • Educational Assistance Center [310]
Ventura County Behavioral Health Alcohol • Outpatient Alcohol and/or Other Drugs [39829]
Ventura County Behavioral Health Center--Fillmore [28497]
Ventura County Behavioral Health Center--Ventura [28838]
Ventura County Behavioral Health Dept
    Alcohol/Drug Programs/New Start for Moms [40340]
    Simi Valley Center [40802]
Ventura County Coalition Against Household Violence [8920]
Ventura County Dept of Alcohol/Drug Progs [40341]
    Ventura Center [40912]
Ventura Recovery Center Inc • A Community Recovery Center [40852]
Ventura Unified School District • Deaf and Hard of Hearing Program [311]
Venture Dialysis Center • DaVita [23432]
Ventures Assertive Community Treatment [30531]
Vera French Community Mental Health Center [29850]
    Pine Knoll Health Care Facility [29851]
Vera House [9991], [27842]

Verde Valley Community Hospice [18787]
Verde Valley Guidance Clinic [28140]
Verde Valley Guidance Clinic Inc [39378]
Verde Valley Guidance Clinic, Inc. [8684]
Verde Valley Medical Center [28141]
Verde Valley Physical Therapy Center, Inc. [38030]
Verde Valley Sanctuary [8730]
Verdugo Hills Hospital [13057]
Verdugo Hospice Care Center [18962]
Veridian Behavioral Health/SRHC [43457]
Veritacare [16987]
Veritas Therapeutic Community Inc
    Family Outpatient Programs [46927]
    Lucy Rudd House [46367]
    Re-entry [46928]
    Young Mothers/Infants/Toddlers Program [46929]
Verma M Krishna • DBA Psychological Medicine Clinic [47532]
Vermilion Hospital [33540]
Vermillion Coalition Against Domestic Violence [10388]
Vermont Achievement Center [8575]
Vermont Center for Cognitive Behavior Therpy [11294]
Vermont Center for the Deaf and Hard of Hearing, Inc. [843]
Vermont Center for Reproductive Medicine • Women's Health Care Service/FAMC [22278]
Vermont Department of Health • SIDS Information and Counseling Program [36550]
Vermont Department of Libraries • Special Services Unit [3841]
Vermont Regional Hemophilia Center [12605]
Vermont Respite House [21669]
Vermont Speech and Language Pathology [3567]
Vermont Sports Medicine Center
    Killington Medical Clinic [39115]
    Rutland [39116]
Vermont State Hospital [33897]
Vernon Addictive Disorders Clinic [43848]
Vernon County Domestic Abuse Program [10741]
Vernon Dialysis Center • DaVita [23184]
Vernon Hills Sports Medicine of Lake Forest Hospital [38415]
Vernon J. Harris East End Community Health Center [7366]
Vernon Parish Schools [454]
Versailles Medical Center [7099]
Vershire Center [31055]
Vesta [30284]
    Extended Care Facility [30303]
VESTA Healthcare Corp. [13275]
Vesta, Inc. - Lenham Region [30298]
Vesta, Inc. - Odenton Region [30302]
Vesta, Inc.--Waldorf Region [30314]
Vet Affairs/Edward Hines Jr Hospital • Substance Abuse Section [42707]
Vet Center
    Aberdeen Outstation [51976]
    Albany NY [52032]
    Albuquerque NM [52026]
    Alexandria VA [52124]
    Amarillo TX [52101]
    Anchorage AK [51858]
    Annapolis MD [51977]
    Arecibo PR [52084]
    Atlanta GA [51933]
    Austin TX [52102]
    Babylon NY [52033]
    Baltimore MD [51978]
    Bangor ME [51971]
    Baton Rouge LA [51968]
    Bay Pines CA [51914]
    Beckley WV [52136]
    Bellingham WA [52129]
    Billings MT [52009]
    Biloxi MS [52002]
    Binghamton NY [52034]
    Birmingham AL [51854]
    Bloomfield NJ [52021]
    Boise ID [51943]
    Boston MA [51984]
    Boulder CO [51902]
    Brockton MA [51985]
    Bronx NY [52035]
    Brooklyn NY [52036]
    Brooklyn Park MN [51999]

    Buffalo NY [52037]
    Caribou ME [51972]
    Charleston WV [52137]
    Charlotte NC [52048]
    Chattanooga TN [52095]
    Cheyenne WY [52152]
    Chicago Heights IL [51947]
    Chico CA [51875]
    Chinle AZ [51862]
    Cincinnati OH [52056]
    Clearwater FL [51915]
    Colton CA [51877]
    Columbia SC [52088]
    Columbus OH [52058]
    Commerce CA [51878]
    Concord CA [51879]
    Corona CA [51880]
    Corpus Christi TX [52103]
    Culver City CA [51881]
    Dallas TX [52105]
    Dayton OH [52060]
    Daytona Beach FL [51917]
    Dearborn MI [51992]
    Denver CA [51904]
    Des Moines IA [51961]
    Detroit MI [51993]
    DuBois PA [52073]
    Duluth MN [52000]
    El Paso TX [52106]
    Elkton MD [51981]
    Erie PA [52074]
    Escanaba MI [51994]
    Eugene OR [52068]
    Eureka CA [51882]
    Evanston IL [51949]
    Evansville IN [51956]
    Everett WA [52130]
    Fairbanks AK [51859]
    Fairfield CA [51883]
    Fairhaven MA [51986]
    Fargo ND [52054]
    Farmington NM [52027]
    Fayetteville AR [51870]
    Fayetteville NC [52049]
    Fort Lauderdale FL [51918]
    Fort Myers FL [51919]
    Fort Wayne IN [51957]
    Fort Worth TX [52107]
    Fresno CA [51884]
    Gainesville FL [51920]
    Grand Rapids MI [51995]
    Grants Pass [52069]
    Green Bay WI [52147]
    Greensboro NC [52050]
    Greenville NC [52051]
    Greenville SC [52089]
    Harrisburg PA [52075]
    Henderson NV [52015]
    Hilo HI [51939]
    Honolulu HI [51940]
    Hopi Vet Center Outstation 2 [51863]
    Houston TX [52110]
    Huntington WV [52140]
    Huntsville AL [51855]
    Hyannis MA [51987]
    Indianapolis IN [51958]
    Jackson MS [52003]
    Jacksonville FL [51922]
    Johnson City TN [52096]
    Kenai Vet Center Satellite [51860]
    Key Largo FL [51924]
    Knoxville TN [52097]
    Lakewood NJ [52023]
    Laredo TX [52111]
    Las Cruces NM [52029]
    Las Vegas NV [52016]
    Lawton OK [52064]
    Lewiston ME [51973]
    Lexington KY [51965]
    Lincoln NE [52013]
    Louisville KY [51966]
    Lowell MA [51988]
    Lubbock TX [52112]
    Macon GA [51935]
    Madison WI [52149]
    Manchester NH [52020]
    Manhattan KS [51963]
    Marietta GA [51936]

Martinsburg WV [52141]
McAllen TX [52113]
McKeesport PA [52077]
Melbourne FL [51925]
Memphis TN [52098]
Merrillville IN [51959]
Miami FL [51926]
Vet Center Mid Atlantic • Towson MD [51983]
Vet Center
Middletown NY [52039]
Midland TX [52115]
Milwaukee WI [52150]
Minot ND [52055]
Mission Viejo CA [51887]
Missoula MT [52012]
Mobile AL [51856]
Modesto CA [51888]
Montgomery AL [51857]
Morgantown WV [52143]
Nashville TN [52099]
Norfolk VA [52125]
Norristown PA [52078]
North Charleston SC [52090]
Vet Center Northeast • Philadelphia PA [52079]
Vet Center
Norwich CT [51909]
Oak Park IL [51951]
Oakland CA [51889]
Oklahoma City OK [52065]
Omaha NE [52014]
Orland Park IL [51952]
Orlando FL [51927]
Vet Center Outstation 1 • Cambridge MD [51980]
Vet Center Outstation
Bismark ND [52053]
Parkersburg WV [52144]
Rockford IL [51954]
Saint Croix VI [52122]
Saint Thomas VI [52123]
Vet Center
Palmdale CA [51890]
Parma OH [52062]
Pensacola FL [51928]
Peoria IL [51953]
Philadelphia PA [52080]
Phoenix AZ [51866]
Pittsburgh PA [52081]
Pocatello ID [51944]
Ponce PR [52085]
Pontiac MI [51996]
Portland ME [51974]
Portland OR [52070]
Prescott AZ [51867]
Princeton WV [52145]
Provo UT [52118]
Pueblo CO [51907]
Raleigh NC [52052]
Rapid City SD [52093]
Readjustment Counseling Service [45766]
Reno NV [52017]
Richmond VA [52126]
Roanoke VA [52127]
Rochester NY [52042]
Rohnert Park CA [51892]
Sacramento CA [51893]
Saginaw MI [51997]
Saint Louis MO [52007]
Saint Petersburg FL [51929]
Salem OR [52071]
Salt Lake City UT [52119]
San Antonio TX [52117]
San Diego [51894]
San Francisco CA [51895]
San Jose CA [51896]
San Marcos CA [51897]
Santa Fe NM [52031]
Sarasota FL [51930]
Vet Center Satellite • Cedar Rapids IA [51960]
Vet Center
Savannah GA [51937]
Scranton PA [52082]
Seattle WA [52132]
Sepulveda CA [51898]
Shreveport LA [51970]
Silver Spring MD [51982]
Sioux City IA [51962]
Sioux Falls SD [52094]
South Burlington VT [52120]

Spokane WA [52133]
Springfield IL [51955]
Springfield MA [51989]
Springfield MO [52008]
Springvale ME [51975]
Staten Island NY [52043]
Syracuse NY [52044]
Tacoma WA [52134]
Tallahassee FL [51931]
Tampa FL [51932]
Temecula CA [51899]
Toledo OH [52063]
Tucson AZ [51868]
Tusla OK [52066]
Ventnor NJ [52025]
Ventura CA [51900]
Victorville CA [51901]
Virginia Beach VA [52128]
Warwick RI [52087]
Watertown NY [52045]
West haven CT [51911]
Wheeling WV [52146]
White Plains NY [52046]
White River Junction VT [52121]
Wichita KS [51964]
Williamsport PA [52083]
Wilmington DE [51912]
Worcester MA [51990]
Yakima WA [52135]
Vet Centers • Colorado Springs CO [51903]
Veteran Healthcare Administration • Edward Hines,
Jr. Veterans Affairs Hospital [4031]
Veterans Administration Medical Center • Chemical
Dep Rehab Prog/Outpt Clinic [46343]
Veterans Administration New Mexico • Healthcare
Services/Albuquerque [46244]
Veterans Administration • PRRTP [46275]
Veterans Affairs [29509]
Veterans Affairs - Akron Community Based
Outpatient Clinic [16833]
Veterans Affairs Ann Arbor Health Care System
[4217]
Veterans Affairs Ann Arbor Healthcare System
[30505]
    Cancer Program [5366]
    PTSD Clinical Team [51752]
Veterans Affairs Bennington Community Based
Outpatient Clinic [32640]
Veterans Affairs Black Hills Health Care System
[17629]
The Veterans Affairs Black Hills Health Care System
• Fort Meade Campus [51647]
Veterans Affairs Black Hills Health Care System •
Fort Meade Veterans Affairs Medical Center •
Multiple Sclerosis Center [34711]
The Veterans Affairs Black Hills Health Care System
• Hot Springs Campus [51648]
Veterans Affairs Black Hills Health Care System -
Hot Springs Campus [17630]
Veterans Affairs Black Hills Health Care Systems
    Fort Meade Campus [32225]
    Hot Springs Campus [32228]
Veterans Affairs Black Hills Healthcare System
    Fort Meade Campus • PTSD Residential
    Program [51814]
    Hot Springs Campus • PTSD Domiciliary
    [51815]
Veterans Affairs Boston Health Care System
    Brockton Campus [4150]
    Jamaica Plain Campus [4151]
Veterans Affairs Boston Healthcare System
    Brockton Division [30353], [51583]
    Jamaica Plain Division [30348], [51584]
    PTSD Clinical Team [51748], [51750]
    West Roxbury Division [30476], [51586]
    West Spinal Care Center, Roxbury Division
    [4152]
    Women's Stress Disorder Treatment Team
    [51749]
Veterans Affairs Butler Health Care [51635]
Veterans Affairs Butler Healthcare [32000]
Veterans Affairs - Canton Outpatient Clinic [16868]
Veteran's Affairs Caribbean Healthcare System
[32137], [35655]
Veterans Affairs Caribbean Healthcare System--San
Juan Division • PTSD Clinical Team [51810]
Veterans Affairs Caribbean Medical Center • Spinal
Cord System of Care [4424]

Veterans Affairs Carson Valley Outpatient Clinic
[31040]
Veterans Affairs Central California Health Care
Services • Veterans Affairs Castle OPC [28383]
Veterans Affairs Central California Health Care
System [28508]
    Multiple Sclerosis Center [34534]
Veterans Affairs Central Iowa Health Care System •
Multiple Sclerosis Center [34582]
Veterans Affairs Central Iowa Healthcare System
    PTSD Clinical Team [51731]
    PTSD Domiciliary [51733]
Veterans Affairs Central Texas Healthcare System •
PTSD Program [51830]
Veterans Affairs CMOP - Dallas [18033]
Veterans Affairs • Connecticut Healthcare System
[41451]
Veterans Affairs Connecticut Healthcare System
    Danbury Clinic [28986]
    Newington Campus [29027], [51547]
    PTSD Clinical Team [51704]
    PTSD Residential Rehabilitation Program
    [51703]
    Substance Abuse PTSD Team [51705]
    West Haven Campus [51548]
    West Haven Division • Cancer Program [4912]
Veterans Affairs Consolidated Mail Outpatient
Pharmacy [17614]
Veterans Affairs Consolidated Mail Outpatient
Pharmacy-Dallas [18034]
Veterans Affairs Eastern Colorado Health Care
System [28890], [51545]
Veterans Affairs Eastern Kansas Health Care
System
    Colmery-O'Neil Veterans Affairs Medical Center
    [51572]
    Dwight D. Eisenhower Veterans Affairs Medical
    Center [51571]
Veterans Affairs Eastern Kansas Healthcare System
    PTSD Clinical Team [51734]
    Specialized Inpatient PTSD Unit [51735]
Veterans Affairs Edward Hines, Jr. Hospital • Cancer
Program [5097]
Veterans Affairs Greater Los Angeles (GLA) Health-
care System [51539]
Veterans Affairs Greater Los Angeles Health Care
System • Multiple Sclerosis Clinic [34535]
Veterans Affairs Greater Los Angeles Healthcare
System • Cancer Center [4802]
Veterans Affairs Gulf Coast Health Care System
[30745]
Veterans Affairs Gulf Coast Medical Center • Pensa-
cola Clinic [29262]
Veterans Affairs Gulf Coast Veterans Health Care
System [51593]
Veterans Affairs Gulf Coast Veterans Healthcare
System • PTSD Program [51759]
Veterans Affairs Health Care System • Cancer
Program [5862]
Veterans Affairs Health Care System--El Paso TX
[51658]
Veterans Affairs Health Care System--Iowa City •
PTSD Clinical Team [51732]
Veterans Affairs Health Care System--Pittsburgh PA
• H. John Heinz III Progressive Care Center
[51640]
Veterans Affairs Healthcare Center, Fort Knox
[30014]
Veterans Affairs Healthcare Center, Grayson [29992]
Veterans Affairs Healthcare Center--New Albany
[29792]
Veterans Affairs Healthcare Center, Newburg
[30071]
Veterans Affairs Healthcare Center, Shively [30072]
Veterans Affairs Healthcare System of Ohio [16880]
Veterans Affairs Healthcare System of Pittsburgh •
Dialysis Center [26566]
Veterans Affairs Hilo Community Based Outpatient
Clinic [29516]
Veterans Affairs Hospital Based Home Care [12857]
Veterans Affairs Hudson Valley Health Care System
• Castle Point Campus • Spinal Care Center
[4322]
Veterans Affairs Hudson Valley Health Care System,
Montrose • Franklin Delano Roosevelt Campus
[4323]
Veterans Affairs Hudson Valley Healthcare System--
Castle Point Campus [51614]

Veterans Affairs Hudson Valley Healthcare System
Castle Point Campus [31302]
PTSD Program [51782]
Veterans Affairs Hudson Valley Healthcare System--
Montrose Campus [51615]
Veterans Affairs Hudson Valley Healthcare System
Montrose Campus [31394]
PTSD Domiciliary [51783]
Veterans Affairs Illiana Health Care System [29606],
[51563]
Veterans Affairs Illiana Healthcare System • PTSD
Clinical Team [51723]
Veterans Affairs Kauai Community Based Outpatient
Clinic [29532]
Veterans Affairs Kona Community Based Outpatient
Clinic [29529]
Veterans Affairs Lahontan Valley Outpatient Clinic
[31024]
Veterans Affairs - Lima Community Based Outpatient
Clinic [16966]
Veterans Affairs Loma Linda Healthcare System
[51538]
Jerry L. Pettis Memorial Cancer Care Program
[4791]
PTSD Clinical Team [51691]
Women's Stress Disorder Treatment Team
[51692]
Veterans Affairs Long Beach Health Care System
Multiple Sclerosis Center [34536]
Spinal Cord Injury/Disorder Health Care Group
[3929]
Veterans Affairs Long Beach Healthcare System
Cancer Program [4794]
PTSD Clinical Team [51693]
Veterans Affairs - Lorain Community Based
Outpatient Clinic [16969]
Veteran's Affairs Los Angeles Healthcare System •
Pain Management [35343]
Veterans Affairs - Mansfield Community Based
Outpatient Clinic [16974]
Veterans Affairs Maryland Health Care System •
Cancer Program [5293]
Veterans Affairs Maryland Healthcare System
PTSD Clinical Team [51745], [51747]
PTSD Day Hospital [51746]
Veterans Affairs Maui Community Based Outpatient
Clinic [29526]
Veterans Affairs Med/Reg Office Center • Substance
Abuse Treatment Services [49749]
Veterans Affairs Medical Center [39530], [41212],
[42001]
Addiction Treatment Program [48313]
Addictive Disorders Services [45235]
Addictive Disorders Treatment Program [45397]
Veterans Affairs Medical Center--Albany • Cancer
Program [5557]
Veterans Affairs Medical Center, Albany • Multiple
Sclerosis Center [34656]
Veterans Affairs Medical Center--Albuquerque •
Cancer Program [5552]
Veterans Affairs Medical Center, Albuquerque •
Multiple Sclerosis Center [34640]
Veterans Affairs Medical Center • Alcohol and Drug
Treatment Program [40588]
Veterans Affairs Medical Center--Alexandria •
Cancer Program [5240]
Veterans Affairs Medical Center--Alexandria LA •
PTSD Clinical Team [51740]
Veterans Affairs Medical Center, Alexandria •
Multiple Sclerosis Center [34589]
Veterans Affairs Medical Center
Amarillo TX [51654]
Anaheim Community Based Outpatient Clinic
[28371]
Ann Arbor MI [51587]
Anniston/Oxford Clinic [28012]
Anthem Community Based Outpatient Clinic
[28128]
Veterans Affairs Medical Center Asheville [31504]
Veterans Affairs Medical Center • Asheville NC
[51619]
Veterans Affairs Medical Center--Asheville NC •
PTSD Clinical Team [51788]
Veterans Affairs Medical Center, Ashville • Multiple
Sclerosis Center [34665]
Veteran's Affairs Medical Center • Audio and Speech
Pathology [3135]
Veterans Affairs Medical Center--Augusta • Cancer

Program [5014]
Veterans Affairs Medical Center
Bath NY [51609]
Battle Creek MI [51588]
Veterans Affairs Medical Center--Battle Creek MI
PTSD Clinical Team [51753]
PTSD Residential Rehabilitation Program
[51754]
Veterans Affairs Medical Center--Bay Pines FL
PTSD Clinical Team [51707]
PTSD Domiciliary [51708]
Veterans Affairs Medical Center, Bay Pines •
Multiple Sclerosis Center [34561]
Veterans Affairs Medical Center--Beckley [18497]
Veterans Affairs Medical Center
Beckley WV [51672]
Bellemont Community Based Outpatient Clinic
[28130]
Birmingham AL [51527]
Veterans Affairs Medical Center--Birmingham AL •
PTSD Clinical Team [51680]
Veterans Affairs Medical Center-Birmingham •
Cancer Program [4729]
Veterans Affairs Medical Center, Birmingham •
Multiple Sclerosis Center [34509]
Veterans Affairs Medical Center • Boise ID [51562]
Veterans Affairs Medical Center--Boise ID
PTSD Clinical Team [51720]
PTSD Evaluation and Brief Treatment Unit
[51721]
Veterans Affairs Medical Center • Boston Healthcare
System Brockton Div [44435]
Veterans Affairs Medical Center--Bronx • Cancer
Program [5562]
Veterans Affairs Medical Center--Bronx NY • PTSD
Clinical Team [51779]
Veterans Affairs Medical Center • Brookings Clinic
[31933]
Veterans Affairs Medical Center Brooklyn [31281]
Veterans Affairs Medical Center, Brooklyn • Multiple
Sclerosis Center [34657]
Veterans Affairs Medical Center, Buffalo • Multiple
Sclerosis Center [34658]
Veterans Affairs Medical Center--Butler [17273]
Veterans Affairs Medical Center • Canandaigua NY
[51613]
Veterans Affairs Medical Center--Canandaigua NY •
PTSD Clinical Team [51781]
Veterans Affairs Medical Center
Captain James A. Lovell Federal Health Care
Center [51566]
Caribbean Healthcare System [51644]
Chalmers P. Wylie Veterans Affairs Ambulatory
Care Center [51628]
Chemical Dependency Treatment Program
[40268]
Veterans Affairs Medical Center--Cheyenne [18649]
Veterans Affairs Medical Center--Cheyenne WY •
PTSD Clinical Team [51853]
Veterans Affairs Medical Center, Chicago--Lakeside
• Multiple Sclerosis Center [34574]
Veterans Affairs Medical Center, Chicago--Westside
• Multiple Sclerosis Center [34574]
Veterans Affairs Medical Center • Childersburg Com-
munity Based Outpatient Clinic [27885]
Veterans Affairs Medical Center - Chillicothe [16871]
Veterans Affairs Medical Center • Chillicothe OH
[51625]
Veterans Affairs Medical Center--Chillicothe OH •
PTSD Clinical Team [51795]
Veterans Affairs Medical Center Cincinnati [31697]
Veterans Affairs Medical Center • Cincinnati OH
[51626]
Veterans Affairs Medical Center--Cincinnati OH
PTSD Clinical Team [51796]
PTSD Day Hospital [51797]
Veterans Affairs Medical Center--Coatesville [17289]
Veterans Affairs Medical Center • Coatesville PA
[51636]
Veterans Affairs Medical Center--Coatesville PA
PTSD Clinical Team [51805]
PTSD Domiciliary [51806]
Veterans Affairs Medical Center • Cottonwood Com-
munity Based Outpatient Clinic [28142], [28160]
Veterans Affairs Medical Center - Dayton Campus
[16928]
Veterans Affairs Medical Center--Dayton • Cancer
Center [5716]

Veterans Affairs Medical Center, Dayton • Multiple
Sclerosis Center [34676]
Veterans Affairs Medical Center • Dayton OH
[51629]
Veterans Affairs Medical Center--Dayton OH
PTSD Clinical Team [51799]
PTSD Day Hospital [51800]
Veterans Affairs Medical Center--Decatur • Cancer
Program [5023]
Veterans Affairs Medical Center • Delray Beach
Clinic [29151]
Veterans Affairs Medical Center, Denver • Multiple
Sclerosis Center [34546]
Veterans Affairs Medical Center, Durham • Multiple
Sclerosis Center [34666]
Veterans Affairs Medical Center • Durham NC
[51620]
Veterans Affairs Medical Center--Durham NC •
PTSD Clinical Team [51789]
Veterans Affairs Medical Center, East Orange •
Multiple Sclerosis Center [34638]
Veterans Affairs Medical Center--Erie [17314]
Veterans Affairs Medical Center • Erie PA [51637]
Veterans Affairs Medical Center--Fargo • Cancer
Program [5672]
Veterans Affairs Medical Center • Fargo ND [51623]
Veterans Affairs Medical Center--Fayetteville •
Cancer Care Program [4749]
Veterans Affairs Medical Center • Fayetteville NC
[51621]
Veterans Affairs Medical Center--Fayetteville NC •
PTSD Clinical Team [51790]
Veterans Affairs Medical Center • Fort Smith Com-
munity Based Outpatient Clinic [28272]
Veterans Affairs Medical Center-Fresno • Cancer
Program [4780]
Veterans Affairs Medical Center
Gadsden Clinic [27934]
Grand Junction CO [51546]
Veterans Affairs Medical Center--Grand Junction CO
• PTSD Clinical Team [51702]
Veterans Affairs Medical Center - Great Lakes
Health Care System [18634]
Veterans Affairs Medical Center • Hackensack Clinic
[31135]
Veterans Affairs Medical Center--Hampton [18310]
Veterans Affairs Medical Center • Hampton VA
[51666]
Veterans Affairs Medical Center--Hampton VA
PTSD Clinical Team [51835]
PTSD Domiciliary [51836]
Veterans Affairs Medical Center
Hancock Clinic [30561]
Harrison Community Based Outpatient Clinic
[28281]
Hot Springs Community Based Outpatient Clinic
[28288]
Veterans Affairs Medical Center--Houston • Cancer
Program [6004]
Veterans Affairs Medical Center - Hunter Holmes
McGuire [18373]
Veterans Affairs Medical Center Huntington [18520],
[32912]
Veterans Affairs Medical Center • Huntington WV
[51673]
Veterans Affairs Medical Center--Huntington WV •
PTSD Clinical Team [51846]
Veterans Affairs Medical Center • Huntsville Clinic
[27953]
Veterans Affairs Medical Center, Indianapolis •
Multiple Sclerosis Center [34579]
Veterans Affairs Medical Center • Iowa City IA
[51570]
Veterans Affairs Medical Center - James H. Quillen
[17744]
Veterans Affairs Medical Center
Jasper Clinic [27962]
Jefferson Barracks Division [51598]
John Cochran Division [51599]
Veterans Affairs Medical Center--Kansas City •
Cancer Program [5451]
Veterans Affairs Medical Center • Kansas City MO
[51596]
Veterans Affairs Medical Center--Kansas City MO •
PTSD Clinical Team [51763]
Veterans Affairs Medical Center
Konawa Clinic [31887]
Lansing Clinic [30587]

Veterans Affairs Medical Center--Lebanon [17375]
Veterans Affairs Medical Center, Lebanon • Multiple Sclerosis Center [34698]
Veterans Affairs Medical Center • Lebanon PA [51638]
Veterans Affairs Medical Center--Lebanon PA • PTSD Clinical Team [51807]
Veterans Affairs Medical Center • Lexington KY [51575]
Veterans Affairs Medical Center--Lexington KY
  PTSD Clinical Team [51737]
  PTSD Residential Rehabilitation Program [51738]
Veterans Affairs Medical Center - Louis A. Johnson [18508]
Veterans Affairs Medical Center--Louisville • Cancer Program [5229]
Veterans Affairs Medical Center, Manchester • Multiple Sclerosis Center [34631]
Veterans Affairs Medical Center • Manchester NH [51603]
Veterans Affairs Medical Center Manhattan [31434]
Veterans Affairs Medical Center • Marion IL [51565]
Veterans Affairs Medical Center--Marion IL • PTSD Clinical Team [51725]
Veterans Affairs Medical Center--Martinsburg [18525]
Veterans Affairs Medical Center • Martinsburg WV [51674]
Veterans Affairs Medical Center--Martinsburg WV
  PTSD Clinical Team [51847]
  PTSD Domiciliary [51848]
Veterans Affairs Medical Center
  Mattoon Community Based Outpatient Clinic [29644]
  Memphis TN [51650]
Veterans Affairs Medical Center--Memphis TN
  PTSD Clinical Team [51818]
  PTSD Domiciliary [51819]
Veterans Affairs Medical Center
  Menominee Clinic [30600]
  Mental Health Rehabilitation Program [50602]
  MH 116 Northern Arizona VA Healthcare [39459]
  MH Outpatient Recovery Services [39299]
  MH RRTP [45297]
  MHRRTP Program [48314]
  Miami FL [51554]
Veterans Affairs Medical Center, Miami • Multiple Sclerosis Center [34562]
Veterans Affairs Medical Center-Minneapolis • Cancer Program [5413]
Veterans Affairs Medical Center • Minneapolis MN [51591]
Veterans Affairs Medical Center--Minneapolis MN • PTSD Clinical Team [51757]
Veterans Affairs Medical Center, Minneapolis • Multiple Sclerosis Center [34614]
Veterans Affairs Medical Center
  Mobile Outpatient Clinic [27987]
  Morristown Clinic [31150]
  New Orleans LA [51577]
Veterans Affairs Medical Center, New Orleans • Multiple Sclerosis Center [34590]
Veterans Affairs Medical Center, New York • Multiple Sclerosis Center [34659]
Veterans Affairs Medical Center--North Chicago IL • PTSD Clinical Team [51727]
Veterans Affairs Medical Center, North Chicago • Multiple Sclerosis Center [34576]
Veterans Affairs Medical Center--Northport • Cancer Program [5602]
Veterans Affairs Medical Center, Northport • Multiple Sclerosis Center [34660]
Veterans Affairs Medical Center • Northport NY [51617]
Veterans Affairs Medical Center, Ohio • Multiple Sclerosis Center [34677]
Veterans Affairs Medical Center, Oklahoma City • Multiple Sclerosis Center [34679]
Veterans Affairs Medical Center • Oklahoma City OK [51631]
Veterans Affairs Medical Center--Oklahoma City OK • PTSD Clinical Team [51802]
Veterans Affairs Medical Center
  Outpatient Subst Abuse Treatment Prog [43282]
  Outpatient Treatment Program [50315]
  Palm Desert Community Based Outpatient Clinic [28690]

Palo Alto Health Care System
  Livermore Division [51537]
  Menlo Park Division [51541]
Paragould Clinic [28338]
Paterson Clinic [31161]
Veterans Affairs Medical Center--Philadelphia [17427]
Veterans Affairs Medical Center, Philadelphia • Multiple Sclerosis Center [34699]
Veterans Affairs Medical Center • Philadelphia PA [51639]
Veterans Affairs Medical Center--Philadelphia PA • PTSD Clinical Team [51808]
Veterans Affairs Medical Center • Pineville LA [51578]
Veterans Affairs Medical Center, Pittsburgh • Multiple Sclerosis Center [34700]
Veterans Affairs Medical Center--Port Saint Lucie • Saint Lucie County PTSD Clinical Team [51712]
Veterans Affairs Medical Center--Portland • Cancer Program [5804]
Veterans Affairs Medical Center • Portland OR [51632]
Veterans Affairs Medical Center--Portland OR • PTSD Clinical Team [51803]
Veterans Affairs Medical Center--Providence [17553]
Veterans Affairs Medical Center Providence • Cancer Program [5893]
Veterans Affairs Medical Center • Providence RI [51645]
Veterans Affairs Medical Center--Providence RI • PTSD Clinical Team [51811]
Veterans Affairs Medical Center • Regional Office Center [51678]
Veterans Affairs Medical Center and Regional Office--Wilimington • Cancer Program [4919]
Veterans Affairs Medical Center • Saint Cloud MN [51592]
Veterans Affairs Medical Center--Salem [18383]
  Cancer Program [6086]
Veterans Affairs Medical Center, Salem • Multiple Sclerosis Center [34732]
Veterans Affairs Medical Center • Salem VA [51667]
Veterans Affairs Medical Center--Salem VA
  PTSD Clinical Team [51838]
  Specialized Inpatient PTSD Unit [51839]
Veterans Affairs Medical Center, Salt Lake City • Multiple Sclerosis Center [34725]
Veterans Affairs Medical Center
  Samuel S. Stratton [51607]
  San Francisco CA [51544]
Veterans Affairs Medical Center--San Francisco • Cancer Program [4845]
Veterans Affairs Medical Center • San Francisco Clinic [28772]
Veterans Affairs Medical Center--San Francisco
  PTSD Clinical Team [51698]
  Substance Abuse PTSD Team [51699]
Veterans Affairs Medical Center - San Juan [17532]
Veterans Affairs Medical Center--San Juan • Cancer Program [5886]
Veterans Affairs Medical Center
  Santa Barbara Community Based Outpatient Clinic [28803]
  Santa Fe Springs Community Clinic [28811]
  Santa Rosa Clinic [28817]
  Sault Sainte Marie Clinic [30583]
Veterans Affairs Medical Center--Sheridan [18662]
Veterans Affairs Medical Center
  Sheridan WY [51679]
  Shoals Area (Florence) Clinic [28043]
  Spokane WA [51669]
Veterans Affairs Medical Center--Spokane WA • PTSD Clinical Team [51844]
Veterans Affairs Medical Center
  Subst Abuse Residential Rehab Treatment Prog [48696]
  Substance Abuse Program [46930]
  Substance Abuse Programs [40645]
  Substance Abuse Rehabilitation Program [41552]
  Substance Abuse Residential Rehab [47490]
  Substance Abuse Services [43699], [50295]
  Substance Abuse Treatment [41155], [45742]
  Substance Abuse Treatment Center [48004]
  Substance Abuse Treatment Prog [45539]

  Substance Abuse Treatment Program [42082], [42091], [43670], [45591], [47646], [48369], [48881], [49841], [50187], [50245]
  Substance Abuse Treatment Programs [42319]
  Substance Abuse Treatment Unit [48445]
  Substance Use Disorder Program [45805]
  Syracuse NY [51618]
Veterans Affairs Medical Center--Syracuse NY • PTSD Clinical Team [51787]
Veterans Affairs Medical Center • Tomah WI [51677]
Veterans Affairs Medical Center--Tomah WI • PTSD Residential Rehabilitation Program [51852]
Veterans Affairs Medical Center, Topeka • Multiple Sclerosis Center [34585]
Veterans Affairs Medical Center • Tuscaloosa AL [51529]
Veterans Affairs Medical Center--Tuscaloosa • Multiple Sclerosis Center [34510]
Veterans Affairs Medical Center, Tuskegee • Multiple Sclerosis Center [34511]
Veterans Affairs Medical Center/TVHs • Substance Abuse Treatment Program [49151]
Veterans Affairs Medical Center/University of Texas Health Science Center • Multiple Sclerosis Center [34721]
Veterans Affairs Medical Center
  Veterans Affairs Maryland Health Care System [51581]
  Victorville Clinic [28839]
  Vista Clinic [28841]
Veterans Affairs Medical Center--Waco TX • PTSD Residential Rehabilitation Program [51832]
Veterans Affairs Medical Center--Washington DC • PTSD Clinical Team [51706]
Veterans Affairs Medical Center, Washington • Multiple Sclerosis Center [34553]
Veterans Affairs Medical Center • West Palm Beach FL [51557]
Veterans Affairs Medical Center, West Roxbury • Multiple Sclerosis Center [34604]
Veterans Affairs Medical Center--White River Junction [18239]
Veterans Affairs Medical Center
  White River Junction VT [51665]
  Wilimington DE [51549]
Veterans Affairs Medical Center Wilkes-Barre [32132]
Veterans Affairs Medical Center--Wilkes Barre [17508]
Veterans Affairs Medical Center--Wilkes-Barre • Cancer Program [5880]
Veterans Affairs Medical Center
  Wilkes Barre PA [51643]
  Women's Stress Disorder Treatment Team [51794]
Veterans Affairs Medical System--East • Multiple Sclerosis Center of Excellence [34595]
Veterans Affairs Miami Medical Center • Outpatient Subst Abuse Clinic OSAC [41802]
Veterans Affairs - Middletown Community Based Outpatient Clinic [16998]
Veterans Affairs Montana Health Care System • Multiple Sclerosis Center [34624]
Veterans Affairs Montana Healthcare System [30936]
  Fort Harrison MT [51600]
Veterans Affairs Nebraska-Western Iowa Health Care System
  Grand Island Division [30986]
  Lincoln Division [31000]
  Omaha Division [31010]
Veterans Affairs Nebraska--Western Iowa Healthcare System • Community-Based Outpatient Clinic • PTSD Clinical Team [51766]
Veterans Affairs Nebraska--Western Iowa Medical Center • PTSD Clinical Team [51767]
Veterans Affairs New Jersey Health Care System
  Cancer Program [5508]
  East Orange Campus [31123]
    Spinal Care Center [4301]
  Lyons Campus [4302], [31146]
Veterans Affairs New Jersey Healthcare System
  East Orange Campus • PTSD Unit [51770]
  PTSD Clinical Team [51771]
  PTSD Residential Rehabilitation Program [51772]
  Women's Trauma Recovery Program [51773]
Veterans Affairs New Mexico Healthcare System

Term [41474]
Vigo County Adult Outpatient Addictions [29822]
Vigo County Lifeline, Inc. [50899]
Villa Center Inc • The Villa [40723]
Villa Esperanza Services [7806]
Villa of Fairview Park • DaVita [26115]
Villa of Great Northern • DaVita [26116]
Villa Maria Continuum [34179]
Villa Marie School [8231]
Villa of St. John • DaVita [25285]
Villa Santa Maria [34311]
Villa Veritas Foundation Inc • Alcoholism Inpatient Rehabilitation [46738]
Villa of Waterbury • DaVita [25251]
Villa of Wentzville • DaVita [25301]
The Village at Angle Lake [32850]
Village Care Plus, Inc. [16570]
Village • CASA Work Perinatal Program [47548]
Village for Family and Children Inc.--Albany Avenue, Hartford [33246]
Village for Family and Children Inc. • Village North [33247]
Village for Family and Children Inc.--Wethersfield Avenue, Hartford [33248]
Village Hospice [20317]
Village II Dialysis Center • Fresenius Medical Care [27041]
Village • LIFE Program [41803]
The Village Network [34385]
The Village Network of Akron [34371]
The Village Network of Mount Vernon/Knox County [34380]
The Village Network of Wooster • Boys' Village Campus [34389]
Village Oaks Kidney Disease Clinic • Fresenius Medical Care [27229]
The Village Sleep Lab [36827]
The Village South [6510]
Village South Inc [41804]
Village Therapy Works [3516]
Village Virgin Islands/Westcare [49752]
The Villages of Indiana [34124]
The Villages of Indiana--Elkhart [33453]
The Villages of Indiana--Evansville [33457]
The Villages of Indiana--Gary [33468]
The Villages of Indiana, Inc. [34130]
The Villages of Indiana--Kokomo [33478]
The Villages of Indiana--Portage [33486]
The Villages of Indianapolis [33476]
Villages West [28206]
Ville Platte Mental Health Center [30177]
Ville Platte • Office of Behavioral Health [43908]
Vince Carter Sanctuary • Adult Residential [41582]
Vincennes Dialysis & At Home • DaVita [24244]
Vincennes Veterans Affairs Community Based Outpatient Clinic [29827]
Vincent P Dole Institute of Treatment and • Research for Opiate Dependency [46932]
Vineland Developmental Center [8276]
Vineland Public Schools [552]
Vineland RC • Dialysis Center [25524]
Vineland Veterans Affairs Clinic [31170]
The Vines Hospital of Ocala [29246]
Vinland National Center • Inpatient Program/Extended Care/Outpatient [45188]
Vintage Healthcare Services [14957]
Viola M. Berard [32185]
Violence Free Crisis Line [9752]
Violence Intervention Network--Smith County [10514]
Violence Intervention Program, Inc.--New York [9963]
Violence Intervention Program--Oneonta [9971]
Violence Intervention Project, Inc.--Algoma [10685]
Violence Intervention Project--Thief River Falls [9640]
Violence Prevention Center--Grand Marais [9598]
Violence Prevention Center of Southwestern Illinois [9194]
Violence Recovery Program--Fenway Community Health Center [9470]
VIP Community Services
    Community Residence [46462]
    Medically Supervised Outpatient Prog [46463]
    Mens Residential Drug Program [46464]
    Opioid Treatment Program [46465]
    Womens Residence [46466]
VIP Drug and Alcohol Eduction Center [40280]

VIP Health Care Services--Richmond Hill [16610]
VIP Healthcare Services--Spring Valley [16632]
Virgin Health Corporation [14176]
Virgin Island State Office of Special Education [847]
Virgin Islands Library for the Visually and Physically Handicapped [3842]
Virgin Valley Hospice-Mesquite [20424]
Virginia Beach Dialysis Center • DaVita [27582]
Virginia Beach Family Medicine [7373]
Virginia Beach Psychiatric Center [33910]
Virginia Beach • Psychiatric Center [49860]
Virginia Center for Reproductive Medicine [22291]
Virginia Clifford Hospice Center • Hospice of Northwest Ohio [20901]
Virginia Commonwealth University • Adult Sickle Cell Program [36442]
Virginia Commonwealth University Health System Medical College of Virginia Hospitals • Department of Human and Molecular Genetics [12363]
    Pain Management [35755]
Virginia Commonwealth University Medical Center AIDS Clinical Trials Unit [36]
    Renal Dialysis Unit [27557]
Virginia Commonwealth University Sports Medicine Center [39134]
Virginia Department for the Blind and Vision Impaired • Virginia Library and Resource center [3850]
Virginia Department for the Deaf and Hard of Hearing [3607]
Virginia Department of Health • Division of Women's and Infants' Health [36553]
Virginia Department of Rehabilitation Services • Deaf and Hard of Hearing Services [3608]
Virginia Garcia Memorial Health Center [7124]
Virginia Health Center [49835]
Virginia Hospital Center [49765]
    Oncology Services [6053]
Virginia Hospital • Sleep Laboratory [37905]
Virginia IVF and Andrology [22292]
Virginia League for Planned Parenthood • Richmond Health Center [12050]
Virginia M Mejia LCSW CADC [42954]
Virginia Mason Clinic [12476]
Virginia Mason Medical Center • Cancer Center [6118]
Virginia Mason Medical Center--Lindemann Pavilion [4487]
Virginia Mason Medical Center
    Pain Management [35764]
    Pain Management Clinic [35765]
    Physical Medicine and Rehabilitation [35766]
    Sleep Disorders Center [37943]
Virginia Mason Medical Center Transplant [27643]
Virginia Mason Multiple Sclerosis Center [34740]
Virginia Neurology & Sleep Centers [37906]
Virginia Polytechnic Institute and State University • Cardiac Therapy and Intervention Center [39121]
Virginia School for the Deaf and the Blind-Staunton [858], [3740]
Virginia Sports Medicine Institute [39120]
Virginia Sudden Infant Death Syndrome Alliance [36554]
Virginia Treatment Center for Children [33907]
Virginia's Hospice Care [21732]
Virgos Home Health Care, Inc. [14933]
Virtua Health • Cancer Program [5522]
Virtua Health, Inc. [16238]
Virtua Home Care at West Jersey [16267]
Virtua Home Care at West Jersey/Community Nursing Services [16244]
Virtua Memorial Hospital Burlington County • Fox Chase Cancer Center [5525]
Virtua Memorial Hospital • Screening and Crisis Intervention Program [51113]
Visalia Dialysis • DaVita [23061]
Vishnia & Associates, Inc. • Professional Nursing Service [16922]
Vision Behavioral Health Service LLC [47411]
Vision Behavioral Health Services [47545]
Vision Health Care Group, Inc. • Sleep Health Center [36828]
Vision Health Care, Inc. [17934]
Vision Homecare Services, Inc. [16545]
Vision Share [35150]
Visionary Pathway Eating Disorder Programs [11067]

VisionQuest Nonprofit Corp • Subst Abuse Intensive Outpatient Prg [47300]
Visions Adolescent Treatment Center [40198]
Visions Health Systems, LLC [14459]
Visions of Hope Inc [47469]
Visions Treatment Center LLC • Visions at Latigo [40199]
Visiting Angels Home Health Care Inc.--Los Angeles [13162]
Visiting Angels--Jacksonville [13822]
The Visiting Nurse Association [16881]
Visiting Nurse Association of Albany, Inc. [16338]
Visiting Nurse Association of Arkansas • Saint Vincent Infirmary Medical Center [12869]
Visiting Nurse Association of Boston [15484]
Visiting Nurse Association of Brooklyn, Inc. [16426]
Visiting Nurse Association of California [19003]
Visiting Nurse Association of Cape Cod--Falmouth/West Side [15495]
Visiting Nurse Association of Cape Cod, Inc. [15502]
Visiting Nurse Association of Central Pennsylvania, Inc. [17336]
Visiting Nurse Association of Cleveland [16890]
Visiting Nurse Association of Eastern Massachusetts [15543]
Visiting Nurse Association of Good Samaritan Health System [17376]
Visiting Nurse Association of Greater Rhode Island [21191]
Visiting Nurse Association of Greater Youngstown Area [17090]
Visiting Nurse Association Hospice of Monroe County [17305]
Visiting Nurse Association Hospice and Palliative Care of Southern California [18907]
Visiting Nurse Association & Hospice of Southwestern Vermont [18233]
Visiting Nurse Association of Hudson Valley [16650]
Visiting Nurse Association, Inc.--Oak Park [15764]
Visiting Nurse Association of the Inland Counties-Banning [18892]
Visiting Nurse Association of the Inland Counties-Barstow [18893]
Visiting Nurse Association of the Inland Counties-Murrieta [18977]
Visiting Nurse Association of the Inland Counties-Palm Desert [18985]
Visiting Nurse Association of the Inland Counties-Victorville [19070]
Visiting Nurse Association of the Inland Counties-Yucca Valley [19083]
Visiting Nurse Association of Lancaster County, Inc. [17368]
Visiting Nurse Association of Long Island, Inc. [16470]
Visiting Nurse Association of Mid-Ohio [16975]
Visiting Nurse Association of the Midlands Hospice [20401]
Visiting Nurse Association of Northern New Jersey [20482]
Visiting Nurse Association--Omaha [16127]
Visiting Nurse Association of Omaha and Council Bluffs - Council Bluffs Branch [15071]
Visiting Nurse Association, Private Duty and Hospice [15028]
Visiting Nurse Association of St. Clare's [16272]
Visiting Nurse Association of Southeast Missouri [2804]
Visiting Nurse Association of Southeastern Connecticut, Inc. [13551]
Visiting Nurse Association of Southeastern MA, Inc. [15493]
Visiting Nurse Association of Southeastern Massachusetts [15537]
Visiting Nurse Association of Southeastern Massachusetts, Inc. [17544]
Visiting Nurse Association of Southern Worcester County Inc. [13546]
Visiting Nurse Association of the Treasure Coast [14383], [14441]
Visiting Nurse Association of Western New York [16678]
Visiting Nurse Association of Wisconsin [18599]
Visiting Nurse Association of Wisconsin - Green Bay Branch [18572]
Visiting Nurse Association of Wisconsin - Hartford Branch [18574]

Visiting Nurse Association of Wisconsin - Hartland [18576]
Visiting Nurse Association of Wisconsin - Kenosha [18577]
Visiting Nurse Association of Wisconsin - Lake Geneva Branch [18580]
Visiting Nurse Association of Wisconsin - Manitowoc County [18635]
Visiting Nurse Association of Wisconsin - Oshkosh [18616]
Visiting Nurse Association of Wisconsin - Sheboygan Branch [18617]
Visiting Nurse Association of Wisconsin - South Shore Branch [18564]
Visiting Nurse Association of Wisconsin - Walnut Avenue Branch [18600]
Visiting Nurse Group, Inc. [17428]
Visiting Nurse & Health Services, Inc. [16236]
Visiting Nurse and Health Services--Trinity Hospice [16208]
Visiting Nurse Health System--Atlanta [14483]
Visiting Nurse Health System--Fayetteville [14528]
Visiting Nurse Health System--Kennesaw [14538]
Visiting Nurse Health System--Norcross [14568]
Visiting Nurse Hospice [20613]
Visiting Nurse and Hospice Care of Santa Barbara [19037]
Visiting Nurse and Hospice Care Services of Northern Carroll [20451]
Visiting Nurse and Hospice Care of Southwest Connecticut [19167]
Visiting Nurse & Hospice of Fairfield County [19175]
Visiting Nurse Hospice & Health Care [20896]
Visiting Nurse & Hospice Home [19630]
Visiting Nurse & Hospice Home--Ft. Wayne [19600]
Visiting Nurse Service of Greater Rhode Island [17542]
Visiting Nurse Service, Inc.--Akron [16834]
Visiting Nurse Service of New York--Rehab Services [3081]
Visiting Nurse Services and Good Samaritan Hospice [15613]
Visiting Nurse Services/Hospice Central Indiana [19617]
Visiting Nurse Services of Michigan--Lansing [15712]
Visiting Nurse Services of Newport & Bristol Counties [17548]
Visiting Nurse Services of the Northwest [18439]
Visiting Nurses Association of Greater New Orleans, Inc. [15331]
Visiting Nurses Association--Longwood [13867]
Visiting Nurses Association--Orlando [14301]
Visiting Nurses Association of Pottstown and Vicinity [21147]
Visiting Nurses Association of the Rockford Area [14916]
Visiting Nurses of Nevada [16161]
Visiting Nursing Association [15112]
Visiting Professionals, Inc.--Columbia [17578]
Visiting Professionals, Inc.--Mauldin [17605]
Visiting Professionals, Inc.--Sumter [17624]
VISN 1: Veterans Affairs New England Healthcare System [4153]
VISN 21: Sierra Pacific Network [3934]
Vista Balboa [28760]
Vista Campus Behavioral Crisis Services [29163]
Vista Care--Amarillo [21381]
Vista Care-Warner Robins [19434]
Vista Community Clinic [6376]
Vista Counseling Center [28498]
Vista Del Mar Boys Group Home [33162]
Vista Del Mar Child and Family Services [33995]
Vista Del Mar Girls' Group Home [33996]
Vista Guidance Centers of Barstow [28400]
Vista Health--Fort Smith [33112]
Vista Health Services--Arkansas Psychiatric Care [28236]
Vista Health-Victory Memorial Hospital • Cancer Program [5130]
Vista Home Health Services, Inc.--Northridge [13216]
Vista Home Health Services--Miami [14177]
Vista Maria [34221]
Vista Maria/Girls Care Program [44722]
Vista Park Center [32735]
Vista Physical Medicine [2046]
Vista Rehab of Mesquite [39084]

VistaCare--Albuquerque [20525]
VistaCare--Austin [21394]
VistaCare-Blue Bell [21058]
VistaCare--Brendan Way, Greenville [21245]
VistaCare/Carillion [21525]
VistaCare--Carlsbad [20531]
VistaCare Center at Lovelace [20526]
VistaCare Center at Wesley Woods [19353]
VistaCare-Clovis [20533]
VistaCare-Columbus Georgia [19376]
VistaCare--Corpus Christi [21425]
VistaCare--Dallas [21438]
VistaCare--Douglasville [19381]
VistaCare-Evansville [19596]
VistaCare--Griffin [19391]
VistaCare--Hobbs [20537]
VistaCare Hospice-Bogart [19365]
VistaCare Hospice--Phoenix [18818]
VistaCare Hospice-Southborough [20003]
VistaCare Hospice-Wheatridge [19133]
VistaCare--Houston [21492]
VistaCare--Indianapolis [19618]
VistaCare--Kerrville [21504]
VistaCare--Lawrenceville [19401]
VistaCare--Montgomery [18747]
VistaCare--Newnan [19410]
VistaCare--Ogden [21630]
VistaCare--Phenix City [18754]
VistaCare-Roswell [20543]
VistaCare-Salt Lake City [21654]
VistaCare--San Angelo [21549]
VistaCare--San Antonio [21558]
VistaCare-San Marcos [21563]
VistaCare-South Ogden [21657]
VistaCare-Sparks [20429]
VistaCare--Temple [21574]
VistaCare--Terre Haute [19655]
VistaCare--Terrell Road, Greenville [21476]
VistaCare--Waco [21589]
VistaCare--Westwood [20012]
Visiting Nurse Association Space Coast [13887]
VITA Eating Disorders Program [11126]
Vital Air Medical--Cody [18650]
Vital Air Medical--Powell [18656]
Vital Air Medical--Worland [18667]
Vital Care Home Health [14430]
Vital Care of Rhode Island [17543]
Vital Changes Treatment Inc [50087]
Vital Hospice-Hammond [19845]
Vital Plus Home Health Inc. [13058]
Vital Sign Home Health Care [15743]
Vital Solutions Home Health Agency, Inc. [13640]
Vital Support Home Health Care Agency, Inc.--Elkins Park [17309]
Vital Support Home Health Care Agency, Inc.--Feasterville Trevose [17323]
VitalCare Health Services/Respiratory [16168]
Vitalife Home Health Care [14178]
Vitalistic Therapeutic Center [31987]
Vitality Center • Residential Treatment [45826]
Vitality • Footprints Counseling [45878]
Vitality Healthcare, Inc. [14841]
Vitality Homecare Supplies [16427]
Vitality Lake Tahoe [40812]
    Vitality Unlimited [40813], [40814], [40815]
Vitality • Restoration Counseling Services [45852]
Vitality Ruby View • Counseling Service [45827]
Vitality • Silver Sage Counseling Services [45883]
VITAS Baylor All Saints Medical Center • Hospice Inpatient Unit [21465]
VITAS - Frankfort Hospital Hospice • Inpatient Unit [21133]
Vitas Healthcare • Corp. [20818]
VITAS Healthcare Corporation-Saint Louis [20338]
VITAS Hospice, Atlanta Metro [19354]
VITAS Innovative Hospice of Brevard County [19253]
VITAS Innovative Hospice Care of Brevard County-N Brevard [19263]
VITAS Innovative Hospice Care of Broward County [19220]
VITAS Innovative Hospice Care of Central Florida [19251]
VITAS Innovative Hospice Care of Central Florida Kissimmee Satellite Ofc. [19244]
VITAS Innovative Hospice Care • Chicagoland Central Satellite Office [19505]
VITAS Innovative Hospice Care of Chicagoland

Northwest [19538]
VITAS Innovative Hospice Care of Chicagoland-S Joliet [19532]
VITAS Innovative Hospice Care of Chicagoland S-Tinley Pk. [19578]
VITAS Innovative Hospice Care of Cincinnati Dayton Satellite [20870]
VITAS Innovative Hospice Care of Cleveland [20805]
VITAS Innovative Hospice Care of Coastal Cities [19063]
VITAS Innovative Hospice Care-Collier [19266]
VITAS Innovative Hospice Care--Columbus [20830]
VITAS Innovative Hospice Care of Dade-Monroe Tavernier [19325]
VITAS Innovative Hospice Care of Dallas [21439]
VITAS Innovative Hospice Care of Delaware [19182]
Vitas Innovative Hospice Care-Delaware [19179]
VITAS Innovative Hospice Care of the East Bay [19075]
VITAS Innovative Hospice Care of Fairfield [19168]
VITAS Innovative Hospice Care of Fort Worth [21466]
VITAS Innovative Hospice Care of Greater Washington [19189]
Vitas Innovative Hospice Care of Hartford [19144]
VITAS Innovative Hospice Care of Houston [21493] North Satellite Office [21494]
VITAS Innovative Hospice Care--Independence [20302]
Vitas Innovative Hospice Care of the Inland Empire [19012]
Vitas Innovative Hospice Care-Inland Empire [19013]
VITAS Innovative Hospice Care of the Inland Empire • Satellite Office [18900]
VITAS Innovative Hospice Care of Kansas City-Shawnee Mission [19777]
Vitas Innovative Hospice Care-LA & Ventura County [18897]
VITAS Innovative Hospice Care-LaSalle [19533]
VITAS Innovative Hospice Care • Mercy Fitzgerald Hospital [21076]
VITAS Innovative Hospice Care of Miami - Dade • Satellite Office [19258]
VITAS Innovative Hospice Care of Milwaukee [21871]
VITAS Innovative Hospice Care of New Jersey North [20476]
VITAS Innovative Hospice Care of New Jersey Shore [20466]
VITAS Innovative Hospice Care of New Jersey West [20484]
VITAS Innovative Hospice Care of Northern VA [21742]
Vitas Innovative Hospice Care of Orange County [18944]
VITAS Innovative Hospice Care of the Palm Beaches [19200]
VITAS Innovative Hospice Care of Philadelphia [21059]
VITAS Innovative Hospice Care of Sacramento Valley and Foothalls [19008]
VITAS Innovative Hospice Care of San Antonio [21559]
VITAS Innovative Hospice Care of San Diego [19021]
Vitas Innovative Hospice Care of San Fernando Valley [18921]
Vitas Innovative Hospice Care of San Francisco Bay Area [18979]
VITAS Innovative Hospice Care of San Gabriel Cities [18914]
Vitas Innovative Hospice Care-Solano County [18925]
VITAS Innovative Hospice Care of Southeast Michigan [20125]
VITAS Innovative Hospice Care of Waterbury [19150]
VITAS Innovative Hospice - Inpatient Unit--Cincinnati [20819]
VITAS Innovtive Hospice Care of Palm Beach Satellite Office [19334]
VITAS Inpatient Hospice Unit
    Aventura Medical Center [19193]
    Florida Medical Center [19221]
    Fort Lauderdale Nursing and Rehabilitation [19222]

HCR Manor Care [19336]
Hearthstone Assisted Living [21500]
Hialeah Hospital [19259]
VITAS Inpatient Hospice Unit at Kennedy Memorial Hospitals Unv Med Ctr Stratford [20498]
VITAS Inpatient Hospice Unit at the Lutheran Home [21859]
VITAS Inpatient Hospice Unit
    Memorial Hospital Pembroke [19295]
    North Shore Medical Center [19260]
VITAS Inpatient Hospice Unit at One Elizabeth Place [20837]
VITAS Inpatient Hospice Unit-Stockbridge [19423]
VITAS Inpatient Unit--San Antonio [21560]
VITAS Mercy Hospital Hospice--Chicago • Inpatient Unit [19506]
VITAS Saint James Hospital Hospice • Inpatient Unit [19508]
Viva Healthcare [14179]
Vivian B. Adams School [7725]
Vivid Visions [9063]
VMT Home Health Agency [13577]
VNA of Cape Cod Hospice [20002]
VNA Care Hospice, Inc-Rose Monahan Hospice Home [20018]
VNA Care Hospice, Inc.-Southborough [20004]
VNA Care Hospice, Inc. • Stanley Tippett House [19981]
VNA Care Hospice Inc.--Worcestser [20019]
VNA Care Network--Danvers [15488]
VNA Care Network--Gloucester [15496]
VNA Care Network, Inc.--Worcester [15568]
VNA Care Network--Leominster [15509]
VNA Care Network--Needham Heights [15521]
VNA Care Network--Southborough [15544]
VNA of Care New England [17557]
VNA of Central Jersey Hospice Program [20502]
VNA of the Central Valley, Inc. [13179]
VNA of Chittenden & Grand Isle Counties, Inc. [18234]
VNA Community Care Services--Coatesville [17290]
VNA Community Care Services--Reading [17463]
VNA of Cordele, Inc.--Americus [14473]
VNA of Cordele, Inc.--Cordele [14511]
VNA of Cordele, Inc.--Oglethorpe [14569]
VNA of Cordele, Inc.--Warner Robins [14604]
VNA of Fox Valley: VNA Hospice [19484]
VNA Health Care • Hospice and Palliative Care [19147]
VNA Home Health Care [19905]
VNA Home Health Care--South Portland [15401]
VNA Home Health and Hospice Services, Inc.-- Manchester [20444]
VNA Home Health and Hospice-Wellspan [21181]
VNA Home Health - Wellspan--George St., York [17518]
VNA Home Health - Wellspan - Gettysburg Branch [17464]
VNA Home Health - Wellspan--Pine Grove Commons, York [17519]
VNA Home Health - Wellspan - Red Lion Office [17465]
VNA HomeCare, Hospice-Michigan City [19632]
VNA Hospice Care-Saint Louis [20339]
VNA Hospice of Greater • Lowell [19975]
VNA Hospice at Home [19101]
VNA Hospice House-Vero Beach [19330]
VNA Hospice of Monroe County [21079]
VNA Hospice of Northeast Pennsylvania [21088]
VNA & Hospice of Northern Berkshire Inc. [19984]
VNA Hospice and Palliative Care Center of Lackawanna Co. [17400]
VNA Hospice and Palliative Care Center of Lackawanna County [21124]
VNA Hospice of Rockford • Hospice of Rockford [19570]
VNA & Hospice of Southern California [12948]
VNA and Hospice of Southern California [19014]
VNA-Hospice of Southern Carroll County [20457]
VNA and Hospice of Southwestern Vermont Healthcare [21660]
VNA & Hospice (VNAH) of Cooley Dickinson [19988]
VNA and Hospice of VT/NH-Springfield [21668]
VNA and Hospice of VT/NH--West Lebanon [20456]
VNA Hospice, Western PA [21064]
VNA of Mercer County Hospice [20509]
VNA of Middlesex - East/Visiting Nurse Hospice [15552]

VNA Services and Foundation, Western Pennsylvania--Butler [17274]
VNA Services and Foundation - Western Pennsylvania--Ford City [17326]
VNA Services and Foundation - Western Pennsylvania--Vandergrift [17498]
VNA of Southern Worcester County, Inc. [15558]
VNA of Southwest Georgia--Blakely [14492]
VNA of Southwest Georgia--Donalsonville [14519]
VNA of Southwest Georgia, Inc.--Bainbridge [14491]
VNA of Venango County, Inc. [21089]
VNACare Hospice, Inc. [19956]
VNACJ Community Health Center, Inc. [6984]
VNS Home Health Services--Narragansett [17546]
VNS Home Health Services - Westerly Office [17559]
VNSNY Hospice Care-Bronx [20556]
VNSNY Hospice Care-Brooklyn [20559]
VNSNY Hospice Care-Queens [20568]
VNSYNY Hospice Care - New York City [20588]
VOA Group Home • Huntsville CMHC [28069]
Vocal Image Pros, P.C. [2165]
Vocal Point Therapies Inc. [2965]
Vocational Industries [8612]
Vocational Transition Center [31374]
The Voice Institute [1786]
Voices Against Violence--Framingham [9479]
Voices Against Violence--Plymouth [9814]
Voices Against Violence--Saint Albans • Laurie's House [10548]
Voices of Hope [9776]
Volta Program • Substance Abuse Treatment Center [43634]
Volunteer Behavioral Health Care System [32282]
Volunteer Behavioral Healthcare • The Guidance Center [49152]
Volunteer Behavioral Healthcare System
    Cumberland Mountain Mental Health Center [49066]
    Reality House [49061]
    RHEA County Mental Health Center [49068]
    Valley Ridge [49116]
Volunteer Emergency Families for Children • Runaway and Homeless Youth Program [36248]
Volunteer and Information Agency [50952]
Volunteer Information Center/HELPLINE [51348]
Volunteer Treatment Center Inc [49055]
Volunteers of America [29310], [49425]
Volunteers of America--Aberdeen SD • Runaway and Homeless Youth Program [36201]
Volunteers of America Alaska
    ARCH [39324]
    Assist [39318]
Volunteers of America
    Brandon Center [8957]
    Care Crisis Line [51441]
Volunteers of America Dakotas [49025]
    Heisler Treatment Center [49026]
Volunteers of America, Dakotas • Runaway and Homeless Youth Program [36202]
Volunteers of America Delaware Valley [31172]
Volunteers of America • Delaware Valley Inc [45954]
Volunteers of America--Denver, CO • Runaway and Homeless Youth Services [35861]
Volunteers of America of Greater Baton Rouge [30131]
Volunteers of America - Greater New York - Runaway and Homeless Youth Program [36125]
Volunteers of America
    Greater Ohio [47733]
    Hello House [44424]
Volunteers of America/InAct [48220]
Volunteers of America Inc
    Freedom House [43700]
    Maud Booth House [43701]
    Third Step Program [43702]
Volunteers of America of Indiana Inc [43118], [43119]
    Hope Hall [43040]
Volunteers of America, Kentucky • Runaway and Homeless Youth Program [35969]
Volunteers of America of Los Angeles
    Hollywood Center [40175]
    Veterans Transitional Housing [40176]
Volunteers of America--North Louisiana • Runaway and Homeless Youth Program [35977]
Volunteers of America Northern New England • Runaway and Homeless Youth Program [35988]

Volunteers of America Northern Rockies • The Gathering Place [50603]
Volunteers of America of Oregon • Day Treatment Program [48221]
Volunteers of America Oregon--Family Center [10253]
Volunteers of America Oregon • Mens Residential Center [48222]
Volunteers of America
    Outpatient Treatment [40177]
    Project Rebound [44425]
Volunteers of America--Sheridan WY • Runaway and Homeless Youth Program [36282]
Volunteers of America--Sioux Falls, SD • Street Outreach Services • Runaway and Homeless Youth Program [36203]
Volunteers of America Southeast Inc • Georgia [42177]
Volunteers of America • Southwest Safehouse [8960]
Volunteers of America, Spokane • Runaway and Homeless Youth Program [36258]
Volunteers of America/SWCC Inc • Hawley Center for Supportive Living [39799]
Volunteers of America Texas Inc
    Avenue J Facility [49343]
    LIGHT Program [49344]
    LIGHT San Antonio [49533]
    McGovern Campus [49419]
    McGovern Campus/Lavender [49420]
    Riverside Treatment Center [49345]
Volunteers of America/Utah
    Adult Detoxification Center [49702]
    Center for Women and Children [49641]
Volunteers of America, Utah • Homeless Youth Resource Center • Runaway and Homeless Youth Program [36238]
Volunteers of America
    Volunteers of America/Detox [40590]
    Womens Recovery Center [45315]
    WYSTAR Outpatient and Men Residential [50604]
Volunteers of American Delaware Valley [9823]
Volunteers of American Home Health Services [12827]
Volusia County Exceptional Student Education [346]
Volver a Casa Home Health Services [18076]
Voorhees Pediatric Rehabilitation Services [8277]
Voorhees Sleep Lab • University Services [37367]
VOTC Inc
    Visions of the Cross/Outpatient [40434]
    Visions of the Cross/Residential [40435]
VRN Home Health, Inc. [16169]

W

W B Health Care [47470]
W David Holden, Counselor [47229]
W and G Enterprises • Alcohol Education/Recovery Services [39706]
W. G. Hefner VA Medical Center [4340]
W House Foundation Inc [44295]
W. Ross MacDonald School [675]
W. Ross McDonald School [3732]
W.A. Foote Memorial Hospital/dba Allegiance Health • Sleep Disorders Center [37209]
Wabash County Hospital • Cancer Program [5179]
Wabash County Hospital--Salisbury [15060]
Wabash General Hospital--Wabash [14866]
Wabash Miami Home Health [15039]
Wabash Valley Alliance Inc [43019], [43185]
    Outpatient Services [43132]
Wabash Valley Hospital [29830]
    Bi--County Domestic Violence Program [9264]
Wabash Valley Hospital--Crawfordsville [33449]
Wabash Valley Hospital--Delphi [33450]
Wabash Valley Hospital Inc • Outpatient Services [42984], [43161]
Wabash Valley Hospital, Inc. [29763]
    Elmwood House [29764]
    Gregory House [29765]
    Outpatient Service [29711], [29713], [29783], [29807]
Wabash Valley Hospital--Lafayette [33479]
Wabash Valley Hospital--Monticello [33483]
Wabash Valley Hospital--Rensselaer [33487]
Wabash Valley Hospital Riverside [29831]
Wabash Valley Hospital--West Lafayette [33442]

Wabaunsee County Health Department • Mental Health Center of East Central Kansas [29905]
Waccamaw Center for Mental Health--Conway [32198]
Waccamaw Center for Mental Health--Kingstree [32206]
Waccamaw Community Hospital • Cancer Program [5910]
Waco Center for Youth [34455]
Waco Veterans Affairs Medical Center [32567]
Waconia Dialysis • Fresenius Medical Care [25093]
Waddell Center for Multiple Sclerosis [34678]
Wade Family Medical Center [7060]
Wadley Inspirations [32559]
Wadley Regional Medical Center • Cancer Program [6032]
Wadsworth Dialysis
    DaVita [26224]
    Fresenius Medical Care [26225]
Wadsworth-Rittman Hospital [17063]
Wagner Dialysis of Sioux Valley Hospital • Dialysis Center [26800]
Wahiawa Dialysis Center • Fresenius Medical Care [23862]
Wahiawa General Hospital [14644]
Wahiawa Middle School [42286]
Wahkiakum Chemical Dependency Services [49922]
Wahkiakum County Mental Health [51430]
Waianae Coast Comprehensive Health Center [6627]
Waianae Coast Comprehensive Health • Center Malama Recovery Services [42290]
Waianae Dialysis • Liberty Dialysis [23863]
Waimanalo Health Center [6629]
Waimea Elementary and Intermediate School [386]
Waipahu Dialysis • Liberty Dialysis [23865]
Wake Dialysis Clinic • Fresenius Medical Care [25931]
Wake Forest Cardiac Rehabilitation Program • Wake Forest University [38838]
Wake Forest Center for Reproductive Medicine--Beckley, West Virginia [22298]
Wake Forest Dialysis Center • DaVita [25932]
Wake Forest University Baptist Medical Center
    Burn Center [4600]
    Cancer Care Program [5667]
    Center for Reproductive Medicine [22203], [22204]
    Cystic Fibrosis Center [7634]
Wake Forest University • Baptist Medical Center • Department of Pediatrics • Clinical Genetics Services [12311]
Wake Forest University Baptist Medical Center Transplant Program [25982]
Wake Forest University
    Elkin Dialysis Center [25861]
    King Dialysis Center [25893]
    Multiple Sclerosis Center [34667]
Wake Forest University School of Medicine • Hemophilia Center [12571]
Wake Forest University • School of Medicine • Pain Management [35597]
Wake Forest University Sports Medicine • CompRehab Outpatient Rehabilitation Center • Wake Forest University Baptist Medical Center [38839]
Wake Forest University • Statesville Dialysis Center Inc. [25958]
WakeMed Cary Hospital [4341]
WakeMed Health and Hospitals [16771]
WakeMed Home Health [4342]
WakeMed N Healthplex • Physicians Office Pavillion [4343]
WakeMed Outpatient Rehab, Wake Forest Rd. [4344]
WakeMed Outpatient Rehabilitation, Cary [4345]
WakeMed Outpatient Rehabilitation, Clayton [4346]
WakeMed Rehab [4347]
WakeMed Rehab Hospital [4348]
WakeMed Zebulon/Wendell Outpatient [4349]
Waking the Village [35849]
Walden Behavioral Care [11096]
Walden - Sierra, Inc. [9456]
Walden Sierra • Outpatient [44311]
Waldo County General Hospital [2350]
Waldo County Healthcare, Inc. [19889]
Waldron & Kern, Inc. [18017]
Walker Center [42320], [42333], [42381]
Walker Methodist Health Center [2715]

Walker Recovery Center Inc [39266]
Walker Wellness Clinic • Eating Disorders Program [11288]
Walkers Point Community Clinic [7436]
Walker's Point Youth and Family Center • Runaway and Homeless Youth Program [36273]
Wall Youth Center and Community Services [46208]
Walla Walla Community Hospice [21780]
Walla Walla Crisis Response Team [51475]
Walla Walla General Hospital [18482]
    Sleep Disorders Center [37944]
Walla Walla Mental Health • Inland Counseling Center [51476]
Wallace Dialysis • DaVita [25967]
Wallowa Valley Center for Wellness • Alcohol and Drug Program [48097]
Walls Regional Hospital [17843]
Walnut Avenue Women's Center [8904]
Walnut Creek Dialysis Center & At Home • DaVita [23065]
Walnut Creek Dialysis Center • DaVita [23066]
Walnut Creek Fertility [21951]
Walnut Hill Dialysis Center • Fresenius Medical Care [27042]
Walnut Medical Services--Burnham [17268]
Walnut Medical Services--Everett [17316]
Walnut Medical Services--Johnstown [17352]
Walnut Street Community Health Center [6795]
Walsenburg Dialysis • Fresenius Medical Care [23143]
Walter B Jones • Alcohol and Drug Abuse Treatment Center [47370]
Walter B. Jones Alcohol and Drug Treatment Center [31541]
Walter DUI and Counseling Services [42460]
Walter Hoving Home [40380]
Walter P. Carter Center [33557]
Walter Reed Army Medical Center
    Cancer Program [4925]
    National Capital Consortium Program • Pain Management [35376]
    Sleep Disorders Center [36765]
Walter Reuther Psychiatric Hospital [33603]
Walter S. Christopher School [7947]
Walterboro Dialysis • DaVita [26780]
Walton County Public Schools [1888]
Walton Dialysis Center [23761]
Walton Family Health Center [7014]
Walton Rehabilitation Hospital [4011], [35419]
Walton West Transitional Living Center [4012]
Walworth County Department of Human Services [51504]
Walworth County Health and Human Services [50385]
WAPI Community Services [50144]
Ward County Mental Health Center [32517]
Ware Visiting Nurses Service, Inc. [14607]
Warm Springs Counseling Center [29542]
Warm Springs Counseling Center West [29548]
Warm Springs Home Health, Inc. [13005]
Warnecke Professional Counseling [42133]
Warner Dialysis Center [24301]
Warren Center for Communication and Learning [2348]
Warren Consolidated Schools [507]
Warren County Council on Domestic Violence • Harmony Place [10569]
Warren County Mental Health [29874]
Warren County Schools [633], [758]
Warren Dialysis Center • American Renal Associates [26135]
Warren G. Murray Developmental Center, Centralia [7932]
Warren Hills Dialysis • Fresenius Medical Care [25968]
Warren Hospital • Cancer Program [5535]
Warren State Hospital [33814]
Warren-Washington Association for Mental Health, Inc. [31356]
Warren/Yazoo Chemical Dependency Center [45425]
Warren/Yazoo Mental Health Service • Vicksburg Center [45426]
Warrensburg Health Center [7044]
Warrensburg Veterans Affairs Clinic [30913]
Warrensville Developmental Center [8414]
Warrensville Heights PD Dialysis • DaVita [26229]

Warrington Speech Language Pathology Services LLC [3384]
Warsaw Dialysis Center • Renal Advantage Inc. [25969]
Warsaw Veterans Affairs Clinic [31487]
Warwick Manor Behavioral Health Inc [44246]
Warwick Manor Outpatient Services [44350]
Waryas House • Abilities First Inc [47003]
Wasatch Artificial Kidney Center [27427]
Wasatch County School District [836]
Wasatch Mental Health Center [32610]
Wasatch Mental Health • Crisis Line [51404]
Wasatch Mental Health Youth Services • Park View School [32611]
Washakie Clinic [7456]
Washburn Child Guidance Center [30687]
Washington Adventist Hospital [44364]
    Cancer Program [5315]
Washington Behavioral Health [49871]
Washington Center for Eating Disorders and Adolescent Obesity [11085]
Washington Center for Reproductive Medicine [22297]
Washington County HD Adol Outpatient East [44342]
Washington County Health Department • Adult Comprehensive Treatment Services [44296]
Washington County Health System • John R. Marsh Cancer Center [5305]
Washington County Hospice & Palliative Care Program [20571]
Washington County Hospital Association Home Healthcare [15448]
Washington County Industries [30116]
Washington County Mental Health--Berlin [32641]
Washington County Mental Health Center
    Arioli Avenue Intermediate Care Program [32632]
    Children and Youth Services [32667]
    Group Home [32668]
    Kynock Street Intermediate Care [32633]
Washington County Mental Health Center--Montpelier [32669]
Washington County Mental Health Center • Outpatient [33027]
Washington County Mental Health Services [51255]
    Community Developmental Services [8574]
Washington County Mental Health Services--Marietta [31801]
Washington County Psychotherapy Associates [50959]
Washington County Regional Medical Center [1905]
Washington County Service Center--Sandersville [29491]
Washington County Youth Service Bureau
    Boys and Girls Club [49738]
    Runaway and Homeless Youth Program [36241]
Washington Courthouse • Fresenius Medical Care [26230]
Washington DC Vet Center • Washington DC [51913]
Washington DC Veterans Affairs Medical Center [51550]
    Cancer Program [4926]
    Southeast Community Clinic [29102]
Washington Dialysis Facility • DaVita [23832]
Washington Fertility Center [22293]
Washington Hospital Center
    The Burn Center [4532]
    Cancer Institute [4927]
    Dept of Psychiatry/Inpatient Service [41553]
    Hearing and Speech Center [1538]
    National Rehabilitation Hospital Program • Pain Management [35377]
    Outpatient Behavioral Health Services [41554]
    Section of Nephrology [23228]
Washington Hospital • Sleep Center [37713]
Washington Memorial Library • Middle Georgia Library for the Blind and Physically Handicapped [3781]
Washington Nursing Dialysis • DaVita [23229]
Washington Parish • Addictive Disorders Clinic [43816]
Washington Parish Dialysis • DaVita [24496]
Washington Pastoral Counseling Service • Substance Abuse Services [44381]
Washington Regional Home Health [12845]
Washington Regional Hospice [18846]

Washington Regional Medical Center
 Cancer Program [4750]
 Sleep Disorders Center [36656]
Washington Regional Transplant Community [35256]
Washington School for the Deaf [869]
Washington School District [840]
Washington Square Dialysis • DaVita • Dialysis
 Facility [25299]
Washington State Department of Health • Maternal
 Child Health Office [36556]
Washington State School for the Blind [3742]
Washington State Services for Children with Deaf--
 Blindness [3634]
Washington State University • Speech and Hearing
 Clinic [3633]
Washington Street Behavioral Health [29080]
Washington Street Hope Center Inc [43856]
Washington Talking Book and Braille Library [3851]
Washington Township Center for Sleep Disorders
 [36716]
Washington Township Health Care District • Cancer
 Program [4777]
Washington University • John L. Trotter Multiple
 Sclerosis Center [34622]
Washington University Medical Center
 Center for Advanced Medicine • Women's
  Health Center--Ultrasound/Genetics [12266]
 Saint Louis Children's Hospital • Department of
  Pediatrics Division of Genetics and Genomic
  Medicine [12267]
Washington University
 Multidisciplinary Sleep Medicine Center [37295]
 Pain Management [35533]
Washington University School of Medicine
 Adult Cystic Fibrosis Center [7591]
 AIDS Clinical Trials Unit [15]
 Barnes Hospital • Adult Comprehensive Sickle
  Cell Disease Center [36373]
 Barnes--Jewish Hospital
  Division of Reproductive Endocrinology and
   Infertility [22148]
  Siteman Comprehensive Cancer Center
   [4684]
Washington University • School of Medicine • MDA/
 ALS Center [130], [34826]
Washington University School of Medicine
 Saint Louis Children's Hospital
  Down Syndrome Center [10821]
  Sickle Cell Disease Center [36374]
Washington University Sports Medicine Clinic
 [38652]
Washington Women's Shelter, Inc. [10323]
Washoe Sleep Disorders Center [37324]
Washtenaw County Community Mental Health
 Center [51033]
Washtenaw County Hearing Impaired Program [481]
Washtenaw Library for the Blind and Physically
 Disabled at AADL [3813]
Wasila Vet Center • Wasilla AK [51861]
Wasueon Dialysis • DaVita [26231]
Watauga Behavioral Health Services [32325]
Watauga Kidney Dialysis Facility • Fresenius Medi-
 cal Care [25822]
Watauga Medical Center Home Health [16698]
Watauga Medical Center • Jones Cancer Center
 [5628]
Watauga Orthopaedics [39031]
Waterbury Day Treatment Center and Alternative
 Care [32684]
Waterbury Heights Dialysis • DaVita [23186]
Waterbury Hospital Health Center • Cancer Program
 [4911]
Waterbury Hospital Psychiatric Center [50738]
Waterbury Public Schools • Hard of Hearing/Deaf
 Program [335]
Waterford Country School, Inc. [34056]
Waterfront Counseling in Blaine [49905]
Waterloo Veterans Affairs Clinic [29902]
Water's Edge Community Health Center • Outpatient
 Eating Disorder Treatment Program [11110]
Watershed of the Palm Beaches [41569]
Watershed Treatment Center [41566]
Watertown Memorial Hospital Association, Inc.
 [18637]
Watkins Kiyoka [47402]
Watson Clinic Center for Rehabilitative Medicine
 [1629]

Watson Clinic Kidney Center • Dialysis Facility
 [23365]
Watson Clinic LLP • Center for Cancer Care and
 Research [4958]
Watson Clinic, LLP • Watson Clinic Sleep Disorders
 Center [36829]
Watsonville Community Hospital [13438]
Watts Health Care Centers [6323]
Watts Healthcare Corp Inc • House of Uhuru
 [40178]
Waubonsee Community College • Access Center for
 Students with Disabilities [413]
Waukegan Public Schools [414]
Waukesha County • Dept of Health and Human
 Services [50554]
Waukesha Memorial Hospital, Inc. [18639]
 Regional Cancer Center [6178]
Waukesha Memorial Hospital
 Pain Rehabilitation Program [35777]
 Pro Health Care Behavioral Medicine Center •
  Eating Disorder Programs [11312]
 ProHealth Care Sleep Disorders Center [37986]
Waupaca Kidney Center • Dialysis Facility [27798]
Waupun Regional Dialysis [27799]
Wausau District Public Schools [894]
Wausau Health Services [50557]
Wausau Hospital • Cancer Program [6179]
Wausau Kidney Center • Dialysis Facility [27801]
Wausau Medical Center, SC [39189]
Waushara County Clinical Services [50558]
Wauwatosa School District [895]
Waverly Children's Home [8447]
Waverly Dialysis • DaVita [26485]
Waverly Health Center [2211], [15113]
Waves Early Intervention Program [8516]
Way Back Inc [40591]
Way Back Inn Inc [42423], [42590], [42778]
 Grateful House [42825]
 Maywood House [42772]
A Way Out [10271]
Way Station Inc [44274]
Way Station, Inc. [30286]
Way Station, Inc.--Howard County [30277]
Way Station, Inc. • Residential Crisis Program
 [30287]
Wayne Behavioral Health Network [31382]
Wayne Community Health Center, Inc. [7318]
Wayne Counseling Center Inc [46212]
Wayne County Board of Education • Special
 Programs [883]
Wayne County Dialysis • Nephrology Center of
 Detroit [24886]
Wayne County Hospital ESRD • ESRD [24258]
Wayne County Kidney Center • Fresenius Medical
 Care [26238]
Wayne County Mental Health Center [30079]
 Hotline [51166]
Wayne County Outpatient Services [50347]
Wayne County Protective Agency [9114]
Wayne County Public Schools [618]
Wayne County Regional Library for the Blind and
 Physically Handicapped [3814]
Wayne General Hospital Home Health [15982]
Wayne Health Care • Cancer Center [4697]
Wayne Health Services and Supplies, Inc. [17080]
Wayne M. Winnick and Associates [38805]
Wayne Memorial Hospital • Cancer Center [5832]
Wayne Metropolitan Community Action Agency •
 Runaway and Homeless Youth Program [36028]
Wayne State University
 AIDS Clinical Trials Unit [14]
 Detroit Medical Center • Pain Management
  [35518]
 Harper University Hospital • Adult MDA Clinic
  [34821]
 Neurogenetics Clinic [12255]
Wayne State University Physicians Group [22131]
Wayne State University
 The School of Medicine • Department of Neurol-
  ogy • Comprehensive Clinical and Research
  Multiple Sclerosis Center [34608]
 University Health Center • Community Program
  for Clinical Research on AIDS [56]
Wayne Substance Abuse Services • Chemical
 Dependency Outpatient [46767]
Wayne T Patrick Hospice House • Hospice & Com-
 munity Care [21275]
Wayne Therapeutic Rehabilitation [30080]

Wayne Uplift [10040]
Waynesboro Dialysis Unit • Hattiesburg Clinic
 [25168]
Waynesboro Family Clinic [47333]
Waynesburg Dialysis • DaVita • Dialysis Facility
 [26603]
Waynesville Dialysis Center • DaVita [25846]
Waypoint • Domestic Violence Program and Shelter
 [9321]
Waypoint Home Health Care [14436]
Wayside [9490]
Wayside Academy School [30416]
Wayside Community Counseling [30420]
Wayside Family Treatment Incarnation Family Con-
 nections [9620]
Wayside Hospice/Parmenter • VNA & Comm Care
 [20009]
Wayside House Inc [41638], [45298]
Wayside Metrowest Counseling Center [30385]
Wayside Youth and Family Support Network [30386]
 Runaway and Homeless Youth Program [36005]
WB Health Care Services, Inc. [13680]
WBIII Inc [43059]
WCA Hospital [3037]
 CD Inpatient Rehabilitation Program [46735]
WCA Hospital Center [37449]
WCA Hospital • Outpatient Chemical Dependency
 Program [46736]
WCHS Inc [40251]
 Vancouver Treatment Solutions [50246]
WCHS of Texas • DBA Hemphill Treatment Services
 [49346]
We Care Arundel Health Service Inc [44288]
We Care Counseling Center [45252]
We Care Health Services Inc [44307]
We Care Hospice Services, LLC [13347]
We Care Services for Children [1085], [28456]
We Kare Medical Equipment, Inc [13163]
Weatherford Dialysis Center • Fresenius Medical
 Care [27391]
WEAVE, Inc. [8878]
Weaver Counseling [48398]
Weaverville Dialysis Center • DaVita [25971]
Weber Human Services [32599], [49651]
 Day Treatment [32600]
 Men's Residential [32601]
 Women's Residential [32602]
 Youth Residential [32603]
Weber Valley Dialysis and At Home • DaVita
 [27408]
Webster Comfort Care Home, Inc. [20614]
Webster County Victim Assistance Program [9700]
Webster Wellness Professionals • Eating Disorder
 and Weight Control Services [11127]
Wecare Home Care [16192]
Weckler and Associates Ltd [42693], [42774]
Wedge Medical Center [48572], [48573], [48574]
Wedgewood Christian Services • Summit Progr/
 Residential Intensive Outpatient [44824]
Wedgwood Christian Services--Grand Rapids
 [34227]
Wedgwood Christian Services--Wyoming [34238]
Wedgwood Christian Youth and Family Services
 [34228]
Wedgwood Recovery Program • Wedgwood
 Christian Services [34229]
Wediko Children's Services [34297]
Wee Speak [2169]
Wee Speech [2110]
Wee Talk LLC--Cookeville [3425]
Wee Talk--Montclair [1187]
Wee Talk Speech and Language Services [3376]
Weeks Medical Center-Home Health and Hospice
 Services [20439]
Weeks and Vietri • Counseling and Community
 [42352]
Weems Community Mental Health Center
 Clarke County Office [45414]
 Kemper County Office [45373]
 Leake County Office [45365]
 Neshoba County Office [45412]
 Newton County Office [45374]
 Scott County Office [45377]
 Smith County Office [45415]
 Weems Life Care [45406]
Weinland House [29708]
Weinstein Hospice-Yad V'Lev [19355]
Weirton Medical Center [18546]

Pain Clinic [35772]
Sleep Center [37961]
Weisman Children's Rehabilitation Hospital [2927]
Weisman Kaplan House [44193]
Weiss Memorial Hospital Hospice Care [19507]
Weiss Renal Center • Dialysis Facility • Good Samaritan Hospital [25783]
Weisskopf Child Evaluation Center [2288]
Wekiva Springs [41714]
Wekiva Springs Center for Women [29189]
Wekiva Springs Wellness Center [11033]
Wel Mor Psychological Group Inc • DBA South Coast Counseling and Psych [39601], [39973]
Welch & McLoy Therapy Services [1675]
Welcome House Inc [49303]
Weld County Health Department Prenatal Clinic [6411]
The Weldon Center for Rehabilitation • Children's Rehabilitation Services [8149]
Welkind Rehabilitation Hospital • Speech Pathology and Audiology Department [2901]
Well-Care Home Health, Inc.--Houston [18015]
Well Of Hope Community Development Cor [46129]
Well Spoken Speech--Language Pathology [1963]
Wellbound of Austin • Satellite Health [26959]
Wellbound of Emeryville • Satellite Healthcare [22677]
Wellbound of Frederick LLC • Satellite Health [24687]
Wellbound of Lafayette [24192]
Wellbound of Menlo Park • Satellite Healthcare [22805]
Wellbound of Mercer • Dialysis Center • Satellite Healthcare [25441]
Wellbound of Milpitas LLC • Satellite Healthcare [22809]
Wellbound of Modesto • Satellite Healthcare [22818]
Wellbound of Sacramento • Satellite Health [22925]
Wellbound of San Francisco • Satellite Healthcare [22965]
Wellbound of San Jose • Satellite Healthcare [22978]
Wellbound of San Mateo • Satellite Healthcare [22987]
Wellbound of Santa Rosa • Satellite Healthcare [23010]
Wellbound/Satellite Dialysis
Evanston Dialysis Center [24086]
Houston Dialysis Center [27183]
Wellbound of South Leandro • Satellite Healthcare [22983]
Wellbound of Stockton LLC • Satellite Healthcare [23028]
Wellbound of Vallejo • Satellite Healthcare [23053]
Wellcare--Burgaw [16702]
Wellcare--Elizabethtown [16720]
Wellcare Home Care--S 17th St., Wilmington [16800]
Wellcare Home Health--Ashton Dr., Wilmington [16801]
Wellcare--Jacksonville [16743]
Wellcare--Supply [16787]
Wellcare--Whiteville [16797]
Wellcome Manor Family Services [45158]
Wellesley Dialysis • DaVita • Dialysis Center [24811]
Wellesley Therapeutic Services [2536]
Wellington Circle Dialysis Center & At Home • DaVita [24778]
Wellington Orthopaedic and Sports Medicine [38864]
Wellington Regional Medical Center • Cancer Program [5003]
Wellmont Bristol Regional Medical Center • Nicewonder Cancer Center [5921]
Wellmont Holston Valley Medical Center • Christine LaGuardia Phillips Cancer Center [5935]
Wellmont Hospice House [21311]
Wellmont Rehabilitation & Sports Clinic [39128]
Wellness Care Home Health--Miami Gardens [14195]
Wellness County [2809]
Wellness Home Care [15646]
Wellness Home Health Care Agency, Inc. [14224]
Wellness Plan, North Health Center [6855]
Wellness Recovery Center [28637]
Stanislaus County Behavioral Health [28638]
Wellness Resource Center [41567]
Wellness Specialist Corporation [14847]
Wellness Supports [31583]

Wellness in the Valley [51193]
WellOne Primary Medical and Dental Care [7218]
Wellplace Inc • Monroeville [48475]
Wells Center [42713]
Mason County [42699]
Wells House Inc • Residential and Outpatient Treatment [44297]
Wells River Health Center [7341]
Wellsboro Laurel Health Center [7191]
Wellspan Behavioral Health • Edgar Square [48715]
Wellspan Dialysis--York [26619]
Wellspan Multiple Sclerosis Center [34701]
Wellspan Pharmacy [17520]
Wellspring Alliance for Families • SAFE Haven [9415]
Wellspring Foundation [28970]
Wellspring Health Center • Pain Clinic [35524]
Wellspring Healthcare Services [14695]
Wellspring Inc [49011]
Mens Program [43936]
Outpatient Services [43937]
Womens Program [43938]
Wellspring • Journey House [43703]
WellSpring Resources [42384]
Wellsprings Inc [49012]
WellSprings Ranch [10922]
WellStar Cobb Hospital Homecare [14553]
WellStar Cobb Hospital • Oncology Program [5015]
Wellstar Community Hospice [19361]
WellStar Health System • WellStar Cancer Program [5032]
WellStar Kennestone Hospital • Cancer Center [5033]
WellStar Sleep Disorders Center • Windy Hill Hospital [36866]
Wellstar Windy Hill Hospital [29469]
Wellstone Regional Hospital [43125]
Wellsville Community Based Outpatient Clinic [16656]
Wellsville Veterans Affairs Clinic [31489]
Welsh Mountain Medical and Dental Center [7171]
Welsh Therapy and Associates [2358]
Wenatchee Valley Clinic • Sports Medicine Center [39155]
Wenatchee Valley Medical Center
Cancer Care Program [6130]
Sleep Medicine Center [37945]
Wendell Foster Campus for Developmental Disabilities [8056]
Wendell Johnson Speech and Hearing Clinic [2208]
Wenden Recovery Services Inc [45266], [45268], [45351]
Wendover Mental Health Center [31047]
Wenger Physical Therapy, Inc. [38631]
Wentworth-Douglass Hospital
Medical Genetics Clinic [12274]
Seacoast Cancer Center [5494]
Wentworth--Douglass Hospital • Speech Therapy [2881]
Wentworth Homecare & Hospice, LLC [20433]
Wentworth Supervised Apartments [32143]
Wenwood House [33990]
Wernersville State Hospital [33823]
Wernle Children's Home, Inc. [34134]
Wescare HomeHealth Providers Inc. [13422]
Weslaco Dialysis Center
Diversified Specialty Institutes [27394]
Fresenius Medical Care [27395]
Wesley Chapel Dialysis • DaVita [23568]
Wesley Health System, LLC [15966]
Wesley Home Health [38470]
Wesley Rehabilitation Hospital [2251], [15159]
Wesley Rehabilitation Hospital, an affiliate of HealthSouth [38471]
Wesley Shelter, Inc. [10103]
Wesley Sleep Center [37269]
Wesley Spectrum Services [48612]
Washington Office [48679]
Wesley Woods Geriatric Hospital [1832]
Wesleyan Hospice-Georgetown [21471]
West Alabama Mental Health Center [27897], [27909], [39239]
Choctaw County Office [27876]
Hale County Office [27936]
West Albany Dental and Medical Center [6580]
West Allis Memorial Hospital • Cancer Program [6180]
West Baton Rouge CAD [43886]

West Beach Dialysis Center • DaVita [23468]
West Bend Public Schools [896]
West Bergen Center for Children and Youth [31165]
West Bergen Mental Health • Substance Abuse Services [46151]
West Bergen Mental Healthcare--Oakland [31157]
West Bergen Mental Healthcare--Ridgewood [31167]
West Bexar County Kidney Disease Center • Fresenius Medical Care [27350]
West Billings Physical Therapy and Sports Medicine [38679]
West Bloomfield Dialysis • DaVita [24990]
West Boca Dialysis Center • Fresenius Medical Care [23244]
West Branch Pulmonary Clinic, P.C. [37210]
West Broadway Dialysis & At Home • DaVita [24421]
West Broadway Dialysis • Fresenius Medical Care • Dialysis Facility [24422]
West Brook Recovery Center LLC [44825]
West Calcasieu Cameron Hospital Home Health Agency [15371]
West Care Health System Home Health & Hospice [16788]
West Center Behavioral Health--Lebanon [31079]
West Central Behavioral Health [45905]
West Central Behavioral Health Counseling Center of Claremont [31053]
West Central Behavioral Health Counseling Center of Newport [31087]
West Central Family Mental Health Service [28615]
West Central Georgia Regional Hospital [33374]
West Central Human Service Center
Chemical Dependency Program [47560]
Crisis and Emergency Services [51185]
West Central Mental Health Center [29836]
West Central Mental Health Center, Inc. [28867]
West Central Speech Services [3694]
West Chester University • Speech, Language Clinic [3385]
West Chicago Dialysis Center • Fresenius Medical Care [24106]
West Coast Children's Center [28484]
West Coast Counseling Services Inc • West Coast Counseling Center [40047]
West Coast Cued Speech Program [308]
West Coast Cued Speech Programs • Information Services, National Cued Speech Association [1351]
West Coast Dialysis Center, LLC [22766]
West Coast Hearing and Balance Center--Camarillo [1072]
West Coast Hearing and Balance Center--Oxnard [1216]
West Coast Hearing and Balance Center--Simi Valley [1323]
West Coast Hearing and Balance Inc.--Thousand Oaks [1337]
West Coast Home Health Care Agency [14256]
West Coast Nursing Ventura Inc. [13385]
West Coast Outpatient Services Inc [39947]
West Coast Outpatient Svc Inc [39948]
West Coast Speech, Language, and Diagnostic Center [1276]
West Coast Spine [3935]
West Cobb Speech and Language Services [1871]
West Columbia Sports Medicine [39020]
West County Medical Clinic • Substance Abuse Program [40048]
West County Medical Corporation [40049]
West Denver Child and Family Center [28891]
West Elk Grove Dialysis Center • DaVita [22676]
West End Behavioral Healthcare System [51424]
West End Health Center [31698]
West End Medical Centers, Inc. [6585]
West End Outreach Services • Forks Community Hospital [49965]
West End Outreach Services /Oak Street Center • Branch of Forks Community Hospital [50060]
West Florida Community Care Center [33326]
West Florida Dialysis • DaVita [23476]
West Florida Hospital
Cancer Program [4983]
Sleep Disorders Center [36830]
West Florida Public Library • Talking Book Library [3769]
West Florida Rehabilitation Institute [1723]
Rehabilitation Institute [3998]

West Fulton County Mental Health Center [29357]
West George Dialysis--LaGrange • Renal Advantage Inc. [23729]
West Georgia Dialysis & At Home • DaVita [23655]
West Georgia Health System • Enoch Callaway Cancer Clinic [5028]
West Georgia Hospice [19398]
West Georgia Medical Center [1873]
West Georgia Medical Center Home Care [14539]
West Haven Board of Education [337]
West Haven Mental Health Clinic [33267]
West Haven Veterans Affairs Medical Center • Multiple Sclerosis Program [34549]
West Hawaii Community Health Center [6622]
West Hawaii Domestic Abuse Shelter [9137]
West Hills Hospital [33649]
West Hills Hospital and Medical Center • Grossman Burn Center [4526]
West Hills Lodge Inc [45257]
West Houston Dialysis Center [27184]
West Iredell Dialysis Center • Wake Forest University [25959]
West Irondequoit School District [599]
West Jefferson Medical Center [15327]
    Cancer Center [5253]
    Rehab Center [4069]
West Jefferson Mental Health Center [30158]
West Kendall Dialysis Center • Fresenius Medical Care [23409]
West Kentucky Easter Seal Center [8057]
West Kentucky Orthopaedics and Sports Medicine [38477]
West Knox Health Center [7262]
West Lafayette Veterans Affairs Clinic [29832]
West Lakes Sleep Center [36987]
West Linn Dialysis Center • DaVita [26361]
West Marriage/Family Counseling Inc [42326]
West Michigan Cancer Center [4681]
West Michigan Reproductive Institute • Assisted Reproductive Technology Program [22132]
West Michigan Sports & Rehabilitation Clinic [38590]
West Michigan Therapy Inc [44938]
    Transitional Living Center [44940]
West Midtown Medical Group
    Methadone Maintenance Treatment Prog [46933]
    Substance Abuse/Alcohol Treatment [46934]
West Mount Houston Dialysis Center [27185]
West Nassau Dialysis Center Inc. [25797]
West Newton Hearing Center [2537]
West Oakland Health Center--Mental Health Department [28683]
West Oakland Health Council • Community Recovery Center East [40310]
West Oakland Health Council, Inc. • West Oakland Health Center [6336]
West Oaks Hospital [33874], [51384]
West Oaks Hospital Inc • Chemical Dependency Services [49421]
West Oregon University • Office of Disability Services [685]
West Palm Beach Health Center [6569]
West Palm Beach Veterans Affairs Medical Center [29322]
    Okeechobee Clinic [29248]
    Vero Beach Clinic [29316]
    Women's Stress Disorder Treatment Team Outpatient [51714]
West Park Dialysis Care [27186]
West Park Rehabilitation [38944]
West Penn Allegheny Health System • Jones Institute for Reproductive Medicine of Eastern Medical School [22237]
West Pensacola Dialysis Center • DaVita [23477]
West Perrine Health Center [6538]
West Pettigrew Dialysis Center • Fresenius Medical Care [25856]
West Philadelphia Dialysis • Dialysis Facility • DaVita [26540]
West Plains Veterans Affairs Clinic [30916]
West Point Sleep Laboratory • North Mississippi Medical Center [37270]
West Ranch, Marshall [30873]
West Region Sleep Center [37595]
West Sacramento Dialysis Clinic • DaVita [23072]
West Saint Paul Dialysis • DaVita [25094]
West St. Paul Dialysis • Fresenius Medical Care [25095]

West Salem Clinic [7147]
West Salem Clinic - Mental Health • Northwest Human Services [31977]
West Seattle Kidney Center • Dialysis Facility • Northwest Kidney Center [27644]
West Side Catholic Center [10138]
West Side Community Health Services, Inc. • La Clinica [6874]
West Side School [34330]
West Side Sports Physical Therapy [38806]
West Sound Treatment Center [50063]
West Suburban Hospital Medical Center
    Cancer Program [5117]
    Snoring and Sleep Disorders Center [36937]
West Suburban Speech Clinic [2095]
West Tallahassee Dialysis • DaVita • Dialysis Facility & At Home [23524]
West Tampa Dialysis • DaVita • Dialysis Facility [23540]
West Tennessee Healthcare • Pathways Behavioral Health Services [33842]
West Tennessee School for the Deaf [752]
West Texas A&M University • Speech and Hearing Clinic [3475]
West Texas Centers for Mental Health/Mental Retardation [32556]
West Texas Counseling and
    Rehabilitation Program of Amarillo [49208]
    Rehabilitation Program of Dallas [49304]
    Rehabilitation Program of Irving [49427]
    Rehabilitation Program of Midland [49467]
    Rehabilitation Program of Odessa [49473]
    Rehabilitation Program of Plano Inc [49492]
    Rehabilitation Program of San Angelo [49509]
    Rehabilitation Program of Temple [49553]
West Texas Rehabilitation Center [8527]
West Texas Renal Care Center • Dialysis Facility [27312]
West Texas Services for the Deaf Inc. [3452]
West Texas VA Health Care System [4466]
West Texas VA Healthcare Services • Substance Abuse Treatment Program [49248]
West Texas Veterans Affairs Health Care System [17828], [51655]
West Texas Veterans Affairs Healthcare System • Big Spring [32414]
West Union Dialysis Center • DaVita [24311]
West Valley Dialysis Clinic [27431]
West Valley Mental Health Center [28424]
West Valley Sleep Disorders Center [36717]
West Valley Vet Center • Peoria AZ [51865]
West Vancouver Community Health Centre • Be Real Clinic [10923]
West Virginia ARH, Inc. [18498]
West Virginia Bureau for Public Health • Office of Maternal, Child, and Family Health • Research, Evaluation and Planning Division • SIDS Program [36557]
West Virginia Department of Education • West Virginia Services to Children Who are Deafblind [3654]
West Virginia Dialysis • DaVita [27680]
West Virginia Library Commission • Special Libraries • Blind and Physically Handicapped Services [3854]
West Virginia Rehabilitation Center [8609]
West Virginia School for the Blind Library [3855]
West Virginia Schools for Deaf and Blind [881]
West Virginia Schools for the Deaf and the Blind [3743]
West Virginia University
    ALS Center [157]
    Center for Reproductive Medicine [22299]
West Virginia University, Charleston • Cystic Fibrosis Center [7697]
West Virginia University Hospital • Renal Dialysis Center [27684]
West Virginia University Hospitals • Cancer Program [6139]
West Virginia University Hospitals - East Home Health Care [18503]
West Virginia University Hospitals • MDA Clinic [34908]
West Virginia University Medical Center • School of Medicine • Mary Babb Randolph Cancer Center • Hemophilia Treatment Center [12613]
West Virginia University

Robert C. Byrd Health Sciences Center • School of Medicine • Department of Pediatrics-Genetics [12373]
    School Of Medicine • Mountain State Cystic Fibrosis Center [7698]
West Windsor Psychotherapy and Addiction Counseling [46145]
West Women's and Children's Shelter [10254]
West Yavapai Guidance Clinic [28193]
WestArk RSVP [28273]
Westbank Chronic Renal Ctr. • DaVita • Dialysis Facility [24562]
Westborough Dialysis Center • DaVita [23020]
Westborough State Hospital [33585]
WestBridge Community Services [31084]
Westbrook Health Services • Amity Detox and Treatment Center [50335]
Westbrook Health Services--Harrisville [32905]
Westbrook Health Services, Inc.--Ravenswood [32933]
Westbrook Health Services, Inc.--Saint Marys [32936]
Westbrook Health Services--Parkersburg [32926]
Westbrook Health Services--Spencer [32937]
Westbrook Health Services • Wood County/Substance Abuse Services [50336]
WestCare Arizona [35799]
WestCare--Atlanta GA [35913]
WestCare California Inc [39871], [39903]
WestCare DUI Program [43637]
WestCare Florida Inc Davis Bradley • Outpatient Treatment Services [41923]
WestCare Foundation • Runaway and Homeless Youth Program [36070]
Westcare Gulfcoast Florida Inc • North County Office [41599]
Westcare Henderson • Safe House [45833]
Westcare Home Health and Hospice [20747]
WestCare, Inc. • Runaway and Homeless Youth Program [36071]
WestCare Kentucky [43521]
    Community Involvement Center [43760]
Westcare Nevada Inc
    Community Triage [45853]
    Harris Springs Ranch [45854]
    Substance Abuse Treatment [45855]
    Women and Children Campus [45856]
Westchester Artificial Kidney Center • Dialysis Unit [25657]
Westchester Cardiac Rehabilitation [38819]
Westchester Community Opportunity Prog
    Greenburgh Open Door Add Recov Clinic [47191]
    Mount Vernon Open Door Program [46799]
    New Rochelle Outreach Center [46803]
Westchester County Medical Center • Burn Center [4598]
Westchester Day Treatment Center [31346]
Westchester Division of Montefiore LTHHCP [16451]
Westchester Institute for Human Development • Speech and Hearing Center [3140]
Westchester Medical Center
    Behavioral Health Center • Crisis Intervention Unit [51154]
    Dialysis Clinic Inc. Extension [25794]
Westchester Medical Center--Nephrology [25795]
Westchester Medical Center • Sleep Center [37450]
Westchester Medical Group Center For Heart And Health [38084]
Westchester Youth Services/Children's Village • Runaway and Homeless Youth Program [36126]
Westcoast Counseling and Treatment Center [49904]
Westend Clinic Inc [45633]
Westerly Hospital • Cancer Care Program [5897]
Western AR Counseling • Adolescent [39523]
Western Arizona Regional Medical Center [12783]
Western Arkansas Counseling and Guidance [28248]
Western Arkansas Counseling and Guidance Center
    Crawford County Clinic [28359]
    Franklin County Clinic [28335]
Western Arkansas Counseling and Guidance Center, Inc. [28274]
Western Arkansas Counseling and Guidance Center
    Logan County Clinic [28339]
    NEW Clubhouse [28275]
    Polk County Clinic [28322]

Therapeutic Children's Homes [28276]
Western Audiology [1225]
Western Baptist Hospital • Cancer Program [5234]
Western Carolina Center • J.Iverson Riddle Developmental Center [8386]
Western Carolina Treatment Center [47218]
Western Carolinians Criminal Justice • Women At Risk Program [47219]
Western Clinical Health Services • DBA Riverside Treatment Center [40466]
Western Community Dialysis Center LLC • American Renal Associates [23496]
Western Health Harbor City Clinic [39905]
Western Highlands Network [31505]
Western Hills Southwest Dialysis • DaVita [26054]
Western Hills Speech Clinic [3226]
Western Home Care Inc. [12915]
Western Illinois Kidney Center [23996]
Western Illinois University
    AOD Resource Center [42757]
    Speech-Language-Hearing Clinic [2066]
Western Iowa Sleep • Sleep Center [36988]
Western Judicial Services Inc [39483], [41975], [41978]
Western Kentucky Drug and Alcohol
    Intervention Services Inc [43547]
    Intervention Services Inc/Mayfield [43710]
    Intervention Services Inc/Paducah [43749]
    Intervention Services Inc/Princeton [43767]
Western Kentucky Hearing and Audiology Services [2258]
Western Kentucky Orthopaedic Associates [38472]
Western Kentucky Speech and Swallowing [2259]
Western Lake Counseling and • DUI Programs LLC [42672]
Western Maryland Center • Renal Division [24694]
Western Maryland Health System • Behavioral Health Services [44240]
Western Maryland Health System Home Care [15432]
Western Maryland Health System-Hospice Services [19921]
Western Maryland Health System • Renal Dialysis Unit [24674]
Western Maryland Recovery Services [44241]
Western Massachusetts Kidney Center • Fresenius Medical Care [24804]
Western Medical Center, Anaheim • Behavioral Health Services [28372]
Western Medical Center Santa Ana Renal Transplant [22995]
Western Mental Development Clinic [30728]
Western Mental Health Center, Birmingham [29110]
Western Mental Health Clinic--Canby • Canby Community Hospital [30670]
Western Mental Health Clinic--Granite Falls [30682]
Western Mental Health Clinic--Ivanhoe • Divine Providence Hospital [30689]
Western Mental Health Clinic--Marshall [30695]
Western Mental Health Clinic--Redwood Falls [30710]
Western Mental Health Institute [33838]
Western Michigan University • Speech Pathology and Audiology Department • Charles Van Riper Language, Speech, and Hearing Clinic [2614]
Western Missouri Mental Health Center [30865]
    Kansas City Suicide Prevention Line [51056]
Western Montana Addiction Services
    Carol Graham [45714]
    Ravalli County [45701]
    Share House [45715]
    Teen Recovery Center [45716]
    Turning Point [45717]
    WMAS Adolescent [45718]
Western Montana Mental Health Center--Addiction Services [30934]
Western Montana Mental Health Center--Anaconda [30918]
Western Montana Mental Health Center
    Beaverhead County Office [30935]
    Child and Family Services Network [30958]
    Lake County Office [30962]
    Lincoln County Office [30955]
Western Montana Mental Health Center--Missoula [30959]
Western Montana Mental Health Center
    Riverfront Counseling [30945]
    Sanders County Office [30968]

Silver House [30930]
Sinopah House [30951]
Stillwater Therapeutic Services [30952]
Turning Point [30960]
Western Montana Sports Medicine and Fitness Center [38684]
Western Montana Tri County • Addictions Services [45677]
Western Neurological Associates • Multiple Sclerosis Center [34726]
Western New Mexico Counseling [31197]
Western New York AKC Kenmore Unit [25693]
Western New York Artificial Kidney Center--Buffalo [25637]
Western New York Children's Psychiatric Center [8363]
    Day Treatment Center [33732]
Western North Carolina Community Health Services • Interlace [10015]
Western Pacific Med Corp
    Western Pacific Fullerton Medical [39875]
    Western Pacific Glendale Medical [39891]
    Western Pacific Lancaster [39992]
    Western Pacific North Hollywood Med [40277]
    Western Pacific Panorama Medical [40357]
    Western Pacific Reseda Medical [40445]
    Western Pacific Stanton Medical [40820]
    Western Pacific Van Nuys Medical [40899]
    Western Pacific Ventura Medical [40913]
Western Pacific Norwalk Medical Clinic [40283]
Western Pennsylvania Hospital
    Burn--Trauma Center [4625]
    Cancer Institute [5863]
Western Pennsylvania School for Blind Children [3734]
Western Pennsylvania School for the Deaf [711]
Western Plains Medical Complex • Neurodiagnostic and Sleep Disorder Center [37015]
Western Psychiatric Institute/Clinic • Narcotic Addiction Treatment Program [48613]
Western Psychological and Counseling Services PC [48076], [48116], [50247]
Western Region SIDS Resources, Inc. [36502]
Western Sierra Medical Mobile Clinic [6301]
Western Skies Dialysis Inc. [22428]
Western State Hospital [8047]
Western State Hospital--Hopkinsville [33522]
Western State Hospital--Staunton [33909]
Western State Hospital--Tacoma [33915]
Western Texas Lions Eye Bank Alliance [35249]
Western Tidewater CSB • Outpatient Services [49848]
Western Tidewater Mental Health Center [32793]
Western Washington Alcoho/Drug Treatment Center [50222]
Western Wayne Family Health Center--Inkster [6849]
Western Wayne Family Health Center--Taylor [6859]
Western Youth Services--Anaheim [28373]
Western Youth Services--Fountain Valley [28500]
Western Youth Services, Laguna Hills [28555]
Western Youth Services, Mission Viejo [28625]
Western Youth Services, San Juan Capistrano [28783]
Western Youth Services, Santa Ana [28798]
Westfall Associates • Chemical Dependence Outpatient [47056]
Westfield Crisis Team [51002]
Westfield Laurel Health Center [7192]
Westgate McGuinness Therapy Services [1837]
Westhab, Inc. • Runaway and Homeless Youth Program [36127]
Westhab Special Needs Housing [10011]
Westhampton Dialysis Center • American Renal Associates [27558]
Westlake Daly City Dialysis Center • DaVita [22656]
Westlake Dialysis Center • Fresenius Medical Care [26235]
Westlake Village Family Services [40948]
Westland Dialysis • Davita [24993]
Westminster Dialysis Center • Fresenius Medical Care [27187]
Westminster Dialysis • DaVita [23146]
Westminster House II [29859]
Westminster House, Inc. • Behavioral Health Resources [29860]
Westminster Rescue Mission [44389]
Westmoreland Intermediate Unit [701]

Westmoreland Regional Hospital [17329]
Westmoreland Sleep Medicine [37714]
Weston Dialysis Center • DaVita [23558]
Westport Dialysis Center • Diversified Specialty Institutes [25231]
Westside Dialysis Center • Innovative Dialysis Systems [22793]
Westside Health Center [7142]
Westside Health Services [6431]
Westside Healthcare [38151]
Westside Home Health Inc. [13164]
Westside Methadone Treatment Program [40646]
Westside Regional Medical Center • Cancer Center [4984]
Westside Sleep Center [37633]
Westside Sober Living Centers Inc • Promises Residential Treatment Center [40179]
Westside Voice and Swallowing Disorders [3082]
Westview Behavioral Health Services [48966]
Westview Dialysis & At Home • DaVita [24181]
Westview Hospital • Outpatient Rehabilitation [2166]
Westville Family Medicine [7122]
Westwind Eating Disorder Recovery Centre [11075]
Westwood Behavioral Health Center Inc [47874]
Westwood Behavioral Health Center, Inc.--Paulding [31824]
Westwood Behavioral Health Center, Inc.--Van Wert [31850]
Westwood Dialysis Center & At Home • DaVita [27645]
Westwood Dialysis Center • Fresenius Medical Care [24813]
Westwood Lodge Hospital [33586], [44603]
Wetzel County Home Care [18529]
Wewahitchka Medical Center [6571]
Wexford Missaukee Intermediate School District [484]
Weyland Consultation Services [40934]
W.G. Bill Hefner VA Medical Center [16778]
W.G. (Bill) Hefner Veterans Affairs Medical Center [31590]
W.G. Bill Hefner Veterans Affairs Medical Center
    Specialized Inpatient PTSD Unit [51791]
    Women's Trauma Recovery Program [51792]
WG Hefner Veterans Affairs Medical Center [51622]
Whaley Children's Center [34224]
Wharton Kidney Center [27396]
Whatcom County Mental Health Program [51428]
Whatley Health Service--Oakman [6196]
Whatley Health Services--Eutaw [6184]
WHCHC--Keiki Health Center [6624]
Wheat Ridge Regional Center [7844]
Wheaton Dialysis Center • DaVita [24738]
Wheaton Franciscan
    All Saints Dialysis East [27775]
    All Saints Dialysis West [27776]
Wheaton Franciscan Health/All Saints • Mental Health and Addiction Care [50514]
Wheaton Franciscan Healthcare--Saint Francis Hospital • Cancer Program [6168]
Wheaton Franciscan Healthcare--Saint Joseph Regional Medical Center • Cancer Program [6169]
Wheaton Franciscan Home Health and Hospice [21860]
Wheaton Franciscan Home Health & Hospice, Inc.--Milwaukee [18601]
Wheaton Franciscan Home Health & Hospice, Inc.--Racine [18621]
Wheeler Clinic [29042]
    Emergency Services [50735]
Wheeler Clinic Helpline [50724]
Wheeler Clinic Inc
    Hartford Outpatient [41411]
    Intensive Daytime Outpatient [41461]
    Intensive Evening Treatment [41462]
Wheeling Clinic [3661]
Wheeling Clinic - Visiting Nurses Association of Medical Park [18551]
Wheeling Dialysis Center [27694]
Wheeling Hospital [3662]
    Schiffler Cancer Center [6143]
    Sports Medicine Center [39170]
Whidbey General Hospital [18426]
    Cancer Program [6097]
    Whidbey Island Sleep Center [37946]
Whidbey Home Medical [18440]
Whidbey Island Dialysis Center • DaVita [27621]
White Bird Clinic [7128], [51252]

Chrysalis Program [48109]
White Bridge Dialysis • Dialysis Center & At Home • DaVita [26912]
White Buffalo Calf Women's Society, Inc. [10377]
White Center Public Health Center [7390]
White County Domestic Violence Prevention [8783]
White County Mental Health Center [50799]
White County Mental Health/Substance Abuse Clinic [29389]
White Deer Run [48271]
    Altoona [48276]
    Harrisburg [48399]
    Lancaster [48434]
    Lewisburg [48451]
    New Castle [48482]
    Williamsport [48703]
    York [48716]
White Earth Battered Women's Service [9626]
White Earth Substance Abuse Program [45343]
White Flint Recovery Inc [44340]
    Eastern Shore Inc [44351]
White Glove Community Care [16428]
White Haven Center [8491]
White Horse Ranch [11203]
White Horse Ranch LLC [47962]
White House Clinic [6738]
White Lane Dialysis • DaVita [22598]
White Memorial Medical Center • Cecilia Gonzalez De La Hoya Cancer Center [4803]
White Mountain Mental Health Center [31080]
White Mountain Safe House for Victim's of Domestic Violence [8721]
White Oaks Dialysis, Home Training & At Home • DaVita [26055]
White Oaks Knolls for Men [29666]
White Oaks Outpatient Services • Human Service Center [29667]
White Picket Fence Counseling Center • Eating Disorders and Food Addictions [11034]
White Plains Dialysis & At Home • DaVita [25804]
White Plains Hospital Center [16675]
    Dickstein Cancer Treatment Center [5625]
White Plains Hospital and Medical Center • MDA Clinic [34845]
White Plains Public Schools [3153]
White River Battered Women's Shelter, Inc. [8779]
White River Junction Veterans Affairs Medical Center [32687]
    PTSD Clinical Team [51834]
White River Medical Center Behavioral Health [28239]
White River Rural Health Center, Inc. • Augusta Medical and Dental Clinic [6258]
White Rose Hospice • Memorial Hospital [21182]
White Sky Hope Center • Rocky Boy Clinic [45687]
Whitesburg Dialysis • DaVita [24449]
Whitesburg DUI Service Agency • Alcohol and Drug Treatment and Education Center [43796]
Whiteside Dialysis Facility • DaVita [24095]
Whiteside Manor [40467]
    Mens Annex [40468]
    Mens Program [40469]
    Wilshire House [40470]
Whiting Dialysis Center • Fresenius Medical Care [25528]
Whitman Walker Clinic/Mental Hlth and Addiction Treatment Service [41555]
Whitman--Walker Clinic Victim Services [9038]
The Whitney Academy [8121], [34188]
Whitney M Young Jr Health Center Inc
    FACTS [46344]
        Methadone Medical Maintenance Prog [46345]
        Methadone Treatment Clinic MMTP [46346]
Whitney M. Young, Jr. Health Center [7007]
Whitney Sleep Center [37240]
Whitten Center [8501]
Whittier Area Regional Deaf Program [315]
Whittier Hearing Center Inc. [1364]
Whittier Kidney Dialysis Center [23077]
Whittier Rehabilitation Hospital [2485], [15475]
Whittier Street Health Center [44558]
Whittier Street Health Center Committee, Inc. • Whittier Street Health Center [6825]
Whole Child Pediatrics [6487]
Whole Person Recovery Center [47561]
WI Community Mental Health Counseling Centers Inc [50410], [50466]
Wichita and Affiliated Tribes of Oklahoma [47907]

Wichita Area Sexual Assault Center [9381]
Wichita Child Guidance Center [8039]
Wichita Children's Home • Runaway and Homeless Youth Program [35964]
Wichita Dialysis Center & At Home • DaVita [24358]
Wichita Falls Intermediate School District [831]
Wichita Falls Regional Day School for the Deaf [832]
Wichita Home Health Service, Inc. [18191]
Wichita Public Library • Talking Books Section [3797]
Wichita Treatment Center [43513]
Wicomico Behavioral Health [44352]
Wicomico County Board of Education [462]
Wiggins Dialysis Unit [25169]
Wikes Regional Medical Center Home Care [16765]
Wilbarger General Hospital Dialysis of Vernon [27385]
Wilbur D. Mills Center • Substance Abuse Treatment Center [28351]
Wilbur Mills Center [39575]
Wilcox County Mental Retardation Service Center [29488]
Wild Acre Inns, Inc. [30321]
Wild Acres [29202]
Wild Iris--Coleville [8805]
Wild Iris Family Shelter Services [8797]
Wild Iris--Lone Pine [8832]
Wild Iris--Mammoth Lakes [8845]
Wilder Healthcare Center [27893]
Wilderness Treatment Center [45710]
Wildwood Dialysis Center • Innovative Dialysis Systems [26219]
Wilford Hall Medical Center • Cancer Program [6007]
Wilkes-Barre General Hospital • Wyoming Valley Health Care System • Cancer Program [5881]
Wilkes Regional Dialysis Center [25920]
Wilkins Center of Greenwich Connecticut [11008]
Will County Health Department • Will County Community Health Center [6672]
Will County Mental Health Center • Intervention Program [50852]
Will--Grundy Center for Independent Living [2051]
Willamette Falls Hospice [21018]
Willamette Falls Hospital • Cancer Program [5796]
Willamette Family Treatment Services
    Buckley House [48110]
    Carlton Unit [48111]
    Womens Residential [48112]
Willamette Orthopedic Group • Pain Clinic [35639]
Willamette Sleep Center [37634]
Willamette Valley Hospice [21033]
Willamette Valley Kidney Center • Diversified Specialty Institutes [26336]
Willamette Valley Medical Center • Cancer Program [5792]
Willamette Valley Treatment Center Inc [48245]
Willapa Counseling Center--Long Beach [51448]
Willapa Counseling Center/Long Beach [50003]
Willapa Counseling Center/Raymond [50077]
Willapa Counseling Center--Raymond • North Pacific County Crisis [51460]
Willapa Counseling Center--South Bend • North Pacific County Crisis [51469]
William Beaumont Army Medical Center--El Paso • Cancer Program [5986]
William Beaumont Hospice [20131]
William Beaumont Hospital • Department of Anatomic Pathology • Genetics Clinic [12256]
William Beaumont Hospital, Home services Center [15867]
William Beaumont Hospital • In Vitro Fertilization Program [22133]
William Beaumont Hospital, Royal Oak • Beaumont Sleep Evaluation Services [37211]
William Beaumont Hospital--Royal Oak
    Cancer Treatment Center--Royal Oak [5395]
    Transplant Center [24964]
William Beaumont Hospital • Speech-Language Pathology Department [2640]
William Beaumont Hospital--Sterling Heights • Dialysis Center [24980]
William Beaumont Hospital--Troy • Cancer Program [5400]
William Center [844]
William Childs Hospice House [19285]
William D. Partlow Developmental Center [7730]

William F. Ryan Community Health Center • Ryan Center [7032]
William F. Walker Professional Counseling Center [32374]
William J McCord • Adolescent Treatment Facility [48968]
William Jennings Bryan Dorn Veterans Administration Hospital [32197], [51646]
William Jennings Bryan Dorn Veterans Affairs Medical Center [17579]
William Jennings Bryan Dorn • Veterans Affairs Medical Center [48922]
William Jennings Bryan Dorn Veterans Affairs Medical Center
    Cancer Program [5905]
    Multiple Sclerosis Center [34708]
William Newton Hospital • Winfield Healthcare Center [2252]
William Osler Health System • Eating Disorders Clinic [11244]
William Paterson University • Communication Disorders Department • Speech and Hearing Clinic [2954]
William R. Courtney State Veterans Home [18171]
William R. Sharpe Jr. Hospital [33920]
William S Hall Psychiatric Institute • Adolscent Recovery Program [48923]
William S. Middleton Memorial Veterans Affairs Hospital • Multiple Sclerosis Center [34746]
William S. Middleton Memorial Veterans Affairs Medical Center [51675]
William S. Middleton Memorial Veterans Hospital [18582], [32989]
William S. Middleton Veterans Affairs Hospital • PTSD Clinical Team [51849]
William S Middleton Veterans Hospital • Addictive Disorders Treatment Program [50453]
William W. Backus Hospital • Cancer Program [4906]
William W. Fox Developmental Center [7950]
Williams Counseling [41168]
Williams House 1 and 2 [39794]
Williams Medical Equipment [16729]
Williams Street Dialysis • DaVita [23787]
Williamsburg County Department on Alcohol and Drug Abuse [48954]
Williamsburg Dialysis and At Home • DaVita [27586]
Williamsburg Place • The William J Farley Center [49866]
Williamson County Dialysis • Dialysis Center • DaVita [26838]
Williamson Medical Center • Cancer Program [5929]
Williamson Treatment Center Inc [50354]
Williamsport Dialysis Clinic • North Central Pennsylvania Dialysis Clinics [26484]
Williamsport YWCA Helpline [51302]
Williamstown Dialysis • DaVita [24450]
Williamsville Wellness [49800]
Willie Ross School for the Deaf [2489]
Willingway Hospital • Substance Abuse Services [42159]
Willis Center/Footsteps Supportive • Housing Program [44622]
Willis Intermediate School District [833]
Willis Knighton Home Health of LA [15367]
Willis Knighton Hospice of Louisiana [19880]
Willis Knighton Med Center--Transplant [24586]
Willis-Knighton Medical Center • Cancer Center [4675]
Willis Knighton Medical Center • Dialysis Center [24587]
Willis-Knighton Rehabilitation Institute [2342]
Willis/Knighton South Hospital • Behavioral Medicine Institute Inpt [43901]
Willis W Hudson Center [44353]
Williston VA Outpatient Clinic [4359]
Williston Veterans Affairs Clinic [31641]
Willmar Regional Treatment Center [33610]
Willough at Naples [11035], [41815]
A Willow Bends Inc [41071]
Willow Creek Day Treatment Center [31772]
Willow Creek Treatment Center [28818]
Willow Creek Treatment Center/NVS [304]
Willow Crest Hospital [33777]
Willow Dialysis Center • DaVita [26237]
Willow Domestic Violence Center [9367]
Willow Home Care, LTD [14908]
Willow Springs Center [34291]

Willow Station Dialysis • Fresenius Medical Care - Greeley [23124]
Willow Tree Hospice [21171]
Willowbrook Dialysis Center--Wayne [25526]
Willowbrook Dialysis--Houston • DaVita [27188]
Willowbrook Home Health Care, Inc.--Dickson [17663]
Willowbrook Home Health Care, Inc.--Franklin [17671]
Willowbrook Home Health Care, Inc.--Hendersonville [17678]
Willowbrook Home Health Care, Inc.--Lewisburg [17721]
Willowbrook Home Health Care, Inc.--Murfreesboro [17749]
Willowbrook Home Health Care, Inc.--Springfield [17774]
Willowbrook Home HealthCare, Inc.--Nashville [17763]
Willowbrook Hospice, Inc. [21333]
Willowbrooke at Tanner [42178]
Willowglen Academy [8626], [34489]
Willowglen Academy North [34492]
Willowglen Academy Wilson [34494]
Willsand Home Health Agency, Inc. [14180]
WilMed Hospice [20769]
Wilmer Hall Children's Home • Murray School [7720]
Wilmington Hospice Care Center [20766]
Wilmington Hospital • Center for Pain Management [35373]
Wilmington Mental Health Center [29081]
Wilmington Treatment Center [47527]
    Outpatient Services [47528]
Wilmington Veterans Affairs Clinic [31612]
Wilmington Veterans Affairs Medical Center
    Dover Outpatient Clinic [29061]
    Georgetown Outpatient Clinic [29065]
    Multiple Sclerosis Center [34551]
Wilmot Clinic [6282]
Wilmot Community Health Center [6254]
WilPower, Inc. [29656]
Wilrose Palliative Care [13290]
Wilshire Dialysis Center • DaVita [22794]
Wilshire Treatment Center Inc [40180]
Wilson County Schools [636]
Wilson County Special Education [757]
Wilson Crisis Center [51181]
Wilson Hospice • Wilson Memorial Hospital [20892]
Wilson In Home, Inc. [14626]
Wilson Medical Center • Cancer Care Program [5664]
Wilson Memorial Hospital [17039]
Wilson Sleep Center [37596]
Wilton Public Schools [339]
Winchelsea Speech and Language Services [1048]
Winchester Addiction Services PLC [49870]
Winchester Dialysis • DaVita [27587]
Winchester Hospital • Cancer Program [5360]
Winchester Hospital Home Care [15564]
Winchester Hospital • Sleep Disorders Center [37142]
Winchester Medical Center [18410]
    Cancer Program [6089]
Winchester Physical Therapy and Sports Medicine [39137]
Wind River Dialysis Center [27814]
WIND Youth Center • Runaway and Homeless Youth Program [35850]
Windber Hospice [21175]
Windber Medical Center [17512]
Windham Community Memorial Hospital • Eastern Connecticut Sleep Program [36756]
Windham Dialysis Center • DaVita [23175]
Windmoor Healthcare [33297]
W.I.N.D.O.W. Victim Services [9601]
Windows of Opportunity • Rehabilitation Services Inc [42591]
Windsong Home Health Agency [18175]
Windsor Community Health Center [7066]
Windsor County Community Services [32689]
Windsor Hospital [33751]
Windsor House [32151]
    Community Healthlink, Inc. [30492]
Windsor Laurelwood Center for • Behavioral Medicine [47885]
Windsor Regional Hospital • Essex County Regional Burn Unit [4618]

Windward Abuse Shelter [9151]
Windward Dialysis Center • Fresenius Medical Care [23856]
Windwood Psychiatric Hospital • Windwood Behavioral Health Services [33388]
Windy City Orthopedics and Sports Medicine [38370]
Wing Memorial Hospital [33579]
Wing Memorial Hospital and Medical Centers Home Care [15534]
Wings Adolescent Treatment Services [45183]
Wings Family Supportive Services [9582]
Wings of Hope Hospice and • Palliative Care, Inc. [20023]
Wings Program Inc. [9241]
Wings of Refuge Inc • Wings of Recovery/Nonresidential [40181]
Wings Speech and Language Center [1210]
Wingspan Anti-Violence Project [8741]
Winifred Masterson Burke Rehabilitation Hospital [4324]
Winkler County Mental Health Center [32490]
Winmar Diagnostics Sleep Wellness Center [37502]
Winn Way Mental Health Center--Central Access [50802]
Winnebago Mental Health Institute [33952]
Winnemucca Mental Health Center [31048]
Winneshiek County Memorial Hospital [15075]
Winneshiek Medical Center Hospice [19684]
Winnie Palmer Hospital for Women and Children • Hughes Center for Fetal Diagnostics [12188]
Winning Wheels, Inc. [4032]
Winnipeg Children's Hospital • Burn Unit [4557]
Winnsboro Mental Health Center [30178]
Winona Area Hospice Services [20217]
Winona Counseling Clinic • Chemical Dependency Services [45352]
Winona Health Services • Dialysis Facility [25097]
Winslow Family Physician [38713]
Winslow Guidance Associates Inc [39518]
Winston County Schools [194]
Winston L. Prouty Center for Child Development [8573]
Winston Preparatory School [3083]
Winston Salem OPC Satellite • Outpatient Clinic [47546]
Winston Salem Veterans Affairs Clinic [31618]
Winter Garden Children's Health Center [6573]
Winter Garden Dialysis • DaVita [23560]
Winter Garden Family Health Center [6574]
Winter Haven Audiology [1797]
Winter Haven Dialysis • DaVita • Dialysis Center [23563]
Winter Haven Hospital [1798]
Winter Park [19337]
Winter Park Dialysis • DaVita [23565]
Winter Park Hemodialysis • DaVita [23566]
Winter Park Physical Therapy [38300]
Winters Healthcare Foundation [6380]
Winthrop Hill [4086]
Winthrop-University Hospital • Cancer Program [5589]
Winthrop University Hospital
    Dialysis Center [25704]
    Dialysis Center at Bethpage [25578]
    Dialysis Center at Glen Cove [25673]
Winthrop-University Hospital Home Health Agency [16525]
Winthrop University Hospital • Sleep Disorders Center [37451]
Winthrop University Hospital at Sun Harbor [25772]
Winton Road Dialysis • Dialysis Facility • DaVita [26056]
Winyah Community Hospice [21213]
Winyah Community Hospice Care - Columbia [21224]
Winyah Community Hospice Care--Florence • Amedisys [21235]
Winyah Community Hospice Care--Greenville • Amedisys [21246]
Winyah Community Hospice Care-Orangeburg • Amedisys [21268]
Winyah Community Hospice Care-Pawleys Island • Amedisys [21269]
Winyah Community Hospice Care-Spartanburg • Amedisys [21282]
Winyah Community Hospice Care--Walterboro • Amedisys [21286]

WIRCCA Victim Services [9238]
Wiregrass Mental Health Board Inc./dba Spectracare [33086]
Wiregrass Mental Health Board, Inc. • dba Spectra-Care [27904]
Wiregrass Rehabilitation Center [7711]
Wisconsin Association for Homeless and Runaway Services • Runaway and Homeless Youth Program [36274]
Wisconsin Center for the Blind and Visually Impaired [3744]
Wisconsin Community Services Inc • DBA Unlimited Potential [50487]
Wisconsin Department of Public Instruction • Wisconsin Educational Services Program for the Deaf and Hard of Hearing [3663]
Wisconsin Dialysis Inc.--East [27733]
Wisconsin Dialysis Inc.--Fitchburg Clinic [27713]
Wisconsin Division of Public Health • SIDS Program [36559]
Wisconsin Fertility Institute [22303]
Wisconsin IV Affiliates, LLC [18588]
Wisconsin Office for the Deaf and Hard of Hearing • Division of Disability and Elder Services [3665]
Wisconsin School for the Deaf [884]
Wisconsin Sleep [37987]
Wisconsin Talking Book and Braille Library [3856]
Wisconsin Tissue Bank [35268]
Wisconsin Veteran Home at Union Grove [18636]
Wise Choices Inc [43060]
Wise County Behavioral Health [32711]
Wise County Children and Youth Services [32712]
Wise Regional Health System [17891]
    Dialysis Center [27044]
    North Texas Cancer Center [4712]
WISEPlace--Steps to Independence [8902]
Wishing Well Clubhouse [28892]
Wishing Well Enterprises [28893]
WISR Ministries Inc • Save Our Siblings [40245]
Wissahickon Hospice [21049]
Wissahickon Hospice, UPHS [17249]
Wistar R and R Program Inc • Wistar Redemption and Recovery [40311]
Wistar Womens R & R Program Inc [40312]
With Friends, Inc. • Runaway and Homeless Youth Program [36137]
WJB Dorn Veterans Affairs Medical Center • PTSD Clinical Team [51813]
WKM Healthcare, Inc. [17935]
WNL Speech Therapy Services [3657]
Woburn Dialysis • DaVita • Dialysis Center [24818]
WOL and MED Back and Neck Pain Center--Dallas [35740]
WOL and MED Back and Neck Pain Center--Denton [35741]
Wolfner Library for the Blind and Physically Handicapped [3817]
Wolfson Children's Rehabilitation Services [1615]
WOMAN, Inc. [8892]
Womancare [9430]
Womankind, Inc. • Support Systems for Battered Women [9621]
Womankind Inc. • Support Systems for Battered Women • Fairview Ridges Hospital [9589]
Woman's Christian Association Hospital • Cancer Program [5585]
Woman's Christian Association Hospital - Dialysis Unit [25692]
Woman's Christian Association Hospital • Sports Medicine Center [38788]
Woman's Home Care [15275]
Woman's Hospital • Cancer Program [5244]
A Woman's Place [10273]
Woman's Place [9698]
A Woman's Place, Inc. [8969]
A Woman's Place of Merced County [8848]
Womanshelter/Companeras [9481]
Womanspace [48279]
Womanspace, Inc. [9847]
Womansplace [10296]
Women Against Abuse [10306]
Women Are Safe, Inc. [10393]
Women Aware, Inc.--New Brunswick [9840]
Women Aware, Inc.--Paducah • Merryman House [9398]
Women and Children First [8769]
Women and Children's Center [6772]
Women and Children's Hospital of Buffalo

Lung and Cystic Fibrosis Center [7627]
Transplant/Dialysis Center [25638]
Women and Children's Hospital
Kid's Team [8069]
Robert Warner Rehabilitation Center • Down
Syndrome Clinic [10837]
Women in Community Services Inc • Residence for
Girls 13 to 18 [45767]
Women in Crisis Carbon County [10292]
Women in Distress of Broward County, Inc. [9049]
Women Empowered Against Violence [9039]
Women Escaping a Violent Environment [10366]
Women and Families Center [35866]
Sexual Assault Crisis Service [8998]
Women Helping Battered Women [10540]
Women Helping Women, Inc.--Cincinnati [10133]
Women Helping Women--Jamaica [9935]
Women Helping Women--Lanai City [9153]
Women Helping Women--Wailuku [9157]
Women of Hope Resource Center Inc [45935]
Women In Safe Home--Muskogee [10204]
Women and Infants Hospital - In Vitro Fertilization
Program [22241]
Women and Infants Hospital - Medical Genetics
Services [12331]
Women and Infants Hospital • Project Link [48882]
Women and Infants Hospital of Rhode Island -
Program in Women's Oncology [5894]
Women in Need [10468]
Women in Need of God's Shelter [9108]
Women in Need Inc • Casa Rita Outpatient Clinic
[46467]
Women in Need, Inc. [10268]
Women in New Recovery [39411]
Women Recovering from Addictions Program
[43815]
Women in Safe Homes--Ketchikan [8666]
Women in Transition [10307]
Women on the Way Recovery Center [39919]
Women of Worth Recovery House [39640]
Womencare Shelter [10608]
Women's Action and Resource Center [10107]
Women's Aid in Crisis [10673]
Women's Aid Service, Inc. [9562]
Women's and Behavioral Health Center [6456]
Women's Center for Advancement [9783]
Women's Center of Beaver County [10264]
Women's Center of Brazoria County [10439]
Women's Center--Carbondale [9198]
Women's Center of East Texas [10485]
Womens Center of Greater Cleveland [47706]
Women's Center of Greater Danbury [8991]
Women's Center High Desert, Inc. • Women's
Shelter Network [8875]
The Women's Center, Inc. [9170]
Women's Center Inc.--Bloomsburg [10265]
Women's Center--Marquette • Harbor House [9556]
Women's Center of Mid-Minnesota [9587]
Women's Center of Montgomery County [10285]
Women's Center of Rhode Island [10338]
Women's Center of San Joaquin [8914]
Women's Center and Shelter of Greater Pittsburgh
[10309]
Women's Center of Southeastern Connecticut [9001]
Women's Center of Tarrant County, Inc. [10462]
Women's Center--Waukesha [10742]
Women's and Children's Alliance [9163]
Womens and Childrens Center for Inner Healing
[39331]
Women's and Children's Community Health Center
[6541]
Women's and Children's Crisis Shelter, Inc. [8928]
Women's and Children's Horizons • Pathways of
Courage [10710]
Women's and Children's Hospital • Rapides
Regional Medical Center • MDA Clinic [34806]
The Women's Circle [10385]
Women's Clinic, Ltd. • Infertility/In Vitro Fertilization
Program [22238]
Women's Community Association [9858]
The Women's Community, Inc. [10743]
Women's Crisis Center--Covington [9386]
Women's Crisis Center of Greater Newburyport •
Jeanne Geiger Crisis Center [9494]
Women's Crisis Center--Maysville [9394]
Women's Crisis Center of South Arkansas [8754]
Women's Crisis Center of Taney County, Inc. [9663]
Women's Crisis Center--Tillamook [10260]

Women's Crisis Center - YCC [10526]
Women's Crisis & Family Outreach Center •
Violence Prevention Institute [8941]
Women's Crisis Services of LeFlore County, Inc.
[10209]
Women's Crisis Shelter--Vernal [10535]
Women's Crisis Support--Santa Cruz [8905]
Women's Crisis Support Team • Safe Home Network
[10233]
Women's Crisis Support--Watsonville [8925]
Women's Fertility Center [22172]
Womens First Step House Inc • Yellowstone [39757]
A Women's Fund [9255]
Women's Group Home [32664]
Women's Haven [10196]
Women's Health Center of Springfield [7339]
Women's Health Clinic [7113]
Weight Preoccupation Program [11076]
Women's Health Services in Clinton County [6702]
Women's Help Center [10286]
Womens Home Inc [49766]
Women's Hospital [22081]
Women's Information Service Inc. [9520]
Womens Institute for Family Health [48575]
Womens Odyssey Organization Inc [39682]
Women's Place [9757]
Women's Project [8770]
Women's Protective Services of Lubbock, Inc.
[10486]
Women's Rape Crisis Center [10541]
Womens Recovery Association
The Center [39670]
San Mateo County/Elms House [40684]
San Mateo County/Laurel House [40685]
Womens Recovery Services [40789]
Women's Residential Center--24 Hour [6511]
Women's Resource Center--Beckley [10671]
Women's Resource Center--Dillon [9745]
Women's Resource Center to End Domestic
Violence, Inc. [9106]
Women's Resource Center of Glasgow [9746]
Women's Resource Center--Lawrence [9485]
Women's Resource Center of the New River Valley
[10587]
Women's Resource Center--Newport [10335]
Women's Resource Center--Norman [10205]
Women's Resource Center of Northern Michigan,
Inc. [9567]
Women's Resource Center--Oceanside [8862]
Women's Resource Center--Racine [10730]
Women's Resource Center--San Luis Rey [8897]
Women's Resource Center--Scranton [10315]
Women's Resource Center, Traverse City [9578]
Women's Resource Center--Watertown [10389]
Women's Resource Center of Winona [9646]
Women's Resource and Crisis Center of Galveston
County [10464]
Women's Resource and Rape Assistance Program
[10405]
Women's Resources of Monroe County, Inc. [10272]
Women's Rural Advocacy Program of Lyon County
[9609]
Women's Rural Advocacy Program of Redwood
County [9632]
Women's Rural Advocacy Program of Yellow
Medicine County [9600]
The Women's Safehouse [9725]
Women's Safety and Resource Center [10226]
Women's Service and Family Resource Center
[10192]
Women's Services • The Greenhouse [10297]
Women's Shelter of Central Arkansas [8756]
Women's Shelter of East Texas, Inc. • Family Crisis
Center [10493]
Women's Shelter Inc. [9633]
Women's Shelter Program, Inc. [8896]
Women's Shelter Rape Crisis Center of Lawrence
County [10300]
Women's Shelter of South Texas [10452]
Women's Specialty and Fertility Center [21952]
Women's Specialty Health Centers [22063]
Women's Therapy Center Institute [11169]
Women's Therapy Service of Montclair LLC [11150]
Women's Transitional Living Center [8863]
Womens Treatment Center [42592]
Women's Tri-County Help Center, Inc. [10169],
[31670]
Womens Wellbriety Center [45191]

WomenSafe, Inc.--Chardon [10131]
WomenSafe, Inc.--Middlebury [10544]
WOMENSPACE [10230]
Wonderful Care Home Health [14181]
Woniya Kini Behavioral Services [45244]
Wood County Hospital Sleep Disorders Center
[37597]
Wood County Human Services • Outpatient [50567]
Wood County Schools [879]
Wood River Health Services, Inc. [7216]
Woodbine Developmental Center [8283]
Woodbourne Center [34174]
Woodbridge Child & Diagnostic Treatment Center
[34298]
Woodbridge Developmental Center [8284]
Woodbury Dialysis Center • Fresenius Medical Care
[25421]
Woodbury Dialysis • DaVita [25098]
Wooddale Mental Health [30132]
Woodglen Recovery Junction Inc [39876], [39877]
Daylight Again [39878]
Woodhaven Dialysis Center [26378]
Woodhull Medical Center
Div of Chemical Dep/Dept of Psych [46541]
Division of Addiction Psychiatry [46542]
Woodland Center--Gallipolis [31770]
Woodland Center--Jackson [31780]
Woodland Center--Pomeroy [31825]
Woodland Centers [8185]
Benson Clinic [30662]
Woodland Centers, Inc. [51219]
Woodland Centers
Litchfield Clinic [30692]
Montevideo Clinic [30702]
Olivia Clinic [30705]
Outpatient Chemical Dependency Treatment
[45347]
Saint Francis Halfway House [30660]
Woodland Centers--Willmar [30733]
Woodland Dialysis Services, LLC [23079]
Woodland Hills [34247]
Woodland Hills/Calabasas Speech and Language
Center [1369]
Woodland Hills • Chisholm House - Community
Transition Program [34248]
Woodland Hills Neighborhood youth Services
[34249]
Woodland Hospice and Morey Bereavement Center
[20096]
Woodland Memorial Hospital [13453]
Sleep Disorders Center [36718]
Woodlands Behavioral Healthcare [30525], [30648]
The Woodlands Dialysis Center • DaVita [27359]
The Woodlands Sports Medicine Centre [39100]
Woodlands Treatment Center [34136]
Woodlawn Home Health Care [15048]
Woodlawn Organization Substance Abuse •
Services/Entry House [42593]
Woodlawn Pediatric Home Program • DaVita
[23965]
Woodmere Dialysis LLC • Rehabilitation and Health-
care Center [25806]
Woodridge Home Dialysis and At Home • DaVita
[24110]
Woodridge Hospital [33843]
Woodridge Interventions • All Alcohol Substance
Abuse Progs on Site [42970]
Woodridge of Missouri LLC • DBA Piney Ridge
Center [45674]
Woodridge Psychological Associates [47483]
Woodroe Place [28530]
Woodrow Wilson Rehabilitation Center [8585]
Woodrow Wilson Rehabilitation Center for Com-
munication Services [3583]
Woods Memorial Hospital District [17668]
Woods Memorial Regional Dialysis Center [26835]
Woods at Parkside [47734]
Woods Services [8469]
Woodside Guidance Center [31496]
Woodstock General Hospital • Youth Eating
Disorders Program [11245]
Woodstone Treatment Facility [10924]
Woodville Dialysis Center • American Renal Associ-
ates [27398]
Woodward Children's Center [8316]
Woodward Counseling Inc [44794], [44973]
Woodward Resource Center [8021]
Wooster Community Hospital [17081]

Cancer Program [5764]
Sleep Disorders Center [37598]
Wooster Veterans Affairs Clinic [31860]
Worcester County Health Department • Alcohol and Other Drug Services [44361]
Worcester Public Library • Talking Book Library [3803]
Worcester State College • Speech, Language and Hearing Clinic [2548]
Worcester State Hospital [33587]
Worcester Youth Guidance Center • Community Healthlink, Inc. [30493]
Worchester County Health Department, Berlin • Runaway and Homeless Youth Program [35995]
Word and Brown Hearing Center at Providence [1213]
Word House Inc • Focus Consultation Services [50316]
Word of Life Evangelistic Ministry Inc • Word of Life Program [40805]
Word Works, Speech--Language Pathologists Inc. [1209]
Work Physiology Laboratory • Ohio University [38852]
Working tor the Lord Ministry • Drug Prevention Program [44901]
Workshops [7709]
World First Class Home Health--Hallandale [13718]
World First Class Home Health, Inc.--Aventura [13583]
World First Class Home Health--Pembroke Park [14317]
World Home Care Services Corporation [13681]
Worldwide health Group of Palm Beach [14457]
Worldwide Health Group [14182]
The Wounded Healer Inc [46136]
Wrentham Developmental Center [8162]
Wright and Filippis Inc. [15786]
Wright Medical Group Inc. [35218]
Wright Patterson Medical Center • 74th Medical Group • Cancer Program [5765]
Wright Patterson Medical Center - Hemodialysis Department [26239]
Wright State University School of Medicine • Children's Medical Center • Cystic Fibrosis Center [7643]
Wrightstown Speech Pathology Services Inc. [3358]
Wrightsville Dialysis • DaVita [23839]
WTCSB Franklin Center [49786]
WTCSB Smithfield Center [49842]
Wuesthoff Brevard Homecare [14442]
Wuesthoff Health System • Cancer Program [4987]
Wuesthoff Hospice & Palliative Care [19331]
Wuesthoff Medical Center, Rockledge [14359]
Wuesthoff Pain Management Center [35400]
Wuesthoff Rehabilitation Network [1743]
Wyandot Center for Community Behavioral Health-care [8027]
Wyandot Mental Health Center [50920]
Wyandotte Central Dialysis • DaVita [24328]
Wyandotte County Dialysis • DaVita [24329]
Wyandotte Veterans Affairs Community Based Outpatient Clinic [29936]
Wyandotte West Dialysis • DaVita • Dialysis Facility [24330]
Wylds Road Dialysis • DaVita [23617]
Wynne Health Center [6283]
Wyoming Behavioral Institute [33953], [51523]
Wyoming Counseling and Outreach Services [50589]
Wyoming County Domestic Violence Project [10000]
Wyoming Department of Education • Special Programs Unit: Outreach for the Deaf/Hard of Hearing [3692]
Wyoming Department of Education Special Services • Wyoming Resource Library for the Deaf and Hard of Hearing [3689]
Wyoming Department of Education • Wyoming Deaf--Blind Project [3696]
Wyoming Department of Health • Maternal and Child Health • Perinatal Program [36560]
Wyoming Health Council • Wyoming Migrant Health Program [7450]
Wyoming Kidney Center • Dialysis Facility [27810]
Wyoming Migrant Health Program [7453]
Wyoming Recovery [50573]
Wyoming State Hospital [33040]
Wyoming State Training School [8633]

Wyoming Valley • Alcohol and Drug Services Inc [48614], [48697]
Wyoming Valley, LLC • Sleep Disorders Center [37715]
Wythe County Community Hospital • Circle Home Care [18413]

X

Xcellent Home Health Care [14249]
XI Hospice, Inc-Emmett Branch [19458]
XI Hospice Inc-Meridian Branch [19459]
XL Hospice Corp.--Fallon [20408]
XL Hospice, Inc.--Payette [19475]
Xtreme Medical, Inc. [13361]
Xytex Cord Blood Bank [35015]

Y

Y Medical Associates, Inc. [18021]
Y & S Home Health Services [14183]
Yadkin County Family Domestic Violence Program [10105]
Yadkin Dialysis Center • Wake Forest University [25983]
Yadkin Valley Extended Services [47511]
Yadkin Valley Home Health • Hugh Chatham Memorial Hospital [16721]
YAI National Institute for People with Disabilities [8338]
Yakama Nation Comprehensive Community • Alcoholism Program [50227]
Yakety Yak Speech--Language Pathologists Inc. [1622]
Yakima Dialysis Center & At Home • DaVita [27661]
Yakima Pediatric Associates [7396]
Yakima Regional Home Health and Hospice [18489]
Yakima Regional Medical and Cardiac Center • Cancer Program [6131]
Yakima School District 7 [870]
Yakima Sexual Assault Unit [10669]
Yakima Sleep Center [37947]
Yakima Valley Farm Workers Clinic • Child & Adolescent Crisis Intervention [51480]
Yakima Valley Farm Workers Clinic--Grandview • Child & Adolescent Crisis Intervention [51443]
Yakima Valley Farm Workers Clinic, Inc. [7393]
Yakima Valley Farm Workers Clinic--Toppenish • Child & Adolescent Crisis Intervention [51473]
Yakima Valley Memorial Home Care and Hospice [18490]
Yakima Valley Memorial Hospital [18491]
Yakima Valley Memorial Hospital - Community Cancer Program [6132]
Yakima Valley Memorial Hospital • Department of Maternal Health Services • Central Washington Genetics Program [12372]
Yakima Valley School • Division of Developmental Disabilities [8604]
Yakima Veterans Affairs Mental Health Outreach Clinic [32884]
Yakutat Tribal Social Servies [28127]
Yale Behavioral Health Services [29000]
Yale Crowberg Learning Center Inc [43514]
Yale--New Haven Hospital • Yale Comprehensive Cancer Center [4902]
Yale-New Haven Organ Transplant Center • Yale-New Haven Hospital [23170]
Yale Reproductive Endocrinology and Infertility--Guilford [21976]
Yale Reproductive Endocrinology and Infertility--Westport [21977]
Yale Sleep Medicine [36757]
Yale Sports Medicine Center [38196]
Yale University • IVF Program [21978]
Yale University School of Medicine • Adult Cystic Fibrosis Center [7493]
Yale University • School of Medicine • Department of Genetics [12174]
Yale University School of Medicine • Department of Internal Medicine • Musculoskeletal Disorders Core Center [162]
Yale University
School of Medicine
Department of Internal Medicine New England Program for AIDS Clinical Trials [44]

Department of Neurology MDA/ALS Center [34774]
Yale University School of Medicine
Department of Pediatrics • Center of Research Translation [163]
Multiple Sclerosis Clinic [34550]
Pediatric Cystic Fibrosis Center [7494]
Yale University • School of Medicine • Sickle Cell Disease Center [36314]
Yale University School of Medicine • Yale-New Haven Hemophilia Center [12498]
Yale Veterans Affairs Clinic [30655]
Yamhill Community Action Partnership • Runaway and Homeless Youth Program [36174]
Yamhill County • Family and Youth Programs [48147]
Yamhill County Mental Health and Human Services [31951]
Yampa Valley Psychotherapists [41315]
Yana House [42594]
Yandeivi Home Health Care [14184]
Yap Memorial Hospital • Department of Health Services [39201]
Yauco Dialysis Center • Fresenius Medical Care [26658]
Yavapai County Health Department [6245]
Yavapai Dialysis • Fresenius Medical Care [22489]
Yavapai Family Advocacy Center [8724]
YC Home Health Care Services [14449]
YCO Clinton Inc [48051]
Ye Home Health Care Corporation [14185]
Yellen and Associates [1202]
Yellow Hawk Tribal Health Center Behav • Health Program [48174]
Yellowbrick Treatment Center [11057]
Yellowstone Boys and Girls Ranch [34278]
Yellowstone Dialysis Center • University of Utah • Dialysis Program [23887]
Yellowstone Medical Center [4258]
Yellowstone Recovery • Boston House [39758]
Yerington Mental Health Center [31049]
Yerington Paiute Tribe [45885]
YES Community Counseling Center • Outpatient Chemical Dependency [46774]
Yes House [48094]
Yeshiva University
Albert Einstein College of Medicine
Children's Evaluation and Rehabilitation Center [8301]
Rose F. Kennedy Center Down Syndrome Clinic [10838]
YFA Connections [50188]
YFS Home Health Care [14186]
YI Maine • Bridge Program [44041]
Yired Home Health Care, Inc. [14187]
YMCA of Dallas, Community Services • Urban Outreach • Runaway and Homeless Youth Program [36234]
YMCA Domestic Violence Center [8637]
YMCA of Greater • CD Outpatient [46543]
YMCA of Honolulu
Aiea Intermediate School [42188]
Central Middle School [42217]
Dole Middle School [42218]
Ilima Intermediate School [42190]
Kalakaua Middle School [42219]
Kapolei High School [42253]
Kapolei Middle School [42254]
Kawananakoa Middle School [42220]
McKinley High School [42221]
Moanalua Middle School [42222]
Stevenson Middle School [42223]
Waipahu Intermediate School [42299]
YMCA of Long Island • YMCA Family Services [46589]
YMCA Outreach Services [42224]
School Based/Aiea High School [42189]
School Based/Campbell High School [42191]
School Based/Farrington High School [42225]
School Based/Leilehua High School [42287]
School Based/Moanalua High School [42226]
School Based/Nanakuli High School [42291]
School Based/Roosevelt High School [42227]
School Based/Waianae High School [42292]
School Based/Waipahu High School [42300]
YMCA Safeplace Services • Runaway and Homeless Youth Program [35970]
YMCA Youth and Family Services [35851]

YN Home Care Services, Inc. [13780]
Yoakum County Mental Health Center [32446]
Yolo Community Care Continuum
    Farm House [28470]
    Supportive Housing/Vocational Services [28471]
Yolo County Alcohol Drug and Mental Health
    Services [40964]
Yolo County Department of Alcohol, Drug and
    Mental Health [28847]
Yolo County Department of Alcohol, Drug, and
    Mental Health Services [28472]
Yolo County • Dept of Alcohol/Drug/Mental Health
    Service [39777], [40947]
Yolo Family Service Agency--Davis [28473]
Yolo Family Service Agency--West Sacramento
    [28848]
Yolo Hospice [18916]
Yolo Wayfarer Center Christian Mission • Walters
    House [40965]
Yonkers Dialysis Center • DaVita [25810]
Yonkers East Dialysis Center • DaVita [25811]
York County Community Health [6784]
York County Dialysis Center • Fresenius Medical
    Care [24607]
York County Shelter Programs Inc [43910]
York County Treatment Center [48935]
York General Dialysis Services [25347]
York General Hospital [2861]
York Hospital
    Cottage Program [44089]
    Crisis Intervention Services [51304]
York Hospital Department of Palliative Care [21183]
York Hospital--Hospital Drive, York • Cancer Care
    Program [5279]
York Hospital--S George Street, York • Cancer
    Center [5884]
York Hospital • Sleep Center [37716]
Yorktown Artificial Kidney Center • Dialysis Facility •
    Dialysis Clinic, Inc. [25812]
Yorktowne Psychological and Addiction • Services
    [48717]
Yorkville Dialysis Center [25740]
Yorkville Dialysis Center LLC [24111]
Yosemite Street Dialysis Center • DaVita [22801]
You Can Health Services • You Can Alcohol and
    Drug Counseling [40182]
Y.O.U., Inc. • Crisis Center [51004]
Y.O.U., Inc. Family Services [50997]
Young Adult Guidance Center Inc. • Runaway and
    Homeless Youth Program • Emergency Shelter
    [35914]
Young House Family Services, Inc. [34137]
Young Medical Equipment/Toledo I.V. Care [16986]
Young People Matter • Runaway and Homeless
    Youth Program [35915]
Young Talkers [3407]
Young Women's Christian Association of Northeast
    Louisiana [50950]
Youngstown Developmental Center [8425]
Youngstown Hearing and Speech Center [3262]
Youngstown Home Care • Centers for Dialysis Care
    [26185]
Your Community in Unity [10522]
Your Empowering Solutions Inc [40471]
Your Family Home Health Care Services, Inc.
    [13789]
Your Human Resource Center [47820], [47832],
    [47845], [47890]
Your Nurse Home Healthcare, LLC [13859]
Your Safe Haven [10276]
Youth Advocates of Sitka • Runaway and Homeless
    Youth Program [35792]
Youth Alternative Home Association • Runaway and
    Homeless Youth Program [36283]
Youth Alternatives Ingraham, Inc. [30232]
Youth Alternatives Ingraham • Runaway and Home-
    less Youth Program [35989]
Youth Bridge [39531], [39538], [39562], [39572]
    Runaway and Homeless Youth Program [35803]
Youth Care, Inc. [32580]
Youth Care of Utah [49610]
Youth Challenge of Connecticut
    Long Term Male Residential Center [41412]
    Mission for Women [41413]
Youth Challenges [31841]
Youth Consultation Service • Department of Addic-
    tion Service [45976]
Youth Continuum • Douglas House Shelter •

Runaway and Homeless Youth Program [35867]
Youth Council • Substance Abuse Treatment [45917]
Youth Crisis Center • Runaway and Homeless Youth
    Program [35900]
Youth Crisis Shelter [32900]
Youth Crisis Stabilization Program [50955]
Youth Development, Albuquerque • Runaway and
    Homeless Youth Program [36087]
Youth Development Services • Runaway and Home-
    less Youth Program [36284]
Youth Eastside Services
    Bellevue Main Facility [49896]
    Lake Washington Branch [49994]
    Redmond Branch [50079]
Youth Emergency Services Inc • House Girls Cot-
    tage [50585]
Youth Emergency Services, Inc. [33043]
Youth Emergency Services, Omaha • Runaway and
    Homeless Youth Program [35959]
Youth Emergency Services • Runaway and Home-
    less Youth Program [35959], [36285]
Youth Emergency Shelter [28308]
Youth Evaluation and Treatment Centers [7743]
Youth-Family-Adult Connections • Runaway and
    Homeless Youth Program [36259]
Youth and Family Alternatives Administration •
    Runaway and Homeless Youth Program [35901]
Youth and Family Alternatives--Bartow • George W.
    Harris, Jr. Runaway and Youth Crisis Shelter
    [35902]
Youth and Family Alternatives--Brooksville •
    Runaway and Homeless Youth Program [35903]
Youth and Family Assistance Crisis Intervention and
    Suicide Prevention Center [50667]
Youth and Family Counseling Agency of • Oyster
    Bay/East Norwich Inc [46971]
Youth and Family Counseling • Runaway and Home-
    less Youth Program [36235]
Youth and Family Enrichment Services Crisis Center
    [50691]
Youth and Family Enrichment Services Inc • Insights
    Adol Substance Abuse Program [39776], [40441]
Youth and Family Project Runaway Program •
    Crossroad [36275]
Youth and Family Services [39828]
Youth & Family Services--Augusta [30191]
Youth and Family Services of Canadian County •
    Runaway and Homeless Youth Program [36161]
Youth and Family Services--Fort Lauderdale [29158]
Youth and Family Services Inc
    Counseling Center [49013]
    Substance Abuse Program/Skowhegan [44060]
Youth and Family Services, Inc.--Fairfield [28496]
Youth and Family Services, Modesto [28639]
Youth and Family Services of North Central
    Oklahoma Inc [47934]
Youth and Family Services of North Central
    Oklahoma • Runaway and Homeless Youth
    Program [36162]
Youth and Family Services of • Washington County
    Inc [47914]
Youth and Family Services, Skowhegan • Runaway
    and Homeless Youth Program [35990]
Youth and Family Services
    Substance Abuse Programs [40884]
    Substance Abuse Services [40885]
Youth Focus, Inc.
    Runaway and Homeless Youth Program [36138]
    Teen Crisis Line [51167]
Youth Focus Residential Treatment Center [34363]
Youth Habilitation (Quinte)--Belleville [11246]
Youth Home [7761]
Youth Home, Inc. [28309]
Youth Link • Runaway and Homeless Youth Program
    [36040]
Youth Moving On • Hillsides Home for Children
    [28700]
Youth in Need, Inc. • Runaway and Homeless Youth
    Program [36060]
Youth Network Council • Runaway and Homeless
    Youth Program [35941]
Youth Oasis • Runaway and Homeless Youth
    Program [35978]
Youth Opportunities Upheld Inc • Structured
    Outpatient Services [44623]
Youth Organizations Umbrella • Runaway and
    Homeless Youth Program [35942]
Youth Outreach Services [42779]

Austin [42595]
Irving Park [42596]
Runaway and Homeless Youth Program [35943]
The Youth Recovery Center • Valley View Hospital
    [41196]
Youth Service Bureau of Illinois Valley • Runaway
    and Homeless Youth Program [35944]
Youth Service Bureau of Monroe County • Runaway
    and Homeless Youth Program [35953]
Youth Service Bureau of • Saint Tammany [43822]
Youth Service Bureau • Runaway and Homeless
    Youth Program [35945]
Youth Service Bureau of Saint Joseph County, Inc. •
    Runaway and Homeless Youth Program [35954]
Youth Service Project Inc [42597]
Youth Services Inc. • Runaway and Homeless Youth
    Program [36187]
Youth Services--La Selva Beach • Tyler House
    [28551]
Youth Services--Muskegon [30610]
Youth Services Network • Runaway and Homeless
    Youth Program [35946]
Youth Services for Oklahoma County • Runaway
    and Homeless Youth Program [36163]
Youth Services--Santa Cruz [28810]
Youth Services of Southern Wisconsin
    Briarpatch • Runaway and Homeless Youth
        Program [36276]
    Runaway and Homeless Youth Program [36277]
Youth Services for Stephens County • Runaway and
    Homeless Youth Program [36164]
Youth Services System, Inc. • Runaway and Home-
    less Youth Program [36264]
Youth Services of Tulsa • Runaway and Homeless
    Youth Program [36165]
Youth Services--Watsonville [28844]
Youth Shelter Jacksonstreet • Runaway and Home-
    less Youth Program [36175]
Youth and Shelter Services • Runaway and Home-
    less Youth Program [35960]
Youth Shelters and Family Services, Santa Fe •
    Runaway and Homeless Youth Program [36088]
Youth Support Systems [49716]
Youth Town of TN Inc [49176]
Youth in Transition School [2386]
Youth Villages • Runaway and Homeless Youth
    Program [36208]
YouthCare Residential Treatment Center for
    Troubled Teens [34457]
YouthCare • Runaway and Homeless Youth Program
    [36260]
Youthville [33517]
Youthville--Dodge City [34144]
Youthville Family Consultation Service [43515]
Youthville--Newton [34146]
Yoya's Home Health Care [14188]
Ypsilanti Dialysis & At Home • DaVita [24996]
Yuba City Dialysis Center • DaVita [23084]
Yucaipa Dialysis Center • DaVita [23085]
Yukon Government • Department of Education [899]
Yukon-Koyukuk Mental Health & Alcohol Program •
    Edgar Nollner Health Center [28092]
Yukon- Koyukuk Mental Health Program
    Huslia Counseling Center [28096]
    Nulato Counseling Center [28112]
    Ruby Counseling Center [28117]
Yukon/Koyukuk School District [220]
Yukon Kuskokwim Delta Regional Hospital [12742]
    Akiachak Native Community Village Clinic
        [12735]
    Chefornak Community Health Clinic [12744]
    Chevak Community Health Clinic [12745]
    Crimet Phillips Senior Clinic [12762]
    Crooked Creek Community Health Clinic
        [12747]
    Edith Kawagly Memorial Clinic [12736]
    Eek Community Health Clinic [12748]
    Emmonak Subregional Clinic [12749]
    Hooper Bay Community Health Clinic [12753]
    Kasigluk Community Health Clinic [12754]
    Kathleen Daniel Memorial Clinic [12778]
    Kipnuk Community Health Clinic [12757]
    Kotlik Community Health Clinic [12759]
    Kwigillingok Community Health Clinic [12761]
    Mount Village Clinic [12764]
    Napakiak Clinic [12765]
    Napaskiak Clinic [12743]
    Nunapitchuk Clinic [12766]

Pilot Station Clinic [12768]
Quinhagak Clinic [12769]
Russian Mission Clinic [12770]
Saint Mary's Subregional Clinic [12771]
Sarah S. Nicholai Memorial Clinic [12760]
Scammon Bay Clinic [12772]
Sleetmute Clinic [12773]
Theresa Elia Memorial Clinic [12763]
Toksook Bay Subregional Clinic [12776]
Tuluksak Clinic [12777]
Tununak Clinic [12779]
Yukon-Kuskokwim Health Corp. [6209]
Yukon Kuskokwim Health Corp.--Behavioral Health [50630]
Yukon Kuskokwim Health Corporation
   Behavioral Health Program [28079]
   Crisis Respite Center [28080]
Yukon-Kuskokwim Health Corporation • Phillips Ay-agnirvik Treatment Center [39320]
Yukon Kuskokwim Health Corporation • Transitional Living Program [28081]
Yuma Community Based Outpatient Clinic [3882]
Yuma Treatment Center [39521]
Yuma Vet Center • Yuma AZ [51869]
YWCA--Arnold • Domestic Violence Services [9440]
YWCA--Batavia • Domestic Violence Program of Genesee County [9896]
YWCA--Billings - Gateway House [9737]
YWCA--Billings - Gateway House Sexual Violence/Victims Services [9738]
YWCA of Boulder County [8939]
YWCA Bradford [10266]
YWCA--Burlington • Domestic Violence Shelter and Sexual Assault Program [9319]
YWCA--Charleston • Resolve Family Abuse Program [10672]
YWCA--Cincinnati • Alice Paul House [10134]
YWCA of Clark County • Safe Choice [10665]
YWCA of Cleveland • Domestic Violence Outreach Program [10139]
YWCA of Cobb County [9118]
YWCA--Cortland • Aid to Women Victims of Violence [9917]
YWCA Crisis Service--Lewiston [50824]
YWCA Crisis Service--Manchester [9812]
YWCA Crisis Services--Clarkston [51433]
YWCA/Daybreak Resources for Women and Children--Worcester [9509]
YWCA--Dayton • Shelter Services [10144]
YWCA--Detroit • Interim House [9531]
YWCA Domestic Violence Program--Lawrence [9486]
YWCA--Dubuque • Domestic Violence Program [9333]
YWCA--Elizabeth • Project: Protect [9825]
YWCA - Enid, Oklahoma [10198]
YWCA of Essex and West Hudson • Adolescent Center for Excellence [9844]
YWCA Evanston/North Shore [9226]
YWCA--Evansville • Domestic Violence Shelter [9274]
YWCA Family Violence Prevention Program--Wheeling [10683]
YWCA Family Violence Program and Shelter--Lihue [9155]
YWCA--Flint • Domestic and Sexual Assault Services [9536]
YWCA--Fort Wayne • Women's Shelter and Outreach Services [9276]
YWCA of Freeport [9227]
YWCA--Fullerton • Beyond Shelter [8816]
YWCA Genesis Program--Richmond [9305]

YWCA of Glendale • Domestic Violence Project [8818]
YWCA Greater Harrisburg [10281]
YWCA of Greater Memphis [10420]
YWCA of Greater Pittsburgh [10310]
YWCA Greater Portland Oregon [10255]
YWCA - Hanover, Pennsylvania [10280]
YWCA of Hudson County • Women Rising, Inc. [9833]
YWCA - Jamestown, New York [9937]
YWCA--Janesville • Alternatives to Violence [10707]
YWCA of Kalamazoo • Domestic Assault Program [9549]
YWCA of Kitsap County [10610]
YWCA--Knoxville • Victim Advocacy Program [10413]
YWCA--Kokomo • Family Intervention Center [9292]
YWCA--Lafayette • Domestic Violence Intervention and Prevention Program [9294]
YWCA--Lancaster • Sexual Assault Prevention and Counseling Center [10290]
YWCA of Lewiston/Clarkston [9178]
YWCA--Lexington • Spouse Abuse Center [9392]
YWCA--Lynchburg • Domestic Violence Prevention Center [10578]
YWCA--Lynnwood • Pathways For Women [10626]
YWCA/Marjaree Mason Center, Inc. [8815]
YWCA Mercy Home [9747]
YWCA of Metropolitan Chicago [9215]
YWCA of the Middle Rio Grande [9859]
YWCA - Missoula, Montana [9758]
YWCA of Mohawk Valley • Rape Crisis and Domestic Violence Services [9997]
YWCA of New Castle County • Helping Hearts [9013]
YWCA - New Orleans, Louisiana [9421]
YWCA of Niagara [9940]
YWCA of North Central Indiana [43206]
YWCA Northcentral Pennsylvania • Wise Options [10327]
YWCA Northeastern New York [9985]
YWCA of Northwest Louisiana [9416]
YWCA--Oklahoma City • Crisis Intervention Services [10206]
YWCA--Portland • Women's Shelter and Fair Harbor Emergency Shelter for Girls [9435]
YWCA--Poughkeepsie • Battered Women's Services [9980]
YWCA - Protective Shelter for Battered Persons [10151]
YWCA--Pueblo • Family Crisis Shelter [8980]
YWCA Residence--Buffalo [9913]
YWCA--Richmond • Women's Advocacy Program [10590]
YWCA of Rochester and Monroe County [9982]
YWCA of Saint Joseph County [9308]
YWCA--Saint Joseph • Shelter for Abused Women and their Children [9714]
YWCA of Saint Paul [9639]
YWCA--Salt Lake City • Women In Jeopardy Program [10533]
YWCA--San Diego • Domestic Violence Service [8884]
YWCA of the Sauk Valley [9251]
YWCA--Seattle • Downtown Women's Shelter [10654]
YWCA Sexual Assault Center--Saint Louis [9726]
YWCA Shelter and Domestic Violence Program--Nashville [10430]
YWCA--Shreveport • Family Violence Program [9425]
YWCA of South Hampton Roads • Women In Crisis Program [10582]

YWCA--Spokane • Alternatives to Domestic Violence [10658]
YWCA--Springfield • Arch Program [9504]
YWCA Support and Safe House--Rock Springs • Green River Office [10763]
YWCA--Tacoma • Women's Support Shelter [10663]
YWCA--Toledo • Battered Women Shelter [10177]
YWCA of the Tonawandas • Domestic Violence Program [9968]
YWCA--Topeka • Battered Women's Task Force [9378]
YWCA of the Upper Lowlands, Inc. [10363]
YWCA--Utica • Hall House [9998]
YWCA of Walla Walla [10666]
YWCA of Wenatchee Valley [10668]
YWCA of West Central Michigan • Domestic Crisis Center [9538]
YWCA--West Palm Beach • Harmony House [9084]
YWCA--Westfield • New Beginnings [9507]
YWCA--Wichita • Women's Crisis Center/Safehouse [9382]
YWCA Women's Advocates--Pocatello [9184]
YWCA Women's and Children's Alliance--Boise [9164]
YWCA-Women's Emergency Shelter Program--Santa Rosa • Safe House [9378]
YWCA Women's Resource Center--Clayton [9668]
YWCA Yakima [10670]
YWCA--York • Access - York, Inc. [10328]

Z

Zablocki Veterans Affairs Medical Center [50488]
Zacharias Sexual Abuse Center [9232]
Zale Lipshy University Hospital - Cancer Program [5980]
Zanesville City Schools Special Education [664]
Zanesville Dialysis & At Home • Dialysis Facility • DaVita [26244]
Zapata Independent School District [834]
Zapata Mental Health Center [32573]
Zarman Surgical Supply, Inc. [16513]
Zebra Inc • DBA Cheyenne Center Inpatient Services [49422]
Zeeba Sleep Center [37325]
Zeigler Outpatient [27988]
Zelden Physical Therapy [2312]
Zen Hospice Project [19027]
Zenith Home Care [13650]
Zepf Community Mental Health Center [31847]
Zephyrhills Dialysis • DaVita • Dialysis Facility [23569]
Zephyrhills Family Health Center [6576]
Zeta House [34414]
ZG International Healthcare Division/dba Pacific Oasis Hospice [18958]
Ziba Hospice [19064]
Zintkala Waste Win Oti [10376]
Zion Recovery [43237], [43247]
Zions Cross Road Dialysis [27498]
Zion's Way Hospice [21639]
Zona Seca Inc
   Alcohol and DA Counseling Agency [40739]
   Youth and Family Treatment Center [40010]
Zoom Sports [39066]
Zouves Fertility Center [21953]
Zufall Health Center [6971]
Zukoski Outpatient [39230]
Zumbro Valley Mental Health Center [30714]
   Community Support Program [30715]
   Crisis Receiving Unit [30716]
   Pacing Recovery Effectively Program [45283]
   Recovery Basics [45284]
   Right to Recovery [45285]
   Thomas House [30717]
Zuni Presbyterian Homes [8596]
Zuni Public Schools [566]

CPSIA information can be obtained
at www.ICGtesting.com
Printed in the USA
FFOW01n1241120614
5893FF

9 781569 959619